Nutraceuticals and Functional Foods in Human Health and Disease Prevention

Nutraceuticals and Functional Foods in Human Health and Disease Prevention

Edited by
Debasis Bagchi
Harry G. Preuss
Anand Swaroop

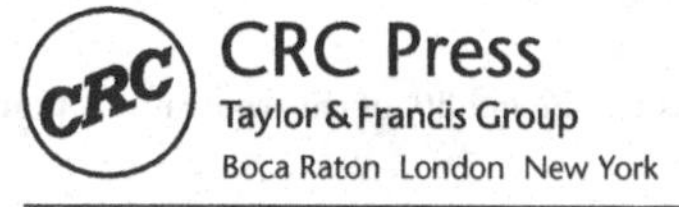

CRC Press is an imprint of the
Taylor & Francis Group, an **informa** business

CRC Press
Taylor & Francis Group
6000 Broken Sound Parkway NW, Suite 300
Boca Raton, FL 33487-2742

First issued in paperback 2021

Version Date: 20150819

ISBN 13: 978-1-03-209826-5 (pbk)
ISBN 13: 978-1-4822-3721-4 (hbk)

Visit the Taylor & Francis Web site at
http://www.taylorandfrancis.com

and the CRC Press Web site at
http://www.crcpress.com

Dedicated to my beloved uncle R.P. Lahiri

Debasis Bagchi

Contents

SECTION VII Hypertension

SECTION VIII Immune Health

SECTION IX Cancer

SECTION X Ocular Health and Vision

SECTION XI Prostate Health

SECTION XII Sleeping Disorders

SECTION XIII Wound Healing

SECTION XIV Hair and Skin Health

SECTION XV Fertility and Sexual Health

SECTION XVI Cosmeceuticals

SECTION XVII Exercise and Physical Health

SECTION XVIII Sickle Cell Anemia

SECTION XIX Role of Probiotics in Gastrointestinal and Dental Health

Preface

Nutraceuticals and functional foods are becoming increasingly popular in the world's marketplace. The global nutraceuticals market reached $142.1 billion in 2011 and is expected to reach $204.8 billion by 2017 [1]. There are two main reasons for this overwhelming response: (1) skyrocketing pharmaceutical and healthcare costs and their adverse events and (2) cost and the broad-spectrum efficacy of nutraceuticals and functional foods in a variety of disease scenarios. Nutritionists are constantly advocating to the world's population how proper nutrition and exercise can help in maintaining good health. Although it is important to mention that a significant number of nutraceuticals and functional foods have demonstrated their efficacy, a large number of supplements are still surviving on false claims. Government regulatory agencies are doing a great job in keeping a continued vigil on these nutraceuticals and functional food supplements.

In this book, we have streamlined 39 chapters as follows.

We focus on certain basic aspects, including (1) global food habits and trends, (2) the safety and toxicology of nutraceuticals and functional foods, and (3) how food addiction or overindulgence of food may lead to a variety of disease states. A snapshot has been provided to visualize how supplements may help in a variety of disease prevention strategies. We intentionally emphasize the safety and toxicology chapter so that people may understand the aspects of risk and benefit and why government regulatory agencies are so critical to these nutraceutical supplements.

Five chapters in Section II highlight obesity, diabetes, and metabolic syndrome and the diverse roles of nutraceuticals and functional foods in attenuating the harmful scenario of metabolic syndrome. Section III focuses on the role of nutrition in improving cardiovascular health. Section IV discusses how anti-inflammatory phytochemicals and probiotics can help against arthritis, inflammation, and joint disorders.

Section V, which contains three chapters, highlights how polyunsaturated fatty acids and selected phytochemicals can prevent regular and age-induced brain dysfunctions. Chapter 14 is dedicated to the use of phytochemicals in Alzheimer's and Parkinson's diseases, as well as regular stress. Furthermore, mental disorders may be partially protected by nutraceuticals, as is discussed in Chapter 15.

Section VI covers pulmonary diseases and dysfunctions. Chapter 16 discusses the roles of pro-, pre-, and synbiotics for the management of pulmonary diseases, while Chapter 17 covers the protective roles of antioxidants and nutraceuticals. Section VII covers hypertension in two dedicated chapters. Professor Mark Houston highlights the benefits of nutrition and nutraceuticals in the treatment of hypertension. Chapter 19, written by the editors, and Dr. Nicholar V. Perricone et al. discusses the effects of dietary fibers on sugar-induced blood pressure elevations in hypertension. Section VIII highlights immune health and the beneficial role of phytochemicals.

Cancer is covered by two eminent scientists in two different chapters. Chapter 21, written by Dr. Michael J. Spinella of Dartmouth Medical School and Kelly C. Heim, deals with diverse natural products. Chapter 22 covers *Helicobacter pylori*, the most abundant deadly bacteria responsible for gastric and stomach cancer. That chapter discusses how phytochemicals may help in eradicating *H. pylori*. In Section X, three distinguished professors from the University of Colorado focus on ocular health. In the next section, Professor Shigeo Horie from Juntendo Hospital, Japan, discusses prostrate health in Chapter 24. Sleep disorder and therapy are major challenges worldwide, and this problem is extensively discussed in Section XII by Professor Lindseth of the University of North Dakota in Chapter 25. The other major worldwide problem is diabetic wounds, and the role of fermented papaya in improving diabetic wounds are discussed in Chapter 26 in Section XIII.

Hair and skin health is covered in three dedicated chapters in Section XIV. Chapters 27 and 28 discuss how proper nutrition and nutraceuticals can promote hair growth and prevent hair loss and alopecia. Chapter 29 discusses how herbal therapy can prevent skin wrinkling.

Fertility and sexual health are discussed next in Chapters 30 and 31. Various mechanistic explorations and discussions are covered. The inclusion of nutraceuticals in cosmeceuticals is discussed in Section XVI. The importance of exercise and physical health and the roles of nutraceuticals and antioxidants are highlighted in Section XVII. Different nutraceuticals in the prevention of sickle cell anemia are discussed in Section XVIII.

Finally, Section XIX discusses the roles of probiotics in gastrointestinal and dental health in five dedicated chapters.

Overall, we expect that our readers will benefit from the versatile chapters and the current state of knowledge presented in this book.

REFERENCE

1. A new market report from Transparency Market Research, Albany, NY. Breaking News June 26, 2013—Nutraceuticals Product Market Forecast to Reach $204.8 Billion by 2017. http://www.nutraceuticalsworld.com/contents/view_breaking-news/2013-06-26/nutraceuticals-product-market-forecast-to-reach-2048-billion-by-2017/?sthash.IHVA513G.mjjo (accessed May 22, 2015).

Editors

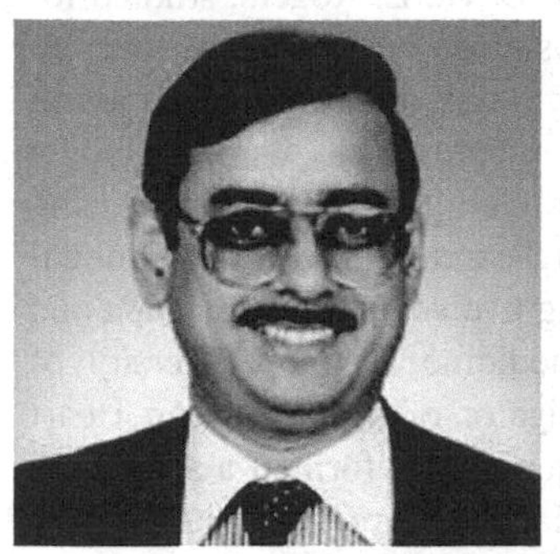

Debasis Bagchi, PhD, MACN, CNS, MAIChE, earned his PhD in medicinal chemistry in 1982. He is a professor in the Department of Pharmacological and Pharmaceutical Sciences at the University of Houston College of Pharmacy, Houston, Texas, and the chief scientific officer of Cepham Research Center, Piscataway, New Jersey. Dr. Bagchi is an adjunct faculty member at Texas Southern University, Houston, Texas. He served as the senior vice president of research and development of InterHealth Nutraceuticals Inc, Benicia, California, from 1998 until February 2011, and then as director of innovation and clinical affairs of Iovate Health Sciences, Oakville, Ontario, until June 2013. Dr. Bagchi received the Master of American College of Nutrition Award in October 2010. He is past chairman of the International Society of Nutraceuticals and Functional Foods, immediate past president of the American College of Nutrition, Clearwater, Florida, and past chair of the Nutraceuticals and Functional Foods Division of the Institute of Food Technologists, Chicago, Illinois. He serves as a distinguished advisor for the Japanese Institute for Health Food Standards, Tokyo, Japan. Dr. Bagchi is a member of the Study Section and the Peer Review Committee of the National Institutes of Health, Bethesda, Maryland.

Dr. Bagchi has published 304 papers in peer-reviewed journals and 26 books and holds numerous patents. He has delivered invited lectures at various national and international scientific conferences and organized workshops, and group discussion sessions. He is a member of the Society of Toxicology, a member of the New York Academy of Sciences, a fellow of the Nutrition Research Academy, and a member of the TCE stakeholder Committee of the Wright Patterson Air Force Base, Ohio. He is the associate editor of the *Journal of Functional Foods*, *Journal of the American College of Nutrition*, and *Archives of Medical and Biomedical Research* and also serves as an editorial board member of numerous peer-reviewed journals, including *Antioxidants & Redox Signaling*, *Cancer Letters*, *Toxicology Mechanisms and Methods*, and *The Original Internist*.

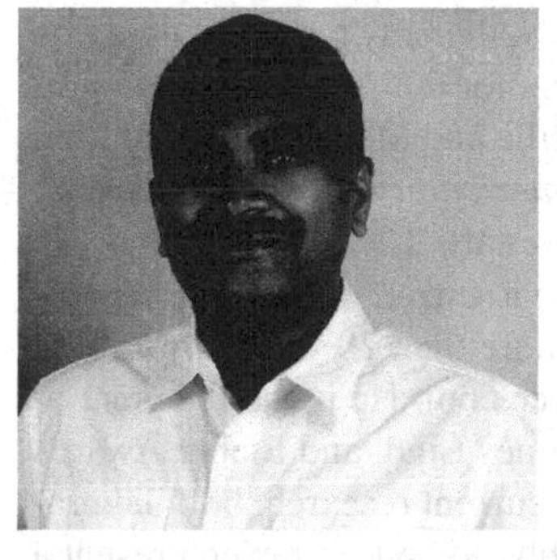

Dr. Anand Swaroop earned his MS in biochemistry in 1986 and PhD in chemistry in 1997. He has gathered over two decades of diversified global management experience in phytopharmaceuticals, global regulations on nutraceuticals and functional foods, chemicals and pharmaceutical ingredients, outsourcing and supply chain management, business development, market research, and strategic planning. He has worked in various multinational pharmaceutical companies, including Alembic Ltd. (Vadodara, India), Cadila Laboratories Ltd. (Ahmedabad, India), Nandesari Rasayanee Ltd. (Vadodara, India), Dai-Ichi Laboratories Ltd. (Hyderabad, India), and Yag Mag Labs Pvt. Ltd. (Hyderabad, India) in senior management positions. Currently, he is the founder president of Cepham Inc., Yag Mag Inc., and RALLIFE Inc. (Piscataway, New Jersey) and Cepham Life Sciences Inc. (Maryland). Dr. Swaroop has several peer-reviewed publications. He is a member of the American Chemical Society (ACS), the American Association of Pharmaceutical Scientists (AAPS), the American Society of Pharmacognosy (ASP), the Council for Responsible Nutrition (CRN), the American Botanical Council (ABC), and the Natural Products Association (NPA). Dr. Swaroop has organized and chaired numerous sessions in the annual meetings of the Institutes of Food Technologists (IFT) and the International Society of Nutraceuticals and Functional Foods (ISNFF) and other scientific meetings. He has also delivered invited lectures in various national and international scientific conferences, organized workshops, and group discussion sessions.

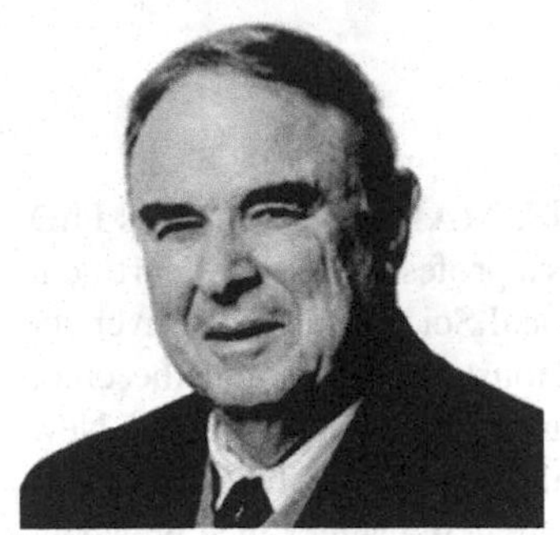

Harry G. Preuss, MD, MACN, CNS, earned his BA and MD from Cornell University, Ithaca, New York, and New York City, New York; trained for three years in internal medicine at Vanderbilt University Medical Center under Dr. David E. Rogers; studied for two years as a fellow in renal physiology at Cornell University Medical Center under Dr. Robert F. Pitts; and spent two years in clinical and research training in nephrology at Georgetown University Medical Center under Dr. George E. Schreiner. During his training years, he was a special research fellow of the National Institutes of Health (NIH). Following five years as an assistant and associate (tenured) professor of medicine at the University of Pittsburgh Medical Center, where he became an established investigator of the American Heart Association, he returned to Georgetown Medical Center. He subsequently performed a six-month sabbatical in molecular biology at the NIH in the laboratories of Dr. Maurice Burg. Dr. Preuss is now a tenured professor in four departments at Georgetown University Medical Center—biochemistry, physiology, medicine, and pathology.

His bibliography includes more than 240 peer-reviewed, original medical research papers, 200 general medical contributions (chapters, review articles, etc.), 7 patents, and more than 250 abstracts. Dr. Preuss has written, edited, or coedited nine books and three symposia published in well-established journals. In 1976, Dr. Preuss was elected to membership in the American Society for Clinical Investigations on his first attempt. He is currently an advisory editor for many journals. His previous government appointments included four years on the Advisory Council for the National Institute on Aging, two years on the Advisory Council of the Director of the NIH (NIA Representative), and two years on the Advisory Council for the Office of Alternative Medicine of the NIH. He has been a member of many other peer research review committees for the NIH and the American Heart Association and was recently a member of the National Cholesterol Education Program of the NHLBI and clinical study section JH-07 of the NIH.

Dr. Preuss was elected the ninth Master of the American College of Nutrition (ACN). He is a former chairman of two ACN councils—Cardiovascular/Aging and Dietary Supplements/Functional Foods. After a brief stint on the board of directors of the ACN, Dr. Preuss spent three years as secretary-treasurer and three consecutive years as vice president, president-elect, and became president in 1998. In 2008 and 2010, he was twice reelected president of the ACN, the only person to hold this office more than once. Dr. Preuss is a member of the board of directors for the Alliance for Natural Health (ANH-USA) and was made a member of the ANH-INT Scientific and Medical collaboration group. Dr. Preuss wrote the nutrition section for the *Encyclopedia Americana* and is past president of the Certification Board for Nutrition Specialists (CBNS) that gives the CNS certification. He was chairman of the Institutional Review Board (IRB) at Georgetown University, which reviews all clinical protocols at Georgetown University Medical Center, for more than 20 years. Dr. Preuss is currently chairman of the Scientific Advisory Board for NutraSpace.com. He is the recipient of the Harold Harper Lectureship Award (ACAM), William B. Peck, James Lind, and Bieber Awards for his research and activities in the medical and nutrition fields. His current research, both laboratory and clinical, centers on the use of dietary supplements to favorably influence or even prevent a variety of medical perturbations, especially those related to obesity, insulin resistance, and cardiovascular disorders. Lately, he has also researched the ability of many natural products to overcome various infections, including those resistant to antibiotics. He won through a vote of his peers the coveted Charles E. Ragus Award of the ACN for publishing the best research paper in their journal in 2006 and the ACN Award for 2010 given to an outstanding senior investigator in nutrition. In 2014, he received the Jonathan Emord Awards for his research in the fields of medicine, nutrition, and integrative medicine.

Contributors

Mohd Fasih Ahmad
Accredited Consultants Private Limited
New Delhi, India

Faruq Ahmed
Algae Biotechnology Laboratory
School of Agriculture and Food Sciences
The University of Queensland
Brisbane, Queensland, Australia

Faisal Alsenani
Algae Biotechnology Laboratory
School of Agriculture and Food Sciences
The University of Queensland
Brisbane, Queensland, Australia

Muhannad Alsyouf
Department of Urology
Loma Linda University
Loma Linda, California

Wataru Aoi
Laboratory of Health Science
Graduate School of Life and Environmental Sciences
Kyoto Prefectural University
Kyoto, Japan

Debasis Bagchi
Department of Pharmacological and Pharmaceutical Services
University of Houston
Houston, Texas

Kathryn Birkenbach
Institute of Human Nutrition
Columbia University Medical Center
New York, New York

Gene Bruno
Academic Administration
Huntington College of Health Sciences
Knoxville, Tennessee

Maria Grazia Cagetti
Department of Health Science
WHO Collaborating Centre of Milan for Epidemiology and Community Dentistry
University of Milan
Milan, Italy

Guglielmo Campus
Department of Health Science
WHO Collaborating Centre of Milan for Epidemiology and Community Dentistry
University of Milan
Milan, Italy

and

Department of Surgery, Microsurgery and Medical Sciences
School of Dentistry
University of Sassari
Sassari, Italy

Runu Chakraborty
Department of Food Technology and Biochemical Engineering
Jadavpur University
Kolkata, India

Gaëlle Champeil-Potokar
Department of Human Nutrition (AlimH)
National Institute for Research in Agronomy
Jouy-en-Josas, France

Archana Chatterjee
Department of Pediatrics
Sanford School of Medicine
and
Sanford Children's Specialty Clinic
University of South Dakota
Sioux Falls, South Dakota

Jae-Suk Choi
Department of Bio-Food Materials
Silla University
Busan, South Korea

Ock K. Chun
Department of Nutritional Sciences
University of Connecticut
Storrs, Connecticut

Dallas Clouatre
Glykon Technologies
Seattle, Washington

Fabio Cocco
Department of Health Science
WHO Collaborating Centre of Milan for Epidemiology and Community Dentistry
University of Milan
Milan, Italy

and

Department of Chemistry and Pharmacy
University of Sassari
Sassari, Italy

Lipi Das
Department of Food Technology and Biochemical Engineering
Jadavpur University
Kolkata, India

B. Demmig-Adams
Department of Ecology and Evolutionary Biology
University of Colorado
Boulder, Colorado

Isabelle Denis
NBO Unit
Department of Human Nutrition (AlimH)
National Institute for Research in Agronomy
Jouy-en-Josas, France

Ryan Dickerson
Department of Surgery
Comprehensive Wound Center
Wexner Medical Center
The Ohio State University
Columbus, Ohio

Antonio Di Mauro
Department of Pediatrics
University of Bari
Bari, Italy

Gert Folkerts
Division of Pharmacology
Utrecht Institute for Pharmaceutical Sciences
Utrecht University
Utrecht, the Netherlands

Johan Garssen
Division of Pharmacology
Utrecht Institute for Pharmaceutical Sciences
Utrecht University
and
Nutricia Research
Utrecht, the Netherlands

Eric Gumpricht
Research Scientist
Isagenix International
Chandler, Arizona

Mash Hamid
Department of Public Health, Epidemiology and Biostatistics
University of Birmingham
Birmingham, United Kingdom

Kelly C. Heim
Department of Research and Development
Pure Encapsulations, Inc.
Sudbury, Massachusetts

Brian Helland
Northern Plains Center for Behavioral Research
University of North Dakota
Grand Forks, North Dakota

Shigeo Horie
Department of Urology
Graduate School of Medicine
Juntendo University
Tokyo, Japan

Mark Houston
School of Medicine Vanderbilt University
and
Hypertension Institute of Nashville
Saint Thomas Medical Group and Health Services
Saint Thomas Hospital
Nashville, Tennessee

J.R. Ifland
The Victory Meals Program, LLC
Houston, Texas

Cassim Igram
Knowledge House Publishers
Vernon Hills, Illinois

Ngozi Awa Imaga
Department of Biochemistry
College of Medicine
University of Lagos
Lagos, Nigeria

Flavia Indrio
Department of Pediatrics
University of Bari
Bari, Italy

Urmila Jarouliya
School of Studies in Biotechnology
Jiwaji University
Gwalior, India

Nimisha Kankan
Gyan Devi Balika Inter College
Bhadohi, Uttar Pradesh, India

Mayuree Kanlayavattanakul
School of Cosmetic Science
Mae Fah Luang University
Chiang Rai, Thailand

Raj K. Keservani
School of Pharmaceutical Sciences
Rajiv Gandhi Proudyogiki Vishawavidyalaya
Madhya Pradesh, India

Rajesh K. Kesharwani
Department of Biotechnology
National Institute of Technology
Telangana, India

Mi-Ryung Kim
Department of Bio-Food Materials
Silla University
Busan, South Korea

Priyamvadah Kinth
National Institute of Science, Technology and Development Studies
Council of Scientific and Industrial Research
New Delhi, India

Edmund Y. Ko
Department of Urology
Loma Linda University
Loma Linda, California

Zwe-Ling Richard Kong
Department of Food Science
National Taiwan Ocean University
Keelung, Taiwan, People's Republic of China

Sang Gil Lee
Department of Nutritional Sciences
University of Connecticut
Storrs, Connecticut

Michelle Lightfoot
Department of Urology
Loma Linda University
Loma Linda, California

Glenda Lindseth
Northern Plains Center for Behavioral Research
University of North Dakota
Grand Forks, North Dakota

Nattaya Lourith
School of Cosmetic Science
Mae Fah Luang University
Chiang Rai, Thailand

Atreyi Maiti
Department of Biomedical Laboratory Sciences and Management
Vidyasagar University
West Bengal, India

M.T. Marcus
School of Nursing
University of Texas at Austin
Austin, Texas

Palma Ann Marone
Department of Pharmacology and Toxicology
Virginia Commonwealth University
Richmond, Virginia

Neetu Mishra
Centre of Food and Technology
University of Allahabad
Uttar Pradesh, India

Paulin Moszczyński
Private Department of Internal Medicine in Brzesko
Tarnowska College
Tarnów, Poland

Ashley Murray
Minnesota State Community and Technical College
Detroit Lakes, Minnesota

Yuji Naito
Department of Molecular Gastroenterology and Hepatology
Graduate School of Medical Science
Kyoto Prefectural University of Medicine
Kyoto, Japan

Kanti Bhooshan Pandey
Centre of Food and Technology
University of Allahabad
Uttar Pradesh, India

Nicholas V. Perricone
College of Human Medicine
Michigan State University
East Lansing, Michigan

S.K. Polutchko
Department of Ecology and Evolutionary Biology
University of Colorado
Boulder, Colorado

Kartick C. Pramanik
Department of Biomedical Sciences
Cancer Biology Center
Texas Tech University Health Sciences Center
Amarillo, Texas

Harry G. Preuss
Departments of Biochemistry, Medicine and Pathology
Georgetown University Medical Center
Washington, DC

Satish Kumar Ramraj
Department of Radiation Oncology
Oklahoma University Health Sciences Center
Oklahoma City, Oklahoma

Giuseppe Riezzo
Laboratory of Nutritional Pathophysiology
National Institute for Digestive Diseases I.R.C.C.S. "Saverio de Bellis"
Bari, Italy

Syed Ibrahim Rizvi
Department of Biochemistry
University of Allahabad
Uttar Pradesh, India

K.M. Rourke
Polytechnic Institute
The State University of New York
Albany, New York

Sashwati Roy
Department of Surgery
Comprehensive Wound Center
Wexner Medical Center
The Ohio State University
Columbus, Ohio

Seil Sagar
Division of Pharmacology
Utrecht Institute for Pharmaceutical Sciences
Utrecht University
Utrecht, the Netherlands

Peer M. Schenk
Algae Biotechnology Laboratory
School of Agriculture and Food Sciences
The University of Queensland
Brisbane, Queensland, Australia

Anil K. Sharma
Department of Pharmaceutics
Delhi Institute of Pharmaceutical Sciences and Research
New Delhi, India

Kathryn (Kay) Sheppard
Private Practice
Palm Bay, Florida

Swati Singh
Department of Pharmacognosy
Sardar Bhagwan Singh PG Institute of Biomedical Sciences
Uttarakhand, India

Virendra Singh
Department of Pharmaceutics
Roorkee College of Pharmacy
Uttarakhand, India

Michael J. Spinella
Department of Pharmacology and Toxicology
Dartmouth Medical School
Hanover, New Hampshire

and

The Norris Cotton Cancer Center
Lebanon, New Hampshire

J.J. Stewart
Department of Ecology and Evolutionary Biology
University of Colorado
Boulder, Colorado

Clare Stradling
Public Health, Epidemiology and Biostatistics
University of Birmingham
and
Heart of England NHS Foundation Trust HIV Service
Birmingham, United Kingdom

Anand Swaroop
Corporate Management
Cepham Inc.
Piscataway, New Jersey

Zbigniew Tabarowski
Department of Experimental Hematology
Institute of Zoology
Jagiellonian University
Krakow, Poland

Shahrad Taheri
Department of Medicine
Weill Cornell Medical College
New York, New York

and

Department of Medicine
King's College London
London, United Kingdom

W.C. Taylor
School of Public Health
University of Texas
Houston, Texas

G. Neil Thomas
Department of Public Health, Epidemiology and Biostatistics
University of Birmingham
Birmingham, United Kingdom

and

Institute of Public Health, Social and Preventive Medicine
Heidelberg University
Mannheim, Germany

Elnaz Vaghef-Mehrabany
Department of Nutrition, Biochemistry and Diet Therapy
Tabriz University of Medical Sciences
Tabriz, Iran

Leila Vaghef-Mehrabany
Department of Clinical Nutrition
Tehran University of Medical Sciences
Tehran, Iran

Terrence M. Vance
Department of Nutritional Sciences
University of Connecticut
Storrs, Connecticut

Krista Varady
Department of Kinesiology and Nutrition
University of Illinois at Chicago
Chicago, Illinois

Arul Venkatesan
Department of Biotechnology
School of Life Sciences
Pondicherry University
Pondicherry, India

H. Theresa Wright
Renaissance Nutrition Center, Inc.
Norristown, Pennsylvania

Section I

Introduction

1 Global Food Habits and Trends
An Overview

Priyamvadah Kinth and Nimisha Kankan

CONTENTS

1.1 INTRODUCTION

"Eat healthy and live healthy" is one of the essential requirements for long life. Unfortunately, today's world has adapted to a system of consumption of foods, which has several adverse effects on health. Diseases like coronary artery disease and diabetes mellitus have seen a profound rise in developing countries, and such unhealthy junk food consumption is one of the notable factors to their contribution. Junk food simply means an empty calorie food. An empty calorie food is a high-calorie or calorie-rich food that lacks micronutrients such as vitamins, minerals, or amino acids, and fiber but has high energy (calories). These foods do not contain the nutrients that your body needs to stay healthy. Hence, these foods, which have poor nutritional value, are considered unhealthy and may be called as junk food.[1] Because of the following factors, junk food looks more appealing over healthy food (Figure 1.1).

This change in lifestyle has brought about a dramatic nutrition transition characterized by a decrease in the consumption of traditional foods and an increasing reliance on processed, store-bought foods imported from the South. There is significant and valid concern for the health implications of consuming increased amounts of these fat- and sugar-rich foods. Obesity is a key target for nutritional interventions aimed at chronic disease prevention due to the fact that excess body weight is linked to a number of deleterious health effects, including increased risk of coronary heart disease, ischemic stroke, hypertension, dyslipidemia, type 2 diabetes mellitus, joint disease, cancer, asthma, and a host of other chronic conditions.[2]

1.2 NUTRITION TRANSITION FROM "FIT TO FAT"

Wealth and poverty have profound effects on diets, nutrition, and health. Economic factors have a far broader influence on global eating habits than might be expected from the analysis of dietary trends in developed nations. As incomes rise and populations become more urban, societies enter different stages of what has been called the nutrition transition. Generally, diets high in complex carbohydrates and fiber give way to more varied diets with a higher proportion of fats, saturated fats, and sugars. These shifts in diet structure accompany demographic shifts

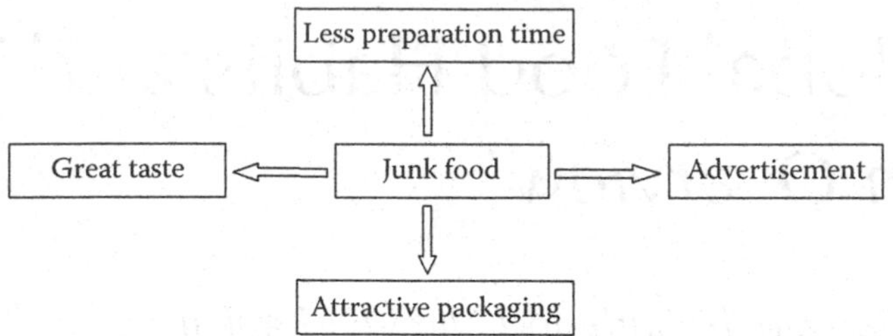

FIGURE 1.1 Appealing factors of junk food.

associated with higher life expectancies and reduced fertility rates. An associated epidemiological transition also takes place as patterns of disease shift away from infectious and nutrient deficiency diseases toward higher rates of coronary heart disease and some types of cancers. The nutrition transition has also been associated with a higher prevalence of obesity, particularly childhood obesity, and noninsulin-dependent diabetes. Food imports, fast foods, and a rising consumption of sugars and animal fats are sometimes held to be responsible for rising global rates of obesity and associated chronic diseases.[3]

The eating habits of our parents, grandparents, and great-grandparents would be completely unrecognizable to many of us today. Our experiences of shopping and cooking have been transformed as have our attitudes toward health, table manners, "foreign" foods, waste, and choice. Today, fast food chains are a global phenomenon and the idea of eating only three meals a day is a thing of the past. We graze our way through the day, nibbling on crisps or chocolate to keep us going between meals. Obesity is on the rise in many developed and developing countries. From cookery programs on television to recipes in magazines and on websites, we are bombarded with advice on what and how to cook.[4]

The global problem of consuming junk food on a large scale and its impact on health needs emphasis and health education that can greatly contribute to its limited consumption and switching over to healthy eating habits for a better living.[1]

Food habits may change because of varying reasons like

- Rapid urbanization
- Availability of different food products
- Alterations in life circumstances force individuals to change
- The influence of rising income and poverty on eating patterns
- Technology change in our kitchens
- Modes of transport supplying our shops
- By the media and government
- By trade and migration

The dietary changes that characterize the "nutrition transition" include both quantitative and qualitative changes in the diet. The adverse dietary changes include shifts in the structure of the diet toward a higher energy density diet with a greater role for fat and added sugars in foods, greater saturated fat intake (mostly from animal sources), reduced intakes of complex carbohydrates and dietary fiber, and reduced fruit and vegetable intakes (Table 1.1). These dietary changes are compounded by lifestyle changes that reflect reduced physical activity at work and during leisure time. At the same time, however, poor countries continue to face food shortages and nutrient inadequacies.[5]

Until the decade following World War II, the majority of fats available for human consumption were animal fats, milk, butter, and meat. The past five decades have seen a revolution in the

TABLE 1.1
Changes in Dietary Pattern

Nutrients	Paleolithic Diet	Modern Diet
Protein	30%–40%	10%–20%
Carbohydrates	35%	60%–70%
Sugars	2%–3%	15%
Fats	30%–35%	30%–35%
Saturated fats	7.5%	15%–30%
Trans-fat	<1%	5%–10% of fats
Omega-6/omega-3	2:1	10–20:1

Source: Sydney-Smith, M.A., *Nutrition Medicine: Genes, Nutrition & Health*, www.nutritionmedicine.org/Files/Genes_Nutrition.ppt.

production and processing of oilseed-based fats. "Urbanization" was the major reason in association of urban residence and diet structure. A large literature review shows that urban as opposed to rural diets are characterized by the consumption of superior and polished grains (rice or wheat, rather than corn or millet), more fats and animal products, more sugar, more processed foods, and more foods consumed away from home.

1.3 GLOBAL HEALTH ISSUES

Because of changes in dietary and lifestyle habits—a phenomenon that can be linked to the whole globalization process—developing countries now face a fast "epidemiological accumulation" of noncommunicable and infectious diseases and must cope with urgent and competing health priorities. Noncommunicable diseases (NCDs)—especially cardiovascular diseases, cancers, chronic respiratory diseases, and diabetes—caused 60% deaths globally in 2005 (approximately 35 million deaths). Total deaths from NCDs are projected to increase by a further 17% over the next 10 years. By 2020, it is predicted that NCDs will account for 80% of the global burden of disease, causing 7 out of every 10 deaths in developing countries. This places a considerable (double) burden on limited health budgets, particularly in emerging economies (Figures 1.2 and 1.3).[7]

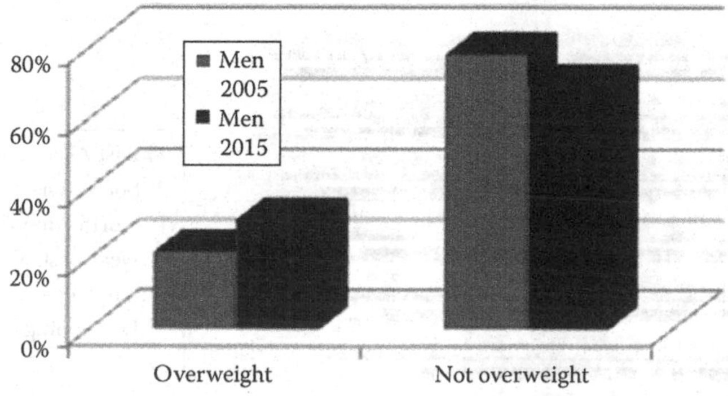

FIGURE 1.2 Projected prevalence of overweight males in India aged 30 years or more, 2005 and 2015. (From WHO, WHO report, http://www.who.int/dietphysicalactivity/publications/trs916/en/gsfao_global.pdf.)

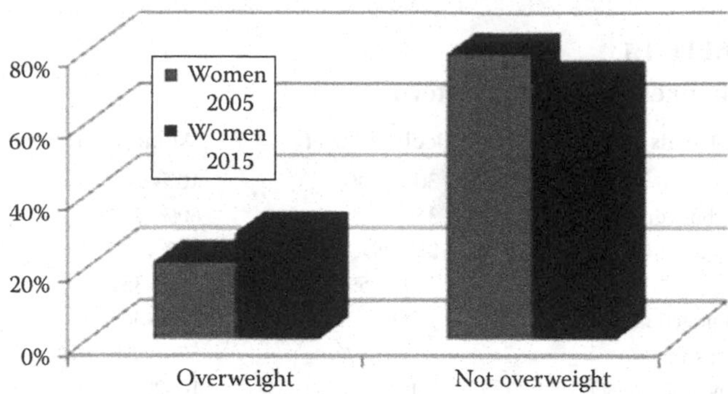

FIGURE 1.3 Projected prevalence of overweight females in India aged 30 years or more, 2005 and 2015. (From WHO, WHO report, http://www.who.int/dietphysicalactivity/publications/trs916/en/gsfao_global.pdf.)

1.4 FOOD CONSUMPTION PATTERN

Changes in agricultural practice over the past 50 years have increased the world's capacity to provide food for its people through increases in productivity, greater diversity of foods, and less seasonal dependence. Food availability has also increased as a consequence of rising income levels and falling food prices. This has resulted in considerable changes in food consumption over the past 50 years. In terms of calories arising from different major food commodities, large differences may be seen between the developing and industrial countries. While developing countries between 1963 and 2003 revealed large increases in the available consumption of calories from meat (119%), sugar (127%), and vegetable oils (199%), only vegetable oil consumption was seen to increase appreciably (105%) in industrial countries over these four decades. China, as a prime example of a populous developing country, showed even more dramatic changes in this 40-year period, especially in vegetable oils (680%), meat (349%), and sugar (305%). In both developing and industrial countries (and again notably in China), declines were seen for pulses and roots and tubers between 1963 and 2003.[8] Figure 1.4 shows the food consumption pattern in kcal/person/day.

The diet of poor people in rural or urban settings in Asia during the 1960s was simple and rather monotonous: rice with a small amount of vegetables, beans, or fish. Today, their eating is transformed. It is common for people in these settings to regularly consume complex meals at any number of away-from-home food outlets—Western or indigenous. The overall composition of diets in the developing world is shifting rapidly, particularly with respect to fat, caloric sweeteners, and animal source foods.[9]

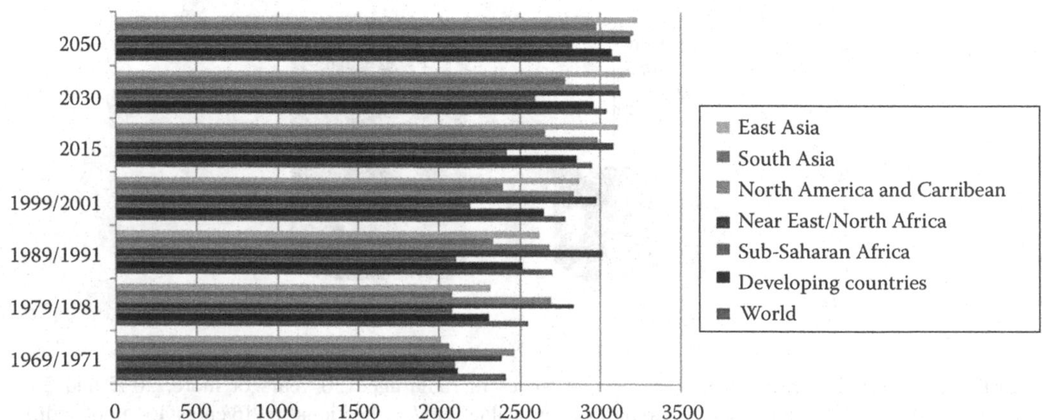

FIGURE 1.4 Per capita food consumption (kcal/person/day).

1.5 CONCLUSION

Nutrition transition is an integral part of life in the developing world, and coming with it is a massive increase in obesity and associated problems. It is important when considering future food policy that a sustainable pattern of food consumption be considered, ensuring a sufficient supply of staples and of micronutrient-rich foods without encouraging excessive consumption of energy-dense, nutrient-poor foods. Food policies will only be effective if they are developed with input from both the agricultural and health sectors, thereby enabling the development of coherent policies that will ultimately be beneficial to agriculture, human health, and the environment.

It is critical that effective investments and social regulations are found that will enhance the components of lifestyle, reduce obesity and diabetes, and provide for a healthier population. In particular, it is important to focus on changes that affect poor people, who are least able to incur the costs of the resultant health burden. The food industry in general has yet to see that its cooperation is critical to improving global health—through the identification of effective society-level measures to increase the relative intake levels of fruit, vegetables, and high-fiber products, replacing the intake of caloric sweeteners and fat.

REFERENCES

1. Ashakiran DR. 2012. Fast foods and their impact on health. *Journal of Krishna Institute of Medical Sciences University* 1:7–15.
2. Sheehy T, Roache C, and Sharma S. 2013. Eating habits of a population undergoing a rapid dietary transition: Portion sizes of traditional and non-traditional foods and beverages consumed by Inuit adults in Nunavut, Canada. *Nutrition Journal* 12:1–11.
3. Drewnowski A and Popkin BM. 1997. The nutrition transition: New trends in the global diet. *Nutrition Reviews* 55:31–43.
4. British Library. *Changes in Eating Habits*. http://www.bl.uk/learning/citizenship/foodstories/Accessible/eatinghabits/changesineatinghabits.html (accessed September 21, 2014).
5. WHO. Global and regional food consumption patterns and trends. http://www.who.int/dietphysicalactivity/publications/trs916/en/gsfao_global.pdf (accessed September 24, 2014).
6. Sydney-Smith MA. *Nutrition Medicine: Genes, Nutrition & Health*. www.nutritionmedicine.org/Files/Genes_Nutrition.ppt (accessed September 21, 2014).
7. Neeha VS and Kinth P. 2013. Nutrigenomics research: A review. *Journal of Food Science and Technology* 50:415–428.
8. Kearney J. 2010. Food consumption trends and drivers. *Philosophical Transactions of the Royal Society B* 365:2793–2807.
9. Popkin BM. 2004. The nutrition transition and the global shift towards obesity. *Diabetes Voice* 49:38–40.

2 Safety and Toxicity of Functional Foods and Nutraceuticals

Palma Ann Marone and Kathryn Birkenbach

CONTENTS

2.1 INTRODUCTION

The Food and Agriculture Organization (FAO) of the United Nations predicts that the world population will reach 9.1 billion people by 2050, 34% higher than it is today (FAO, 2014). In order to ensure the ability to adequately nourish such a global community, a safe, healthy, affordable, and logistically available food supply is common to the development and advancement of all countries. On the consumer level, nutrition ranks second in consideration close behind taste and affordability in the selection of food. To this end, foods, as necessities to all people, are now and will be increasingly called upon to not only provide basic nutrition, but to have a positive effect on health and subsequently, longevity and quality of life. While all foods may be functional in terms of offering physiological benefits and various food ingredients and botanicals have been used for centuries as cultural remedies, the term "Functional Foods" is defined more recently according to the Academy of Nutrition *and* Dietetics as "a food that provides additional health benefits that may reduce disease risk and/or promote good health." Similarly, while the Japanese government was among the first to create this class of foods circa 1980 to distinguish foods on their ability to promote health as an additive benefit to providing basic nutritional needs, the U.S. Food and Drug Administration (U.S. FDA) does not have a regulatory category for foods of functional status. For this reason, the safety and toxicity of these foods is indistinguishable from a regulatory standpoint from those for any food and/or food ingredients in the United States. Nonetheless, a distinct difference arises in relation to the health claims for which they are marketed and claims themselves an important vehicle for informing consumers of the potential health benefits of a given nutrient and the awareness of good nutrition overall.

2.1.1 Classification of Functional Foods

Beyond maintaining survival, functional foods and beverages are intended to optimize a healthy lifestyle. In the United States, the earliest concept of foods as advantageous in the maintenance and management of health extends from the early 1900s when incorporation of iodine into salt was found beneficial in the treatment of goiter. Along with a balanced diet, including a variety of foods, and regular physical activity, a growing number of foods within its respective categories is gaining consideration for its benefits to health and well-being. With the understanding that food science is an advancing continuum and new nutritional combinations are being realized constantly, processed and/or unprocessed functional foods are generally grouped into three categories: (1) foods fortified with nutritional ingredients intended to treat deficiency-based disease; (2) foods containing microorganisms beneficial in promoting healthy internal flora (usually intestinal); and (3) foods that support normal metabolic pathways through physiological enzymatic influence, including genetically modified foods (Williams, 2008). Examples of specific products that have already found common use include soluble and insoluble dietary fibers for digestive and cardiac health; fatty acids and phytoestrogens for cardiac, mental, and immune health; probiotics for digestive health; and vitamins and minerals for metabolic support and cartilage and bone health. Newer functional foods are becoming increasingly better known and utilized and include such examples as carotenoids, isothiocyanates, phytoesters/sterols, polyphenols, and flavonoids as antioxidants for a wide spectrum of physiological support for their anti-inflammatory, antimicrobial, and antimutagenic properties in foods and beverages (Gaur and Agnihotri, 2014). More recently, the use of zinc in the prevention and treatment of colds and flu has gained attention, as its importance in maintaining health of the immune system is well established (Haase and Rink, 2014). The Institute of Food Technologists (IFT) review (IFT, 2005) remains an excellent review of functional foods' role and opportunities.

2.2 REGULATORY STANDARDS FOR FUNCTIONAL FOODS

Food is the most heterogeneous category of consumer product available to humans and the one to which they are most often exposed. Unlike other products that are manufactured under carefully controlled environments, defined by distinct chemical entities, purity and manufacture, commercially available under strict standards, food and its potential nutrient content is a complex mixture, reliant upon variable parameters such as environment and growth conditions, animal feed and supply systems, storage conditions, transportation, handling, processing, and packaging. Considering this in conjunction with the infinitely vast myriad of components a natural botanical may contain, the means of assuring safety from "farm to fork" become challenging and ever-changing. With this understanding, some basic and globally harmonized regulatory processes for purposing functional foods under a variety of uses have become standard. Trends of the industry are gravitating toward specialization to the tailored nutritional needs of a specific culture, and more exclusively, individual. Nutrigenomics, or personalized nutrition, is the application of the human genome to nutrition and personal health for the purpose of providing individual dietary recommendations (IFT, 2005). New market products specifically designed for children and seniors are also spurring the regulatory process due to the special nutritional needs and sensitivities of these populations.

Functional foods and beverages are regulated as part of the larger context of food, drink, chewing gum, and any components thereof by the U.S. FDA. However, the United States Environmental Protection Agency (U.S. EPA) safeguards human health and the natural environment through environmental/antipollution and pesticide regulations (Pollution Prevention, Toxic Substances, Clean Air, Clean Air and Safe Drinking Water Acts), thereby indirectly influencing food safety. As defined, the current Food and Drug and Cosmetics (FD&C) Act under the jurisdiction of the FDA considers food to be inherently safe, without the need for premarket approval (Sections 201(f); 401(a)(1)) presuming that the food is uncontaminated. While the original Food and Drug Act of 1906 forbade the marketing of any food containing substances injurious to health, it is the 1938 revision (FD&C Act, now including cosmetics) that detailed the standards of food safety, including the criteria for quality and adulteration. This legislation placed the burden of safety on the manufacturer when food is marketed outside of its point of origin, particularly that across state lines. The contents of food were distinguished between those naturally present (pesticide residues) and those that were added (food/color additives for taste, aroma, and nutritive value) depending on their intended use. The FD&C Act was again revised in 1958 to include the Food Additives Amendment, most notably for incorporation of the directorate that the "... Food and Drug Administration shall not approve for use in food any chemical additive found to induce cancer in man, or, after tests, found to induce cancer in animals" (Merrill, 1997). The "Delaney Clause," as it has come to be known, prohibits the use of any food additive known to be carcinogenic in man (Sections 409, 512, 721).

Of additional importance is the distinction of Generally Recognized as Safe (GRAS), which eliminates the need for premarket approval of such products from the FDA by virtue of their history and/or condition of use and the readily available information evaluated by scientists qualified by their training and experience, on any substance intended to be a component of food (U.S FDA http://www.fda.gov/Food/IngredientsPackagingLabeling/GRAS/ucm094040.htm) (Sections 201(s), 409; 21 CFR 570.3 and 21 CFR 570.30). Any intentionally added food ingredient that is not GRAS is considered either a food additive or a color additive (color additives are not eligible for GRAS status). Since that time, the "GRAS List" has been modified from an FDA GRAS affirmation process (1972) to one of the notifications (1997). This distinction moves the onus of safety from the FDA to the manufacturer by way of toxicological testing through regulation-approved safety guidelines (Neltner et al., 2011). The U.S. FDA's Redbook II and the Organization of Economic Cooperative and Development (OECD) provide standardized guidelines for safety testing of food additives for human and pet foods for member countries.

Recommended study designs and data for preclinical genotoxicity, general short- and long-term toxicity, developmental and reproductive toxicity studies, and pharmacokinetic and metabolism studies, the extent of which varies from low and intermediate safety concern levels to clinical studies when the safety concern level is high, are reviewed in the United States by the Center of Food Safety and Applied Nutrition within the FDA. Added clarifications to food safety regulation include the Dietary Supplement Health and Education Act of 1994 (DSHEA), which defines dietary supplements as food apart from drugs and offers premarket recommendations for new dietary ingredients (NDIs). In addition, guidance for the manufacturing methods and requirements for processed foods and dietary supplements, along with the critical control points identifying the potential hazards of food manufacture, handling, processing, and distribution for food ingredients and food packaging are regulated under the current Good Manufacturing Practices (cGMP) and Hazard Analysis and Critical Control Points (HACCP), respectively. Most recently, sweeping legislation in the form of the Food Safety Modernization Act (U.S. FDA, 2011) was implemented to enforce FDA food safety standards applicable to the United States and foreign manufacturers producing, packaging, and distributing food for U.S. consumption. Timelines for the complete implementation of the current law regarding preventive controls for human and animal foods, produce safety, the foreign supplier verification program and third-party accreditation, sanitary transport, and for intentional adulteration are now being imposed (http://www.fda.gov/Food/GuidanceRegulation/FSMA).

U.S. regulatory food safety standards have continually been adapted and revised, harmonized efforts among regulatory agencies within the international community, to ensure a safe global food supply from "farm to fork." The International Organization for Standardization (ISO) has implemented a global food management safety system (ISO 22000; FSSC 22000) used by its member countries to certify quality measures for manufacturing and processing under the original 1995 HACCP regulations. Working together with the FAO, the World Health Organization (WHO), and the Codex Alimentarius Commission, the International Food Safety Authorities Network (INFOSAN) includes a 181-country network conferencing under Pan-American and Pan-European as well as Asian-Pacific regions to adopt guidelines for food safety. International consortia and commissions such as the European Food Safety Authority (EFSA), the Joint FAO/WHO Expert Committee on Food Additives (JECFA), the European Action on Latin America Functional Foods (EULAFF), the OECD, and others now coordinate efforts to harmonize global food safety guidelines (Table 2.1).

Beyond internationally coordinated efforts, the definition and regulation of functional foods have advanced at the level of individual nations and regions. In Canada, Agriculture and Agri-Food Canada with Health Canada recognizes foods of health benefit through labeling and health claims in a manner similar to that of the United States. In the European Union (EU), regulation released in 1997 defined "novelty foods" as those not used prior to May 1997 (EC Reg. 258/1997; EC, 1997). Its 2013 revision (EC, 2013) was intended to restore consumer confidence by controlling fraud and misinformation and encouraging healthy dietary habits. Under this revision, manufacturers must simplify the procedure for notifying consumers of the presence of nanomaterials and their safe usage. In Asia, specific directives included the "Food *for* Specified Health Use" (FOSHU) standard created by the Japanese Ministry of Health, Labor and Welfare in 1991, which allowed functional food producers to make health claims on authorized product labels. In China, the Ministry of Health implemented the Control of Health Food in 1996 to recognize foods with health benefits. Further, the Chinese Ministry of Health regulates functional foods through China's State Food and Drug Administration, while Indonesia and others recognize functional foods through Ministries of Health.

In addition, individual industry consortia such as the International Organization of the Flavor Industry (IOFI) along with the Flavor and Extract Manufacturers Association (FEMA), the International Association of Color Manufacturers (IACM), the American Spice Trade Association, the Renewable Citrus Products Association, the U.S. Department of Agriculture (USDA), the Grocery Manufacturers Association, and many others in the United States and worldwide work together to assess new products and safety for their respective industry. EFSA has published a QPS (Qualified Presumption of Safety) listing of botanicals considered safe in the EU. Assisting is the joint BelFrit guideline listing of approximately 1000 botanicals that may or may not be used in dietary supplements based on available efficacy and safety data. BelFrit, an example of the specificity of some safety laws according to nation, is considered legally binding in Italy, whereas for other members such as France and Belgium, the guideline is a recommendation.

TABLE 2.1
Listing of the Major International Food Safety Groups

Africa

National Agency for Food and Drug Administration Ministry of Health

Americas

European Action on Latin America Functional Foods
Latin America Functional Foods (EULAFF)

- Argentina
  - Minister of Economy
    - Secretariat of Agriculture, Livestock, Fishing and Food
      - National Food Safety and Quality Service (SENASA). Servicio Nacional de Sanidad y Calidad Agroalimentaria
- Canada
  - Minister of Agriculture
    - Agriculture and Agri-Food Canada
      - Canadian Food Inspection Agency (CFIA)
    - Minister of Health
      - Health Canada
        - Health Products and Food Branch
        - Guelph Food Technology Centre (Canada)
- The United States
  - U.S. Food and Drug Administration (U.S. FDA)
    - Center for Food Safety and Applied Nutrition (CFSAN)
  - International Food Protection Training Institute (IFPTI)
  - Joint Expert Committee on Food Additives (JECFA)
  - United States Department of Agriculture (USDA)
    - Under Secretary for Food Safety
      - Food Safety and Inspection Service (FSIS)
  - NSF International

Asia

Asia-Pacific Economic Cooperation Food Safety Cooperation Forum (APEC-FSCF)
Food Safety Cooperation Working Group (FSCWG)

- China
  - General Administration of Quality Supervision, Inspection and Quarantine
  - State Food and Drug Administration
- India
  - Food Safety and Standards Authority of India
- Philippines
  - Food & Drug Administration (Philippines)
- South Korea
  - Ministry of Food and Drug Safety (MFDS)
  - Minster for Health, Welfare and Family Affairs
    - Ministry for Health, Welfare and Family Affairs
      - Office for Healthcare Policy

Europe

- Multinational
  - European Union
    - Committee on the Environment, Public Health and Food Safety (EU)
    - European Food Safety Authority
    - SAFEFOODS

(Continued)

TABLE 2.1 (*Continued*)
Listing of the Major International Food Safety Groups

- Food Safety Promotion Board
- Advisory Group of the European Commission

- Germany
    - Federal Ministry of Food, Agriculture and Consumer Protection
        - Bundesamtfür Verbraucherschutz und Lebensmittelsicherheit
        - Bundesanstaltfür Landwirtschaft und Ernährung
- Ireland
    - Food Safety Authority of Ireland
- Netherlands
    - Ministry of Economic Affairs, Agriculture and Innovation (ELI)
        - nieuwe Voedselen Waren Autoriteit (nVWA)
        - Rijks Kwaliteits instituutvoor Land-en Tuinbouwproducten (RiKILT)
        - Rijksinstituutvoor Volksgezondheiden Milieu (RiVM)
    - Stichting Voedingscentrum Nederland
- Norway
    - Minister of Agriculture and Food
        - Norwegian Ministry of Agriculture and Food *Landbruks- og matdepartementet*
            - Norwegian Food Safety Authority *Mattilsynet*
- Spain
    - Health Department of the Generalitatde Catalunya
        - Catalan Food Safety Agency
- The United Kingdom
    - Department for Environment, Food and Rural Affairs
        - Animal Health
        - Pesticides Safety Directorate
        - U.K. Government Decontamination Service
        - Veterinary Medicines Directorate
    - Food Standards Agency
        - Advisory committee on the microbiological safety of food

Oceania

- Multinational
    - Food Standards Australia New Zealand (FSANZ)
- Australia
    - Minister for Agriculture, Fisheries and Forestry
        - Department of Agriculture (DAFF)
            - Australian Quarantine and Inspection Service (AQIS)
            - Biosecurity Australia
    - Government of New South Wales
        - Minister for Primary Industries (NSW)
            - New South Wales Food Authority
    - Australian International Food Security Centre (AIFSC)
- New Zealand
    - Minister for Food Safety
        - New Zealand Food Safety Authority (NZFSA)

International

- Conference for Food Protection
- Institute of Food and Agricultural Sciences
- Institute of Food Technologists
- International Association for Food Protection

(*Continued*)

TABLE 2.1 (*Continued*)
Listing of the Major International Food Safety Groups

- International Food Information Council
- International Life Sciences Institute
- World Health Organization
- Food and Agriculture Organization of the United Nations
- International Organization for Standardization
- HACCP International-Hazard Analysis and Critical Control Points
- International Food Safety Authorities Network (INFOSAN)
- Joint FAO/WHO Expert Committee on Food Additives (JECFA)
- Office of Economic Cooperation and Development (OECD)

2.2.1 Functional Food Labeling Regulation

The purpose of food labeling is to facilitate informed choices on the part of the consumer to optimize consumption of a nutritional diet. In addition, contents of a dietary label allow for sensitive individuals to ascertain the possible hazards associated with intolerance to particular ingredients. With consumers becoming more aware of the importance of nutrition to health, food labels are being increasingly used to make informed decisions through comparison of what is actually being consumed to what the consumer knows about nutrition and health. Label components contain information (top to bottom) for serving size, calories from fat, and the amount of individual nutrients in percent of daily values with appropriately sized type commensurate with importance. However, the current standard nutritional facts label, which has been unchanged in more than 20 years of use, can be misleading in informing consumers of true nutritional impact, often reflecting quantities of food significantly smaller than those that would realistically be consumed in one sitting. Changes to the current nutrition facts label have thus recently been proposed by FDA "to expand and highlight the information they (consumers) most need when making food choices." To this end, the first changes will include updating serving sizes of foods such as potato chips and ice cream to reflect *actual* quantities likely to be consumed at one time, as opposed to what *should* be eaten. Associated with this is enlarging in bold the caloric contents/serving type for healthy weight maintenance; dual listings for the actual quantities of an ingredient metrically along with the traditional percentage, now shifted to the left for visual ease; eliminating the "calories from fat" to include only the *type* of fat; updating the daily values for sodium and dietary fiber; adding a line item for potassium and vitamin D to highlight the established link of these micronutrients to bone health and to prompt consumer awareness to add these nutrients to their diet; and including a line item for added sugar content (http://www.fda.gov/Food/GuidanceRegulation/GuidanceDocumentsRegulatoryInformation/LabelingNutrition/ucm385663). Most recently, the FDA has extended the calorie content requirement of foods and beverages, to be displayed "clearly and conspicuously," to supermarkets, restaurants, convenience stores, movie theaters, vending machines (exempting transportation venues), and other eating establishments with 20 or more locations. Additional nutritional information (i.e. fats, sugars, minerals, etc.) must be made available on request.

2.2.2 Regulation of Functional Food Health Claims

As described in detail later, the FDA recognizes three categories of claims that are defined by statute or regulation for conventional foods and dietary supplements: health claims, nutrient content claims, and structure/function claims. Each of these, by definition, requires the following two essential and truthful components: (1) a substance—usually a food or food component or dietary supplement—and (2) a disease or health-related condition as a target for the product's beneficial use.

a. *Health claims*: Through the Nutrition Labeling and Education Act of 1990 (NLEA), food labeling allows for health claims that characterize a relationship between a food, a food component, or dietary ingredient and the risk of a disease on the basis of evidence in the scientific literature and scientific agreement (e.g. "adequate calcium throughout life may reduce the risk of osteoporosis"). "The Food and Drug Administration Modernization Act of 1997 (FDAMA) provides for the use of a health claim in food labeling to be authorized by submission of a notification to FDA of a claim based on an 'authoritative statement' from certain scientific bodies of the U.S. Government or the National Academy of Sciences." This path is unavailable for dietary supplements. An interim qualification for review of heath claims when there is "emerging evidence for a relationship between a food substance (a food, food component, or dietary ingredient) and reduced risk of a disease or health-related condition, but the evidence is not well enough established to meet the significant scientific agreement standard required for FDA to issue an authorizing regulation."
b. *Nutrient content claims* describe the level of nutrient in the product with such terms as "low," "high," "lite," "reduced," etc. In quantitative comparison, these claims ensure that these terms are used consistently and accurately. These claims apply only to those nutrients that have an established Daily Value as defined by the food labeling guide.
c. *Structure/function claims* are statements that address the role of a specific substance in maintaining normal healthy structures or functions of the body (IFT, 2005). The Dietary Supplement Health and Education Act of 1994 established regulatory requirements and procedures for using three types of structure/function claims: (i) Those that describe the role of a nutrient or dietary ingredient intended to affect the normal structure or function of the human body, for example "calcium builds strong bones"; (ii) "Those that characterize the means by which a nutrient or dietary ingredient acts to maintain such structure or function, for example, 'fiber maintains bowel regularity'"; and (iii) Those that support generalized well-being or as part of a benefit related to a nutrient deficiency (vitamin D for the treatment of rickets). Unlike health claims, structure/function claims are not subject to premarket review and authorization by the FDA (http://www.fda.gov/Food/IngredientsPackagingLabeling/LabelingNutrition/ucm111447.htm).

With the understanding that there is no regulatory recognition of functional food status by the U.S. FDA, the consumer is often left to evaluate claims of health promotion independently. When applicable, these statements are often used as a marketing tool where premarket approval is not needed.

In 2006, the European Commission adopted regulation on nutrition and health claims made on foods, laying down harmonized rules across the EU (http://ec.europa.eu/food/food/labelling-nutrition/claims/index_en.htm). More recently in 2008 and in its revision (EU, 2013), Novel Food Nutrition added emphasis on labeling regulation for the application of nanomaterials, the assessment of traditional foods from third countries, and the criteria for risk assessment in novel food authorization. The use of cloned animals in food production remains to be considered. However, newer regulation addresses the use of enzyme technologies in food, and along with it, EFSA has agreed to consider intestinal and immune health claim status for pre- and probiotics, previously unattainable in the EU (EU, 2013; McCartney, 2014).

2.3 EVALUATION OF FUNCTIONAL FOODS

In the United States, functional foods, food additives, and color additives follow similar safety requirements. Safety is established on the basis of purpose of use, the food to which the food product is added, its proposed concentration level, and the population for which it is intended (Kotsonis et al., 2010). The manufacturers of functional foods and their bioactive components, in order to support health claims and garner consumer confidence, must demonstrate both science-based efficacy and safety in processes that are weighed in time and cost for benefit. While the criteria for evaluating efficacy and the factors influencing bioavailability are beyond the scope of this review, and excellent discussions on biomarkers and pharmacological processes are available at IFT (2005) and Ghosh et al. (2015), it is noteworthy to indicate that the chemical and physical form of a given food, even subtly, may profoundly influence the absorption and thus its utilization/bioactivity. These factors, as a result, may profoundly influence a food's cumulative level of exposure and safety. Closer scrutiny of dose level is warranted as a higher bioavailability results in the need for lower doses for effect, particularly in sensitive individuals. Examples of such changes include physical changes (encapsulation, coatings, emulsifiers, buccoadhesive strip melts, and gummy delivery systems) for convenience and ease of use; chemical changes (heating, oxidation, states, pasteurization, irradiation, detergents, and others [vitamins C and E, curcumin additions as antioxidants]); processing aids, including disinfectants and preservatives (ethanol, ozone, chlorine, lactic acid), for microbial control; enhancements of color, texture, and taste for appeal (anthocyanin, capsaicin, gum arabic, carrageenan); and fortification technologies (addition of vitamin D to milk to prevent rickets; niacin to flour to prevent pellegra). Bioavailability ultimately plays a large role in the success of a product since consumers unable to feel the benefit of the functional food likely will not accept it (IFIC, 2013).

2.3.1 Exposure and Concern Level

The concept of exposure and safety level arose out of modification to the 1958 FD&C from the ideas that food additives at any level should be without harm, that safety of a food additive, and thereby its proposed functionality, is not absolute, and that purity and exposure level are important criteria in the assessment of food additive safety. Safety is determined such that the expected exposure is lower than the acceptable daily intake (ADI) and that all dietary sources of a given ingredient must be considered in formulating a cumulative assessment (Alger et al., 2013).

Exposure, as determined by the Estimated Daily Intake (EDI), is dependent upon the daily intake of the food to which the substance is added, and the concentration of that substance in the food developed from food consumption surveys and modeling intake data (Kruger et al., 2014). The FDA considers the maximal intended use levels to calculate the highest level of exposure (dose) possible, oftentimes resulting from the sum of a given additive being used in more than one food. Because the additive may be available for another purpose, all sources, including those of nonfood usage (migration from surfaces/containers/packaging), must be considered. The FDA maintains a database with this information (www.fda.gov/Food/IngredientsPackagingLabeling/PackagingFCS/CEDI/default.htm). With these data in hand, safety for intended use, as required by the United States and global regulatory agencies, is dependent on the EDI being less than the ADI (WHO, 1989). In turn, the ADI is generally based on in vivo long-term preclinical toxicological studies, oftentimes in rodent, for which a No-Adverse-Effect Level (NOAEL) with a 100-fold safety factor accounting for the uncertainty in variance of species (10×) and individuals (10×) for human use is determined.

Structure–activity relationships resulting from the known physical and chemical behaviors of functional groups incorporated into food additives and the duration of exposure are the basis for determining concern level and the degree of toxicological testing appropriate for the given food. Categories for concern include those of (1) low concern—requiring in vitro or short-term or acute testing of 1-month duration or less; (2) intermediate concern—requiring a 1–3-month testing duration in rodents and nonrodents, some reproductive assessment and short-term tests for carcinogenicity potential; and (3) high concern—long-term (1-year duration) testing in rodent and nonrodent, with multigenerational reproduction studies. More recently, quantitative structure–activity relationships (QSAR), in silico model, and high-throughput screening have been proposed for identifying bioactivity and the toxicological potential of chemicals in foods and packaging (Hartung and Hoffmann, 2009; Lattanzio et al., 2009; Price and Chaudhry, 2014; Schilter et al., 2014), and these, along with traditional toxicological methods of safety evaluation, have served to complement and extend regulatory review (EFSA, 2014b).

2.3.2 Safety and Toxicological Determinants

Safety determinants for food additive petitions and GRAS notifications for their respective purpose have relied on thorough assessment of any and all information available on the given test product. Components of a safety review traditionally have included review of the existing literature; analysis of the neat test substance by verifiable and validated chemical protocols, with comparison to all similar classed chemical compounds; determination of the exposure levels with possible accumulated risk over time; and performance and integration of available published and unpublished toxicological and pharmacological studies (in vitro and in vivo; clinical and preclinical) (Kruger et al., 2014).

Performance of preclinical toxicological and pharmacological studies is mandated through Good Laboratory Practice (GLP) to ensure reproducible, reliable results under global regulatory guidelines. First adopted in New Zealand and Denmark in 1972, in the United States by the FDA (1978) and U.S. EPA (1979/1980), and later the EU (1987), the OECD has helped endorse GLP compliance through their present 34 member countries. Since that time, the OECD guidelines for the testing of chemicals (Sections 1–5) were instituted and, over the ensuing years, have been continually adapted and refined (http://www.oecd.org/chemicalsafety/testing/oecdguidelinesforthetestingofchemicals.htm) for the chemical properties, the influence on the environment, and the potential health effects in in vitro and in vivo systems of a given test substance.

Along with the OECD health effects guidelines, FDA's Center of Food Safety and Applied Nutrition and Center for Drug Evaluation and Research (CDER) is responsible for compliance with FDA Redbook II, Toxicological Principles for the Safety Assessment of Food Ingredients, Section IV (Guidelines for Toxicity Studies—Genotoxicity, Acute/Subchronic/Chronic, Reproductive Toxicity) in the United States. In addition, the *International Conference on Harmonization of Technical Requirements for Registration of Pharmaceuticals for Human Use* (ICH, formed 1990) (Safety Sections S1A–S10) unites the regulatory authorities and pharmaceutical industry of Europe, Japan, and the United States to coordinate scientific and technical aspects of drug registration (http://www.ich.org/products/guidelines/safety/article/safety-guidelines.html) when the functional food has a product health claim.

Preclinical safety testing processes performed for either premarket approval (NDI) or premarket exemption (GRAS) are fundamentally similar. While a manufacturer intending to market a New Dietary Ingredient must submit to the FDA documented evidence establishing that the NDI is reasonably expected to be safe as used in the dietary supplement at least 75 days before introduction of the product into commerce, both NDIs and GRAS notifications require carefully planned, product-specific designed studies in toxicology to ensure that a NOAEL is obtained and is sufficiently high to assure safety.

Similarly, just as GLP helps to ensure a standardized rigor for the individual studies, the degree of testing will depend on the available information and potential safety concern. Generally, testing to assure food and beverage safety falls into three categories by requirement: (1) characterization of the test product; (2) preclinical toxicology and pharmacology under accepted guidelines; and (3) clinical testing, when warranted. GRAS determination is accompanied by a peer-reviewed published manuscript as documented verification of its safety review and approval by an expert scientific panel, qualified by knowledge and experience, for its intended use.

2.3.2.1 Analytic Characterization of Functional Foods

Inherent safety is a requirement of foods and GRAS products are safe by virtue of their history of use. Nonetheless, foods by their ecologic origin are not pure and derived fundamentally of plant origin, inherently subject to variability of soils and climate. Food impurities include residues from soils in the raw product, through the manufacturing and handling process, to packaging leachates. The ability to assess impurities is important to manufacture brand as it gives indication of food quality, the hygienic rigor under which the food is produced, and its freshness. Contaminants in the form of heavy metals (lead, cadmium), pesticides (dioxin), microbial (pathogenic bacteria, i.e. *Salmonella*, viruses, parasites, and marine poisons), and natural plant constituent hazards (mycotoxins, aflotoxins; Alexander et al., 2012) should be determined prior to market. Adulteration, considered by the FDA as the addition of injurious substances not inherent in food, often for the purposes of increasing product weight for economic gain, may be determined analytically, but awareness of an incident most usually lags behind the analytic methods in place for proactive prevention. An example of economically motivated adulteration with serious toxicological consequences was the introduction of melamine to infant formula and pet food in China in 2007. The addition of melamine to form melamine cyanurate leading to kidney stones and renal failure was widely documented (Gossner et al., 2009; WHO, 2008). Thus, it is important for manufacturers to both anticipate and identify any possible impurities/contaminants and in cooperation with regulatory bodies through scientific consensus in order to determine acceptable levels of risk. Food Chemicals Codex (FCC) and the EU Regulation No. 231/2012 food additives listed in Annexes II and III to Regulation (EC) No. 1333/2008 (food additives) along with the JECFA, specify acceptable levels of quality and purity of food-grade ingredients in the United States and EU, respectively (EC, 2012, http://www.fda.gov/Food/GuidanceComplianceRegulatoryInformation/GuidanceDocuments/ChemicalContaminantsandPesticides/default.htm). Recent considerations for food contaminants include the ability to detect and measure antibiotic and steroid hormone implants used in veterinary foodstuffs (http://www.fda.gov/AnimalVeterinary/GuidanceComplianceEnforcement/GuidanceforIndustry/ucm042450.htm), and identification of $^{131,133}I$; $^{134,137}Cs$; and ^{90}Sr radioactivity as occurred in the Fukushima Diichi nuclear disaster of 2011 (U.S. FDA). For this reason, any monograph addressing product safety is required to detail the analytic method suitable to the unique processing of the food chemical since the conditions and techniques utilized in one laboratory may yield different results for purity and contaminants in another.

The process of characterization of the test product, the most fundamental of requirements, requires documentation of the precise, complete chemical method/profile, including substantiation on the part of the manufacturer of the product's potency, purity, and stability, and the ability through current agricultural and GMPs, and thus permits reliable reproduction of the same product on a large scale while keeping impurities to the lowest level reasonably achievable. Pertinent guidelines for the determination of chemical preparation in foods include Section 1, Physical Chemical Properties (http://www.oecd-ilibrary.org/environment/oecd-guidelines-for-the-testing-of-chemicals-section-1-physical-chemical-properties_20745753); residue chemistry in field crops and groundwater leaching and ecotoxicology, Section 2, Effects on Biotic Systems (http://www.oecd-ilibrary.org/environment/oecd-guidelines-for-the-testing-of-chemicals-section-2-effects-on-biotic-systems_20745761) and Section 5 (Other) as needed; and biodegradation and accumulation, Section 3, Degradation and Accumulation (http://www.oecd-ilibrary.org/environment/oecd-guidelines-for-the-testing-of-chemicals-section-3-degradation-and-accumulation_2074577x).

Analytic support during the course of a toxicological study is critical for the verification of the validity of the study and the subsequent ability to determine a NOEL, NOAEL, or low-effect level (LOEL) for the product. In addition to quantifying the neat test product, assessment for dose formulation homogeneity, stability, and dose verification using a quantifiable, reproducible method against a known standard makes allowances for incorporation of the active ingredient into the vehicle or heterogeneous dietary mix, *under the conditions of the study*. Similarly, pharmacokinetic and toxicokinetic biochemical analysis from blood and/or target tissue during a toxicological study gives indication of the absorption, distribution, metabolism, and elimination (ADME) of the active test product and may be used to illuminate its bioactivity and efficacy, mechanism, and/or mode of action.

2.3.2.2 Regulatory and Preclinical Assessment

The 2011 FDA Food Safety Modernization Act was promulgated to ensure a safe food supply. Incumbent upon the manufacturer is the responsibility to produce a safe, high-quality product, and to that end preclinical studies remain a most useful tool to evaluate the safety of functional foods. The need for acute, short-term and/or repeated-dose, long-term studies along with genotoxic and reproductive toxicity evaluation is determined by the concern level of the test product (Faqi, 2013; Kruger et al., 2014) and is available at: http://www.oecd-ilibrary.org/environment/oecd-guidelines-for-the-testing-of-chemicals-section-4-health-effects_20745788 and http://www.fda.gov/Food/GuidanceRegulation/GuidanceDocumentsRegulatoryInformation/IngredientsAdditivesGRASPackaging/ucm2006826.htm.

Genotoxicity studies, required as part of the standard battery of tests for NDIs and GRAS, are a preliminary screen for carcinogenicity, clinical studies, and long-term toxicology testing. As such, this initial line of toxicity testing satisfies the Delaney prohibition and elimination of known carcinogens in food or color additives to the food supply. Three levels (gene, chromosome, and genome) of information on the mutagenic potential of a product may be determined through in vitro or in vivo tests designed to detect agents that can induce genetic damage directly or indirectly (Kirsch-Volders et al., 2011; Mazzoleni et al., 2009). Gene mutations, structural chromosomal aberrations, recombinations, and numerical changes may elicit effects in germ cells for heritable defects or in somatic mutations for their role in malignancy. For this reason, one test does not detect more than one endpoint, hence the need for a genotoxic battery of tests. The in vitro Ames test (ICH S2R1, 2011; OECD TG 471, 1997a; U.S. FDA, 2007a) for mutagenicity in bacteria remains the industry standard for recommended preliminary Tier I testing for its rapid, inexpensive concordance to carcinogens (specificity) (EFSA Scientific Committee, 2011b). This test, in combination with the in vitro mammalian micronucleus test (OECD TG 487, 2010a) for clastogenicity, is most efficient in detecting all relevant genotoxic carcinogens (Kirkland et al., 2005, 2011). It is notable to mention that dietary supplements are often composed of natural ingredients, so it is particularly useful when performing these tests to have an analytic profile of the test product for purity and contaminants as they can interfere with plating and solubility. Food product solubility is a particular concern for oil/fat products as their interaction with the indicator bacterial lipid bilayer predisposes to false positives (low specificity). Recommended Tier II genotoxicity testing (EFSA Scientific Committee, 2011b; ICH, 2011) includes the in vivo mammalian micronucleus test (OECD TG 474, 2014) to investigate the positive results obtained with in vitro testing. The in vivo mammalian micronucleus test can be incorporated into a standard subchronic toxicology study in rodents for efficiently applying three R (replacement, reduction, refinement) testing for animal usage.

Acute toxicity studies (OECD TG 425, 2008a; U.S. FDA, 1993a), defined by their single, usually oral dosages, generally have higher dose levels for the determination of target organ specificity and overall survival (LD50). Limit testing (1000 mg/kg/day) is acceptable for products with anticipated low toxicity and may be most useful in genetically modified product testing where availability of the test product is at a premium.

Repeated-dose toxicology studies (US FDA, 2003a,b,c, 2006; 2007b; ICH, S4 1998, S1, S1A-1CR2, 1995, 1997, 2008, 2013, 1995, 1997, 2008; OECD TGs 407, 408, 409 451, 452, 453, 2008b, 1998a,b, 2009a,b,c), considered subacute (<1 month), subchronic (1–3 months), and chronic (>3 months) (Eaton and Klaasen, 2001), typically consisting of a control and three test groups with dose levels approximately 90%, 50%, and 10%–25% of the maximal tolerated dose, are used for the determination of a NOAEL, NOEL, or LOEL. Sensitivity to the test material as well as availability of an ample historical database will influence species selection. Rodents are most often used as the preferred species for most routes of exposure. Similarly, limited test product availability such as the case in nanoparticulate products or genetically modified foods may also play a role in species selection, with smaller rodents (i.e. mice) being chosen for conservation of test material. As the level of toxicological concern rises, usage of dogs and rabbits become the second, confirmatory species, with rabbits more common in teratologic and developmental studies. When possible, the oral route of administration is often preferred for dietary supplements as this is the route most closely resembling that used by humans. Dosage is well controlled as long as the dietary concentration of the test product is adjusted for weekly body weight. The maximum recommended test product in the diet is 5% (Borzelleca, 1992; Hayes, 2008; Kruger et al., 2014) in order to maintain nutritional balance over time and individual dietary ingredients in various natural and purified formulas may be tailored to suitably complement the test product. For example isocaloric diets are available when the test product, such as a fat or oil, adds caloricity for comparison with the control. Dietary certification is recommended to assure consistency in formulation over time and batch, and the choice of powdered meal over pellets assures greater accuracy in food consumption measurement during the course of the study. Measurement of the test product in drinking water is considered less accurate due to unavoidable leakage. End-of-study pathological endpoints of clinical chemistry, hematology, coagulation, and urinalysis along with anatomic pathology tissue weight and histological evaluation are recommended, considered definitive, assessments for the determination of safety.

Additional clinical analyses coordinate with anticipated effects of the given test product may be performed and may include quantitative assessments in lipid profiles (LDL, HDL), hormone levels (estrogen, testosterone), heart enzymes (creatine kinase-MB, malondialdehyde), to name a few. Standard histological evaluation of lymphoid organs and bone marrow will satisfy Type 1 immunotoxicity screening, while more detailed Type II level testing incorporating challenge with a known antigen (ICH, 2005a; U.S. FDA, 1993b) is used when indicated. Procurement of blood and target organs for toxicokinetic and metabolic (ICH, 1994a,b; U.S. FDA, 1993c) determination, performance of functional observational battery with motor activity screening for possible neurologic effects (Boucard et al., 2010; Moser, 2011; OECD TG 424, 1997c; U.S. FDA, 2000c), and ophthalmological assessment are also recommended as terminal endpoints when no other such information is available. Familiar in vivo and in vitro pharmacological models widely used for proof-of-concept support standardized guideline testing for such disorders as metabolic syndrome—dyslipidemia, obesity/eating disorders, and diabetes; cardiovascular function—shock, hemorrhage, heart failure, hypertension, atherosclerosis; immune enhancement/suppression—inflammation, and arthritis; gastrointestinal disorders—ulcer, diarrhea, abdominal pain and bloating, irritable bowel syndrome, and emesis; central nervous system function—cognition/memory, insomnia, and pain; and osteoporosis, calcium supplementation, and bone loss, among others (ICH, 2000, 2005b) and provide a sound basis for clinical studies.

Safety concern is heightened when foods are intended for consumption by juveniles (e.g. baby formulas), during pregnancy, and by men and women of reproductive potential. These products generally warrant reproductive and developmental toxicity testing for food additives and GRAS products in order to identify foods that are systemically absorbed or cross the placenta to impair reproduction and/or embryonic, fetal, and neonatal development and function. Studies for the prenatal and postnatal period divided into three segments of fertility (parental generation), reproductive performance and development (parental and filial generations) under OECD (TGs 414, 415, 416, 421, 422, 443, 1983, 2001a,b, 1995, 1996, 2011), ICH, (S5R2, 2000b) and Redbook II (U.S. FDA 2000a,b) guidelines may be structured to incorporate developmental, endocrine, neurological (OECD TG 426, 2007), and immunological effects for as long as two generations in a tiered approach (Güngörmüş and Kılıç, 2012).

Extension of in vitro methods in risk assessment from chemicals to functional foods and beverages has resulted in increasingly efficient, cost-effective preliminary screening in the evaluation of complex mixtures for their mechanistic processes and structure–function relationships. Traditional in vitro models to mimic the in vivo condition for acute eye and skin sensitivity and irritation cytotoxicity (EpiSkin; skin penetration), phototoxicity (EpiDerm, 3T3 cells) are now adapted and regulatorily approved for metabolic stability (human hepatocytes) and intestinal absorption through the development of reliable biomarkers and toxicological endpoints (Martin and Avrelija, 2012). Cell, tissue, and organ culture along with ex vivo techniques can identify and characterize the physiological processes of absorption, distribution, metabolism, and excretion in toxicokinetic models to simulate compartmentalization through cell membranes (CACO-2) and tissue-blood partitioning for absorption; identify metabolites and their bioactivity through microbial effects (gut) for metabolism; and signify clearance (enzymatic activity), kinetics, and saturability (active site models) for distribution and elimination. Eisenbrand remains an excellent review of the applicability of in vitro techniques to food (Eisenbrand et al., 2002).

2.3.2.3 Clinical Assessment

While not a general requirement of functional food regulatory dossiers, clinical trials under Good Clinical Practice guidelines (ICH, 1996) are advised in accordance with health claim status (U.S. FDA, 1993d; Regulation (EC) No. 1924/2006, 2007, 2011) and are invaluable in securing consumer confidence for product efficacy. Health claims based on generally acceptable scientific proof (i.e. calcium is good for bone health) need no study. However, claims associated with a specific product that relate to a function (i.e. product is good for bone health) or to the reduction of a risk of disease (i.e. product reduces the risk of osteoporosis) must be substantiated by reliable scientific evidence. Yet before undertaking these costly, population-structured and highly regulated studies, thorough preclinical assessments are typically recommended. Indeed, studies are usually performed for premarket approval where preclinical trials and history of use ensure their safe and efficient design. Clinical studies incorporate placebo-controlled, randomized, double-blind design, often of a target population. Protocols are closely scrutinized by the FDA's CFSAN for rationale and objective, including results of all available preclinical and ADME studies, the chemical composition of the product, and its proposed physiological effect, and the suitability/expertise of the primary investigator under which the study is performed, granting that no known hazards to study subjects exist. Study preparation and conduct is highly regulated for selection criteria of subjects (informed consent), with the study design including proposed test product doses and amount consumed, duration, criteria of clinical assessment, and data management and reporting (published and unpublished). Dietary protocols addressing the more common health concerns of obesity/weight management (satiety), metabolic syndrome and diabetes, cardiovascular health (Estruch et al., 2013; Hasler, 1998), bone health (National Dairy Council, 2014), mental acuity (Selhub et al., 2014), and allergies (immunological support/therapy) (Wang and Sampson, 2013) are among the most common and well utilized for the general population.

Benefits for the potential treatment of individual disorders for specific populations are the target of many functional foods. The percentage of the world's population over the age of 60 is expected to double from 11% to 22% between 2000 and 2050, making the elderly the fastest growing target group and the one with greatest financial resources to invest in staying healthy. Serving this and other demographics provide ever-expanding market possibilities both in the United States and worldwide. Among the target groups of expanding health potential for which clinical safety studies are adapted: (1) the elderly, defined by EFSA as persons over 65 years of age. These individuals have an interest in maintaining/improving cognitive, bone, immune and eye health, and lean body mass; (2) athletes, who would focus on protein utilization and maximal muscle performance, energy enhancement, joint and bone health; (3) children, for focus on immune support, cognitive development, and healthy snacking; and (4) overweight/obese persons, as the prevalence of obesity has increased by more than 40% in the last 10 years, particularly in children (Krebs and Jacobson, 2003). This fourth group is of particular interest for studies related to the regulation of metabolic disease, weight control/satiety (e.g. fat and glucose burners and binders, intestinal biota/prebiotics and probiotics), and behavioral control with healthy dietary choices (lifestyle changes).

2.4 NOVEL CONSIDERATIONS IN FUNCTIONAL FOOD SAFETY

2.4.1 Foods Derived from Genetically Modified Organisms

Among the most current considerations in food safety, the class of foods originating from genetically modified organisms (GMOs) is the most poorly defined and heavily contested in the regulatory setting. Genetically engineered plants, the majority being corn, soybean, canola, and cotton, are ubiquitous in the food chain as they are often primary ingredients in the formulation of sauces, soups, sweeteners, thickeners, condiments, and derivatives thereof. The safety of foods derived from plants genetically engineered for consumption by both humans and animals must meet the same regulatory requirements as those from traditionally bred plants and is regulated in the United States by the three agencies: U.S. EPA for pesticide usage; FDA for foods; and the USDA for meat and poultry. The FDA considers most GM crops to be "substantially equivalent" and historically similar to non-GM crops under a 1992 policy and, as such, these products are usually designated as GRAS without the need for premarket approval under the Federal FD&C Act. It is only upon the introduction of a transgenic gene producing a protein substantially different in structure and function from the natural plant, with the possibility of harm to the consumer, that the FDA will require premarket approval. Responsibility of safety, particularly for toxicity and allergenicity, lies with the crop developers under the determination of "substantial equivalence" first developed under the OECD and WHO/FAO for voluntary premarket approval by the FDA on an individual product basis (OECD, 1993). Labeling is voluntary, although the FDA has issued guidance to the industry to avoid misbranding (U.S. FDA, 2001). Fundamentally, as determined by the FDA to date, no genetically bioengineered food has been shown to be any more hazardous (including allergenic) or less nutritious than those traditionally grown. Yet consumer confidence in GMOs remains uncertain due to possible unforeseen consequences of their expanded use outside the regulatory realm. Furthermore, delays in reporting these changes may arise from unintended alterations in genotype, chemical composition, phenotype, toxin and allergen development. For this reason, manufacturer commitment to vigilance in GMO food safety is of particular importance to maintaining consumer confidence. The present toxicology safety testing guidelines are the same as for non-GMO products. As stated under EFSA EC Regulation 1829/2003 (1), the GMO and derived products are compared to the (non-GM) conventional counterpart and any identified differences are assessed (EFSA Panel on Genetically Modified Organisms [GMO], 2010a,b; EFSA, 2014a) with added accountability for environmental impact and allergenicity (http://www.efsa.europa.eu/en/gmo/gmoguidance.htm). Practically, as the safety assessment of GM crops focuses on comparison to the nearest isogenic relative using agronomic performance metrics and compositional analysis to determine if the particular genetic modification produces unintended effects, difficulty may arise when production costs and product quantity needs cannot be met for limit doses in acute and repeated-dose studies (2000 mg/kg/day). Consideration for the presence of transgenic proteins and the possibility of allergenicity will often necessitate the use of specified soy-free diets for toxicological studies.

2.4.2 Foods Derived from the Use of Nanotechnology

Engineered nanotechnology (particulate size 1–100 nm) is widely used in diverse functional food additives and dietary supplements. In food agriculture, nanotechnology is utilized for delivering pesticides and fertilizers during cultivation, while in food processing, nanosensors are employed for detecting pathogens and nanoemulsions are utilized for decontamination, to name a few examples. Furthermore, nanotechnology is also used in packaging (e.g. encapsulation) as well as in food contact substances (e.g. cutting boards, plastic containers) for its expected advantages in absorption and bioactivity (Sekhon, 2014; Figure 2.1). Compared with standard-sized ingredients, nanomaterials possess altered physical and chemical properties, including changes in solubility, which are expected to increase absorption and chemical reactivity (Warheit and Donner, 2010) with profoundly different safety risks. These findings are borne out by their potential for exaggerated pathologic tissue response from their increased surface area-to-mass ratio as the size of the particle decreases. Studied by electron microscopy, nanoparticulates have the capacity to intercalate into and between cells to disrupt cellular structures and function in all vital organs of deposition (Hubbs et al., 2011). Alternatively, products may be genetically engineered to be inherently safer. Potatoes engineered to produce less acrylamide when cooked are among the first GM crops to reportedly *increase* the safety of a food product directly upon preparation (Drahl and Morrison, 2014; Rommens et al., 2008).

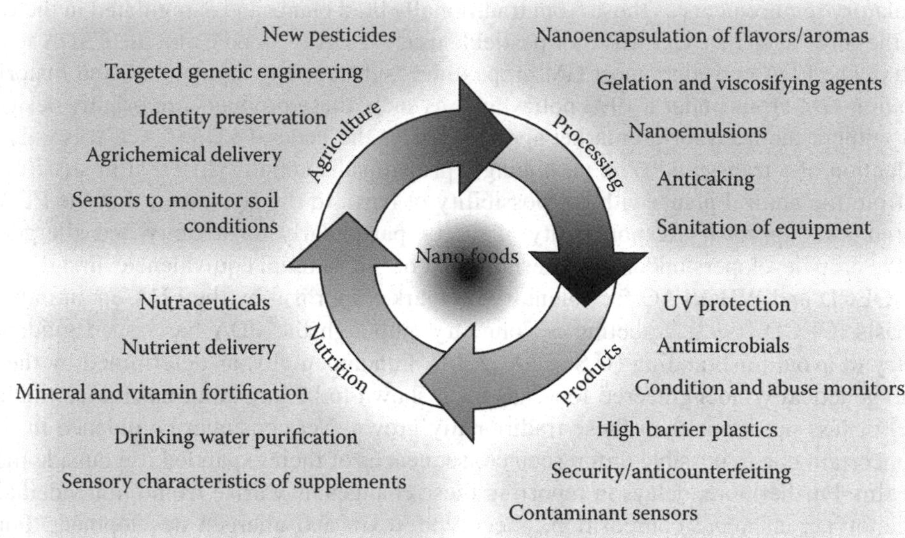

FIGURE 2.1 **(See color insert.)** Food nanotechnology applications in the food production, processing, and delivery pipeline. (From Saba, N., et al., *Polymers*, 6(8), 2247, 2014.)

Commensurate with the routine incorporation of these products, regulatory oversight supporting its responsible development has recently been implemented under three new guidelines. Updated originally from FDA's Working Party on Manufactured Nanomaterials (WPMN) task force in 2007 (U.S. FDA, 2014a), they include the consideration involving the usage of nanotechnology; the effects of the technology on food and food contact materials; and the use of nanotechnology in animal feed (http://www.fda.gov/ScienceResearch/SpecialTopics/Nanotechnology/default.htm). Generally, "the FDA does not make a categorical judgment that nanotechnology is inherently safe or harmful, and will continue to consider the specific characteristics of individual product." This stance reflects an acknowledgment of the great impact any regulation may have on this diverse group of products and the possibility for disincentive of innovation (Burdock and Matulka, 2014). Nonetheless, basic questions remain: How are these foods classified, and is it appropriate to incorporate nanomaterials into organic foods, for example? As with any other food additive or GRAS product, subsequent to self-identification of the nano-product, safety remains the responsibility of the manufacturer. Similarly, the FDA recommends individual product consultation prior to marketing. Presently, there is no labeling requirement for products containing nanosized materials; therefore, consumers are advised to remain aware of developments and new products available in the industry in order to avoid misinformation. In the United States, as current safety testing of these products is indistinguishable from other food testing, the regulatory focus of this industry is on the appropriate application of the current OECD and FDA Redbook II guidelines to uniquely and adequately address these novel products. Europe and Canada were among the first to address nanotechnology in foods through regulation EFSA (EFSA Scientific Committee, 2011a) and Health Canada, respectively, and more comprehensively through OECD (2013). While the FDA has recognized the need to treat nanomaterials differently by promulgating first guidance for manufacturers to distinguish them from macro-sized products (U.S. FDA, 2014), practically, the standard safety assessment remains similar to those of GM and food additive products: preliminary FDA consultation and the comparison of traditional pharmacological absorption, distribution, metabolism, and elimination, genotoxicity and toxicity (a repeated-dose 90-day toxicity) studies with the same studies of the non-nano form, when applicable and appropriate, contingent upon known comparable dosages. Regulatory and consumer interest group oversight of nanoparticulates in food remains an ongoing issue and will likely require the careful cooperation of food safety authorities and advocates throughout the world (Pray and Yaktine, 2009) as the industry continues to grow and increase its food chain footprint.

2.4.3 Beverages and Energy Enhancers

The methods used for the assessment of nutrients and efficacy in foods are generally applicable to beverages, with recent guidance distinguishing these products as conventional foods. Beverages have their own regulatory and labeling requirements apart from those of liquid dietary supplements (U.S. FDA, 2014b). Functionally, many of these products are marketed as high-performance energy enhancers, the primary components of which are often caffeine, creatinine, or taurine. Of particular interest are caffeine/guarana-containing stimulants, now under close regulatory review for widespread use as additives in foods, candies, chewing gum, energy drinks, and colas. The FDA has aggressively sought to investigate the safety of such components, with the goal of limiting consumption by children and sensitive populations (Goetz, 2013; Mitchell et al., 2014). The Code of Federal Regulations provides that in cola beverages the level of caffeine is not to exceed 0.02% by volume, or about 70 mg caffeine/12 oz can. Although this level is presumed by the FDA to be safe as GRAS without the need of further safety testing, the Code does not limit how much caffeine can be included as a dietary supplement (Stewart and Stevenson, 2013), nor does it require a manufacturer to precisely divulge caffeine content on product labels (A. Wallace Hayes, communication). This scenario oftentimes leads to higher levels of ingestion by the consumer, as evidenced by the typical caffeine levels of 70–200 mg present in most energy drinks (Weise, 2008). Similarly, creatinine, believed to provide energy directly to muscle via the formation of adenosine triphosphate, and taurine, an amino acid purportedly used to support neurological development, are newcomers to an as-yet unknown, unregulated space (Mejia, 2014). More regulatory guidance followed by analytic recommendations and standards are expected from FDA.

2.4.4 Hemp and Marijuana

Another topic of growing regulatory importance in food application and safety is the utilization of marijuana (*Cannabis sativa*) and hemp, a variety of cannabis grown for its fiber and seed, as a medicinal treatment and dietary supplement. Since the 1996 California legalization of marijuana for medical purposes, a growing number of states have ratified the possession and legal use in specified and limited quantities of marijuana and hemp for both medicinal and, more recently, recreational use. Legally, hemp is available only as an import, mainly through Canada, China, and Europe, though its cultivation is currently allowed in select states (Colorado and Kentucky) (Gardner, 2014). Even as U.S. federal restrictions remain, state laws make way for easing restrictions on its cultivation and availability. This, along with wider public acceptability, has garnered the attention of the FDA for federal oversight (http://www.fda.gov/NewsEvents/Testimony/ucm402061.htm). Marijuana is presently classified by the Controlled Substances Act as a Schedule I drug (1970), the most tightly restricted drug class, due to its content of tetrahydrocannibinol (THC) and other psychotropic drugs. However, the FDA is currently considering an unprecedented classification downgrading at the request of the Drug Enforcement Agency (DEA) following analysis of the safety and efficacy of the compound. Marijuana/hemp seed oil is used traditionally for the treatment of pain, nausea associated with chemotherapy, glaucoma, neurological disorders, and epilepsy, and it is now poised for availability as a dietary supplement to the general public as a muscle relaxant, sleep and anxiety aid, schizophrenia treatment, and cosmetic and skin care emollient, among other applications. It has been available clandestinely for decades in North America in nutritional processed foods as diverse as baked goods, yogurts, cereals, frozen desserts, condiments, pasta, burgers, and pizza as well as beverages such as milk, beer, and coffee (Small, 2004). With the continued erosion of its traditional taboo, the compound has become highly sought after for its medicinal purposes, particularly for its promise in suppressing the seizures of children's epilepsy. Acceptance of marijuana as a therapy for children has further been fueled by cultivation of a strain known as Charlotte's Web, bred to contain very low levels of the psychoactive compound THC, with high levels of the non-psychoactive, isomeric component, cannabidiol (CBD). Because this strain does not elicit the psychoactive effects of more traditional high-THC strains, it is generally regarded as more safe, particularly for children. Compounding the assessment of safety is the fact that baking, brewing, and processing create a reduction in active ingredients, making actual effective doses difficult to establish under uncontrolled environments. The unknown strength of popular dosages has, very recently (2014), been implicated in two reported deaths indirectly linked to the side effects of the marijuana intoxication when used for recreation, though the compound is considered of low toxicity with no reported deaths when used under medical supervision (Calabria et al., 2010). Though the FDA has provided no timeline as to its guidance on marijuana, its high demand, ease of growth and availability, and creative use in foods would lend itself to prompt action.

2.5 POTENTIAL UNDESIRABLE EFFECTS ASSOCIATED WITH FUNCTIONAL FOODS

Surveys conducted by the International Food Information Council (IFIC, 2013) indicate that 90% of all Americans agree that functional foods provide a benefit to health and are interested in learning more about the association. Given the anticipated 6% global market increase between 2015 and 2018, there is strong indication that this opinion is shared by the international community. Consequently, the exchange among greater numbers of countries, manufacturers and products in the United States and worldwide has necessitated enhanced quality measures and the identification and management of potential harmful by-products, influences, and outcomes in the food supply. The following section describes some of the more common potential adverse factors that threaten the safety and quality of functional foods and beverages. For this reason, these functional foods, intended and originally purposed for their health advantages, may be ultimately responsible for *negative* impacts on health.

2.5.1 ALLERGENS

As foods become more processed to include high nutrient value for functional advantage, food allergens are becoming increasingly common and difficult to avoid. Specifically, the addition of proteins and fortification nutrients accompanied by chemicals intended for the purposes of enhancing rapid growth, production, and distribution to a growing worldwide population has the potential to adversely affect an ever larger demographic. Food allergies among children have risen nearly 50% from the period from 1997 through 2011 in the United States (Jackson et al., 2013), with severe reactions increasing sevenfold over the past decade in Europe (European Academy of Allergy and Clinical Immunology [EAACI, 2009]).

An allergenic food is defined by its ability to provoke an immunologic reaction in a sensitive individual upon its specific ingestion, and allergenic food intolerance is suspected in approximately 5% of children and 3%–4% of adults in developed countries (Branum and Lukacs, 2009; Rona et al., 2007). The most common allergenic foods in descending order of prevalence are milks, yeast, eggs and grains (wheat), fish/shellfish, tree nuts, and legumes (peanuts and soy).

Generally, there are two types of food allergies: the rarer immediate-onset IgE allergies, found largely in children and occurring within seconds of exposure; and the more common delayed-onset IgG allergies, appearing hours to days after exposure (see Kruger et al., 2014 for review).

A few of the most relevant for the food industry due to their ubiquitous, often masked off-label, usage in prepared foods are mentioned in the following.

IgE milk food allergy is the most common and can mimic symptoms of gastrointestinal disorder such as diarrhea, bloating, cramping, and excess gas, as well as provoke the more common systemic allergic symptoms of skin rash, pruritus, asthma, rhinitis, and, more severely, swelling (anaphylaxis). Unlike lactose intolerance, which is caused by low production of lactase and affects as much as 75% of the human population, allergic reactions to milk are produced by its casein protein. Adverse reactions to milk products can therefore be a combination of the two simultaneous but separate physiological events of lactose intolerance and casein allergy. Presently, a number of fermented milks and lactose-free milk products are available to ease the discomfort associated with milk intolerances and can be essential sources of nutrition. Probiotic dairy foods with lactic acid bacteria (yogurts) as well as soy-free dairy products are associated with positive health benefits, particularly for immune and gastrointestinal health. These products have been reported to colonize the gut with beneficial bacteria, and a growing body of evidence suggests that such symbiotic microflora, particularly when provided in infancy, have a long-lasting role in the protection against gastrointestinal infections, prevention of obesity, reduction of serum cholesterol levels, and promotion of antimutagenic activity (Shiby and Mishra, 2013).

Digestive discomfort is also prevalent in wheat allergies. Symptoms include abdominal cramping, weight loss, diarrhea, constipation, bloating, diverticulitis, as well as generalized sinusitis, fatigue, and at its worst, anemia, depression, and in children, possible attention and behavioral problems. Wheat allergies are oftentimes associated with a spectrum of gastrointestinal disorders including gluten sensitivity, celiac disease (hereditary) and possibly irritable bowel disease, and involve the gluten protein gliadin as the causative allergen. Distinguishing between these maladies is the subject of careful clinical determination as they may not be discrete entities, though it is generally thought that gluten sensitivity is a less severe condition than the others. Currently, the subject of active study, the reader is referred to excellent reviews on the clinical response to gluten challenge (Biesiekierski et al., 2013; Bruins, 2013). Wheat and gluten grain (wheat, rye, barley, and oats) is significant for its ubiquitous use in breads/baked products and cereals, and, as the staple of most diets the world over, the potential exists for increased allergic outcomes and subsequently, health costs over a larger proportion of the world's population. In anticipation of this possibility, the gluten-free market, which is still in its early growth, was expected to grow 31% (up from 15% of North American consumers) from 2011 to 2014.

Aside from the more common, known food allergens, other foods—particularly herbals and botanicals—may inadvertently result in unexpected, severe adverse health outcomes, though the specific offending component is more difficult to distinguish and often remains unknown. In the case of botanicals like tree nuts and peanuts, their diverse chemical compositions originating from various soils, growth environments and climates, there remains the capacity to trigger undesirable health effects from any one of their basic constituents, known and unknown. Fundamentally, any of the minerals or vitamins, including the interactions of proteins with lipids and polysaccharides (Fremont et al., 2004), of natural or processed origin introduced anywhere along the food chain, have the potential to likewise trigger allergic hypersensitivity.

Food allergies are unique to the given individual and treatment begins with identification and removal of the offending food allergen. Elimination of the suspected causative food from the diet is usually performed under the supervision of a qualified health-care provider, particularly when the suspected allergen is an essential part of the diet for a given individual (e.g. a growing child).

2.5.2 Natural and Unintended Contaminants

The risks to health for foodborne contaminants and impurities, though oftentimes unidentifiable and difficult to manage, can, depending on the contaminant, be alleviated through manufacture and supplier process surveillance (HACCP regulation). This, combined with consumer awareness, selection, and proper end-stage food preparation, offers the best, most efficient means of avoiding unwanted food outcomes. Most common categories of contaminants include heavy metals, microbial contamination, pesticide residues, and molds and mycotoxins, any and all of which may be both of natural and/or of human origin. Such potential toxicants have been well documented and are briefly discussed here, with reference to excellent reviews for the reader's interest.

2.5.2.1 Heavy Metals

The most prevalent heavy metal contaminants with the potential to negatively impact food safety and human health are arsenic, lead, cadmium, and mercury. Symptoms of heavy metal toxicity include initial nonspecific gastrointestinal distress, nausea, and vomiting, which progress to cognitive, motor, language, and behavioral difficulties, and later to shock, anemia, and kidney failure in more severe cases. Exposure typically occurs via contact with contaminated soil, water, and air. Environmental deposits may be of natural origin (e.g. inherent plant constituents such as alkaloids) (Alexander et al., 2012; Goyer and Clarkson, 2001) or the result of human activities such as farming, industrial exhausts, and smoking. Bioaccumulation of these elements from high-level exposures from drinking water, air, and plant and animal foodstuffs can result in toxicity from foods derived from them. Excellent detailed reviews are available (Kotsonis et al., 2001; Morais et al., 2012). This issue has been of particular concern in recent years due to reports of rising arsenic and cadmium levels in rice and higher incidence of consequent poisoning, prompting many manufacturers to magnify screening efforts for these metals in their products.

The FDA recommends eating a variety of foods to avoid excessive exposure from any one food. The most recent guidance for heavy metals in foods comes from EFSA's Panel on Contaminants in the Food Chain (CONTAM), which promulgated Regulation 315/93/EEC (http://www.efsa.europa.eu/en/topics/topic/metals.htm) in 2007 to establish maximal allowable levels of nonradioactive lead, cadmium, uranium, and tin, as well as to propose standard methods of sampling and analysis based on previous joint FAO/WHO Expert Committee assessment. Generally, the EU sets maximum levels with the goal of reducing the presence of metals as well as other contaminants in food to as low as reasonably achievable by means of good manufacturing or agricultural practices. Though definitive regulatory standards have been established for mercury, the FDA has not advised on maximum acceptable levels of other heavy metals in the food supply. However, the FDA continues to monitor their prevalence and health impact, particularly during pregnancy (http://www.fda.gov/Food/FoodborneIllnessContaminants/Metals/default.htm). Awareness of food origins, making good food choices, and avoiding foods more likely to contain metals (e.g. high trophic–level oceanic fish and seafood, canned foods, and foods grown with phosphate-based fertilizers more apt to contain higher levels of cadmium), are the first precautions against metal contamination. Treatment for severe cases involves the administration of chelating agents such as calcium disodium edetate, dimercaprol, penicillamine, or ethylenediaminetetraacetic acid (EDTA) to form complexes with the toxic metals in body tissues and allow their excretion in urine.

2.5.2.2 Pesticides and Herbicides

Pesticides and herbicides, either natural or synthetic, are used throughout the food production process from growth to transport and storage, and residuals levels of these compounds may remain present in end-product raw functional foods. The EPA sets maximum allowable limits (tolerances) on pesticides in food based on the evaluation of environmental and potential health risks. The FDA monitors and enforces pesticide tolerances in raw agricultural goods and processed foods while maximal levels for meat, poultry, and some egg products are monitored and enforced by the USDA for both domestic and imported foods. Tolerances and exemptions for pesticide chemical residues in food appear in U.S. Code of Federal Regulations 40 CFR Part 180 (http://www.fda.gov/Food/GuidanceComplianceRegulatoryInformation/GuidanceDocuments/ChemicalContaminantsandPesticides/default.htm). In the EU, pesticides must be scientifically proven to be efficacious without harm to human health and without any effect on the environment. Regulatory guidance, including maximum tolerances, is periodically updated on http://ec.europa.eu/food/plant/pesticides/index_en.htm.

The most common chemical (synthetic) pesticides used in the food industry are organophosphates, carbamates, organochlorides, and pyrethroids, all of which are neuroactive and toxic at high levels. Common herbicides that may be pre-plant, pre-emergent, or post-emergent chemicals of the auxin, photosystem, or essential nutrient (amino acid, lipid) inhibitor varieties have the capacity to remain in the soil for extended periods of time.

Biopesticides and herbicides (natural products of plant, animal or bacterial origin) are also used for the control of specific target organisms. One form of biopesticide is xenoestrogens, derived from exogenous estrogen-like hormones found in soils and farm animals and originating from food processing and packaging (e.g. bisphenol A*). According to recent reports, synthetic xenoestrogens have the capacity to adversely increase estrogen levels in wildlife and humans, may remain in the body longer than estrogens produced endogenously, and are capable of producing hormonal imbalances in humans and animals (Diamanti-Kandarakis et al., 2009).

Judicious food choices and care in handling and preparation are highly efficient means of reducing the risk of illness from pesticide and herbicide residue. Organic foods, grown without the use of synthetic pesticides and herbicides, have been shown to contain smaller amounts of residues than produce grown conventionally, but they often come with higher prices. The easiest, most cost-effective means to substantially reduce pesticide/herbicide residue is through proper handling of foods by thorough washing, peeling/skinning, and cooking.

2.5.2.3 Molds, Mycotoxins, and Natural Plant Toxins

Molds, particularly certain species of the *Penicillium* and *Aspergillus* genera, are used to human advantage in fermented food products such as surface-ripened and rind-washed cheeses, as well as blue cheeses and soy sauce. They are used for the production of citric acid, lactic acid, and many enzymes, and are also utilized as critical components of the fermentation process in the beverage and wine-making industries, for example. Indeed, they are responsible for most of the distinctive tastes and appearances of these products (Molimard and Spinnler, 1996).

Frequently, however, the natural but unwanted presence of molds in plant-related agriculture is undesirable and has the potential to produce severe human and veterinary adverse health effects, regardless of the crop in which they are found. Mycotoxins, the toxic by-products of mold spores, are diverse in their chemical composition and grow under damp (>12%–15% moisture), aerated conditions. Disease occurs in humans through direct consumption of contaminated harvest grain or as a result of eating animal products contaminated through animal feed. Of the more common mycotoxins, aflatoxins, which originate from *Aspergillus flavus* and *Aspergillus parasiticus*, are best documented for their known association with liver and kidney disease potential carcinogenicity. Aflatoxins contaminate many dietary staples such as groundnuts (peanuts/peanut butter), rice, seeds (cottonseed), grains (corn), and milks. Like most disease-producing molds, aflatoxins are of greatest concern in developing countries where wet weather and poor drying conditions at harvest contribute to mold growth. The prevalence of aflatoxin, previously undetermined throughout the world, is now being studied as an international health concern (Kong et al., 2014). Other mycotoxins with the capacity to produce disease include citrinin (fermentation products, grains, rice); ergot alkaloids (fescue, beef cattle), fumonisins (feed, beef and dairy cattle), ochratoxin A (animal feed, grains, nuts, cocoa, coffee); patulin (fruits, grains); trichothecenes/T-2 (cereal grains, dairy cattle), deoxynivalenol or vomitoxin (animal feed, beef and dairy cattle); and zearalenon (corn, wheat, grains; mimics estrogen; cows, swine) (Bennett and Klich, 2003; Kruger et al., 2014; http://www.extension.org/pages/11768/mold-and-mycotoxin-issues-in-dairy-cattle:-effects-prevention-and-treatment#.VIiwDzHF-ZA). Prevention of spore growth is best accomplished through rapid postharvest drying, removal of air, and dry, cool storage. Once infiltration has occurred, the use of binders acting as absorbent materials (activated carbon; aluminosilicates—clay, bentonite, montmorillonite, zeolite,

* After an extensive 4-year review, the FDA has recently concluded that current levels of bisphenol A used in packaging are safe.

phyllosilicates; complex glucomannans; peptidoglycan indigestible carbohydrates—cellulose, polysaccharides in the cell walls of yeast and bacteria; and synthetic polymers—cholestryamine and polyvinylpyrrolidone and derivatives), to limit toxin effects have proven useful. The presence of molds and their potential toxic effects is considered less common in functional processed foods than in those consumed as raw ingredients. In Western countries where oversight of food storage and preservation is generally more comprehensive, incidence of mold-produced illness is more commonly restricted to immunosuppressed individuals and to areas that have experienced natural disasters such as hurricanes and floods (Brandt et al., 2006). It is important to note that noninfectious allergens on mold spores of raw food products may also provoke intolerance and hypersensitivity, which must be clinically separated from toxicity.

2.5.2.4 Microbiological Agents in Food

While the intentional addition of some "good" bacteria to processed foods (e.g. *Lactobacillus* in dairy products) defines its functionality, unintended biological contamination transmitted through food during the harvesting and manufacturing process remains a significant source of human disease. Infectious disease resulting from microorganisms in food may be either invasive through the introduction and replication of the organisms themselves and their preformed toxins (e.g. botulinum), or through the release of enterotoxins from the colonizing species (e.g. *Salmonella*) (Kotsonis et al., 2001; Kruger et al., 2014). Briefly, the most common foodborne pathogens include Gram-positive *Listeria monocytogenes*, found most often in sensitive populations and resulting from poultry, beef, and raw milk contamination; *Clostridium perfringes*, found commonly in meat and fish; *Clostridium botulinum*, a neurotoxin found in honey and improperly canned fruits and vegetables; *Staphylococcus aureus*, the most common of food infections resulting from improper human handling and preparation of uncooked foods (e.g. salads, bakery products); and *Bacillus cereus*, a toxin produced when foods such as leftovers are kept too long unrefrigerated. Gram-negative microorganisms include pathogenic *Escherichia coli* (O157:H7 strain, primarily), found in undercooked or unpasteurized beef and milk and contaminated water/feces; *Campylobacter jejuni* found in raw and undercooked poultry, unpasteurized milk and contaminated water; *Yersinia enterocolitica*, found in pigs and meat, unpasteurized milk, and contaminated water; and *Salmonella,* a common pathogenic bacteria with over 50 serotypes found most often in wildlife feces-contaminated eggs, poultry, meat, unpasteurized milk or juice, cheese, contaminated raw fruits and vegetables (Kruger et al., 2014; Mahony et al. 2014).

Viruses have been reported as responsible for over 67% of food-related infections, with increasing transmission through food and water as the world population grows (Atreya, 2004). Of the more common viruses, norovirus (Norwalk Virus) is the pathogen most commonly associated with stomach influenza, accounting for over 60% of all enteroviral etiologies (Hall et al., 2013). Typical routes of norovirus transmission include consumption of contaminated produce, shellfish, and foods handled by infected individuals (symptomatic and/or asymptomatic). A second example of a foodborne viral agent, *Rotavirus,* originates from improper handling of raw foods and salads. This pathogen commonly afflicts children and is transmitted by the fecal/oral route.

Bacterial and viral foodborne illnesses present as mild to severe acute gastrointestinal distress accompanied by nausea, vomiting, diarrhea, loss of appetite, severe abdominal cramps, and fever. They are rarely life threatening and in most cases are cleared within 4–7 days. However, in older adults, infants, immunocompromised persons, and persons with chronic diseases, symptoms may progress to more serious septicemia and shock, depending on the infection. Proper food handling, preparation, storage, and refrigeration can prevent many of these occurrences. The Centers for Disease Control and Prevention (CDC) considers foodborne illness a serious and underreported health issue. In an effort to reduce the health and financial consequences of foodborne disease, the CDC urges consumers in large cities to report adverse events through social media soon after they occur. Health authorities can then track and respond to complaints in an effort to enhance surveillance of products from food suppliers and preparers (Harris et al., 2014).

Prions, another form of pathogenic agent that may be transmitted through food, are infectious proteins capable of inducing misfolding and aggregation of specific normal cellular proteins known as prion proteins. Abnormal folding of these susceptible proteins leads to proteins capable of neurodegenerative spongiform encephalopathies (CDC, http://www.cdc.gov/ncidod/dvrd/prions/). The resulting disease is termed bovine spongiform encephalopathy (BSE, also known as mad cow disease) when it affects beef and dairy cattle and as scrapie when affecting sheep and goats (Colby and Prusiner, 2011), and though the prions that cause the disease are most commonly found in neural tissue, any organ may be affected. The disease, known in humans as Creutzfeldt–Jakob disease and variants, may be transmitted through the consumption of infected animal products. Following a long latency period, the progression of Creutzfeldt–Jakob disease is rapid and fatal. According to the National Institutes of Health, prion proteins, denoted PrP, are most likely associated with the cellular import of copper ions, cell signaling, the formation of cell synapses, and cell protection (U.S. National Library of Medicine, 2008). Since 1997 the FDA, along with WHO and the USDA, has prohibited the use of mammalian animal proteins, particularly brains and spinal cords from high-risk cattle, in *all* animal feeds. Though human cases of classical Creutzfeldt–Jakob disease and variant Creutzfeldt–Jakob disease are rare, BSE has been reported in Japan, Brazil, Canada, the United Kingdom, the United States, Ireland, Switzerland, France, Liechtenstein, Luxembourg, the Netherlands, Portugal, and Denmark. The occurrence of prions in some countries has led to changes in consumer dietary preferences, particularly because aberrant proteins cannot be destroyed by cooking. For example sales of tongue and other organ meats have spiked in Japan following the recent relaxation of restrictions on the importation of beef.

2.5.3 Marine Foods and Toxins

A vast array of marine-derived nutrients has exhibited significant health benefits ranging from cardioprotective and anti-inflammatory effects to improvements in cognitive function. As sources of the omega-3 fatty acids docosahexaenoic acid (DHA) and eicosapentaenoic acid (EPA), oils from fish and algae are well known for their substantiated heart and mental health benefits. Numerous marine compounds have also been identified for their bioactive antioxidant qualities, most notably the carotenoids and phenolic compounds found in crustaceans, seaweed, and a variety of compounds isolated from microalgae and fish protein hydrolysates. In addition, various polysaccharides, including fucoidans derived from algae and chitin derived from crustacean shells, have demonstrated both antiviral and antitumor activity in mammals (Lordan et al., 2011). Consumption of health-promoting marine-derived foods has been recommended and encouraged for all persons, but they are particularly beneficial for pregnant women and young children due to their positive effects on prenatal and postnatal neural development.

Increased consumption of fish and shellfish has, however, recently prompted concerns by the FDA for communication of the safety of these foodstuffs, particularly for consumption during pregnancy and childhood (Lunder, 2014), and the agency is currently considering updates to its nearly 20-year old recommendations for manufacturers and consumers (http://www.fda.gov/Food/GuidanceRegulation/GuidanceDocumentsRegulatoryInformation/Seafood/ucm2006751.htm). Though shark, tilefish, swordfish, king mackerel, and canned tuna are fishes traditionally associated with the threat of high levels of mercury, other species of fresh and salt water fish and seafood may also contain levels far in excess of the recommended limit for safe mercury ingestion. This limit, originally calculated by the EPA in 1999, was updated by the World Health Organization in 2003 to 1.6 μg/kg body weight/week (http://www.epa.gov/mercury/advisories.htm; http://www.fda.gov/Food/FoodborneIllnessContaminants/Metals/ucm393070.htm), but as fish consumption becomes more prevalent in an increasingly populated world, this figure is currently being reconsidered. Ironically, since mercury is neuro-, nephro-, and immunotoxic, any potential health benefits of marine-derived foods could be negated by exposure to this toxic substance, as reported most markedly in children (Bose-O'Reilly et al., 2010).

In addition to the potential risks of mercury exposure, adverse outcomes associated with fish and seafood ingestion include food-induced anaphylactic allergic reactions, and less commonly, seafood toxin-induced neurological poisoning. Confounding the classification of negative health effects arising from seafood is the fact that seafood toxin poisoning in its milder form may frequently mimic allergic reaction. In exoskeleton-containing shellfish, cross-reactivity of the tropomyosin protein has been identified as the major allergen associated with IgE-mediated hypersensitivity. Marine allergy prevalence in the general population is estimated at 0.5%–2.5%, with shrimp, crab, lobster, clam, oyster, and mussel as causative agents in order of decreasing frequency. Shellfish allergies are most prevalent in Asia, most likely due to comparatively high reliance on seafood as a major component of the diet in this area. Overall, the condition is less common in children in spite of the observation that affected children have higher IgE levels than affected adults, suggesting a decreased sensitivity with age (Woo and Bahna, 2011).

Seafood toxins may be produced by the fish itself, the plankton or algae consumed by the fish, or by the action of bacteria on muscle histidines to produce histamine by the fish (Kruger et al., 2014; Woo and Bahna, 2011). Generally, the greatest toxicological impact arises the five types of shellfish poisoning (James et al., 2010) as well as from fish-borne scombroid poisoning, as these are most prevalent (Hungerford, 2010). As excellent reviews are available under these titles, only a brief synopsis is presented here.

Scombroid poisoning is the most widespread fish poisoning and has been linked to the action of bacteria on muscle histidines. Its causative agents are improperly preserved abalone, tuna, mackerel, and other sea fish, and it typically presents with symptoms including diarrhea, nausea, and gastrointestinal distress, with respiratory failure occurring in its most severe forms.

Of the five classified adverse shellfish reactions, diarrhetic shellfish poisoning, occurring with the consumption of mussels, scallops, clams, and oysters, is the most innocuous. The causative toxins, which include okadaic acid, pectenotoxins, and dinophysistoxin-1, are generated by unicellular marine dinoflagellates that proliferate during summer blooms (Lee et al., 1989). Presenting symptoms include flu-like gastrointestinal cramping, vomiting, and nausea, accompanied by fever and chills (Woo and Bahna, 2011). Shellfish poisoning also includes the more severe amnesic, neurotoxic, paralytic, and azaspiracid disease entities. Paralytic shellfish poisoning is the best characterized and most widespread. Though most prevalent on the east and west coasts of North America, these incidents occur worldwide, causing various degrees of neurologic dysfunction, from numbness to neuromuscular and respiratory paralysis. The toxins from the amnesic, neurotoxic, and paralytic varieties are heat-/acid-stable tetrahydropurines, of which at least 12 are known. The most common and well characterized include saxitoxins (paralytic), brevetoxin (neurotoxic), and domoic acid (amnesic) from dinoflagellates (paralytic, neurotoxic) and phytoplankton (amnesic). Less is known about azaspiracid intoxication, which principally affects areas of western Europe and Africa. Arising from a polyether marine toxin, it is considered to be of dinoflagellate origin (Wang, 2008). Marine neurotoxins more common to Asia include ciguatoxins, produced by the microalgae; *Gambierdiscus toxicus*, found in sea bass, snapper, grouper, and others; and tetrodotoxin, found in puffer fish. All of these toxins accumulate in fish liver and act to adversely affect sodium channel permeability. Less common are poisonings from fish roe, moray eels, sea urchins, and sea turtles, any of which may occur as a result of various toxins specific to the organism, or seasonally, as a result of algal bloom–derived bioaccumulation (Kotsonis et al., 2001).

The presence of bacteria, bacterial toxins, and viruses in fish and seafood may also result in adverse reactions upon consumption of contaminated raw or undercooked food. Foodborne pathogens such as Norwalk virus, bacteria including *Vibrio vulnificus*, and bacterial toxins such as botulism toxin produced by *Clostridium botulinum* and Staphylococcal enterotoxin produced by *Staphylococcal aureus* bacteria are all common sources of coastal contamination and possible causes of severe illness. The intestinal symptoms of infectious contamination may mimic toxin-induced disease; however, unlike the presence of pathogenic microorganisms, toxins do not alter the taste and appearance of food and are not inactivated by standard cooking or food processing techniques (http://www.fda.gov/Food/GuidanceRegulation/GuidanceDocumentsRegulatoryInformation/Seafood/ucm2018426.htm).

The United States imports about 90% of the seafood it consumes, primarily originating from Asia, which produces over 89% of all global seafood. Of this quantity imported by the United States, about half is the product of aquaculture, and only 2% is inspected by FDA. Increasing demand has increased aquacultivation over 8% since 1970 making it the fastest growing area of food production (Grainger, 1999). In coordination, the FDA has enhanced its monitoring of hazards associated with seafood, more closely regulating imports through the new Foreign Safety Verification and Imported Seafood Safety Programs as components of the Food Safety Modernization Act (http://www.fda.gov/Food/GuidanceRegulation/ImportsExports/Importing/ucm248706.htm). As these directorates become fully operational, more stringent regulatory oversight is expected in the near future. One area of concern is that of fish and seafood fraud, which occurs primarily for economic gain, but creates the potential for severe health consequences. A 2009 U.S. Government Accounting Office (GAO) report has identified seafood mislabeling as a widespread issue; according to the FDA, as much as 70% of fish sold in restaurants and grocery stores in the United States is mislabeled or substituted. Many laboratories now perform taxonomic DNA identification as a quality control measure, as mislabeling of the geographical origin of wild-caught marine products as a substitute for aquaculture-produced food is difficult to detect. In addition to mislabeling, other forms of fraud include overstating food quantity (adulteration). Adverse health consequences most commonly arise due to scombroid fish poisoning, the presence of ciguatera toxins, and allergic reactions among susceptible individuals. The consumer is advised to be aware of the food source, avoid unfamiliar suppliers, and report any health-related issue to advocacy groups such as Oceana.

2.5.4 Plant Toxins and Bioactives

The natural existence of many plant toxins generally does not pose a risk to human health when consumed as part of a balanced diet. However, when they are consumed in large amounts as part of a diet based on limited food sources (e.g. veganism), some plant components have the ability to produce undesirable health effects. Among the more common plant toxins are lectins, glycoalkaloids of the *Solanaceae* family, and cyanogenic glycodies, star anise, and xanthine alkaloids, described briefly later. However, this list is by no means exhaustive, and many other examples have been documented.* Lectins are hemagglutinens found in fruits and dry legumes such as apples, bananas, cucumbers and sweet peppers, soybeans, lentils, lima beans and kidney beans, and are capable of causing gastrointestinal distress. Glycoalkaloids of the *Solanaceae* family, found in spoiled potatoes and tomatoes, may cause abdominal cramping, nausea, vomiting, and diarrhea, progressing in severe cases to neurologic signs of drowsiness, apathy, restlessness, tremors, and confusion, and cyanogenic glycosides, which are found in apricots, apples, almonds, lima beans, soy, spinach, bamboo shoots, and cassava, cause headache, nausea, and vomiting, along with death from respiratory distress in most severe cases. Star anise, which is used in beverages and derived from *Illicium anisatum* found in teas, may cause diarrhea and vomiting, as well as possible kidney disease, respiratory paralysis, and death. Finally, xanthine alkaloids from the *Theobroma* genus in teas and coffees may cause symptoms related to the hyperactivity of the central nervous and cardiovascular system.

Unlike the agents used in food processing or synthetic growth enhancement (e.g. xenoestrogens, see Section 2.5.2.3), phytoestrogens are hormones of natural plant origin and are commonly present as nonsteroidal polyphenol lignans, flavonoids (hops), stilbenes (resveratrol), and isoflavones in foods (Cos et al., 2003; Dai and Mumper, 2010). Lignans are found in vegetables, fruits, nuts, and seeds, while isoflavones (family *Leguminosae*) are estrogen-like hormones found in dairy products, grains, and soy products. Animals that graze on phytoestrogen-containing plants or are fed soy and grains will transmit these hormones through their meat and milk. Phytoestrogen-containing fruits, vegetables, herbs, and seeds (e.g. apples, cherries, peas, potatoes, tomatoes, soy, parsley, licorice, sage,

* See, for example, furocoumarin in citrus fruits and certain vegetables, oxalic acid in spinach and root vegetables, etc. (Dolan et al., 2010).

sesame, and flaxseed) in the diet have the potential to increase estrogen hormone levels in humans. Other, more commonly known plant bioactives include phytosterols and stanols (e.g. soybean, vegetable oils), which inhibit absorption of dietary cholesterol; inhibitors of various enzymes including proteases, lipases, and amylases; milk toxicants (snakeroot; Panter and James, 1990); and oxalates (rhubarb).

2.6 FOOD PROCESSING, PRESERVATION, PACKAGING, AND PREPARATION

Overall, as the number of processes involved in getting a particular food from farm to fork increase, so do the potential for contamination and possible health consequences. Generally, functional foods incorporate many processing procedures (ingredient extraction, fortification, preservation, etc.) and, as such, the numerous steps in manufacturing allow for possible entry of contamination along the way. Processing and packaging of functional food and beverage products have significant capacity to influence their sensory appeal and, depending on the method and food type, cause undesirable changes in taste, aroma, texture, and color by way of changes to its microstructure through leachability (Wang and Bohn, 2012). Ideally, food processing and packaging are intended to preserve the natural ingredients in raw materials to the greatest extent possible while maintaining an inert barrier against disease-causing agents. Processing has traditionally included thermal and nonthermal treatments used to prepare, enhance (e.g. Maillard reaction), or preserve (e.g. sterilize) solid and liquid food products. Similarly, preparation of some foods may lead to the formation of toxic acrylamides (e.g. from potatoes, cereals, coffee); polycyclic aromatic hydrocarbons and phenolic compounds (cured meats); heterocyclic amines (charred meat); and lipid polymerization and oxidation products resulting from high fat/oil heating, many of which have been shown to be mutagenic and carcinogenic. Preparation must be considered together with the beneficial effects of food processing on food safety, flavor, preservation, and convenience. These treatments often result in a loss of ingredient bioactivity. Newer methods of processing technologies, such as microencapsulation, have proven useful in minimizing microstructural modifications. Microencapsulation provides the advantage of protection of core ingredients from degradation or reaction while offering the option of controlled release (Gray and Morton, 1981; Sultanbawa, 2011; Wang and Bohn, 2012).

Increasingly, food packaging must meet longer shelf life and adhere to international safety and quality standards. An active barrier, including the addition of antimicrobial coatings in the form of bioactive packaging, will protect against product spoilage (water and water vapor; oil and grease; oxygen and aroma) and influence visual appeal (clear vs. opaque) at the same time, reflecting on brand image. However, barrier safety and greater upstream food processing must be weighed against the potentially heightened risks of introducing residues of processing aids such as reagents, solvents, and catalysts. Similarly, synergies in flavors have been used to maximize antimicrobial properties (Sultanbawa, 2011). Most recently, the use of mild heat stress combined with a low concentration of preservatives has proven effective in providing a safe, high-quality food. These techniques include nonthermal processing, high-pressure processing, and pulsed electric field active packaging. The growing use of nanotechnology in food design and food packaging has led to a safety, environmental, and regulatory guidance in the United States and Europe (Duncan, 2011; EFSA Scientific Committee, 2011b; OECD, 2010b, 2012; Panagiotou and Fisher, 2013; Rizvi et al., 2010; Sekhon, 2010; U.S. FDA, 2012a).

2.7 FUNCTIONAL FOOD: PRESENT AND FUTURE TRENDS

Current and ongoing growth areas for the functional food and beverage industry will continue to develop uses for GMO, botanical/natural and marine products with sensory appeal, many using nanotechnologies. At the same time, national and international food and law agencies enhance and advance surveillance of the distribution of these foods, and all foods that continue to be plagued by threats of adulteration and bioterrorism (Kruger et al., 2014).

In conjunction with relaxed laws and taboos, the near future holds promise for hemp/marijuana and their derivatives for the treatment of neurological disease. Fundamentally, gaining the physiological understanding required for individualized nutrition and biochemical nutrition for targeted populations, particularly for the control of brain–body communications in obesity and mental health, will make great contributions to global health.

With an eye toward feeding a growing world population, entrepreneur-led, process-oriented advancements in agriculture technology are emerging to vastly improve farm production and efficiency. Robotics is being utilized for lettuce harvesting, and software is being developed for calculations of grass production per head of cattle. Meanwhile, meat and poultry substitutes are reducing the use of chemicals, hormones, and foodborne illness. With droughts in California expected to impact future agriculture and therefore food availability, Ag-tech in both the United States and worldwide is expected to dwarf even the high-tech communications industry in its growth and influence.

Further on the horizon is the formal cultivation of edible insects as an emerging sustainable, nutritious food resource of the twenty-first century. While already accepted in developing areas of the world where cattle beef is not available, the use of insects as food protein in Western countries remains unpopular. Nonetheless, crickets, among other species, are already being cultivated and harvested in powder extracts, optimizing land usage and reducing environmental impact. The potential for a plentiful, renewable, environmentally and economically beneficial protein food source makes entomophagy a sound alternative to food shortages if consumer preferences, regulatory support, and cooperation can be established, particularly in wealthier, developed countries (Van Huis et al., 2013).

2.8 EXTERNAL EVENTS INFLUENCING THE FOOD SUPPLY: CONCLUSIONS

The capacity to impact the quality and safety of the food supply is increasingly influenced by globalization and the international interdependence of manufacturing, communication, transportation, and technological advances. Countries are becoming more efficient at recognizing the need for, and understanding the importance of, good nutrition for the progress of its society. Yet even with this interdependence, one in nine people in the world continues to suffer from hunger, nearly half of whom are children (Rooney, 2014). Many more live with daily food insecurity, compromised quality, and micronutrient insufficiency. Unfortunately, civil instability and acute dietary crises in the most vulnerable of populations may also result from interdependence. Factors such as social unrest, bioterrorism, climate changes, dissolution of natural habitats (rainforest), macro- and microeconomic volatility, and fuel/transportation costs resulting in out-of-reach food prices are just a few obstacles that will negatively impact the ability of the food industry to benefit all peoples. Through awareness, education, and surveillance, consumers, manufacturers, suppliers, and global consortia alike have a responsibility to inform good policy decisions in order to ensure that the functional food and beverage industry remains safe and of high quality for its greatest obligation, the accessibility to and for all people.

REFERENCES

Alexander, J., Benford, D., Boobis, A., Eskola, M., Fink-Gremmels, J., Fürst, P., Heppner, C., Schlatter, J., and van Leeuwen, R. (2012). Special issue: Risk assessment of contaminants in food and feed. *EFSA J, 10*(10), 1–12.

Alger, H. M., Maffini, M. V., Kulkarni, N. R., Bongard, E. D., and Neltner, T. (2013). Perspectives on how FDA assesses exposure to food additives when evaluating their safety: Workshop proceedings. *Compr Rev Food Sci Food Saf, 12*(1), 90–119. doi: 10.1111/j.1541-4337.2012.00216.x.

Atreya, C. D. (2004). Major foodborne illness causing viruses and current status of vaccines against the diseases. *Foodborne Pathog Dis, 1*(2), 89–96. doi: 10.1089/153531404323143602.

Bennett, J. W. and Klich, M. (2003). Mycotoxins. *Clin Microbiol Rev, 16*(3), 497–516.

Biesiekierski, J. R., Peters, S. L., Newnham, E. D., Rosella, O., Muir, J. G., and Gibson, P. R. (2013). No effects of gluten in patients with self-reported non-celiac gluten sensitivity after dietary reduction of fermentable, poorly absorbed, short-chain carbohydrates. *Gastroenterology, 145*(2), 320–328,e323. doi: 10.1053/j.gastro.2013.04.051.

Borzelleca, J. F. (1992). Macronutrient substitutes: Safety evaluation. *Regul Toxicol Pharmacol, 16*(3), 253–264.

Bose-O'Reilly, S., McCarty, K. M., Steckling, N., and Lettmeier, B. (2010). Mercury exposure and children's health. *Curr Probl Pediatr Adolesc Health Care, 40*(8), 186–215. doi: 10.1016/j.cppeds.2010.07.002.

Boucard, A., Betat, A. M., Forster, R., Simonnard, A., and Froget, G. (2010). Evaluation of neurotoxicity potential in rats: The functional observational battery. *Curr Protoc Pharmacol*, Chapter 10, Unit 10, 12. doi: 10.1002/0471141755.ph1012s51.

Brandt, M., Brown, C., Burkhart, J., Burton, N., Cox-Ganser, J., Damon, S., Falk, H. et al. (2006). Mold prevention strategies and possible health effects in the aftermath of hurricanes and major floods: U.S. Department of Health and Human Services, Centers for Disease Control and Prevention. *MMWR, 55*(RR08), 1–27.

Branum, A. M. and Lukacs, S. L. (2009). Food allergy among children in the United States. *Pediatrics, 124*(6), 1549–1555. doi: 10.1542/peds.2009-1210.

Bruins, M. J. (2013). The clinical response to gluten challenge: A review of the literature. *Nutrients, 5*(11), 4614–4641. doi: 10.3390/nu5114614.

Burdock, G. A. and Matulka, R. A. (2014). Nanotechnology: The regulatory impact. *World Food Ingred*, (September), 56–59.

Calabria, B., Degenhardt, L., Hall, W., and Lynskey, M. (2010). Does cannabis use increase the risk of death? Systematic review of epidemiological evidence on adverse effects of cannabis use. *Drug Alcohol Rev, 29*(3), 318–330. doi: 10.1111/j.1465-3362.2009.00149.x.

Colby, D. W. and Prusiner, S. B. (2011). Prions. *Cold Spring Harb Perspect Biol, 3*(1), a006833. doi: 10.1101/cshperspect.a006833.

Cos, P., De Bruyne, T., Apers, S., Vanden Berghe, D., Pieters, L., and Vlietinck, A. J. (2003). Phytoestrogens: Recent developments. *Planta Med, 69*(7), 589–599. doi: 10.1055/s-2003-41122.

Dai, J. and Mumper, R. J. (2010). Plant phenolics: Extraction, analysis and their antioxidant and anticancer properties. *Molecules, 15*(10), 7313–7352. doi: 10.3390/molecules15107313.

Diamanti-Kandarakis, E., Bourguignon, J. P., Giudice, L. C., Hauser, R., Prins, G. S., Soto, A. M., Zoeller, R. T., and Gore, A. C. (2009). Endocrine-disrupting chemicals: An Endocrine Society scientific statement. *Endocr Rev, 30*(4), 293–342. doi: 10.1210/er.2009-0002.

Dolan, L. C., Matulka, R. A., and Burdock, G. A. (2010). Naturally occurring food toxins. *Toxins (Basel), 2*(9), 2289–2332. doi: 10.3390/toxins2092289.

Drahl, C. and Morrison, J. (2014). Modified spud gains approval. *Chem Eng News, 92*(46), 6.

Duncan, T. V. (2011). Applications of nanotechnology in food packaging and food safety: Barrier materials, antimicrobials and sensors. *J Colloid Interface Sci, 363*(1), 1–24. doi: http://dx.doi.org/10.1016/j.jcis.2011.07.017.

Eaton, D. L. and Klaasen, C. D. (2001). Principles of toxicology. In Curtis, D. K. (Ed.), *Casserett and Doull's Toxicology. The Basic Science of Poisons* (6th edn., pp. 11–34). New York: McGraw-Hill.

EC. (2012). COMMISSION REGULATION (EU) No 231/2012. Laying down specifications for food additives listed in Annexes II and III to Regulation (EC). 22.3.2012. L 83/1. http://www.mpeda.com/Aquaculture/EC-Regulation.pdf. Accessed December 5, 2014. No 1333/2008 of the European Parliament and of the Council.

EC. (2013). http://ec.europa.eu/food/safety/novel_food/legislation/index_en.htm. Accessed December 4, 2014.

EFSA Panel on Genetically Modified Organisms (GMO). (2010a). Guidance on the environmental risk assessment of genetically modified plants. *EFSA J, 8*(11), 1–111.

EFSA Panel on Genetically Modified Organisms (GMO). (2010b). Scientific opinion on the assessment of potential impacts of genetically modified plants on non-target organisms. *EFSA J, 8*(11), 1–72.

EFSA Scientific Committee. (2011a). Guidance on the risk assessment of the application of nanoscience and nanotechnologies in the food and feed chain. *EFSA J, 9*(5).

EFSA Scientific Committee. (2011b). Scientific opinion on genotoxicity testing strategies applicable to food and food safety assessment. *EFSA J, 9*(9), 1–69.

Eisenbrand, G., Pool-Zobel, B., Baker, V., Balls, M., Blaauboer, B. J., Boobis, A., Carere, A. et al. (2002). Methods of in vitro toxicology. *Food Chem Toxicol, 40*(2–3), 193–236.

Estruch, R., Ros, E., Salas-Salvadó, J., Covas, M., Corella, D., Arós, F., Gómez-Gracia, E. et al. (2013). Primary prevention of cardiovascular disease with a mediterranean diet. *N Engl J Med, 368*(14), 1279–1290. doi: doi:10.1056/NEJMoa1200303.

European Academy of Allergy and Clinical Immunology (EAACI). (2009). Allergies growing at alarming rate among children and teenagers: One out of two adults will suffer of a chronic allergic disease in 2015. Zurich, Switzerland: EAACI.

European Commission. (EC). 1997. REGULATION (EC) No 258/97 OF THE EUROPEAN PARLIAMENT AND OF THE COUNCIL of 27 January 1991 concerning novel foods and novel food ingredients. 14.2.97.No L 43/ 1. Brussels. http://eur-lex.europa.eu/LexUriServ/LexUriServ.do?uri=OJ:L:1997:043:0001:0006:EN:PDF. Accessed December 4, 2014.

European Food Safety Authority (EFSA). (2014a). GMO Publications. http://www.efsa.europa.eu/en/gmo/gmoscdocs.htm

EFSA. (2014b). Modern methodologies and tools for human hazard assessment of chemicals. *EFSA J, 12*(4), 1–87. Accessed December 14, 2014.

Faqi, A. (Ed.). (2013). *A Comprehensive Guide to Preclinical Drug Development* (1st edn.). London, U.K.: Academic Press.

Food and Agriculture Association (FAO). (2014). How to feed the world in 2050. Retrieved November 7, 2014. www.fao.org/fileadmin/templates/wsfs/docs/expert_paper/How_to_Feed_the_World_in_2050.pdf.

Fremont, S., Sanchez, C., Errahali, Y., Mouecoucou, J., Metche, M., Mejean, L., and Nicolas, J. P. (2004). Food allergy: effect of proteins-lipids and proteins-polysaccharides interactions. *Eur Ann Allergy Clin Immunol, 36*(3), 82–87.

Gardner, R. (2014). What studies say about Hemp CBD. *Nutr Outlook*, November 18, 34–38.

Gaur, S. and Agnihotri, R. (2014). Green tea: a novel functional food for the oral health of older adults. *Geriatr Gerontol Int, 14*(2), 238–250. doi: 10.1111/ggi.12194.

Ghosh, D., Bagchi, D., and Konishi, T. (2015). *Clinical Aspects of Functional Foods and Nutraceuticals*. Boca Raton, FL: CRC Press.

Goetz, G. (2013). FDA to investigate safety of added caffeine. *Food Safety News*, April 30, 2013.

Gossner, C. M., Schlundt, J., Ben Embarek, P., Hird, S., Lo-Fo-Wong, D., Beltran, J. J., Teoh, K. N., and Tritscher, A. (2009). The melamine incident: Implications for international food and feed safety. *Environ Health Perspect, 117*(12), 1803–1808. doi: 10.1289/ehp.0900949.

Goyer, R. A. and Clarkson, T. W. (2001). Toxic effects of metals. In Klaassen, D. and Watkins, J. B. (Eds.), *Casarett and Doull's Essentials of Toxicology* (2nd edn., pp. 811–867). New York: McGraw-Hill.

Grainger, R. (1999). Global Trends in Fisheries and Aquaculture. In: *Proceedings of a Workshop: Trends and Future Challenges for U.S. National Ocean and Coastal Policy*, Cicin-Sain, B., Knecht, R.W. and Foster N. (eds.), 22 January, 1999, Washington D.C., pp. 21–25.

Gray, J. I. and Morton, I. D. (1981). Some toxic compounds produced in food by cooking and processing. *J Hum Nutr, 35*(1), 5–23.

Güngörmüş, C. and Kılıç, A. (2012). The safety assessment of food additives by reproductive and developmental toxicity studies. In El-Samragy, Y. (Ed.), *Food Additive* (pp. 31–48). Rijeka, Croatia: Intech.

Haase, H. and Rink, L. (2014). Zinc signals and immune function. *BioFactors, 40*(1), 27–40. doi: 10.1002/biof.1114.

Hall, A. J., Lopman, B. A., Payne, D. C., Patel, M. M., Gastañaduy, P. A., Vinjé, J., and Parashar, U. D. (2013). Norovirus disease in the United States. *Emerg Infect Dis, 19*(8), 1198–1205.

Harris, J. K., Mansour, R., Choucair, B., Olson, J., Nissen, C., and Bhatt, J. (2014). Health department use of social media to identify foodborne illness—Chicago, Illinois, 2013–2014. *Morbid Mortal Wkly Rep, 63*(32), 681–685.

Hartung, T. and Hoffmann, S. (2009). Food for thought… on in silico methods in toxicology. *Altex, 26*(3), 155–166.

Hasler, C. M. (1998). Functional foods: Their role in disease prevention and health promotion. *Food Technol, 52*(2), 57–62.

Hayes, A. W. (Ed.) (2008). *Principles and Methods of Toxicology* (5th edn.). Boca Raton, FL: CRC Press.

Hubbs, A. F., Mercer, R. R., Benkovic, S. A., Harkema, J., Sriram, K., Schwegler-Berry, D., Goravanahally, M. P. et al. (2011). Nanotoxicology—A pathologist's perspective. *Toxicol Pathol, 39*(2), 301–324. doi: 10.1177/0192623310390705.

Hungerford, J. M. (2010). Scombroid poisoning: A review. *Toxicon, 56*(2), 231–243. doi: 10.1016/j.toxicon.2010.02.006.

International Conference on Harmonization (ICH). (1994a). Note for guidance on toxicokinetics: The assessment of systemic exposure in toxicity studies. Guideline S3A. European Medicines Agency (EMA), CPMP/ICH/384/95.

ICH. (1994b). Pharmacokinetics: Guidance for repeated dose tissue distribution studies. Guideline S3B. CPMP/ICH/385/95.

ICH. (1995). Guideline on the need for carcinogenicity studies of pharmaceuticals Guidelines S1A. EMA/536328/2013. http://www.ich.org/fileadmin/Public_Web_Site/ICH_Products/Guidelines/Safety/S1A/Step4/S1A_Guideline.pdf. Accessed on line May 28, 2015.

ICH. (1997). Testing for carcinogenicity of pharmaceuticals Guideline. S1B. http://www.ich.org/fileadmin/Public_Web_Site/ICH_Products/Guidelines/Safety/S1B/Step4/S1B_Guideline.pdf. Accessed on line May 28, 2015.

ICH. (1998). Duration of chronic toxicity testing in animals (rodent and non rodent toxicity testing). Guideline S4.

ICH. (2000). Safety pharmacology studies for human pharmaceuticals. Guideline S7A. CPMP/ICH/539/00.

ICH. (2005a). Immunotoxicity studies for human pharmaceuticals. Guideline S8. EMEA/CHMP/167235/2004-ICH.

ICH. (2005b). The non-clinical evaluation of the potential for delayed ventricular repolarization (QT interval prolongation) by human pharmaceuticals. Guideline S7B. CHMP/ICH/423/02.

ICH. (2008). Dose selection for carcinogenicity studies of pharmaceuticals. Guideline S1C(R2).http://www.ich.org/products/guidelines/safety/article/safety-, guidelines.html, Accessed on line May 28, 2015.

ICH. (2011). Genotoxicity testing and data interpretation for pharmaceuticals intended for human use. Guideline S2(R1). EMA/CHMP/ICH/126642/2008.

ICH. (2013). Rodent carcinogenicity studies for human pharmaceuticals. Guideline S1. Concept paper. 2013. http://www.ich.org/products/guidelines/safety/article/safety-guidelines.html. Accessed on lin May 28, 2015.

International Food Information Council (IFIC). (2013). Functional foods consumer survey. Executive Research Report (pp. 1–7).

International Food Technologists (IFT). (2005). *Functional Foods: Opportunities and Challenges*. Chicago, IL: IFT Foundation.

Jackson, K. D., Howie, L. D., and Akinbami, L. J. (2013). Trends in allergic conditions among children: United States, 1997–2011. http://www.cdc.gov/nchs/data/databriefs/db121.htm.

James, K. J., Carey, B., O'Halloran, J., van Pelt, F. N., and Skrabakova, Z. (2010). Shellfish toxicity: Human health implications of marine algal toxins. *Epidemiol Infect, 138*(7), 927–940. doi: 10.1017/S0950268810000853

Kirkland, D., Aardema, M., Henderson, L., and Muller, L. (2005). Evaluation of the ability of a battery of three in vitro genotoxicity tests to discriminate rodent carcinogens and non-carcinogens I. Sensitivity, specificity and relative predictivity. *Mutat Res, 584*(1–2), 1–256. doi: 10.1016/j.mrgentox.2005.02.004.

Kirkland, D., Reeve, L., Gatehouse, D., and Vanparys, P. (2011). A core in vitro genotoxicity battery comprising the Ames test plus the in vitro micronucleus test is sufficient to detect rodent carcinogens and in vivo genotoxins. *Mutat Res, 721*(1), 27–73. doi: 10.1016/j.mrgentox.2010.12.015.

Kirsch-Volders, M., Decordier, I., Elhajouji, A., Plas, G., Aardema, M. J., and Fenech, M. (2011). In vitro genotoxicity testing using the micronucleus assay in cell lines, human lymphocytes and 3D human skin models. *Mutagenesis, 26*(1), 177–184. doi: 10.1093/mutage/geq068.

Kong, W., Wei, R., Logrieco, A. F., Wei, J., Wen, J., Xiao, X., and Yang, M. (2014). Occurrence of toxigenic fungi and determination of mycotoxins by HPLC-FLD in functional foods and spices in China markets. *Food Chem, 146*, 320–326. doi: 10.1016/j.foodchem.2013.09.005.

Kotsonis, F. N., Burdock, G. A., and Flamm, G. (2001). Food toxicology. In Klaassen, D. (Ed.), *Casarett and Doull's Toxicology: The Basic Science of Poisons* (6th edn., pp. 1049–1088). New York: McGraw-Hill.

Kotsonis, F. N., Burdock, G. A., and Flamm, G. (2010). Food toxicology. In Klaassen, D. and Watkins, J. B., III (Eds.), *Casarett and Doull's Essentials of Toxicology* (2nd edn., pp. 399–407). New York: McGraw-Hill.

Krebs, N. F. and Jacobson, M. S. (2003). Prevention of pediatric overweight and obesity. *Pediatrics, 112*(2), 424–430.

Kruger, C. L., Reddy, C. S., Conze, D. B., and Hayes, A. W. (2014). Food safety and foodborne toxicants. In Hayes, A. W. and Kruger, C. L. (Eds.), *Hayes' Principles and Methods of Toxicology* (6th edn., pp. 621–675). Boca Raton, FL: CRC Press.

Lattanzio, V., Kroon, P. A., Linsalata, V., and Cardinali, A. (2009). Globe artichoke: A functional food and source of nutraceutical ingredients. *J Funct Foods, 1*(2), 131–144.

Lee, J., Igarashi, T., Fraga, S., Dahl, E., Hovgaard, P., and Yasumoto, T. (1989). Determination of diarrhetic shellfish toxins in various dinoflagellate species. *J Appl Phycol, 1*(2), 147–152. doi: 10.1007/BF00003877.

Lordan, S., Ross, R. P., and Stanton, C. (2011). Marine bioactives as functional food ingredients: Potential to reduce the incidence of chronic diseases. *Marine Drugs, 9*(6), 1056–1100. doi: 10.3390/md9061056.

Lunder, S. (November 3, 2014). EWG and 18,000 supporters call for FDA to improve seafood consumption advice for pregnant women and children. http://www.ewg.org/testimony-official-correspondence/ewg-and-18000-supporters-call-fda-improve-seafood-consumption. Retrieved December 3, 2014.

Mahony, J., Collins, B., Cornelissen, A., and van Sinderen, D. (2014). Exploring phage ecology, genetics and impact in food fermentations. In Bai, J. A. and Ravishankar, R. V. (Eds.), *Beneficial Microbes in Fermented and Functional Foods* (pp. 73–94). Boca Raton, FL: CRC Press.

Martin, T., and Avrelija, C. (2012). Application of gut cell models for toxicological and bioactivity studies of functional and novel foods. *Foods,* 1:40:51. doi: 10.3390/foods1010040.

Mazzoleni, G., Di Lorenzo, D., and Steimberg, N. (2009). Modelling tissues in 3D: The next future of pharmaco-toxicology and food research? *Genes Nutr, 4*(1), 13–22. doi: 10.1007/s12263-008-0107-0.

McCartney, E. (2014). Food safety re-evaluations dominate trends. *World Food Ingred* (September), 60–62.

Mejia, C. D. (2014). Energy drink ingredients demand proper characterization. *World Food Ingred* (September), 74–75.

Merrill, R. A. (1997). Food safety regulation: Reforming the delaney clause. *Ann Rev Public Health, 18*(1), 313–340. doi: 10.1146/annurev.publhealth.18.1.313.

Mitchell, D. C., Knight, C. A., Hockenberry, J., Teplansky, R., and Hartman, T. J. (2014). Beverage caffeine intakes in the U.S. *Food Chem Toxicol, 63*, 136–142. doi: 10.1016/j.fct.2013.10.042.

Molimard, P. and Spinnler, H. E. (1996). Review: Compounds involved in the flavor of surface mold-ripened cheeses: Origins and properties. *J Dairy Sci, 79*(2), 169–184. doi: http://dx.doi.org/10.3168/jds.S0022-0302(96)76348-8.

Morais, S., Garcia e Costa, F., and de Lourdes Pereira, M. (2012). Heavy metals and human health, environmental health—Emerging issues and practice. http://www.intechopen.com/books/environmental-health-emerging-issues-and-practice/heavy-metals-and-human-health. Accessed December 3, 2014.

Moser, V. C. (2011). Functional assays for neurotoxicity testing. *Toxicol Pathol, 39*(1), 36–45. doi: 10.1177/0192623310385255.

National Dairy Council. (2014). Dairy food consumption is associated with bone health in adults: Science summary. Retrieved November 19, 2014. http://www.nationaldairycouncil.org/Research/ResearchSummaries/Documents/DMI%20FactSheet_BoneHealth_FNL.pdf. Accessed December 12, 2014.

Neltner, T. G., Kulkarni, N. R., Alger, H. M., Maffini, M. V., Bongard, E. D., Fortin, N. D., and Olson, E. D. (2011). Navigating the U.S. Food Additive Regulatory Program. *Compr Rev Food Sci Food Safety, 10*(6), 342–368. doi: 10.1111/j.1541-4337.2011.00166.x.

Organization for Economic Cooperation and Development (OECD). (1983). Guideline for the testing of chemicals. Section 4 (Part 415): Health effects: One-generation reproduction toxicity study.

OECD. (1993). Safety evaluation of foods derived by modern biotechnology: Concepts and principles. Paris Cedex 16, France.

OECD. (1995). Guideline for the testing of chemicals. Section 4 (Part 421): Health effects: Reproduction/developmental toxicity screening test. July 1995.

OECD. (1996). Guideline for the testing of chemicals. Section 4 (Part 422): Health effects: Combined repeated dose toxicity study with the reproduction/developmental screening test. March 1996.

OECD. (1997a). Guideline for the testing of chemicals. Section 4 (Part 471): Health effects: Bacterial reverse mutation test. July 1997.

OECD. (1997b). Guideline for the testing of chemicals. Section 4 (Part 474): Health effects: Mammalian erythrocyte micronucleus test. July 1997.

OECD. (1997c). Guideline for the testing of chemicals. Section 4 (Part 424): Health effects: Neurotoxicity study in rodents. July 1997.

OECD. (1998a). Guideline for the testing of chemicals. Section 4 (Part 408): Health effects: Repeated dose 90-day oral toxicity study in rodents. September 1998.

OECD. (1998b). Guideline for the testing of chemicals. Section 4 (Part 409): Health effects: Repeated dose 90-day oral toxicity study in non-rodents. September 1998.

OECD. (2001a). Guideline for the testing of chemicals. Section 4 (Part 414): Health effects: Prenatal developmental toxicity study. January 2001.

OECD. (2001b). Guideline for the testing of chemicals. Section 4 (Part 416): Health effects: Two-generation reproduction toxicity study. January 2001.

OECD. (2007). Guideline for the testing of chemicals. Section 4 (Part 426): Health effects: Developmental neurotoxicity study. October 2007.

OECD. (2008a). Guideline for the testing of chemicals. Section 4 (Part 425); Health effects: Acute oral toxicity: Up-and-down procedure. October 2008.

OECD. (2008b). Guideline for the testing of chemicals. Section 4 (Part 407): Health effects: Repeated dose 28-day oral toxicity study in rodents. October 2008.

OECD. (2009a). Guideline for the testing of chemicals. Section 4 (Part 451): Health effects: Carcinogenicity studies. September 2009.

OECD. (2009b). Guideline for the testing of chemicals. Section 4 (Part 452): Health effects: Chronic toxicity studies. September 2009.

OECD. (2009c). Guideline for the testing of chemicals. Section 4 (Part 453): Health effects: Combined chronic toxicity/carcinogenicity studies. September 2009.

OECD. (2010a). Guideline for the testing of chemicals. Section 4 (Part 487): Health effects: in vitro mammalian cell micronucleus test. July 2010. doi: 10.1787/9789264091016-en.

OECD. (2010b). Guidance manual for the testing of manufactured nanomaterials: OECD's sponsorship programme; first revision. Environment directorate joint meeting of the chemicals committee and the working party on chemicals, pesticides and biotechnology. ENV/JM/MONO(2009)20/REV. Accessed Online: October 4, 2013. Available at: http://search.oecd.org/officialdocuments/displaydocumentpdf/?cote= Mejia env/jm/mono(2009)20/rev&doclanguage=en.

OECD. (2011). Guideline for the testing of chemicals. Section 4 (Part 443): Health effects: Extended one-generation reproductive toxicity study. July 2011. doi: 10.1787/9789264122550-en.

OECD. (2012). Guidance on sample preparation and dosimetry for the safety testing of manufactured nanomaterials. Series on the Safety of Manufactured Nanomaterials. No. 36 JT03332780. ENV/JM/MONO(2012)40.

OECD. (2013). Working Party on Nanotechnology. Regulatory frameworks for nanotechnology in foods and medical products. Summary results of a survey activity. Directorate for Science, Technology and Industry. Committee for Scientific and Technological Policy. DSTI/STP/NANO(2012)22/FINAL. March 21, 2013.

OECD. (2014). Guideline for the testing of chemicals. Section 4 (Part 474): Health effects: Mammalian erythrocyte micronucleus test. September 2014. doi: 10.1787/9789264224292-en.

Panagiotou, T. and Fisher, R. J. (2013). Producing micron- and nano- size formulations for functional foods applications. *Funct Foods Health Dis, 3*(7), 274–289.

Panter, K. E. and James, L. F. (1990). Natural plant toxicants in milk: A review. *J Anim Sci, 68*(3), 892–904.

Pray, L. and Yaktine, A. (2009). *Nanotechnology in Food Products: Workshop Summary* (Inst. Med of the Natl Acad Ed.). Washington, DC: The National Academy Press.

Price, N. and Chaudhry, Q. (2014). Application of in silico modelling to estimate toxicity of migrating substances from food packaging. *Food Chem Toxicol, 71*, 136–141. doi: 10.1016/j.fct.2014.05.022.

Rizvi, S. S. H., Moraru, C. I., Bouwmeester, H., and Klampers, F. W. H. (2010). Nanotechnology and food safety. In Boisrobert, S., Oh. C., Stjaponovic, A., and Lelieveld, H. (Eds.), *Ensuring Global Food Safety: Exploring Global Harmonization* (pp. 263–279). London, U.K.: Academic Press.

Rommens, C. M., Yan, H., Swords, K., Richael, C., and Ye, J. (2008). Low-acrylamide French fries and potato chips. *Plant Biotechnol J, 6*(8), 843–853. doi: 10.1111/j.1467-7652.2008.00363.x.

Rona, R. J., Keil, T., Summers, C., Gislason, D., Zuidmeer, L., Sodergren, E., Sigurdardottir, S. T. et al. (2007). The prevalence of food allergy: A meta-analysis. *J Allergy Clin Immunol, 120*(3), 638–646. doi: 10.1016/j.jaci.2007.05.026.

Rooney, B. (2014). 1 in 9 goes hungry worldwide. *CNN Money.* http://money.cnn.com/2014/09/15/news/un-hunger-report/, Accessed December 4, 2014.

Schilter, B., Benigni, R., Boobis, A., Chiodini, A., Cockburn, A., Cronin, M. T., Lo Piparo, E., and Worth, A. (2014). Establishing the level of safety concern for chemicals in food without the need for toxicity testing. *Regul Toxicol Pharmacol, 68*(2), 275–296. doi: 10.1016/j.yrtph.2013.08.018.

Sekhon, B. S. (2010). Food nanotechnology—An overview. *Nanotechnol Sci Appl, 3*, 1–15.

Sekhon, B. S. (2014). Nanotechnology in agri-food production: An overview. *Nanotechnol Sci Appl, 7*, 31–53. doi: 10.2147/NSA.S39406.

Selhub, E. M., Logan, A. C., and Bested, A. C. (2014). Fermented foods, microbiota, and mental health: Ancient practice meets nutritional psychiatry. *J Physiol Anthropol, 33*, 2. doi: 10.1186/1880-6805-33-2.

Shiby, V. K. and Mishra, H. N. (2013). Fermented milks and milk products as functional foods—A review. *Crit Rev Food Sci Nutr, 53*(5), 482–496. doi: 10.1080/10408398.2010.547398.

Small, E. (2004). Narcotic plants as sources of medicinals, nutraceuticals, and functional foods. In: Hou FF, Lin HS, Chou MH, Chang TW (eds). *Proceedings of the International Symposium on the Development of Medicinal Plants*, Hualien District Agricultural Research and Extension Station, Taiwan, pp. 11–66.

Stewart, N. and Stevenson, K. (2013). CRN expands its self-regulatory initiatives with recommended guidelines for caffeine-containing supplements. Retrieved December 10, 2013. http://crnusa.org/caffeine/.

Sultanbawa, Y. (2011). Plant antimicrobials in food applications: Minireview. In Méndez-Vilas, A. (Ed.), *Science Against Microbial Pathogens: Communicating Current Research and Technological Advances* (pp. 1084–1093). Badajoz, Spain: Formatex Research Center.

U.S. FDA (U.S. Food and Drug Administration). (2014). FDA response to the Fukushima Dai-ichi Nuclear Power Facility incident. Last modified: July 30, 2014. http://www.fda.gov/newsevents/publichealthfocus/ucm247403.htm. Accessed December 12, 2014.

U.S. FDA (U.S. Food and Drug Administration). (1993a). *Toxicological Principles for the Safety Assessment of Direct Food Additives Used in Foods. Draft Redbook II.* Chapter IV.C.2. Acute oral toxicity tests.

U.S. FDA (U.S. Food and Drug Administration). (1993b). *Toxicological Principles for the Safety Assessment of Direct Food Additives Used in Food. Draft Redbook II.* Chapter V.D. Immunotoxicity studies.

U.S. FDA (U.S. Food and Drug Administration). (1993c). *Toxicological Principles for the Safety Assessment of Direct Food Additives Used in Food. Draft Redbook II.* Chapter V.B. Metabolism and Pharmacokinetic studies.

U.S. FDA (U.S. Food and Drug Administration). (1993d). *Toxicological Principles for the Safety Assessment of Direct Food Additives Used in Food. Draft Redbook II.* Chapter VI.A. Clinical evaluation of food ingredients.

U.S. FDA (U.S. Food and Drug Administration). (2000a). *Toxicological Principles for the Safety Assessment of Food Ingredients. Redbook 2000.* Chapter IV.C.9a. Guidelines for reproduction studies. July 2000.

U.S. FDA (U.S. Food and Drug Administration). (2000b). Toxicological Principles for the Safety Assessment of Food Ingredients. Redbook 2000. Chapter IV.C.9b. Guidelines for developmental toxicity studies. July 2000.

U.S. FDA (U.S. Food and Drug Administration). (2000c). *Toxicological Principles for the Safety Assessment of Food Ingredients. Redbook 2000.* Chapter IV.C.10. Neurotoxicity studies. July 2000.

U.S. FDA (U.S. Food and Drug Administration). (2001). Draft Guidance for Industry: Voluntary labeling indicating whether foods have or have not been developed using bioengineering; Draft Guidance. Accessed November 20, 2014. http://www.fda.gov/Food/GuidanceRegulation/GuidanceDocumentsRegulatoryInformation/ucm059098.htm.

U.S. FDA (U.S. Food and Drug Administration). (2003a). *Toxicological Principles for the Safety Assessment of Food Ingredients. Redbook 2000.* Chapter IV.C.3a. Short-term toxicity studies with rodents. November 2003.

U.S. FDA (U.S. Food and Drug Administration). (2003b). *Toxicological Principles for the Safety Assessment of Food Ingredients. Redbook 2000.* Chapter IV.C.4a. Subchronic toxicity studies with rodents. November 2003.

U.S. FDA (U.S. Food and Drug Administration). (2003c). *Toxicological Principles for the Safety Assessment of Food Ingredients. Redbook 2000.* Chapter IV.C.5b. One-year toxicity studies with non-rodents. November 2003.

U.S. FDA (U.S. Food and Drug Administration). (2006). *Toxicological Principles for the Safety Assessment of Food Ingredients. Redbook 2000.* Chapter IV.C.6. Carcinogenicity studies with rodents. January 2006.

U.S. FDA (U.S. Food and Drug Administration). (2007a). *Toxicological Principles for the Safety Assessment of Food Ingredients. Redbook 2000.* Chapter IV.C.1. Short-term tests for genetic toxicity. July 2007.

U.S. FDA (U.S. Food and Drug Administration). (2007b). *Toxicological Principles for the Safety Assessment of Food Ingredients. Redbook 2000.* Chapter IV.C.5a. Chronic toxicity studies with rodents. July 2007.

U.S. FDA (U.S. Food and Drug Administration). (2011). FDA Food Safety Modernization Act, 111–353 C.F.R.

U.S. FDA (U.S. Food and Drug Administration). (2012). Draft Guidance for Industry: Assessing the effects of significant manufacturing process changes, including emerging technologies on the safety and regulatory status of food ingredients and food contact substances, including food ingredients that are color additives. Accessed December 4, 2013. http://www.fda.gov/Food/GuidanceRegulation/GuidanceDocumentsRegulatoryInformation/IngredientsAdditivesGRASPackaging/ucm300661.htm.

U.S. FDA (U.S. Food and Drug Administration). (2014a). Guidance for Industry: Considering whether an FDA-regulated product involves the application of nanotechnology. U.S. Department of Health and Human Services Food and Drug Administration, Office of the Commissioner. June 2014. http://www.fda.gov/RegulatoryInformation/Guidances/ucm257698.htm. Accessed December 4, 2014.

U.S. FDA (U.S. Food and Drug Administration). (2014b). Guidance for Industry. Distinguishing liquid dietary supplements from beverages. Center for Food Safety and Applied Nutrition. U.S. Department of Health and Human Services. January 2014.

U.S. National Library of Medicine. (2008). Genetics Home Reference: Prion Disease. Retrieved December 12, 2014. http://ghr.nlm.nih.gov/condition/prion-disease#definition. Accessed December 12, 2014.

Van Huis, A., Van Itterbeeck, J., Klunder, H., Mertens, E., Halloran, A., Muir, G., and Vantomme, P. (2013). *Edible Insects: Future Prospects for Food and Feed Security.* Rome, France: Food and Agriculture Organization of the United Nations.

Wang, D. (2008). Neurotoxins from marine dinoflagellates: A brief review. *Marine Drugs, 6*(2), 349–371.

Wang, J. and Sampson, H. A. (2013). Oral and sublingual immunotherapy for food allergy. *Asian Pac J Allergy Immunol, 31*(3), 198–209.

Wang, L. and Bohn, T. (2012). Health-promoting food ingredients and functional food processing technology. In Bouayed, J. (Ed.), *Nutrition, Well-Being and Health.* Retrieved. http://www.intechopen.com/books/nutrition-well-being-and-health/health-promoting-food-ingredientsdevelopment-and-processing. Accessed December 4, 2014.

Warheit, D. B. and Donner, E. M. (2010). Rationale of genotoxicity testing of nanomaterials: Regulatory requirements and appropriateness of available OECD test guidelines. *Nanotoxicology, 4*, 409–413. doi: 10.3109/17435390.2010.485704.

Weise, E. (2008). Petition calls for FDA to regulate energy drinks. *USA Today.* http://usatoday30.usatoday.com/news/health/2008-10-21-energy-drinks_N.htm. Accessed December 4, 2014.

Williams, J. (2008). Factoring safety into functional foods. *Food Saf Mag, 14*(6), 42.

Woo, C. K. and Bahna, S. L. (2011). Not all shellfish "allergy" is allergy! *Clin Transl Allergy, 1*(1), 3. doi: 10.1186/2045-7022-1-3.

World Health Organization (WHO). (1989). Guidelines for simple evaluation of food additive intake. CAC/GL 3-1989. *Codex Alimentarius* (pp. 1–18). Geneva, Switzerland: WHO.

WHO. (2008). *Toxicological and Health Aspects of Melamine and Cyanuric Acid.* Geneva, Switzerland: WHO.

3 Functional Foods in the Treatment of Processed Food Addiction and the Metabolic Syndrome

J.R. Ifland, Harry G. Preuss, M.T. Marcus, K.M. Rourke, W.C. Taylor, H. Theresa Wright, and Kathryn (Kay) Sheppard

CONTENTS

3.1 INTRODUCTION

As the obesity epidemic rages on without effective treatment, the food addiction model has gained attention as a new approach to treatment. Growing acceptance of the concept of food addiction is supported by well-documented similarities in neuro-functioning between overeating and classic drug addiction in sensitized craving and reward pathways, heightened reactivity to substance-related cues, and suppression of cognitive centers. These neuro-anomalies manifest in patterns of behavior described in addiction diagnostic criteria by the American Psychiatric Association in their Diagnostic and Statistical Manual for Mental Illnesses (DSM). There are also other similarities between chemicals addiction and processed food addiction, including prominence of cravings, genetic anomalies, family patterns, behavioral patterns, congenital defects, extensive consequences, age of onset issues, and addiction-promoting business practices (tobacco, alcohol, and processed foods) related to advertising, availability, and pricing particularly to children (Ifland et al., 2012).

Not surprisingly, both drug and processed food addiction are treated through abstinence from addictive substances, avoidance of cues related to the addictive substances, and recovery techniques such as meetings, sponsors, reading, and meditation. Addiction is a complex brain disease characterized by craving, seeking, and use that persists despite potentially devastating consequences. Replacing cravings with healthy food choices and rational thought patterns is a core goal of recovery.

The discovery of abstinence from addictive substances for addiction treatment and the founding of Alcoholics Anonymous is credited to Bill Wilson in the 1930s. Similarly, Abstinent Food Plans for the treatment of overeating have now spread to 12-step groups such as Food Addicts in Recovery Anonymous (FA) and Food Addicts Anonymous (FAA).

With growing interest in functional foods, it is appropriate to look at Abstinent Food Plans as a functional food approach to the treatment of chronic overeating of processed foods and the associated metabolic syndrome. This chapter describes the evidence for functional food plans used in the treatment of the metabolic syndrome.

Useful definitions for this chapter include substance addiction, functional foods, and metabolic syndrome. According to the American Society of Addiction Medicine,

> Addiction is a primary, chronic disease of brain reward, motivation, memory and related circuitry. Dysfunction in these circuits leads to characteristic biological, psychological, social and spiritual manifestations. This is reflected in an individual pathologically pursuing reward and/or relief by substance use and other behaviors.
>
> Addiction is characterized by inability to consistently abstain, impairment in behavioral control, craving, diminished recognition of significant problems with one's behaviors and interpersonal relationships, and a dysfunctional emotional response. Like other chronic diseases, addiction often involves cycles of relapse and remission. Without treatment or engagement in recovery activities, addiction is progressive and can result in disability or premature death (American Society of Addiction Medicine, 2014).

According to the Academy of Nutrition and Dietetics, functional foods can include the following:

- Conventional foods such as grains, fruits, vegetables, and nuts
- Modified foods such as yogurt, cereals, and orange juice
- Medical foods such as special formulations of foods and beverages for certain health conditions
- Foods for special dietary use such as infant formula and hypoallergenic foods (Denny, 2014)

This chapter addresses functional foods under the first category.

According to the Mayo Clinic, the metabolic syndrome includes

> a cluster of conditions—increased blood pressure, a high blood sugar level, excess body fat around the waist and abnormal cholesterol levels—that occur together, increasing your risk of heart disease, stroke and diabetes (Mayo.Clinic, 2014).

3.2 METHODS

Three methods were used to collect data for this chapter: searches of PubMed, data extraction from the USDA Economic Service, and qualitative data from 12-step food addiction literature. PubMed was accessed between 2005 and 2014 with searches for combinations of words including addiction, obesity, overweight, diet, weight loss, dopamine, serotonin, opiates, endocannabinoids, endorphins, leptin, ghrelin, orexin, craving, reward sensitivity, instrument transfer, diabetes, bariatric surgery, sugar, dietary fat, fructose, dairy, caffeine, cardiovascular, validation, DSM, paleolithic diet, and Mediterranean Diet. Articles that described an aspect of addiction to processed foods were downloaded and reviewed. Of the 4180 articles over an extended period of time, 80 papers were selected for this article based on their relevance to food addiction and food plans used to treat food addiction.

Qualitative data were extracted from 78 stories of recovery from processed food addiction found in the manuals of two food addiction fellowships, FA and FAA. These 12-step fellowships are non-profit organization models on Alcoholics Anonymous. Members abstain from addictive foods in the same way that recovering alcoholics abstain from alcohol. The stories are solicited nationally within the United States from members of the fellowships. Editorial committees made up of experienced fellowship members select the stories for inclusion in the manual.

3.3 RESULTS

3.3.1 Results from PubMed for Research Related to Food Addiction and Functional Food Plans

3.3.1.1 Introduction to PubMed Results

Three patterns emerge from PubMed results. There is addiction symptomatology in overeating, specific processed foods are used in the addictive overeating, and when those foods are eliminated, satiation improves. Research into diabetes, Mediterranean, and Paleo diets demonstrates that unprocessed foods, specifically proteins combined with unprocessed vegetables, fruits, and starches as well as cold-pressed oils, are effective at treating the metabolic syndrome and promoting satiety (Jonsson et al., 2009, 2010; Lindeberg et al., 2007). There is a body of literature that shows characteristics of addiction in overeating as sensitized craving and reward neuro-pathways that suppress cognitive functions and inhibition when activated. There is further evidence for peripheral signaling that exacerbates this neurotransmitter and suppressive activity (Volkow et al., 2012). There is also evidence for addictive properties in processed foods including sweeteners, flour, salt, processed fats, dairy, and caffeine (Wright and Ifland, 2014).

3.3.1.2 Evidence for the Efficacy of Diabetes, Mediterranean, and Paleo Diets

There is evidence that diets that eliminate some range of processed foods are associated with improvements in the metabolic syndrome, specifically diabetes, blood pressure, and overweight.

One study compared a diabetes diet with the Paleo diet. The diabetes diet included "vegetables, root vegetables, dietary fiber, whole-grain bread and other whole-grain cereal products, fruits and berries, and decreased intake of total fat with more unsaturated fat. … Salt intake was recommended to be kept below 6 g per day" (Jonsson et al., 2009). By comparison, the Paleolithic diet included "lean meat, fish, fruit, leafy and cruciferous vegetables, root vegetables, eggs and nuts, while excluding dairy products, cereal grains, beans, refined fats, sugar, candy, soft drinks, beer and extra addition of salt" (Jonsson et al., 2009). In the two meal plans, the Paleolithic diet had fewer addictive foods than did the diabetes diet.

Compared to the diabetes diet, the Paleolithic diet showed improved measures for diabetes, cholesterol, blood pressure, weight, BMI, and waist circumference. In another study, the Paleolithic diet was also found to be more satisfying than the diabetes diet (Jonsson et al., 2013). Cravings are important to the processed food addiction model. Carbohydrate cravings are found more in diabetics with poor control than diabetics with good control (Yu et al., 2013).

Another study compared the Paleolithic with the Mediterranean diet. Similar to the earlier studies, the Paleolithic diet was based on lean meat, fish, fruit, vegetables, root vegetables, eggs, and nuts. The Mediterranean diet was based on whole grains, low-fat dairy products, vegetables, fruit, fish, and oils and margarines (Jonsson et al., 2010). The Paleolithic diet was as satiating as the Mediterranean group but consumed less energy per day. In yet another study, the Paleolithic diet controlled glucose better than the Mediterranean diet (Lindeberg et al., 2007).

As compared to either the diabetes or Mediterranean diet, the Paleolithic diet showed improved efficacy in satiation, which is critical in the treatment of food addiction. The improved results in the management of the metabolic syndrome in the Paleolithic diet are consistent with what is known about the effects of sugar and salt (Preuss and Clouatre, 2012; Preuss and Preuss, 2014).

3.3.1.3 Outcomes and Food Plans

In Table 3.1, food plans are ranked according to the number of addictive foods included in the plan. The *idealized* plan eliminates all foods for which there is evidence of addictive properties (Jonsson et al., 2009; Lindeberg et al., 2007; Putnam and Allshouse, 1999; Wright and Ifland, 2014).

In a food addiction model, the progressive reduction in addictive foods may be the most important change from the standard American diet to an ideal abstinent food plan. Although the standard deviations in the data are large, there is a meaningful reduction in addictive foods from the diabetes and Mediterranean diets to the Paleo and abstinent diets. From the table, a reader might see that the ideal abstinent food plan could work best to relieve cravings because it eliminates all addictive foods such as sweetened beverages, cereals, and dairy. In the qualitative evidence taken from the food addiction 12-step literature, it is the elimination of craving foods that precedes control over overeating. It is significant to note that higher satiation was found in the Paleolithic diet, which eliminated more craving foods than the diabetes diet (Jonsson et al., 2009). As satiation can be related to cravings, there is evidence that reducing processed foods reduces cravings.

Of course, there are a number of other reasons for improvements in health besides reduction in cravings. Some of the eliminated foods such as sugar have been shown to remove minerals from the body in the process of digestion (Eaton and Eaton, 2000; Tsanzi et al., 2008). Some eliminated foods are considered to be inflammatory (Michaelsson et al., 2014; Schwander et al., 2014; Shriner, 2013; Spreadbury, 2012). Wheat and dairy may impede digestion and promote irritable bowel syndrome (Carroccio et al., 2011). Sweeteners and salt are associated with a broad range of disease (Preuss and Clouatre, 2012; Preuss and Preuss, 2014). However, in a food addiction model, the cessation of cravings is a prerequisite for reduced use of these harmful processed foods.

If the issue with the American diet were simply that people should know to eat healthier foods, there would not be an epidemic of the metabolic syndrome. However, as the issue with poor choices

TABLE 3.1
Results of Eliminating Addictive Foods

Plan	Food (g/day)			Results
	Sweetened Drinks	Cereals	Diary	
Ideal abstinent	0	0	0	Cessation of overeating, cravings, and metabolic syndrome.
Paleolithic	56 ± 121 12 ± 35	18 ± 52 12 ± 20	45 ± 119 16 ± 32	Improved blood pressure, cholesterol, improved satiation.
Diabetes	48 ± 90	172 ± 96	183 ± 123	Less robust than Paleolithic. Diabetes epidemic persists.
Mediterranean	141 ± 231	268 ± 96	287 ± 193	Less robust than Paleolithic. Heart disease persists.
American	645	215	88.6	Epidemic of metabolic syndrome.

appears to be one of the addictions, then it seems appropriate to address craving reduction as the core goal. As the abstinent food plan appears to accomplish this, it becomes helpful to discuss challenges in its implementation.

3.3.1.4 Evidence for the Neurological Basis of Processed Food Addiction

Brain imaging technology introduced in the 1990s gave insight into the origins of addictive behaviors. With scanning technology such as magnetic resonance imaging (MRI) and positron emission topography, addictions could be defined as the presence of specific dysfunctions in the brain (Wang et al., 2004). These dysfunctions appear as hyperactivation of craving, reward-sensitive, and instrument transfer (*take-action*) pathways simultaneous with the suppression of inhibition and decision-making centers that fail to curb drug and processed food taking.

The literature describing neuro-adaptations in addictive overeating is extensive. A number of recent review articles articulate these findings comprehensively (D'Addario et al., 2014; Kelley et al., 2005; Kringelbach and Stein, 2010; Stice et al., 2013; Wang et al., 2014). An exhaustive description of the findings is well beyond the scope of this chapter. Nonetheless, an understanding of food addiction as a disorder of the brain is essential in comprehending how abstinent food plans could effectively treat addictive overeating. In this model, success in applying functional food plans to overeating results from reconditioning and stabilizing sensitized craving and reward-seeking pathways by disassociating eating from craving.

There is general agreement that the neuro-dysfunction found in addictive overeating is the result of Pavlovian conditioning in response to repeated use of addictive foods as well as repeated exposure to processed food cues (Volkow et al., 2012). Peptides originating elsewhere in the body exacerbate feeding neuro-dysfunction (Sobrino Crespo et al., 2014). In addition, other conditions such as stress and hunger can enhance cravings and reward sensitivity. The evidence helps explain the irrational eating behavior that leads to overweight.

The craving pathways activated in addictions include dopamine, opiate, serotonin, endorphin, and endocannabinoid neurotransmitters. Of all the craving pathways, the dopamine pathway in the nucleus accumbens is perhaps the best understood (Wang et al., 2014). Sugar more than fat has been implicated in excessive dopamine activation (van de Giessen et al., 2013). In a rat antagonist study, both sucrose and fructose cues and ingestion activate both D1 and D2 circuitry but differently (Pritchett and Hajnal, 2011). Excessive fat intake has been linked to downregulated dopamine receptors, which suggests the progression of tolerance (Tellez et al., 2013). Dopamine production in the striata has also shown tolerance in an fMRI study as receptor activity decreased with repeat consumption of ice cream (Burger and Stice, 2012). Dopamine tolerance to sugar was also found in rats (Alsio et al., 2010).

Four other craving pathways are also susceptible to Pavlovian conditioning in response to processed food cues. The opiate pathways encode positive responses to sugar and fat within ventral striatal medium spiny neurons (Kelley et al., 2002). Euphoric endorphins have been found to be released excessively in the nucleus accumbens both in people with alcoholism and in those with sweet preference as well as their children (Fortuna, 2010). Evidence for the impact of sugar on serotonin was found in that "elevated blood glucose levels catalyze the absorption of tryptophan through the large neutral amino acid (LNAA) complex and its subsequent conversion into the mood-elevating chemical serotonin" (Fortuna, 2012). Endocannabinoid functioning has been found to integrate many of the functions described earlier (Karatsoreos et al., 2013). Endocannabinoids impact 22 neuro-processes (D'Addario et al., 2014). Recently, dietary fats have been shown to activate endocannabinoid pathways in the gut and that this was necessary for rats to develop a preference for fat (DiPatrizio et al., 2013). The evidence shows a complex of craving neuro-pathways, conditioned to respond to processed food cues.

The reward-sensitive pathways stimulate food seeking and are also vulnerable to Pavlovian conditioning. The pathways include long-recognized connections between the amygdala and the hypothalamus that play a crucial role in developing learning that drives addictive overeating. An associated cue can acquire strong motivational properties by being paired with food under conditions of hunger. Cues are powerful enough to override satiety and cause eating in sated rats. Neuro-pathways through which cues control feeding behavior describe maladaptive conditioned control of eating that contributes to eating disorders (Petrovich and Gallagher, 2003).

The instrument transfer pathways translate cravings and reward seeking into action. These pathways are also susceptible to Pavlovian conditioning. They include two anatomically and functionally distinct processes. The first is a goal-directed process that is based in the prefrontal cortex and dorsomedial striatum and encodes the causal relationship between an action and the motivational value of the outcome. The second process is a dorsolateral striatum–based habit function that learns associations between actions and antecedent stimuli (Schwabe and Wolf, 2011).

At the same time when craving, reward-seeking, and instrument transfer pathways respond to processed food cues, a parallel reaction is seen in the suppression of *control* pathways including executive decision making, memory, learning, and inhibition (Volkow et al., 2012). There is general consensus in the field that even though cravings, reward seeking, and instrument transfer are well conditioned to respond to processed food cues, this would not be enough to explain chronic overeating. The suppression of control pathways is needed for the addictive behavior to take place (O'Doherty et al., 2006).

In addition to cravings, stimulation, and suppression of *brakes*, food-related peptides enhance reactions. These include leptin (Grosshans et al., 2012), insulin (Jastreboff et al., 2013; Kroemer et al., 2013), orexin (Ho and Berridge, 2013), and ghrelin (Folgueira et al., 2014; Kroemer et al., 2013). These peptides originate elsewhere in the body including adipose tissue, pancreas, gut, and liver. They travel to the brain and can contribute at multiple points to the excitation of the earlier-described pathways (Sobrino Crespo et al., 2014).

Other factors that can exacerbate sensitivity include stress (Meye and Adan, 2014), prior drug use (Orsini et al., 2014), and hunger (Witt et al., 2014).

In summary, the research reveals vulnerability to developing food addiction through Pavlovian conditioning to crave, seek, and take action for processed food rewards simultaneous with the suppression of neuro-circuits that would otherwise exert rational control. The reactions are exacerbated by peripherally generated peptides and by conditions such as hunger and stress. The extensive similarity between neuro-dysfunction found in drug addiction and addictive eating offers a rationale for the application of addiction treatment protocols of abstinence, cue avoidance, and support to overeating.

3.3.1.5 Evidence for Addictive Properties in Foods

It has been shown that processed foods and cues cause the cascade of neuro-reaction described earlier while bland foods do not (Beaver et al., 2006; Guerrieri et al., 2008; Pelchat et al., 2004; Stice et al., 2008). The words for processed foods include hedonic, palatable, calorie dense, and excitatory. These foods fall into six general categories of sweeteners, flour, excessive salt, processed fat, dairy, and caffeine.

Sweeteners: These include sugar and any products that include the word "sugar." Sweeteners also include any product with the word syrup, including high-fructose corn syrup. Words ending in "itol" and "ose" are also sweeteners as are stevia and artificial sweeteners. The research literature has found addictive properties for sugar in the form of tolerance and withdrawal in rats (Avena et al., 2012) and heightened cue responsivity in humans (Yau and Potenza, 2013). Fructose has also been found to have addictive properties (Lustig, 2013). Sugar and fructose have been found to correlate with heart disease (Preuss and Preuss, 2014; Yudkin, 1988).

Flour: This category includes any carbohydrate that has been ground into a powder including wheat, rye, kamut, spelt, barley, bean, and lentil flours. A morphine peptide has been isolated from wheat, and a gluteomorphine has been discovered in gluten (Fanciulli et al., 2005; Fukudome and Yoshikawa, 1992; Huebner et al., 1984; Takahashi et al., 2000). The acellular properties of ground carbohydrates contribute to rapid breakdown, absorption, and inflammation (Spreadbury, 2012).

Salt: Research shows that salt has addictive properties (Cocores and Gold, 2009; Tekol, 2006). It has also been shown to be associated with the metabolic syndrome (Preuss and Clouatre, 2012).

Fat: Fat consumption triggers addictive activity (Ziauddeen et al., 2013) and has shown a withdrawal syndrome (Sharma et al., 2013).

Dairy: This includes cheese, cream, sour cream, and butter. The findings of addictive properties for fat shown earlier also apply here. In addition, milk has been shown to have a numbing effect in rats (Blass and Shide, 1994). A casomorphine has been isolated from milk and is the only peptide that when injected peripherally stimulates the craving neuro-pathways (Bray, 2000).

Caffeine: Caffeine use is a diagnosis in the DSM-V (Thomasius et al., 2014). The research on the addictive properties of caffeine shows both tolerance and a withdrawal syndrome (Bernstein et al., 2002).

Volume: There is a general caveat in food addiction recovery that any food that the client loses control over should be eliminated from the diet (p. 271) (Food Addicts Anonymous, 2010). This is supported by research showing that gastric distension activates the craving pathways that are also sensitized in drug addicts (Wang et al., 2006).

In summary, there is evidence for addictive properties in processed foods. This evidence supports the concept of processed food addiction as a substance-based use disorder rather than a behavioral disorder. With this evidence, the use of functional food plans that eliminate these foods gains credibility. As will be seen in the next sections, reductions in the use of these specific foods appear to result in diminishment of cravings, which is the goal of addiction recovery.

3.3.2 Food Disappearance Data from the USDA Economic Service

The USDA Economic Service food disappearance data shows how much food disappears into the U.S. economy and thus includes consumption as well as waste. Between 1970 and 1997, the years of the development of the obesity epidemic in the United States, the data showed significant increases in the annual per capita consumption of foods with addictive properties as shown in Table 3.2 (Putnam and Allshouse, 1999).

This dramatic increase in use points to the possibility of addictive properties for these foods and the need to eliminate them in a food plan addressing food addiction.

3.3.3 Qualitative Data from 12-Step Food Addiction Literature

3.3.3.1 Introduction to 12-Step Food Addiction Literature

A review of the literature from 12-step groups FAA and FA yielded descriptions of a classic substance addiction syndrome in terms of loss of control over the use of processed foods, implementation of abstinent food plans, and recovery (Food Addicts Anonymous, 2010; Food Addicts in Recovery Anonymous, 2013).

TABLE 3.2
Increase in the U.S. Annual per Capita Consumption of Addictive Foods from 1970 to 1997

Processed Food	Increase in 1970–1997 (Pounds per Capita)	Total in 1997 (Pounds per Capita)
Corn and wheat flour	50.8	172.8
Sweeteners	31.8	154.1
High-fructose corn syrup	61.9	62.4
High-fat dairy	20.4	36.7
Frozen potatoes (French fries)	30.5	59.0

3.3.3.2 Conformance to DSM-V Addiction Diagnostic Criteria

The 12-step literature yielded examples of addictive behavior according to the addiction diagnostic criteria found in the DSM-V. The foods used in the loss of control are described as sweets, candy, cakes, molasses, bread, crackers, pasta, starchy foods, gravy, catsup, baked beans, canned fruit, ice cream, cheese, butter, and grease with sodas, diet sodas, sweet tea, and coffee. This is consistent with the research described earlier showing addictive properties for processed foods.

Representative examples of behavior for each of the DSM-V addiction criteria are shown later as excerpted from the manuals of the food addiction 12-step fellowships (Food Addicts Anonymous, 2010; Food Addicts in Recovery Anonymous, 2013).

Criterion 1. Unintended use: "I remember following the instructions I'd once been given in a behavior modification class. I was supposed to cut a cookie into small pieces so I could savor it. I obediently put two cookies on a plate, laid out a placemat, fork and knife and divided each one into eight pieces. I fully tasted every bite and then got up and ate the whole bag. I did things like that all the time." (p. 24) (Food Addicts in Recovery Anonymous, 2013).

Criterion 2. Failed attempts to cut back: "I would diet and take off the weight, but the same cycle repeated itself endlessly." (p. 54) (Food Addicts in Recovery Anonymous, 2013).

Criterion 3. Time spent: "My mother says that she couldn't turn her back on me. Baby aspirin, Aspergum, and laxatives tasted sweet to me, and she had to hide them all. I spent a lot of time looking for them." (p. 178) (Food Addicts in Recovery Anonymous, 2013).

Criterion 4. Cravings: "From morning to night, I fought my cravings for food." (p. 169) (Food Addicts in Recovery Anonymous, 2013).

Criterion 5. Failure to fulfill roles: "Instead of calling on customers for my work, I drove here and there, bingeing in my car." (p. 23) (Food Addicts in Recovery Anonymous, 2013).

Criterion 6. Problems in relationships: "I had a wonderful husband and four children, but during that terrible time, I didn't want to live." (p. 51) (Food Addicts in Recovery Anonymous, 2013).

Criterion 7. Activities given up: "I had access to an unlimited food plan and to nearby late-night cafes. I spent a lot of time eating alone in my room. The more I ate, the more depressed and isolated I became." (p. 201) (Food Addicts in Recovery Anonymous, 2013).

Criterion 8. Hazardous use: "I knew from experience that when I binged, I got sleepy and would pass out. Now I was in my car, and I was scared. How was I going to eat all the food and get home without falling asleep behind the wheel?" (p. 139) (Food Addicts Anonymous, 2010).

Criterion 9. Use in spite of consequences: "Bingeing gave me terrible headaches and stomach pains. I couldn't take off my shoes until I was ready for bed because my feet were so swollen I couldn't get them on again. The skin on my legs felt like it was going to split. I had high cholesterol and high blood pressure, and my joints hurt from arthritis." (p. 51) (Food Addicts in Recovery Anonymous, 2013).

Criterion 10. Tolerance: "At that point, I could not limit how much I ate for even one day." (p. 22) (Food Addicts in Recovery Anonymous, 2013).

Criterion 11. Withdrawal: "My initial reaction was an overwhelming hunger, which made no sense because I had just eaten. Then came crabbiness, followed by nausea and a headache so terrible that I had to take a nap." (p. 150) (Food Addicts in Recovery Anonymous, 2013).

In summary, the loss of control that conforms to the DSM-V addiction diagnostic criteria is supported by qualitative data related to eating behavior associated with processed foods.

3.3.3.3 Abstinent Food Plans

Both the 12-step food addiction recovery fellowships advocate eliminating sugars, flours, and any foods that trigger volume eating. FA does not advocate specific abstinence beyond this (p. 427) (Food Addicts in Recovery Anonymous, 2013). In addition to sugars, flours, and trigger foods, FAA advocates eliminating caffeine and reducing salt, particularly for members with high blood pressure. Its food plan combines proteins with unprocessed vegetables, fruits, and starches as well as cold-pressed oils (pp. 271–285) (Food Addicts Anonymous, 2010).

Foods listed in the FAA food plan include (p. 276) (Food Addicts Anonymous, 2010) the following:

Protein: Beef, pork, goat, poultry, eggs fish, and shellfish, low or normal-fat dairy, tofu, and tempeh.

Starch: Unprocessed starches including sweet potato, winter squash, beans, brown rice, quinoa, buckwheat.

Vegetable: Any vegetable including asparagus, onion, broccoli, cauliflower, cabbage, carrots, celery, beets, lettuce, spinach, peppers, eggplant, tomato, cucumber, summer squash, zucchini, etc.

Fruit: Apple, pear, plum, peach, apricot, nectarine, strawberry, blueberry, raspberry, orange, grapefruit, tangerine, pineapple, melon.

Cold-pressed oils: Olive, avocado, flaxseed, coconut, sesame, sunflower, pumpkin seed, etc.

Foods eliminated from the FAA abstinent food plan include (pp. 271–273) (Food Addicts Anonymous, 2010) the following:

Sweeteners: Any sugar or syrup. Words ending in –itol such as mannitol and sorbitol. Words ending in –ose such as sucrose and dextrose. Artificial sweeteners.

Flour: Any carbohydrate that has been ground into a powder including flours ground from grains, beans, quinoa, or buckwheat. This includes corn starch.

Wheat in any form: Including close relatives such as kamut, spelt, and rye.

Excessive salt: Very salty foods include olives and excessive salting of otherwise abstinent foods.

Fats: Processed fats, fried foods, cheese, and cream.

Some foods may be categorized as either abstinent or non-abstinent depending on the addict's ability to each them normally, that is in measured quantities.

Nuts and seeds: Some practitioners exclude them because of their fat content and because nuts are a common allergic food.

3.3.3.4 Other Eliminated Foods

These foods are not necessarily eliminated from all 12-step food plans. However, some practitioners and sponsors eliminate them.

Dairy: May be excluded because its composition of fat, sugar (lactose), and casomorphine may make dairy addictive. They also may create cross-cravings for ice cream and cheese, which are commonly abused foods. Dairy may also be eliminated because it is a common allergic food.

Soy: May be excluded because it is a common allergic food and because its protein content is not high enough to offset carbohydrate servings.

Gluten: In addition to wheat and its close relatives, barley and corn may be eliminated because of the gluteomorphine found in gluten.

Puffed grains found in puffed cereal and rice cakes may be eliminated if the client loses control over them.

Potato: May be eliminated because of cross-cravings to commonly abused foods such as French fries, potato chips, and baked potatoes loaded with sour cream and cheese. Potatoes are also a low-nutrient food.

3.3.3.5 Recovery through Abstinent Food Plans

The two fellowships describe recovery in terms of being able to avoid the behaviors described earlier in the DSM addiction diagnostic criteria. Representative examples include the following:

Criterion 1. Unintended use: Food addicts in recovery report planned, weighed, and measured food (p. 207) (Food Addicts in Recovery Anonymous, 2013).
Criterion 2. Failed attempts to cut back: Fellowship members report long-term stable weight (p. 25) (Food Addicts in Recovery Anonymous, 2013).
Criterion 3. Time spent: In recovery, participants describe time for activities, career, and family (p. 163) (Food Addicts Anonymous, 2010).
Criterion 4. Cravings: Release from cravings, and obsession is a commonly described state when abstaining from processed foods (p. 205) (Food Addicts in Recovery Anonymous, 2013).
Criterion 5. Failure to fulfill roles: The stories contain reports of new careers and frequently a return to complete an education (p. 196) (Food Addicts in Recovery Anonymous, 2013).
Criterion 6. Problems in relationships: Members report on repaired family relationships, new spouses, and healthy children (p. 196) (Food Addicts in Recovery Anonymous, 2013).
Criterion 7. Activities given up: A frequent description of engagement in fellowship meetings and service activities is found in the stories (p. 151) (Food Addicts Anonymous, 2010).
Criterion 10. Tolerance: The authors of the stories report eating the same amount of food daily for years (p. 22) (Food Addicts in Recovery Anonymous, 2013).
Criterion 8. Hazardous use, Criterion 9. Use in spite of consequences, and Criterion 11. Withdrawal: The descriptions of recovery did not include reports of these behaviors.

3.3.3.6 Summary of 12-Step Literature

The 12-step literature describes behavior that is consistent with drug and alcohol addiction according to the DSM-V. It also describes the use of food plans that abstain from processed foods for which there is evidence of addictive properties. Finally, the literature describes a reduction in the DSM-V-defined addictive behavior after implementation of an abstinent food plan.

3.3.4 Summary of the Results

Throughout the results section, three themes are repeated. (1) The results describe an addiction syndrome in overeating. The evidence carries through from brain anomalies related to cravings and suppression of cognition to loss of control in eating behaviors as described in the 12-step literature according to the DSM-V addiction diagnostic criteria. (2) There are processed foods that are used in addictive eating for which there is evidence of addictive properties. (3) The loss of control seems to abate when processed foods are eliminated in abstinent food plans. The "Discussion Section" that follows builds on these results to bridge evidence to practice.

3.4 DISCUSSION

Through the lens of the food addiction model, a number of points can be drawn together from the "Results Section" to understand how to use functional food plans in the treatment of obesity and the metabolic syndrome. Cravings cessation is the key. Bridging research to clinical practice is accomplished by describing challenges in the implementation of abstinent food plans especially in terms of the scope of abstinence and cue avoidance.

3.4.1 Issues in Implementing an Abstinent Food Plan

The key issue in designing treatment plans for addictions is to match severity of disease with the scope of recovery program (McLellan et al., 1983). In this regard, implementing an abstinent food plan in a Westernized food environment has important challenges. As in all addictions, successful treatment depends on a Pavlovian reconditioning of the craving neuro-pathways (O'Brien et al., 1988). This is accomplished both by reducing cravings stimulation through the elimination of substances of abuse and by avoiding cues as well as engaging in activities that stabilize craving and reward pathways in the brain.

3.4.1.1 Food Addiction vs. Drug and Alcohol Addiction

Comparing food versus drug addiction illuminates the particular challenges of recovery from food addiction. Basic protocols in food addiction parallel classic drug and alcohol addiction treatment and aim to reduce cravings triggered by cues. In recovery from food addiction, the goal is to recondition craving and reward pathways to disassociate cravings from eating. Unprocessed foods that do not trigger cravings constitute an abstinent food plan and make disassociation possible. Avoidance of stimulating food environments is also critical.

Compared to the issues of trigger avoidance in drug and alcohol treatment, processed food addiction treatment is much more difficult. In drug and alcohol recovery, there is a reasonably good chance that clients can avoid accidental reintroduction and cues that can trigger relapse. By going to support meetings and making new friends, recovering addicts can avoid the people and places associated with the addiction.

By contrast, in processed food addiction, there is a much lower chance for successful avoidance of reintroduction and triggering because of the prevalence of addictive ingredients and cues in Westernized societies. The level of exposure to cues for processed food cues in the United States is multiples of the level of exposure to other substances of abuse such as alcohol or tobacco, particularly among children but also among adults (Powell et al., 2013; Scully et al., 2014; Terry-McElrath et al., 2014).

As a result, there are a number of reasons that food addiction is harder to treat than drug and alcohol addiction, which are given in the following:

1. Cueing for processed foods is more intense. Alcohol, tobacco, and recreational drug cues are easily avoided in most workplace settings, but processed food and drink cues are rampant and virtually unavoidable in break-rooms, vending machines, conference rooms, and workplace events. Advertising on television, print media, highways, and increasingly the Internet is ubiquitous. Cues are cited as the most common reason that overeaters relapse (Berthoud, 2004; Crowley et al., 2014).
2. Processed food ingredients are commonly mixed into prepared foods making accidental ingestion a hazard of recovery. This also makes it difficult to find *clean* prepared foods.
3. Combinations of processed foods are generally formulated into commercial products such as fast-food meals that combine sweetener, flour, processed fat, excessive salt, dairy, and caffeine. The range of substances activates a range of craving pathways creating de facto poly-substance use.

4. Health professionals are generally unaware of processed food addiction and are unable to educate or support clients in abstinence protocols.
5. In households where the addiction has affected children, adults are unable to withstand children's demands to keep processed foods in the house. The younger a person starts an addiction, the harder it is to treat.
6. Processed food addicts may be physically, emotionally, and mentally compromised because of obesity, diabetes, depression, heart disease, stroke, fatigue, sleep disorders, ADD, etc. Their diminished states make it difficult to overcome stimulating food environments, purchase, and prepare abstinent food meal after meal.
7. Great effort is required to replace processed foods with abstinent foods. Learning, planning, shopping, cooking, and cleaning up mean that processed food addicts have to master new jobs that are not required of drug and alcohol addicts.
8. The process of recovery from food addiction requires food addicts to be in intensely triggering food environments such as grocery stores and even their own kitchens.
9. Because food addiction can start in utero and continue unabated to adulthood, food addicts are more severely conditioned and more vulnerable to reintroduction and cues. They may lack coping mechanisms for stress and intense emotions.

These multiple barriers to recovery suggest that programs of recovery from processed food addiction should be more comprehensive to compensate for increased likelihood of accidental reintroduction and exposure to cues. The three legs of recovery described later are abstinence from addictive foods, avoidance of cues, and recovery activities. In each case, comprehensive recovery strategies are offered.

3.4.1.2 Achieving Effective Abstinence: Adequate Elimination of Addictive Foods

Adequate elimination of cravings foods from a Westernized diet is essential to recondition neuropathways to the point that they can be exposed to a cue and not react with cravings. However, achieving an adequate degree of abstinence can be challenging for several reasons.

1. Delusion is an element of the addiction syndrome (Ferrari et al., 2008). The broad range of addictive foods encourages denial. Many food addicts simply cannot believe that they need to eliminate so many foods (p. 92) (Food Addicts in Recovery Anonymous, 2013).
2. Support groups are inconsistent about which foods to eliminate (Rozanne, 2005). Media and health professionals do not teach abstinence food plans.
3. In a society in which people consume an average of over 1 pound per person per day of processed foods (Ifland et al., 2009), abstaining from these foods sets recovering food addicts outside of mainstream culture. Recovering food addicts also do not have the disease profiles commonly found in consumers of processed foods and thus have less in common with their friends, family, and colleagues.

Given the likelihood of accidental relapses and cue exposures, a comprehensively abstinent client is likely to have more protective conditioning than a client who is routinely using a food that has even minor addictive qualities.

Another important reason to advocate for comprehensive abstinence is the severity of the consequences of relapse. As seen in the DSM-V diagnostic criteria, food addiction is a disease that when active can severely damage its victims in all aspects of their lives. The grave consequences of relapse justify comprehensive abstinence as a risk reduction strategy.

In summary, the recommendation to comprehensively eliminate addictive foods in abstinent food plans is supported by research, likelihood of cue exposure, and management of risk of relapse. Sweeteners, flour, excessive, salt, processed fats, dairy, and caffeine are eliminated at a minimum. Gluten, high-sugar fruits, nuts, olives, puffed cereals, and soy are also candidates for elimination. Any other food that the client eats excessively can be considered as a personal binge food and should be eliminated.

3.4.1.3 Adequate Reduction in Exposure to Craving Cues

As discussed earlier, cues have been shown to effectively trigger relapse, and processed food cues are highly prevalent in Western society. Processed food advertising is pervasive including television, Internet, newsprint, and highway signage (Cohen, 2008). Brightly lit vending machines are common in gas stations, workplaces, schools, and transportation centers. Grocery stores and restaurants are heavily cued with sights, sounds, smells, samples, many choices, low prices, and bright packaging (Cohen and Babey, 2012). Workplaces may broadcast the availability of addictive foods in the break-room. Workplace parties with sweets may be frequent. Even the home and people can be craving triggers (Hetherington, 2007). These cues present a serious challenge to maintaining a non-craving, rational state of mind.

Conducting a trigger inventory and developing avoidance strategies are two important exercises for new clients. Severely addicted clients may need to hire a shopper/cook for a few weeks to reduce exposure during the process of disassociating cravings from eating.

3.4.1.4 Effective Level of Recovery Activities

The activities of the 12-step food addiction recovery groups include meetings, prayer, meditation, conversation, reading, writing, phone calling, etc. Their effectiveness has been shown in long-term recovery from alcoholism (Witbrodt et al., 2014). Mindfulness-based stress reduction has been shown to be effective in addiction treatment (Marcus et al., 2009). All of these activities are aimed at stabilizing neuro-pathways and reducing cravings as well as filling time previously spent in the addiction.

Food addiction treatment groups have evolved so that, today, there are more comprehensive programs. For example FA requires abstinence from sugar, flour, wheat, and no milk in coffee and tea, caffeine, etc. A member must have 90 days of abstinence in order to share at a meeting. FA offers intense weekly programs called "A Way of Life" (AWOL) to develop personality management skills, but members must have a sponsor in order to participate in an AWOL (Food Addicts in Recovery Anonymous, 2014).

Residential treatment is also available. However, some centers appear to be treating food addiction as a behavioral issue. The research suggests that food addiction is a substance use disorder that responds to abstinence protocols based on the elimination of addictive foods.

3.4.2 Summary of Discussion

Employing classic addiction recovery techniques in the treatment of overeating provides a novel and valuable method for an epidemic that has been resistant to improvement. The key issues in treatment are reducing the likelihood of exposure to cues and addictive ingredients and the appropriate depth of abstinence, cue avoidance, and recovery.

3.5 CONCLUSION

There is compelling research evidence that food addiction is a substance use disorder involving a number of processed foods. These include sweeteners, flour, excessive salt, processed fats, dairy, and caffeine. There is also evidence in the research and 12-step literature that abstaining from these foods results in reduced cravings in a pattern similar to that of abstinence from alcohol and drugs of abuse. The evidence also shows that reducing or eliminating processed foods is associated with improvements in the metabolic syndrome.

Treating addictions in general is difficult with recurring relapse, a common feature. Food addiction presents special challenges, but recognition of the need for a very comprehensive approach is the key to success.

Although much is known in recovery circles about managing food addiction, research is needed to establish best practices. Studies would be useful into treatment protocols, development of optimal food plans, withdrawal management, and cue avoidance.

REFERENCES

Alsio, J., Olszewski, P. K., Norback, A. H., Gunnarsson, Z. E., Levine, A. S., Pickering, C., and Schioth, H. B. (2010). Dopamine D1 receptor gene expression decreases in the nucleus accumbens upon long-term exposure to palatable food and differs depending on diet-induced obesity phenotype in rats. *Neuroscience*. doi: S0306-4522(10)01294-7 [pii] 10.1016/j.neuroscience.2010.09.046 [doi].

American Society of Addiction Medicine. (2014). Definition of addiction. Retrieved December 9, 2014, from http://www.asam.org/for-the-public/definition-of-addiction.

Avena, N. M., Bocarsly, M. E., and Hoebel, B. G. (2012). Animal models of sugar and fat bingeing: Relationship to food addiction and increased body weight. *Methods Mol Biol*, 829, 351–365. doi: 10.1007/978-1-61779-458-2_23.

Beaver, J. D., Lawrence, A. D., van Ditzhuijzen, J., Davis, M. H., Woods, A., and Calder, A. J. (2006). Individual differences in reward drive predict neural responses to images of food. *J Neurosci*, 26(19), 5160–5166.

Bernstein, G. A., Carroll, M. E., Thuras, P. D., Cosgrove, K. P., and Roth, M. E. (2002). Caffeine dependence in teenagers. *Drug Alcohol Depend*, 66(1), 1–6.

Berthoud, H. R. (2004). Mind versus metabolism in the control of food intake and energy balance. *Physiol Behav*, 81(5), 781–793.

Blass, E. M. and Shide, D. J. (1994). Some comparisons among the calming and pain-relieving effects of sucrose, glucose, fructose and lactose in infant rats. *Chem Senses*, 19(3), 239–249.

Bray, G. A. (2000). Afferent signals regulating food intake. *Proc Nutr Soc*, 59(3), 373–384.

Burger, K. S. and Stice, E. (2012). Frequent ice cream consumption is associated with reduced striatal response to receipt of an ice cream-based milkshake. *Am J Clin Nutr*, 95(4), 810–817. doi: 10.3945/ajcn.111.027003.

Carroccio, A., Brusca, I., Mansueto, P., Soresi, M., D'Alcamo, A., Ambrosiano, G., … Di Fede, G. (2011). Fecal assays detect hypersensitivity to cow's milk protein and gluten in adults with irritable bowel syndrome. *Clin Gastroenterol Hepatol*, 9(11), 965–971, e963. doi: 10.1016/j.cgh.2011.07.030.

Cocores, J. A. and Gold, M. S. (2009). The salted food addiction hypothesis may explain overeating and the obesity epidemic. *Med Hypotheses*, 73(6), 892–899. doi: S0306-9877(09)00484-8 [pii] 10.1016/j.mehy.2009.06.049 [doi].

Cohen, D. A. (2008). Obesity and the built environment: Changes in environmental cues cause energy imbalances. *Int J Obes (Lond)*, 32(Suppl 7), S137–S142. doi: ijo2008250 [pii] 10.1038/ijo.2008.250.

Cohen, D. A. and Babey, S. H. (2012). Contextual influences on eating behaviours: Heuristic processing and dietary choices. *Obes Rev*, 13(9), 766–779. doi: 10.1111/j.1467-789X.2012.01001.x.

Crowley, N., Madan, A., Wedin, S., Correll, J. A., Delustro, L. M., Borckardt, J. J., and Karl Byrne, T. (2014). Food cravings among bariatric surgery candidates. *Eat Weight Disord*. doi: 10.1007/s40519-013-0095-y.

D'Addario, C., Micioni Di Bonaventura, M. V., Pucci, M., Romano, A., Gaetani, S., Ciccocioppo, R., … Maccarrone, M. (2014). Endocannabinoid signaling and food addiction. *Neurosci Biobehav Rev*. doi: 10.1016/j.neubiorev.2014.08.008.

Denny, S. (2014). What are functional foods? Retrieved September 25, 2014, from http://www.eatright.org/Public/content.aspx?id=6442472528.

DiPatrizio, N. V., Joslin, A., Jung, K. M., and Piomelli, D. (2013). Endocannabinoid signaling in the gut mediates preference for dietary unsaturated fats. *FASEB J*, 27(6), 2513–2520. doi: 10.1096/fj.13-227587.

Eaton, S. B. and Eaton, S. B., III. (2000). Paleolithic vs. modern diets—Selected pathophysiological implications. *Eur J Nutr*, 39(2), 67–70.

Fanciulli, G., Dettori, A., Demontis, M. P., Tomasi, P. A., Anania, V., and Delitala, G. (2005). Gluten exorphin B5 stimulates prolactin secretion through opioid receptors located outside the blood-brain barrier. *Life Sci*, 76(15), 1713–1719.

Ferrari, J. R., Groh, D. R., Rulka, G., Jason, L. A., and Davis, M. I. (2008). Coming to terms with reality: Predictors of self-deception within substance abuse recovery. *Addict Disord Their Treat*, 7(4), 210–218. doi: 10.1097/ADT.0b013e31815c2ded.

Folgueira, C., Seoane, L. M., and Casanueva, F. F. (2014). The brain–stomach connection. *Front Horm Res*, 42, 83–92. doi: 10.1159/000358316.

Food Addicts Anonymous. (2010). *Food Addicts Anonymous*. Port St. Lucie, FL: Food Addicts Anonymous, Inc.

Food Addicts in Recovery Anonymous. (2013). *Food Addicts in Recovery Anonymous*. Woburn, MA: Food Addicts in Recovery Anonymous.

Food Addicts in Recovery Anonymous. (2014). AWOL updates. Retrieved November 24, 2014, from http://www.foodaddictsphonemeetings.org/AWOL-Updates.html.

Fortuna, J. L. (2010). Sweet preference, sugar addiction and the familial history of alcohol dependence: Shared neural pathways and genes. *J Psychoactive Drugs*, 42(2), 147–151.

Fortuna, J. L. (2012). The obesity epidemic and food addiction: Clinical similarities to drug dependence. *J Psychoactive Drugs*, 44(1), 56–63.

Fukudome, S. and Yoshikawa, M. (1992). Opioid peptides derived from wheat gluten: Their isolation and characterization. *FEBS Lett*, 296(1), 107–111.

Grosshans, M., Vollmert, C., Vollstadt-Klein, S., Tost, H., Leber, S., Bach, P., … Kiefer, F. (2012). Association of leptin with food cue-induced activation in human reward pathways. *Arch Gen Psychiatry*, 69(5), 529–537. doi: 10.1001/archgenpsychiatry.2011.1586.

Guerrieri, R., Nederkoorn, C., and Jansen, A. (2008). The interaction between impulsivity and a varied food environment: Its influence on food intake and overweight. *Int J Obes (Lond)*, 32(4), 708–714.

Hetherington, M. M. (2007). Cues to overeat: Psychological factors influencing overconsumption. *Proc Nutr Soc*, 66(1), 113–123.

Ho, C. Y. and Berridge, K. C. (2013). An orexin hotspot in ventral pallidum amplifies hedonic 'liking' for sweetness. *Neuropsychopharmacology*, 38(9), 1655–1664. doi: 10.1038/npp.2013.62.

Huebner, F. R., Lieberman, K. W., Rubino, R. P., and Wall, J. S. (1984). Demonstration of high opioid-like activity in isolated peptides from wheat gluten hydrolysates. *Peptides*, 5(6), 1139–1147.

Ifland, J. R., Preuss, H. G., Marcus, M. T., Rourke, K. M., Taylor, W. C., Burau, K., … Manso, G. (2009). Refined food addiction: A classic substance use disorder. *Med Hypotheses*, 72(5), 518–526. doi: S0306-9877(08)00642-7 [pii] 10.1016/j.mehy.2008.11.035 [doi].

Ifland, J. R., Preuss, H. G., Marcus, M. T., Rourke, K. M., Taylor, W. C., and Lerner, M. (2012). The evidence for refined food addiction. In D. Bagchi and H. G. Preuss (Eds.), *Obesity: Epidemiology, Pathophysiology and Prevention* (2nd edn., pp. 53–72). Boca Ratan, FL: CRC Press.

Jastreboff, A. M., Sinha, R., Lacadie, C., Small, D. M., Sherwin, R. S., and Potenza, M. N. (2013). Neural correlates of stress- and food cue-induced food craving in obesity: Association with insulin levels. *Diabetes Care*, 36(2), 394–402. doi: 10.2337/dc12-1112.

Jonsson, T., Granfeldt, Y., Ahren, B., Branell, U. C., Palsson, G., Hansson, A., … Lindeberg, S. (2009). Beneficial effects of a Paleolithic diet on cardiovascular risk factors in type 2 diabetes: A randomized cross-over pilot study. *Cardiovasc Diabetol*, 8, 35. doi: 10.1186/1475-2840-8-35.

Jonsson, T., Granfeldt, Y., Erlanson-Albertsson, C., Ahren, B., and Lindeberg, S. (2010). A paleolithic diet is more satiating per calorie than a mediterranean-like diet in individuals with ischemic heart disease. *Nutr Metab (Lond)*, 7, 85. doi: 10.1186/1743-7075-7-85.

Jonsson, T., Granfeldt, Y., Lindeberg, S., and Hallberg, A. C. (2013). Subjective satiety and other experiences of a Paleolithic diet compared to a diabetes diet in patients with type 2 diabetes. *Nutr J*, 12, 105. doi: 10.1186/1475-2891-12-105.

Karatsoreos, I. N., Thaler, J. P., Borgland, S. L., Champagne, F. A., Hurd, Y. L., and Hill, M. N. (2013). Food for thought: Hormonal, experiential, and neural influences on feeding and obesity. *J Neurosci*, 33(45), 17610–17616. doi: 10.1523/jneurosci.3452-13.2013.

Kelley, A. E., Bakshi, V. P., Haber, S. N., Steininger, T. L., Will, M. J., and Zhang, M. (2002). Opioid modulation of taste hedonics within the ventral striatum. *Physiol Behav*, 76(3), 365–377.

Kelley, A. E., Baldo, B. A., Pratt, W. E., and Will, M. J. (2005). Corticostriatal-hypothalamic circuitry and food motivation: Integration of energy, action and reward. *Physiol Behav*, 86(5), 773–795. doi: 10.1016/j.physbeh.2005.08.066.

Kringelbach, M. L. and Stein, A. (2010). Cortical mechanisms of human eating. *Forum Nutr*, 63, 164–175. doi: 10.1159/000264404.

Kroemer, N. B., Krebs, L., Kobiella, A., Grimm, O., Pilhatsch, M., Bidlingmaier, M., … Smolka, M. N. (2013). Fasting levels of ghrelin covary with the brain response to food pictures. *Addict Biol*, 18(5), 855–862. doi: 10.1111/j.1369-1600.2012.00489.x.

Kroemer, N. B., Krebs, L., Kobiella, A., Grimm, O., Vollstadt-Klein, S., Wolfensteller, U., … Smolka, M. N. (2013). (Still) longing for food: Insulin reactivity modulates response to food pictures. *Hum Brain Mapp*, 34(10), 2367–2380. doi: 10.1002/hbm.22071.

Lindeberg, S., Jonsson, T., Granfeldt, Y., Borgstrand, E., Soffman, J., Sjostrom, K., and Ahren, B. (2007). A Palaeolithic diet improves glucose tolerance more than a Mediterranean-like diet in individuals with ischaemic heart disease. *Diabetologia*, 50(9), 1795–1807. doi: 10.1007/s00125-007-0716-y.

Lustig, R. H. (2013). Fructose: It's "alcohol without the buzz". *Adv Nutr*, 4(2), 226–235. doi: 10.3945/an.112.002998.

Marcus, M. T., Schmitz, J., Moeller, G., Liehr, P., Cron, S. G., Swank, P., ... Granmayeh, L. K. (2009). Mindfulness-based stress reduction in therapeutic community treatment: A stage 1 trial. *Am J Drug Alcohol Abuse*, 35(2), 103–108. doi: 10.1080/00952990902823079.

Mayo Clinic. (2014). Metabolic syndrome. Retrieved December 9, 2014, from http://www.mayoclinic.org/diseases-conditions/metabolic-syndrome/basics/definition/con-20027243.

McLellan, A. T., Luborsky, L., Woody, G. E., O'Brien, C. P., and Druley, K. A. (1983). Predicting response to alcohol and drug abuse treatments. Role of psychiatric severity. *Arch Gen Psychiatry*, 40(6), 620–625.

Meye, F. J. and Adan, R. A. (2014). Feelings about food: The ventral tegmental area in food reward and emotional eating. *Trends Pharmacol Sci*, 35(1), 31–40. doi: 10.1016/j.tips.2013.11.003.

Michaelsson, K., Wolk, A., Langenskiold, S., Basu, S., Warensjo Lemming, E., Melhus, H., and Byberg, L. (2014). Milk intake and risk of mortality and fractures in women and men: Cohort studies. *BMJ*, 349, g6015. doi: 10.1136/bmj.g6015.

O'Brien, C. P., Childress, A. R., Arndt, I. O., McLellan, A. T., Woody, G. E., and Maany, I. (1988). Pharmacological and behavioral treatments of cocaine dependence: Controlled studies. *J Clin Psychiatry*, 49(Suppl), 17–22.

O'Doherty, J. P., Buchanan, T. W., Seymour, B., and Dolan, R. J. (2006). Predictive neural coding of reward preference involves dissociable responses in human ventral midbrain and ventral striatum. *Neuron*, 49(1), 157–166.

Orsini, C. A., Ginton, G., Shimp, K. G., Avena, N. M., Gold, M. S., and Setlow, B. (2014). Food consumption and weight gain after cessation of chronic amphetamine administration. *Appetite*, 78, 76–80. doi: 10.1016/j.appet.2014.03.013.

Pelchat, M. L., Johnson, A., Chan, R., Valdez, J., and Ragland, J. D. (2004). Images of desire: Food-craving activation during fMRI. *Neuroimage*, 23(4), 1486–1493.

Petrovich, G. D. and Gallagher, M. (2003). Amygdala subsystems and control of feeding behavior by learned cues. *Ann N Y Acad Sci*, 985, 251–262.

Powell, L. M., Harris, J. L., and Fox, T. (2013). Food marketing expenditures aimed at youth: Putting the numbers in context. *Am J Prev Med*, 45(4), 453–461. doi: 10.1016/j.amepre.2013.06.003.

Preuss, H. G. and Clouatre, D. (2012). Sodium, chloride, and potassium. In J. Werman (Ed.), *Present Knowledge in Nutrition* (10th edn., pp. 475–492). Washington, DC: ILSI Press.

Preuss, H. G. and Preuss, J. M. (2014). Strategies for the prevention of Type II diabetes. In M. Rothkopf, M. Nusbaum, and L. Haverstick (Eds.), *Metabolic Medicine and Surgery* (1st edn., pp. 183–206). Boca Raton FL: CRC Press.

Pritchett, C. E. and Hajnal, A. (2011). Obesogenic diets may differentially alter dopamine control of sucrose and fructose intake in rats. *Physiol Behav*, 104(1), 111–116. doi: 10.1016/j.physbeh.2011.04.048.

Putnam, J. and Allshouse, J. (1999). Food consumption, prices and expenditures. *Econ Res Serv Stat Bull*, 965, 1970–1997.

Rozanne, S. (2005). *Beyond Our Wildest Dreams*. Rio Rancho, NM: Overeaters Anonymous.

Schwabe, L. and Wolf, O. T. (2011). Stress-induced modulation of instrumental behavior: From goal-directed to habitual control of action. *Behav Brain Res*, 219(2), 321–328. doi: 10.1016/j.bbr.2010.12.038.

Schwander, F., Kopf-Bolanz, K. A., Buri, C., Portmann, R., Egger, L., Chollet, M., ... Vergeres, G. (2014). A dose–response strategy reveals differences between normal-weight and obese men in their metabolic and inflammatory responses to a high-fat meal. *J Nutr*. doi: 10.3945/jn.114.193565.

Scully, P., Macken, A., Leddin, D., Cullen, W., Dunne, C., and Gorman, C. O. (2014). Food and beverage advertising during children's television programming. *Irish J Med Sci*. doi: 10.1007/s11845-014-1088-1.

Sharma, S., Fernandes, M. F., and Fulton, S. (2013). Adaptations in brain reward circuitry underlie palatable food cravings and anxiety induced by high-fat diet withdrawal. *Int J Obes (Lond)*, 37(9), 1183–1191. doi: 10.1038/ijo.2012.197.

Shriner, R. L. (2013). Food addiction: Detox and abstinence reinterpreted? *Exp Gerontol*, 48(10), 1068–1074. doi: 10.1016/j.exger.2012.12.005.

Sobrino Crespo, C., Perianes Cachero, A., Puebla Jimenez, L., Barrios, V., and Arilla Ferreiro, E. (2014). Peptides and food intake. *Front Endocrinol (Lausanne)*, 5, 58. doi: 10.3389/fendo.2014.00058.

Spreadbury, I. (2012). Comparison with ancestral diets suggests dense acellular carbohydrates promote an inflammatory microbiota, and may be the primary dietary cause of leptin resistance and obesity. *Diabetes Metab Syndr Obes*, 5, 175–189. doi: 10.2147/dmso.s33473.

Stice, E., Figlewicz, D. P., Gosnell, B. A., Levine, A. S., and Pratt, W. E. (2013). The contribution of brain reward circuits to the obesity epidemic. *Neurosci Biobehav Rev*, 37(9 Pt A), 2047–2058. doi: 10.1016/j.neubiorev.2012.12.001.

Stice, E., Spoor, S., Bohon, C., Veldhuizen, M. G., and Small, D. M. (2008). Relation of reward from food intake and anticipated food intake to obesity: A functional magnetic resonance imaging study. *J Abnorm Psychol*, 117(4), 924–935. doi: 2008-16252-017 [pii] 10.1037/a0013600.

Takahashi, M., Fukunaga, H., Kaneto, H., Fukudome, S., and Yoshikawa, M. (2000). Behavioral and pharmacological studies on gluten exorphin A5, a newly isolated bioactive food protein fragment, in mice. *Jpn J Pharmacol*, 84(3), 259–265.

Tekol, Y. (2006). Salt addiction: A different kind of drug addiction. *Med Hypotheses*, 67(5), 1233–1234.

Tellez, L. A., Medina, S., Han, W., Ferreira, J. G., Licona-Limon, P., Ren, X., ... de Araujo, I. E. (2013). A gut lipid messenger links excess dietary fat to dopamine deficiency. *Science*, 341(6147), 800–802. doi: 10.1126/science.1239275.

Terry-McElrath, Y. M., Turner, L., Sandoval, A., Johnston, L. D., and Chaloupka, F. J. (2014). Commercialism in US elementary and secondary school nutrition environments: Trends from 2007 to 2012. *JAMA Pediatr*, 168(3), 234–242. doi: 10.1001/jamapediatrics.2013.4521.

Thomasius, R., Sack, P. M., Strittmatter, E., and Kaess, M. (2014). Substance-related and addictive disorders in the DSM-5. *Z Kinder Jugendpsychiatr Psychother*, 42(2), 115–120. doi: 10.1024/1422-4917/a000278.

Tsanzi, E., Light, H. R., and Tou, J. C. (2008). The effect of feeding different sugar-sweetened beverages to growing female Sprague-Dawley rats on bone mass and strength. *Bone*, 42(5), 960–968.

van de Giessen, E., la Fleur, S. E., Eggels, L., de Bruin, K., van den Brink, W., and Booij, J. (2013). High fat/carbohydrate ratio but not total energy intake induces lower striatal dopamine D2/3 receptor availability in diet-induced obesity. *Int J Obes (Lond)*, 37(5), 754–757. doi: 10.1038/ijo.2012.128.

Volkow, N. D., Wang, G. J., Fowler, J. S., Tomasi, D., and Baler, R. (2012). Food and drug reward: Overlapping circuits in human obesity and addiction. *Curr Top Behav Neurosci*, 11, 1–24. doi: 10.1007/7854_2011_169.

Wang, G. J., Tomasi, D., Convit, A., Logan, J., Wong, C. T., Shumay, E., ... Volkow, N. D. (2014). BMI modulates calorie-dependent dopamine changes in accumbens from glucose intake. *PLoS ONE*, 9(7), e101585. doi: 10.1371/journal.pone.0101585.

Wang, G. J., Tomasi, D., Volkow, N. D., Wang, R., Telang, F., Caparelli, E. C., and Dunayevich, E. (2014). Effect of combined naltrexone and bupropion therapy on the brain's reactivity to food cues. *Int J Obes (Lond)*, 38(5), 682–688. doi: 10.1038/ijo.2013.145.

Wang, G. J., Volkow, N. D., Thanos, P. K., and Fowler, J. S. (2004). Similarity between obesity and drug addiction as assessed by neurofunctional imaging: A concept review. *J Addict Dis*, 23(3), 39–53. doi: 10.1300/J069v23n03_04.

Wang, G. J., Yang, J., Volkow, N. D., Telang, F., Ma, Y., Zhu, W., ... Fowler, J. S. (2006). Gastric stimulation in obese subjects activates the hippocampus and other regions involved in brain reward circuitry. *Proc Natl Acad Sci USA*, 103(42), 15641–15645.

Witbrodt, J., Ye, Y., Bond, J., Chi, F., Weisner, C., and Mertens, J. (2014). Alcohol and drug treatment involvement, 12-step attendance and abstinence: 9-year cross-lagged analysis of adults in an integrated health plan. *J Subst Abuse Treat*, 46(4), 412–419. doi: 10.1016/j.jsat.2013.10.015.

Witt, A. A., Raggio, G. A., Butryn, M. L., and Lowe, M. R. (2014). Do hunger and exposure to food affect scores on a measure of hedonic hunger? An experimental study. *Appetite*, 74, 1–5. doi: 10.1016/j.appet.2013.11.010.

Wright, H. T. and Ifland, J. R. (2014). Obesity epidemic: Understanding addiction in managing overeating. *Behav Health Nutr Newsl, Acad Nutr Diet*, 32(2), 1, 3–6.

Yau, Y. H. and Potenza, M. N. (2013). Stress and eating behaviors. *Minerva Endocrinol*, 38(3), 255–267.

Yu, J. H., Shin, M. S., Kim, D. J., Lee, J. R., Yoon, S. Y., Kim, S. G., ... Kim, M. S. (2013). Enhanced carbohydrate craving in patients with poorly controlled Type 2 diabetes mellitus. *Diabet Med*, 30(9), 1080–1086. doi: 10.1111/dme.12209.

Yudkin, J. (1988). Sucrose, coronary heart disease, diabetes, and obesity: Do hormones provide a link? *Am Heart J*, 115(2), 493–498.

Ziauddeen, H., Chamberlain, S. R., Nathan, P. J., Koch, A., Maltby, K., Bush, M., ... Bullmore, E. T. (2013). Effects of the mu-opioid receptor antagonist GSK1521498 on hedonic and consummatory eating behaviour: A proof of mechanism study in binge-eating obese subjects. *Mol Psychiatry*, 18(12), 1287–1293. doi: 10.1038/mp.2012.154.

4 Nutraceuticals and Their Role in Human Health
A Review

Runu Chakraborty and Lipi Das

CONTENTS

4.1 INTRODUCTION

The term "nutraceutical" was coined from "nutrition" and "pharmaceutical" by Stephen De Felice, founder and chairman of the Foundation for Innovation in Medicine, Cranford, NJ, in 1989. According to De Felice, nutraceutical can be defined as "a food (or a part of food) that provides medical or health benefits, including the prevention and or treatment of a disease" (Das et al., 2012). This emerging class of product occupies an intermediate position between food and medicine. European medicine law has defined nutraceuticals as a medicine for two reasons:

1. It can be used for the prevention, treatment, or cure of a disease condition.
2. It can be administered with a view to restoring, correcting, or modifying physiological functions in human beings (Pandey et al., 2010).

Nutraceuticals may range from isolated nutrients, herbal products, dietary supplements, and diets to genetically engineered *designer* foods and processed products such as cereals, soups, and beverages (Dureja et al., 2003; Malik, 2008). Nutraceuticals cover most of the therapeutic areas such as antiarthritic, cold and cough, sleeping disorders, digestion and prevention of certain cancers, osteoporosis, blood pressure, cholesterol control, pain killers, depression, diabetes, cardiovascular disease, and other chronic and degenerative diseases such as Parkinson's and Alzheimer's diseases. Nutraceuticals are found in a mosaic of products emerging from (a) the food industry, (b) the herbal and dietary supplement market, (c) pharmaceutical industry, and (d) the newly merged pharmaceutical/agribusiness/nutrition conglomerates. Table 4.1 depicts some of the most common nutraceuticals available in the market.

TABLE 4.1
Nutraceuticals Available in Market

Brand Name	Components	Function
Z-trim	Wheat	Zero-calorie fat replacer
Linumlife	Lignan extract flax	Maintains prostate health
Fenulife	Fenugreek galactomannan	Controls blood sugar
Teamax	Green tea extract	Potent antioxidant
Marinol	ω-3 FA, DHA, EPA	Heart protection
Clarinol	CLA	Weight loss ingredient
Cholestaid	Saponin	Reduces cholesterol
Betatene	Carotenoids	Immune function
Soylife	Soybean Phytoestrogen	Maintains bone health
Xangold	Lutein esters	Maintains eye health
Premium probiotics	Probiotics	Controls intestinal disorder

4.2 CLASSIFYING NUTRACEUTICALS

Broadly, nutraceuticals can be classified into two groups (Pandey et al., 2010):

1. Potential nutraceuticals
2. Established nutraceuticals

A potential nutraceutical could become an established one only after efficient clinical data of its health and medical benefits are obtained. It is to be noted that much of the nutraceutical products still lay in the *potential* category. Nutraceuticals can further be classified on the basis of food sources, mechanism of action, and chemical nature as follows:

- On the basis of food sources, nutraceutical substances can be grouped as plants, animals, and microbial sources.
- In case of classification by mechanism of action, nutraceuticals can be grouped as those having antioxidant, antibacterial, antihypertensive, anti-inflammatory, anticarcinogenic, anti-aggregate, influence on blood or lipid profile, osteoprotective, and so on. This classification is based on the proven or purported physiological properties of the nutraceutical substances.
- On the basis of chemical nature, nutraceuticals can be grouped as the following:
    - Carbohydrates and their derivatives
    - Fatty acids and lipid structures
    - Microorganisms
    - Proteins and amino acid structures
    - Phenolic compounds
    - Isoprenoid derivatives
    - Minerals

The food sources used as nutraceuticals are all natural and can be categorized as follows:

1. Dietary fiber
2. Probiotics and prebiotics
3. Polyunsaturated fatty acids
4. Antioxidant vitamins

5. Polyphenols
6. Spices
7. Minerals

In the next sections, a brief description of the nutraceuticals based on food sources with respect to their roles in human diseases is given.

4.3 DIETARY FIBER

Dietary fiber is defined as the plant part that is not hydrolyzed by enzymes secreted by the human digestive tract, but digested by microflora in the gut. Dietary fibers mostly include non-starch polysaccharides such as celluloses, hemicelluloses, gums, and pectins as well as oligosaccharides like lignin, resistant dextrins, and resistant starches. Food rich in dietary fiber mainly comprises whole grain food, vegetables, fruits, legumes, and nuts (Anderson et al., 2009). Dietary fibers are divided into two forms: (1) insoluble dietary fiber, which includes celluloses, some hemicelluloses, and lignins having bulking action and are fermented to a limited extend in the colon. (2) Soluble dietary fiber, which includes β-glucans, pectins, gums, mucilages, and hemicelluloses that are viscous and fermented in the colon. Foods containing fibers mostly have about one-third insoluble and two-third soluble fiber portions (Wong and Jenkins, 2007; Lattimer and Haub, 2010). In colon, dietary fiber increases fecal bulking due to increased water retention, increased transit time, and increased fecal bacterial mass caused by soluble fiber fermentation. The fiber also promotes the growth of Bifidobacteria in the gut (Das et al., 2012). A good intake of dietary fiber lowers the risk of several diseases like coronary heart disease (Liu et al., 1999), stroke (Steffen et al., 2003), hypertension (Whelton et al., 2005), diabetes (Montonen et al., 2003), obesity (Lairon et al., 2005), and certain gastrointestinal disorders (Petruzziello et al., 2006). Again, increase in the intake of high fiber food improves serum lipoprotein values (Brown et al., 1999), lowers blood pressure level (Keenan et al., 2002), improves blood glucose control for diabetes (Anderson et al., 2004), aids weight loss (Birketvedt et al., 2005), and promotes regularity (Cummings, 2001). Dietary fiber's ability to decrease body weight could be contributed to several factors: (1) soluble fiber when fermented in the large intestine creates a feeling of satiety, (2) dietary fiber may decrease energy absorption by way of diluting a diet's energy availability while maintaining other important nutrients, and (3) dietary fiber may decrease a diet's metabolizable energy (Lattimer and Haub, 2010). This is attributed to the fact that fat digestibility decreases as dietary fiber intake increases. Increased fiber content decreases the glycemic index of foods, which in turn leads to a smaller increase in the blood glucose level (Post et al., 2012). Many studies again showed conflicting results in this respect. The recommended dietary fiber intake for children and adults is estimated to be 14 g/1000 kcal (USDA, 2005). Several case histories have reported that consumption of excessive amounts of dietary fiber causes diarrhea (Saibil, 1989).

4.4 PROBIOTICS AND PREBIOTICS

A probiotic can be defined as live microorganism, which when administered in adequate amounts has beneficial effect on the host animal. Species of lactobacillus and bifidobacterium are most commonly used in the manufacture of probiotic products for their known effects on human health as well as their "generally recognized as safe" status (O'Bryan et al., 2013). Apart from these, yeast, *Escherichia coli*, and some bacilli can also be considered as probiotics.

Most common probiotic food in the market now are yogurt, cheese, fermented and unfermented milks, fruit juice, smoothies, cereals, nutrition bars, and infant/toddler formulas. Other than food, probiotics are also sold as dietary supplements, medical foods, and drugs. Probiotic milk can be tolerated by lactose-intolerant individuals, possibly because these fermented products contain the microbial β-galactosidase, which functions in the small intestine to support lactose hydrolysis (de Vrese et al., 1999).

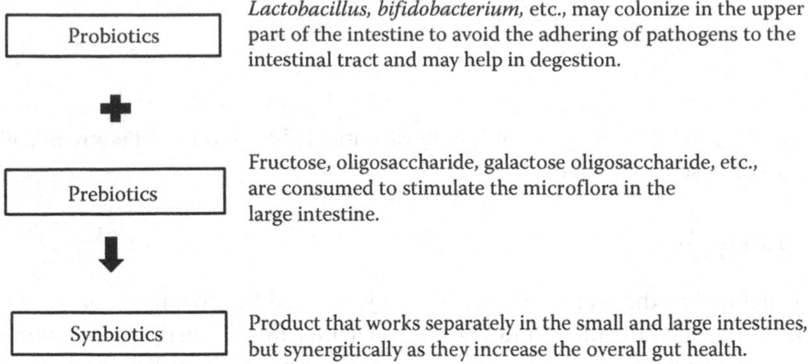

FIGURE 4.1 Synergistic relationship of probiotics and prebiotics.

Administration of probiotics reduces the symptoms of antibiotic-associated diarrhea or due to rotavirus (Gill and Guarner, 2004). Specific strains of lactic acid bacteria, when consumed in certain numbers, can modulate aspects of both natural and acquired immune responses. Probiotic therapy can lower the risk of colon cancer by reducing the concentration of the cancer-promoting enzymes and putrefactive metabolites in the gut (de Vrese and Schrezenmeir, 2008). There are several mechanisms proposing the lowering of cholesterol by probiotics (O'Bryan et al., 2013). There are evidences that administration of probiotics decreases the risk of systemic conditions, such as allergy, asthma, and several other infections of the ear and urinary tract (Das et al., 2012). It also normalizes the stool in subjects suffering from obstipation and irritable colon.

Prebiotics are dietary ingredients that beneficially affect the host by selectively altering the composition or metabolism of the gut microbiota. These are short-chain polysaccharides that have unique chemical structures that are not digested by humans; in particular, fructose-based oligosaccharides that exist naturally in food and are also added in food. Vegetables like chicory roots, banana, tomato, and alliums are rich in fructo-oligosaccharides. Some other examples of these oligosaccharides are raffinose and stachyose, found in beans and peas. The health benefits of the prebiotics are mostly indirect. They generally promote the lactobacillus and bifidobacterial growth in the gut, thus helping in metabolism (Gibson, 1999; Hord, 2008). Synbiotics refer to nutritional supplements combining probiotics and prebiotics in a form of synergism. This term is used for products in which the prebiotic compound selectively favors the probiotic compound (Schrezenmeir and de Vrese, 2001). A clear relationship between the probiotics, prebiotics, and synbiotics is shown in Figure 4.1.

4.5 OMEGA FATTY ACIDS

Essential fatty acids are crucial to the body's function and are introduced externally through the diet. Polysaturated fatty acids or PUFAs have two main subdivisions: omega-3 (*n*-3) fatty acids and omega-6 (*n*-6) fatty acids based on the location of the last double bond. Omega-3 fatty acids mostly consist of α-linolenic acid (ALA), eicosapentaenoic acid (EPA), docosahexaenoic acid (DHA). ALA is the precursor of EPA and DHA. On the other hand, omega-6 fatty acids mainly consist of linoleic acid (LA), γ-linolenic acid (GLA), and arachidonic acid (ARA), LA being the parent fatty acid of this group. EPA and DHA are found mainly in fatty fishes such as mackerel, salmon, herring, trout, bluefin tuna, and fish oils (Ackman, 2008). Principal sources of ALA are mainly flaxseed, soybeans, canola, some nuts (e.g. walnuts), and red/black currant seeds. LA occurs mainly in vegetable oils, for example corn, safflower, soybean, and sunflower (White, 2008). ARA is found in animal products such as meat, poultry, and eggs as well as algae and other aquatic plants. Omega-3 fatty acids have been shown to be beneficial at various stages of life. Infant formulas nowadays contain DHA along with ARA, which closely mimic the breast milk. Omega fatty acids regulate a wide variety of

TABLE 4.2
Different Dietary Fatty Acids, Their Sources, and Effects on Human Health

Name	Omega-3	Omega-6	Omega-9
Type	Polyunsaturated	Polyunsaturated	Monounsaturated
Dietary source	*Oils*: canola, flax, soybean. *Nuts*: walnut *Fish*: sea fishes (herring, mackerel, salmon, trout, tuna). *Other*: algae, eggs	*Oils*: canola, corn, olive, peanut, safflower, soybean, sunflower. *Nuts*: almonds, cashews, hazelnuts, peanuts, pecans, walnuts. *Others*: eggs	*Oils*: canola, olive, safflower, sunflower. *Nuts*: almonds, cashews, hazelnuts, peanuts, pecans, walnuts, pistachios, macadamias. *Others*: avocados, egg, poultry
Positive health effect	Brain development, heart health, cholesterol, mood	Heart health, cholesterol	Heart health, cholesterol, blood sugar control

biological functions ranging from blood pressure and blood clotting to the development and functioning of the brain and nervous system, important roles in immune regulation and inflammation (Calder, 2009; Wall et al., 2010). In general, eicosanoids derived from *n*-6 PUFA are proinflammatory, while eicosanoids derived from *n*-3 PUFA are anti-inflammatory (Patterson et al., 2012). Present-day dietary changes in the intake of *n*-6 and *n*-3 show striking increases in the (*n*-6) to (*n*-3) ratio (~15:1), which are associated with greater metabolism of the *n*-6 compared with *n*-3 fatty acids leading to chronic inflammatory diseases such as nonalcoholic fatty liver disease, cardiovascular disease, obesity, inflammatory bowel disease, rheumatoid arthritis, and Alzheimer's disease. By increasing the ratio of (*n*-3):(*n*-6) fatty acids in the diet, reductions may be achieved in the incidence of these chronic inflammatory diseases. A third kind of dietary fatty acid is omega-9 or monosaturated fats. These may induce several positive health outcomes like reduction of cardiovascular disease, increase in HDL cholesterol, increasing metabolism, and elimination of plaque from the arteries. The dietary sources and health effects of omega-3, -6, and -9 are given in a comparative chart in Table 4.2.

4.6 ANTIOXIDANT VITAMINS

The principal micronutrient antioxidants of the body like vitamin E (α-tocopherol), vitamin C (ascorbic acid), and β-carotene can scavenge free radicals. Body cannot manufacture these micronutrients, so they should be supplied in the diet. These vitamins are present in nature in a number of fruits and vegetables. Vitamins act singly or synergistically in the prevention of a number of oxidative reactions leading to degenerative diseases like cancer, cardiovascular diseases, and cataracts (Elliot, 1999). Vitamin E, which comprises of tocopherols together with tocotrienols, functions as an in vivo antioxidant, protecting tissue lipids from free radical attack (Meydani, 2000). α-Tocopherol acts either by donating a hydrogen radical to remove the free lipid radical, reacting with it to form nonradical products, or simply by trapping the lipid radical. In several studies, researchers found that tocotrienols have 40–60 times more powerful antioxidation properties than tocopherol in cells (Serbinova et al., 1991), while some others found much higher initial uptake of tocotrienol by cells of up to 70 times more than α-tocopherol (Saito et al., 2004). Vitamin E and selenium have a synergistic role against lipid peroxidation. Vitamin C is considered as the most important antioxidant in extracellular fluids (Sies and Stahl, 1995). It is a reducing agent and can reduce and thereby neutralize reactive oxygen species (Padayatty et al., 2003). It also acts by interacting with other antioxidants. Glutathione is important in recycling oxidized vitamin C, and vitamin C itself is crucial to the regeneration of lipid-bound vitamin E (AHRQ, 2003). Carotenoids like lycopene, β-carotene, lutein, and zeaxanthin are known to be the most efficient singlet oxygen quencher in the biological systems. At low concentrations found in most tissues under physiological conditions, β-carotene was found to inhibit oxidation (Das et al., 2012).

4.7 POLYPHENOLS

Polyphenols are natural compounds that are widely found in a large number of fruits and vegetables. About 8000 or more polyphenols have been identified from plant sources. Some of the most common classes of polyphenols in food are flavonoids, phenolic acids, stilbenes, and lignans. Polyphenolic compounds in diet affect human health by their antioxidant, antimicrobial, anti-inflammatory, vasodilating, and prebiotic properties (Landete, 2012). Beneficial effects of plant polyphenols on human health (Figure 4.2) have been proved by various epidemiological studies. Some of the widely studied polyphenols on human health are resveratrol from red wine (Ahn et al., 2008; Szkudelska et al., 2009), epigallocatechin from green tea (Li et al., 2006; Potenza et al., 2007; Bose et al., 2008), curcumin from turmeric (Ejaz et al., 2009), chlorogenic acid from coffee (Onakpoya et al., 2011), cocoa polyphenols (Andújar et al., 2012), quercetin from different sources of fruits and vegetable (Kim et al., 2007; Rivera et al., 2008; Egert et al., 2009; Lee and Mitchell, 2012), and many more. The mechanism followed by the polyphenols on human diseases is via numerous cellular processes like gene expression, apoptosis, platelet aggregation, intercellular signaling, and related machinery. Research studies have shown that polyphenols present in tea, cocoa, red wine, fruit juices, and olive oil influence carcinogenesis by interacting with carcinogens, mutagens, and other reactive intermediates, controlling the proteins associated with cell cycle, preventing oxidation, and modulating the expression of certain genes associated with cancer (Calomme et al., 1996; Duthie and Dobson, 1999; van Erk et al., 2005; García-Lafuente et al., 2009). Mechanisms by which polyphenols may have an influence on cardiovascular diseases are antioxidant, antiplatelet, and anti-inflammatory properties, inhibiting LDL oxidation, increasing HDL, and improving endothelial function (Aviram et al., 2000; García-Lafuente et al., 2009). Quercetin, cocoa flavonoids, tea catechins, red wine, and purple grape juice have shown to contribute in reducing cardiovascular diseases (Stein et al., 1999; Wan et al., 2001; Maeda et al., 2003; Lin et al., 2007; Desch et al., 2010). Numerous studies have reported the antidiabetic property of polyphenols. The mechanism followed here is like inhibition of glucose absorption by the gut or by peripheral tissues (Pandey and Rizvi, 2009). Polyphenols such as catechins, epicatechins, epigallocatechins from tea, isoflavones from soybean, tannic acid, glycyrrhizin from licorice root, chlorogenic acid, and saponins decrease the intestinal transport of glucose (Pandey and Rizvi, 2009). The theory behind human aging is the immense production of free radicals/oxidative stress in the body. Antioxidant polyphenolic compounds have a deleterious effect on the free radicals and hence on aging. Anthocyanin from grape fruits, resveratrol from grapes, and catechin from green tea and other fruit and vegetables having high levels of flavonoids have reported to exert preventive effects against aging (Seeram et al., 2003; Markus and Morris, 2008; Maurya and Rizvi, 2008; Shukitt-Hale et al., 2008). Regular intake of flavonoids has a reducing effect on certain age-related disease like dementia, Alzheimer's, and Parkinson's disease. Flavonoids act against the neurodegenerative disease by ways of protecting vulnerable neurons, enhancing existing neuronal functions, and by stimulating neuronal regeneration (Youdim and Joseph, 2001). *Ginkgo biloba* extracts have neuroprotective functions (Bastianetto et al., 2000), and citrus flavanone tangeretin are potential agent against Parkinson's disease (Datla et al., 2001). Apart from these, epidemiological studies revealed association of apple and soy isoflavone genistein intake with better lung function in asthmatic patients (Woods et al., 2003; Smith et al., 2004). The health effects of polyphenols depend on the amount consumed and their bioavailability.

4.8 HERBS AND SPICES

Spices and herbs are used from long back both in cuisines and in age-old therapeutics. On one hand, they add to the flavor and aroma of food, and on the other hand, they can be used as herbal medicines on a number of human chronic diseases. Epidemiological studies have revealed that many of these herbs and spices in their minute amounts possess antioxidative, chemopreventive, antimutagenic, anti-inflammatory, or immune-stimulating properties, which help in reducing human diseases like cancer, cardiovascular diseases, diabetes, gastrointestinal diseases, and other metabolic diseases.

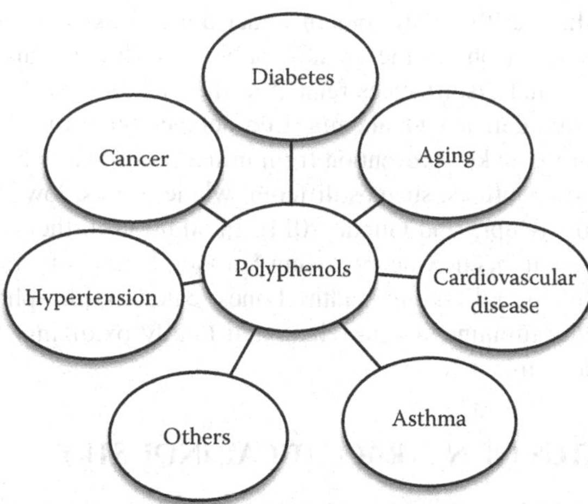

FIGURE 4.2 Beneficial effects of dietary plant polyphenols on human health. (From Pandey, K.B. and Rizvi, S.I., *Oxidat. Med. Cell. Longe.*, 2, 270, 2009.)

Chemoprevention helps in the prevention of cancer by different spice-derived nutraceuticals. In this regard, the potential of turmeric (curcumin), red chili (capsaicin), cloves (eugenol), ginger (zerumbone), fennel (anethole), kokum (gambogic acid), fenugreek (diosgenin), black cumin (thymoquinone), and ursolic acid from rosemary has been established (Aggarwal et al., 2008). These spicy nutraceuticals have shown great potential for modulating multiple targets such as transcription factors, growth factor receptors, inflammatory mediators, and other targets involved in tumor progression (Sung et al., 2012). A considerable number of human and animal experiments have been carried out on the antidiabetic property of spices. Some of the spices or their bioactive compounds extensively studied for their antidiabetic properties are fenugreek, turmeric, garlic, onion, and cumin (Srinivasan, 2005). One of the active components identified in fenugreek for its antidiabetic and antidyslipidemic effects on animal models is the amino acid 4-hydroxyisoleucine (Broca et al., 1999; Narender et al., 2006; Jaiswal et al., 2012). Hypoglycemic potency of garlic and onion has been attributed to their sulfur compounds (Augusti and Sheela, 1996). Studies revealed that in human red blood cell membranes, lipid peroxidation is inhibited by curcumin from turmeric, capsaicin from chili, and eugenol from clove (Salimath et al., 1986; Nagashima, 1989). These bioactive compounds also possess anti-inflammatory properties as is indicated by several animal studies (Srinivasan, 2005). Spices and herbs play a major role in their antimicrobial effects. In vitro studies suggest that the extracts from dietary spices and medicinal herbs possess antibacterial activities against several food-borne pathogens like *Bacillus cereus*, *Listeria monocytogenes*, *Staphylococcus aureus*, *E. coli*, *Salmonella anatum*, *Aspergillus*, *Candida*, and other species (Arora and Kaur, 1999; Shan et al., 2007). The antimicrobial property of the spices is mainly due to the essential oil fraction present in it (Srinivasan, 2005; Panpatil et al., 2013).

4.9 MINERALS

Minerals are inorganic substances essential for the human body to carry out certain physiological functions. Each and every mineral plays a key role in human activities. Minerals are broadly divided into two groups, that is the major minerals or the macro minerals and the trace minerals or the micro minerals. Macro minerals are major as their daily requirement to an individual is 100 mg or more, whereas micro minerals have their daily requirement of less than 20 mg for an individual (Soetan et al., 2010). Some of the most common macro minerals are calcium, sodium, chlorine, phosphorus, magnesium, potassium, and sulfur, and some such micro minerals are zinc, copper, iron, magnesium, chromium, cobalt, selenium, iodine, and molybdenum. Minerals generally differ from other nutrients in the fact that they remain intact during digestion and other physiological functions. Mineral deficiency is one of the greatest public health concerns in most countries giving rise to certain diseases and disturbances related to the metabolism. Mineral deficiencies may lead to osteoporosis (calcium deficiency), anemia (iron deficiency), arthritis (boron), goiter (iodine deficiency), and many more. The key prevention from mineral nutrient deficiencies is to consume a variety of foods in modest quantities, such as different whole grains, low-fat dairy, meat, and different vegetables and fruits (Gupta and Gupta, 2014). In addition to their role in maintaining the body electrolyte balance (sodium, chloride, potassium), minerals have others functions like forming blood in the body (iron, copper), building healthy bones (calcium, phosphorus, magnesium, fluoride), maintaining a healthy immune system (zinc), and finally oxidizing the excess free radicals produced in the body (selenium).

4.10 CURRENT STATUS OF NUTRACEUTICAL INDUSTRY

Nutraceutical is the most emerging and fastest growing segment in today's food and pharmacological industries. The growth of the nutraceutical market is attributed to the increasing trend of consumer propensity toward preventive care. World demand for nutraceutical ingredients expands about 7% annually to $29 billion in 2014, serving a $236 billion global nutritional product industry (Shinde et al., 2014). The United States, Europe, and Japan are the most developed nutraceutical markets, while India, China, and Brazil have huge potential for growth. Some of major food and pharmaceutical companies that have gained popularity in nutraceutical market recently are Kellogg, Heinz, Quaker oats, Unilever, Cargill, Glaxo-SmithKline, Danone, Nestle, and General Mills.

Research and development is at the peak in this emerging nutraceutical field. In spite of having promising effects in human disease prevention, appropriate regulations should be worked out by health and food professionals to provide the ultimate therapeutic benefits to the mankind. In this respect certain quality control tests like composition and safely limits of the natural components, their processing conditions are critically important. Extensive research on product safety and efficacy is required, which includes toxicity test, effects of supplementation, and in vitro and in vivo studies (Andlauer and Fürst, 2002; Dev et al., 2011, Das et al., 2012).

4.11 CONCLUSION

With the advent of hectic life schedule and aging population, human beings are now more prone to meet nutrition requirements daily. Apart from this, people are also nowadays opting for healthy foods rather than the costly medications. Thus, the popularity of nutraceuticals is on the rise. Most of the nutraceuticals have proven to have health benefits, and their consumption (within their recommended limit) will keep away diseases to maintain good health. For example dietary fibers have pronounced effect on controlling gastrointestinal disorders, probiotics have beneficial effects on colon cancer, consumption of omega-3 fatty acids reduces the risk of cardiovascular diseases, polyphenols are effective against cancer and cardiac neurodegenerative diseases, and spices are proven to have antioxidant, antimicrobial, and anti-lipidemic agents. The present accumulated knowledge of nutraceuticals represents undoubtedly great challenge for the food and pharmacy professionals. However, an individual's susceptibility to any particular disease predominantly depends upon genetic predisposition and lifestyle disorders. So, response of nutraceuticals can vary from person to person.

REFERENCES

Ackman, R.G. 2008. Fatty acids in fish and shellfish. In *Fatty Acids in Foods and Their Health Implications*, ed. C.K. Chow, pp. 155–185. London, U.K.: CRC Press.

Aggarwal, B.B., Kunnumakkara, A.B., Harikumar, K.B., Tharakan, S.T., Sung, B., and Anand P. 2008. Potential of spice-derived phytochemicals for cancer prevention. *Planta Medica*, 74:1560–1569.

Ahn, J., Cho, I., Kim, S., Kwon, D., and Ha, T. 2008. Dietary resveratrol alters lipid metabolism-related gene expression of mice on an atherogenic diet. *Journal of Hepatology*, 49(6):1019–1028.

AHRQ. 2003. *Effect of Supplemental Antioxidants Vitamin C, Vitamin E, and Coenzyme Q10 for the Prevention and Treatment of Cardiovascular Disease.* Rockville, MD: Agency for Healthcare Research and Quality, U.S. Department of Health and Human Services (Southern California–RAND Evidence-Based Practice Center, Santa Monica, CA), www.ahrq.gov.

Anderson, J.W., Baird, P., Davis, Jr R.H., Ferreri, S., Knudtson, M., Koraym, A., Waters, V., and Williams, C.L. 2009. Health benefits of dietary fibre. *Nutrition Reviews*, 67(4):188–205.

Anderson, J.W., Randles, K.M., Kendall, C.W.C., and Jenkins, D.J.A. 2004. Carbohydrate and fiber recommendations for individuals with diabetes: a quantitative assessment and meta-analysis of the evidence. *The Journal of American College of Nutrition*, 23:5–17.

Andlauer, W. and Fürst, P. 2002. Nutraceuticals: A piece of history, present status and outlook. *Food Research International*, 35:171–176.

Andújar, L., Recio, M.C., Giner, R.M., and Ríos, J.L. 2012. Cocoa polyphenols and their potential benefits for human health. *Oxidative Medicine and Cellular Longevity*, 2012:1–23.

Arora, D.S. and Kaur, J. 1999. Antimicrobial activity of spices. *International Journal of Antimicrobial Agents*, 12:257–262.

Augusti, K.T. and Sheela, C.G. 1996. Antiperoxide effect of S-allyl cysteine sulfoxide, an insulin secretagogue in diabetic rats. *Experientia*, 52:115–119.

Aviram, M., Dornfeld, L., Rosenblat, M., Volkova, N., Kaplan, M., Coleman, R., Hayek, T., Presser, D., and Fuhrman, B. 2000. Pomegranate juice consumption reduces oxidative stress, atherogenic modifications to LDL, and platelet aggregation: Studies in humans and in atherosclerotic apolipoprotein E-deficient mice. *American Journal of Clinical Nutrition*, 71:1062–1076.

Bastianetto, S., Zheng, W.H., and Quirion, R. 2000. The *Ginkgo biloba* extract (EGb 761) protects and rescues hippocampal cells against nitric oxide-induced toxicity: Involvement of its flavonoid constituents and protein kinase C. *Journal of Neurochemistry*, 74:2268–2277.

Birketvedt, G.S., Shimshi, M., Erling, T., and Florholmen, J. 2005. Experiences with three different fibre supplements in weight reduction. *Medical Science Monitor*, 11:15–18.

Bose, M., Lambert, J.D., Ju, J., Reuhl, K.R., Shapses, S.A., and Yang, C.S. 2008. The major green tea polyphenol, (–) epigallocatechin-3-gallate, inhibits obesity, metabolic syndrome, and fatty liver disease in high-fat-fed mice. *The Journal of Nutrition*, 138:1677–1683.

Broca, C., Rene, G., Pierre, P., Yves, S., Manteghetti, M., Tournier, M., Masiello, P., Gomis, R., and Ribes, G. 1999. 4-Hydroxyisoleucine: Experimental evidence of its insulinotropic and antidiabetic properties. *American Journal of Physiology*, 277:E617–E623.

Brown, L., Rosner, B., Willett, W.W., and Sacks, F.M. 1999. Cholesterol lowering effects of dietary fiber: A meta-analysis. *American Journal of Clinical Nutrition*, 69:30–42.

Calder, P.C. 2009. Polyunsaturated fatty acids and inflammatory processes: New twists in an old tale. *Biochimie*, 91:791–795.

Calomme, M., Pieters, L., Vlietinck, A., and Vanden Berghe, D. 1996. Inhibition of bacterial mutagenesis by Citrus flavonoids. *Planta Medica*, 62:222–226.

Cummings, J.H. 2001. The effect of dietary fibre on fecal weight and composition. In *Dietary Fibre in Human Nutrition*, ed. G. Spiller, pp. 183–252. Boca Raton, FL: CRC Press.

Das, L., Bhaumik, E., Raychaudhuri, U., and Chakraborty, R. 2012. Role of nutraceuticals in human health. *Journal of Food Science and Technology*, 49:173–183.

Datla, K.P., Christidou, M., Widmer, W.W., Rooprai, H.K., and Dexter, D.T. 2001. Tissue distribution and neuroprotective effects of citrus flavonoid tangeretin in a rat model of Parkinson's disease. *Neuroreport*, 12:3871–3875.

de Vrese, M. and Schrezenmeir, J. 2008. Probiotics, prebiotics and synbiotics. *Advances in Biochemical Engineering/Biotechnology*, 111:1–66.

de Vrese, M., Sieber, R., and Stransky, M. 1999. Lactose malabsorption and eating yogurt. *Schweizerische medizinische Wochenschrift*, 129:253–254.

Desch, S., Schmidt, J., Kobler, D., Sonnabend, M., Eitel, I., Sareban, M., Rahimi, K., Schuler, G., and Thiele, H. 2010. Effect of cocoa products on blood pressure: Systematic review and meta-analysis. *American Journal of Hypertension*, 23:97–103.

Dev, R., Kumar, S., Singh, J., and Chauhan, B. 2011. Potential role of nutraceuticals in present scenario: A review. *Journal of Applied Pharmaceutical Science*, 1:26–28.

Dureja, H., Kaushik, D., and Kumar, V. 2003. Developments in nutraceuticals. *Indian Journal of Pharmacology*, 35:363–372.

Duthie, S.J. and Dobson, V.L. 1999. Dietary flavonoids protect human colonocyte DNA from oxidative attack *in vitro*. *European Journal of Nutrition*, 38:28–34.

Egert, S., Bosy-Westphal, A., Seiberl, J., Kürbitz, C., Settler, U., Plachta-Danielzik, S., Wagner, A.E. et al. 2009. Quercetin reduces systolic blood pressure and plasma oxidised low density lipoprotein concentrations in overweight subjects with a high-cardiovascular disease risk phenotype: A doubleblinded, placebo-controlled cross-over study. *British Journal of Nutrition*, 102:1065–1074.

Ejaz, A. Wu, D. Kwan, P., and Meydani, M. 2009. Curcumin inhibits adipogenesis in 3T3-L1 adipocytes and angiogenesis and obesity in C57/BL mice. *The Journal of Nutrition*, 139:919–925.

Elliot, J.G. 1999. Application of antioxidant vitamins in foods and beverages. *Food Technology*, 53:46–48.

García-Lafuente, A., Guillamón, E., Villares, A., Rostagno, M.A., and Martínez, J.A. 2009. Flavonoids as anti-inflammatory agents: Implications in cancer and cardiovascular disease. *Inflammation Research*, 58:537–552.

Gibson, G.R. 1999. Dietary modulation of human gut microflora using the prebiotics Oligofructose and Inulin. *Journal of Nutrition*, 129:1438S–1441S.

Gill, H.S. and Guarner, F. 2004. Probiotics and human health: A clinical perspective. *Postgraduate Medical Journal*, 80:516–526.

Gupta, U.C. and Gupta, S.C. 2014. Sources and deficiency diseases of mineral nutrients in human health and nutrition: A review. *Pedosphere*, 24:13–38.

Hord, N.G. 2008. Eukaryotic microbiotic crosstalk: Potential mechanisms for health benefits of prebiotics and probiotics. *Annual Review of Nutrition*, 28:215–231.

Industry ARC. October 10, 2013. *Global Functional Food and Nutraceuticals Market (2013–2018)*.

Jaiswal, N., Maurya, C.K., Venkateswarlu, K. Sukanya, P., Srivastava, A.K., Narender, T., and Tamrakar, A.K. 2012. 4-Hydroxyisoleucine stimulates glucose uptake by increasing surface GLUT4 level in skeletal muscle cells via phosphatidylinositol-3-kinase-dependent pathway. *European Journal of Nutrition*, 51:893–898.

Kim, E.K., Kwon, K.B., Song, M.Y., Han, M.J., Lee, J.H., Lee, Y.R., Lee, J.H., Ryu, D.G., Park, B.H., and Park, J.W. 2007. Flavonoids protect against cytokine-induced pancreatic β-cell damage through suppression of nuclear factor κB activation. *Pancreas*, 35:el–e9.

Keenan, J.M., Pins, J.J., Frazel, C., Moran, A., and Turnquist, L. 2002. Oat ingestion reduces systolic and diastolic blood pressure in patients with mild or borderline hypertension: A pilot trial. *Journal of Family Practice*, 51:369–375.

Lairon, D., Arnault, N., Bertrais, S., Planells, R., Clero, E., Hercberg, S., and Boutron-Ruault, M.-C. 2005. Dietary fiber intake and risk factors for cardiovascular disease in French adults. *American Journal of Clinical Nutrition*, 82:1185–1194.

Landete, J.M. 2012. Updated knowledge about polyphenols: Functions, bioavailability, metabolism, and health. *Critical Reviews in Food Science and Nutrition*, 52:936–948.

Lattimer, J.M. and Haub, M.D. 2010. Effects of dietary fiber and its components on metabolic health. *Nutrients*, 2:1266–1289.

Lee, J. and Mitchell, A.E. 2012. Pharmacokinetics of quercetin absorption from apples and onions in healthy humans. *Journal of Agricultural Food Chemistry*, 60:3874–3881.

Li, C., Allen, A., Kwagh J., Doliba, N.M., Qin, W., Najafi, H., Collins, H.W., Matschinsky, F.M., Stanley, C.A., and Smith, T.J. 2006. Green tea polyphenols modulate insulin secretion by inhibiting glutamate dehydrogenase. *The Journal of Biological Chemistry*, 281:10214–10221.

Lin, J., Rexrode, K.M., Hu, F., Albert, C.M., Chae, C.U., Rimm, E.B., Stampfer, M.J., and Manson, J.E. 2007. Dietary intakes of flavonols and flavones and coronary heart disease in US women. *American Journal of Epidemiology*, 165:1305–1313.

Liu, S., Stampfer, M.J., Hu, F.B., Giovannucci, E., Colditz, G.A., Hennekens, C.H., and Willett, W.C. 1999. Whole-grain consumption and risk of coronary heart disease: results from the nurses' health study. *American Journal of Clinical Nutrition*, 70:412–419.

Maeda, K., Kuzuya, M., Cheng, X.W., Asai, T., Kanda, S., Tamaya-Mori, N., Sasaki, T., Shibata, T., and Iguchi, A. 2003. Green tea catechins inhibit the cultured smooth muscle cell invasion through the basement barrier. *Atherosclerosis*, 166:23–30.

Malik, A. 2008. The potentials of nutraceuticals. In *The Prolongation of life,* ed. E. Metchinkoff, 1907, pp. 151–183. New York: Putmans Sons.

Markus, M.A. and Morris, B.J. 2008. Resveratrol in prevention and treatment of common clinical conditions of aging. *Journal of Clinical Interventions in Aging*, 3:331–339.

Maurya, P.K. and Rizvi, S.I. 2008. Protective role of tea catechins on erythrocytes subjected to oxidative stress during human aging. *Natural Products Research*, 14:1–8.

Meydani, M. 2000. Effect of functional food ingredients: Vitamin E modulation of cardiovascular diseases and immune status in the elderly. *American Journal of Clinical Nutrition*, 71:1665S–1668S.

Montonen, J., Knekt, P., Jarvinen, R., Aromaa, A., and Reunanen, A. 2003. Whole-grain and fiber intake and the incidence of type 2 diabetes. *American Journal of Clinical Nutrition*, 77:622–629.

Nagashima, K. 1989. Inhibitory effect of eugenol on Cu2+-catalysed lipid peroxidation I human erythrocyte membrane. *International Journal of Biochemistry*, 21:745–749.

Narender, T., Puri, A., Shweta, S., Khaliq, T., Saxena, R., Bhatia, G., and Chandra, R. 2006. 4-Hydroxyisoleucine an unusual amino acid as antidyslipidemic and antihyperglycemic agent. *Bioorganic and Medicinal Chemistry Letters*, 16:293–296.

O'Bryan, C., Pak, D., Crandall, P.G., Lee, S.O., and Ricke, S.C. 2013. The role of prebiotics and probiotics in human health. *Journal of Probiotics and Health*, 1:1–8.

Onakpoya, I., Terry, T., and Ernst, E. 2011. The use of green coffee extract as a weight loss supplement: A systematic review and meta-analysis of randomised clinical trials. *Gastroenterology Research and Practice*, 2011:1–6.

Padayatty, S., Katz, A., Wang, Y., Eck, P., Kwon, O., Lee, J., Chen, S., Corpe, C., Dutta, A., Dutta, S.K., and Levine, M. 2003. Vitamin C as an antioxidant: Evaluation of its role in disease prevention. *The Journal of the American College of Nutrition*, 22:18–35.

Pandey, K.B. and Rizvi, S.I. 2009. Plant polyphenols as dietary antioxidants in human health and disease. *Oxidative Medicine and Cellular Longevity*, 2:270–278.

Pandey, M., Verma, R.K., and Saraf S.A. 2010. Nutraceuticals: new era of medicine and health. *Asian Journal of Pharmaceutical and Clinical Research*, 3:11–15.

Panpatil, V.V., Tattari, S., Kota, N., Nimgulkar, C., and Polasa, K. 2013. In vitro evaluation on antioxidant and antimicrobial activity of spice extracts of ginger, turmeric and garlic. *Journal of Pharmacognosy and Phytochemistry*, 2:143–148.

Patterson, E., Wall, R., Fitzgerald, G.F., Ross, R.P., and Stanton, C. 2012. Health implications of high dietary omega-6 polyunsaturated fatty acids. *Journal of Nutrition and Metabolism*, 2012:1–16.

Petruzziello, L., Iacopini, F., Bulajic, M., Shah, S., and Costamagna, G. 2006. Review article: Uncomplicated diverticular disease of the colon. *Alimentary Pharmacology and Therapeutic*, 23:1379–1391.

Post, R.E., Mainous III, A.G., King, D.E., and Simpson, K.N. 2012. Dietary fiber for the treatment of type 2 diabetes mellitus: A meta-analysis. *The Journal of the American Board of Family Medicine*, 25:16–23.

Potenza, M.A., Marasciulo, F.L., Tarquinio, M., Tiravanti, E., Colantuono, G., Federici, A., Kim, J.A., Quon, M.J., and Montagnani, M. 2007. EGCG, a green tea polyphenol, improves endothelial function and insulin sensitivity, reduces blood pressure, and protects against myocardial I/R injury in SHR. *American Journal of Physiology*, 292:E1378–E1387.

Rivera, L., Morón, R., Sánchez, M., Zarzuelo, A., and Galisteo, M. 2008. Quercetin ameliorates metabolic syndrome and improves the inflammatory status in obese Zucker rats. *Obesity*, 16:2081–2087.

Saibil, F. 1989. Diarrhea due to fiber overload. *The New England Journal of Medicine*, 320:599.

Saito, Y., Yoshida, Y., Nishio, K., Hayakawa, M., and Niki, E. 2004. Characterization of cellular uptake and distribution of vitamin E. *Annals of the New York Academy of Sciences*, 1031:368–375.

Salimath, B.P., Sundaresh, C.S., and Srinivas, L. 1986. Dietary components inhibit lipid peroxidation in erythrocyte membrane. *Nutrition Research*, 6:1171–1178.

Schrezenmeir, J. and de Vrese, M. 2001. Probiotics, prebiotics and synbiotics-approaching a definition. *American Journal of Clinical Nutrition*, 73:361S–364S.

Seeram, N.P., Cichewicz, R.H., Chandra, A., and Nair, M.G. 2003. Cyclooxygenase inhibitory and antioxidant compounds from crabapple fruits. *Journal of Agricultural and Food Chemistry*, 51:1948–1951.

Serbinova, E., Han, D., and Packer, L. 1991. Free radical recycling and intramembrane mobility in the antioxidant properties of alpha-tocopherol and alpha-tocotrienol. *Free Radical Biology and Medicine*, 10:263–267.

Shan, B., Cai, Y.Z., Brooks, J.D., and Corke H. 2007. The in vitro antibacterial activity of dietary spice and medicinal herb extracts. *International Journal of Food Microbiology*, 117:112–119.

Shinde, N., Bangar, B., Deshmukh, S., and Kumbhar, P. 2014. Nutraceuticals: A review on current status. *Research Journal of Pharmacy and Technology*, 7:110–113.

Shukitt-Hale, B., Lau, F.C., and Joseph, J.A. 2008. Berry fruit supplementation and the aging brain. *Journal of Agricultural and Food Chemistry*, 56:636–641.

Sies, H. and Stahl, W. 1995. Vitamins E and C, a-carotene, and other carotenoids as antioxidants. *American Journal of Clinical Nutrition*, 195:1315S–1321S.

Smith, L.J., Holbrook, J.T., Wise, R., Blumenthal, M., Dozor, A.J., Mastronarde, J., and Williams, L. 2004. Dietary intake of soy genistein is associated with lung function in patients with asthma. *Journal of Asthma*, 41:833–843.

Soetan, K.O., Olaiya, C.O., and Oyewole, O.E. 2010. The importance of mineral elements for humans, domestic animals and plants: A review. *African Journal of Food Science*, 4:200–222.

Srinivasan, K. 2005. Role of spices beyond food flavoring: nutraceuticals with multiple health effects. *Food Reviews International*, 21:167–188.

Steffen, L.M., Jacobs, D.R. Jr., Stevens, J., Shahar, E., Carithers, T., and Folsom, A.R. 2003. Associations of whole-grain, refined grain, and fruit and vegetable consumption with risks of all-cause mortality and incident coronary artery disease and ischemic stroke: The atherosclerosis risk in communities (ARIC) study. *American Journal of Clinical Nutrition*, 78:383–390.

Stein, J.H., Keevil, J.G., Wiebe, D.A., Aeschlimann, S., and Folts, J.D. 1999. Purple grape juice improves endothelial function and reduces the susceptibility of LDL cholesterol to oxidation in patients with coronary artery disease. *Circulation*, 100:1050–1055.

Sung, B., Prasad, S., Yadav, V.R., and Aggarwal, B.B. 2012. Cancer cell signalling pathways targeted by spice-derived nutraceuticals. *Nutrition and Cancer*, 64:173–197.

Szkudelska, K., Nogowski, L., and Szkudelski, T. 2009. Resveratrol, a naturally occurring diphenolic compound, affects lipogenesis, lipolysis and the antilipolytic action of insulin in isolated rat adipocytes. *The Journal of Steroid Biochemistry and Molecular Biology*, 113:17–24.

U.S. Department of Agriculture (USDA), U.S. Department of Health and Human Services. 2005. *Dietary Guidelines for Americans*. Washington, DC: USDA.

van Erk, M.J., Roepman, P., van der Lende, T.R., Stierum, R.H., Aarts, J.M., van Bladeren, P.J., and van Ommen, B. 2005. Integrated assessment by multiple gene expression analysis of quercetin bioactivity on anticancer-related mechanisms in colon cancer cells in vitro. *European Journal of Nutrition*, 44:143–156.

Wall, R., Ross, R.P., Fitzgerald, G.F., and Stanton, C. 2010. Fatty acids from fish: The anti-inflammatory potential of long chain omega-3 fatty acids. *Nutrition Reviews*, 68:280–289.

Wan, Y., Vinson, J.A., Etherton, T.D., Proch, J., Lazarus, S.A., and Kris-Etherton, P.M. 2001. Effects of cocoa powder and dark chocolate on LDL oxidative susceptibility and prostaglandin concentrations in humans. *American Journal of Clinical Nutrition*, 74:596–602.

Whelton, S.P., Hyre, A.D., Pedersen, B., Yi, Y., Whelton, P.K., and He, J. 2005. Effect of dietary fiber intake on blood pressure: A metaanalysis of randomized, controlled clinical trials. *Journal of Hypertension*, 23:475–481.

White, P.J. 2008. Fatty acids in oilseeds (vegetable oils). In *Fatty Acids in Foods and Their Health Implications*, ed. K.C. Chow, pp. 227–262. New York: CRC Press.

Wong, J.M. and Jenkins, D.J. 2007. Carbohydrate digestibility and metabolic effects. *Journal of Nutrition*, 137:2539S–2546S.

Woods, R.K., Raven, J.M., Wolfe, R., Ireland, P.D., Thien, F.C.K., and Abramson, M.J. 2003. Food and nutrient intakes and asthma risk in young adults. *American Journal of Clinical Nutrition*, 78:414–421.

Youdim, K.A. and Joseph, J.A. 2001. A possible emerging role of phytochemicals in improving age-related neurological dysfunctions: A multiplicity of effects. *Free Radical Biology and Medicine*, 30:583–594.

Section II

Obesity, Diabetes, and Metabolic Syndrome

5 Dietary Factors in Promoting Healthy Lifestyle

A New Prospect of Neuroendocrine in Obesity

Zwe-Ling Richard Kong

CONTENTS

ABBREVIATIONS

AgRP agouti-related peptide
AD Alzheimer's disease
BBB blood–brain barrier
BMI body mass index
CART cocaine and amphetamine-regulated transcript
CLA conjugated linoleic acid
CR calorie restriction
CVD cardiovascular disease
DHA docosahexaenoic acid
DM diabetes mellitus
EDC endocrine-disrupting chemicals
EPA eicosapentaenoic acid
GnRH gonadotropin-releasing hormone
HFD high-fat diet

IL interleukin
INKT invariant natural killer T cells
LH luteinizing hormone
MS metabolic syndrome
NFAT calcineurin/nuclear factor of activated T cells
POMC proopiomelanocortin
POPs persistent organic pollutants
PPARγ peroxisome proliferator–activated receptor gamma
ROS reactive oxygen species
TNFα tumor necrosis factor alpha
T2D type 2 diabetes
WAT white adipose tissue
WHR waist-to-hip ratio

5.1 INTRODUCTION

Obesity has become a global pandemic, and it is one of the important medical problems worldwide today. It is associated with a number of acute and chronic medical complications, including MS, CVD, T2D, AD, arthritis, stroke, respiratory and gastrointestinal disorder, and infertility. The occurrence of the obesity and related systemic disorders are linked with high individual-dependent risk factors, including genetic profile, diet behavior, environmental stress, and gut microbiome. On the other hand, traditional weight loss treatments, usually involving calorie restriction or reduction of fat intake, in fact, have generally very limited success. In this chapter, from the viewpoint of dietary factors, we will review the updated knowledge of obesity regarding human health, focusing on emerging prospect of interplay among brain function, neuroendocrine, adipokines, and immunological regulation.

5.2 EPIDEMIOLOGY, PATHOLOGY, AND PREVALENCE

5.2.1 Obesity, Body Weight, and Waist-to-Hip Ratio

Despite the enormous medical implications of obesity, effective prevention and treatment strategies are still unsolvable. It is important to distinguish the term "obesity", used to describe excess body fat from other forms of overweight. Weight is measured in relation to height as BMI: it is a relatively simple measure and a valuable tool, but has several disadvantages. There is a lack of consensus regarding the values that should be used to define "overweight" or "obese" [1]. Obesity results from the hypertrophy, and hyperplasia of adipocytes, and is generally thought to be the result of both genetic and environmental influences. Being overweight or obese has become highly prevalent in western countries, and the populations are rapidly growing up in the developing world. A prospective cohort study [2] was conducted to evaluate the independent utility of body fat percentage and other obesity indices in predicting mortality and CVD. Results, in contrast, of higher BMI and WHR were associated with an increased risk of both mortality and CVD outcomes, and WHR might be the best indicator.

More than one-third of adults and 17% of youth in the United States are obese. There was a significant decrease in obesity among children (2–5-year old) and a significant increase in obesity among women aged 60 years and older [3,4], as shown in Figure 5.1.

Obesity has become a major global health challenge. The rise in obesity has led to widespread calls for monitoring changes in overweight prevalence in all populations recently. The global, regional, and national prevalence of overweight and obesity in children and adults during 1980–2013 revealed some findings [5]. Worldwide, the proportion of adults with a BMI increased substantially in children and adolescents in both developed and developing countries.

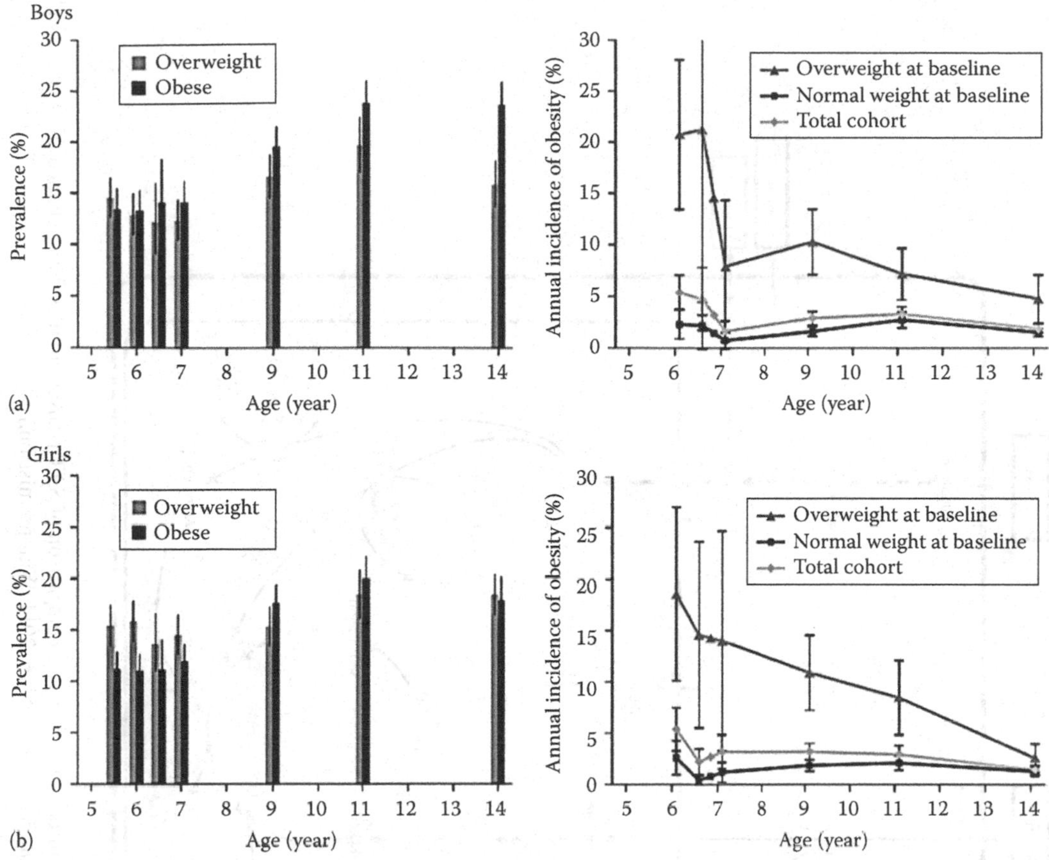

FIGURE 5.1 Prevalence and incidence of obesity between kindergarten and eighth grade for boys (a) and girls (b). The black vertical lines and I bars represent 95% confidence intervals. (Adapted from Cunningham, S.A. et al., *N. Engl. J. Med.*, 370(5), 403, 2014. With permission.)

5.2.2 Proteomics, Genetics, and Epigenetics

Body WAT has a major role in the progression of obesity [6]. Decreasing glutaminolysis and alterations have been reported in the obese subjects compared to lean subjects. The mechanism for the changes in the plasma level of glutamate, pyruvate, and α-ketoglutarate in obese subjects are shown in Figure 5.2.

Accumulating investigations contributed to characterize the age-dependent changes either at both gene and protein expression level [7]. Increasing attention on environment modifications in aging, increasingly oxidized and eventually dysfunctional as a function of age. The modification is irreversible and may alter protein function. Obesity occurs because of an interaction between an extrinsic obesogenic environment and intrinsic genetics. Evidence suggests that environmental epigenetics may serve as a biomarker or a target for intervention [8]. Occurrence of differential methylation in visceral adipose tissue of obese men is responsible for metabolic disturbances [9]. The pathways were related to structural components of the cell membrane, inflammation, immune response, and cell cycle regulation. High methylation potential is associated with diet, genotype, protein, and metabolite levels [10]. Some identified key SNPs in genes demonstrating the genetic basis of the methylation potential. Individual plasma metabolites also correlated with plasma proteins, BMI, group age, and gender. The impact of epigenetic processes of TNF-α and paraoxonase promoters in the susceptibility to stroke was revealed, when considering body composition and dietary intake [11].

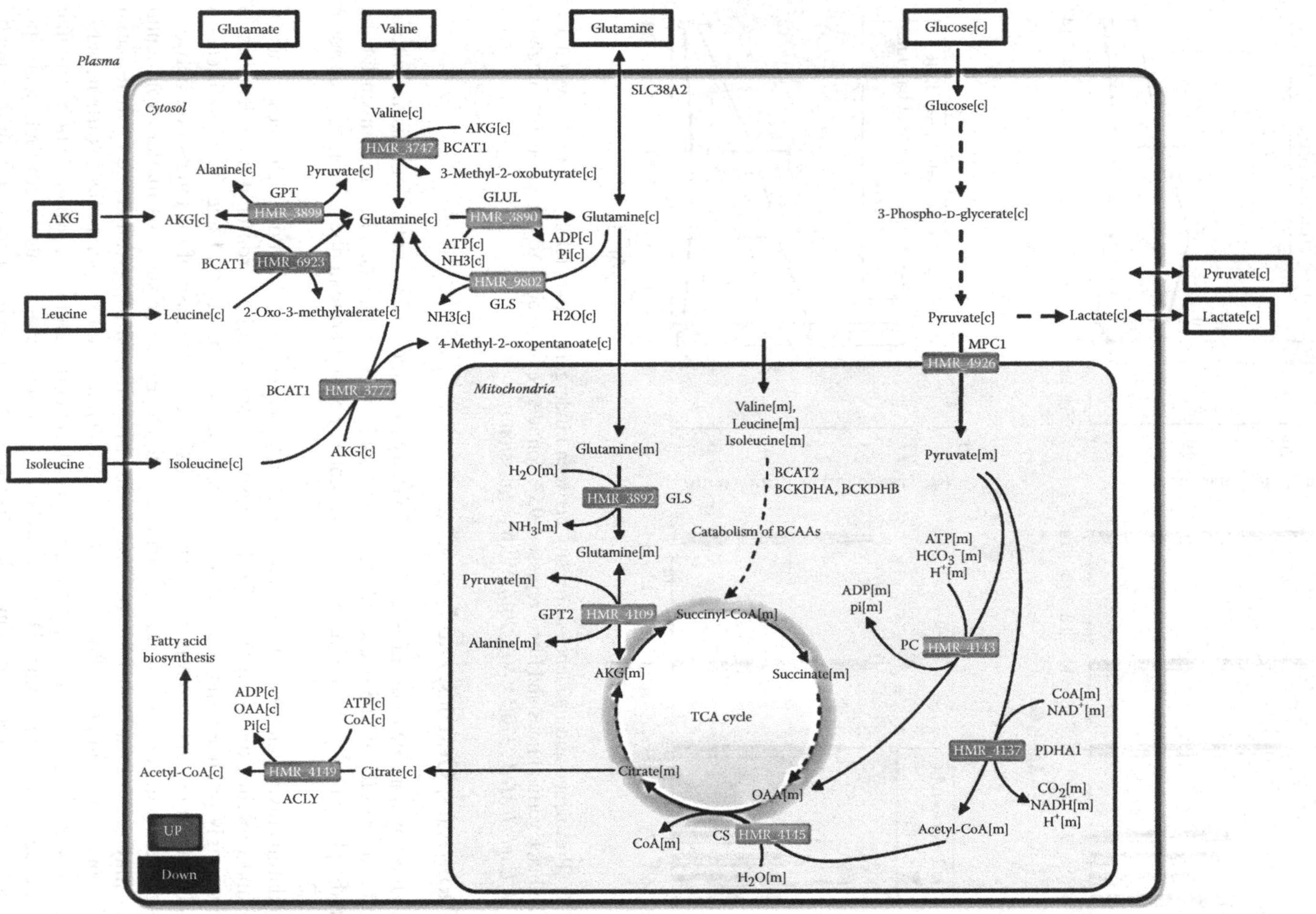

FIGURE 5.2 Abnormalities in the mitochondria of the SAT were identified through the pairwise comparison of SAT transcriptomics data obtained from obese and lean male and female subjects. (Adapted from Mardinoglu, A. et al., *J. Proteome Res.*, 13(11), 5106, 2014. With permission.)

It is believed that mammalian aging can be delayed by genetic, dietary, and pharmacologic approaches. This is against the following backdrop: the elderly population is dramatically increasing and aging is the greatest risk factor for chronic diseases driving both morbidity and mortality [12]. Obesity contributes to both peripheral and central inflammation and is often associated with aging. Leptin is involved in age-dependent changes in response to systemic inflammation [13]. Increased expression of the endogenous immune regulator microRNA146a in aged animals has been confirmed, which suggests a role for these mediators in counteracting brain inflammation. Weight gain often accompanies with aging issue, the divergent influences of chronological aging on body weight is shown in Figure 5.3 [14]. The changes in whole brain weight and serum macrophage colony-stimulating factor levels correlated better with body weight than with chronological aging problem. A decrease in brain cytokines and brain plasminogen activator inhibitor levels correlated also better with chronological aging than with body weight. These findings show that the influences of both aging and body weight are distinct in: various cytokines/hormones, the central nervous system, and the peripheral tissue compartments.

Obesity has bad effects on the brain and cognitive function in the elderly. Aging exacerbates HFD-induced decrease in neurovascular function via increased NADPH-oxidase-derived ROS production. It significantly enhances capillary rarefaction in the brain, probably contributing to cognitive decline observed in aged obese individuals [15]. The emerging key peptide, sirtuins, is involved

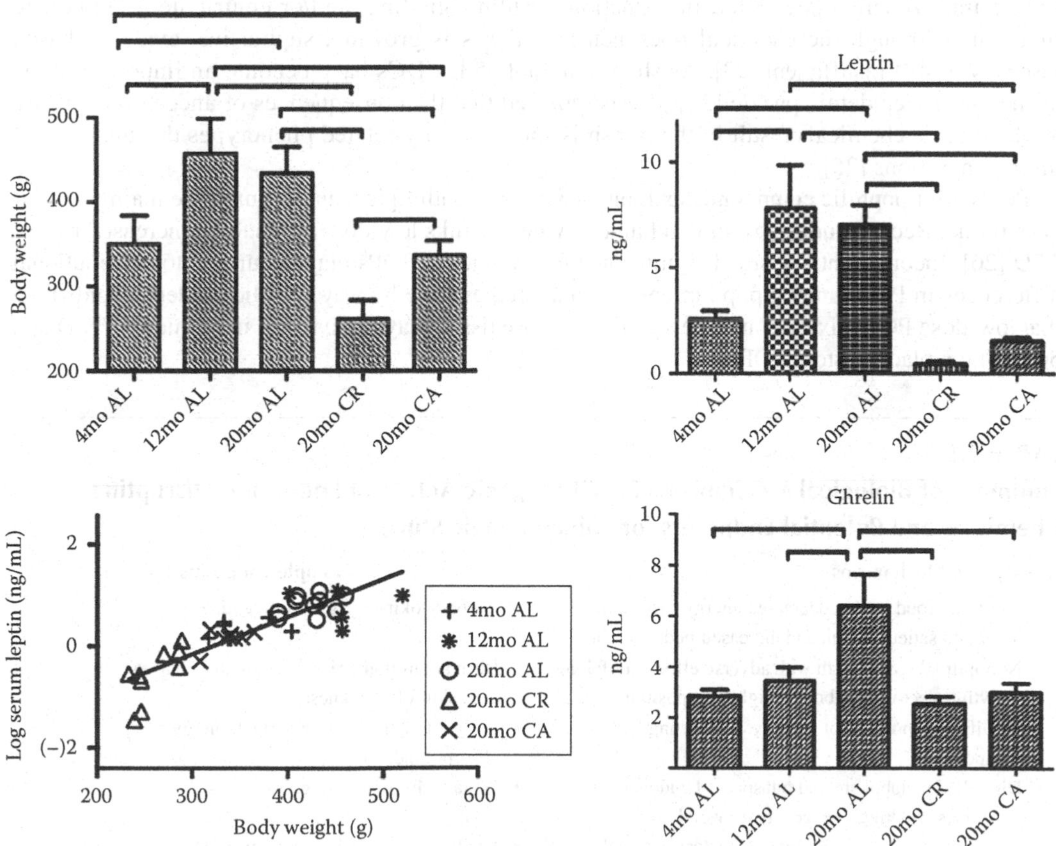

FIGURE 5.3 Body weight and blood levels of gastrointestinal hormones. Upper left panel shows effects of aging and diet on body weight. Upper right panel shows effects on serum leptin levels [14]. Lower left panel shows relation for serum leptin and body weight. Lower right panel shows effects of aging and diet on serum ghrelin levels. Values are means ± standard error. (Adapted from Banks, W.A. et al., *J. Gerontol. A: Biol. Sci. Med. Sci.*, 476380, 2014. With permission.)

in longevity of life. A lot of evidence now indicates that sirtuins suppress a variety of age-related pathologies and prolong health life span [16].

5.2.3 Emerging Countries, Dietary Factors, and Obesogens

CR with adequate nutrition extends life span in model organisms from yeast to mammals, lowers the deterioration of biological functions, and reduces the risk of many age-related diseases. The positive effects of CR include regulation of energy metabolism, oxidative stress, insulin sensitivity, inflammation, and triggering of autophagy of neuroendocrine glands. The antiaging effect of CR was confirmed including PPAR, AMP-activated protein kinase, insulin/insulin growth factor-1, and sirtuins [17]. Recent trends in childhood overweight in the transition countries of Eastern and Central Europe were reported [18]. Prevalence of childhood overweight was very similar in those of Central and Eastern European countries. There is a remarkable evidence of obesity-related comorbidities in BRICS countries [19]. This was reported in China in the period of transition from scarcity and extensive undernutrition to emerging nutrition-related diseases, 1949–1992 [20]. Economic progress and the longer-term food supply changed greatly. Diet composition shifted greatly during this period.

Chemical exposure also complicates the role of obesity in the etiology of DM [21]. The prevalence of obesity has increased dramatically worldwide in the last three decades. Several studies suggest a link between EDCs' exposure and obesity [22]. In fact, many contaminants have been found to deregulate endocrine function, insulin signaling, and/or contribute to adipocyte function. Although the chemical obesogen hypothesis is growing, supportive, evidence-based research is still insufficient [23]. As shown in Table 5.1, EDCs have become an important issue of the obesity epidemic puzzle [24]. It was reported that the consequences of ancestral exposure to obesogenic chemicals result in the transmission of obesity-related phenotypes through at least three generations [25].

POPs are lipophilic compounds, exhibit easy uptake with lipids, and accumulate mainly in adipose tissue. Recent studies reveal that human evidence links low-dose POPs to an increased risk of T2D [26]. Inconsistent statistical significance for individual POPs may occur due to distributional differences in POPs among populations. Animal studies have by way of solid evidence confirmed that low-dose POP mixtures are obesogenic. Adipose tissue plays a dual role in promoting T2D and providing a place to store POPs.

TABLE 5.1
Summary of Biological Mechanisms for Obesogenic Action of Endocrine-Disrupting Chemicals and Potential Endpoints for Epidemiologic Study

Obesogenic Mechanisms	Example Endpoints
• Increased food intake, decreased energy expenditure, disrupted satiety signal, and increased body weight	• Adipocytokines (e.g. serum leptin)
• Nonoptimal size at birth with adverse effect on lifelong growth trajectory and body weight/composition	• Birth anthropometrics, adipose distribution (e.g. skinfold thickness)
• Modified disposition of adipocytes affecting body composition	• Body fat distribution (e.g. dual-energy x-ray absorptiometry)
• Disturbed metabolism and transport of endogenous hormones resulting in excess body weight	• Gonadal hormones (e.g. estrogen)
• Dysfunction of glucose/lipid homeostasis or insulin resistance	• Insulin (e.g. oral glucose tolerance test)
• Changes in epigenetic regulation of adipogenesis, appetite and satiety signaling, and glucose/lipid metabolism	• DNA methylation, histone modification, or expression of genes involved in metabolism or adipogenesis

Source: Adapted from Romano, M. et al., *Curr. Epidemiol. Rep.*, 1(2), 57, 2014. With permission.

5.3 COMPLICATIONS: IMMUNE SYSTEM AND CELL BIOLOGICAL INSIGHTS

5.3.1 Adipocyte Differentiation

Adipogenesis is a multistage and complicated process beginning with mesenchymal cells capable of forming muscle, bone, or adipose tissue. Adipose tissue is formed as a result of a long-term process called adipogenesis. There is inflammation and progressive infiltration by macrophages as obesity develops, that link to metabolic disease and immune response, and the signaling pathways [27]. The recent studies demonstrate that calcineurin is a critical effector of a calcium-dependent pathway that acts to inhibit adipocyte differentiation. Moreover, constitutively active NFAT mutant preadipocyte inhibits its differentiation into mature adipocytes. Cells expressing NFAT lose contact-mediated growth inhibition and are protected from apoptosis following growth factor deprivation [28]. The first, and best characterized, model of adipogenesis in vitro is the 3T3-L1 mouse fibroblast cell line. When confluent/growth-arrested 3T3-L1 cells are subjected to the adipogenic hormone, dexamethasone, and insulin, they undergo a defined genetic program of terminal differentiation and give rise to mature morphologically distinct adipocytes [29]. It is dependent on the sequential activation of transcription factors including PPAR, which leads to changes in the gene expression [30].

5.3.2 Metabolic Syndrome

Obesity is associated with endothelial dysfunction and arterial stiffness from as early as the first decade of human life. This is probably mediated partially by low-grade inflammation associated with adipokines. WAT is a major endocrine/secretory organ, which releases a wide range of adipokines [31]. A decrease in motor nerve conduction velocity with progression of diabetes was presented in obese diabetic rats. Observation of hypotestosteronemia and erectile dysfunction in obese T2D rats has been reported [32].

It was revealed that the brain macrostructure was not associated with MS. In early manifest of MS, brain tissue decline can be detected. Serum HDL cholesterol, triglycerides, BMI, and diastolic blood pressure were independent factors in brain tissue integrity [33]. In contrast, MS was associated with decreased gray and white matter peak height. Chronic microinflammation is a hallmark of many aging-related neurodegenerative diseases as well as MS-trigger diseases. Recent research indicates that long-term/chronic caloric excess can lead to hypothalamic microinflammation. Hypothalamus microinflammation has a fundamental role in translating overnutrition and aging into complex outcomes [34]. Obesity is associated with depression. Evidence shows that brain-derived neurotrophic factor (BDNF), but not body weight, correlated with a reduction in depression scale scores in men with MS [35]. As shown in Figure 5.4, deficiency of BDNF is involved in the mechanism of depression. Weight reduction would improve depressive symptoms via increasing BDNF levels in obese men.

5.3.3 Immunology: iNKT and Macrophage

Diet-induced obesity results in lymphatic dysfunction and impaired T-cell function [36]. Interleukin-1β is one of the key proinflammatory cytokines that contributes to the generation of insulin resistance and diabetes. It was revealed that a regulatory mechanism controlled diet-induced insulin resistance, with E3 ubiquitin ligase playing a critical role for. It regulates IL-1β expression and this regulation has implications for diseases like T2D [37]. It is characterized by insulin resistance and chronic low-grade inflammation, conditions that are the consequences of the complex interplay between adipocytes and immune cells, as shown in Table 5.2. The links between obesity and gut microbiota have given rise to an emerging new field of interest [38].

The elderly exhibit increased susceptibility to a number of inflammatory or degenerative pathologies. Aging is similarly thought to be associated with increased prevalence [39]. Impairment of

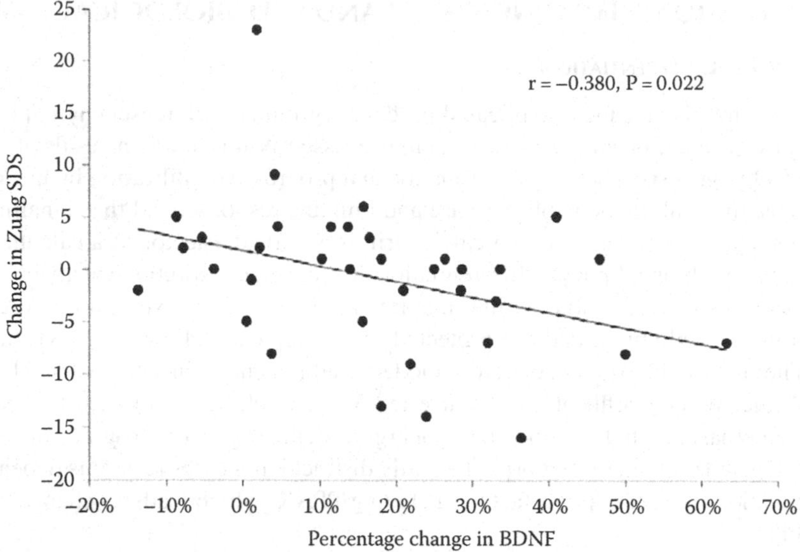

FIGURE 5.4 Relationship between the percentage changes in BDNF and changes in the Zung Self-Rating Depression Scale (Zung SDS) score; r = −0.380, P = 0.022. (Adapted from Lee et al. *Diab. Met. Synd.*, 6, 18, 2014. With permission.)

immune defenses might be aggravated by chronic infections and malnutrition during aging [40]. There is a pathophysiological link between macrophages, obesity, and insulin resistance, which highlights the dynamic immune cell response of adipose tissue for inflammation [41]. The general view in obesity is that there is an imbalance in the ratio of M1/M2 macrophages, leading to chronic inflammation and the propagation of metabolic dysfunction. However, there is emerging evidence revealing a more interesting scenario of different macrophage profiles [42,43]. Polarized microglial and macrophage populations in brain repair after acute injury, and point to the therapeutic approaches targeting cerebral inflammation should shift from broad suppression of microglia and macrophages [44].

The central nervous system has an immune privilege protected by the BBB and maintained by the glia. As shown in Table 5.3, it is also known that in homeostatic conditions, peripheral immune cells are able to penetrate down to the deepest regions of brain without altering the structural integrity of the BBB [45].

EPA and DHA, the bioactive components of fish oil, exert immunomodulatory properties. In in vivo study [46], they establish that fish oil can boost B-cell-mediated immunity in obesity. Additionally, immune cells recognize β-glucans through a cell surface receptor Dectin-1. The β-glucan from *Saccharomyces cerevisiae* induces the expression of immune regulatory cytokines (IL-10, TGF-β1, and IL-2). Furthermore, the innate immune response induced by low-dose β-glucan is regulatory in nature and can be exploited to modulate T-cell response to β cell for inducing an effective protection [47]. The combination of white rice with β-glucan-rich barley could play a beneficial role in preventing and treating obesity and other obesity-related metabolic diseases [48,49]. Gamma-tocotrienol attenuates high-fat diet–induced obesity and insulin resistance by inhibiting adipose inflammation and M1 macrophage recruitment [50]. Oxidized LDL regulates macrophage gene expression also through ligand activation of PPARγ [51].

iNKT cells subsets classified by surface receptors are enriched in lean adipose tissue where they produce IL-10. As shown on Figure 5.5, during obesity, adipose iNKT cells are depleted, representing the loss of an important regulatory population, adipose tissue becomes an chronic inflammatory environment [52]. A bidirectional cross talk between iNKT [53] and adipocytes mediated by leptin modulates the susceptibility for T cell [54]. The adipose iNKT cells induced an anti-inflammatory

TABLE 5.2
Potential Role of Selected Adipokines in Insulin Resistance and Inflammation

Adipokine	Source	Role in Insulin Resistance and Inflammation
Leptin	Adipocytes	Induces JAK/STAT signaling
		Enhances NFκB- and JNK-mediated gene transcription
		Stimulates TNF-α and IL-6 production
		Activates monocytes and macrophages
		Enhances proinflammatory Th1 and suppresses anti-inflammatory Th2 cytokines
Adiponectin	Adipocytes	Inhibits NFκB activation and TNF-α production
		Promotes the production of anti-inflammatory cytokines
		Decreases macrophage IFN-γ secretion
		Promotes anti-inflammatory M2 phenotypic of macrophages
		Inhibits oxLDL-induced endothelial cell proliferation
IL-6	Adipocytes	Induces JAK/STAT signaling
	Macrophages	Promotes SOCS-3 induction
	T cells	Increases energy expenditure when acting centrally
TNF-α	Adipocytes	Induces NFκB- and JNK-mediated gene transcription
	Macrophages	Increases hepatic lipogenesis
	T and B cells	
Resistin	Macrophages	Enhances IL-6 and TNF-α secretion
	Adipocytes (unknown)	Activates JNK, p38 MAPK, and SOCS-3 signaling when acting centrally
RBP4	Adipocytes	Interferes with GLUT4 expression and IRS-1 phosphorylation
	Macrophages	
Visfatin	Monocytes	Induces proinflammatory cytokine production
	Macrophages	
	Dendritic cells	
	Adipocytes (unknown)	
Chemerin	Adipocytes	Regulates adipocyte maturation
	B cells	Interferes with IRS-1 phosphorylation
	Neutrophils	May act toward or against inflammation
Adipsin	Adipocytes	Alternative complement activation
	Monocytes	
	Macrophages	
Omentin-1	Stromal vascular cells	Exerts insulin-mimetic effects
		Attenuates NFκB activation

Source: Adapted from Paragh, G. et al., Dynamic interplay between metabolic syndrome and immunity, in: J. Camps, ed., *Oxidative Stress and Inflammation in Non-communicable Diseases—Molecular Mechanisms and Perspectives in Therapeutics*, Springer International Publishing, Switzerland, 2014, pp. 171–190. With permission.

phenotype of macrophages through the production of IL-2, and also controlled the number, proliferation, and suppressor function of regulatory T cells in adipose tissue. Thus, iNKT cells in adipose tissue are unique regulators of immunological homeostasis in adipose tissue [55].

Restoring iNKT cells, or activating them in obese mice, leads to improved glucose handling, insulin sensitivity, and even weight loss, and hence represents an exciting therapeutic highway to be explored for restoring homeostasis in obese adipose tissue.

TABLE 5.3
Monocyte Recruitment through Intact Brain Barriers

Barriers	Macrophage Locations	CNS Status
Brain endothelium (BBB)	Perivascular macrophages at postcapillary levels	Homeostasis
	Recruited and crossing through capillary endothelium	Neuroinflammation
Choroid plexus (B-SCFB)	Macrophages in choroid plexus stroma	Homeostasis
	Monocyte/macrophage in CSF (25% in humans)	Homeostasis
	Recruitment through the fenestrated endothelium	Neuroinflammation
Blood-leptomeninges (B-LMB)	Resting macrophages in leptomeningeal spaces	Homeostasis
	M1-activated macrophages	Neuroinflammation
Spinal cord (B-SCB)	Macrophages recruitment from CSF	Neuroinflammation
	M2-activated macrophages from CPt	Response to injury
Retina (B-RB)	Reparative macrophages recruited by pigmented epithelium	Response to injury and inflammation

Source: Adapted from Corraliza, I., *Front. Cell. Neurosci.*, 8, 262, 2014. With permission.

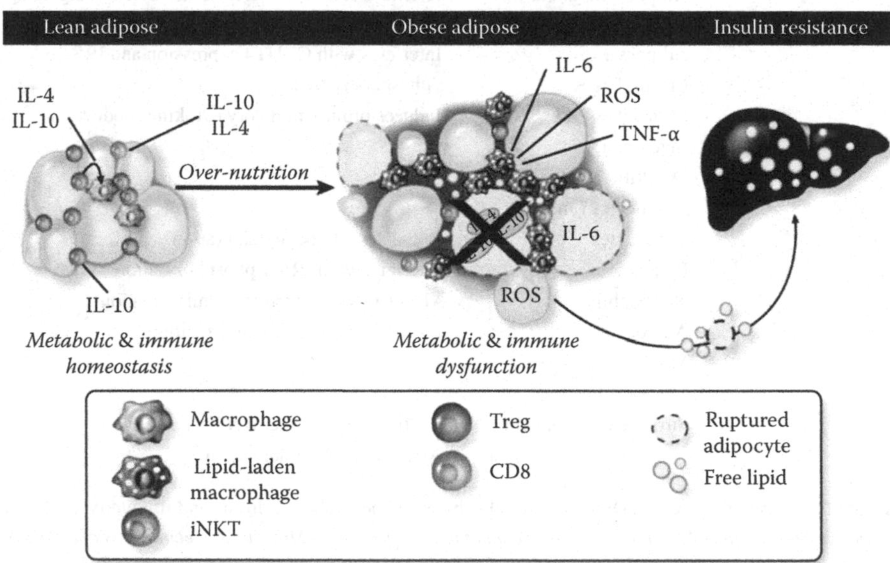

FIGURE 5.5 **(See color insert.)** The role of iNKT cells in lipid handling and metabolic regulation. (Adapted from Lynch, L., *Immunology*, 142(3), 337, 2014. With permission.)

5.3.4 Mitochondrial Stress: NF-κB and PPARγ

The mitochondrial energy-transducing capacity is essential for the maintenance of neuronal function, and the impairment of energy metabolism and redox homeostasis is a hallmark of brain aging. It is particularly accentuated in the early stages of neurodegenerative diseases [56]. Impairment of this regulatory device is critical for aging and the early stages of neurodegenerative diseases. It was confirmed that metabolic signaling, transcriptional regulation, and mitochondrial function control the cellular energy levels during brain aging and neurodegeneration. Increasing evidence shows that mitochondrial dysfunction in the prediabetic/insulin-resistant state contributes to neurodegenerative diseases, obesity, insulin sensitivity, and cancer [57]. Inductions of mitochondrial uncoupling proteins promote fatty acid oxidation and resistance to obesity. Understanding of brain development, senescence, and disease have emerged from the recognition of structural and functional plasticity within the mammalian brain. The role of BDNF that mediate neurogenesis, as well as synaptic and dendritic plasticity in psychiatric disorders, has revealed unforeseen neuronal regulatory mechanisms. The role of mitochondria decline in regulating synaptic transmission, cognitive function, and memory in the aging brain [58].

Metabolic and immune responses are highly integrated and interdependent. In obesity and diabetes, there are firm links between inflammatory mediators. NFκB plays a key role in inflammatory and immune responses. Peripheral blood mononuclear cells in obese patients are in a proinflammatory state with an increase in intranuclear NFκB binding [59]. TNFα and adiponectin are antagonistic in stimulating NFκB activation. In 3T3-L1 adipocytes model, they further stimulate the formation of additional inflammatory cytokines, along with adhesion molecules that promote endothelial dysfunction and downstream modulate specific MS [60]. TNFα induces oxidative stress, which leads to oxidized low-density lipoprotein and triggers dyslipidemia, insulin resistance, hypertension, endothelial dysfunction, and atherogenesis. Oxidative stress levels are elevated in obesity correlated with fat accumulation. Overall, serum concentrations of TNFα and IL-6 were significantly correlated with weight, BMI, and visceral adipose tissue [61], which are important pathogenic mechanisms of obesity-associated MS.

The innate immune system activation in adipose tissue promotes an increase in the production and release of proinflammatory cytokines that contributes to the triggering of the systemic acute-phase response, which is characterized by the elevation of acute-phase protein levels [62]. The PPARγ co-activator 1α plays a key role in regulating mitochondrial biogenesis and energy homeostasis. Overexpression favored a shift from incomplete to complete beta-oxidation and enables muscle mitochondria to better cope with a high lipid load [63]. These reflecting a fundamental metabolic benefit of exercise training and upregulation of PPARγ co-activator 1α may as an effective strategy for preventing insulin resistance or obesity. Host inflammation response mechanisms are largely shared by the body's different tissues. Recently, special attention has been paid to the possible linkages among chronic periodontitis and other chronic systemic diseases [64].

Adipose tissue inflammation was proposed as a central mechanism connecting obesity with MS and complications such as T2D, arterial hypertension, and ischemic heart disease [65]. Accumulating evidence indicates that the obese state is characterized by chronic low-grade inflammation. Fat tissue releases numerous bioactive molecules, such as adipokines that affect whole-body homeostasis. The deregulated production of adipokines seen in obesity is linked to the pathogenesis of various disease processes [66]. It was suggested that systemic autophagy insufficiency could be a factor in the progression from obesity to diabetes, and autophagy modulators have therapeutic potential against diabetes associated with obesity and inflammation [67].

CLA has been reported to increase voluntary activities in mice. CLA acts as a potential exercise mimetic, resulting in increased voluntary activity and improving muscle metabolisms in both normal and obese animals [68]. The anti-inflammatory activity of fucoxanthin was confirmed by significantly increased IL-10 and decreased TNF-α production. The combination of the antioxidants had more antioxidant and anti-inflammatory effects than when they were applied alone [69], and may via the Nrf2-mediated pathway [70]. Figure 5.6 shows the effects of fucoxanthin on body weights [71]. Supplementation of fucoxanthin is a promising strategy for blocking macrophage-mediated inflammation and inflammation-induced obesity and its associated complications. *Sargassum polycystum* powder treatment also had a positive effect on the inhibition of weight gain and shows a promising value in preventing obesity [72].

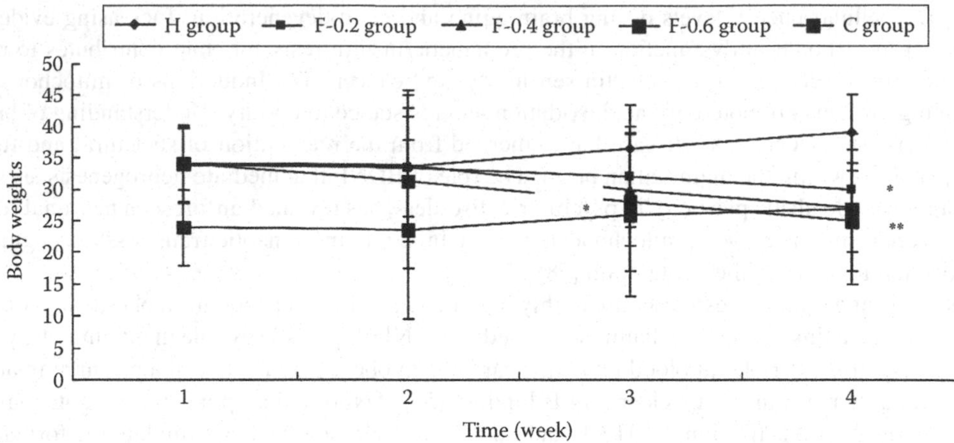

FIGURE 5.6 Effects of fucoxanthin on body weights of mice. Values are shown as means ± SEM. *P < 0.05 vs. H group, **P < 0.01 vs. H group. (Adapted from Tan, C. and Hou, Y.-H., *Inflammation*, 37(2), 443, 2014. With permission.)

5.4 BRAIN FUNCTION CROSS TALK BETWEEN ADIPOSITY AND ENDOCRINE

5.4.1 Adipokine Endocrinology

Adipocytes act not only as a fuel storage depot but also as a critical endocrine organ that secretes a variety of signaling molecules into the circulation. Adipocytes serve also as an important source of proinflammatory molecules, including leptin, TNFα, and IL-6, as well as anti-inflammatory molecules. A number of adipokines, including IL-1β, IL-6, MCP-1, MIF, TNFα, leptin, and adiponectin, are somehow linked to the inflammatory response. A high leptin concentration, in particular, is found in obese individuals and is strongly associated with vascular changes related to early atherosclerosis [73]. The adipokine resistin displays potent proinflammatory properties by strongly upregulating IL-6 and TNFα, which were abrogated by NFκB inhibitor. An increasing number of researchers of the MS assume that many mechanisms are involved in the impact of complex pathophysiology of neurotrophins, such as disorders of the HPG axis, the chronic subclinical infections, proinflammatory cytokines, the effect of adipocytokines, and/or psychoemotional stress. Its potential role in the control of obesity was recently acknowledged [74].

Adipose tissue apoE expression is distinct from circulating apoE, on systemic substrate metabolism and adipose tissue inflammatory state. ApoE is highly expressed in adipose tissue where it is important for modulating adipocyte lipid flux and gene expression in isolated adipocytes. Adipocyte triglyceride synthesis in the presence of apoE-containing was markedly impaired. Adipose tissue macrophage inflammatory activation was markedly diminished with suppression of adipose tissue apoE expression [75]. One good example, the CLA performed as an antioxidant, promotes at least in part, NFκB activation and subsequent induction of IL-6, which are partly responsible for suppression of PPARγ target gene expression and insulin sensitivity in mature human adipocytes [76].

5.4.2 Cognitive Impairment and Intestinal Microbiome

Aging-associated cellular processes such as oxidative stress and inflammation are accelerated in obesity. Aging has been implicated to alter leptin and insulin sensitivity in rodents [77]. Weight loss is strongly associated with PD and impacts symptoms and disease progression. An inverse relation was revealed between change in body weight and physical activity level [78]. Meta-analysis showed that overweight might be a potential risk factor of PD. A causal role of overweight/obesity in PD development could have important therapeutic implications [79,80], see Figure 5.7. MS is also associated with both schizophrenia and antipsychotic medication. Both cytokine and adipokine alterations in patients with schizophrenia treated with clozapine were reported [81]. Clozapine-induced hyperglycemia and insulin resistance occur in a manner mostly independent of weight gain and may be due to an increase in hepatic phosphorylase activity and increased key enzyme expression level of G6Pase [82].

In addition to the traditional etiological pathways, the role of the intestinal microbiome in cognitive function has been suggested and warrants further investigation [83,84]. Chronic functional bowel syndrome enhances gut–brain axis dysfunction, neuroinflammation, and cognitive impairment, and vulnerability to dementia has been confirmed [85]. Pathogenic gut microbiota-related systemic inflammation may trigger neuroinflammation, enhancing dysfunctional brain regions including hippocampus and cerebellum.

5.4.3 Obesity and Infertility: HPG axis, Kisspeptin, and Sex Hormone

Reproduction is sensitive to body energy situation; the increasing prevalence of obesity and the clinical evidence on male fertility (spermatogenesis) have raised considerable concerns. Conditions of low leptin levels observed in negative energy balance and mutations of leptin or leptin receptor genes are characterized by decreased fertility. Nutritional stress, especially HFD, has a profound deleterious impact on metabolic and gonadotropic function as well as neuroendocrine reproductive senescence in the male [86]. The kisspeptin regulates reproduction by stimulating GnRH neurons via the kisspeptin receptor GPR54. It was also confirmed that impaired kisspeptin signaling decreases metabolism and promotes glucose intolerance and obesity [87]. In addition to reproduction, kisspeptin signaling influences BW, energy expenditure, and glucose homeostasis in a partially sex steroid independent manner. It was revealed that alterations in kisspeptin signaling might contribute, directly or indirectly, to obesity, diabetes, or metabolic dysfunction.

Obesity-related factors may contribute to the process of reproductive dysfunction via the dysregulation/damage of the epigenetic machinery. The obesity-induced microenvironment may influence gene expression levels. The activities of the different enzymes have been implicated in epigenetic control to induce changes in DNA methylation, posttranslational histone modifications, and non-coding RNAs expression. These epigenetic dysregulations/modification can change the activities of several genes that are involved in the reproductive pathways. The effect of obesity-related factors on reproduction is shown in Figure 5.8. Both obesity and overweight are significantly involved in several reproductive pathologies contributing to infertility in men and women. Epidemiological studies demonstrate that factors secreted by the adipose tissue and gut in an obesity state can directly induce reproductive disturbances [88].

Increased leptin does not cross brain BBB because of transport system eventually affecting HPG axis and altering sex hormone levels in obese infertile males. It may negatively influence Leydig cell testosterone synthesis by inhibiting the conversion of 17OH progesterone into testosterone. Leptin acts on epithelial cells of the accessory male genital glands directly and on the spermatozoa via spermatozoa leptin receptors. Adipocytes release various adipocytokines, as shown in Figure 5.9. Cytokines by increasing ROS may affect DNA integrity in spermatozoa, resulting in poor pregnancy outcome, and are capable of reducing ova-penetrating ability of spermatozoa [89].

The adipocyte-derived hormone leptin, as a key hormone in energy homeostasis, regulates neuroendocrine function, also including reproduction. It has a permissive role in the initiation of puberty and maintenance of the HPG axis [90], see Figure 5.10. Leptin stimulates POMC/CART neurons

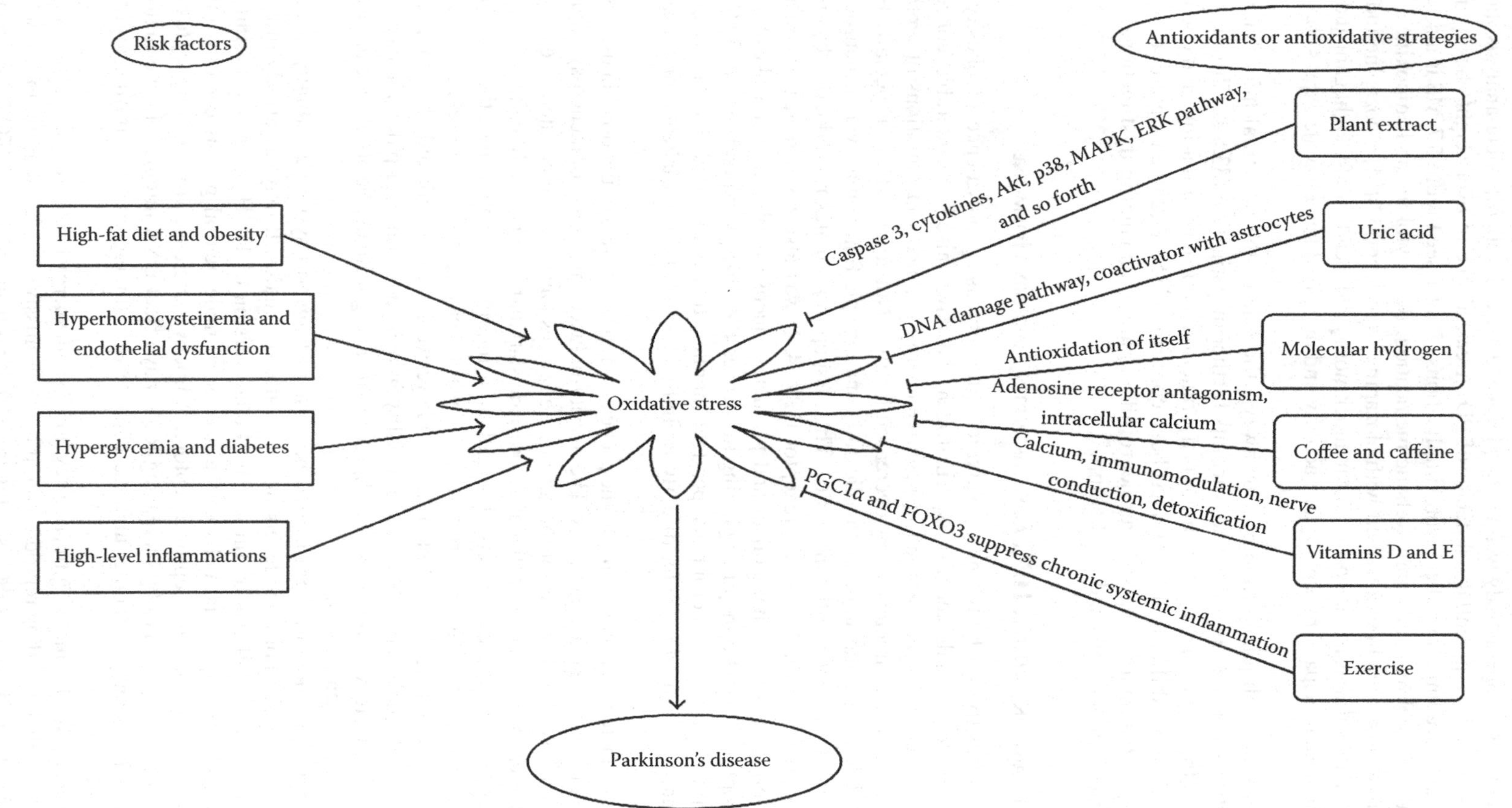

FIGURE 5.7 Summary of this review about oxidative stress and Parkinson's disease. (Adapted from Zhang, P. and Tian, B., *Oxidat. Med. Cell. Long.*, 2014, 729194, 2014. With permission.)

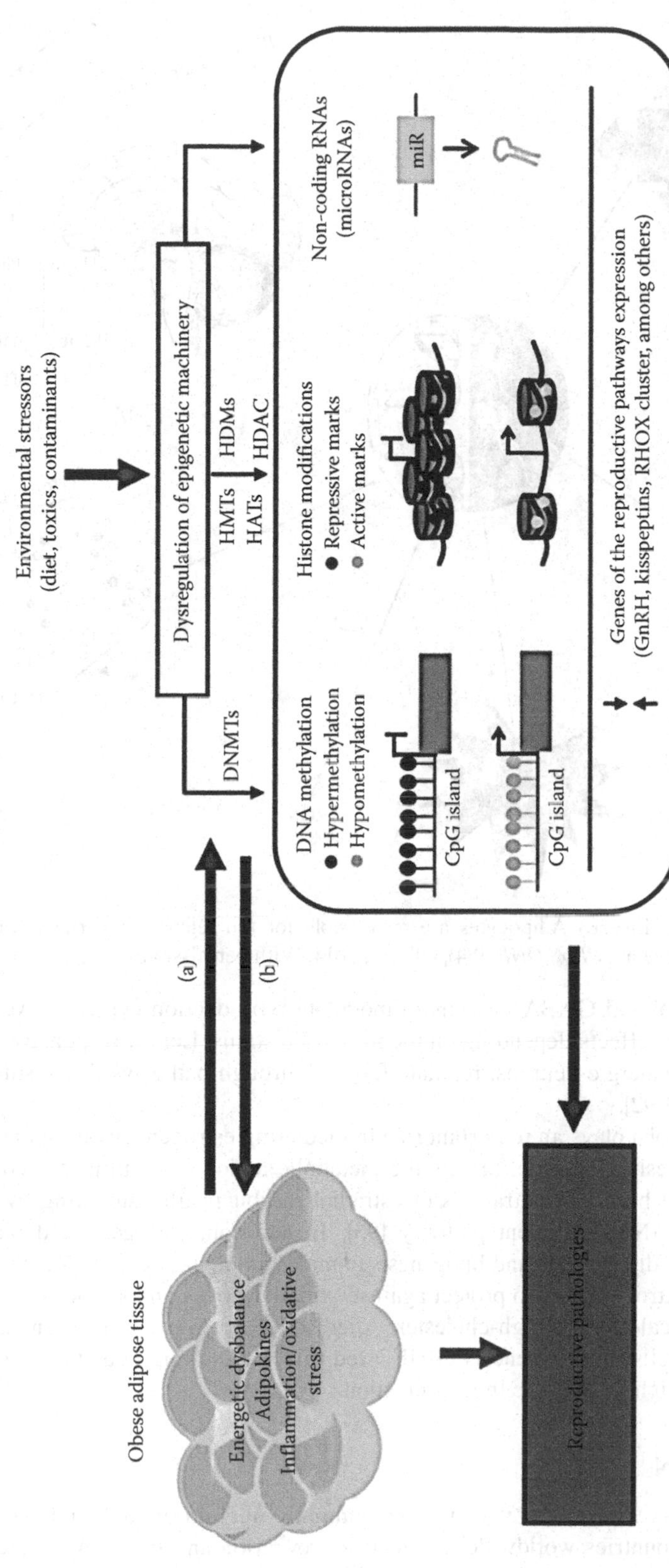

FIGURE 5.8 Effects of obesity-related factors on reproductive pathologies. (Adapted from Crujeiras, A.B. and Casanueva, F.F., *Hum. Reprod.*, 21, 249, 2015. With permission.)

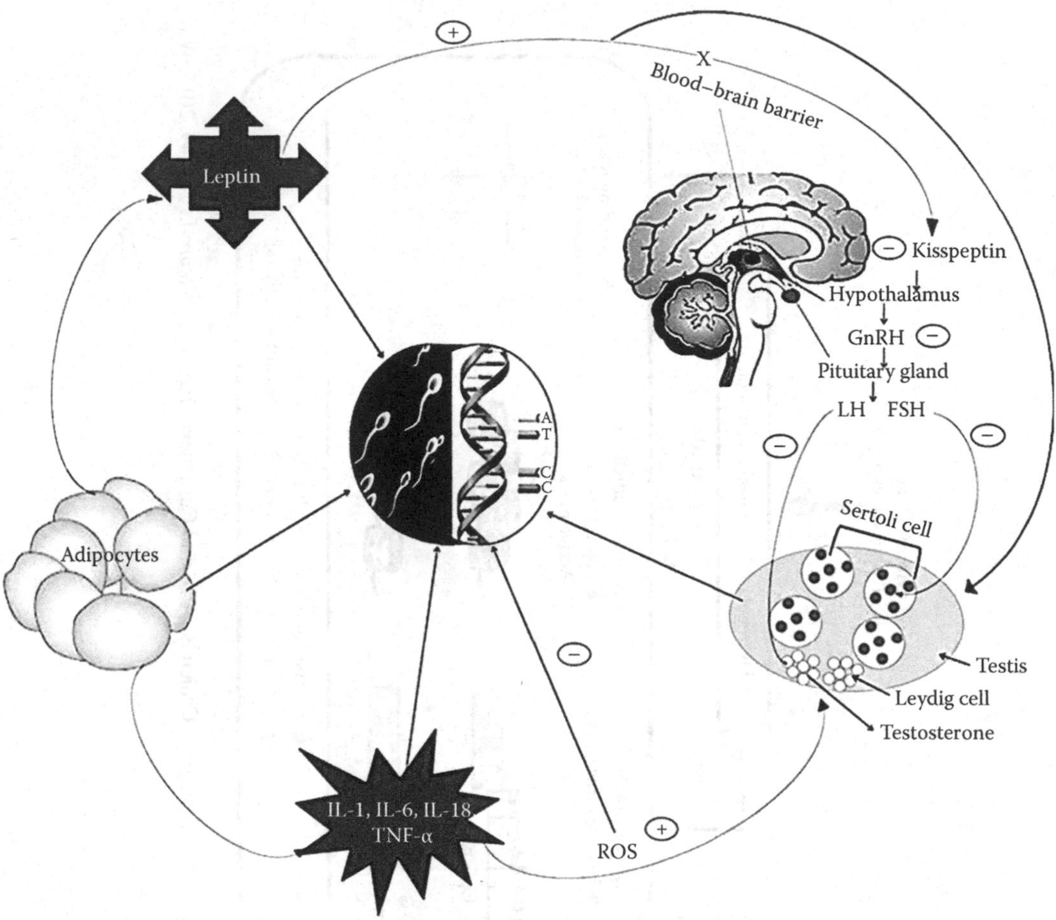

FIGURE 5.9 **(See color insert.)** Adipocytes are responsible for the release of various adipocytokines. (Adapted from Shukla, A. et al., *PLoS ONE*, 9(4), e94433, 2014. With permission.)

and inhibits AgRP/NPY and GABA neurons to modulate reproduction centrally. At the ovaries, leptin can have different effects depending on the metabolic status. Leptin-responsive GABAergic neurons, but not glutamatergic neurons, regulate fertility through pathways that result in reduced kisspeptinergic tone [91,92].

Estrogen receptor alpha plays an important role in mediating estrogen signaling and is involved in osteoporosis and obesity. Estradiol affects the metabolic action of insulin in a concentration-dependent manner, and high concentrations of estradiol inhibit insulin signaling by modulating phosphorylation via a JNK-dependent pathway [93]. In addition, estrogens and phytoestrogen genistein also regulate adipogenesis and lipogenesis in males and females [94]. Recent studies have also shown that resveratrol appears to protect against oxidative stress and steroidogenesis collapse in mice fed with high-calorie and high-cholesterol diet [95]. Resveratrol may attenuate detrimental effects on Leydig cells steroidogenesis in HFD-fed mice, and its upregulations of antioxidant defense mechanisms might play a role in its protection.

5.5 CONCLUSION

The proportion of adults with a BMI increased substantially in children and adolescents in developed and developing countries worldwidely. Effective prevention and treatment strategies toward enormous medical implications of obesity are still lacking. Aging (oxidative stress, epigenetic

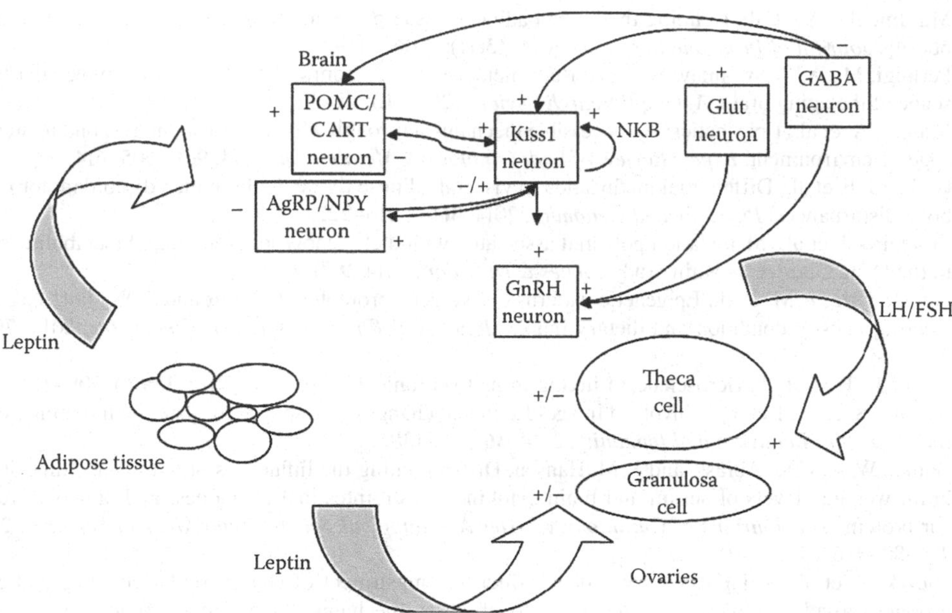

FIGURE 5.10 Schematic illustration of the interactions of leptin with the hypothalamic–pituitary–gonadal axis. (Adapted from Chou, S.H. and Mantzoros, C., *J. Endocrinol.*, 223(1), T49, 2014. With permission.)

modification, and eventually dysfunction) or hypertrophy (overweight or obese), or EDCs exposure (deregulated endocrine function) is associated with increased different adipokines profile, which are linked to a higher risk for insulin resistance, CVD, DM, infertility as well as neurodegenerative diseases. Here, we propose that obese tissue may get activated via cell–cell interaction due to sustained cell proliferation and size enlargement, which triggers progressive mitochondria stress, then inflammation, proinflammatory cytokines, and related adipokine secreting from adipocyte. These complicated mechanisms are involved in immune response, gut microbiome, gene expression, intracellular signal transduction, as well as the interplay between neuroendocrine and adipocytokines.

Finally, a new approach to this problem may be a calorie restriction/low glycemic index/low fat/high dietary fiber and enriched antioxidants diet; this has a salutary effect on insulin level after a meal. It may be a practical and safe approach in the prevention and treatment of obesity and related complications. From the viewpoint of dietary factors in promoting healthy lifestyle, a new prospect of suitable regulating neuroendocrine in obesity will be one important consideration. Hereby, any bioactive ingredient can prevent or ameliorate obesity-induced diseases; for public health benefit, we may suggest it as a health beneficial dietary supplement.

REFERENCES

1. Sweeting, H., Measurement and definitions of obesity in childhood and adolescence: A field guide for the uninitiated. *Nutrition Journal*, 2007. **6**(1): 32–38.
2. Myint, P.K. et al., Body fat percentage, body mass index and waist-to-hip ratio as predictors of mortality and cardiovascular disease. *Heart*, 2014. 100: 1613–1619.
3. Ogden, C.L. et al., Prevalence of childhood and adult obesity in the united states, 2011–2012. *JAMA*, 2014. **311**(8): 806–814.
4. Cunningham, S.A., M.R. Kramer, and K.M.V. Narayan, Incidence of childhood obesity in the United States. *New England Journal of Medicine*, 2014. **370**(5): 403–411.
5. Ng, M. et al., Global, regional, and national prevalence of overweight and obesity in children and adults during 1980–2013: A systematic analysis for the Global Burden of Disease Study 2013. *The Lancet*, 2014. **384**(9945): 766–781.

6. Mardinoglu, A. et al., Defining the human adipose tissue proteome to reveal metabolic alterations in obesity. *Journal of Proteome Research*, 2014. **13**(11): 5106–5119.
7. Perluigi, M., A.M. Swomley, and D.A. Butterfield, Redox proteomics and the dynamic molecular landscape of the aging brain. *Ageing Research Reviews*, 2014. **13**: 75–89.
8. Majnik, A. et al., Epigenetics: An accessible mechanism through which to track and respond to an obesogenic environment. *Expert Review of Endocrinology & Metabolism*, 2014. **9**(6): 605–614.
9. Guénard, F. et al., Differential methylation in visceral adipose tissue of obese men discordant for metabolic disturbances. *Physiological Genomics*, 2014. **46**(6): 216–222.
10. Monteiro, J. et al., Methylation potential associated with diet, genotype, protein, and metabolite levels in the Delta Obesity Vitamin Study. *Genes & Nutrition*, 2014. **9**(3): 1–19.
11. Gómez-Uriz, A.M. et al., Epigenetic patterns of two gene promoters (TNF-α and PON) in stroke considering obesity condition and dietary intake. *Journal of Physiology and Biochemistry*, 2014. **70**(2): 603–614.
12. Kennedy, B.K. et al., Geroscience: Linking aging to chronic disease. *Cell*, 2014. **159**(4): 709–713.
13. Koenig, S. et al., Leptin is involved in age-dependent changes in response to systemic inflammation in the rat. *Brain, Behavior, and Immunity*, 2014. **36**: 128–138.
14. Banks, W.A., C.K. Abrass, and K.M. Hansen, Differentiating the influences of aging and adiposity on brain weights, levels of serum and brain cytokines, gastrointestinal hormones, and amyloid precursor protein. *The Journals of Gerontology Series A: Biological Sciences and Medical Sciences*, 2014: 476380–476387.
15. Tucsek, Z. et al., Aging exacerbates obesity-induced impairment of neurovascular coupling and cerebromicrovascular rarefaction: Implications for the pathomechanism of vascular cognitive impairment (665.2). *The FASEB Journal*, 2014. **28**(1 Suppl.).
16. Giblin, W., M.E. Skinner, and D.B. Lombard, Sirtuins: Guardians of mammalian healthspan. *Trends in Genetics*, 2014. **30**(7): 271–286.
17. Testa, G. et al., Calorie restriction and dietary restriction mimetics: A strategy for improving healthy aging and longevity. *Current Pharmaceutical Design*, 2014. **20**(18): 2950–2977.
18. Bodzsar, E.B. and A. Zsakai, Recent trends in childhood obesity and overweight in the transition countries of Eastern and Central Europe. *Annals of Human Biology*, 2014. **41**(3): 263–270.
19. Shukla, A., K. Kumar, and A. Singh, Association between obesity and selected morbidities: A study of BRICS countries. *PLoS ONE*, 2014. **9**(4): e94433.
20. Du, S.F. et al., China in the period of transition from scarcity and extensive under nutrition to emerging nutrition-related non-communicable diseases, 1949–1992. *Obesity Reviews*, 2014. **15**: 8–15.
21. Whaley, P., Childhood obesity and the environment, in *Controversies in Obesity*, D.W. Haslam, A.M. Sharma, and C.W. le Roux (eds.), Springer, London, U.K., 2014, pp. 97–102.
22. Gaissert, C., K. Subramany, and B. Sampoli Benitez, Can bisphenol-A migrating from canned food contribute to the obesity epidemic? (959.10). *The FASEB Journal*, 2014. **28**(1 Suppl.).
23. Simmons, A., J. Schlezinger, and B. Corkey, What are we putting in our food that is making us fat? Food additives, contaminants, and other putative contributors to obesity. *Current Obesity Reports*, 2014. **3**(2): 273–285.
24. Romano, M., D. Savitz, and J. Braun, Challenges and future directions to evaluating the association between prenatal exposure to endocrine-disrupting chemicals and childhood obesity. *Current Epidemiology Reports*, 2014. **1**(2): 57–66.
25. Chamorro-García, R. and B. Blumberg, Transgenerational effects of obesogens and the obesity epidemic. *Current Opinion in Pharmacology*, 2014. **19**(0): 153–158.
26. Lee, D.-H. et al., Chlorinated persistent organic pollutants, obesity, and type 2 diabetes. *Endocrine Reviews*, 2014. **35**(4): 557–601.
27. Emanuela, F. et al., Inflammation as a link between obesity and metabolic syndrome. *Journal of Nutrition and Metabolism*, 2012, 476–380.
28. Vigilanza, P. et al., Modulation of intracellular glutathione affects adipogenesis in 3T3-L1 cells. *Journal of Cellular Physiology*, 2011. **226**(8): 2016–2024.
29. Griffin, M.J. et al., Early B-cell Factor-1 (EBF1) is a key regulator of metabolic and inflammatory signaling pathways in mature adipocytes. *Journal of Biological Chemistry*, 2013. **288**(50): 35925–35939.
30. Vigouroux, C. et al., Molecular mechanisms of human lipodystrophies: From adipocyte lipid droplet to oxidative stress and lipotoxicity. *The International Journal of Biochemistry & Cell Biology*, 2011. **43**(6): 862–876.
31. Sun, C. et al., Effects of early-life environment and epigenetics on cardiovascular disease risk in children: Highlighting the role of twin studies. *Pediatric Research*, 2013. **73**(4–2): 523–530.

32. Katsuda, Y. et al., Diabetic complications in obese type 2 diabetic rat models. *Experimental Animals*, 2014. **63**(2): 121–132.
33. Sala, M. et al., Microstructural brain tissue damage in metabolic syndrome. *Diabetes Care*, 2014. **37**(2): 493–500.
34. Tang, Y., S. Purkayastha, and D. Cai, Hypothalamic microinflammation: A common basis of metabolic syndrome and aging. *Trends in Neurosciences*, 2015. **38**(1): 36–44.
35. Lee, I.T. et al., Brain-derived neurotrophic factor, but not body weight, correlated with a reduction in depression scale scores in men with metabolic syndrome: A prospective weight-reduction study. *Diabetology & Metabolic Syndrome*, 2014. **6**(1): 1–7.
36. Albano, N.J. et al., Abstract 146: Diet-induced obesity results in lymphatic dysfunction and impaired T cell function. *Plastic and Reconstructive Surgery*, 2014. **133**(3S): 161–162.
37. Yang, S. et al., The E3 ubiquitin ligase Pellino3 protects against obesity-induced inflammation and insulin resistance. *Immunity*, 2014. **41**(6): 973–987.
38. Paragh, G. et al., Dynamic interplay between metabolic syndrome and immunity, in *Oxidative Stress and Inflammation in Non-communicable Diseases—Molecular Mechanisms and Perspectives in Therapeutics*, J. Camps (ed.), Springer International Publishing, Switzerland, 2014, pp. 171–190.
39. Hajishengallis, G., Aging and its impact on innate immunity and inflammation: Implications for periodontitis. *Journal of Oral Biosciences*, 2014. **56**(1): 30–37.
40. Shekarabi, M. and F. Asgari, Aging immunity and infection, in *Immunology of Aging*, A. Massoud and N. Rezaei (eds.), Springer, Berlin, Germany, 2014, pp. 231–238.
41. McNelis, J.C. and J.M. Olefsky, Macrophages, immunity, and metabolic disease. *Immunity*, 2014. **41**(1): 36–48.
42. Kraakman, M.J. et al., Macrophage polarization in obesity and type 2 diabetes: Weighing down our understanding of macrophage function? *Frontiers in Immunology*, 2014. **5**: 470–476.
43. Exley, M.A. et al., Interplay between the immune system and adipose tissue in obesity. *Journal of Endocrinology*, 2014. **223**(2): R41–R48.
44. Hu, X. et al., Microglial and macrophage polarization—New prospects for brain repair. *Nature Reviews Neurology*, 2015. 11: 56–64.
45. Corraliza, I., Recruiting specialized macrophages across the borders to restore brain functions. *Frontiers in Cellular Neuroscience*, 2014. **8**: 262.
46. Teague, H., M. Harris, and S. Shaikh, EPA and DHA increase the frequency of murine B cell subsets and restore antibody production in obesity upon stimulation with a T-independent antigen (382.5). *The FASEB Journal*, 2014. **28**(1 Suppl.).
47. Karumuthil-Melethil, S. et al., Fungal β-glucan, a Dectin-1 ligand, promotes protection from type 1 diabetes by inducing regulatory innate immune response. *The Journal of Immunology*, 2014. **193**(7): 3308–3321.
48. Dong, J.-L. et al., Effect of oat soluble and insoluble β-glucan on lipid metabolism and intestina lactobacillus in high-fat diet-induced obese mice. *Journal of Food and Nutrition Research*, 2014. **2**(8): 510–516.
49. Aoe, S. et al., Effect of cooked white rice with high β-glucan barley on appetite and energy intake in healthy Japanese subjects: A randomized controlled trial. *Plant Foods for Human Nutrition*, 2014. **69**(4): 325–330.
50. Zhao, L. et al., Gamma-tocotrienol attenuates high-fat diet-induced obesity and insulin resistance by inhibiting adipose inflammation and M1 macrophage recruitment. *International Journal of Obesity*, 2015. 39: 438–446.
51. Babaev, V.R. et al., Macrophage mall deficiency suppresses atherosclerosis in low-density lipoprotein receptor–null mice by activating peroxisome proliferator-activated receptor-γ-regulated genes. *Arteriosclerosis, Thrombosis, and Vascular Biology*, 2011. **31**(6): 1283–1290.
52. Lynch, L., Adipose invariant natural killer T cells. *Immunology*, 2014. **142**(3): 337–346.
53. Winkels, H. et al., Atherosclerosis: Cell biology and lipoproteins focus on iNKT cells and CD40/CD40L in atherosclerosis and metabolic disorders. *Current Opinion in Lipidology*, 2014. **25**(5): 408–409.
54. Venken, K. et al., A bidirectional crosstalk between iNKT cells and adipocytes mediated by leptin modulates susceptibility for T cell mediated hepatitis. *Journal of Hepatology*, 2014. **60**(1): 175–182.
55. Lynch, L. et al., Regulatory iNKT cells lack expression of the transcription factor PLZF and control the homeostasis of Treg cells and macrophages in adipose tissue. *Nature Immunology*, 2015. **16**(1): 85–95.
56. Yin, F., A. Boveris, and E. Cadenas, Mitochondrial energy metabolism and redox signaling in brain aging and neurodegeneration. *Antioxidants & Redox Signaling*, 2014. **20**(2): 353–371.
57. Sadler, N.C. et al., Activity-based protein profiling reveals mitochondrial oxidative enzyme impairment and restoration in diet-induced obese mice. *PLoS ONE*, 2012. **7**(10): e47996.

58. Picard, M. and B.S. McEwen, Mitochondria impact brain function and cognition. *Proceedings of the National Academy of Sciences*, 2014. **111**(1): 7–8.
59. Dandona, P. et al., Insulin suppresses the expression of amyloid precursor protein, presenilins, and glycogen synthase kinase-3β in peripheral blood mononuclear cells. *The Journal of Clinical Endocrinology & Metabolism*, 2011. **96**(6): 1783–1788.
60. Ikeda, R. et al., Brazilian propolis-derived components inhibit TNF-α-mediated downregulation of adiponectin expression via different mechanisms in 3T3-L1 adipocytes. *Biochimica et Biophysica Acta (BBA)—General Subjects*, 2011. **1810**(7): 695–703.
61. Lasselin, J. et al., Adipose inflammation in obesity: Relationship with circulating levels of inflammatory markers and association with surgery-induced weight loss. *The Journal of Clinical Endocrinology & Metabolism*, 2013. **99**(1): E53–E61.
62. Rodríguez-Hernández, H. et al., Obesity and inflammation: Epidemiology, risk factors, and markers of inflammation. *International Journal of Endocrinology*, 2013. **2013**: 11.
63. Ouchi, N. et al., Adipokines in inflammation and metabolic disease. *Nature Reviews Immunology*, 2011. **11**(2): 85–97.
64. Bullon, P., H.N. Newman, and M. Battino, Obesity, diabetes mellitus, atherosclerosis and chronic periodontitis: A shared pathology via oxidative stress and mitochondrial dysfunction? *Periodontology*, 2000, 2014. **64**(1): 139–153.
65. Mraz, M. and M. Haluzik, The role of adipose tissue immune cells in obesity and low-grade inflammation. *Journal of Endocrinology*, 2014. **222**(3): R113–R127.
66. Ohashi, K. et al., Role of anti-inflammatory adipokines in obesity-related diseases. *Trends in Endocrinology & Metabolism*, 2014. **25**(7): 348–355.
67. Lim, Y.-M. et al., Systemic autophagy insufficiency compromises adaptation to metabolic stress and facilitates progression from obesity to diabetes. *Nature Communications*, 2014. **5**: 4934.
68. Kim, Y. et al., Molecular mechanisms of conjugated linoleic acid (CLA) on muscle metabolism in adult onset inactivity-induced obese mice (1045.46). *The FASEB Journal*, 2014. **28**(1 Suppl.).
69. Molina, N. et al., Comparative effect of fucoxanthin and vitamin C on oxidative and functional parameters of human lymphocytes. *International Immunopharmacology*, 2014. **22**(1): 41–50.
70. Zheng, J. et al., Fucoxanthin enhances the level of reduced glutathione via the Nrf2-mediated pathway in human keratinocytes. *Marine Drugs*, 2014. **12**(7): 4214–4230.
71. Tan, C. and Y.-H. Hou, First evidence for the anti-inflammatory activity of fucoxanthin in high-fat-diet-induced obesity in mice and the antioxidant functions in PC12 cells. *Inflammation*, 2014. **37**(2): 443–450.
72. Awang, A. et al., Anti-obesity property of the brown seaweed, *Sargassum polycystum* using an in vivo animal model. *Journal of Applied Phycology*, 2014. **26**(2): 1043–1048.
73. Blüher, M., Adipose tissue dysfunction contributes to obesity related metabolic diseases. *Best Practice & Research Clinical Endocrinology & Metabolism*, 2013. **27**(2): 163–177.
74. Enciu, A.-M., M. Gherghiceanu, and B.O. Popescu, Triggers and effectors of oxidative stress at blood–brain barrier level: Relevance for brain ageing and neurodegeneration. *Oxidative Medicine and Cellular Longevity*, 2013. **2013**: 297512.
75. Huang, Z.H. et al., Selective suppression of adipose tissue ApoE expression impacts systemic metabolic phenotype and adipose tissue inflammation. *Journal of Lipid Research*, 2015. **56**(2): 215–226.
76. Maria, P.M.-G., R. Tamas, and R. Mercedes, Biology and therapeutic applications of peroxisome proliferator-activated receptors. *Current Topics in Medicinal Chemistry*, 2012. **12**(6): 548–584.
77. Filippi, B.M. and T.K.T. Lam, *Leptin and aging. Aging* (Albany, NY), 2014. **6**(2): 82–83.
78. Vikdahl, M. et al., Weight gain and increased central obesity in the early phase of Parkinson's disease. *Clinical Nutrition*, 2014. **33**(6): 1132–1139.
79. Chen, J. et al., Meta-analysis: Overweight, obesity, and Parkinson's disease. *International Journal of Endocrinology*, 2014. **2014**: 7.
80. Zhang, P. and B. Tian, Metabolic syndrome: An important risk factor for Parkinson's disease. *Oxidative Medicine and Cellular Longevity*, 2014. **2014**: 729194–729201.
81. Klemettilä, J.-P. et al., Cytokine and adipokine alterations in patients with schizophrenia treated with clozapine. *Psychiatry Research*, 2014. **218**(3): 277–283.
82. El-Seweidy, M.M. et al., Chronic effects of clozapine administration on insulin resistance in rats: Evidence for adverse metabolic effects. *Pathology—Research and Practice*, 2014. **210**(1): 5–9.
83. Caracciolo, B. et al., Cognitive decline, dietary factors and gut–brain interactions. *Mechanisms of Ageing and Development*, 2014. **136–137**: 59–69.
84. Rusinek, H. and A. Convit, Obesity: Cerebral damage in obesity-associated metabolic syndrome. *Nature Reviews Endocrinology*, 2014. **10**(11): 642–644.

85. Daulatzai, M., Chronic functional bowel syndrome enhances gut–brain axis dysfunction, neuroinflammation, cognitive impairment, and vulnerability to dementia. *Neurochemical Research*, 2014. **39**(4): 624–644.
86. Sánchez-Garrido, M.A. et al., Obesity-induced hypogonadism in the male: Premature reproductive neuroendocrine senescence and contribution of kiss1-mediated mechanisms. *Endocrinology*, 2014. **155**(3): 1067–1079.
87. Tolson, K.P. et al., Impaired kisspeptin signaling decreases metabolism and promotes glucose intolerance and obesity. *The Journal of Clinical Investigation*, 2014. **124**(7): 3075–3079.
88. Crujeiras, A.B. and F.F. Casanueva, Obesity and the reproductive system disorders: Epigenetics as a potential bridge. *Human Reproduction Update*, 2014.
89. Shukla, K.K. et al., Recent scenario of obesity and male fertility. *Andrology*, 2014. **2**(6): 809–818.
90. Chou, S.H. and C. Mantzoros, 20 years of leptin: Role of leptin in human reproductive disorders. *Journal of Endocrinology*, 2014. **223**(1): T49–T62.
91. Martin, C. et al., Leptin-responsive GABAergic neurons regulate fertility through pathways that result in reduced kisspeptinergic tone. *The Journal of Neuroscience*, 2014. **34**(17): 6047–6056.
92. Ratra, D.V. and C.F. Elias, Chemical identity of hypothalamic neurons engaged by leptin in reproductive control. *Journal of Chemical Neuroanatomy*, 2014. **61–62**: 233–238.
93. Nagira, K. et al., Altered subcellular distribution of estrogen receptor α is implicated in estradiol-induced dual regulation of insulin signaling in 3T3-L1 adipocytes. *Endocrinology*, 2006. **147**(2): 1020–1028.
94. Behloul, N. and G. Wu, Genistein: A promising therapeutic agent for obesity and diabetes treatment. *European Journal of Pharmacology*, 2013. **698**(1–3): 31–38.
95. Wang, H.J. et al., Resveratrol appears to protect against oxidative stress and steroidogenesis collapse in mice fed high-calorie and high-cholesterol diet. *Andrologia*, 2015. **47**(1): 59–65.

6 Health Effects and Weight Loss Benefits of Calorie Restriction Dietary Regimens

Eric Gumpricht and Krista Varady

CONTENTS

6.1 INTRODUCTION

Since the seminal rat studies by Clive McCay at Cornell University in the 1930s, scientists have reported life span extension and amelioration of age-associated pathologies by calorie restriction (CR) (McCay et al. 1935). Similar CR benefits have also been expanded to nonhuman primates in some (Colman et al. 2014; Weindruch and Walford 1982), but not all studies (Mattison et al. 2012). These promising results from laboratory animals are now targeting CR regimens as a strategic dietary option for safe and effective weight loss and cardiometabolic improvement in humans. The relevance of examining potential benefits of CR in humans is twofold: (1) public health statistics reveal that approximately 35% of American adults are classified as obese (Ogden et al. 2014) with a similar number classified as overweight, and (2) the potential benefits of CR have been most studied and best characterized in subjects with one or more metabolic dysfunctions associated with an increased risk for developing cardiovascular disease.

CR may be defined as a reduction of energy intake of 10%–50% of baseline energy requirements with adequate provision of essential nutrients. Some clinical studies have designed CR dietary regimens based upon the reduction of a specific number of calories (such as a 500 kcal deficit/day), whereas others target caloric goals as a percentage of restricted intake (frequently 20%–25%). Much of the information gathered on clinical, biochemical, and physiological effects of CR has been obtained from an increasing number of intervention studies including Comprehensive Assessment of the Long-term Effects of Reducing Intake of Energy (CALERIE), a multicenter research program funded by National Institutes of Aging to evaluate CR in a nonobese population. Other studies are prospective in nature with data obtained from individuals undergoing self-imposed CR (Fontana et al. 2004) or through controlled, albeit unintentional, decreases in food availability such as experienced by subjects in the Biosphere 2 experiment. Overall, results from both these study designs indicate that CR interventions may improve biomarkers associated with increased risk for cardiovascular disease, especially in obese individuals (Sung and Dyck 2012).

Despite promising results, several obstacles exist for CR prior to any recommendation or endorsement for weight loss or modification of cardiometabolic status. First, the safety of long-term adherence to CR regimens is not clearly established due to obvious logistic and economic limitations inherent in conducting randomized, long-term, strict dietary-enforced studies. Also, it is unclear if these dietary approaches are beneficial or indeed harmful under specific diseases or practiced in certain populations. Finally, while CR is effective for weight loss in some individuals, many people find this type of dieting difficult as it requires vigilant and daily calorie considerations (Das et al. 2007), increased frustration with daily dietary limitations, and consequently, poor adherence in free-living subjects. Unfortunately, these limitations make traditional CR rather impractical as a long-term and feasible strategy for weight loss, weight maintenance, and reduced cardiovascular risk modification for the large number of individuals.

Due to limitations inherent in traditional CR, several laboratories have modified and proposed alternative CR regimens to overcome obstacles of adherence and improve suitability for real-world compliance. One alternative strategy is intermittent fasting (IF). From an historical and scientific perspective, a relatively obscure publication using laboratory rats merits special acknowledgment: Carlson and Hoelzel (1946) for considering the feasibility and health benefits of IF noted "a general improvement following intermittent fasting seemed equal to that following less prolonged fasts." Moreover, they hypothesized that a more realistic method of CR in humans would be equivalent to an IF intervention. IF also has a long history of practice by various religions including Muslims during Ramadan, where followers abstain from food or water from 12 to 14 h/day over the religion's holy month (see Lam and Ravussin 2014; Trepanowski et al. 2011, for excellent overviews of IF and religious adherents). In contrast to the daily restriction of calories required by CR, IF offers the individual more flexibility by restricting calorie intake only 1–2 days/week with the remaining days allowing for *ad libitum* consumption. Furthermore, depending on the desired goal of IF, this strategy need not result in a reduction in caloric intake. A third CR regimen currently investigated for promoting weight loss and improving cardiovascular disease risk factors is alternate-day fasting (ADF). Perhaps the first study to clinically investigate ADF was initiated by the Spanish physician Eduardo Vallejo (Vallejo 1956), who oversaw that a 3-year study of healthy, elderly men provided a diet alternating 900 kcal every other day with *overconsumption* (2300 kcal) resulting in stable body weight (apparently, this study has been mischaracterized as an example of CR due to an error in translation; see Johnson et al. (2006)). Daily dietary intake patterns associated with ADF are distinguished by either *feed days* where subjects eat *ad libitum* or *fast days* providing significantly reduced calorie consumption (Varady and Hellerstein 2007). These CR regimens are not mutually exclusive and indeed have been combined, altered, and compared to assess their impact on obesity-related health risk factors while improving adherence and suitability for the individual. An example of a comparative daily dietary consumption pattern among these CR strategies is presented in Figure 6.1.

What follows is a comparative overview of the health effects of CR regimens on major physiological and clinical pathways implicated in obesity-related cardiometabolic dysfunctions. With a few notable exceptions, this discussion will neither focus on CR effects in specific diseased populations, in non-adults, nor compare CR interventions combined with other lifestyle-modifying behaviors such as exercise. Also, this discussion will not consider very low-calorie diets as these dietary plans are not safe, sustainable, or recommended as a strategy for long-term weight loss.

6.2 EFFECTS OF CALORIE RESTRICTION REGIMENS ON BODY COMPOSITION

Observational reports on the effects of CR have included individuals under either experimentally imposed CR or those intentionally adhering to a CR lifestyle. An example of the first category are subjects participating in the Biosphere 2 project for 2 years under a closed ecosystem environment (Walford et al. 2002). Under a forced reduction in calorie intake of approximately 20%–30%, these subjects experienced 17% and a 16% reduction in body mass index (BMI), with much of the changes

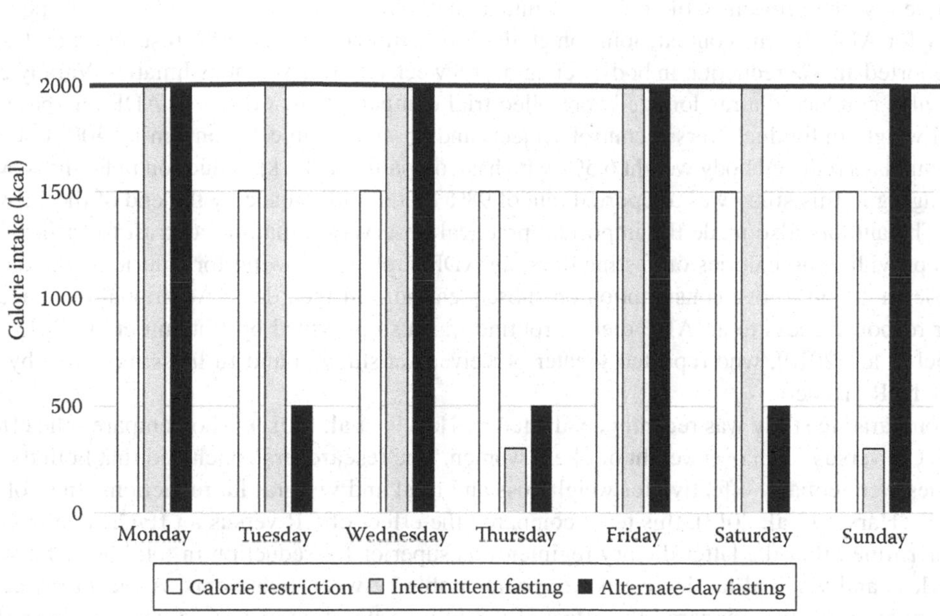

FIGURE 6.1 Calorie restriction (CR) interventions targeted for health benefits and weight loss. Depicted in the figure are three calorie restriction regimens and a representative example of daily caloric intake and distribution over a week. The horizontal bar at 2000 kcal is an assumption of daily caloric needs of a hypothetical individual. Traditional CR studies frequently target a 25% reduction in calories; during intermittent fasting (IF), the individual may consume *ad libitum* 4–6 days/week; finally, during alternate-day fasting (ADF), individuals may alternate *ad libitum* dietary intake with low-calorie fast days.

in body composition attributable to a reduction in fat mass. Studies of individuals voluntarily adhering to CR have also been conducted. Here, Fontana et al. (2004) compared Calorie Restriction Society members who self-imposed 30% CR (years practicing averaging 6.5 years) against healthy, aged-matched controls and reported that CR individuals had a BMI > 20% less than that of controls and the CR men had a total % body fat of only 6.7% versus 22.4% in control men. These observational studies have stimulated a significant number of intervention studies evaluating CR under more scientifically controlled conditions.

Beginning with CALERIE trials, clinical interventions have determined the effects of 20%–25% CR on body weight and composition. Short-term (4–24 weeks) CR regimens typically result in weight loss from 4% to 14% (Buchowski et al. 2012). In contrast, studies of either longer duration (6–12 months) or imposing greater CR (up to 50% energy restriction) unsurprisingly yielded greater weight loss (Heilbronn et al. 2006; Larson-Meyer et al. 2006), and a parallel decrease in total body fat (Heilbronn et al. 2006; Tam et al. 2012). Interestingly, two 12-month studies of 20% CR achieved almost identical weight loss of ≈10% (Hofer et al. 2008; Racette et al. 2006) which was particularly striking considering that the latter study documented only an 11.5% restriction of calories. These studies suggest that long-term adherence to CR is achievable and resulted in significant loss in body weight and fat mass. However, despite these successes compliance with traditional CR continued to prove difficult as food limitations are required every day. Therefore, consideration of IF and ADF strategies, as well as novel combination approaches (Klempel et al. 2012; Kroeger et al. 2012), have been adopted. Heilbronn et al. (2005b) conducted the first study determining the feasibility and effectiveness of ADF on several parameters related to longevity and reported normal-weight men and women who fasted (no calories) every other day for 22 days lost 2.5% body weight and 4% fat. The authors also noted, however, increased hunger in these subjects leading to the conclusion that ADF was unlikely to result in any extended compliance. Consequently, the allowance of some food intake on fasting days has provided a novel, modified strategy for ADF. In this context, Johnson et al. (2007) allowing for an 80% restriction on fasting days reported an 8% reduction in body weight over 8 weeks in overweight asthmatics. Varady et al. (2009) also conducted a randomized controlled trial comparing the effects of ADF on obese and normal-weight individuals versus control subjects and observed subjects consuming 400–600 kcal on fasting days reduced body weight 6.5%, which accompanied a 3.6 kg reduction in fat mass. Most encouraging in this study was a reported rate of 98% dietary adherence by the end of the 12-week study. The authors also made the important practical observation that, in contrast to earlier ADF studies providing no calories on fasting days, an ADF strategy allowing for calorie intake on fast days does not lead to overconsumption on subsequent normal feed days. Additional evidence for greater responsiveness to an ADF dietary routine was also provided by Bhutani et al. (2013) and Klempel et al. (2010), who reported greater perceived satisfaction and fullness measures by this modified CR protocol.

A comparative study was recently conducted by Harvie et al. (2011), who compared the effects of 25% CR versus IF in overweight or obese women. The researchers concluded that both dietary strategies were equally effective for weight loss and total and visceral fat reductions. In a follow-up study (Harvie et al. 2013), this team compared the effect of CR versus an IF/CR combination and determined that the latter dietary regimen was superior for reduction in total body fat while weight loss and visceral fat decreases were comparable between treatments. A recent review by Barnosky et al. (2014) compared the effect of CR to incorporation of fasting days as either IF or ADF on several biomarkers associated with an increased risk of developing type 2 diabetes. In agreement with Harvie's studies, these reviewers concluded that ADF protocols typically resulted in greater weight loss than IF. Moreover, the authors suggested that clinicians may preferentially recommend ADF dietary strategies for facilitating more rapid weight loss, whereas those seeking a slower pattern of weight loss may advocate IF as their method of choice. This greater potential for weight loss in ADF versus IF is not surprising considering that the former strategy requires 3–4 days/week of significant calorie reduction in contrast to IF, which requires only 1–2 days/week calorie reduction.

Because excessive visceral fat mass is a characteristic hallmark of the obese individual, a prime storage depot for generation of pro-inflammatory mediators, and insulin resistance contributing to vascular dysfunction (Lim and Meigs 2014), several investigators have assessed the impact of CR on visceral fat. As part of CALERIE trials, Tam et al. (2012) observed a significant 28% decrease in visceral fat from individuals following a 25% CR diet for 6 months. Most studies incorporating either IF, ADF, or an IF/CR combination described more modest visceral fat decreases of 4%–7% (Barnosky et al. 2014). Finally, several studies from Varady's laboratory (Klempel et al. 2012, 2013a; Varady et al. 2009) and Harvie et al. (2011) all point to a significant reduction in visceral fat by ADF and IF interventions. As the primary goal of CR-induced weight loss in the obese individual is the reduction of visceral fat and the low-grade inflammation associated with obesity, these CR regimens offer significant potential benefits as a lifestyle-modifying intervention against increased overall cardiovascular risk.

6.3 EFFECTS OF CALORIE RESTRICTION REGIMENS ON PLASMA LIPIDS

The deliberate target of dyslipidemia (elevated plasma lipids) is a primary intervention strategy for reducing cardiovascular risks, particularly when these risk factors are comorbid. Observational studies of subjects adhering to CR regimens exhibit several benefits in lipid profiles compared to control subjects. For example Fontana et al. (2004) determined that Calorie Restriction Society members had total cholesterol and triglyceride levels in the lowest 10% and 5th percentiles for age-matched controls and 20-year-olds, respectively. Interestingly, controlled CR regimens have elicited mixed results on plasma lipid concentrations. Several short-term CR interventions reported no lipid-lowering effects in nonobese subjects (Buchowski et al. 2012; Velthuis-te Wierik et al. 1994), whereas longer-term studies reported a considerable lipid-lowering effect (Fontana et al. 2007; Harvie et al. 2011; Lefevre et al. 2009; Verdery and Walford 1998). Improvements in HDL-C have also been reported by some authors (Lefevre et al. 2009; Velthuis-te Wierik et al. 1994), but not others (Harvie et al. 2011). It is frequently hypothesized that a threshold of weight loss may be necessary to effectively modulate lipid responses to specific CR interventions and perhaps discrepancies in these studies are at least partly attributable to study length.

The addition of fasting days enhances the lipid-lowering effects of CR. For example, IF (Harvie et al. 2011; Teng et al. 2013), ADF (Varady et al. 2009, 2013), and combination of IF/CR approaches (Klempel et al. 2012; Kroeger et al. 2012) have all demonstrated significant lipid-lowering effects. The mechanism(s) responsible for lipid lowering by CR regimens is unclear, but plausible physiological mechanisms include an increased gene expression of SIRT1 which stimulates the oxidation of free fatty acids (FFAs) (Kulkarni et al. 2013). This elevated circulation of FFAs may in turn reduce VLDL secretion and hepatic cholesterol biosynthesis (Kudchodkar et al. 1977). An additional factor may be via the modulation of adipokines as recently suggested by Kroeger et al. (2012).

Several researchers have postulated that a heretofore underappreciated cardiovascular risk factor is LDL particle size (Rizzo et al. 2009). For example several investigators have noted a significant association between the incidence of heart disease and smaller LDL particle size (Gardner et al. 1996; Nishikura et al. 2014), presumably due to the smaller LDL to more efficiently transport into the arterial wall where they may undergo oxidative modification resulting in rapid uptake by macrophages (Krauss 2001). Consequently, several laboratories have determined the effect of CR regimens on the physical–chemical properties of this lipoprotein. Current results indicate that both traditional CR and ADF interventions increase LDL particle size (Bhutani et al. 2013; Klempel et al. 2013a; Varady et al. 2009). Because the clinical importance and the role of LDL particle size as an independent risk factor for cardiovascular disease is unknown, additional studies are warranted.

Although results of interventions with CR on plasma lipid profiles are mixed, most studies investigating CR protocols support improved blood lipid profiles. Additional studies will be required to determine factors responsible for the observed variability and, most importantly whether CR-induced alterations in lipid profiles can translate into a reduced risk for cardiovascular events.

6.4 EFFECTS OF CALORIE RESTRICTION REGIMENS ON INSULIN AND GLUCOSE

Numerous studies in rodents provide evidence for improved glucose and insulin response by CR (Roth et al. 2001). Studies have similarly reported that CR humans exhibit lower plasma glucose concentrations and greater insulin sensitivity (Fontana et al. 2007; Walford et al. 2002), and attenuation of obesity-associated elevated glucose and insulin concentrations may provide protection against metabolic dysfunctions. However, most interventions with CR have found no impact on fasting glucose levels (Harvie et al. 2011; Larson-Meyer et al. 2006; Williams et al. 1998). Moreover, in one of the first ADF studies, researchers noted worsening of glucose clearance in women, but not men, after the 22-day intervention suggesting a potential gender-specific response in glucose responsiveness (Heilbronn et al. 2005a). As follow-up, they also found no effect on glucose levels (Heilbronn et al. 2005b, 2006). In contrast, studies with ADF or IF/CR generally report a significant reduction in plasma fasting glucose (Eshghinia and Mohammadzadeh 2013; Klempel et al. 2012; Varady et al. 2009, 2013). Explanations for apparent discrepancies in these studies are unknown, although one obvious difference in protocols reporting no effect versus glucose-lowering response was that the former studies allowed no provisions for calorie intake, whereas studies reporting glucose lowering provided 240–600 kcal.

Despite an inconsistent effect of CR interventions on glucose concentrations, most studies do report significant reductions (11%–41%) in plasma insulin concentrations (Barnosky et al. 2014;

Heilbronn et al. 2006). These findings not only are indicative of improved insulin sensitivity but also imply an improved glycemic response independent of glucose concentrations. Barnosky et al. (2014) noted that in six IF and ADF studies, consistent improvements in insulin sensitivity were determined in both normoglycemic and prediabetic subjects. As one example, a comparison between CR and IF/CR conducted by Harvie et al. (2013) noted greater improvements in insulin sensitivity from the IF/CR protocol compared to 25% CR. These researchers also speculated that the greater response may be attributable to the greater body fat reduction in these individuals as a consequence of better adherence to the IF/CR protocol. Finally, it is possible that studies failing to demonstrate improved glucose and insulin homeostasis by CR regimens may be due to either an insufficient study duration or the normoglycemic status of study subjects.

It is unknown what mechanisms may be responsible for the attenuation of the glucose response and improved insulin sensitivity noted by some CR interventions, or whether these potential cardiometabolic benefits are simply attributed to weight loss following these dietary plans (Barnosky et al. 2014). Relatedly, it is possible that CR-induced weight loss improves insulin secretory patterns (Henry et al. 1988), which, in addition to the improved β-cell function could modulate insulin levels and lower plasma glucose (Utzschneider et al. 2004). Further studies will be necessary to elucidate the precise effects of CR regimens on glucose and insulin homeostasis and whether these changes allow for better glycemic control in both diabetic and nondiabetic individuals.

6.5 EFFECTS OF CALORIE RESTRICTION REGIMENS ON BLOOD PRESSURE

In view of the significant contribution of hypertension as a primary risk factor for the development of cardiovascular disease, CR has been investigated as a potential ameliorative strategy to reduce blood pressure. Cohort studies of both Biosphere 2 subjects (Walford et al. 2002) and Calorie Restriction Society members (Fontana et al. 2004) suggest a potent hypotensive effect of CR where subjects in the latter study displayed remarkably low blood pressure (average: 99 ± 10 mm Hg and 61 ± 6 mm Hg for systolic and diastolic pressures, respectively) after 3–15 years of self-imposed CR. This hypotensive effect by CR, however, has generally not been reported in normotensive individuals. For example neither a short-term 4-week study (Buchowski et al. 2012) nor a longer-term CALERIE study by Lefevre et al. (2009) detected any changes in the blood pressure of individuals placed on a 25% CR diet.

Results with IF and ADF have also produced mixed results on blood pressure. Heilbronn et al. (2005b) examining 22 days of ADF found no effect on blood pressure, and a study by Varady et al. (2009) reported that systolic, but not diastolic, blood pressure was significantly reduced in both males and females. In contrast, a recent randomized controlled trial from the same laboratory noted reductions in both blood pressure measurements among both genders (Varady et al. 2013). Other studies have also failed to detect any effect of ADF on blood pressure (Klempel et al. 2012, 2013a,b). It should be noted that all the subjects in the earlier-mentioned studies were normotensive and an additional explanation for the positive results in the randomized controlled trial was due to its increased study length (12 weeks) versus other studies (8 weeks).With this caveat, it will be of interest to better document the effects of ADF and IF strategies as potential blood pressure–modifying strategies in hypertensive individuals.

There are several pathways affected by CR that may alter vascular tone and potentially influence blood pressure profiles. For example as noted earlier, CR regimens significantly improve insulin sensitivity and reduce circulating insulin levels, physiological effects associated with reduced blood pressure. Also, it is possible that sympathetic nervous activity is improved by CR. Finally, CR interventions increase endothelial nitric oxide synthase activity that may augment generation of nitric oxide, a potent vasodilating signaling molecule (Civitarese et al. 2007; Yousefi et al. 2014). Future studies should focus on the effects of CR regimens on hypertensive individuals, independent of weight status.

6.6 EFFECTS OF CALORIE RESTRICTION ON OXIDATIVE STRESS AND INFLAMMATORY MEDIATORS

The accumulative effect of oxidative damage to key biological macromolecules (proteins, lipids, DNA) as an integral component of the aging process is the central tenet of the free radical theory of aging (Harman 1957). A wealth of data from experimental animal models supports a significant reduction in oxidative stress during CR (Sohal and Weindruch 1996). This CR-mediated reduction in oxidative stress may be attributed to several factors, including: (1) inhibition of reactive oxygen species (ROS) generation, (2) modulation of antioxidant/anti-inflammatory defense systems, (3) a combination of these stimulatory or inducible processes, and (4) a hormetic effect by which CR stimulates adaptive cellular responses resulting from an initial, mildly toxic or oxidative environment (Allard et al. 2008; Lam and Ravussin 2014; Omodei et al. 2013). Because modification of oxidative damage by CR is one plausible mechanism for its potential antioxidative effects in rodents, several clinical studies have addressed CR regimens on biomarkers of oxidative stress.

Earlier studies evaluating CR on indices of oxidative stress have yielded mixed results. Dandona et al. (2001) placed obese subjects on 1000 kcal/day for 4 weeks and noted a significant reduction in oxidative damage to leukocytes. In contrast, Loft et al. (1995) subjecting normal-weight individuals to 20% CR for 10 weeks observed no protection against DNA damage. The influence of traditional CR on oxidative stress has also been determined in several CALERIE trials. Heilbronn et al. (2006) and Civitarese et al. (2007) both observed significant reductions in DNA damage, but not in protein carbonyls after 6 months of 25% CR. In contrast, Meydani et al. (2011) found a decrease in protein carbonyls. These latter authors also observed CR-mediated enhancement of antioxidant defenses by increasing glutathione peroxidase (GPX) activity but no effect on either catalase or superoxide dismutase (SOD). Also, Buchowski et al. (2012), in a unique study protocol targeting overweight and obese women, measured at multiple intervals the effect of 25% CR on oxidative stress biomarkers and found a significant and rapid reduction (within 5 days) of isoprostanes to similar levels measured in normal-weight individuals. In a long-term (1-year) intervention by Hofer et al. (2008) with 20% CR, there was approximately 36% and 49% reductions in RNA and DNA damage, respectively. Finally, in an intriguing *ex vivo* study, Omodei et al. (2013) cultured cells from both calorie-restricted subjects (members of the Caloric Restriction Society) and subjects consuming a typical U.S. diet and found that those cells incubated from serum collected from the CR individuals exhibited increased resistance to hydrogen peroxide damage and a significant elevation in antioxidant defenses (SOD2 and GPX1), providing additional evidence that attenuation of oxidative stress may be one mechanism responsible for reported CR benefits.

Incorporation of IF or ADF dietary strategies may also suppress oxidative stress suggesting a potential mechanism implicated in cardiovascular risk reduction by CR. Corroboration of the anti-oxidative effects of ADF have been reported by some researchers (Teng et al. 2013), but not others (Kroeger et al. 2012). Also, an extensive 6-month elaborate study by Harvie et al. (2011) comparing IF and 25% CR protocols suggested that IF incorporating about 540 kcal on 2 days/week had greater impact on reducing oxidative stress. Johnson et al. (2007) examining the effect of ADF in overweight asthmatics also found a significant reduction of a battery of oxidative stress biomarkers including protein carbonyls, 4-hydroxynonenal, and isoprostanes along with the elevation in the circulating antioxidant uric acid. Interestingly, these authors noted that oxidative stress markers were reduced on both the fasting day (consisting of 320–380 kcal of a meal replacement shake) and on *ad libitum* consumption days.

Finally, it is unclear what factors are responsible for these rather discordant results although there are several possibilities. For instance, there are many methodological differences in oxidative stress biomarker measurements. Also, the selection of these biomarkers may be differentially impacted such that free radical–mediated oxidation of lipids, for example, may not occur concomitantly or temporally compared with other targeted macromolecules. Furthermore, the magnitude of weight and/or fat loss, along with the dietary antioxidant intake and status (adequate versus inadequate), may also significantly influence the extent of CR modification of oxidative stress pathways. Additional studies with multiple oxidative stress biomarkers may also be necessary to fully delineate precise effects of CR regimens on oxidative stress and how modification of oxidative stress may contribute to potential clinical improvements in humans.

Low-grade inflammation has long been implicated in the pathogenesis and promotion of obesity (Hotamisligil et al. 1993). This inflammation is associated with increased levels of pro-inflammatory marker proteins such as C-reactive protein (CRP), interleukin-6 (IL-6), and tumor necrosis factor alpha (TNF-α) (Hotamisligil et al. 1993; Pradhan et al. 2001). Because inflammation may provide an essential link between obesity and cardiometabolic disorders, interest in the potential amelioration of inflammation by CR regimens has been the subject of increased interest among clinicians and basic scientists. Reports on the effect of CR in a cohort of long-term calorie-restricted individuals by Fontana et al. (2004) found circulating CRP levels that were fivefold less compared to control subjects. However, some clinical CR interventions with 25% CR for 6 months failed to influence circulating levels of CRP, IL-6, and TNF-α (Larson-Meyer et al. 2006; Tam et al. 2012). Tam et al. (2012) commented on potential factors responsible for the failure of CR to affect the status of these inflammatory mediators: no evidence for low-grade inflammation in the subjects at study onset, and/or an insufficient level of obesity in these subjects. More studies have measured these cytokines using IF and ADF dietary approaches. Interventions with ADF have led to decreases in CRP (Harvie et al. 2011; Varady et al. 2013), IL-6, and TNF-α (Kroeger et al. 2012). Significant decreases in TNF-α were also observed in overweight asthmatics (Johnson et al. 2007). IF as part of Ramadan also resulted in decreases of IL-6 and CRP in both males and females (Aksungar et al. 2007). Finally, an IF/CR combination significantly reduced IL-6 and TNF-α, but not CRP, in obese subjects (Kroeger et al. 2012).

Mechanisms implicated for a potential anti-inflammatory effect of CR regimen include reduced adiposity and secretion of pro-inflammatory mediators, reduced oxidative stress, and increased insulin sensitivity. As has been described for several cardiometabolic risk factors, it is possible that there may be a threshold for weight loss in CR studies necessary for effectively modifying cytokine concentrations. Alternatively, it is possible that for many obese subjects there is insufficient cause for characterization of a whole-body *inflammatory* state. Further studies, perhaps selecting individuals with a greater inflammatory profile may be required to fully evaluate any potential anti-inflammatory effect of CR regimens in humans.

6.7 EFFECTS OF CALORIE RESTRICTION REGIMENS ON PLASMA TOXINS

Studies in CR rodents have alterations in detoxification pathways that commensurate with an increased protection against age-associated pathologies (Cho et al. 2003; Feuers et al. 1989; Hart et al. 1992). Modulation of these pathways may influence several physiological and biochemical-mediated mechanisms affecting the detoxification of xenobiotics such as: (1) a reduction in fat stores by CR resulting in their increased mobilization from diminishing fat depots, (2) increased metabolism of released toxins, and/or (3) increased or more efficient urinary or biliary toxin excretion. There is extensive evidence for the mobilization of persistent organic pollutants such as polychlorinated biphenyls (PCBs) from adipose depots into the circulation of subjects during weight loss (De Roos et al. 2012). However, only Walford et al. (1999) have reported on the effects of a CR protocol on *total PCBs* in their study of Biosphere 2 subjects. Although the interrelationships among weight and fat reductions and toxin status may be an important component of the observed benefits of CR regimens, studies investigating this research area are woefully lacking. In this context, a long-term study is under way to determine the effect of an IF/CR combination approach on total and individual PCB congener plasma concentrations. In a recently published abstract of the results (Gumpricht et al. 2014), the authors reported that obese men and women following this regimen lost substantial weight and body fat, which was associated with a significant increase in circulating PCBs. Coincidental to this weight loss–associated toxin mobilization was an improvement in total antioxidant capacity and a reduction in oxidative stress. Unfortunately, because of methodological constraints in human PCB analysis, this study did not measure either urinary or biliary excretion of PCB metabolites; thus, no direct evidence for increased detoxification of these toxins was obtained. Clearly, further studies are warranted to fully assess the effects of CR regimens on patterns of detoxification pathways, enzymes responsible for detoxification, and the physiological consequences of weight loss–induced toxin release.

6.8 SUMMARY

In summary, accumulating evidence from observation studies of CR-practicing individuals and an increasing number of intervention studies strongly support that both weight loss and improvement in a variety of biomarkers associated with age- and obesity-related risk factors may be significantly modified by CR regimens (Figure 6.2). Future studies should continue to address not only the potential benefits of these regimens in obese individuals but also their potential efficacy, safety, and toxicity concerns for long-term adherence under specific disease populations as well as in nonobese subjects. Mechanistic-based targets are also needed to precisely define those pathways most affected by CR interventions. Finally, as a potential nutritional therapeutic treatment for weight loss and reduced risk of cardiovascular disease, CR regimens also need to be explored from both psychosocial (Incollingo Belsky et al. 2014) and demographic (DeLany et al. 2014) perspectives.

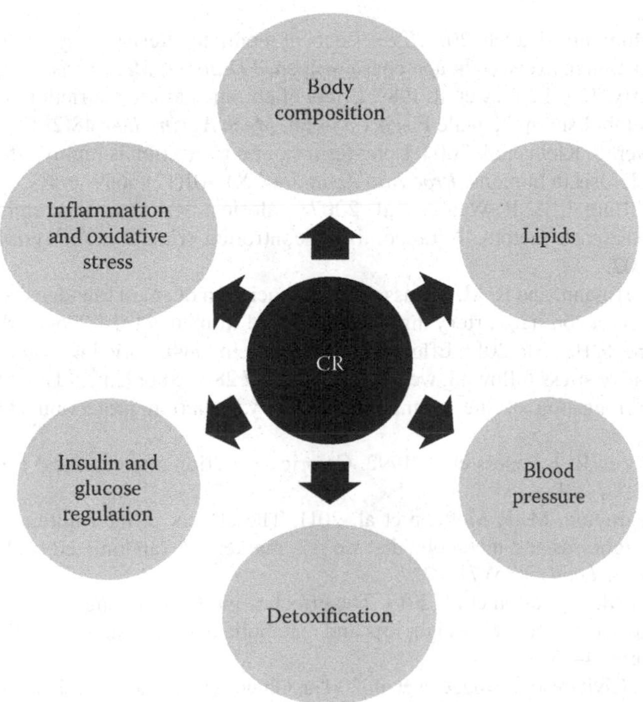

FIGURE 6.2 Potential metabolic and physiological pathways modified by CR regimens.

REFERENCES

Aksungar, F. B., A. E. Topkaya, and M. Akyildiz. 2007. Interleukin-6, C-reactive protein and biochemical parameters during prolonged intermittent fasting. *Ann Nutr Metab* 51(1):88–95.

Allard, J. S., L. K. Heilbronn, C. Smith et al. 2008. In vitro cellular adaptations of indicators of longevity in response to treatment with serum collected from humans on calorie restricted diets. *PLoS ONE* 3(9):e3211.

Barnosky, A. R., K. K. Hoddy, T. G. Unterman et al. 2014. Intermittent fasting vs daily calorie restriction for type 2 diabetes prevention: A review of human findings. *Transl Res.* 164(4):302–311.

Bhutani, S., M. C. Klempel, C. M. Kroeger et al. 2013. Effect of exercising while fasting on eating behaviors and food intake. *J Int Soc Sports Nutr* 10(1):50.

Buchowski, M. S., N. Hongu, S. Acra et al. 2012. Effect of modest caloric restriction on oxidative stress in women, a randomized trial. *PLoS ONE* 7(10):e47079.

Carlson, A. J. and F. Hoelzel. 1946. Apparent prolongation of the life span of rats by intermittent fasting. *J Nutr* 31:363–375.

Cho, C. G., H. J. Kim, S. W. Chung et al. 2003. Modulation of glutathione and thioredoxin systems by calorie restriction during the aging process. *Exp Gerontol* 38(5):539–548.

Civitarese, A. E., S. Carling, L. K. Heilbronn et al. 2007. Calorie restriction increases muscle mitochondrial biogenesis in healthy humans. *PLoS Med* 4(3):e76.

Colman, R. J., T. M. Beasley, J. W. Kemnitz et al. 2014. Caloric restriction reduces age-related and all-cause mortality in rhesus monkeys. *Nat Commun* 5:3557.

Dandona, P., P. Mohanty, W. Hamouda et al. 2001. Inhibitory effect of a two day fast on reactive oxygen species (ROS) generation by leucocytes and plasma ortho-tyrosine and meta-tyrosine concentrations. *J Clin Endocrinol Metab* 86(6):2899–2902.

Das, S. K., C. H. Gilhooly, J. K. Golden et al. 2007. Long-term effects of 2 energy-restricted diets differing in glycemic load on dietary adherence, body composition, and metabolism in CALERIE: A 1-y randomized controlled trial. *Am J Clin Nutr* 85(4):1023–1030.

De Roos, A. J., C. M. Ulrich, A. Sjodin et al. 2012. Adiposity, body composition, and weight change in relation to organochlorine pollutant plasma concentrations. *J Expo Sci Environ Epidemiol* 22(6):617–624.

DeLany, J. P., J. M. Jakicic, J. B. Lowery et al. 2014. African American women exhibit similar adherence to intervention but lose less weight due to lower energy requirements. *Int J Obes (Lond)* 38(9):1147–1152.

Eshghinia, S. and F. Mohammadzadeh. 2013. The effects of modified alternate-day fasting diet on weight loss and CAD risk factors in overweight and obese women. *J Diabetes Metab Disord* 12(1):4.

Feuers, R. J., P. H. Duffy, J. A. Leakey et al. 1989. Effect of chronic caloric restriction on hepatic enzymes of intermediary metabolism in the male Fischer 344 rat. *Mech Ageing Dev* 48(2):179–189.

Fontana, L., T. E. Meyer, S. Klein et al. 2004. Long-term calorie restriction is highly effective in reducing the risk for atherosclerosis in humans. *Proc Natl Acad Sci USA* 101(17):6659–6663.

Fontana, L., D. T. Villareal, E. P. Weiss et al. 2007. Calorie restriction or exercise: Effects on coronary heart disease risk factors. A randomized, controlled trial. *Am J Physiol Endocrinol Metab* 293(1):E197–E202.

Gardner, C. D., S. P. Fortmann, and R. M. Krauss. 1996. Association of small low-density lipoprotein particles with the incidence of coronary artery disease in men and women. *JAMA* 276(11):875–881.

Gumpricht, E., E. Ward, F. He et al. 2014. Effects of a high-protein low-calorie intermittent fast diet on plasma toxins and oxidative stress following weight loss. *Faseb J* 28(1):Supplement LB435, CA.

Harman, D. 1957. Prolongation of the normal life span by radiation protection chemicals. *J Gerontol* 12(3):257–263.

Hart, R. W., M. W. Chou, R. J. Feuers et al. 1992. Caloric restriction and chemical toxicity/carcinogenesis. *Qual Assur* 1(2):120–131.

Harvie, M. N., M. Pegington, M. P. Mattson et al. 2011. The effects of intermittent or continuous energy restriction on weight loss and metabolic disease risk markers: A randomized trial in young overweight women. *Int J Obes (Lond)* 35(5):714–727.

Harvie, M., C. Wright, M. Pegington et al. 2013. The effect of intermittent energy and carbohydrate restriction v. daily energy restriction on weight loss and metabolic disease risk markers in overweight women. *Br J Nutr* 110(8):1534–1547.

Heilbronn, L. K., A. E. Civitarese, I. Bogacka et al. 2005a. Glucose tolerance and skeletal muscle gene expression in response to alternate day fasting. *Obes Res* 13(3):574–581.

Heilbronn, L. K., L. de Jonge, M. I. Frisard et al. 2006. Effect of 6-month calorie restriction on biomarkers of longevity, metabolic adaptation, and oxidative stress in overweight individuals: A randomized controlled trial. *JAMA* 295(13):1539–1548.

Heilbronn, L. K., S. R. Smith, C. K. Martin et al. 2005b. Alternate-day fasting in nonobese subjects: Effects on body weight, body composition, and energy metabolism. *Am J Clin Nutr* 81(1):69–73.

Henry, R. R., G. Brechtel, and K. Griver. 1988. Secretion and hepatic extraction of insulin after weight loss in obese noninsulin-dependent diabetes mellitus. *J Clin Endocrinol Metab* 66(5):979–986.

Hofer, T., L. Fontana, S. D. Anton et al. 2008. Long-term effects of caloric restriction or exercise on DNA and RNA oxidation levels in white blood cells and urine in humans. *Rejuvenation Res* 11(4):793–799.

Hotamisligil, G. S., N. S. Shargill, and B. M. Spiegelman. 1993. Adipose expression of tumor necrosis factor-alpha: Direct role in obesity-linked insulin resistance. *Science* 259(5091):87–91.

Incollingo Belsky, A. C., E. S. Epel, and A. J. Tomiyama. 2014. Clues to maintaining calorie restriction? Psychosocial profiles of successful long-term restrictors. *Appetite* 79:106–112.

Johnson, J. B., D. R. Laub, and S. John. 2006. The effect on health of alternate day calorie restriction: Eating less and more than needed on alternate days prolongs life. *Med Hypotheses* 67(2):209–211.

Johnson, J. B., W. Summer, R. G. Cutler et al. 2007. Alternate day calorie restriction improves clinical findings and reduces markers of oxidative stress and inflammation in overweight adults with moderate asthma. *Free Radic Biol Med* 42(5):665–674.

Klempel, M. C., S. Bhutani, M. Fitzgibbon et al. 2010. Dietary and physical activity adaptations to alternate day modified fasting: Implications for optimal weight loss. *Nutr J* 9:35.

Klempel, M. C., C. M. Kroeger, S. Bhutani et al. 2012. Intermittent fasting combined with calorie restriction is effective for weight loss and cardio-protection in obese women. *Nutr J* 11:98.

Klempel, M. C., C. M. Kroeger, E. Norkeviciute et al. 2013a. Benefit of a low-fat over high-fat diet on vascular health during alternate day fasting. *Nutr Diabetes* 3:e71.

Klempel, M. C., C. M. Kroeger, and K. A. Varady. 2013b. Alternate day fasting (ADF) with a high-fat diet produces similar weight loss and cardio-protection as ADF with a low-fat diet. *Metabolism* 62(1):137–143.

Krauss, R. M. 2001. Atherogenic lipoprotein phenotype and diet–gene interactions. *J Nutr* 131(2):340S–343S.

Kroeger, C. M., M. C. Klempel, S. Bhutani et al. 2012. Improvement in coronary heart disease risk factors during an intermittent fasting/calorie restriction regimen: Relationship to adipokine modulations. *Nutr Metab (Lond)* 9(1):98.

Kudchodkar, B. J., H. S. Sodhi, D. T. Mason et al. 1977. Effects of acute caloric restriction on cholesterol metabolism in man. *Am J Clin Nutr* 30(7):1135–1146.

Kulkarni, S. R., L. E. Armstrong, and A. L. Slitt. 2013. Caloric restriction-mediated induction of lipid metabolism gene expression in liver is enhanced by Keap1-knockdown. *Pharm Res* 30(9):2221–2231.

Lam, Y.Y. and E. Ravussin. 2014. Periodic fasting and hormesis. In *Hormesis in Health and Disease*, S. I. S. Rattan and Le Bourg, E. (eds.). Boca Raton, FL: CRC Press.

Larson-Meyer, D. E., L. K. Heilbronn, L. M. Redman et al. 2006. Effect of calorie restriction with or without exercise on insulin sensitivity, beta-cell function, fat cell size, and ectopic lipid in overweight subjects. *Diabetes Care* 29(6):1337–1344.

Lefevre, M., L. M. Redman, L. K. Heilbronn et al. 2009. Caloric restriction alone and with exercise improves CVD risk in healthy non-obese individuals. *Atherosclerosis* 203(1):206–213.

Lim, S. and J. B. Meigs. 2014. Links between ectopic fat and vascular disease in humans. *Arterioscler Thromb Vasc Biol* 34(9):1820–1826.

Loft, S., E. J. Velthuis-te Wierik, H. van den Berg et al. 1995. Energy restriction and oxidative DNA damage in humans. *Cancer Epidemiol Biomarkers Prev* 4(5):515–519.

Mattison, J. A., G. S. Roth, T. M. Beasley et al. 2012. Impact of caloric restriction on health and survival in rhesus monkeys from the NIA study. *Nature* 489(7415):318–321.

McCay, C. M., M. F. Crowell, and L. A. Maynard. 1935. The effect of retarded growth upon the length of life span and upon the ultimate body size. *J Nutr* 10:63–79.

Meydani, M., S. Das, M. Band et al. 2011. The effect of caloric restriction and glycemic load on measures of oxidative stress and antioxidants in humans: Results from the CALERIE Trial of Human Caloric Restriction. *J Nutr Health Aging* 15(6):456–460.

Nishikura, T., S. Koba, Y. Yokota et al. 2014. Elevated small dense low-density lipoprotein cholesterol as a predictor for future cardiovascular events in patients with stable coronary artery disease. *J Atheroscler Thromb* 21(8):755–767.

Ogden, C. L., M. D. Carroll, B. K. Kit et al. 2014. Prevalence of childhood and adult obesity in the United States, 2011–2012. *JAMA* 311(8):806–814.

Omodei, D., D. Licastro, F. Salvatore et al. 2013. Serum from humans on long-term calorie restriction enhances stress resistance in cell culture. *Aging (Albany NY)* 5(8):599–606.

Pradhan, A. D., J. E. Manson, N. Rifai et al. 2001. C-reactive protein, interleukin 6, and risk of developing type 2 diabetes mellitus. *JAMA* 286(3):327–334.

Racette, S. B., E. P. Weiss, D. T. Villareal et al. 2006. One year of caloric restriction in humans: Feasibility and effects on body composition and abdominal adipose tissue. *J Gerontol A Biol Sci Med Sci* 61(9):943–950.

Rizzo, M., Kotur-Stevuljevic, J., Berneis, K. et al. 2009. Atherogenic dyslipidemia and oxidative stress: A new look. *Transl Res* 153(5):217–223.

Roth, G. S., D. K. Ingram, and M. A. Lane. 2001. Caloric restriction in primates and relevance to humans. *Ann N Y Acad Sci* 928:305–315.

Sohal, R. S. and R. Weindruch. 1996. Oxidative stress, caloric restriction, and aging. *Science* 273(5271):59–63.

Sung, M. M. and J. R. Dyck. 2012. Age-related cardiovascular disease and the beneficial effects of calorie restriction. *Heart Fail Rev* 17(4–5):707–719.

Tam, C. S., J. D. Covington, E. Ravussin et al. 2012. Little evidence of systemic and adipose tissue inflammation in overweight individuals. *Front Genet* 3:58.

Teng, N. I., S. Shahar, N. F. Rajab et al. 2013. Improvement of metabolic parameters in healthy older adult men following a fasting calorie restriction intervention. *Aging Male* 16(4):177–183.

Trepanowski, J. F., R. E. Canale, K. E. Marshall et al. 2011. Impact of caloric and dietary restriction regimens on markers of health and longevity in humans and animals: A summary of available findings. *Nutr J* 10:107.

Utzschneider, K. M., D. B. Carr, R. L. Hull et al. 2004. Impact of intra-abdominal fat and age on insulin sensitivity and beta-cell function. *Diabetes* 53(11):2867–2872.

Vallejo, E. A. 1956. La dieta de hambre a dı´as alternos en la alimentacio´n de los viejos. *Rev Clin Esp* 63:25–27.

Varady, K. A., S. Bhutani, E. C. Church et al. 2009. Short-term modified alternate-day fasting: A novel dietary strategy for weight loss and cardioprotection in obese adults. *Am J Clin Nutr* 90(5):1138–1143.

Varady, K. A., S. Bhutani, M. C. Klempel et al. 2013. Alternate day fasting for weight loss in normal weight and overweight subjects: A randomized controlled trial. *Nutr J* 12(1):146.

Varady, K. A. and M. K. Hellerstein. 2007. Alternate-day fasting and chronic disease prevention: A review of human and animal trials. *Am J Clin Nutr* 86(1):7–13.

Velthuis-te Wierik, E. J., H. van den Berg, G. Schaafsma et al. 1994. Energy restriction, a useful intervention to retard human ageing? Results of a feasibility study. *Eur J Clin Nutr* 48(2):138–148.

Verdery, R. B. and R. L. Walford. 1998. Changes in plasma lipids and lipoproteins in humans during a 2-year period of dietary restriction in Biosphere 2. *Arch Intern Med* 158(8):900–906.

Walford, R. L., D. Mock, T. MacCallum et al. 1999. Physiologic changes in humans subjected to severe, selective calorie restriction for two years in biosphere 2: Health, aging, and toxicological perspectives. *Toxicol Sci* 52(2 Suppl.):61–65.

Walford, R. L., D. Mock, R. Verdery et al. 2002. Calorie restriction in biosphere 2: Alterations in physiologic, hematologic, hormonal, and biochemical parameters in humans restricted for a 2-year period. *J Gerontol A Biol Sci Med Sci* 57(6):B211–B224.

Weindruch, R. and R. L. Walford. 1982. Dietary restriction in mice beginning at 1 year of age: Effect on lifespan and spontaneous cancer incidence. *Science* 215(4538):1415–1418.

Williams, K. V., M. L. Mullen, D. E. Kelley et al. 1998. The effect of short periods of caloric restriction on weight loss and glycemic control in type 2 diabetes. *Diabetes Care* 21(1):2–8.

Yousefi, B., Z. Faghfoori, N. Samadi et al. 2014. The effects of Ramadan fasting on endothelial function in patients with cardiovascular diseases. *Eur J Clin Nutr* 68(7):835–839.

7 Overview of Novel Herbal Supplements in Diabetes

Neetu Mishra, Kanti Bhooshan Pandey, and Syed Ibrahim Rizvi

CONTENTS

7.1 INTRODUCTION

Diabetes mellitus (DM) is a disease of metabolic dysregulation, primarily of carbohydrate metabolism, characterized by hyperglycemia that results from defects in impaired insulin action, insulin secretion, or both. Uncontrolled diabetes may lead to long-term and life-threatening complications like coronary artery disease, cerebrovascular disease, peripheral vascular disease, nephropathy, neuropathy, retinopathy, morbidity, and/or mortality (Brownlee 2001; Hammes et al. 2011; Wilmot and Idris 2014).

A global increase in the prevalence of DM has been reported in last few decades. As per International Diabetes Federation, the number of individuals with diabetes in 2011 has reached an astounding figure of 366 million, causing 4.6 million deaths each year (Dong et al. 2012). This figure is expected to climb up to 592 million by the year 2035 (IDF Diabetes Atlas 2013). Although DM is a growing health concern in both developed and developing countries since enormous financial burden is associated with it. It has been estimated that there will be approximately 70% increase in DM in developing countries and 20% increase in developed countries by 2030 in which India's diabetic population is expected to reach more than 100 million with the age of onset getting reduced to a range of 40–59 years (IDF Diabetes Atlas 2013; Wang et al. 2013). India and its subcontinent nations including Bangladesh, Nepal, Sri Lanka, and Pakistan have emerged as the epidemic centers of DM in last 2–3 decades. Prevalence of DM in 20–79 age-group population has been reported to be the highest in India after Bangladesh (Whiting et al. 2011).

Currently available cures for DM including sulfonylureas, biguanide, thiazolidinedione, and α-glycosidase inhibitors have restricted use due to long-term unavoidable complications as well as high cost. These medications frequently have side effects including bone loss, weight gain, and increased risk of cardiovascular events (AHFS 2012; Inzucchi 2002). Plant-based medications have attracted a large population of diabetics due to relatively safe and effective oral hypoglycemic properties. Recent studies have shown that some plants or their products having medicinal properties can provide a significant protection against diabetic events (Pandey and Rizvi 2014; Patel et al. 2012; Tiwari et al. 2014).

As per World Health Organization (WHO) data, up to 90% of population in developing countries use plants or its products as traditional medicine for primary health care (WHO 2002). The WHO has listed 2,500 species in India among 21,000 plants around the world, which have been used for medicinal purposes, in which more than 400 possess antidiabetic effect (Modak et al. 2007; Prabhakar and Doble 2011). This chapter is an attempt to provide a review of the plants commonly used for the management of diabetes in the Indian subcontinent.

7.2 INDIAN PLANTS WITH ANTIDIABETIC PROPERTIES

7.2.1 *Syzygium cumini*

English name: Blackberry
Common name: Jamun
Family: Myrtaceae
Parts used: Seeds, leaves, fruit, bark
Syzygium cumini is an evergreen tropical tree being 8–15 m tall, with smooth and glossy oblong opposite leaves having a turpentine smell. It is also known as *Eugenia jambola*. The bark is scaly gray, and the trunk is forked; it has fragrant white flowers in branched clusters at stem tips and purplish-black oval edible berries. The berries have only one seed. The taste is usually acid to fairly sweet and somewhat astringent (Periyathambi 2007). *S. cumini* is found to grow in tropical and subtropical regions of the world. Indian subcontinent and regions of South Asia as Indonesia, Bangladesh, Pakistan, Burma, Nepal, and Sri Lanka produce good amount of *S. cumini* (Ayyanar and Subash-Babu 2012).

The hypoglycemic effect of *S. cumini* may be due to an increased secretion or a diminished degradation of insulin. Phytochemical and pharmacological studies indicate that ethanol extract contains flavonoids, saponins, and traces of phenol and steroids. Saponin appears to be involved in the stimulation of pancreatic cells and subsequent secretion of insulin (Srivastava et al. 2012). *S. cumini* is reported to reduce blood cholesterol, triglycerides, and free fatty acids thereby showing hypolipidemic effect (Sagrawat et al. 2006). This effect was reported to be due to the presence of flavonoids, saponins, and glycoside in the extract, which in turn decreased the activity of enzyme 3-HMG Co-A reductase in liver (Ravi et al. 2005). The seed extract of *S. cumini* also contains ellagic acid that has been shown to reduce blood pressure (Morton 1987).

S. cumini has promising therapeutic value with various phytoconstituents such as tannins, alkaloids, steroids, flavonoids, terpenoids, fatty acids, and vitamins. The seeds of *S. cumini* have been observed to be rich in flavonoids (Ravi et al. 2004). The essential oil of *S. cumini* contains terpenes, ellagic acid, isoquercetin, quercetin, kaempferol, and myricetin in different concentrations (Rastogi and Mehrotra 1990). Leaves contain rich amounts of acylated flavonolglycosides, myricetin, quercetin, esterase, and tannins all of which can be helpful for diabetics. Bark is reported to be rich in betulinic acid, eugenin, β-sitosterol, quercetin, ellagic acid, gallic acid, bergenin, tannins, and flavonoids. Fruits are rich sources of raffinose, glucose, fructose, anthocyanins, and malic acid (Ravi et al. 2004).

Several studies on animal models have shown the reduction in blood sugar level and improvement in the histopathology of pancreatic islets after supplementation of *S. cumini* seeds and seed powder (Singh and Gupta 2007). Oral administration of pulp extract of the fruit of *S. cumini* to diabetic rats showed very significant hypoglycemic activity in 30 min, the action possibly mediated by insulin secretion (Achrekar et al. 1991). In addition, the extract inhibited insulinase activity from liver and kidney (Achrekar et al. 1991). There are a number of studies that report that supplementation of seed extract, leaf extract, fruits, or other parts of the *S. cumini*-reduced blood glucose level, cholesterol, free fatty acids, and restored the redox imbalance in diabetic rats (Chaturvedi et al. 2007; Grover et al. 2002; Wang et al. 2013).

7.2.2 MOMORDICA CHARANTIA

English name: Bitter gourd
Common name: Karela
Family: Cucurbitaceae
Parts used: Fruit, seed, bark, root, leaves, oil

Momordica charantia is found in abundance in Asian and African subcontinents. The plant grows up to 5 m with simple, alternate leaves 4–12 cm across. Fruit part of the plant is often used as vegetable in diet. *M. charantia* is a popular fruit used for the treatment of diabetes and related events in indigenous populations of Asia, South America, India, and East Africa. It contains substances with antidiabetic properties such as charantin, vicine, and polypeptide-p, and antioxidants (Krawinkel and Keding 2006). Several studies have been documented the antidiabetic and hypoglycemic effects of *M. charantia* through various hypothesized mechanisms (Leung et al. 2004).

Shetty et al. (2005) studied the effect of *M. charantia* at 10% level in the diet in streptozotocin (STZ)-induced diabetic rats and have reported the prevention of renal dystrophy by 38%, reduction in glomerular filtration rate by 27%, and an amelioration of about 30% in fasting blood glucose (FBG). Hypoglycemic and lipid-lowering properties of *M. charantia* against rosiglitazone treatment in humans have also been observed (Inayat-ur-Rahman et al. 2009). Studies have shown that the treatment of *M. charantia* repaired damaged β-cells to stimulate/regenerate insulin levels (Saxena and Vikram 2004). *M. charantia* has also been reported to improve sensitivity/signaling of insulin (Wang et al. 2011). Chaturvedi (2012) on the basis of the result of his study proposed that *M. charantia* may inhibit the absorption of glucose by inhibiting glucosidase and suppressing the activity of disaccharidases in the intestine.

Hypoglycemic and antihyperglycemic effects of *M. charantia* have been reported in normal and STZ-diabetic rats (Shabib et al. 1993). It has been proposed that the activity shown by *M. charantia* may be due to the inhibition of glucose-6-phosphatase and stimulation of hepatic glucose-6-phosphate dehydrogenase (Shabib et al. 1993). Histological study performed by Fernandes et al. (2007) documented that the extract of *M. charantia* fruit has the ability to restore the altered architecture of islets of Langerhans.

Sekar et al. (2005) have reported that the treatment of seed extract of *M. charantia* to diabetic rats resulted in significant reduction in blood glucose, glycosylated hemoglobin, lactate dehydrogenase, glucose-6-phosphatase, fructose-1,6-bisphosphatase, and glycogen phosphorylase, and a concomitant increase in the levels of hemoglobin, glycogen, and activities of hexokinase and glycogen synthase, confirming the strong antidiabetic effect of *M. charantia*.

Supplementation of *M. charantia* to STZ-induced diabetic rats showed a strong protection against oxidative stress markers. Experiment on plasma and pancreas tissues of *M. charantia*–supplemented diabetic rats showed a significant reduction in plasma glucose, thiobarbituric acid–reactive substances, lipid hydroperoxides, alpha-tocopherol, and significant improvement in ascorbic acid, reduced glutathione (GSH), and insulin (Sathishsekar and Subramanian 2005).

7.2.3 Trigonella foenum-graecum

English name: Fenugreek
Common name: Methi
Family: Fabaceae
Parts used: Leaves, seeds
Trigonella foenum-graecum L. is cultivated throughout India as well as in some other parts of the world as a semiarid crop (Kavishankar et al. 2011). Its green leaves are used as a vegetable, and the seeds are used as spice in India. It is also used as a food supplement and one of the staple foods in Egypt and Yemen. *T. foenum-graecum* is popular for its pungent aromatic properties and is often used to add flavors in food. Studies on several experimental models have reported *T. foenum-graecum* as an effective antidiabetic agent (Vats et al. 2002; Wang et al. 2013; Zia et al. 2001). Human studies have also confirmed the glucose and lipid-lowering potential of *T. foenum-graecum* (Sharma et al. 1990).

Different studies have demonstrated that *T. foenum-graecum* seed extracts, mucilage of seeds, powder, and leaves can reduce blood glucose and cholesterol levels in human and experimental diabetic animals (Gupta et al. 2001; Vats et al. 2002). The therapeutic potential of *T. foenum-graecum* is primarily due to the presence of saponins (Petit et al. 1995), high-fiber content (Ali et al. 1995), 4-hydroxyisoleucine, and trigonelline, an alkaloid (Raghuram et al. 1994). Extrapancreatic effects of *T. foenum-graecum* have been projected for the hypoglycemic action (Saxena and Vikram 2004).

The activity of creatine kinase in liver, skeletal muscles, and heart of diabetic rats was found to be restored to normal levels by administering seed powder of *T. foenum-graecum* (Genet et al. 1999). *T. foenum-graecum* seeds are also known to possess hypolipidemic or cholesterol-lowering properties (Stark and Madar 1993; Vijayakumar et al. 2010). *T. foenum-graecum* extract given orally produced reduction in blood glucose levels in both normal and diabetic rats (Khosla et al. 1995), which may be due to increased glucose metabolism (Gupta et al. 1999). Enhancement of insulin sensitivity and glucose uptake in peripheral tissues are recorded in *T. foenum-graecum*-supplemented diabetic rats (Singh et al. 2010). A considerable increment of the area of insulin-immunoreactive β-cells and a marked reduction in renal toxicity have been seen in *T. foenum-graecum*-supplemented diabetic rats (Hamden et al. 2010).

7.2.4 Pterocarpus marsupium

English name: Indian Malabar
Common name: Vijayasar
Family: Fabaceae
Parts used: Heartwood, leaves, flowers, bark, gum
Pterocarpus marsupium is one of the most versatile medicinal plants with a wide spectrum of biological activity. It is a medium-to-large deciduous tree that grows up to 30 m in height. It grows well in India and neighboring countries including Nepal and Sri Lanka. Every part of the tree has been known to possess medicinal value. Compositional studies on *P. marsupium* have established it as a good source of secondary plant metabolites.

P. marsupium contains terpenoids and related phenolic compounds, β-sitosterol, lupenol, epicatechin, and aurone glycosides, and isoflavonoids (Kumar and Seshadri 1976; Mitra and Joshi 1983). *P. marsupium* is known for its antidiabetic activity since long (Kameswara et al. 2001). *P. marsupium* has been reported to elicit a plethora of biological activities including antidiabetic (Jahromi and Ray 1993), antihyperlipidemic, antiobesity (Ambujakshi and Ganapathy 2011), anthelmintic, anti-inflammatory (Hougee et al. 2005; Salunkhe et al. 2005), antioxidative, antiulcerative, and antitumorogenic (Grover et al. 2005; Nair et al. 2005).

P. marsupium elicits its antidiabetic effect through multiple mechanisms. It not only exhibits the property of glucose reduction but also possesses β-cell-protective and regenerative properties

(Chakravarty et al. 1980; WHO 1980). Studies done on various experimental models document that administration of *P. marsupium* has shown a nearly complete restoration of normal insulin secretion and regeneration of beta cells (Chakravarty et al. 1980; Manickam et al. 1997). Supplementation of methanolic extract of *P. marsupium* for 7 and 14 days to STZ-diabetic rats showed normalization of STZ-distressed serum glucose by correcting glycosylated hemoglobin (HbA1c), serum protein, insulin, alkaline and acid phosphatases, and albumin levels (Gupta 2009).

Supplementation of *P. marsupium* has been reported to regenerate β-cells, the effect supposed to be due to flavonoid fraction of the plant (Chakravarty et al. 1980). The strong antihyperlipidemic activity shown by *P. marsupium* in many studies could be due to the contribution of marsupin, pterosupin, and liquiritigenin present in the plant (Jahromi and Ray 1993).

7.2.5 Ocimum sanctum

English name: Holy basil
Common name: Tulsi
Family: Lamiaceae
Parts used: Leaves, stem, flower, root, seeds, oil

Ocimum sanctum is reported to grow worldwide. This aromatic plant is native to South Asia. It is an erect, much branched subshrub, 30–60 cm tall with hairy stems and simple opposite green or purple leaves. Chemical and nutritional composition proves *O. sanctum* a plant with diverse potency. Eugenol, the active constituents present in *O. sanctum* L., has been found to be largely responsible for the therapeutic potential. In addition to eugenol, *O. sanctum* leaf oil also contains eugenol, euginal, urosolic acid, carvacrol, linalool, limatrol, and caryophyllene in enough amounts (Pattanayak et al. 2010).

The antidiabetic property of *O. sanctum* was appreciated in Ayurveda. A significant reduction in blood glucose, glycosylated hemoglobin, and urea along with a simultaneous increase in glycogen, hemoglobin, and protein in STZ-induced diabetic rats has been observed when rats were supplemented with the ethanolic extract of *O. sanctum* (Narendhirakannan et al. 2006). The leaf extract of *O. sanctum* L. has been reported to stimulate the physiological pathways of insulin secretion (Hannan et al. 2006). Administration of *O. sanctum* L. extract, 200 mg/kg for 30 days, has been reported to decrease plasma glucose level by 24.4% in STZ-induced model of diabetic rats. In addition to this, moderate correction in the activities of vital enzymes of carbohydrate metabolism has also been observed (Vats et al. 2004).

It has been reported that oral administration of alcoholic extract of leaves of *O. sanctum* significantly lowered blood sugar level in both normal glucose-fed hyperglycemic and STZ-induced diabetic rats and improved the action of exogenous insulin in normal rats (Chattopadhyay et al. 1998). *O. sanctum* is also suggested to be an effective hypocholesterolemic agent. A marked decrease in serum cholesterol, triacylglycerol, and LDL + VLDL cholesterol as compared to untreated cholesterol-fed group was observed in cholesterol-fed (100 mg/kg body weight/day) rabbits when supplemented with *O. sanctum* seed oil (0.8 g/kg body weight/day) for 4 weeks (Trevisan et al. 2006). A similar kind of study performed on normal albino rabbits and supplementation of *O. sanctum* showed lowered levels of serum total cholesterol, triglyceride, phospholipids, LDL cholesterol, and significant boost in the HDL cholesterol and total fecal sterol contents (Sarkar et al. 1994).

Apart from antidiabetic and cardioprotective effects, *O. sanctum* has also been suggested to possess strong anticancer (Prakash and Gupta 2000), antistress (Modak et al. 2007), analgesic (Khanna and Bhatia 2003), anti-inflammatory (Kelm et al. 2000), antioxidant (Trevisan et al. 2006; Yanpallewar et al. 2004), and immunomodulatory properties, which can be correlated with the prevention of late diabetic complication (Mukherjee et al. 2005), Department of Pharmacology, Jamia Hamdard, New Delhi, India.

7.2.6 Gymnema sylvestre

English name: Gymnema
Common name: Gurmar
Family name: Asclepiadaceae
Parts used: Rhizomes, leaves, volatile oils
Gymnema sylvestre is a herb native to the tropical forests of India and Sri Lanka. It is a large climber, with roots at nodes. It is a potent antidiabetic plant used in Ayurvedic preparations since ancient times. Several studies have proved its antidiabetic potential in different animal models (Sugihara et al. 2000). Aqueous extract of *G. sylvestre* caused reversible increase in intracellular calcium and insulin secretion in mouse and human β-cells with type 2 diabetes (Liu et al. 2009). It has been reported that *G. sylvestre* can prevent adrenal hormones from stimulating the liver to produce glucose in mice, thereby reducing blood sugar level (Gholap and Kar 2003). A group of triterpene saponins, known as gymnemic acids (I–XVIII) and gymnemosaponins (I–V), are present in *G. sylvestre*. These phytochemicals are responsible for its pharmacological properties.

Oral administration of *G. sylvestre* is reported to be effective against several etiological factors related to diabetes such as chronic inflammation (Leach 2007), obesity (Preuss et al. 2004), enzymatic defects, and pancreatic B-cell malfunction (Al-Romaiyan et al. 2010). Karthic et al. (2012) have reported that *G. sylvestre* suspension extract has strong antidiabetic potential against many hyperglycemia-induced complications in alloxan-induced diabetic albino rats. The hypoglycemic effect of ethanolic extract of *G. sylvestre* is reported to be due to enhanced effect of insulin, which comes into play by increasing either the pancreatic secretion of insulin from B cells or its release from the bound form (Liu et al. 2009).

Oral administration of *G. sylvestre* to rats has been reported to show antidiabetic potential with increased utilization of glucose and/or by decreasing the mobilization of fat (Karthic et al. 2012). A significant reduction in body weight, plasma proteins, and total hemoglobin levels has also been observed after oral administration of *G. sylvestre* extract (Karthic et al. 2012).

The leaf extract of *G. sylvestre* has been reported to stimulate insulin secretion in vitro utilizing MIN6 B-cell line and isolated human islets of Langerhans (Liu et al. 2009). Aqueous leaf extract showed hypoglycemic and lipid-lowering activity in alloxan-induced diabetic rats at 400–800 mg/kg doses (Mall et al. 2009). The compounds present in the stem of *G. sylvestre* have been reported to show hypoglycemic activity by inhibiting the atrophy of thymus, pancreas, and splencias in alloxan-induced diabetic rats (Wei et al. 2008). Dihydroxy gymnemic triacetate isolated from *G. sylvestre* leaves has been reported to exhibit hypoglycemic and hypolipidemic effects in STZ-induced diabetic rats (Daisy et al. 2009).

7.2.7 Cinnamomum zeylanicum

English name: Cinnamon
Popular name(s): Dalchini
Family name: Lauraceae
Parts used: Leaves, bark
Cinnamomum zeylanicum has a long history to be used both as a spice and as a medicine. *C. zeylanicum* is obtained from the inner bark of the tree and is commonly used as one of the common ingredients in spice mixtures and in various Ayurvedic preparations. Oil extracted from *C. zeylanicum* leaf and bark contains active components including *cinnamaldehyde*, *cinnamyl acetate*, *cinnamyl alcohol*, and *eugenol* and a wide range of other volatile substances. *C. zeylanicum* is rich in fiber, manganese, and calcium too. Therapeutic studies have proved the ability of cinnamaldehyde as a hypoglycemic agent. Cinnamaldehyde inhibits the activity of aldose reductase, the key enzyme involved in the polyol pathway. Inhibition of this enzyme prevents the conversion of glucose to sorbitol, thereby preventing several diabetic complications: cataract, neuropathy, and retinopathy (Lee et al. 2013).

Cinnamaldehyde has also been reported to possess antiadipogenic effects through the modulation of the peroxisome proliferator–activated receptor (PPAR)-γ and AMP-activated protein kinase signaling pathways thus functioning as an antiobesity agent (Huang et al. 2011). *C. zeylanicum* has been proposed to be effective in moderating postprandial glucose response in normal-weight and obese adults (Magistrelli and Chezem 2012). Different mechanisms of action have been reported behind the antidiabetic effect of *C. zeylanicum* including reducing the rate at which the stomach empties after meals, thus reducing the rise in blood sugar after eating. Hlebowicz et al. (2007), in their study, measured gastric-emptying rate after adding *C. zeylanicum* to the rice pudding and observed a lowered gastric emptying rate from 37% to 34.5% and significantly lowered the rise in blood sugar levels after meal.

C. zeylanicum extract has been reported to significantly increase insulin sensitivity, reduce serum and hepatic lipids, and improve hyperlipidemia and hyperglycemia probably by regulating the PPAR-medicated glucose and lipid metabolism (Kim and Choung 2010). A study performed on type 2 diabetic humans, consuming 1 g of *C. zeylanicum* per day, was found to be effective in decreasing blood sugar, triglycerides, and total cholesterol, which indicated that including *C. zeylanicum* in the diet of people with type 2 diabetes may reduce risk factors associated with diabetes (Khan et al. 2003). An intake of 2 g of cinnamon for 12 weeks has been reported to significantly reduce the HbA1c, systolic, and diastolic blood pressures among poorly controlled type 2 diabetic patients (Akilen et al. 2010).

The pancreas-protective and hypoglycemic potential of leaf essential oil from indigenous *C. zeylanicum* in diabetic rats has been observed and found to be ameliorative against oxidative stress and pro-inflammatory environment in the pancreas thereby providing a protective effect on pancreatic β-cells (Lee et al. 2013). Repairing pancreatic β-cells, improving its antioxidative capacity, as well as attenuating cytotoxicity via the inhibition of iNOS and NF-κB activation in diabetic mice are other effects of *C. zeylanicum* supposed to be responsible for its strong antidiabetic effect (Li et al. 2013). In another study conducted on 66 type 2 diabetics in Chinese population, a significantly improved blood glucose control has been observed, which supports that cinnamon supplementation controls glycemic levels in diabetics and prediabetics (Davis and Yokoyama 2011).

7.2.8 Zingiber officinale

English name: Ginger
Popular name(s): Adrak
Family name: Zingiberaceae
Parts used: Root, essential oil

Zingiber officinale is a perennial reed-like plant with annual leafy stems, about a meter tall. It is consumed worldwide in cookeries as a spice and flavoring agent. Due to the strong aroma, *Z. officinale* is used in food, beverages, and dietary supplements since ancient times. The rhizome of *Z. officinale* has been used since antiquity in various traditional systems of medicine among Asian and Arabians to treat sprains, cramps, muscular aches, pains, sore throats, hypertension, and dementia (Haniadka et al. 2013).

Numerous studies have reported the beneficial effect of *Z. officinale* against diabetes and associated events. The extract of *Z. officinale* has been shown to reduce the burden of oxidative stress, lower cytotoxicity, and protect β-cell viability (Račková et al. 2013). Enhancement of insulin sensitivity in adipocytes by *Z. officinale* supplementation has also been observed (Sekiya et al. 2004). *Z. officinale* has been reported to inhibit the key enzymes, which control carbohydrate metabolism associated with diabetes. A significant increase in the activities of pancreatic lipase, amylase, trypsin, and chymotrypsin has been seen after the supplementation of *Z. officinale* to rats for 8 weeks.

Gingerols, the important pungent component in *Z. officinale*, were ascribed to facilitate insulin-independent glucose uptake by enhancing the translocation of glucose transporter (GLUT4) to the muscle cell plasma membrane surface, simultaneously with small increases in total GLUT4 protein expression (Li et al. 2013). Gingerol possesses hypoglycemic property and can improve impaired insulin signaling in arsenic-intoxicated mice (Chakraborty et al. 2012). In a double-blinded, placebo-controlled clinical trial, 1600 mg *Z. officinale* per day when supplemented for 12 weeks to diabetic patients, a significant reduction in insulin, fasting plasma glucose, glycated hemoglobin, triglyceride, total cholesterol, C-reactive protein, and prostaglandin E2 has been observed (Arablou et al. 2014).

Inflammation, a common feature in type 2 diabetes, has been reported to be reversed by *Z. officinale* supplementation. A significant reduction in pro-inflammatory cytokine (IL-6 and TNF-α) level in diabetics has been observed after *Z. officinale* supplementation (Mahluji et al. 2013). Decrease in the levels of total cholesterol and LDL and a substantial reduction in glucose level have been reported in *Z. officinale*–treated diabetic rat models (Chakraborty et al. 2012).

Evidence from in vivo studies has proved that *Z. officinale* exerts the protective power against oxidative stress during diabetes. A diet containing 1% and 2% of *Z. officinale* powder when fed to diabetic rats for 30 days resulted in an increment of GSH and decrease in malondialdehyde content. Activities of superoxide dismutase (SOD), catalase (CAT), glutathione peroxidase, and glutathione reductase have also been restored after *Z. officinale* administration, which were diminished in diabetics (Shanmugam et al. 2011).

7.2.9 Aegle marmelos

English name: Stone fruit, golden apple
Popular name: Bael
Family name: Rutaceae
Parts used: Roots, leaves, fruit, bark, and seeds

Aegle marmelos tree is indigenous to India, but is found to be present in many other Asian countries such as Sri Lanka, Myanmar, Nepal, Bangladesh, Pakistan, Vietnam, and Thailand. The tree is generally large, which grows to about 8–10 m in height. It has a wide trunk with long straight branches and sweet aromatic leaves. The fruits of *A. marmelos* are smooth, woody, and hard, with sweet and aromatic flesh inside.

A. marmelos contains various chemical constituents like steroids, coumarins, and alkaloids in root, wood, bark leaves, and fruits. Some of the well-known bioactive components responsible for the medicinal properties of the plant are aurapten, aegelin, cineol, citral, citronellal, cuminaldehyde, eugenol, fagarine, lupeol, luvangetin, mermelosin, marmelide, marmin, psoralen, skimmianine, umbelliferone, and tannins (Maity et al. 2009). This plant is also rich in vitamins and minerals (Paricha 2004).

The aqueous extract of *A. marmelos* leaves, when administered to alloxan-induced diabetic albino rats, showed strong hypoglycemic and antioxidant activities thereby contributing to long-term management of diabetes (Upadhya et al. 2004). *A. marmelos* has been reported to modulate the activity of enzymatic and nonenzymatic antioxidants and thereby enhance the defense against reactive oxygen species–generated damage in diabetic rats. Histopathological studies also support the protective effect of *A. marmelos* on pancreatic β-cells (Narendhirakannan and Subramanian 2010). The ethanolic extract of *A. marmelos* administered orally for 30 days (150 mg/kg body weight/day) to diabetic rats showed a significant increase in the levels of plasma glucose, vitamin E, ceruloplasmin, and lipid peroxides, and a concomitant decrease in the levels of vitamin C and GSH (Narendhirakannan and Subramanian 2010).

The antihyperlipidemic activity of aqueous extract of *A. marmelos* fruits has also been studied in STZ-induced diabetic Wistar rats (Marzine and Gilbart 2005). The ameliorative effect of *A. marmelos* leaf extract on early stage alloxan-induced diabetic cardiomyopathy in rats has been studied by Bhatti et al. (2011). The extract of *A. marmelos* was found to decrease the levels of FBG, total cholesterol, TBARS, lactate dehydrogenase, and creatine kinase and to increase the levels of GSH, CAT, and SOD dose dependently with a dose of 200 mg/kg body weight.

Umbelliferone, one of the phytoconstituents of *A. marmelos*, has been found to be effective in the restoration of plasma insulin and glucose and in the protection of diabetes-induced alterations in the activities of membrane-bound ATPases (Balakrishnan and Pugalendi 2007). Antihyperlipidemic and antioxidant efficacies of umbelliferone have also been reported (Kumar et al. 2013).

7.3 OTHER EFFECTIVE SUPPLEMENTS HAVING BENEFICIAL EFFECT AGAINST DIABETES

7.3.1 Alpha-Lipoic Acid

Alpha-lipoic acid (ALA) is a disulfide compound, produced in tiny amounts in cells, and serves as a coenzyme in the alpha-ketoglutarate dehydrogenase and pyruvate dehydrogenase mitochondrial enzyme complexes. ALA is known for its potent antioxidant property. Intravenous (i.v.) infusion of ALA has been reported to increase insulin-mediated glucose disposal. ALA had been used for the treatment of diabetes-induced neuropathy (Evans and Goldfine 2000). ALA has also been reported to be protective against diabetic cardiomyopathy (Hegazy et al. 2013). ALA along with omega 3 fatty acid and vitamin E is suggested to be used as an add-on therapy in patients with type 2 DM to improve insulin sensitivity and lipid metabolism (Udupa et al. 2013).

ALA in a dose of 600 mg, parenterally, for 7 days, positively managed the BMI, HbA1C, and cholesterol, which thereby showed tangible beneficial effect on erectile dysfunction and on metabolic disorder during diabetes (Mitkov et al. 2013). ALA has been found to be effective against diabetic distal sensory-motor neuropathy (Ibrahimpasic 2013).

7.3.2 Magnesium

Magnesium-containing enzymes are involved in glucose homeostasis, nerve transmission, RNA, and DNA production (Swaminathan 2003). Deficiency of magnesium has been reported to decrease insulin-mediated glucose uptake (Afridi et al. 2006). Low-level serum and increased excretion of magnesium have been reported in diabetics (Afridi et al. 2006). Reports have supported the effectiveness of magnesium supplementation in the prevention of insulin resistance (Mooren et al. 2011). Two large cohort studies have reported a strong negative correlation between the intake of magnesium and the risk of type 2 diabetes among men aged 40–75 years and women aged 40–65 years (Salmeron et al. 1997a,b).

7.3.3 Manganese

Manganese is a cofactor in several enzymes including those involved in the metabolism of carbohydrates, proteins, and fats, and in the production of bone marrow (Orbea et al. 2002). Alteration in the metabolism of manganese is supposed to be involved in the development of diabetes (Kazi et al. 2008). Appropriate manganese level is required for normal insulin synthesis and secretion (Naga et al. 2006). Ekmekcioglu et al. (2001) have documented that insulin-resistant diabetic patients responded well to oral doses of manganese.

7.3.4 Zinc

Zinc is an essential trace element that is required for normal cell division and apoptosis. It plays an important role in the storage and secretion of insulin, which consequently increases glucose uptake (Forte et al. 2013; Kazi et al. 2008). Importance of zinc in the maintenance and integration of insulin hexamer and its role in the metabolic regulation has been studied (Rungby 2010). Mutation in zinc transporter (ZnT8), a key protein for the regulation of insulin secretion, has been found associated with type 2 diabetes (Wijesekara et al. 2010).

A large body of experimental and clinical evidence has reported alteration of zinc homeostasis in diabetics (Chung et al. 1995; Kazi et al. 2008). Diabetic patients have been found to excrete more zinc through urine, which results in lower values in blood and serum, especially in patients with diabetic nephropathy (Chung et al. 1995). Deficiency of zinc makes diabetics prone to infections and damages the heart, arteries, and other integral parts of the vascular system (Di-Silvestro 2000).

7.3.5 Chromium

Chromium is an essential metal found in traces in human beings, the biological activity of which depends on its state of valency and chemical complexes it forms (Guidotti et al. 2008). Trivalent form of chromium has been shown to have high biological activity for the optimal glucose uptake by cells (Tudan et al. 2011).

Chromium regulates insulin and glucose levels in blood by stimulating insulin signaling pathway and metabolism by regulating GLUT4 translocation in muscle cells (Qiao et al. 2009). Prolonged dietary deficiency of chromium or increased excretion of urinary chromium is reported to cause diabetes (Forte et al. 2013), which may revert back after the supplementation of chromium.

7.3.6 Selenium

Selenium is incorporated into selenoproteins through a complex genetic mechanism encoded by the UGA codon (Papp et al. 2007). Selenium of selenoproteins is thought to participate in various biological functions including thyroid and immune functions and in providing protection against oxidative stress (Papp et al. 2007; Rayman 2000).

Selenium is reported to associate with diabetic prevalence; insulin combined with selenium could significantly lower blood glucose levels and markedly restore the diminished expression of in IRS-1, PI3K, and GLUT4 levels in skeletal muscles of diabetic rats (Xu et al. 2013).

7.4 CONCLUSION

A strong body of evidence suggests that several herbal sources and mineral supplements have strong antidiabetic potential. Indian traditional medicine has thrived for ages and offers many antidiabetic strategies based on the use of plants. While the active principle in many of the herbal-based products has been isolated and characterized, there are still many plants whose active principles have not been identified. Sometimes, the synergistic effect plays an important role, and isolated compounds fail to mimic the effect observed with the whole extract. Studies on herbal supplements offer important clues for the development of antidiabetic drugs.

REFERENCES

Achrekar, S., Kaklij, G.S., Pote, M.S. et al. 1991. Hypoglycemic activity of *Eugenia jambolana* and *Ficus bengalenesis*: Mechanism of action. *In Vivo* 5:143–147.

Afridi, H.I., Kazi, T.G., Kazi, N. et al. 2006. Potassium, calcium, magnesium, and sodium levels in biological samples of hypertensive and nonhypertensive diabetes mellitus patients. *Biol Trace Elem Res* 13:206–224.

AHFS Drug Information. 2012. *Authority of the Board of the American Society of Health-System Pharamacists.* American Hospital Formulary Service, Bethesda, MD.

Akilen, R., Tsiami, A., Devendra, D. et al. 2010. Glycated haemoglobin and blood pressure-lowering effect of cinnamon in multi-ethnic type 2 diabetic patients in the UK: A randomized, placebo-controlled, double-blind clinical trial. *Diab Med* 27:1159–1167.

Ali, L., Kalam, A., Khan, A. et al. 1995. Characterization of the hypoglycemic effects of *Trigonella foenum-graecum* seed. *Planta Med* 61:358–360.

Al-Romaiyan, A., Liu, B., Asare-Anane, H. et al. 2010. A novel *Gymnema sylvestre* extract stimulates insulin secretion from human islets in vivo and in vitro. *Phytother Res* 24:1370–1376.

Ambujakshi, H.R. and Ganapathy, S. 2011. Anti obese activity of *Pterocarpus marsupium* barks extract in experimentally induced obese rats. *Inventi Impact: Nutraceut* 7:15.

Arablou, T., Aryaeian, N., Valizadeh, M. et al. 2014.The effect of ginger consumption on glycemic status, lipid profile and some inflammatory markers in patients with type 2 diabetes mellitus. *Int J Food Sci Nutr* 65:515–520.

Ayyanar, M. and Subash-Babu, P. 2012. *Syzygium cumini* (L.) Skeels: A review of its phytochemical constituents and traditional uses. *J Trop Biomed* 2:240–246.

Balakrishnan, R. and Pugalendi, K.V. 2007. Influence of umbelliferone on membrane bound ATPases in streptozotocin-induced diabetic rats. *Pharmacol Rep* 59:339–348.

Bhatti, R., Sharma, S., Singh, J. et al. 2011. Ameliorative effect of *Aegle marmelos* leaf extract on early stage alloxan-induced diabetic cardiomyopathy in rats. *Pharm Biol* 49:1137–1143.

Brownlee, M. 2001. Biochemistry and molecular cell biology of diabetic complications. *Nature* 414:813–820.

Chakraborty, D., Mukherjee, A., Sikdar, S. et al. 2012. [6]-Gingerol isolated from ginger attenuates sodium arsenite induced oxidative stress and plays a corrective role in improving insulin signaling in mice. *Toxicol Lett* 210:34–43.

Chakravarty, B.K., Gupta, S., Gambhir, S.S. et al. 1980. Pancreatic beta cell regeneration. A novel antidiabetic mechanism of *Pterocarpus marsupium* Roxb. *Ind J Pharmacol* 12:123–127.

Chattopadhyay, D., Sinha, B.K., and Vaid, L.K. 1998. Antibacterial activity of *Syzygium species. Fitoterapia* 69:356–367.

Chaturvedi, A., Bhawani, M.K., Chaturvedi, H. et al. 2007. Effect of ethanolic extract of *Eugenia jambolana* seeds on gastric ulceration and secretion in rats. *Indian J Physiol Pharmacol* 51:131–140.

Chaturvedi, P. 2012. Antidiabetic potentials of *Momordica charantia*: Multiple mechanisms behind the effects. *J Med Food* 15:101–107.

Chung, J.S., Franco, R.J.S., and Curi, R.R. 1995. Renal excretion of zinc in normal individuals during zinc tolerance test and glucose tolerance test. *Trace Elem Electrol* 12:62–67.

Daisy, P., Eliza, J., and Mohamed, F.K.A. 2009. A novel dihydroxy gymnemic triacetate isolated from *Gymnema sylvestre* possessing normoglycemic and hypolipidemic activity on STZ-induced diabetic rats. *J Ethnopharmacol* 126:339–344.

Davis, P.A. and Yokoyama, W. 2011. Cinnamon intake lowers fasting blood glucose: Meta-analysis. *J Med Food* 14:884–889.

Di-Silvestro, R.A. 2000. Zinc in relation to diabetes and oxidative disease. *J Nutr* 130:1509–1511.

Dong, H., Wang, N., Zhao, L., and Lu, F. 2012. Berberine in the treatment of type 2 diabetes mellitus: A systemic review and meta-analysis. *Evid Based Complem Alternat Med* 2012:1–12.

Ekmekcioglu, C., Prohaska, C., Pomazal, K. et al. 2001. Concentrations of seven trace elements in different hematological matrices in patients with type-2 diabetes as compared to healthy controls. *Biol Trace Elem Res* 79:205–219.

Evans, J.L. and Goldfine, I.D. 2000. Alpha-lipoic acid: A multifunctional antioxidant that improves insulin sensitivity in patients with type 2 diabetes. *Diab Technol Ther* 2:401–413.

Fernandes, N.P., Lagishetty, C.V., Panda, V.S., and Naik, S.R. 2007. An experimental evaluation of the antidiabetic and antilipidemic properties of a standardized *Momordica charantia* fruit extract. *BMC Complem Altern Med* 7:29.

Forte, G., Bocca, B., Peruzzu, A. et al. 2013. Blood metals concentration in type 1 and type 2 diabetics. *Biol Trace Elem Res* 13:79–90.

Genet, S., Kale, R.K., and Baquer, N.Z. 1999. Effects of vanadate, insulin and fenugreek (*Trigonella foenum graecum*) on creatine kinase levels in tissues of diabetic rat. *Indian J Exp Biol* 37:200–202.

Gholap, S. and Kar, A. 2003. Effects of *Inula racemosa* root and *Gymnema sylvestre* leaf extracts in the regulation of corticosteroid induced diabetes mellitus: Involvement of thyroid hormones. *Pharmazie* 58:413–415.

Grover, J.K., Vats, V., and Yadav, S.S. 2005. *Pterocarpus marsupium* extract (Vijayasar) prevented the alteration in metabolic patterns induced in the normal rat by feeding an adequate diet containing fructose as sole carbohydrate. *Diab Obes Metab* 7:414–420.

Grover, J.K., Yadav, S., and Vats, V. 2002. Medicinal plants of India with anti-diabetic potential. *J Ethnopharmacol* 81:81–100.

Guidotti, T.L., McNamara, J., and Moses, M.S. 2008. The interpretation of trace element analysis in body fluids. *Indian J Med Res* 13:524–532.

Gupta, A., Gupta, R., and Lal, B. 2001. Effect of *Trigonella foenum-graecum* (fenugreek) seeds on glycaemic control and insulin resistance in type 2 diabetes mellitus: A double blind placebo controlled study. *J Assoc Phys India* 49:1057–1061.

Gupta, D., Raju, J., and Baquer, N.Z. 1999. Modulation of some gluconeogenic enzyme activities in diabetic rat liver and kidney: Effect of antidiabetic compounds. *Indian J Exp Biol* 37:196–199.

Gupta, R.S. 2009. Effect of *Pterocarpus marsupium* in streptozotocin-induced hyperglycemic state in rats: Comparison with glibenclamide. *J Diabetol Croat* 38:39–45.

Hamden, K., Masmoudi, H., Carreau, S., and Elfeki, A. 2010. Immunomodulatory, β-cell, and neuroprotective actions of fenugreek oil from alloxan-induced diabetes. *Immunopharmacol Immunotoxicol* 32:437–445.

Hammes, H.P., Feng, Y., Pfister, F., and Brownlee, M. 2011. Diabetic retinopathy: Targeting vasoregression. *Diabetes* 60:9–16.

Haniadka, R., Saldanha, E., Sunita, V. et al. 2013. A review of the gastroprotective effects of ginger (*Zingiber officinale Roscoe). Food Funct* 4:845–855.

Hannan, J.M., Marenah, L., Ali, L. et al. 2006. *Ocimum sanctum* leaf extracts stimulate insulin secretion from perfused pancreas, isolated islets and clonal pancreatic beta-cells. *J Endocrinol* 189:127–136.

Hegazy, S.K., Tolba, O.A., Mostafa, T.M. et al. 2013. Alpha-lipoic acid improves subclinical left ventricular dysfunction in asymptomatic patients with type 1 diabetes. *Rev Diab Stud* 10:58–67.

Hlebowicz, J., Darwiche, G., Björgell, O. et al. 2007. Effect of cinnamon on postprandial blood glucose, gastric emptying, and satiety in healthy subjects. *Am J Clin Nutr* 85:1552–1556.

Hougee S., Faber, J., Sanders, A. et al. 2005. Selective COX-2 inhibition by a *Pterocarpus marsupium* extract characterized by pterostilbene and its activity in healthy human volunteers. *Planta Med* 71:387–392.

Huang, B., Yuan, H.D., Kim do, Y. et al. 2011. Cinnamaldehyde prevents adipocyte differentiation and adipogenesis via regulation of peroxisome proliferator-activated receptor-γ (PPARγ) and AMP-activated protein kinase (AMPK) pathways. *J Agric Food Chem* 59:3666–3673.

Ibrahimpasic, K. 2013. Alpha lipoic acid and glycaemic control in diabetic neuropathies at type 2 diabetes treatment. *Med Arh* 67:7–9.

Inayat-ur-Rahman, Malik, S.A., Bashir, M. et al. 2009. Serum sialic acid changes in non-insulin-dependent diabetes mellitus (NIDDM) patients following bitter melon (*Momordica charantia*) and rosiglitazone (Avandia) treatment. *Phytomedicine* 16:401–405.

IDF Diabetes Atlas Sixth edition, 2013 online version of IDF Diabetes Atlas: www.idf.org/diabetesatlas. ISBN: 2-930229-85-3.

Inzucchi, S.E. 2002. Oral antihyperglycemic therapy for type 2 diabetes: Scientific review. *JAMA* 287:360–372.

Jahromi, M.A. and Ray, A.B. 1993. Antihyperlipidemic effect of flavonoids from *Pterocarpus marsupium. J Nat Prod* 56:989–994.

Kameswara, R.B., Guiri, R., Kesavulu, M.M., and Apparao, C.H. 2001. Effect of oral administration of bark extracts of *Pterocarpus santalinus* L. on blood glucose level in experimental animals. *J Ethnopharmacol* 74:69–74.

Karthic, R., Nagaraj, S., Arulmurugan, P. et al. 2012. *Gymnema sylvestre* R. Br. suspension cell extract show antidiabetic potential in Alloxan induced diabetic albino male rats. *Asian Pac J Trop Biomed* 2:S930–S933.

Kavishankar, G.B., Lakshmidevi, N., Mahadeva Murthy, S. et al. 2011. Diabetes and medicinal plants—A review. *Int J Pharm Biomed Sci* 2:65–80.

Kazi, T.G., Afridi, H.I., Kazi, N. et al. 2008. Copper, chromium, manganese, iron, nickel, and zinc levels in biological samples of diabetes mellitus patients. *Biol Trace Elem Res* 13:1–18.

Kelm, M.A., Nair, M.G., Stasburg, G.M. et al. 2000. Antioxidant and cyclooxygenase inhibitory phenolic compounds from *Ocimum sanctum* Linn. *Phytomedicine* 7:7–13.

Khan, A., Safdar, M., Ali Khan, M.M. et al. 2003. Cinnamon improves glucose and lipids of people with type 2 diabetes. *Diab Care* 26:3215–3218.

Khanna, N. and Bhatia, J. 2003. Antinociceptive action of *Ocimum sanctum* (Tulsi) in mice: Possible mechanisms involved. *J Ethnopharmacol* 88:293–296.

Khosla, P., Gupta, D.D., and Nagpal, R.K. 1995. Effect of *Trigonella foenum graceum* (fenugreek) on blood glucose in normal and diabetic rats. *Indian J Physiol Pharmacol* 39:173–174.

Kim, S.H. and Choung, S.Y. 2010. Antihyperglycemic and antihyperlipidemic action of *Cinnamomi cassiae* (Cinnamonbark) extract in C57BL/Ks db/db mice. *Arch Pharm Res* 33:325–333.

Krawinkel, M.B. and Keding, G.B. 2006. Bitter gourd (*Momordica Charantia*): A dietary approach to hyperglycemia. *Nutr Rev* 64:331–337.

Kumar, N. and Seshadri, T.R. 1976. A new triterpene from *Pterocarpus santalinus* bark. *Phytochemistry* 9:1877–1878.

Kumar, V., Ahmed, D., Anwar, F. et al. 2013. Enhanced glycemic control, pancreas protective, antioxidant and hepatoprotective effects by umbelliferon-α-D-glucopyranosyl-(2I→1II)-α-D-glucopyranoside in streptozotocin induced diabetic rats. *Springer Plus* 2:639.

Leach, M.J. 2007. *Gymnema sylvestre* for diabetes mellitus: A systematic review. *J Altern Complem Med* 13:977–983.

Lee, C.M., Colagiuri, R., Magliano, D.J., Cameron, A.J., Shaw, J., Zimmet, P. and Colagiuri, S. 2013. The cost of diabetes in adults in Australia. *Diab Res Clin Pract* 99:385–390.

Lee, S.C., Xu, W.X., Lin, L.Y. et al. 2013. Chemical composition and hypoglycemic and pancreas-protective effect of leaf essential oil from indigenous cinnamon (*Cinnamomum osmophloeum Kanehira*). *J Agric Food Chem* 61:4905–4913.

Leung, L., Birtwhistle, R., Kotecha, J. et al. 2004. Pharmacological actions and potential uses of *Momordica charantia*: A review. *J Ethnopharmacol* 93:123–132.

Li, R., Liang, T., Xu, L. et al. 2013. Protective effect of cinnamon polyphenols against STZ-diabetic mice fed high-sugar, high-fat diet and its underlying mechanism. *Food Chem Toxicol* 51:419–425.

Liu, B., Asare-Anane, H., Al-Romaiyan, A. et al. 2009. Characterisation of the insulinotropic activity of an aqueous extract of *Gymnema sylvestre* in mouse beta-cells and human islets of Langerhans. *Cell Physiol Biochem* 23:125–132.

Magistrelli, A. and Chezem, J.C. 2012. Effect of ground cinnamon on postprandial blood glucose concentration in normal-weight and obese adults. *J Acad Nutr Diet* 112:1806–1809.

Mahluji, S., Ostadrahimi, A., Mobasseri, M. et al. 2013. Anti-inflammatory effects of *zingiber officinale* in type 2 diabetic patients. *Adv Pharm Bull* 3:273–276.

Maity, P., Hansda D., Bandyopadhyay, U. et al. 2009. Biological activities of crude extracts of chemical constituents of Bael, *Aegle marmelos* (L.) Corr. *Indian J Exp Biol* 47:849–861.

Mall, G.K., Mishra, P.K., and Prakash, V. 2009. Antidiabetic and hypolipidemic activity of *Gymnema sylvestre* in alloxan induced diabetic rats. *Glob J Biotechnol Biochem* 4:37–42.

Manickam, M., Ramanathan, M., Jahromi, M.A. et al. 1997. Antihyperglycemic activity of phenolics from *Pterocarpus marsupium*. *J Nat Prod* 60:609–610.

Marzine, P.S. and Gilbart, R. 2005. The effect of an aqueous extract of *A. marmelos* fruits on serum and tissue lipids in experimental diabetes. *J Sci Food Agric* 85:569–573.

Mitkov, M.D., Aleksandrova, I.Y., and Orbetzova, M.M. 2013. Effect of transdermal testosterone or alpha-lipoic acid on erectile dysfunction and quality of life in patients with type 2 diabetes mellitus. *Folia Med* (*Plovdiv*) 55:55–63.

Mitra, J. and Joshi, T. 1983. Isoflavonoids from the heart wood of *Pterocarpus marsupium*. *Phytochemistry* 22:2326–2327.

Modak, M., Dixit, P., Londhe, J. et al. 2007. Indian herbs and herbal drugs used for the treatment of diabetes. *J Clin Biochem Nutr* 40:163–173.

Mooren, F.C., Kruger, K., Volker, K. et al. 2011. Oral magnesium supplementation reduces insulin resistance in non-diabetic subjects—A double-blind, placebo-controlled, randomized trial. *Diab Obes Metab* 13:281–284.

Morton, J.F. 1987. *Fruits of Warm Climates*. Creative Resource Systems, Inc., Winterville, NC, 505 p.

Mukherjee, R., Dash, P.K., and Ram, G.C. 2005. Immunotherapeutic potential of *Ocimum sanctum* (L.) in bovine subclinical mastitis. *Res Vet Sci* 79:37–43.

Naga Raju, G.J., Sarita, P., Ramana Murty, G.A.V. et al. 2006. Estimation of trace elements in some anti-diabetic medicinal plants using PIXE technique. *Appl Radiat Isotopes* 64:893–900.

Nair, R., Kalariya, T., and Chanda, S. 2005. Antibacterial activity of some selected Indian medicinal flora. *Turk J Biol* 29:41–47.

Narendhirakannan, R.T. and Subramanian, S. 2010. Biochemical evaluation of the protective effect of *Aegle marmelos* (L.), Corr. leaf extract on tissue antioxidant defense system and histological changes of pancreatic beta-cells in streptozotocin-induced diabetic rats. *Drug Chem Toxicol* 33:120–130.

Narendhirakannan, R.T., Subramanian, S., and Kandaswamy, M. 2006. Biochemical evaluation of antidiabetogenic properties of some commonly used Indian plants on streptozotocin-induced diabetes in experimental rats. *Clin Exp Pharmacol Physiol* 33:1150–1157.

Orbea, A., Ortiz-Zarragoitia, M., Sole, M. et al. 2002. Antioxidant enzymes and peroxisome proliferation in relation to contaminant body burdens of PAHs and PCBs in bivalve molluscs, crabs and fish from the Urdaibai and Plentzia estuaries (Bay of Biscay). *Aquat Toxicol* 13:75–98.

Pandey, K.B. and Rizvi, S.I. 2014. Role of red grape polyphenols as antidiabetic agents. *Integr Med Res* 3:119–125.

Papp, L.V., Lu, J., Holmgren, A. et al. 2007. From selenium to selenoproteins: Synthesis, identity, and their role in human health. *Antioxid Redox Signal* 9:775—806.

Paricha, S. 2004. Bael (*Aegle marmelos*) Natures most natural medicinal fruit. *Orissa Rev* 9:16–17.

Patel, D.K., Prasad, S.K., Kumar, R., and Hemalatha, S. 2012. An overview on antidiabetic medicinal plants having insulin mimetic property. *Asian Pac J Trop Biomed* 2:320–330.

Pattanayak, P., Behera, P., Das, D. et al. 2010. *Ocimum sanctum* Linn. A reservoir plant for therapeutic applications: An overview. *Pharmacogn Rev* 4:95–105.

Periyathambi, R. 2007. Jamun—The potential untapped. *Horticulture* 1:30–32.

Petit, P.R., Sauvaire, Y.D., Hillaire-Buys, D.M. et al. 1995. Steroid saponins from fenugreek seeds extraction, purification, and pharmacological investigation on feeding behavior and plasma cholesterol. *Steroids* 60:674–680.

Prabhakar, P. K. and Doble, M. 2011. Mechanism of action of natural products used in the treatment of diabetes mellitus. *Chin J Integr Med* 17:563–574.

Prakash, J. and Gupta, S.K. 2000. Chemopreventive activity of *Ocimum sanctum* seed oil. *J Ethnopharmacol* 72:29–34.

Preuss, H., Bagchi, D., and Bagchi, M. 2004. Effects of a natural extract of (–)-hydroxycitric acid (HCA-SX) and combination of HCA-SX plus niacin-bound chromium and *Gymnema sylvestre* extract on weight loss. *Diab Obes Metab* 6:171.

Qiao, W., Peng, Z., Wang, Z. et al. 2009. Chromium improves glucose uptake and metabolism through upregulating the mRNA levels of IR, GLUT4, GS, and UCP3 in skeletal muscle cells. *Biol Trace Elem Res* 13:133–142.

Račková, L., Cupáková, M., Tažký, A. et al. 2013. Redox properties of ginger extracts: Perspectives of use of *Zingiber officinale* Rosc. as antidiabetic agent. *Interdiscip Toxicol* 6:26–33.

Raghuram, T.C., Sharma, R.D., Sivakumar, B., and Sahay, K. 1994. Effect of fenugreek seeds on intravenous glucose disposition in non-insulin dependent diabetic patients. *Phytotherapy Res* 8:83–86.

Rastogi, R.M. and Mehrotra, B.N. 1990. Compendium of Indian medicinal plants. *Central Drug Res Inst Lucknow India* 1:388–389.

Ravi, K., Ramachandran, B., and Subramanian, S. 2004. Protective effect of *Eugenia jambolana* seed kernel on tissue antioxidants in streptozotocin induced diabetic rats. *Biol Pharm Bull* 27:1212–1217.

Ravi, K., Rajasekaran, S., and Subramanians, S. 2005. Anti hyperlipidaemic effects of *Eugenia jambolana* seed kernel on streptozotocin induced diabetic rats. *Food Chem Toxicol* 43:1433–1439.

Rayman, M.P. 2000. The importance of selenium to human health. *Lancet* 356:233–241.

Rungby, J. 2010. Zinc, zinc transporters and diabetes. *Diabetologia* 13:1549–1551.

Sagrawat, H., Mann, A.S., and Kharya, M.D. 2006. Pharmacological potential of *Eugenia jambolana*: A review. *Pharmacog Mag* 2:96–105.

Salmeron, J., Ascherio, A., Rimm, E.B. et al. 1997a. Dietary fiber, glycemic load and risk of NIDDM in men. *Diab Care* 20:545–550.

Salmeron, J., Manson, J.E., Stampfer, M.J. et al. 1997b. Dietary fiber, glycemic load, and risk of noninsulin-dependent diabetes mellitus in women. *J Am Med Assoc* 277:472–477.

Salunkhe, V.R., Yadav, A.V., Shete, A.S. et al. 2005. Anti-inflammatory activity of hydrogels of extracts of *Pterocarpus marsupium* and *Coccinia indica*. *Indian Drugs* 42:319–321.

Sarkar, A., Lavania, S.C., Pandey, D.N. et al. 1994. Changes in the blood lipid profile after administration of *Ocimum sanctum* (Tulsi) leaves in the normal albino rabbits. *Indian J Physiol Pharmacol* 38:311–312.

Sathishsekar, D. and Subramanian, S. 2005. Beneficial effects of *Momordica charantia* seeds in the treatment of STZ-induced diabetes in experimental rats. *Biol Pharm Bull* 28:978–983.

Saxena, A. and Vikram, N.K. 2004. Role of selected Indian plants in management of type 2 diabetes: A review. *J Altern Complem Med* 10:369–378.

Sekar, D.S., Sivagnanam, K., and Subramanian, S. 2005. Antidiabetic activity of *Momordica charantia* seeds on streptozotocin induced diabetic rats. *Pharmazie* 60:383–387.

Sekiya, K., Ohtani, A., and Kusano, S. 2004. Enhancement of insulin sensitivity in adipocytes by ginger. *BioFactors* 22:153–156.

Shabib, B.A., Khan, L.A., and Rahman, R. 1993. Hypoglycemic activity of *Coccinia indica* and *Momordica charantia* in diabetic rats: Depression of the hepatic gluconeogenic enzymes glucose-6-phosphatase and fructose-1,6-biphosphatase and elevation of liver and red-cell shunt enzyme glucose-6-phosphate dehydrogenase. *Biochem J* 292:267–270.

Shanmugam, K.R., Mallikarjuna, K., Nishanth, K. et al. 2011. Protective effect of dietary ginger on antioxidant enzymes and oxidative damage in experimental diabetic rat tissues. *Food Chem* 124:1436–1442.

Sharma, R.D., Raghuram, T.C., and Rao, N.S. 1990. Effect of fenugreek seeds on blood glucose and serum lipids in type I diabetes. *Eur J Clin Nutr* 44:301–306.

Shetty, A.K., Kumar, G.S., Sambaiah, K., and Salimath, P.V. 2005. Effect of bitter gourd (*Momordica charantia*) on glycaemic status in streptozotocin induced diabetic rats. *Plant Foods Hum Nutr* 60:109–112.

Singh, A.B., Tamarkar, A.K., Narender, T., and Srivastava, A.K. 2010. Antihyperglycemic effect of an unusual amino acid (4-hydroxyisoleucine) in C57BL/KsJ-db/db mice. *Nat Prod Res* 24:258–265.
Singh, N. and Gupta, M. 2007. Effects of ethanolic extract of *Syzygium cumini* (Linn) on pancreatic islets of alloxan diabetic rats. *Ind J Exp Biol* 45:861–867.
Srivastava, B., Sinha, A.K., Gaur, S. et al. 2012. Study of hypoglycaemic and hypolipidemic activity of *Eugenia Jambolana* pulp and seed extract in streptozotocin induced diabetic albino rats. *Asian J Pharm Life Sci* 2:10–19.
Stark, A. and Madar, Z. 1993. The effect of an ethanol extract derived from fenugreek (*Trigonella foenum-graecum*) on bile acid absorption and cholesterol levels in rats. *Br J Nutr* 69:277–287.
Sugihara, Y., Nojima, H., Matsuda, H. et al. 2000. Antihyperglycemic effects of gymnemic acid IV, a compound derived from *Gymnema sylvestre* leaves in streptozotocin-diabetic mice. *J Asian Nat Prod Res* 2:321–327.
Swaminathan, R. 2003. Magnesium metabolism and its disorders. *Clin Biochem Rev* 13:47–66.
Tiwari, B.K., Pandey, K.B., Jaiswal, N. et al. 2014. Antidiabetic effect of composite extract of leaves of some Indian plants on alloxan induced diabetic Wistar rats. *J Pharm Invest* 44:205–211.
Trevisan, M.T., Vasconcelos Silva, M.G., Pfundstein, B. et al. 2006. Characterization of the volatile pattern and antioxidant capacity of essential oils from different species of the genus *Ocimum*. *J Agric Food Chem* 54:4378–4382.
Tudan, C., Weber, F.X., and Levine, K.E. 2011. The status of trace elements analysis in biological systems. *Bioanalysis* 13:1695–1697.
Udupa, A., Nahar, P., Shah, S. et al. 2013. A comparative study of effects of omega-3 Fatty acids, alpha lipoic Acid and vitamin e in type 2 diabetes mellitus. *Ann Med Health Sci Res* 3:442–446.
Upadhya, S., Shanbhag, K.K., Suneetha, G. et al. 2004. A study of hypoglycemic and antioxidant activity of *Aegle marmelos* in alloxan induced diabetic rats. *Ind J Physiol Pharmacol* 48:476–480.
Vats, V., Grover, J.K., and Rathi, S.S. 2002. Evaluation of anti-hyperglycemic and hypoglycemic effect of *Trigonella foenum-graecum* Linn, *Ocimum sanctum* Linn and *Pterocarpus marsupium* Linn in normal and allox-anized diabetic rats. *J Ethnopharmacol* 79:95–100.
Vats, V., Yadav, S.P., and Grover, J.K. 2004. Ethanolic extract of *Ocimum sanctum* leaves partially attenuates streptozotocin-induced alterations in glycogen content and carbohydrate metabolism in rats. *J Ethnopharmacol* 90:155–160.
Vijayakumar, M.V., Pandey, V., Mishra, G.C., and Bhat, M.K. 2010. Hypolipidemic effect of fenugreek seeds is mediated through inhibition of fat accumulation and up regulation of LDL receptor. *Obesity* (*Silver Spring*) 18:667–674.
Wang, Z., Wang, J., and Chan, P. 2013. Treating type 2 diabetes mellitus with traditional Chinese and Indian medicinal herbs. *Evid Based Complem Alter Med* 2013:1–17.
Wang, Z.Q., Zhang, X.H., Yu, Y. et al. 2011. Bioactives from bitter melon enhance insulin signaling and modulate acyl carnitine content in skeletal muscle in high-fat diet-fed mice. *J Nutr Biochem* 22:1064–1073.
Wei, J.H., Zhen, H.S., Qiu, Q. et al. 2008. Experimental (corrected) study of hypoglycemic activity of conduritol A of stems of *Gymnema sylvestre*. *Zhongguo Zhong Yao Za Zhi* 33:2961–2965.
Whiting, D.R., Guariguata, L., Weil, C., and Shaw, J. 2011. IDF diabetes atlas: Global estimates of the prevalence of diabetes for 2011 and 2030. *Diab Res Clin Pract* 94:311–321.
WHO. 1980. Second Report of the WHO Expert Committee on Diabetes Mellitus. World Health Organization, Geneva, Switzerland. http://whqlibdoc.who.int/trs/WHO_TRS_646.pdf (accessed December 3, 2014).
Wijesekara, N., Dai, F.F., Hardy, A.B. et al. 2010. Beta cell-specific Znt8 deletion in mice causes marked defects in insulin processing, crystallisation and secretion. *Diabetologia* 13:1656–1668.
Wilmot, E. and Idris, I. 2014. Early onset type 2 diabetes: Risk factors, clinical impact and management. *Ther Adv Chronic Dis* 5:234–244.
World Health Organization. 2002. Traditional medicine-growing needs and potential. *WHO Policy Perspect Med* 2:1–6.
Xu, T., Liu, Y., Meng, J. et al. 2013. The combined effects of insulin and selenium in improving insulin signal transduction in skeletal muscles of diabetic rats. *Xi Bao Yu Fen Zi Mian Yi Xue Za Zhi* 29:1245–1250.
Yanpallewar, S.U., Rai, S., Kumar, M. et al. 2004. Evaluation of antioxidant and neuroprotective effect of *Ocimum sanctum* on transient cerebral ischemia and long-term cerebral hypoperfusion. *Pharmacol Biochem Behav* 79:155–164.
Zia, T., Hasnain, S.N., and Hasan, S.K. 2001. Evaluation of the oral hypoglycemic effect of *Trigonella foenum-graecum* in normal mice. *J Ethanopharmacol* 75:191–195.

8 Recommended Diet for Diabetics

Hydrocarbons, Glycemic Impact, Glycemic Load, Glycemic Index, and Mediterranean Diet

Paulin Moszczyński and Zbigniew Tabarowski

CONTENTS

8.1 INTRODUCTION

From ancient times, man has recognized the special role of the diet in health and disease. The effect of a diet is determined by several characteristics, including absorption, metabolism, and degree of interaction with physiological processes.

The global epidemic of diabetes mellitus (DM) is largely driven by the globalization of Western culture and lifestyles. A "westernized" dietary pattern with low fiber and high saturated and trans-fats, refined carbohydrates, sweetened beverages, sodium, and red meat intake has been shown to be associated with an increased type 2 diabetes risk. Specifically, there is now evidence from large-scale observational studies, and from intervention studies, of powerful synergistic interactions between the diet, obesity, coronary heart disease, and exercise in the development of glucose intolerance. It is estimated that >90% of cases of type 2 diabetes in the population could be prevented with the adoption of a prudent diet (high in cereal fiber and polyunsaturated fatty acids [PUFAs] and low in trans-fatty acids and glycemic load), avoidance of overweight and obesity (body mass index [BMI] < 25 kg/m^2), engagement in moderate to vigorous physical activity for at least 0.5 h/day, nonsmoking, and moderate alcohol consumption [1].

8.2 EPIDEMIOLOGY AND CLASSIFICATION OF DM (FIGURE 8.1)

DM is a nutritional disease with genetic and environmental cofactors. The number and prevalence of people with DM is rapidly increasing. International Diabetes Federation estimated that there was 381.8 million people with diabetes in 2013 (Figure 8.1) with a projected increase of 55% to 591.9 million by 2035 [2]. African Americans have a disproportionately high risk for developing DM and DM-associated end-stage renal disease with an estimated prevalence twice than that observed

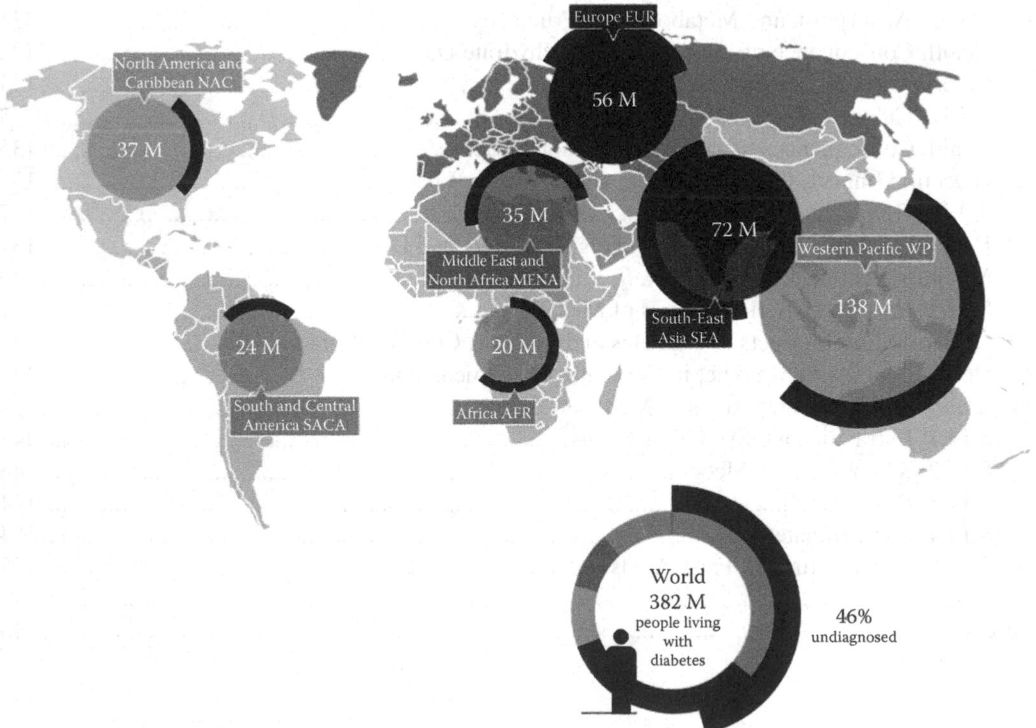

FIGURE 8.1 Number of people with diabetes by IDF Region and whole world (2013). (From IDF Diabetes Atlas, International Diabetes Federation, 2013.)

for their European-American counterparts, but large vessel complications may be less frequent in African Americans with DM when compared with Caucasians [3]. It is suggested that the risk is caused by multiple loci and that these loci are distinct from those identified in other ethnic populations [4]. In Europe, in 2013, the number of people with DM was estimated to be 56 million with an overall estimated prevalence of 8.5%. However, estimated prevalence of DM in 2013 varied widely in the 56 diverse countries from 2.4% in Moldova to 14.9% in Turkey. For Europe, in 2035, a further increase of nearly 10 million people with DM is projected. Structural deprivation may explain part of the regional differences along with individual socioeconomic status or ethnic mixture [5]. The prevalence of DM in Turkish immigrants living in Sweden was higher among females than males (similar to findings from Turkey) while the opposite pattern was found among the Swedish population [6]. Between 1987 and 2009 in Portugal, the prevalence of self-reported DM remained approximately constant in young adults, while it increased in middle-aged and older adults, more than twofold among women and threefold among men [7].

DM is classified into four distinct types: type 1 (due to pancreatic islet β-cell destruction), type 2 (with varying degrees of insulin resistance and/or insulin secretory defects), gestational diabetes mellitus (GDM), and other specific types [8]. Type 2 (T2DM) accounts for about 85%–95% of all disease cases. The highest prevalence of T2DM is in Saudi Arabia and is very high in over 10% of adults in the United States, Switzerland, and Austria. Prevalence is low in Norway, China, and Iceland, but in China the number of patients with T2DM is expected to double in 2030. In the economically advanced countries, the increase will be about 50% in 2030 [9]. More than 1% of the Iranian urban population older than 20 years develops T2DM each year [10].

The important health hazard is the prolonged asymptomatic phase (undiagnosed diabetes mellitus [UDM]) of T2DM. It may last many years. In the course of UDM, unmanaged elevated blood glucose leads to serious and irreversible development of micro- and macrovascular complications [2].

In the United States, up to 41.7% of adults with previously undiagnosed DM have chronic kidney disease. Furthermore, BMI, blood pressure, and other cardiovascular and metabolic markers have been found to be significantly higher in a cohort of people with UDM when compared with diagnosed T2DM subjects. Undiagnosed diabetes has been reported to carry a similar risk of mortality to diagnosed T2DM and is associated with a 1.5- to 3.0-fold higher risk of mortality compared to normoglycemic individuals. Globally, 45.8%, or 174.8 million, of all diabetes cases in adults are estimated to be undiagnosed, ranging from 24.1% to 75.1% across data regions. An estimated 83.8% of all cases of UDM are in low- and middle-income countries. Pacific Island nations have the highest prevalence of UDM [2].

GDM is glucose intolerance discovered during pregnancy. The prevalence of GDM in the United States is 1%–25%, depending on patient demographics and diagnostic thresholds [11]. Pregnant women with GDM are at increased risk for maternal and fetal complications, including preeclampsia, fetal macrosomia (which can cause shoulder dystocia and birth injury), and neonatal hypoglycemia. Frequently, women with prior GDM exhibit tendencies for central obesity, insulin resistance, and glucose intolerance. Women with GDM are also at increased risk for T2DM; approximately 15%–60% of such women will develop T2DM within 5–15 years of delivery [12].

8.3 AN OVERVIEW OF DIABETIC COMPLICATIONS

T2DM is associated with long-term damage, dysfunction, and failure of various organs, especially the heart, eyes, kidneys, nerves, and blood vessels. Cardiovascular disease is the leading cause of mortality among individuals with T2DM, and >50% of patients will die from a cardiovascular event, especially coronary artery disease, but also stroke and peripheral vascular disease [13]. T2DM may be complicated by subclinical myocardial injury [14] and may be associated with the presence and extent of mitral annular calcification (MAC), independent of coronary artery calcium. There are probably additional mechanisms for MAC formation in diabetics patients that are distinct from those related to generalized atherosclerosis [15]. The prevalence of MAC in a cohort of 2032 subjects with T2DM was 14.3% in Caucasians and 8.3% in African Americans.

T2MD individuals develop dyslipidemia characterized by hypertriglycerolemia, reduced HDL cholesterol, and increased levels of small, dense atherogenic low-density lipoprotein (LDL) particles, each of which is a major cardiovascular disease risk factor [16]. Human paraoxonase (PON1) is a calcium-dependent esterase that confers antioxidant properties to HDL. Hyperglycemia, increased lecithin:cholesterol acyltransferase (LCAT) activity, and lower PON-1 activity likely contribute to the impaired antioxidative functionality of HDL [17]. In T2DM, serum PON-1 activity was found to be decreased and has been correlated to higher morbidity and mortality related to cardiovascular complications. The level of serum PON1 activity can be a better predictor than that of HDL for atherosclerotic risk in T2DM patients [18].

Fatty acid composition of serum lipids and adipose tissue triacylglycerols, besides the diet, also influence desaturating enzymes activity (stearoyl-CoA-desaturase, delta-6-desaturase, and delta-5-desaturase), which mediate the metabolism of fatty acids to long-chain PUFAs. Their activities may be related to metabolic risk factors for T2DM and coronary heart disease [19]. Stearoyl-CoA desaturase activity significantly correlates with BMI, waist circumference, triglycerides, and HDL cholesterol levels. There are ethnic differences in stearoyl-CoA desaturase activity, which is 18%–35% higher in white Europeans than in African Caribbeans or Asian Indian women [20].

The frequency of nonalcoholic fatty liver disease positively correlates with that of T2DM. An important role in the pathogenetic mechanism seem to play hepatokines secreted by the steatotic liver that favor potentiating hepatic insulin resistance. In Edinburgh Type 2 Diabetes Study, nonalcoholic fatty liver was stated in 42.6% T2DM patients [21]. Lipasin, known as C19ORF80, RIFL (Re-feeding Induced in Fat and Liver), or ANGPTL8 (angiopoietin-like protein 8) and betatrophin are hepatokines circulating in the blood, regulating lipid metabolism and stimulating proliferation of pancreatic β cells. Lipasin/betatrophin is a nutritionally regulated hepatokine that is increased in T2DM and obesity. Among obese people and T2DM patients, the concentration of lipasin increased by 35% 2 h after meal and positively correlated with BMI, while that of betatrophin positively correlated with levels of total cholesterol, LDL cholesterol and apolipoprotein B. Further studies on the properties of hepatokines should lead to an effective treatment of T2DM since it is already known that they stimulate proliferation and increase the mass of β pancreatic cells in mice.

The advanced glycation end products (AGE)–the AGE receptor (RAGE) interaction was identified as a potential mechanism underlying chronic and inflammatory diseases such as atherosclerosis, T2DM, and kidney disease. AGEs are the derivatives of glucose–protein or glucose–lipid reactions and are mainly generated from the diet (depending on the intensity of heating, cooking time, and oxygenation). Binding of AGEs or other ligands to the RAGE results in cellular activation, that is increased expression of inflammatory mediators and oxidative stress. Accumulated at many sites of the body including the heart and large blood vessels, AGEs induce deleterious effects on tissues and the cardiovascular system. They are generated in T2DM as a result of chronic hyperglycemia and enhanced oxidative stress [120,121]. Accumulation of AGEs in vessel walls may increase arterial stiffness and/or thickness, contributing to a high incidence of cardiovascular disease in patients with T2DM [122].

8.4 RELATIONSHIP BETWEEN OBESITY, METABOLIC SYNDROME, AND T2DM

Obesity and the metabolic syndrome (MetS) are the major and escalating public health and clinical challenge worldwide. By 2030, the respective number of overweight and obese adults is projected to be 1.35 billion and 573 million individuals, respectively, without adjusting for secular trends [22]. Despite growing recognition of the problem, the obesity epidemic continues in the United States, and obesity rates are increasing around the world. The latest estimations are that approximately 34% of adults and 15%–20% of children and adolescents in the United States are obese [23,24]. BMI, abdominal fat distribution, and weight gain are important risk factors for the development of T2DM. It is estimated that 90% of individuals with T2DM are obese [25].

MetS confers a fivefold increase in the risk of T2DM and twofold the risk of developing cardiovascular disease over the next 5–10 years [26].

MetS, according to the Joint Statement Criteria by the American Heart Association/National Heart Lung and Blood Institute and the International Diabetes Federation, is defined by a constellation of interconnected physiological, biochemical, clinical, and metabolic factors that directly increase the risk of cardiovascular disease, T2DM, and all-cause mortality. Insulin resistance, visceral adiposity, atherogenic dyslipidemia, endothelial dysfunction, genetic susceptibility, elevated blood pressure, hypercoagulable state, and chronic stress are the several factors that constitute the syndrome. Adipocytes produce several adipokines that modulate insulin action as well as glucose and lipid metabolism. In patients with T2DM, adiponectin concentrations are closely related to insulin resistance and the components of MetS [27]. Upper body subcutaneous adipocytes generate the majority of circulating free fatty acids while an intra-abdominal fat content has been positively correlated with the splanchnic free fatty acids levels, which may contribute to the liver fat accumulation commonly found in abdominal obesity [28]. Chemerin and apelin are recently discovered adipokines secreted by the enlarged adipose tissue with diverse biological effects that are not well detailed yet [29]. They play a key role in the pathological process of insulin resistance, glucose metabolism, and obesity. It was found that the levels of chemerin and apelin were changed significantly in T2DM with obesity; however, the underlying mechanism involved remains unclear. Chemerin is correlated positively with leptin and negatively with adiponectin levels and may contribute to chronic inflammation and increased oxidative stress in obese individuals, even in the absence of manifest insulin resistance and may represent a novel link between metabolic signals and atherosclerosis [30]. Chemerin is strongly associated with markers of inflammation and components of MetS [31].

8.5 CARBOHYDRATES

The important dietary goal for individuals with T2DM is the establishment of a regular meal pattern with consistent day-to-day carbohydrate intake. The 2010 Dietary Guidelines for Americans specifically recommend to reduce the intake of calories from added sugars, nonnaturally occurring sugars added to food, such as sodas and candies, that are also known as "empty calories" as they provide little or no nutrients yet are high in calories [32]. Meantime, the American people consume 39% of foods containing added sugar and 22% containing both solid fats and added sugar. Solid fat is any fat that is solid at room temperature (which includes naturally occurring fat found in full-fat milk and yogurt, fatty cuts of meat and butter and spreads). The American Heart Association (AHA) has advocated that women and men do not consume more than 100 and 150 kcal/day, respectively, from added sugars. These levels are currently exceeded by over 90% of the adult population in the United States [33].

8.5.1 Types of Carbohydrates

Carbohydrates are for the human body one of the key energy substrates. They provide energy to cells in the body, particularly the brain, which is the only organ in the body completely dependent on carbohydrates. The content and type of carbohydrates in the diet have a significant impact on human health. Medical nutrition therapy, which provides a flexible and individualized approach to diet, emphasizes the role of the total number (rather than the type) of carbohydrate consumed [34].

Carbohydrates are divided into simple carbohydrates (mono- and disaccharides), which include glucose, fructose, sucrose, lactulose, and complex carbohydrates (polysaccharides, oligosaccharides). Carbohydrates that contain more than two simple sugars are called oligosaccharides or polysaccharides, depending upon the length of the structure. Oligosaccharides usually have between 3 and 10 sugar units while polysaccharides or complex carbohydrates can have more than 3000 units. Starch is the most important plant polysaccharide supplied by the diet. Starch derived from different sources varies in the spatial structure of the chain, which comprises a large number of glucose molecules, which makes it slightly different as far as physicochemical properties are concerned. The main components of the diet supplying the polysaccharides are starch grains, rice, and potatoes [35]. The morphological, chemical, and structural properties of basic types of starch and its digestibility can be controlled by critically manipulating the food microstructure, processing techniques, and food composition. Commonly used food processing techniques such as thermal processing, extrusion cooking, and postcooking refrigerated storage alter the physical state of starch (gelatinization, retrogradation, etc.) and its digestibility.

Glucose and fructose are present in products such as honey, fruits, including berries, and vegetables. Fructose has now become a major constituent of our modern diet. High-fructose corn syrup (HFCS) is a fructose–glucose liquid sweetener alternative to sucrose first introduced to the food and beverage industry in the 1970s [36]. The two most important HFCS products of commerce contain 42% fructose (HFCS-42) or 55% fructose (HFCS-55). The glucose-to-fructose ratio in HFCS is nearly 1:1, similar to the ratio found in sucrose, invert sugar, and honey. A similar ratio is also found in many fruits and fruit juices. Soda also called soft drink, pop, soda pop, or carbonated beverage is a beverage that typically contains water usually with a sweetener and a flavoring agent. The sweetener may be sugar, high-fructose corn syrup, fruit juice, sugar substitutes, or some combination of these. Soft drinks may also contain caffeine, colorings, preservatives, and other ingredients.

8.5.2 Absorption and Metabolism

When assessing the carbohydrate absorption and metabolic effects, we are talking about digestible and indigestible carbohydrates [37]. Digestible carbohydrates are fully hydrolyzed in the digestive tract to monosaccharides, and their absorption causes an increase in glucose level in the circulation. Nonabsorbable carbohydrates do not cause an increase in blood glucose because they cannot be hydrolyzed into simple sugars, but can be fermented under the influence of intestinal bacteria. Indigestible carbohydrates with high impact on human health are the components of dietary fiber [38]. Most dietary fiber is not digested or absorbed, so it stays within the intestine where it modulates digestion of other foods and affects the consistency of stool but there are two types of fiber, each of which is thought to have its own benefits.

Soluble fiber consists of a group of substances that is made of carbohydrates and dissolves in water. Examples of foods that contain soluble fiber include fruits, oats, barley, and legumes (peas and beans). Insoluble fiber comes from plant cells walls and does not dissolve in water. Examples of foods that contain insoluble fiber include wheat, rye, and other grains. The traditional fiber, wheat bran, is a type of insoluble fiber.

Dietary fiber is the sum of all soluble and insoluble fiber.

Dietary fibers are applied as food-integrated, as supplement, and as purified substances. The individual dietary fibers differ substance specifically. Dietary fiber preparations such as wheat bran, flax seed, or sugar-beet fiber are useful in the treatment of constipation, colon diverticulosis, and adiposity. Oat bran is preferentially used in hypercholesterolemia. Purified dietary fibers such as cellulose, guar, psyllium, and beta-glucan have an anti-diabetic effect, while all viscous fibers have an antilipemic effect.

Digestion of carbohydrates in the gastrointestinal tract is carried out by many enzymes. In the oral cavity under the influence of salivary amylase, the digestion of starch starts. The result of this action are oligosaccharides with different chain lengths. Their further digestion occurs in the small intestine, where pancreatic amylase works and disaccharides are created such as maltose and isomaltose. Hydrolysis of disaccharides both those arising from the decomposition of poly- and oligosaccharides and those supplied in the diet, saccharose and lactose, takes place under the influence of enzymes present in the intestinal mucosa. Enzymes present in small intestine mucosa: maltase and isomaltase hydrolyze maltose and isomaltose into glucose, saccharase hydrolyzes saccharose into glucose and fructose, whereas lactase hydrolyzes lactose into glucose and galactose. Then, all monosaccharides are absorbed through the intestinal epithelial cells and this process significantly depends on the presence of specific glucose transporter members of GLUT family. Oligosaccharides, (starch) digestion and absorption are augmented appreciably by physical processing of grain or legume and by heating to 100°C for several minutes before its ingestion [39]. Glucose metabolism is influenced by numerous intrinsic rhythms and behaviors, including autonomic, hormonal, and cardiovascular responses to activity, meals, and sleep. The absorbed monosaccharides are transported mainly to the liver. This is the organ responsible for maintaining adequate concentration of sugar glucose in blood to provide inputs to the cells of other tissues [40]. Glycogen stored in the liver is essential to ensure a constant level of glucose in the circulatory system when not supplied with the carbohydrate diet. The decrease in blood glucose level stimulates the synthesis of glucagon by α-cells of pancreatic islands, which in turn activates the breakdown of glycogen in the hepatocytes and then elevation of glucose secretion into the circulatory system, which ensures the appropriate concentration and flow into the cells of peripheral tissues such as fat and muscle tissues, that use glucose for metabolism. Increasing the concentration of glucose in the circulatory system, which occurs after eating a meal containing carbohydrates, is a factor stimulating the synthesis of insulin by the β-cells of pancreatic isles. Insulin is a hormone that regulates glucose uptake by fat and skeletal muscle and heart cells known as insulin-dependent tissues. These cells have on the surface of cell membrane receptors binding insulin. Interaction of insulin with its receptor activates the flux of glucose into the cells of these tissues. The entry of glucose and related hexoses into various cells is possible due to the presence in their membranes of glucose transporters. The family (GLUT) comprises 13 members identified to date differing in tissue expression pattern. GLUT-4 is the major insulin-responsive transporter that is expressed almost exclusively in skeletal muscle, heart muscle, and adipocytes. GLUT-4 is sequestered in specialized vesicles in the cytosol. They are synthesized, released from the Golgi in vesicles, and then move between an intracellular pool and the plasma membrane, where they can facilitate glucose entry [41].

In adipocytes, glucose is used for the synthesis of triglycerides (the compounds composed of glycerol formed from glucose and fatty acids). Skeletal muscle cells capture glucose from the circulatory system and can accumulate it in the form of glycogen, which is a key substrate allowing muscles to produce energy and thus perform physical activity. Glucose present in the circulatory system is still taken up by cells and other tissues. This process can be independent of the presence of insulin (and such tissues are called "insulin independent") and takes place through cell membranes equipped with the specific glucose transporters of the GLUT family. For example GLUT1 transporters are present in cell membranes of red blood while GLUT3 is expressed mainly in neurons and placenta.

The three newly discovered peptides play an important role in carbohydrate metabolism. Preptin is synthesized in pancreatic β-cells, and adropin mainly in the liver and brain, and many peripheral tissues. Irisin is synthesized principally in the heart muscle, along with peripheral tissues, including salivary glands, kidney, and liver. Preptin and adropin regulate carbohydrate metabolism by moderating glucose-mediated insulin release and irisin that is an antiobesitic and antidiabetic hormone regulating adipose tissue metabolism and glucose homeostasis by converting white to brown adipose tissue [42].

8.5.3 Absorption and Metabolism of Fructose

There are two sources of fructose to the body, the exogenous, supplied by the diet, and the endogenous, made from glucose via aldose reductase. The digestion, absorption, and metabolism of fructose differ from those of glucose. Fructose absorption by human adults can be estimated by breath hydrogen test. It increases as a function of dietary fructose concentration, so that for every 10 g increase in fructose dose the number of positive breath hydrogen tests increases by 15% [43]. Fructose is believed to be more slowly absorbed from the gastrointestinal tract than glucose [44], and has no active absorption mechanism in the intestinal mucosa but is slowly and incompletely absorbed by facilitated diffusion. Because of this slow absorption, the increasing effect of fructose in the blood glucose is lower than after ingestion of most other carbohydrate sources. Fructose is transported passively across membranes by a member of glucose transporter family [45].

GLUT5 is the sole transporter specific for fructose with no ability to transport glucose or galactose and does not depend on insulin [44]. The small intestine cells expressing the highest number of GLUT5 in human and animals regulate fructose absorption from dietary sources and, therefore, the availability of fructose to other tissue [46]. The second major fructose transporter is GLUT2, a low-affinity transporter that is also capable of recognizing glucose and galactose. Five other GLUTs may possess varying degrees of fructose selectivity based on sequence homology with GLUT5: GLUT7, GLUT9a/b, GLUT8, GLUT11, and GLUT12 [45,47]. Most of the metabolic effects of fructose are due to its rapid utilization by the liver and bypassing the phosphofructokinase regulatory step in glycolysis, leading to far-reaching consequences to carbohydrate and lipid metabolism. These consequences include increased lipogenesis and VLDL secretion, leading to triglyceridemia, decreased glucose tolerance, and hyperinsulinemia. Acute loading of the liver with fructose causes sequestration of inorganic phosphate in fructose-1-phosphate and diminished ATP synthesis. Hepatic metabolism of fructose favors de novo lipogenesis. In addition, unlike glucose, fructose does not stimulate insulin secretion or enhance leptin production. Because insulin and leptin act as key afferent signals in the regulation of food intake and body weight, this suggests that dietary fructose may contribute to increased energy intake and weight gain. Furthermore, calorically sweetened beverages may enhance caloric overconsumption. Thus, the increase in consumption of HFCS has a temporal relation to the epidemic of obesity, and the overconsumption of HFCS in calorically sweetened beverages may play a role in the epidemic of obesity [44].

8.6 HEALTH CONSEQUENCE OF LOW-/HIGH-CARBOHYDRATE DIETS

Sugar in the diet enhances dietary fat absorption and chylomicrons secretion. This phenomenon contributes quantitatively to the described hypertriglyceridemia that occurs with diets high in carbohydrate and low in fat [48].

Most U.S. adults consume more added sugar than is recommended for a healthy diet. The mean percentage of daily calories from added sugar slightly decreased from 15.7% in 1988–1994 to 14.9% in 2005–2010. Most adults consumed 10% or more of calories from added sugar (71.4%) and approximately 10% consumed 25% or more in 2005–2010. A significant relationship between added sugar consumption and increased risk for cardiovascular disease mortality has been observed [49]. The Recommended Dietary Allowance (RDA) for carbohydrate is set at 130 g/day for adults and children based on the average minimum amount of glucose utilized by brain [35,50]. This level of intake, however, is typically exceeded to meet energy needs while consuming acceptable intake levels of fat and protein. The median intake of carbohydrates is approximately 220–330 g/day for men and 180–230 g/day for women. Carbohydrates should be eaten mainly in the vegetable form; consumption of starchy vegetables (potatoes, rice, corn) should be reduced and fruit can be eaten in moderation. The goal of eating 30 g/day of dietary fiber should be presented so that it can be practically implemented.

Vegan diets are characterized by the increased intake of carbohydrate, fiber, and several micronutrients, in contrast to the American Diabetes Association (ADA) recommended diet [51].

Two randomized trials evaluated the effects of a vegan diet on body weight, blood glucose levels, and plasma lipid levels in individuals with T2DM. In both trials, the vegetarian and vegan diets were rich in carbohydrates but consisted of vegetables, fruit, grains, and legumes, carbohydrate foods particularly rich in fiber and with low glycemic index (GI). Data from many trials show that a diet low in fat and rich in carbohydrates and fiber represents a useful and effective strategy to reduce body weight and improve insulin sensitivity and metabolic abnormalities in patients with T2DM, with satisfactory compliance also in the long run. Changes in insulin sensitivity and enzymatic oxidative stress markers correlated with changes in visceral fat. Probably, the sustainability in the long term is due to the large variety of foods available, the high palatability, and the greater satiating effects [52,53]. The observation made among subjects with T2DM supports the health effectiveness of eating vegetables before carbohydrates. If subjects with T2DM ate vegetables before carbohydrates, their glycemic excursions and incremental glucose peak were significantly lower [54].

In epidemiological studies, consumption of sugar and/or sugar-sweetened beverages has been linked to the presence of unfavorable lipid levels, insulin resistance [55], cardiovascular disease, and MetS [56].

Prospective cohort analyses conducted from 1991 to 1999 among women in the Nurses' Health Study II showed that higher consumption of sugar-sweetened beverages was associated with a greater magnitude of weight gain and an increased risk for the development of T2DM. This was possibly caused by providing excessive calories and large amounts of rapidly absorbable sugars. There were 741 incident cases of T2DM during 716,300 person-years of follow-up [57].

In the study on 2037 employees of a factory in Japan, it was shown that consumption of diet soda was significantly associated with an increased risk for T2DM. Thus, diet soda is not always effective at preventing T2DM even though it is a zero-calorie drink [58]. High carbohydrate intake, mainly from refined grains, was associated with an increased coronary heart disease risk in Chinese adults. Carbohydrate intake accounted for 67.5% of the total energy intake in women and 68.5% in men [59].

Emerging evidence from recent epidemiological and biochemical studies clearly suggests that the high dietary intake of fructose has rapidly become an important causative factor in the development of MetS [60]. Men and women with the highest fructose intakes had higher risk for large waist circumference, hypertension, and higher risk of impaired fasting glucose levels.

The analysis of the risk of incident MetS and T2DM in the Multi-Ethnic Study of Atherosclerosis proved that the consumption of diet soda was associated with significantly greater risks of MetS components and T2DM. Over follow-up, 871 cases of incident MetS (22.5%) and 413 cases of incident T2DM (8.2%) were identified. Fourteen percent consumed ≥1 serving of sugar-sweetened soda daily, whereas 45% never consumed sugar-sweetened soda. Twenty-four percent did not consume either beverage; only 2% reported consuming ≥1 serving of both at least daily [61].

Contrary to these findings, a systematic review and meta-analysis to assess the effect of fructose on postprandial triglycerides showed that fructose in isocaloric exchange for other carbohydrate does not increase postprandial triglycerides [62,63]. Also when 65 overweight or obese individuals were placed on an eucaloric (weight stable) diet for 10 weeks, which incorporated sucrose- or high-fructose corn syrup no change was observed in body weight, blood pressure, total cholesterol, triglycerides, low-density lipoprotein, or apolipoprotein B [33].

Intraportal infusion of small amounts of fructose markedly augmented net hepatic glucose uptake (NHGU) during hyperglycemia and hyperinsulinemia in dogs [64]. In that study, the increased glycolytic flux associated with the inclusion of fructose was probably secondary to an increase in the intracellular glucose 6-phosphate content and in general was secondary to the activation of glucokinase, perhaps with an associated increase in the activity of phosphofructokinase. These experimental results suggest that higher doses of fructose increase the blood glucose level and that only small doses of fructose can have beneficial effects on blood glucose regulation in diabetic animals [65]. Fructose promotes reactive oxygen species formation, which leads to cellular dysfunction and aging, and promotes changes in the brain's reward system, which drives excessive consumption. Thus, fructose can exert detrimental health effects beyond its calories and in ways that mimic those of ethanol, its metabolic cousin. The metabolic analogies argue that fructose should be thought of as "alcohol without the buzz" [66].

Fructose, in the amounts currently consumed enhances lipogenesis and the production of uric acid and worsening blood lipid profile, contributing to obesity, diabetes, fatty liver, and gout, so is hazardous to the health of people [67]. There is a need for increased public awareness of the risks associated with high-fructose consumption and greater efforts should be made to curb the supplementation of packaged foods with high-fructose additives.

Consumption of the different types of starchy foods was assessed among 80,209 adult participants in France. Obtained data suggested that the part of energy intake coming from complex carbohydrates should be increased because only about 43% of the subjects had intakes in line with French Nutritional Guidelines concerning starchy foods [68]. The therapeutic dosages of dietary fiber preparations are 20–40 g/day and of purified fiber substances 10–20 g/day, respectively. The

TABLE 8.1
Some Examples of Fiber Content of Foods in Common Portions

Food Item	Serving Size	Total Fiber/ Serving (g)	Soluble Fiber/ Serving (g)	Insoluble Fiber/ Serving (g)
Raw vegetables				
Carrots, fresh	1.7½ in. long	2.3	1.1	1.2
Celery, fresh	1 cup chopped	1.7	0.7	1.0
Cucumber, fresh	1 cup	0.5	0.2	0.3
Pepper, green, fresh	1 cup chopped	1.7	0.7	1.0
Tomato, fresh	1 medium	1.0	0.1	0.9
Fruits				
Apple, red, fresh w/skin	1 small	2.8	1.0	1.8
Banana, fresh	1/2 small	1.1	0.3	0.8
Grapefruit, fresh	1/2 medium	1.6	1.1	0.5
Orange, fresh flesh only	1 small	2.9	1.8	1.1
Pear, fresh w/skin	1/2 large	2.9	1.1	1.8

For fiber contents in food, please consult the following extensive table of fiber content (total, soluble and insoluble) in foods in common portions.

Source: Anderson, J,W., *Plant Fiber in Foods*, 2nd ed, HCF Nutrition Research Foundation Inc., Lexington, KY, 1990.

usual daily intake of dietary fiber in Europe and the United States amounts to only 15–20 g, while health authorities and nutrition societies recommend a reference value of at least 30 g [38].

Several studies have shown that the adverse metabolic effects of high-carbohydrate diets are neutralized when fiber and carbohydrate are increased simultaneously in the diet for diabetic patients. A high-carbohydrate/high-fiber diet significantly improves blood glucose control and reduces plasma cholesterol levels in T2DM patients compared with a low-carbohydrate/low-fiber diet [69]. In addition, a high-carbohydrate/high-fiber diet does not increase plasma insulin and triglyceride concentrations, despite the higher consumption of carbohydrates. Consequently, products with slowly digestible starch can have health beneficial long-term effects [70], but unfortunately, dietary fiber represents a heterogeneous category, and there is still much to understand as to which foods should be preferred to maximize the metabolic effects of fiber. There are indications that only water-soluble fiber is active on plasma glucose and lipoprotein metabolism in humans. Therefore, in practice, the consumption of legumes, vegetables, and fruits rich in water-soluble fiber should be particularly encouraged (Table 8.1).

8.7 CALORIC INTAKE

Homeostasis of energy is regulated by food intake, genetic factors, and energy expenditure. Energy consumed must equal energy expended by a person to remain at the same body weight [71]. Numerous peripheral signals contribute to the regulation of food intake and energy homeostasis. The energy density of food and short-term hormonal signals (i.e. insulin, leptin, and possibly the orexigenic and anorexigenic peptides, ghrelin) by themselves are insufficient to produce sustained changes in energy balance and body adiposity [72]. Preptin with 34 amino acids, adropin with 43 amino acids, and irisin with 112 amino acids are three newly discovered peptides critical for regulating energy metabolism [42].

Caloric excess induces an inhibition of the further uptake of energy-bearing substrates into muscle, adipose tissue, and the liver, giving rise to the clinical picture of insulin resistance. It is associated with multiple further disturbances of energy metabolism because insulin is the primary regulatory hormone, not only of glucose metabolism, but of fat and protein metabolism as well. Obesity, especially when fatty tissue is mainly abdominally distributed and when combined with physical inactivity, is often associated with high triglyceride levels and low HDL cholesterol levels, impaired glucose tolerance, and/or a high fasting blood glucose concentration, microalbuminuria, hypertension, high fibrinogen levels, subclinical inflammation, nonalcoholic fatty liver disease, and hyperuricemia [73]. There is abundant evidence from animal, human, and in vitro studies to support functional roles for a number of inflammatory factors in obesity-induced insulin resistance [74]. Immunological abnormalities such as inflammation and activation of monocytes and increased levels of inflammatory markers, for example C-reactive protein, plasminogen activator inhibitor-1, and other cytokines, may lead to insulin resistance and to T1DM and T2DM and diabetic complications [74,75].

Studies on both animals and humans have demonstrated a beneficial role of dietary restriction and leanness in promoting health and longevity. Epidemiological studies have found strong direct associations between increasing BMI from 20 to 21 kg/m^2 and risks of developing T2DM, cardiovascular disease, and several types of cancer [76].

A lower energy intake and carbohydrate consumption and less weight gain in Pima Indians were associated with glucose-level regulation (fasting glucose < 5.6 mmol/L) and 2 h glucose < 7.8 mmol/L and incremental area under the curve for insulin during an oral glucose tolerance test. These data indicated a role for peripheral insulin as a negative feedback signal in the regulation of energy intake and body weight [77].

8.7.1 Calorie Counting and Energy Balance

Energy is derived from the oxidation of carbohydrate and protein (4 kcal/g), fat (9 kcal/g), and pure ethyl alcohol (7 kcal/g). Some researches try to explain the regulation of energy balance by the "thrifty genotype" hypothesis, which suggests that, in the early years of life, the diabetic genotype was thrifty in the sense of being exceptionally efficient in utilization of food. In contemporary societies, as food is usually available in unlimited amounts, the "thrifty genotype" no longer provides a survival advantage, but renders its owners more susceptible to obesity and diabetes as a result of response to environmental circumstances and climatic factors. This phenomenon would explain that populations in some areas of the developing world would be at greater risk of obesity and its comorbidities [78].

The current ADA recommendations suggest a range of carbohydrate intake of between 45% and 65% of total calories, protein 10%–20%, total fat ≤ 30%, saturated fatty acids (SFAs) < 7%, monounsaturated fatty acids (MUFAs) up to 20%, and PUFAs up to 10% of total calorie [79] and advocates that women and men should not consume more than 100 and 150 kcal/day, respectively, from added sugars (Table 8.2). These levels are currently exceeded by over 90% of the adult population

TABLE 8.2
Recommendations of the Main Diabetes Associations

Main Source of Calories	Main Diabetes Associations	Joslin Diabetes Center
Carbohydrates	40%–65% of calories	40% of calories
Proteins	10%–20% of calories	30% of calories
Fats	30%–35% of calories	30% of calories

ADA (American Diabetes Association), EASD (European Association for the Study of Diabetes), CAD (Canadian Diabetes Association), Diabetes UK, and Joslin Diabetes Center, Regarding the Percentage of Calories from Carbohydrates, Proteins and Fats in the Diet of Diabetics.

Source: Moszczyński, P. and Rutowski, J., Meal plans for diabetics: Caloric intake, calorie counting and glycemic index, in: Bagchi, D. and Sreejayan, N., *Nutritional and Therapeutic Interventions for Diabetes and Metabolic Syndrome*, Elsevier and Academic Press, pp. 431–442, 2012.

in the United States [66]. Digestible carbohydrates are one of the main sources of dietary energy in infancy and childhood and are essential for growth and development. In infants, minimum carbohydrate (mainly lactose) intake should be 40% of total energy, gradually increasing to 55% energy by the age of 2 years [80].

The study on the influence of frequency and distribution of meals on the lipoprotein levels revealed that the consumption of 4–5 meals/day would seem more advisable than taking of fewer meals [81]. Individuals with a more irregular intake of energy, especially during breakfast and between meals, appeared to have an increased MetS risk. Moreover, increased waist circumference was associated with irregular energy intake during breakfast, evening meal, and daily total energy intake [82].

The first main meal in T2DM should be breakfast. In health, the rise in plasma glucose after lunch is less if breakfast is eaten. In obese T2DM subjects, the rise in plasma glucose was 95% less after lunch when the lunch had been preceded by breakfast, confirming the occurrence of the second meal metabolic effect. The standard breakfast consisted of 50 g muesli, 100 g milk, two slices of toast (56 g), 20 g marmalade, 20 g margarine, and 200 mL orange juice (106 g carbohydrate, 18 g fat, 15 g protein, 646 kcal). The standard lunch comprised a cheese sandwich, 200 mL orange juice, 170 g yogurt, and 150 g jelly (103 g carbohydrate, 30 g fat, 44 g protein, 858 kcal) [83]. The consumption of biscuits with a high content of slowly digestible starch reduces the rate of appearance of exogenous glucose in the first part of the morning and prolongs this release in the late phase of the morning (210 min). These results emphasize that modulation of glucose availability at breakfast is an important factor for metabolic control throughout the morning in healthy subjects due to the lowering of blood glucose and insulin excursions [84].

The aim of the rational development of the diet for diabetics, the Healthy Weight Pyramid, shows the number of calories per serving of the food. On the first level, there are vegetables—serving = 25 cal and fruit serving = 60 cal; one should consume a minimum of 4 servings per day. The second level involved carbohydrates—cereals, grains and seeds, and whole grain bread—4–8 servings, 1 serving = 70 cal. The third level of the pyramid is reserved for skimmed milk products—3–7 servings with a portion of protein = 70 cal. The fourth level—fats: olive oil, vegetable oil such as rich in Ω-3 fatty acids canola oil (oil from the seeds of *Brassica campestris*), nuts, and avocados from 3 to 5 servings per day, 1 serving = 45 cal [85].

8.8 HEALTH CONSEQUENCES OF LOW-/HIGH-CALORIC DIETS

The main fundamental principle of treatment of patients with T2DM is reducing energy intake as well as matching insulin to planned carbohydrate intake [73,86].

Fifty-nine overweight/obese adults with T2DM were randomized to one of two isocaloric diabetic diets for 3 months; big breakfast rich in fat and protein that provided 33% of total daily energy or small breakfast rich in carbohydrates that provided 12.5% of total daily energy. A simple dietary manipulation such as enriching breakfast with energy in the form of protein and fat appeared to confer metabolic benefits and might be a useful alternative for the management of diet in patients with T2DM [87].

The abnormalities underlying T2DM are reversible by reducing dietary energy intake. Eleven people with T2DM (49.5 ± 2.5 years, BMI 33.6 ± 1.2 kg/m^2, nine males and two females) were studied before and after 1, 4, and 8 weeks of a 2.5 MJ (600 kcal)/day diet. Normalization of both β-cell function and hepatic insulin sensitivity in T2DM was achieved by dietary energy restriction alone. This was associated with decreased pancreatic and liver triacylglycerol stores, which was measured using three-point Dixon magnetic resonance imaging [88].

The study to determine the effect of energy contributed by fructose on plasma lipids showed that dietary fructose was associated with increased fasting and postprandial plasma triacylglycerol concentrations in men, but not in women. In the fructose diet, 14% of energy came from added fructose and 3% of energy came from fructose occurring naturally in the foods used in the diet. In the glucose diet, 14% of energy came from added glucose and 3% of energy came from fructose occurring naturally in the foods used in the diet. The crystalline fructose and glucose added to the diets were used in baking and to sweeten breakfast cereals and beverages. Therefore, glucose may be a suitable replacement sugar for women [89].

Another observation of 750 T2DM patients (261 men and 489 women, aged 35–65 years) showed that the substitution of fat for carbohydrate was associated with low concentrations of HbA1c in high calorie–consuming T2DM patients. Calorie intake of 25 kcal/body weight was identified as a cutoff point of the negative effect of dietary carbohydrate and 30 for the positive effect [90].

8.9 GLYCEMIC IMPACT, GLYCEMIC INDEX, AND GLYCEMIC LOAD

8.9.1 Definitions

A lack of values to guide food choices based on the food effects has been a long-standing problem. The American Association of Cereal Chemists recognized the need to "communicate glycemic response in grams per serving of food" and established an ad hoc committee to consider how to express the glycemic impact of foods for consumer use. This committee decided that relative glycemic impact (RGI) should be expressed as glucose equivalents and defined as "the weight of glucose that would induce a glycemic response equivalent to that induced by a given amount of food." Dietary carbohydrates produce different glycemic responses depending not only on their chemical structure but also on particle size, fiber content, and food processing. These differences between carbohydrate-containing foods can be expressed in the GI, which is a measure of the postprandial glucose response, and can be considered an indicator of the quality of food carbohydrates. The GI refers to the glycemic effect of available carbohydrate in food relative to the effect of an equal amount of glucose, so the measurement of GI is equicarbohydrate. The quantity of food used in measuring GI is not necessarily a customary intake, but is one that delivers the same amount of carbohydrate (usually 50 g) as the glucose reference. Glycemic load (GL) is calculated by multiplying the GI of a food with its carbohydrate content and represents both the quality and quantity of carbohydrates. It is calculated indirectly as the product of the average GI of carbohydrate foods consumed and the total carbohydrate intake over a specified time period. GL = GI × P × weight of food, where P is the proportion of available carbohydrate in the food [91,92] (Table 8.3).

Effects of meal composition and food intake on RGI could be better represented by the glycemic glucose equivalent (GGE) content, but not by GI. Correlations between GI and GGE content per serving are highest in food groupings of similar carbohydrate content and serving size, including breads ($r = 0.73$) and breakfast cereals ($r = 0.8$), but low in more varied groups including pulses ($r = 0.66$), fruits ($r = 0.48$), and vegetables ($r = 0.28$) [93]. Low GI is a value ≤ 55, the average 56–69, and high ≥ 70 [83].

8.10 HEALTH EFFECTS OF LOW-GI/LOAD VERSUS HIGH-GI/LOAD DIETS

Many studies purporting to investigate lower GI interventions actually studied lower GL interventions: that unavailable carbohydrate (e.g. dietary fiber), independent of GI, seems to have at least as big an effect on health outcome as GI itself; that lower GI and GL diets are beneficial for health in persons with impaired glucose metabolism, but that it is as yet unclear what they mean for healthy persons; and that the larger the divergence of glucose metabolism from the norm, the larger the effect of lower GI and GL interventions [94].

The incretin gut hormones, glucagon-like peptide-1 (GLP-1) and glucose-dependent insulinotropic polypeptide (GIP), are gut-derived insulinotropic hormones synthesized and released from intestinal L and K cells in response to nutrient ingestion. They control consummatory behavior and glucose homeostasis. Investigators propose using low-GL diets to improve glycemia and insulinemia by changes in

TABLE 8.3
List of Food Products According to GI

The Average GI of 62 Common Food Derived from Multiple Studies by Different Laboratories

Breakfast Cereals		Vegetables		Dairy Products and Alternatives	
Cornflakes	81 ± 6	Potato, boiled	78 ± 4	Milk, full fat	39 ± 3
Wheat flake biscuits	69 ± 2	Potato, instant mash	67 ± 3	Milk, skim	37 ± 4
Porridge, rolled oats	55 ± 2	Potato, french fries	63 ± 5	Ice cream	51 ± 3
Instant oat porridge	79 ± 3	Carrots, boiled	39 ± 4	Yogurt, fruit	41 ± 2
Rice porridge/congee	78 ± 9	Sweet potato, boiled	63 ± 6	Soy milk	34 ± 4
Millet porridge	67 ± 5	Pumpkin, boiled	64 ± 7	Rice milk	86 ± 7
Muesli	57 ± 2	Plantain/green banana	55 ± 6		
		Taro, boiled	53 ± 2		
		Vegetable soup	48 ± 5		
Legumes		Snack Products		Sugar	
Chickpeas	28 ± 9	Chocolate	40 ± 3	Fructose	15 ± 4
Kidney beans	24 ± 4	Popcorn	65 ± 5	Sucrose	65 ± 4
Lentils	32 ± 5	Potato crisps	56 ± 3	Glucose	103 ± 3
Soya beans	16 ± 1	Soft drink/soda	59 ± 3	Honey	61 ± 3
		Rice crackers/crisps	87 ± 2		
High-Carbohydrate Foods		Fruit and Fruit Products			
White wheat bread[a]	75 ± 2	Apple, raw[b]	36 ± 2		
Whole wheat/whole meal bread	74 ± 2	Orange, raw[b]	43 ± 3		
		Banana, raw[b]	51 ± 3		
Specialty grain bread	53 ± 2	Pineapple, raw	59 ± 8		
Unleavened wheat bread	70 ± 5	Mango, raw[b]	51 ± 5		
Wheat roti	62 ± 3	Watermelon, raw	76 ± 4		
Chapatti	52 ± 4	Dates, raw	42 ± 4		
Corn tortilla	46 ± 4	Peaches, canned[b]	43 ± 5		
White rice, boiled[a]	73 ± 4	Strawberry jam/jelly	49 ± 3		
Brown rice, boiled	68 ± 4	Apple juice	41 ± 2		
Barley	28 ± 2	Orange juice	50 ± 2		
Sweet corn	52 ± 5				
Spaghetti, white	49 ± 2				
Spaghetti, whole meal	48 ± 5				
Rice noodles [b]	53 ± 7				
Udon noodles	55 ± 7				
Couscous [b]	65 ± 4				

Data are ±SEM.

[a] Low-GI varieties were also identified.

[b] Average of all available data.

Source: Atkinson, F.S. et al., *Diab. Care*, 31, 2281, 2008.

the incretin axis [95,96]. A decreased GLP-1 secretion may contribute to impaired insulin secretion in T2DM. The incretin responses were significantly higher in individuals after the large meal (and 520 kcal) compared with the small meal (260 kcal) [97]. High-GL diets in weight-maintaining healthy individuals lead to higher postprandial glucose and lower postprandial GLP-1 concentrations. Dietary manipulation of incretin effects would be helpful to modulate the β-cell sensitivity to glucose in obese healthy subjects and in patients with T2DM by giving them a large meal, compared with a small meal [98].

Sucralose is a synthetic organochlorine sweetener that is a common ingredient in the world's food supply. Sucralose interacts with chemosensors in the alimentary tract that play a role in sweet taste sensation and hormone secretion. Both human and rodent studies demonstrated that sucralose may alter glucose, insulin, and GLP-1 levels [99].

The continued intake of high-GL meals is associated with an increased risk of chronic diseases such as obesity, cardiovascular disease, and T2DM. In diabetic patients, evidence from medium-term studies suggests that replacing high-GI diet with a low-GI diet improves glycemic control and, among persons treated with insulin, reduces hypoglycemic episodes. These dietary changes, which can be made by replacing products made with white flour and potatoes with whole-grain and minimally refined cereal products, have also been associated with a lower risk of cardiovascular disease and can be an appropriate component of recommendations for an overall healthy diet [100]. Diet with low fiber and high GL was found to be associated with women's GDM risk [101].

Low-GL and low-GI foods lower postprandial glucose and insulin responses and may be beneficial in weight control by increasing satiety and possibly by promoting fat oxidation at the expense of carbohydrate oxidation [102,103]. The epidemiological literature analysis linking GI and GL diets to coronary heart disease, insulin sensitivity, dyslipidemia, T2DM, and obesity showed that low-GI/-GL diet may protect against heart disease in women and reduce high-density-lipoprotein cholesterol and triacylglycerol levels in both sexes [104]. A low-GI and energy-restricted diet containing moderate amounts of carbohydrates may be more effective than a high-GI and low-fat diet at reducing body weight and controlling glucose and insulin metabolism [105]. In a cross-sectional study of 640 T2DM patients, usual dietary intakes were assessed by validated food frequency questionnaire. GL and carbohydrate intake were found to be positively associated with the risk of hyperglycemia in T2DM patients. After additional adjusting for dietary fiber and protein intakes, the relation of GL with elevated fasting serum glucose and HbA1c level was stable. GI was not significantly associated with either elevated fasting serum glucose or HbA1c [106]. Among Dutch population of 8,855 men and 10,753 women, aged 21–64 years, and free of T2DM and coronary heart disease high-GL and -GI diets, and high carbohydrate and starch intake, were associated with increased risk of cardiovascular diseases only among men [107]. The 6 months lasting study showed that lowering the dietary GI of conventional diets improved glucose tolerance and reduced body weight, in comparison to the conventional diet in women with previous history of GDM. Subjects with higher fasting insulin level in the low-GI group demonstrated the most positive effects in the improvement of their dysglycemia and weight loss [108].

A protein enriched and low-GI diet supplemented with long-chain Ω-3 PUFAs in a real-life clinical setting improved glycemic control and also reduced waist circumference and silent inflammation in overweight or obese patients with T2DM [109]. Moreover, a low-GI and energy-restricted diet containing moderate amounts of carbohydrates may be more effective than a high-GI and low-fat diet at reducing body weight and controlling glucose and insulin metabolism [105]. In diabetic patients, evidence from medium-term studies suggests that replacing high-GI carbohydrates with a low-GI forms improves glycemic control and, among persons treated with insulin, reduces hypoglycemic episodes. These dietary changes, which can be made by replacing products made with white flour and potatoes with whole grain, minimally refined cereal products, have also been associated with a lower risk of cardiovascular disease and can be an appropriate component of recommendations for an overall healthy diet [100]. Diets with a high dietary GI increased the risk of mortality from stroke among Japanese women [103].

The healthy overweight women and men with relatively greater insulin secretion in response to a standard oral glucose tolerance test lost more weight when assigned to a low-GL hypocaloric diet than to a high-GL diet, but there was no differential effect of the two diets on weight loss in individuals who had relatively lower insulin secretion [110].

Elevated plasma total homocysteine acts synergistically with hypertension to exert a multiplicative effect on cardiovascular diseases risk. It has been suggested that diets that enhance diurnal insulin secretion, such as a high-GI and -GL diet, can be expected to increase homocysteine levels. In a group of 1500 free-living young Japanese women, dietary GI, but not GL, was independently and positively associated with serum homocysteine concentration. In this study, dietary intake was assessed using a validated, self-administered, comprehensive diet history questionnaire [111]. Plasma total homocysteine concentration was also independently associated with the occurrence of macular edema in T2DM [112].

8.11 MEDITERRANEAN DIET (FIGURE 8.2)

Optimal eating is associated with increased life expectancy, reduction in lifetime risk of all chronic disease, and amelioration of gene expression. In this context, claims abound for the competitive merits of various diets relative to one another (Table 8.4). A diet of minimally processed foods close to nature, predominantly plants, is decisively associated with health promotion and disease prevention and is consistent with the salient components of seemingly distinct dietary approaches [113]. To help people everywhere understand the Mediterranean Diet Oldways organization (www.oldwayspt.org) promoting healthy eating and drinking developed the Mediterranean Diet Pyramid.

The ADA has made several recommendations regarding the medical nutrition therapy of diabetes; these emphasize the importance of minimizing macrovascular and microvascular complications in people with diabetes. Four types of diets were reviewed for their effects on diabetes: the Mediterranean diet (MedDiet), a low-carbohydrate/high-protein diet, a vegan diet, and a vegetarian diet. Each of the four types of diet has been shown to improve metabolic conditions, but the degree of improvement varies from patient to patient. Therefore, it is necessary to evaluate a

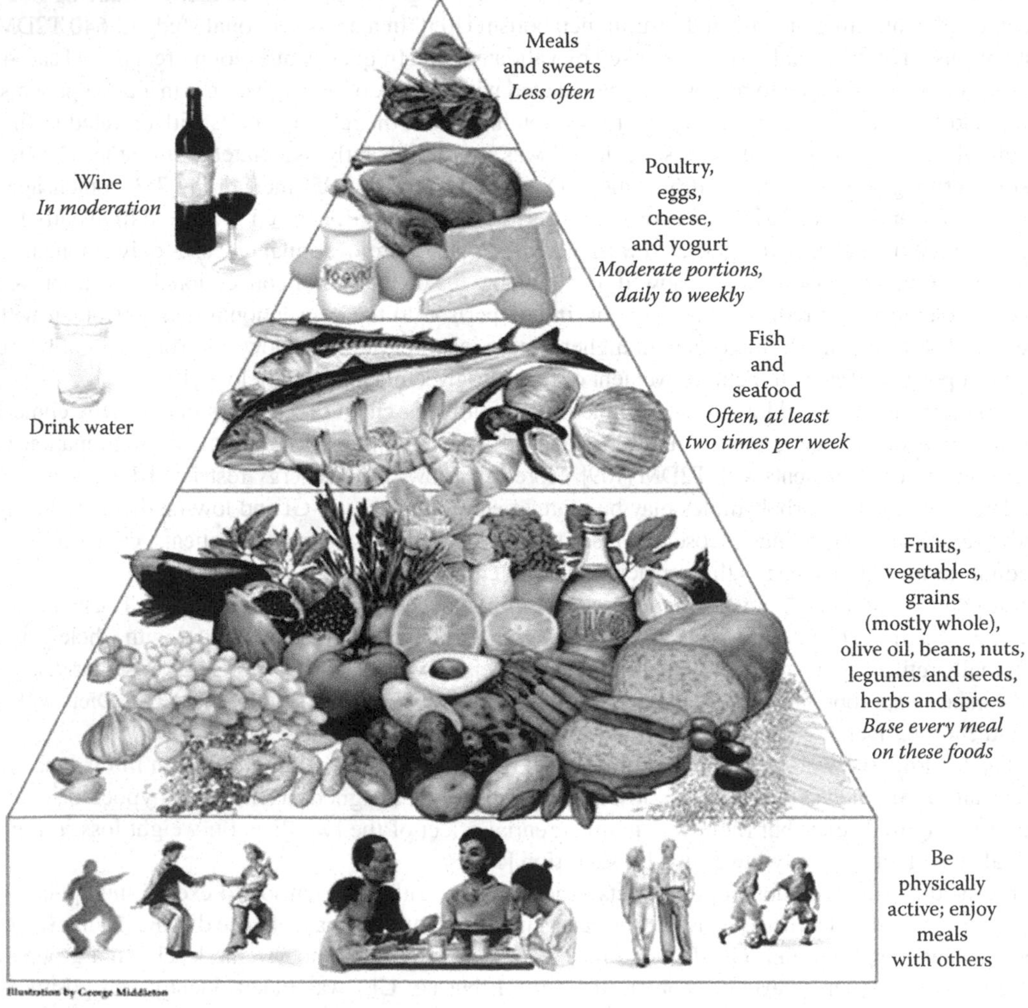

FIGURE 8.2 Mediterranean diet pyramid.

TABLE 8.4
Comparison of Diets

	Hunter-Gatherer	Low-Carbohydrate (Aftws Diet)	Traditional Low-Fat (Ornish Diet)	Traditional Mediterranean
Protein (%)	High (19–35)	Moderate (18–23)	Low (<15)	Moderate (16–23)
Carbohydrates (%)	Moderate (22–40)	Low (4–26)	High (80)	Moderate (50)
Total fat (%)	Moderate (28–47)	High (51–78)	Low (<10)	Moderate (30)
Saturated fat	Moderate	High	Low	Low
Monounsaturated fat	High	Moderate	Low	High
Polyunsaturated fat	Moderate	Moderate	Low	Moderate
Omega-3 fat	High	Low	Low	High
Total fiber	High	Low	High	High
Fruits and vegetables	High	Low	High	High
Nuts and seeds	Moderate	Low	Low	Moderate
Salt	Low	High	Low	Moderate
Refined sugars	Low	Low	Low	Low
Glycemic load	Low	Low	High	Low

Source: O'Keefe, J.H., Jr. and Cordain, L., *Mayo Clin Proc.*, 79, 101, 2004.

patient's pathophysiological characteristics in order to determine the diet that will achieve metabolic improvement in each individual. Many dietary regimens are available for patients with T2DM to choose from, according to personal taste and cultural tradition. It is important to provide a tailor-made diet wherever possible in order to maximize the efficacy of the diet on reducing diabetes symptoms and to encourage patient adherence [114]. The MedDiet has been operationalized through various computational scores (e.g. the MedDiet score for adults and the KIDMED index for children), which are all based on the dietary components that capture its essence.

8.11.1 Various Dietetic Features of MedDiet

The traditional MedDiet, characterized by high consumption of vegetables, fruits, legumes, grains, nuts, and olive oil, moderate consumption of fish and wine, and low consumption of red and processed meat and whole-fat dairy products, is widely recognized as a healthy dietary pattern [115]. The term "MisDiet," implying that all Mediterranean people have the same diet, is a misnomer. The countries around the Mediterranean basin have different diets, religions, and cultures. Their diets differ in the amount of total fat, olive oil, type of meat, and wine intake; milk versus cheese; and fruits and vegetables. Extensive studies on the traditional diet of Greece indicate that the dietary pattern of Greeks consists of a high intake of fruits, vegetables (particularly wild plants), nuts and cereals mostly in the form of sourdough bread rather than pasta; more olive oil and olives; less milk but more cheese; more fish; less meat; and moderate amounts of wine, more so than other Mediterranean countries [116]. When dietary pattern of the traditional MedDiet of southern European populations was examined, it appeared that Crete had the highest frequency of fast-food and sweets consumption whereas Malta had the lowest frequency of fish and vegetable consumption [117]. There was the study that was carried out to compare using MedDiet with a Paleolithic ("Old Stone Age") diet, based on lean meat, fish, fruits, vegetables, root vegetables, eggs and nuts, among 29 patients with ischaemic heart disease plus either glucose intolerance or T2DM. In the Paleolithic group, the strong association between changes in plasma glucose and in waist circumference was established [118]. In patients on the Paleolithic diet, mean values of HbA1c, TG, diastolic blood pressure, weight, BMI, and waist circumference were lower, while mean values for HDL were higher compared to diabetes diet designed in accordance with dietary guideline in patients with T2DM. Dietary GI was slightly lower in the Paleolithic diet (GI = 50) than in the diabetic diet (GI = 55) [119].

8.12 GLYCATION END PRODUCTS IN DIABETES AND DIABETIC COMPLICATIONS

The AGE–RAGE model and investigations of the underlying cellular mechanisms thus may lead to a better understanding of the health benefits of diets (MedDiet, uncooked vegetarian diets), caloric restriction, and intermittent fasting [123].

8.13 HEALTH BENEFITS OF MEDDIET IN RANDOMIZED CLINICAL TRIALS

Although the MedDiet has long been praised for its impact on cardiovascular health, mounting evidence indicates a favorable effect on obesity and T2DM, as well [124]. Emerging data from epidemiological studies have revealed a protective effect of the MetDiet against metabolic complications associated with T2DM [125]. Dietary patterns rich in fruits, vegetables, whole grains, dairy products, and unsaturated fats are also associated with a lower prevalence of MetS [126]. The older subjects at high risk of cardiovascular disease who increased adherence to MedDiets supplemented with virgin olive oil or mixed nuts showed reduced immune cell activation and decreased concentrations of plasma inflammatory biomarkers related to atherogenesis [127].

The impact of the MedDiet on HDL kinetics has been studied of late. Data from this controlled feeding study suggested that the heterogeneous HDL-C response to a traditional MedDiet in men with MetS, independent of weight change, appeared to be primarily determined by individual responses in apoA-I and triglyceride content of the HDL_2 and HDL_3 subfractions [128].

In 901 outpatients with T2DM2, adherence to a MedDiet-type diet was assessed by a nine-point scale. Diabetic patients with the highest scores (6–9) had lower BMI and waist circumferences, a lower prevalence of the MetS, and lower HbA(1c) and post-meal glucose levels than diabetic patients with the lowest scores (0–3) [125].

Five randomized controlled trials have evaluated the effects of a MedDiet, as compared with other commonly used diets, on glycemic control in subjects with T2DM. Improvement of HbA1c levels was greater with a MedDiet and ranged from 0.1% to 0.6% for HbA1c. No trial reported worsening of glycemic control with a MedDiet [129].

In an Italian rural area middle-aged male population aged 45–64 years, free from previous coronary events, the dietary index derived from the Mediterranean habits showed the protective effect of a healthy MedDiet pattern versus the occurrence of fatal coronary heart disease events in individuals aged 20–40 years [130].

MedDiet regimens, including low level of cholesterol and SFAs, effectively improved long-term outcome including death and cerebrovascular events in T2DM patients with coronary artery disease in the Iranian population [131].

Data on health benefits from consumption of fish are still a debatable issue. These effects have mainly been assigned to the long-chain Ω-3 fatty acids docosahexaenoic acid (DHA) and eicosapentaenoic acid (EPA). Even though PUFA shows protective effects against coronary heart disease, there is concern about possible negative health effects from the ingestion of oxidized lipids from fish oils. Lean fish consumption of 75–100 g/day had a beneficial effect on patients with T2DM and was associated with a reduced risk of T2DM by close to 30%, compared to zero consumption [132]. A protective effect from fish consumption was also observed in Japanese men, but not in women (median intake of 63 g/day) [133] and among Chinese middle-aged women (median intake of fish and shellfish ~40 g/day) [134]. Several systematic reviews and meta-studies have concluded that there are indications of geographical differences in observed effects of fish consumption, with studies from Asia showing a protective effect whereas studies from North America/Europe indicating an increased risk of T2DM with fish consumption [135,136]. Data from 18 separate cohorts comprising

540,184 individuals and 25,670 cases of incident T2DM showed that consumption of fish and/or seafood was not significantly associated with T2DM [136]. A MedDiet enriched with fish and other seafood is the main source of human exposure to heavy metals. The fish-eating populations should reduce the quantity of marine fishes to efficiently diminish the exposure to mercury [137,138].

8.14 MULTIFUNCTIONAL COMPOUNDS OF MEDDIET

MedDiet is a rich source of fiber, PUFAs (especially α-linolenic acid), antioxidants (especially resveratrol (RSV) from wine and polyphenols from the olive oil), selenium, vitamin C, vitamin E, and glutathione. It is collection of similar eating habits traditionally followed in at least 16 countries bordering the Mediterranean Sea. Among numerous foodstuffs characterizing the MedDiet, virgin olive oil and nuts are the key foods components that may have the important effect on inflammatory biomarkers related to atherosclerosis, MetS, and T2DM [139,140].

8.14.1 Extra-Virgin Olive Oil and Nuts

Olive and olive oil, a traditional food product with thousands of years of history, are the essential components of MedDiet and are largely consumed all over the world. A MedDiet enriched with extra-virgin olive oil but without energy restrictions reduced T2DM risk among persons with high cardiovascular risk [139]. The health benefits attributed to the MedDiet and its components, such as olive oil, could be explained by a transcriptomic effect on atherosclerosis, inflammation, and oxidative stress–related genes (i.e. ADRB2, IL7R, IFN-γ, MCP1, TNF-α). Gene expression changes toward a protective mode were often associated with an improvement in systemic markers for oxidation and inflammation [142]. MetDiet and virgin olive oil consumption decreased plasma oxidative and inflammatory status and the gene expression related with both inflammation and oxidative stress in peripheral blood mononuclear cells [143].

The European Food Safety Authority released a claim concerning the effectiveness of the ingestion of olive oil polyphenols (5 mg/day) on protecting LDL from oxidation [144].

Nuts (tree nuts and peanuts) are nutrient-dense foods with complex matrices rich in unsaturated fatty and other bioactive compounds: high-quality vegetable protein, fiber, l-arginine, the precursor of nitric oxide, minerals, tocopherols, phytosterols, and phenolic compounds. Peanut seeds are currently widely used as a source of human food ingredients in the United States and in European countries due to their high-quality protein and oil content. By virtue of their unique composition, nuts are likely to beneficially impact health outcomes. Clinical studies with nuts have documented reduced inflammatory cytokine concentrations but no consistent changes of C-reactive protein. Nut consumption also reduced the expression of endothelin 1, a potent endothelial activator, in an animal model of accelerated atherosclerosis [145]. Epidemiological studies have associated nut consumption with a reduced incidence of coronary heart disease and gallstones in both genders and T2DM in women [146]. Consumption of tree nuts revealed strong inverse association with obesity and favorable through weak associations with abdominal obesity and MetS independent of demographic, lifestyle, and other dietary factors [147]. Nuts are energy-dense foods high in total fat (50%–75% by weight), thus perceived as fattening. Nevertheless, epidemiological studies and short-term controlled feeding trials have supported the theory that the inclusion of nuts in the typical diet does not induce weight gain, despite an expected increase in total caloric intake [148]. Results from a recent meta-analysis of clinical trials conclude that nut-enriched diets do not increase body weight, BMI, or waist circumference [149].

8.14.2 Red Wine and Alcohol

The mechanisms responsible for the health effects of wine are extremely complex due to the many different pathways involved. There is controversy as to which component is the most active, alcohol or polyphenolic compounds. Some studies have provided evidence that wine exhibits beneficial properties that are independent of the presence of alcohol, which should be attributed to its polyphenolic content. Red wine polyphenols are a complex mixture of flavonoids. These compounds act as potent antioxidants as they reduce LDL cholesterol oxidation, modulate cell signaling pathways, and reduce platelet aggregation. Red wine contains more polyphenols than white wine (around 10-fold) because during the wine-making process, red wine, unlike white wine, is macerated for weeks with the skin, which is one of the parts of the grape with the highest concentrations of phenolic compounds. It has been suggested that wine phenolics could reduce platelet activity mediated by nitric oxide [150,151].

Comparing the relative risk for T2DM in men drinking alcohol with lifetime abstainers, alcohol was most protective when consumed 22 g/day and became deleterious at just over 60 g/day. Among women, consumption of 24 g/day alcohol was most protective and became deleterious at about 50 g/day [152].

8.14.3 Resveratrol

RSV is a plant-derived polyphenol suggested to have many beneficial health effects, including antioxidant, anti-inflammatory, antiproliferative, proapoptotic, and antiangiogenic ones. It is even speculated that uptake of RSV by red wine consumption could be behind the so-called French paradox meaning the lower incidence of cardiovascular diseases in the French population. These properties, together with good absorption and tolerance, would make it an attractive agent in prevention and treatment of metabolic diseases, especially in T2DM and MetS. RSV consumption significantly decreases systolic and diastolic blood pressure [153] and significantly reduced fasting glucose, insulin, hemoglobin A_{1c}, levels and insulin resistance (measured by using the homeostatic model assessment) in participants with T2DM but no significant effect of RSV on glycemic measures of nondiabetic participants was found [154]. RSV improved flap survival significantly in streptozotocin-induced diabetic Sprague–Dawley albino rats [155]. An experiment assessing the effects of RSV on mitochondrial content and respiration, glyceroneogenesis, and adiponectin secretion in adipose tissue from Zucker diabetic fatty (ZDF) rats was conducted. Five-week-old ZDF rats were fed a chow diet with or without RSV (200 mg/kg body wt) for 6 weeks. The obtained data demonstrate that RSV can induce adipose tissue mitochondrial biogenesis in parallel with increases in glyceroneogenesis and adiponectin secretion [156].

Grape pomace is a natural product rich in dietary fiber and polyphenols. A major part of dietary polyphenols is not absorbed in the small intestine and can interact with colonic microbiota. The influence of grape polyphenols on *Lactobacillus acidophilus* through agar diffusion assays and cultures in liquid media have shown that a grape pomace phenolic extract (1 mg/mL) induced a significant increase in *L. acidophilus* growth [157]. Grape phenolic concentration and composition depend on agro-geographic factors and processing conditions. In humans, grape polyphenols demonstrated effects such as maintenance of endothelial function, increase in the antioxidant capacity, and protection against LDL oxidation. Grape phenolic extracts obtained from *Vitis vinifera* varieties Cabernet Franc and Pinot Noir and Vitis interspecific hybrid varieties Baco Noir and Noiret were highly effective against specific virulence traits of *Streptococcus mutans*, which is a well-known dental pathogen [158]. The scientific data performed in the last years indicate links between periodontitis and atheromatosis, coronary heart disease, and acute coronary events, including myocardial infarction. Potential mechanisms of induction of acute coronary events connected with platelet aggregation induced by specific proteins secreted by *Streptococcus* were noted [159].

8.14.4 Pomegranate

Pomegranate is an ancient fruit that is still part of the diet in the Mediterranean area, the Middle East, and India. Various studies indicated that several compounds present of the pomegranate fruit can be beneficial in T2DM prevention and treatment. Although both in vitro and animal studies show that punicalagin and ellagic, gallic, oleanolic, ursolic, and uallic acids and polyphenols from the pomegranate juice possess an antidiabetic potential, controlled clinical studies on humans are scarce [160]. In one of them, it was found that pomegranate polyphenols reduce lipid peroxidation in patients with T2DM, but with no effects in healthy controls, and specifically modulate liver enzymes in diabetic and nondiabetic subjects [161].

8.14.5 Polyunsaturated Fatty Acids

PUFAs are of particular interest in the nutritional therapy for T2DM, given their potential role in several pathophysiological processes related to cardiovascular disease. As suggested by the known associations among subtypes of dietary fat and T2DM risk, the increased unsaturated fat load of MedDiets was probably instrumental in achieving T2DM risk reduction [162].

The findings from the prospective study (EPIC-Norfolk) of 25,639 individuals aged 40–79 years provided consistent evidence, suggesting a protective role of Ω-6 PUFA substitution for saturated fats for coronary heart disease prevention [163].

Ω-3 PUFAs are beneficial for improving lipid profiles in healthy individuals and among T2DM Chinese patients. They lowered the levels of triglycerides and VLDL cholesterol in the blood [164,165]. The systematic review and meta-analysis of randomized controlled trials comparing dietary or nondietary intake of Ω-3 PUFA with placebo in patients with T2DM was performed. Compared with placebo, Ω-3 PUFA had a statistically significant effect on four different outcomes, reducing levels of (1) triacylglycerol (18 trials, 969 subjects), (2) VLDL cholesterol (7 trials, 238 subjects), (3) VLDL triacylglycerol (6 trials, 178 subjects) but (4) slightly increasing LDL (16 trials, 565 subjects). There were no significant effects on total cholesterol and apolipoproteins levels [169].

Twenty-three randomized controlled trials (1075 participants) have revealed that Ω-3 PUFA supplementation in T2DM patients lowered their blood levels of triglycerides and VLDL cholesterol, but raised LDL cholesterol and had no statistically significant effect on glycemic control or fasting insulin levels [166]. In 234 postmenopausal women, a positive association of PUFA consumption with atherosclerosis progression was observed [167].

Our diet contains a complex mixture of fats and oils consisting of different fatty acids that may affect human health. The Ω-3 are present mainly in linseed oil, nuts, soya beans, wheat, and cold water fish, whereas Ω-6 are present mainly in maize, sunflower, and sesame oil and eating equal amounts of Ω-3 and Ω-6 nutrients provides a more benign health consequence [168,169].

A joint Food and Agriculture Organization of the United Nations/World Health Organization (FAO/WHO) report from 2009 claims that there is convincing evidence that replacing dietary saturated fatty acids (SF) with PUFA decreases the risk of cardiovascular diseases [170]. The report recommends replacing SF in the diet with PUFA. In practice, this may be done by replacing foods such as high-fat dairy products and fatty meat, with foods such as several vegetable oils (but not palm oil and coconut oil), fatty fish, and fish oils.

There is concern about possible negative health effects from the ingestion of oxidized lipids from fish oils [171]. Lipid oxidation in foods is one of the major degradative processes responsible for losses in food quality. It is well known that lipids in edible oils are susceptible to autooxidation and photooxidation during processing and storage [172]. The oxidation of oils is influenced by many factors such as the fatty acid composition (i.e. the degree of unsaturation), oil processing, heat, light, transition metals, and antioxidants. The primary lipid oxidation products, lipid hydroperoxides, may decompose into secondary oxidation products such as the highly reactive and cytotoxic 4-hydroxy-2-alkenals [172]. The oxidation of unsaturated fatty acids results in significant generation of the dietary advanced lipid oxidation end products (ALEs) that are in part cytotoxic and genotoxic compounds. Some of the dietary ALEs, which are absorbed from the gut to the circulatory system, seem to act as injurious chemicals that activate an inflammatory response that affects not only circulatory system but also organs such as liver, kidney, lung, and the gut itself [173]. The screening of oxidative status of commercially available Ω-3 supplements available in Norway and vegetable oils shows that the content of oxidation products varies. Both fresh and heated vegetable oils have been studied. The content of hydroperoxides and alkenals in marine Ω-3 supplements was far higher than in fresh vegetable oils, but after heating, a 2.9–11.2-fold fold increase in alkenals concentration was observed [172]. However, due to a larger intake of vegetable oils in the diet compared to fish oil supplements, the former are the largest source of primary as well as secondary oxidation products in the diet. Despite the biological toxicity of several secondary lipid oxidation products, such as 4-hydroxy-2-alkenals, an upper limit corresponding to a safe dose of these compounds has not been established yet.

8.15 CONCLUSIONS

No specific diet can be recommended to prevent T2DM. A total of 21,372 cases of T2DM from 18 prospective studies, with 20 cohorts, in four world regions were identified. The risk of incident T2DM did not change appreciably considering the geography (the United States, Europe, and Asia), the duration of follow-up (≤10 and >10 years), and type of diets (Mediterranean and DASH, Dietary Approaches to Stop Hypertension, diets). They were equally and consistently associated with a 20% reduced risk of future T2DM [173]. Low-carbohydrate, low-GI, Mediterranean, and high-protein diets are effective in improving various markers of cardiovascular risk in people with T2DM and should be considered in the overall strategy of T2DM management [174]. The ADA has made several recommendations regarding the medical nutrition therapy of T2DM; these emphasize the importance of minimizing macrovascular and microvascular complications in people with T2DM. Four types of diets were reviewed for their effects on diabetes: MedDiet, a low-carbohydrate/high-protein diet, a vegan diet, and a vegetarian diet. Each of the four types of diet has been shown to improve metabolic conditions, but the degree of improvement varies from patient to patient. Therefore, it is necessary to evaluate a patient's pathophysiological characteristics in order to determine the diet that will achieve metabolic improvement in each individual [118].

REFERENCES

1. Perry, I.J. 2002. Healthy diet and lifestyle clustering and glucose intolerance. *Proc Nutr Soc.* 61:543–551.
2. Beagley, J., Guariguata, L., Weil, C., Motala, A.A. 2014. Global estimates of undiagnosed diabetes in adults. *Diabetes Res Clin Pract.* 103:150–160.
3. Crook, E.D., Patel, S.R. 2004. Diabetic nephropathy in African-American patients. *Curr Diab Rep.* 4:455–461.
4. Palmer, N.D., McDonough, C.W., Hicks, P.J., Roh, B.H. et al. 2012. A genome-wide association search for type 2 diabetes genes in African Americans. *PLoS One.* 7(1):e29202. doi: 10.1371/journal.pone.0029202. Epub January 4, 2012.
5. Tamayo, T., Rosenbauer, J., Wild, S.H., Spijkerman, A.M.W. et al. 2014. Diabetes in Europe: An update. *Diabetes Res Clin Pract.* 103:206–217.
6. Satman, I., Omer, B., Tutuncu, Y., Kalaca, S. et al. 2013. TURDEP-II Study Group. Twelve-year trends in the prevalence and risk factors of diabetes and prediabetes in Turkish adults. *Eur J Epidemiol.* 28:169–180.
7. Pereira, M., Carreira, H., Lunet, N., Azevedo, A. 2014. Trends in prevalence of diabetes mellitus and mean fasting glucose in Portugal (1987–2009): A systematic review. *Public Health.* 128:214–221.
8. Kuzuya, T. 2000. Early diagnosis, early treatment and the new diagnostic criteria of diabetes mellitus. *Br J Nutr.* 84(Suppl 2):S177–S181.
9. Ginter, E., Simko, V. 2012. Type 2 diabetes mellitus, pandemic in 21st century. *Adv Exp Med Biol.* 771:42–50.
10. Lotfi, M.H., Saadati, H., Afzali, M. 2014. Prevalence of diabetes in people aged ≥30 years: The results of screening program of Yazd Province, Iran, in 2012. *J Res Health Sci.* 14:87–91.
11. Moyer, V.A., On behalf of the U.S. Preventive Services Task Force. 2014. Screening for gestational Diabetes Mellitus: U.S. Preventive Services Task Force Recommendation Statement. *Ann Intern Med.* 160(6):414–420 doi:10.7326/M13-2905.
12. Kim, C., Newton, K.M., Knopp, R.H. 2002. Gestational diabetes and the incidence of type 2 diabetes: A systematic review. *Diabetes Care.* 25:1862–1868.
13. Laakso, M., Kuusisto, J. 2014. Insulin resistance and hyperglycaemia in cardiovascular disease development. *Nat Rev Endocrinol.* 10:293–302.

14. Yiu, K.H., Zhao, C.T., Chen, Y., Siu, C.W. et al. 2013. Association of subclinical myocardial injury with arterial stiffness in patients with type 2 diabetes mellitus. *Cardiovasc Diabetol.* 12:94. doi: 10.1186/1475-2840-12-94
15. Qasim, A.N., Rafeek, H., Rasania, S.P., Churchill, T.W. et al. 2013. Cardiovascular risk factors and mitral annular calcification in type 2 diabetes. *Atherosclerosis.* 226:419–424.
16. Wan Mahmood, W.A., Draman Yusoff, M.S., Behan, L.A., Di Perna, A. et al. 2013. Association between sleep disruption and levels of lipids in Caucasians with type 2 diabetes. *Int J Endocrinol.* 2013:341506. doi: 10.1155/2013/341506.
17. Kappelle, P.J., de Boer, J.F., Perton, F.G., Annema, W. et al. 2012. Increased LCAT activity and hyperglycaemia decrease the antioxidative functionality of HDL. *Eur J Clin Invest.* 42:487–495.
18. Patra, S.K., Singh, K., Singh, R. 2013. Paraoxonase 1: A better atherosclerotic risk predictor than HDL in type 2 diabetes mellitus. *Diabetes Metab Syndr.* 7:108–111.
19. Warensjö, E., Rosell, M., Hellenius, M.L., Vessby, B. et al. 2009. Associations between estimated fatty acid desaturase activities in serum lipids and adipose tissue in humans: Links to obesity and insulin resistance. *Lipids Health Dis.* 8:37. doi: 10.1186/1476-511X-8-37.
20. Gray, R.G., Kousta, E., McCarthy, M.I., Godsland, I.F. et al. 2013. Ethnic variation in the activity of lipid desaturases and their relationships with cardiovascular risk factors in control women and an at-risk group with previous gestational diabetes mellitus: A cross-sectional study. *Lipids Health Dis.* 12:25. doi: 10.1186/1476-511X-12-25,
21. Bae, J.C., Rhee, E.J., Lee, W.Y. 2011. Combined effect of nonalcoholic fatty liver disease and impaired fasting glucose on the development of type 2 diabetes: A 4-year retrospective longitudinal study. *Diabetes Care.* 34:727–729.
22. Kelly, T., Yang, W., Chen, C.S., Reynolds, K., He, J. 2008. Global burden of obesity in 2005 and projections to 2030. *Int J Obes (Lond).* 32:1431–1437.
23. Mitchell, N.S., Catenacci, V.A., Wyatt, H.R., Hill, J.O. 2011. Obesity: Overview of an epidemic. *Psychiatr Clin North Am.* 34:717–732.
24. Flegal, K.M., Carroll, M.D., Ogden, C.L., Curtin, L.R. 2010. Prevalence and trends in obesity among US adults, 1999–2008. *JAMA.* 303:235–241.
25. Allison, D.B., Saunders, S.E. 2000. Obesity in North America. An overview. *Med Clin North Am.* 84:305–332.
26. Alberti, K.G., Eckel, R.H., Grundy, S.M., Zimmet, P.Z. et al. 2009. Harmonizing the metabolic syndrome: A joint interim statement of the international diabetes federation task force on epidemiology and prevention; National Heart, Lung, and Blood Institute; American Heart Association; World Heart Federation; International Atherosclerosis Society; and International Association for the Study of Obesity. *Circulation.* 120:1640–1645.
27. Mojiminiyi, O.A., Abdella, N.A., Al Arouj, M., Ben Nakhi, A. 2007. Adiponectin, insulin resistance and clinical expression of the metabolic syndrome in patients with Type 2 diabetes. *Int J Obes (Lond).* 31:213–220.
28. Kaur, J. 2014. A comprehensive review on metabolic syndrome. *Cardiol Res Pract.* 2014:943162. Epub March 11, 2014.
29. Yu, S., Zhang, Y., Li, M.Z., Xu, H. et al. 2012. Chemerin and apelin are positively correlated with inflammation in obese type 2 diabetic patients. *Chin Med J (Engl).* 125:3440–3444.
30. Fülöp, P., Seres, I., Lőrincz, H., Harangi, M., Somodi, S., Paragh, G. 2014. Association of chemerin with oxidative stress, inflammation and classical adipokines in non-diabetic obese patients. *J Cell Mol Med.* 18:1313–1320.
31. Lehrke, M., Becker, A., Greif, M., Stark, R. et al. 2009. Chemerin is associated with markers of inflammation and components of the metabolic syndrome but does not predict coronary atherosclerosis. *Eur J Endocrinol.* 161:339–344.
32. Jahns, L., Kranz, S. 2014. High proportions of foods recommended for consumption by United States Dietary Guidance contain solid fats and added sugar: Results from the National Health and Nurition Examination Survey (2007–2008). *Nutr J.* 13(1):23. doi: 10.1186/1475-2891-13-23.
33. Lowndes, J., Sinnett, S., Pardo, S., Nguyen, V.T. et al. 2014. The effect of normally consumed amounts of sucrose or high fructose corn syrup on lipid profiles, body composition and related parameters in overweight/obese subjects. *Nutrients.* 6:1128–1144.
34. Vetter, M.L., Amaro, A., Volger, S. 2014. Nutritional management of type 2 diabetes mellitus and obesity and pharmacologic therapies to facilitate weight loss. *Postgrad Med.* 126:139–152.
35. Carbohydrates in human nutrition. 1998 Report of a Joint FAO/WHO Expert Consultation. Rome, Italy: Food and Agriculture Organization of the United Nations (FAO Food and Nutrition Paper, No. 66).

36. White, J.S. 2008. Straight talk about high-fructose corn syrup: What it is and what it ain't. *Am J Clin Nutr.* 88:1716–1721.
37. Dietary Reference Intakes for Energy, Carbohydrates, Fiber, Fat, Fatty Acids, Cholesterol, Protein, and Amino Acids (Macronutrients). 2005. Washington, DC: The National Academies Press. Retrieved February 8, 2015 from http://nap.edu/openbook/0309085373/html/265.html.
38. Trepel, F. 2004. Dietary fibre: More than a matter of dietetics. I. Preventative and therapeutic uses. *Wien Klin Wochenschr.* 116:511–522.
39. Gray, G.M. 1992. Starch digestion and absorption in nonruminants. *J Nutr.* 122:172–177.
40. Kruszynska, Y.T. 2005. Normal metabolism: The physiology of fuel homeostasis. In *Textbook of Diabetes*, eds. J.C. Pickup and G. Wiliams, Chapter 9, 9.1–9.38. Oxford, U.K.: Blackwell Publishing.
41. Klip, A., Sun, Y., Chiu, T.T., Foley, K.P. 2014. Signal transduction meets vesicle traffic: The software and hardware of GLUT4 translocation. *Am J Physiol Cell Physiol.* 306:C879–C886.
42. Aydin, S. 2014. Three new players in energy regulation: Preptin, adropin and irisin. *Peptides.* 56C: 94–110. doi: 10.1016/j.peptides.2014.03.021
43. Jones, H.F., Burt, E., Dowling, K., Davidson, G., Brooks, D.A., Butler, R.N. 2011. Effect of age on fructose malabsorption in children presenting with gastrointestinal symptoms. *J Pediatr Gastroenterol Nutr.* 52:581–584.
44. Bray, G.A., Nielsen, S.J., Popkin, B.M. 2004. Consumption of high-fructose corn syrup in beverages may play a role in the epidemic of obesity. *Am J Clin Nutr.* 79:537–543.
45. Douard, V., Ferraris, R.P. 2008. Regulation of the fructose transporter GLUT5 in health and disease. *Am J Physiol Endocrinol Metab.* 295:E227–E237.
46. Kim, H.R., Park, S.W., Cho, H.J., Chae, K.A. et al. 2007. Comparative gene expression profiles of intestinal transporters in mice, rats and humans. *Pharmacol Res.* 56:224–236.
47. Manolescu, A., Salas-Burgos, A.M., Fischbarg, J., Cheeseman, C.I. 2005. Identification of a hydrophobic residue as a key determinant of fructose transport by the facilitative hexose transporter SLC2A7 (GLUT7). *J Biol Chem.* 280:42978–42983.
48. Morgantini, C., Xiao, C., Dash, S. Lewis, G.F. Dietary carbohydrates and intestinal lipoprotein production. *Curr Opin Clin Nutr Metab Care.* 17:355–359.
49. Yang, Q., Zhang, Z., Gregg, E.W., Flanders, W.D., Merritt, R., Hu, F.B. 2014. Added sugar intake and cardiovascular diseases mortality among US adults. *JAMA Intern Med.* 174:516–524.
50. Scientific Report of the DGAC on the Dietary Guidelines for Americans. 2015. Part D1–2.: Retrieved February, 7, 2015 from http//www.cnpp.usda.gov/Publications/DietaryGuidelines.
51. Turner-McGrievy, G.M., Barnard, N.D., Cohen, J., Jenkins, D.J. et al. 2008. Changes in nutrient intake and dietary quality among participants with type 2 diabetes following a low-fat vegan diet or a conventional diabetes diet for 22 weeks. *J Am Diet Assoc.* 108:1636–1645.
52. Barnard, N.D., Cohen, J., Jenkins, D.J. et al. 2009. A low-fat vegan diet and conventional diabetes diet in the treatment of type 2 diabetes: A randomized, controlled, 74-wk clinical trial. *Am J Clin Nutr.* 89:1588S–1596S.
53. Kahleova, H., Matoulek, M., Malinska, H., Oliyarnik, O. et al. 2011. Vegetarian diet improves insulin resistance and oxidative stress markers more than conventional diet in subjects with type 2 diabetes. *Diabet Med.* 28:549–559.
54. Imai, S., Fukui, M., Kajiyama, S. 2014. Effect of eating vegetables before carbohydrates on glucose excursions in patients with type 2 diabetes. *J Clin Biochem Nutr.* 54:7–11.
55. Yoshida, M., McKeown, N.M., Rogers, G., Meigs, J.B. et al. 2007. Surrogate markers of insulin resistance are associated with consumption of sugar-sweetened drinks and fruit juice in middle and older-aged adults. *J Nutr.* 137:2121–2127.
56. Dhingra, R., Sullivan, L., Jacques, P.F., Wang, T.J. et al. 2007. Soft drink consumption and risk of developing cardiometabolic risk factors and the metabolic syndrome in middle-aged adults in the community. *Circulation.* 116:480–488.
57. Schulze, M.B., Manson, J.E., Ludwig, D.S., Colditz, G.A. et al. 2004. Sugar-sweetened beverages, weight gain, and incidence of type 2 diabetes in young and middle-aged women. *JAMA.* 292:927–934.
58. Sakurai, M., Nakamura, K., Miura, K., Takamura, T. et al. 2014. Sugar-sweetened beverage and diet soda consumption and the 7-year risk for type 2 diabetes mellitus in middle-aged Japanese men. *Eur J Nutr.* 53:251–258.
59. Yu, D., Shu, X.O., Li, H., Xiang, Y.B. et al. 2013. Dietary carbohydrates, refined grains, glycemic load, and risk of coronary heart disease in Chinese adults. *Am J Epidemiol.* 178:1542–1549.

60. Hosseini-Esfahani, F., Bahadoran, Z., Mirmiran, P., Hosseinpour-Niazi, S. et al. 2011. Dietary fructose and risk of metabolic syndrome in adults: Tehran Lipid and Glucose study. *Nutr Metab (Lond).* 8(1):50. doi: 10.1186/1743-7075-8-50.
61. Nettleton, J.A., Lutsey, P.L., Wang, Y., Lima, J.A. et al. 2009. Diet soda intake and risk of incident metabolic syndrome and type 2 diabetes in the Multi-Ethnic Study of Atherosclerosis (MESA). *Diabetes Care.* 32:688–689.
62. Wang, D., Sievenpiper, J.L., de Souza, R.J., Cozma, A.I. et al. 2014. Effect of fructose on postprandial triglycerides: A systematic review and meta-analysis of controlled feeding trials. *Atherosclerosis.* 232:125–133.
63. Sievenpiper, J.L., Carleton, AJ., Chatha, S., Jiang, H.Y. et al. 2009. Heterogeneous effects of fructose on blood lipids in individuals with type 2 diabetes: Systematic review and meta-analysis of experimental trials in humans. *Diabetes Care.* 32:1930–1937.
64. Shiota, M., Moore, M.C., Galassetti, P., Monohan, M. et al. 2002. Inclusion of low amounts of fructose with an intraduodenal glucose load markedly reduces postprandial hyperglycemia and hyperinsulinemia in the conscious dog. *Diabetes.* 51:469–478.
65. Kwon, S., Kim, Y.J., Kim, M.K. 2008. Effect of fructose or sucrose feeding with different levels on oral glucose tolerance test in normal and type diabetic rats. *Nutr Res Pract.* 2:252–258.
66. Lustig, R.H. 2013. Fructose: It's "alcohol without the buzz". *Adv Nutr.* 4:226–235.
67. Bray, G.A. 2013. Energy and fructose from beverages sweetened with sugar or high-fructose corn syrup pose a health risk for some people. *Adv Nutr.* 4:220–225.
68. Szabo de Edelenyi, F., Julia, C., Courtois, F., Méjean, C. et al. 2014. Starchy food consumption in French adults: A cross-sectional analysis of the profile of consumers and contribution to nutritional intake in a web-based prospective cohort. *Ann Nutr Metab.* 64:28–37.
69. Riccardi, G., Rivellese, A.A. 1991. Effects of dietary fiber and carbohydrate on glucose and lipoprotein metabolism in diabetic patients. *Diabetes Care.* 14:1115–1125.
70. Eelderink, C., Schepers, M., Preston, T., Vonk, R.J. et al. 2012. Slowly and rapidly digestible starchy foods can elicit a similar glycemic response because of differential tissue glucose uptake in healthy men. *Am J Clin Nutr.* 96:1017–1024.
71. Papanek, P.E. 2003. Exercise physiology. In *Physiology Secrets, Questions and Answers Reveal the Secrets to Understanding Physiology,* 2nd edn. H. Raff, pp. 279–308. Philadelphia, PA: Hanley & Belfus.
72. Havel, P.J. 2001. Peripheral signals conveying metabolic information to the brain: Short-term and long-term regulation of food intake and energy homeostasis. *Exp Biol Med (Maywood).* 226:963–977.
73. Pfeiffer, A.F., Klein, H.H. 2014. The treatment of type 2 diabetes. *Dtsch Arztebl In.* 111:68–82.
74. Richardson, V.R., Smith, K.A., Carter, A.M. 2013. Adipose tissue inflammation: Feeding the development of type 2 diabetes mellitus. *Immunobiology.* 218:1497–1504.
75. King, G.L. 2008. The role of inflammatory cytokines in diabetes and its complications. *J Periodontol.* 79(8 Suppl):1527–1534.
76. Fontana, L., Hu, F.B. 2014. Optimal body weight for health and longevity: Bridging basic, clinical, and population research. *Aging Cell.* 13:391–400.
77. He, J., Votruba, S., Venti, C., Krakoff, J. 2011. Higher incremental insulin area under the curve during oral glucose tolerance test predicts less food intake and weight gain. *Int J Obes (Lond).* 35:1495–1501.
78. Prentice, A.M., Rayco-Solon, P., Moore, S.E. 2005. Insights from the developing world: Thrifty genotypes and thrifty phenotypes. *Proc Nutr Soc.* 64:153–161.
79. Bantle, J.P., Wylie-Rosett, J., Albright, A.L., Apovian, C.M. et al. 2008. Nutrition recommendations and interventions for diabetes: A position statement of the American Diabetes Association. *Diabetes Care.* 12(Suppl 1):S61–S78.
80. Stephen, A., Alles, M., de Graaf, C., Fleith, M. et al. 2012. The role and requirements of digestible dietary carbohydrates in infants and toddlers. *Eur J Clin Nutr.* 66:765–779.
81. Ortega, R.M., Redondo, M.R., Zamora, M.J., López-Sobaler, A.M. et al. 1998. Relationship between the number of daily meals and the energy and nutrient intake in the elderly. Effect on various cardiovascular risk factors [Article in Spanish]. *Nutr Hosp.* 13:186–192.
82. Pot, G.K., Hardy, R., Stephen, A.M. March 28, 2014. Irregular consumption of energy intake in meals is associated with a higher cardio-metabolic risk in adults of a British birth cohort. *Int J Obes (Lond).* doi: 10.1038/ijo.2014.51.
83. Moszczyński, P., Rutowski, J. 2012. Meal plans for diabetics: Caloric intake, calorie counting and glycemic index. In *Nutritional and Therapeutic Interventions for Diabetes and Metabolic Syndrome*, eds. D. Bagchi, and N. Sreejayan, pp. 431–442. Elsevier and Academic Press.

84. Vinoy, S., Normand, S., Meynier, A., Sothier, M. 2013. Cereal processing influences postprandial glucose metabolism as well as the GI effect. *J Am Coll Nutr.* 32:79–91.
85. Mayo Clinic Healthy Weight Pyramid Retrieved February, 15, 2015 from http://www.mayoclinic.org/healthy-lifestyle/nutrition-and-healthy-eating/in-depth/healthy-weight-pyramid/art-20045416.
86. Franz, M.J., Boucher, J.L., Evert, A.B. 2014. Evidence-based diabetes nutrition therapy recommendations are effective: The key is individualization. *Diabetes Metab Syndr Obes.* 7:65–72.
87. Rabinovitz, H.R., Boaz, M., Ganz, T., Jakubowicz, D., Matas, Z., Wainstein, J. 2014. Big breakfast rich in protein and fat improves glycemic control in type 2 diabetics. *Obesity.* 22:E46–E54.
88. Lim, E.L., Hollingsworth, K.G., Aribisala, B.S., Chen, M.J., Mathers, J.C., Taylor, R. 2011. Reversal of type 2 diabetes: Normalisation of beta cell function in association with decreased pancreas and liver triacylglycerol. *Diabetologia.* 54:2508–2514.
89. Bantle, J.P., Raatz, S.K., Thomas, W., Georgopoulos, A. 2000. Effects of dietary fructose on plasma lipids in healthy subjects. *Am J Clin Nutr.* 72:1128–1134.
90. Shadman, Z., Khoshniat, M., Poorsoltan, N., Akhoundan, M., Omidvar, M., Larijani, B., Hoseini, S. 2013. Association of high carbohydrate versus high fat diet with glycated hemoglobin in high calorie consuming type 2 diabetics. *J Diabetes Metab Disord.* 12:27.
91. Monro, J.A., Mishra, S. 2010. Glycemic impact as a property of foods is accurately measured by an available carbohydrate method that mimics the glycemic response. *J Nutr.* 140:1328–1334.
92. Monro, J.A., Shaw, M. 2008. Glycemic impact, glycemic glucose equivalents, glycemic index, and glycemic load: Definitions, distinctions, and implications. *Am J Clin Nutr.* 87:237S–243S.
93. Monro, J.A. 2002. Glycaemic glucose equivalent: Combining carbohydrate content, quantity and glycaemic index of foods for precision in glycaemia management. *Asia Pac J Clin Nutr.* 11:217–225.
94. Howlett, J., Ashwell, M. 2008. Glycemic response and health: Summary of a workshop. *Am J Clin Nutr.* 87:212S–216S.
95. Solomon, T.P., Haus, J.M., Kelly, K.R., Cook, M.D. et al. 2010. A low-glycemic index diet combined with exercise reduces insulin resistance, postprandial hyperinsulinemia, and glucose-dependent insulinotropic polypeptide responses in obese, prediabetic humans. *Am J Clin Nutr.* 92:1359–1368.
96. Isken, F., Weickert, M.O., Tschop, M.H., Noqueiras, R. et al. 2009. Metabolic effects of diets differing in glycaemic index depend on age and endogenous glucose-dependent insulinotrophic polypeptide in mice. *Diabetologia.* 52:2159–2168.
97. Vilsbøll, T., Krarup, T., Sonne, J., Madsbad, S. et al. 2003. Incretin secretion in relation to meal size and body weight in healthy subjects and people with type 1 and type 2 diabetes mellitus. *J Clin Endocrinol Metab.* 88:2706–2713.
98. Runchey, S.S., Valsta, L.M., Schwarz, Y., Wang, C., Song, X., Lampe, J.W., Neuhouser, M.L. 2013. Effect of low- and high-glycemic load on circulating incretins in a randomized clinical trial. *Metabolism.* 62:188–195.
99. Schiffman, S.S., Rother, K.I. 2013. Sucralose, a synthetic organochlorine sweetener: Overview of biological issues. *J Toxicol Environ Health B Crit Rev.* 16:399–451.
100. Willett, W., Manson, J., Liu, S. 2002. Glycemic index, glycemic load, and risk of type 2 diabetes. *Am J Clin Nutr.* 76:274S–280S.
101. Zhang, C., Liu, S., Solomon, C.G., Hu, F.B. 2006. Dietary fiber intake, dietary glycemic load, and the risk for gestational diabetes mellitus. *Diabetes Care.* 29:2223–2230.
102. Brand-Miller, J.C., Holt, S.H., Pawlak, D.B., McMillan, J. 2002. Glycemic index and obesity. *Am J Clin Nutr.* 76:281S–285S.
103. Oba, S., Nagata, C., Nakamura, K., Fujii, K. et al. 2010. Dietary glycemic index, glycemic load, and intake of carbohydrate and rice in relation to risk of mortality from stroke and its subtypes in Japanese men and women. *Metabolism* 59:1574–1582.
104. Hare-Bruun, H., Nielsen, B.M., Grau, K., Oxlund, A.L., Heitmann, B.L. 2008. Should glycemic index and glycemic load be considered in dietary recommendations? *Nutr Rev.* 66:569–900.
105. Juanola-Falgarona, M., Salas-Salvadó, J., Ibarrola-Jurado, N., Rabassa-Soler, A. et al. 2014. Effect of the glycemic index of the diet on weight loss, modulation of satiety, inflammation, and other metabolic risk factors: A randomized controlled trial. *Am J Clin Nutr.* 100:27–35.
106. Farvid, M.S., Homayouni, F., Shokoohi, M., Fallah, A., Farvid, M.S. 2014. Glycemic index, glycemic load and their association with glycemic control among patients with type 2 diabetes. *Eur J Clin Nutr.* 68:459–463.
107. Burger, K.N., Beulens, J.W., Boer, J.M., Spijkerman, A.M., van der A.D.L. 2011. Dietary glycemic load and glycemic index and risk of coronary heart disease and stroke in Dutch men and women: The EPIC-MORGEN study. *PLoS One.* 6(10):e25955. doi: 10.1371/journal.pone.0025955.

108. Shyam, S., Arshad, F., Abdul Ghani, R., Wahab, N.A. et al. 2013. Low glycaemic index diets improve glucose tolerance and body weight in women with previous history of gestational diabetes: A six months randomized trial. *Nutr J.* 12:68. doi:10.1186/1475-2891-12-68.
109. Moosheer, S.M., Waldschütz, W., Itariu, B.K., Brath, H., Stulnig, T.M. 2014. A protein-enriched low glycemic index diet with omega-3 polyunsaturated fatty acid supplementation exerts beneficial effects on metabolic control in type 2 diabetes. *Prim Care Diabetes.* pii: S1751–9918(14)00036-9. doi: 10.1016/j.pcd.2014.02.004.
110. Pittas, A.G., Das, S.K., Hajduk, C.L., Golden, J. et al. 2005. A low-glycemic load diet facilitates greater weight loss in overweight adults with high insulin secretion but not in overweight adults with low insulin secretion in the CALERIE Trial. *Diabetes Care.* 28:2939–2941.
111. Murakami, K., Sasaki, S., Uenishi, K. 2014. Japan dietetic students' study for nutrition and biomarkers group. Dietary glycemic index, but not glycemic load, is positively associated with serum homocysteine concentration in free-living young Japanese women. *Nutr Res.* 34:25–30.
112. Li, J., Zhang, H., Shi, M., Yan, L., Xie, M. 2014. Homocysteine is linked to macular edema in type 2 diabetes. *Curr Eye Res.* 39:730–735.
113. Katz, D.L., Meller, S. 2014. Can we say what diet is best for health? *Annu Rev Public Health.* 35:83–103.
114. Khazrai, Y.M., Defeudis, G., Pozzilli, P. 2014. Effect of diet on type 2 diabetes mellitus: A review. *Diabetes Metab Res Rev.* 30(Suppl 1):24–33.
115. Martínez González, M.A., Bes Rastrollo, M., Serra Majem, L., Lairon, D., Estruch, R., Trichopoulou, A. 2009. Mediterranean food pattern and the primary prevention of chronic disease: Recent developments. *Nutr Rev.* 67(Suppl 1):S111–S116.
116. Simopoulos, A.P. 2001. The Mediterranean diets: What is so special about the diet of Greece? The scientific evidence. *J Nutr.* 131(Suppl 11):3065S–3073S.
117. Tourlouki, E., Matalas, A.L., Bountziouka, V., Tyrovolas, S. et al. 2013. Are current dietary habits in Mediterranean islands a reflection of the past? Results from the MEDIS study. *Ecol Food Nutr.* 52:371–386.
118. Lindeberg, S., Jönsson, T., Granfeldt, Y., Borgstrand, E. et al. 2007. A Paleolithic diet improves glucose tolerance more than a Mediterranean-like diet in individuals with ischaemic heart disease. *Diabetologia* 50:1795–1807.
119. Jönsson, T., Granfeldt, Y., Ahrén, B., Branell, U.C. et al. 2009. Beneficial effects of a Paleolithic diet on cardiovascular risk factors in type 2 diabetes: A randomized cross-over pilot study. *Cardiovasc Diabetol.* 8:35. doi: 10.1186/1475-2840-8-35.
120. Jandeleit-Dahm, K., Cooper, M.E. 2008. The role of AGEs in cardiovascular disease. *Curr Pharm Des.* 14:979–986.
121. Yan, S.F., D'Agati, V., Schmidt, A.M., Ramasamy, R. 2007. Receptor for Advanced Glycation Endproducts (RAGE): A formidable force in the pathogenesis of the cardiovascular complications of diabetes and aging. *Curr Mol Med.* 7:699–710.
122. Yoshida, N., Okumura, K., Aso, Y. 2005. High serum pentosidine concentrations are associated with increased arterial stiffness and thickness in patients with type 2 diabetes. *Metabolism* 54:345–350.
123. Michalsen, A., Bierhaus, A., Nawroth, P.P., Dobos, G.J. 2006. A new mechanism for understanding the preventive effects of lifestyle modifications. *Bundesgesundheitsblatt Gesundheitsforschung Gesundheitsschutz.* 49:773–779.
124. Giugliano, D., Esposito, K. 2008. Mediterranean diet and metabolic diseases. *Curr Opin Lipidol.* 19:63–68.
125. Esposito, K., Maiorino, M.I., Di Palo, C., Giugliano, D., Campanian Postprandial Hyperglycemia Study Group. 2009. Adherence to a Mediterranean diet and glycaemic control in type 2 diabetes mellitus. *Diabet Med.* 26:900–907. doi: 10.1111/j.1464-5491.2009.02798.x.
126. Bédard, A., Dodin, S., Corneau, L., Lemieux, S. 2014. Impact of the traditional Mediterranean diet on the Framingham risk score and the metabolic syndrome according to sex. *Metab Syndr Relat Disord.* 12:95–101.
127. Mena, M.P., Sacanella, E., Vazquez-Agell, M., Morales, M. et al. 2009. Inhibition of circulating immune cell activation: A molecular antiinflammatory effect of the Mediterranean diet. *Am J Clin Nutr.* 89:248–256.
128. Richard, C., Couture, P., Desroches, S., Lichtenstein, A.H., Lamarche, B. 2013. Effect of an isoenergetic traditional Mediterranean diet on apolipoprotein A-I kinetic in men with metabolic syndrome. *Nutr J.* 12(1):76. doi: 10.1186/1475-2891-12-76.
129. Esposito, K., Giugliano, D. 2014. Mediterranean diet and type 2 diabetes. *Diabetes Metab Res Rev.* 30(Suppl 1):34–40.

130. Menotti, A., Alberti-Fidanza, A., Fidanza, F. 2012. The association of the Mediterranean Adequacy Index with fatal coronary events in an Italian middle-aged male population followed for 40 years. *Nutr Metab Cardiovasc Dis.* 22:369–375.
131. Mosharraf, S., Sharifzadeh, G., Darvishzadeh-Boroujeni, P., Rouhi-Boroujeni, H. 2013. Impact of the components of Mediterranean nutrition regimen on long-term prognosis of diabetic patients with coronary artery disease. *ARYA Atheroscler.* 9:337–342.
132. Rylander, C., Sandanger, T.M., Engeset, D., Lund, E. 2014. Consumption of lean fish reduces the risk of type 2 diabetes mellitus: A prospective population based cohort study of Norwegian women. *PLoS One.* 9(2):e89845. doi: 10.1371/journal.pone.0089845. eCollection 2014.
133. Nanri, A., Mizoue, T., Noda, M., Takahashi, Y. et al. 2011. Fish intake and type 2 diabetes in Japanese men and women: The Japan Public Health Center-based Prospective Study. *Am J Clin Nutr.* 94:884–891.
134. Villegas, R., Xiang, Y.B., Elasy, T., Li, H.L. et al. 2011. Fish, shellfish, and long-chain n-3 fatty acid consumption and risk of incident type 2 diabetes in middle-aged Chinese men and women. *Am J Clin Nutr.* 94:543–551.
135. Wallin, A., Di Giuseppe, D., Orsini, N., Patel, P.S. et al. 2012. Fish consumption, dietary long-chain n-3 fatty acids, and risk of type 2 diabetes: Systematic review and meta-analysis of prospective studies. *Diabetes Care.* 35:918–929.
136. Wu, J.H., Micha, R., Imamura, F., Pan, A. et al. 2012. Omega-3 fatty acids and incident type 2 diabetes: A systematic review and meta-analysis. *Br J Nutr.* 107(Suppl):2S214–2S227.
137. Moszczyński, P. 2005. Mercury is still dangerous. Part. II. Health effects. *Lek w Polsce.* 10:66–73, in Polish.
138. Moszczyński, P. 2006. Mercury and the risk of coronary heart disease. *Przegl Lek.* 63(Suppl 7):84–87, Review in Polish.
139. Georgoulis, M., Kontogianni, M.D., Yiannakouris, N. 2014. Mediterranean diet and diabetes: Prevention and treatment. *Nutrients.* 6:1406–1423.
140. Urpi-Sarda, M., Casas, R., Chiva-Blanch, G., Romero-Mamani, E.S. et al. 2012. Virgin olive oil and nuts as key foods of the Mediterranean diet effects on inflammatory biomarkers related to atherosclerosis. *Pharmacol Res.* 65:577–583.
141. Salas-Salvad6, J., Bull6, M., Estruch, R., Ros, E. et al. 2014. Prevention of diabetes with Mediterranean diets: A subgroup analysis of a randomized trial. *Ann Intern Med.* 160:1–10.
142. Konstantinidou, V., Covas, M.I., Sola, R., Fitó, M. 2013. Up-to date knowledge on the in vivo transcriptomic effect of the Mediterranean diet in humans. *Mol Nutr Food Res.* 57:772–783.
143. Konstantinidou, V., Covas, M.I., Muñoz-Aguayo, D., Khymenets, O. et al. 2010. in vivo nutrigenomic effects of virgin olive oil polyphenols within the frame of the Mediterranean diet: A randomized controlled trial. *FASEB J.* 24:2546–2557.
144. Castañer, O., Covas, M.I., Khymenets, O., Nyyssonen, K. et al. 2012. Protection of LDL from oxidation by olive oil polyphenols is associated with a downregulation of CD40-ligand expression and its downstream products in vivo in humans. *Am J Clin Nutr.* 95:1238–1244.
145. Brown, A.A., Hu, F. 2001. Dietary modulation of endothelial function: Implications for cardiovascular disease. *Am J Clin Nutr.* 73:673–686.
146. Ros, E. 2010. Health benefits of nut consumption. *Nutrients.* 2:652–682.
147. Jaceldo-Siegl, K., Haddad, E., Oda, K., Fraser, G.E., Sabaté, J. 2014. Tree nuts are inversely associated with metabolic syndrome and obesity: The Adventist Health Study-2. *PLoS One.* 9(1):e85133.
148. Vadivel, V., Kunyanga, C.N., Biesalski, H.K. 2012. Health benefits of nut consumption with special reference to body weight control. *Nutrition.* 28:1089–1097.
149. Flores-Mateo, G., Rojas-Rueda, D., Basora, J., Ros, E., Salas-Salvado, J. 2013. Nut intake and adiposity: Meta-analysis of clinical trials. *Am J Clin Nutr.* 97:1346–1355.
150. Brown, L., Kroon P.A., Das, D.K., Das, S. et al. 2009. The biological responses to resveratrol and other polyphenols from alcoholic beverages. *Alcohol Clin Exp Res.* 33:1513–1523.
151. Ruf, J.C. 1999. Wine and polyphenols related to platelet aggregation and atherothrombosis. *Drugs Exp Clin Res.* 25:125–131.
152. Baliunas, D.O., Taylor, B.J., Irving, H., Roerecke, M. et al. 2009. Alcohol as a Risk Factor for Type 2 Diabetes: A systematic review and meta-analysis. *Diabetes Care.* 32:2123–2132.
153. Liu, Y., Ma, W., Zhang, P., He, S., Huang, D. 2014. Effect of resveratrol on blood pressure: A meta-analysis of randomized controlled trial. *Clin Nutr.* pii: S0261-5614(14)00084-3. doi: 10.1016/j.clnu.2014.03.009.
154. Liu, K., Zhou, R., Wang, B., Mi, M.T. 2014. Effect of resveratrol on glucose control and insulin sensitivity: A meta-analysis of 11 randomized controlled trials. *Am J Clin Nutr.* 99:1510–1519.

155. Ciloglu, N.S., Zeytin, K., Aker, F. 2013. The effects of resveratrol on flap survival in diabetic rats. *J Plast Surg Hand Surg*. 48:234–237.
156. Beaudoin, M.S., Snook, L.A., Arkell, A.M., Simpson, J.A., Holloway, G.P., Wright, D.C. 2013. Resveratrol supplementation improves white adipose tissue function in a depot-specific manner in Zucker diabetic fatty rats. *Am J Physiol Regul Integr Comp Physiol*. 305:R542–R551.
157. Hervert-Hernández, D., Pintado, C., Rotger, R., Goñi, I. 2009. Stimulatory role of grape pomace polyphenols on *Lactobacillus acidophilus* growth. *Int J Food Microbiol*. 136:119–122.
158. Gollücke, A.P. 2010. Recent applications of grape polyphenols in foods, beverages and supplements. *Recent Pat Food Nutr Agric*. 2:105–109.
159. Bochniak, M., Sadlak-Nowicka, J. 2004. Periodontitis and cardiovascular diseases-review of publications. *Przegl Lek*. 61:518–522, Article in Polish.
160. Banihani, S., Swedan, S., Alguraan, Z. 2013. Pomegranate and type 2 diabetes. *Nutr Res*. 33:341–348.
161. Basu, A., Newman, E.D., Bryant, A.L., Lyons, T.J., Betts, N.M. 2013. Pomegranate polyphenols lower lipid peroxidation in adults with type 2 diabetes but have no effects in healthy volunteers: A pilot study. *J Nutr Metab*. 2013:708381.
162. Riserus, U., Willett, W.C., Hu, F.B. 2009. Dietary fats and prevention of type 2 diabetes. *Progr Lipid Res*. 48:44–51.
163. Khaw, K.T., Friesen, M.D., Riboli, E., Luben, R., Wareham, N. 2012. Plasma phospholipid fatty acid concentration and incident coronary heart disease in Men and women: The EPIC-Norfolk prospective study. *PLoS Med*. 9:e1001255.
164. Dai, J., Su, Y.X., Bartell, S., Le, N.A. et al. 2009. Beneficial effects of designed dietary fatty acid compositions on lipids in triacylglycerol-rich lipoproteins among Chinese patients with type 2 diabetes mellitus. *Metabolism*. 58:510–518.
165. Hartweg, J., Farmer, A.J., Perera, R., Holman, R.R., Neil, H.A. 2007. Meta-analysis of the effects of n-3 polyunsaturated fatty acids on lipoproteins and other emerging lipid cardiovascular risk markers in patients with type 2 diabetes. *Diabetologia*. 50:1593–1602.
166. Hartweg, J., Perera, R., Montori, V., Dinneen, S. et al. 2008. Omega-3 polyunsaturated fatty acids (PUFA) for T2DM. *Cochrane Database Syst Rev*. (1):CD003205. doi: 10.1002/14651858.CD003205.pub2.
167. Kalantarian, S., Rimm, E.B., Herrington, D.M., Mozaffarian, D. 2014. Dietary macronutrients, genetic variation, and progression of coronary atherosclerosis among women. *Am Heart J*. 167:627–635.
168. Lands, B., Lamoreaux, E. 2012. Using 3–6 differences in essential fatty acids rather than 3/6 ratios gives useful food balance scores. *Nutr Metab (Lond)*. 9:46. doi: 10.1186/1743-7075-9-46.
169. Lands, B. 2012. Consequences of essential fatty acids. *Nutrients*. 4:1338–1357.
170. FAO. 2009. Fats and fatty acids in human nutrition. *Proceedings of the Joint FAO/WHO Expert Consultation,* November 10–14, 2008, Geneva, Switzerland. *Ann Nutr Metab*. 55:5–300. Summary and recommendations: Retrieved February, 10, 2015 from http://www.who.int/nutrition/topics/FFA_summary_rec_conclusion.pdf
171. Kanner, J. 2007. Dietary advanced lipid oxidation endproducts are risk factors to human health. *Mol Nutr Food Res*. 51:1094–1101.
172. Halvorsen, B.L., Blomhoff, R. 2011. Determination of lipid oxidation products in vegetable oils and marine omega-3 supplements. *Food Nutr Res*. 55. doi: 10.3402/fnr.v55i0.5792.
173. Esposito, K., Chiodini, P., Maiorino, M.I., Bellastella, G., Panagiotakos, D., Giugliano, D. 2014. Which diet for prevention of type 2 diabetes? A meta-analysis of prospective studies. *Endocrine*. 47:107–116.
174. Ajala, O., English, P., Pinkney, J. 2013. Systematic review and meta-analysis of different dietary approaches to the management of type 2 diabetes. *Am J Clin Nutr*. 97:505–516.
175. International Diabetes Federation. IDF Diabetes Atlas, 6th edn. Brussels, Belgium: International Diabetes Federation, 2013. http://www.idf.org/diabetesatlas.
176. Atkinson, F.S., Foster-Powell, K., Brand-Miller, J.C. 2008. International tables of glycemic index and glycemic load values: 2008. *Diab Care*. 31:2281.
177. O'Keefe, J.H. Jr., Cordain, L. 2004. Cardiovascular disease resulting from a diet and lifestyle at odds with our Paleolithic genome: How to become a 21st-century hunter-gatherer. *Mayo Clin Proc*. 79:101–108.
178. Anderson, J.W. *Plant Fiber in Foods*. 2nd ed. HCF Nutrition Research Foundation Inc., PO Box 22124, Lexington, KY 40522, 1990.

9 Antioxidative and Anti-Inflammatory Effects and Health Implications of Berry Polyphenols

Evidence from Compositional and Structural Background to Cell, Animal, and Human Studies

Sang Gil Lee, Terrence M. Vance, and Ock K. Chun

CONTENTS

9.1 INTRODUCTION

Obesity is typically defined according to body mass index (BMI)—the ratio of weight in kilograms to height in meters squared—with a BMI between 25.0 and 29.9 kg/m^2 classified as overweight and 30 kg/m^2 or more as obesity [1]. Obesity represents a major public health problem in the United States, where the prevalence of obesity is among the highest for industrialized countries and has significantly increased during the past few decades. While data from the National Health and Nutrition Examination Survey (NHANES) conducted from 1988 to 1994 [2] and 2003 to 2006 [3] have demonstrated an increase in the average waist circumference and prevalence of abdominal obesity among adults in the United States, data from 2011 to 2012 demonstrate that obesity has become more prevalent among children as well [4]. If current rates of obesity continue, it has been predicted that by 2030, approximately 44% of the U.S. population will be obese [4]. The increased prevalence of obesity has coincided with a significant increase in health-care costs. In 2008, medical expenditures for the care of obese patients were approximately $147 billion and by 2030 are projected to increase to between $390 and $580 billions [4]. For these reasons, many public health efforts have focused on preventing obesity and reducing its prevalence. In addition to greater health-care costs, obesity has been implicated in the development of numerous chronic diseases, including cardiovascular disease, type 2 diabetes, hypertension, and certain types of cancer [5].

The underlying mechanism of the increased risk of chronic disease in obesity has not been clearly elucidated yet and is an area of active research. However, oxidative stress and chronic inflammation are thought to be involved in the development of chronic diseases in obesity [6–8]. Since oxidative stress and chronic inflammation are associated with the development of chronic diseases, it is plausible that antioxidants and anti-inflammatory compounds may reduce the risk of those diseases. One such class of compounds, anthocyanins, are commonly found in red and purple color fruits and vegetables. Anthocyanins represent a broad class of compounds [9]. The unique chemical structures of different anthocyanins suggest that different anthocyanins may exhibit distinct antioxidant and anti-inflammatory effects [10]. Berries are a particularly prominent source of anthocyanins in the diet, and different varieties and species of berries exhibit substantial variation in the amount and types of anthocyanins. Thus, it is possible that the consumption of various anthocyanins in berry may reduce oxidative stress and inflammation, and thereby the risk of obesity-related chronic diseases, differently. Therefore, this review will focus on the relationship between the structure and the function of various berry anthocyanins.

9.2 CHRONIC INFLAMMATION AND OXIDATIVE STRESS IN OBESITY

An association between inflammation and obesity is well established [11]. Inflammation is a coordinated response to harmful stimuli, such as pathogens, cell damage, or irritants [11]. In response to these stimuli, leukocytes are attracted to the source of inflammation, and increases are observed in the systemic circulation of inflammatory cytokines, chemokines, and related proteins, such as tumor necrosis factor (TNF)α, interleukin (IL)-6, fibrinogen, C-reactive protein, monocyte chemotactic protein-1 (MCP-1), and plasminogen activator inhibitor-1 [12]. However, the inflammation associated with obesity is distinctly different from the inflammation during infection or autoimmune disease. One key difference is that in obesity, inflammation is chronic in nature and causes gradual perturbations in metabolic homeostasis over time [12,13]. Obesity-induced inflammation may also affect multiple organ systems. Increases in circulating cytokines from an inflammatory response may precipitate inflammation in multiple organs; some examples include hypothalamic inflammation in the brain, adipocyte enlargement in adipose tissue, steatosis or nonalcoholic fatty liver disease, lipid accumulation in muscle, atherosclerosis, and β-cell failure in pancreatic islets [14].

9.2.1 Chronic Inflammation in Obesity

NF-κB proteins are a family of transcription factors and play an important role in regulating cell growth, differentiation, development, and apoptosis [15]. These transcription factors also regulate a variety of genes involved in inflammation and immunity. The NF-κB pathway is activated primarily through pro-inflammatory receptors such as TNF receptors, toll-like receptor family (TLRs), and various other cytokine receptors. Upstreamed receptors, by various extracellular signals, activate the IkB kinase (IKK), which can phosphorylate IKBα, which is retaining NF-κB in cytosol [12,15,16]. In turn, phosphorylated IKBα is ubiquitinated and degraded by a proteasome, subsequently releasing and allowing the translocation of an NF-κB heterodimer from the cytosol to the nucleus. Translocated NF-κB can bind with specific DNA sequences, called response elements (REs), to express the mRNA of target genes [12,15]. Among various receptors, pattern recognition receptors (PRRs) are receptors that recognize foreign molecules by sensing pathogen-associated molecular patterns [12,13]. They have been implicated in obesity-related inflammation through the

NF-κB pathway. Among various PRRs, toll-like receptor-4 (TLR4) and NOD-like receptor (NLR) are likely key factors for the induction of inflammation in obesity [13,15]. Lipopolysaccharide (LPS), a cell wall component of gram-negative bacteria has been considered one of the causes of chronic inflammation in obesity, as intestinal mucosal barriers in obesity become leaky and bacteria are recognized by TLR4 resulting in the innate immune response [15]. TLR4 also recognizes free fatty acids and promotes an inflammatory response by activating c-Jun N-terminal kinases (JNK) through activator protein 1 and IKBα through NF-κB pathways, respectively. Therefore, a greater concentration of plasma saturated fatty acids, which is often observed in obesity, may contribute to chronic inflammation [13,15].

Changes in the characteristics of adipose tissue resident immune cells are also involved in chronic inflammation. Leukocytes are normally present in metabolic tissues, especially adipose tissue. Macrophages, one of the more prominent leukocytes residing in adipose, consist of two types: M1 macrophages and M2 macrophages. These macrophages are poised to respond to nutrition related signals [17]. M1 macrophages play a pro-inflammatory role, producing IL-1β, IL-6, and TNFα; M2 macrophages play an anti-inflammatory role, producing IL-4 and IL-10. Hypertrophy and hyperplasia of adipocytes enhance a shift in the macrophage profile from M2 to M1 resulting in a pro-inflammatory environment in adipose tissue [17]. Along with the macrophage status in adipose tissue, T-cell accumulation is also considered as a functional role of immunity in obesity [18]. Of T cells, helper T (Th) cells can be characterized into Th1 or Th2, which are induced by interferon (IFN)-δ and by IL-4, respectively. Th1 is a pro-inflammatory T cell secreting IFN-δ, IL-12, and TNFα, but Th2 cell plays an anti-inflammatory role secreting IL-4, 5, 10, and 13 [18]. Therefore, the characteristic of immune cells present in adipose tissue contributes to the chronic inflammatory status in obesity.

9.2.2 Partial Mechanisms of Oxidative Stress Generation by Inflammation in Obesity

Free radicals are highly reactive molecules derived from oxygen, nitrogen, or sulfur, generating reactive oxygen species (ROS), reactive nitrogen species (RNS), and reactive sulfur species [19]. Among them, ROS are a common source of oxidative stress *in vivo*. ROS comprise several fundamental radicals, including superoxide anions (O_2-•), hydroperoxyl radicals (HO_2•), and hydroxyl radicals (•OH). ROS are necessary for a variety of cellular processes and are generated via various pathways, including oxidative phosphorylation, the induction of certain enzymes, and phagocytosis [19]. However, while some levels of ROS are necessary for normal physiological functions, excessive amounts can be toxic and result in oxidative stress.

NF-κB is not the only critical inflammatory transcription factor, but some enzymes that generate ROS are regulated by the NF-κB pathway (Figure 9.1) as target genes, such as NADPH oxidase (NOX), xanthine oxidase (XO), inducible nitric oxide synthase (iNOS), lipoxygenase, and cyclooxygenase (COX)-2. The NOXs are a family of phagocytic enzymes that produce ROS, specifically superoxide, using NADPH as a substrate. Since superoxide dismutase (SOD) is located near NOX, the generated superoxide is subsequently converted to hydrogen peroxide and further metabolized [19].

XO is also regulated by the NF-κB pathway. XO is predominantly located in the liver and is converted from xanthine dehydrogenase (XDH). Both XO and XDH catalyze purine degradation in two steps: converting hypoxanthine to xanthine and then xanthine to uric acid. However, the two enzymes differ in by-products. XDH catalyzes the production of xanthine and uric acid, transferring electron to NAD+ to generate NADH. In contrast, XO has a greater affinity for O_2 compared with NAD+, resulting in the transfer of an electron to O_2, generating superoxide and hydrogen peroxide. XO can be regulated by NF-κB as mentioned earlier, but xanthine oxidase–induced oxidative stress also can cause the activation of NF-κB and increase the expression of genes for inflammatory cytokines, creating a vicious cycle. NOS consists of three isomers: eNOS, which is involved in the regulation of endothelial function; nNOS, which plays a role as a neurotransmitter; and iNOS, which catalyzes the production of RNS from L-arginine. iNOS is up-regulated by the activation of NF-κB by an upstream PRR, such as TLR4. In an oxidative environment, iNOS produces large

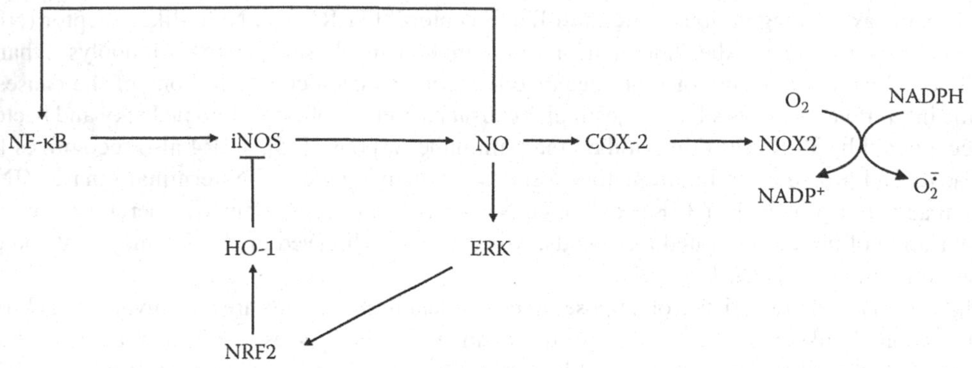

FIGURE 9.1 Mechanism of oxidative stress generated by chronic inflammation and regulation by HO-1. iNOS, COX-2, NOX2, and ERK stand for inducible nitric oxide synthase, cyclooxygenase-2, NADPH oxidase 2, and extracellular signal–regulated kinases, respectively.

amounts of NO that can react with superoxide to form peroxynitrite, which may cause oxidative damage within the cell. It has been reported that in obesity, the binding of saturated fatty acids to TLR4 can activate NF-κB and generate oxidative stress through the up-regulation of iNOS. iNOS signaling can also interact with the COX-2 pathway, one of the well-known inflammatory mediators targeted by NF-κB. COX-2 is involved in the conversion of arachidonic acid to prostaglandin H2 (PGH2) and may generate superoxide by up-regulating NOX activity. Therefore, in obesity, various ROS-generating enzymes interact with each other and inflammatory transcription factors.

9.3 ANTIOXIDANT SYSTEM

Even though some ROS are important for many physiological processes, excessive ROS can lead to oxidative stress *in vivo*. Therefore, a balance between ROS and antioxidants is essential to mitigate the damage from oxidative stress [20]. For this reason, various regulatory systems exist to maintain appropriate levels of ROS. There are different types of antioxidants *in vivo*, including endogenous antioxidants, such as albumin, bilirubin, glutathione (GSH), uric acid, and antioxidant enzymes, such as SOD, catalase (CAT), glutathione peroxidase (GPx), heme oxygenase-1 (HO-1), NAD(P)H: quinone oxidoreductase (NQO1), and dietary antioxidants, including vitamins C and E, carotenoids, and various polyphenol compounds [20].

9.3.1 Enzymatic Antioxidant Defense System

Many antioxidant enzymes are regulated by nuclear factor (erythroid-derived 2)-like 2 (NRF2) at the transcriptional level [21]. NRF2 is retained by Kelch-like ECH-associated protein 1 (Keapl) in cytosol [20]. NFR2 is liberated from Keapl when a primary stress sensor in Keapl (several cysteine residues) triggers conformational changes of Keapl. After NRF2 is released from Keapl, it translocates to the nucleus and binds to antioxidant gene regulatory sequences named antioxidant response elements (AREs) for the upregulation of various antioxidant enzymes [20].

Regulation of ROS by antioxidant enzymes is illustrated in Figure 9.2. SOD is an enzyme that catalyzes the dismutation of a superoxide radical into hydrogen peroxide. Superoxide is a by-product of oxygen metabolism and NOX activity [22,23]. SOD converts superoxide radical to hydrogen peroxide. CAT and GPx can further convert hydrogen peroxide to water. GPx uses reduced GSH for antioxidant activity producing GSSG, which is oxidized GSH. GSSG can be regenerated to 2 GSH by glutathione reductase using NADPH [23]. HO-1 is the enzyme involved in the catabolism of heme in hemoglobin [24]. HO-1 can cleave heme to form biliverdin. The biliverdin is subsequently

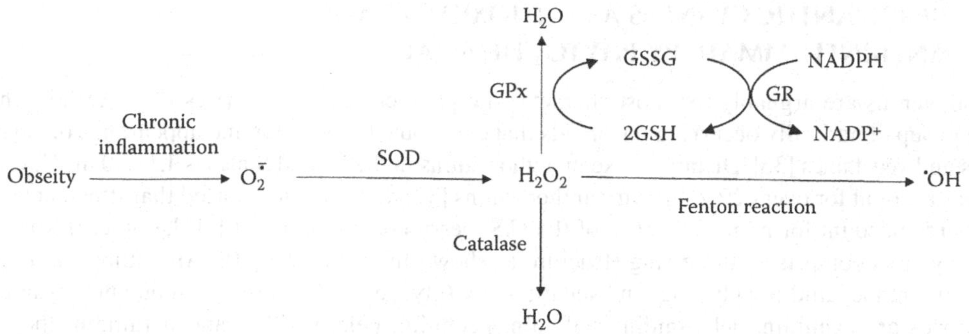

H_2O
GPx
GSSG
NADPH
GR
2GSH
$NADP^+$
Chronic inflammation
Obseity → $O_2^{\bar{\cdot}}$
SOD
H_2O_2
$^{\bullet}OH$
Fenton reaction
Catalase
H_2O

FIGURE 9.2 Systemic regulation of excessively generated ROS by endogenous antioxidant enzymes. SOD, GPx, GSH, GSSG, and GR stand for superoxide dismutase, glutathione peroxidase, reduced glutathione, oxidized glutathione, and glutathione reductase, respectively.

converted to bilirubin by biliverdin reductase. Bilirubin may act as an antioxidant, since bilirubin can be converted to biliverdin by ROS [24]. In addition to producing bilirubin, HO-1 may have antioxidant capacity through its anti-inflammatory effects as illustrated in Figure 10.1. One study showed that the extracellular signal–regulated kinases (ERK) pathway can up-regulate HO-1 expression [21,24,25]. In addition, HO-1 expression suppresses iNOS gene expression leading into the reduction of NO generation and thus inhibits COX-2 activity [21]. Since NOX is up-regulated by COX-2, HO-1 expression can inhibit the generation of superoxide by NOX. NADPH: quinone oxidoreductase (NQO1) can catalyze the detoxification of quinone to hydroquinone, which is less toxic [25]. It also regenerates oxidized vitamin E to antioxidant vitamin E again [26]. These antioxidant enzymes maintain a balanced level of ROS *in vivo*. However, excessive generation of ROS in obesity may overwhelm the capacity of the endogenous antioxidant defense system. Indeed, many studies have found that plasma antioxidant enzymes are decreased [27,28], corresponding to increased oxidative stress in obesity [28]. Therefore, exogenous antioxidants, namely antioxidants derived from the diet, may also play a role in counteracting oxidative stress.

9.3.2 Dietary Antioxidant Intake

Numerous dietary compounds are thought to possess antioxidant activity, including vitamin C, vitamin E, carotenoids, and various polyphenol compounds [29]. Polyphenols are widely distributed and produced as secondary metabolites by various fruits and vegetables and have been known as strong antioxidant and anti-inflammatory compounds [30]. Observational studies have found an inverse association between antioxidant consumption and chronic disease risk [31,32]. In a review by Ness and Powles [33], 9 of 10 ecological studies and 2 of 3 case-control studies have reported an inverse association between fruit and vegetable consumption and cardiovascular disease. Since oxidative stress and chronic inflammation are associated with the risk of obesity related chronic diseases, it is thought that the prevention of chronic diseases is in part attributable to the antioxidants and anti-inflammatory properties of polyphenols in fruits and vegetables [12]. However, a large proportion of the U.S. population does not consume the recommended amount of fruits and vegetables [34]. For this reason, it is necessary to find the way to increase the dietary fruit and vegetable consumption. Berries are one of the most popular fruits in the United States and highly recommended as a bioactive compound source with few calories compared with other popular fruits, such as oranges and bananas [35]. Therefore, encouraging berry consumption maybe a good dietary strategy to lower oxidative stress and inflammation-mediated chronic diseases through increasing the intake of polyphenols of the U.S. population.

9.4 BERRY ANTHOCYANINS AS ANTIOXIDANT AND ANTI-INFLAMMATORY PHYTOCHEMICAL

Anthocyanins are arguably the most characteristic phytochemical of berries [35]. Anthocyanins are a group of naturally occurring flavonoids that contribute to the color and appearance of various fruits and vegetables [36]. Dietary intake of anthocyanins in the United States is 1.5–3.0 mg/day, and berries account for over 42% of dietary anthocyanins [37]. It has been reported that strawberry and blueberry account for more than 60% of the U.S. berry consumption [40]. Like other flavonoids, anthocyanins comprise a three-ring structure as shown in Figure 9.3 [10]. An anthocyanin comprise an anthocyanidin (aglycone) and sugar moiety (glycone). The most common anthocyanidins in berries are cyanidin, delphinidin, malvidin, peonidin, pelargonidin, and petunidin; they are present in combination with various glycones, such as glucose, galactose, xylose, rhamnose, arabinose, rutinose, and sophorose. Thus, a variety of anthocyanins are present in berries [10]. Although berries are well-known sources of anthocyanins, their anthocyanin composition varies considerably. Table 9.1 shows the different composition of anthocyanins in popular berries [39]. For example, delphinidin is the exclusive anthocyanin of black currant, and cranberry contains peonidin derivatives [39]. In addition, chokeberry, blackberry, and elderberry contain cyanidin-based anthocyanins but with different glycones [39]. It has been reported that different anthocyanins have different degrees of antioxidant and anti-inflammatory effects [36,40]. Furthermore, *in vivo*, the absorption, distribution, metabolism, and excretion of anthocyanins depend on their structure.

9.4.1 Structural Differences in the Antioxidant Capacity of Berry Anthocyanins

Anthocyanins have direct antioxidant capacities, which are radical scavenging capacity or the degree of inhibition of oxidation. Several assays have been developed to measure the antioxidant capacity of various substances including food, drug, and biological fluids [41]. Depending on which radicals are used in the assay, various analyses have been developed, including ABTs, DPPH, and

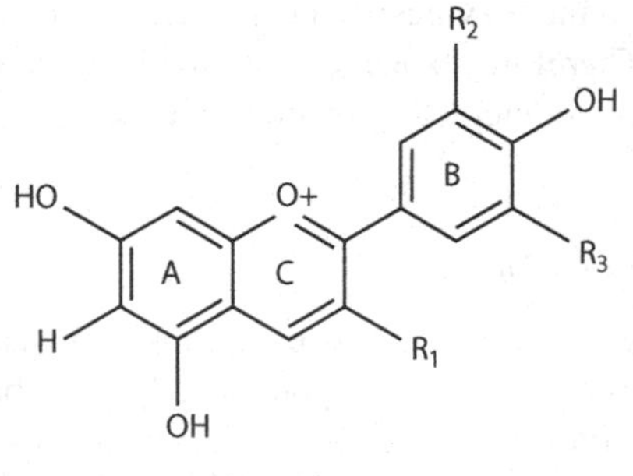

Aglycone	R_2	R_3	Glycone	R_1
Cyanidin	OH	H	Glucoside	Glucose
Delphinidin	OH	OH	Rutinoside	Rutinose
Malvidin	OCH_3	OCH_3	Galactoside	Galactose
Peonidin	OCH_3	H	Arabinoside	Arabinose
Pelargonidin	H	H	Diglucoside	Diglucose
Petunidin	OCH_3	OH	Acylated sugar moietide	Acylated sugar moiety

FIGURE 9.3 Structure of anthocyanins and various derivatives based on the substitution on glycone and aglycone.

TABLE 9.1
Major Anthocyanins of Various Popular Berries

Berry	Major Anthocyanins
Blueberry	Delphinidin-3-galactoside
	Malvidin-3-galactoside
	Delphinidin-3-arabinoside
	Malvidin-3-arabinoside
	Petunidin-3-galactoside
	Malvidin-3-glucoside
Raspberry	Cyanidin-3-sophoroside
	Cyanidin-3-glucoside
Blackberry	Cyanidin-3-glucoside
Strawberry	Pelagonidin-3-glucoside
	Pelagonidin-3-(6″-succinyl-glucoside)
Cranberry	Peonidin-3-galactoside
	Peonidin-3-arabinoside
	Cyanidin-3-galactoside
Black currant	Cyanidin-3-rutinoside
	Delphinidin-3-glucoside
	Delphinidin-3-rutinoside
	Cyanidin-3-glucoside
Chokeberry	Cyanidin-3-galactoside
	Cyanidin-3-galactoside
Elderberry	Cyanidin-3-sambubioside
	Cyanidin-3-glucoside
Mulberry	Cyanidin-3-rutinoside
	Cyanidin-3-glucoside
Bilberry	Delphinidin-3-glucoside
	Delphinidin-3-galactoside
	Delphinidin-3-arabinoside
	Cyanidin-3-glucoside
	Cyanidin-3-galactoside
	Cyanidin-3-arabinoside
	Petunidin-3-glucoside
	Malvidin-3-glucoside

ORAC. The inhibition of lipid or reducing power from ferric iron (Fe^{3+}) to ferrous iron (Fe^{2+}) by anthocyanins is also measured to determine the antioxidant capacity [42].

The number of hydroxyl groups contributes to the direct antioxidant capacity of flavonoids including anthocyanins, since hydroxyl groups can bind with radicals as electron-donating groups [43]. Anthocyanins are identified based on the substitution of hydroxyl, methoxyl, and hydrogen groups at R_2 and R_3 (Figure 9.3) [44]. A methoxyl group substitution yields less antioxidant capacity than a hydroxyl group, but more than substitution with hydrogen. Cyanidin-3-glucoside (cya-3-glc) and cyanidin-3-rutinoside (cya-3-rut) in plum have stronger antioxidant capacity than peonidin-3-glucoside (peo-3-glc) and peonidin-3-rutinoside (peo-3-rut), because cyanidin has a hydroxyl group on R_2, while peonidin has a methoxyl group [45]. In other circumstances, anthocyanins with only one hydroxyl group, such as pelagonidin, had lower antioxidant capacity [46]. Generally, glycosylation decreases the antioxidant capacity of an anthocyanidin. The type of glycones substituted at R_1 also affects the antioxidant capacity of anthocyanins (Figure 9.3). Anthocyanins with R_1 substitutions of rutinosides or diglucosides have less antioxidant capacity compared with those with glucosides, which indicates that the sugar moiety also has an effect on the antioxidant capacity [10].

However, several exceptional results have been shown in some studies. Delphinidin has a greater antioxidant capacity than cyanidin as it has three hydroxyl groups on its B ring. However, delphinidin was a notable exception; it has a relatively lower antioxidant capacity than cyanidin [46]. In one study, the effects of glycosylation were largely dependent on the specific anthocyanidin [46]. For example glycosylation of cyanidin increases its antioxidant capacity, whereas glycosylation of malvidin has the opposite effect. Different analytical methods often show different results. For example the ability of anthocyanins to inhibit LDL oxidation did not agree with their ability to scavenge free radicals [10], which indicates that in this case antioxidant effects were not dependent on the number of hydroxyl groups [10]. Overall, the antioxidant capacity of various anthocyanidins and their glycosides might be attributed to various factors including analytical method, types of radical used in the assay, and experimental conditions.

9.4.2 Structural Differences in the Anti-Inflammatory Effects of Berry Anthocyanins

There are substantial evidences to show the anti-inflammatory effects of berry anthocyanins. Anthocyanins inhibited COX-2 and iNOS expression in RAW 264.7 macrophages treated with LPS. In addition, anthocyanins suppressed the activation of NF-κB-mediated inflammation by inhibiting the degradation of IκB-α. Anthocyanins also inhibited TNFα-induced MCP-1 secretion in human umbilical vein endothelial cells [47]. Those evidences indicate that anthocyanins may ameliorate chronic inflammation in adipose tissue under obesity.

Blackberry anthocyanins have been shown to inhibit NO synthesis in murine monocyte/macrophage J774 cell line [48]. The study demonstrated that the effects were attributed to the attenuation of NF-κB pathway and mitogen-activated protein kinase (MAPK) activities. Since around 90% of the anthocyanins in blackberry are cya-3-glc, this suggests that cya-3-glc contributes to those anti-inflammatory effects [36,48,49]. Another study examined the anti-inflammatory effects of an anthocyanin mixture, consisting of 72% of cya-3-glc, 20% of del-3-glc, and 6% of petunidin-3-glucoside (pet-3-glc). This mixture suppressed iNOS and COX-2 gene expression, and the products of NO and PEG2, as well as the expression of pro-inflammatory cytokine genes, notably TNFα and IL-1β. These effects were attributed to two mechanisms: inhibition of NF-κB pathway and MAPK activities (p38, ERK, and JNK). Cya-3-glc in blackberry extract also showed significant anti-inflammatory effects in ovariectomized rat through suppressing NF-κB pathway and COX-2 expression in hepatic liver, and even increased serum antioxidant capacity [50].

Blueberry polyphenol extract and blueberry anthocyanins also suppressed the expression of pro-inflammatory cytokines, including IL-1β, IL-12, and IL-6 as well as NF-κB translocation in LPS-induced Raw 264.7 macrophages [51]. Malvidin-3-glucoside (mal-3-glc) and malvidin-3-galctoside (mal-3-gal), two anthocyanins prominent in blueberries, inhibit intercellular adhesion molecule 1 (ICAM-1) and vascular cell adhesion protein 1 (VCAM-1) [52] and suppress MCP-1 [52], by preventing the degradation of IKBα. Taken together, these results largely indicate that anthocyanins have anti-inflammatory effects through the inhibition of NF-κB translocation. Furthermore, since ICAM-1, VCAM-1, and MCP-1 are well-known cardiovascular disease mediators, it is possible that blueberry anthocyanins could affect cardiovascular disease.

In an animal study, blueberry supplementation significantly reduced the gene expressions regulated by NF-κB pathway in liver and abdominal adipose tissue in obese Zucker rats [53]. This result indicates that blueberry anthocyanin can be absorbed and regulate the systemic inflammatory status. However, the result of human study is still controversial. Blueberry juice consumption did not alter the plasma pro-inflammatory cytokines and antioxidant enzymes compared with placebo group [54].

One study compared anti-inflammatory effects of 6 anthocyanidins. Delphinidin had the greatest anti-inflammatory properties due to the presence of an ortho-dihydroxyphenyl group on B ring on it. Malvidin did not show as strong anti-inflammatory effect as delphinidin and cyanidin [55].

9.4.3 Structural Differences in the Effects of Berry Anthocyanins on Obesity-Related Disorder

Various berry anthocyanins showed beneficial effects on obesity-related chronic disease such as insulin resistance, diabetes, metabolic syndrome, and dyslipidemia. The db/db C57BL mice fed blackberry supplement showed significantly decreased plasma glucose level and pro-inflammatory cytokine level including TNFα, IL-6 and MCP-1, and hepatic triglyceride (TG) level [56]. Cya-3-glc reduced the accumulation of fat in visceral adipose and liver tissues in KK-*Ay* mice [57]. Cya-3-glc also reduced plasma TG levels in the study, which suggests that cya-3-glc has TG-lowering effect [57]. Berry anthocyanin showed antidiabetic effect in the murine model of type II diabetes. Maqui berry anthocyanin (delphinidin-3-sambubioside-5-glucoside) improved fasting glucose levels and glucose tolerance in hyperglycemic obese C57BL/6J mice fed high fat diet [58]. Delphinidin-rich maqui berry supplement also showed similar results in a crossover intervention study with 10 subjects having moderate glucose intolerance [59]. These studies suggest that delphinidin may have antidiabetic effect through improving glucose tolerance.

A randomized crossover study with 110 overweight and obese female subjects showed positive effect of berries on obesity-related disease [60]. Two different berries were served in the study: bilberry and sea buckthorn. Both berries had slightly but significant positive effects on obesity-related disease markers including the decrease in plasma VCAM-1, plasma TNFα, and waist circumference. However, some markers were changed differently in each group. For example plasma ICAM-1 and fasting plasma glucose concentrations were reduced only in sea buckthorn group [60]. Mixed-berry puree made of bilberry, black currant, cranberries, and strawberry also modified the postprandial plasma glucose response to sucrose in a crossover study with 12 healthy subjects [61]. After the consumption of the berry meal with sucrose, the plasma glucose level was significantly lower by time compared with control meal [61]. The obese Zucker rats fed blueberry with high-fat diet showed decrease in retroperitoneal and epididymal fat mass and plasma fasting insulin. The activity of peroxisome proliferator–activated receptors (PPARs), which is responsible for fat oxidation, was greater in the skeletal muscle of blueberry group compared with control high-fat diet group [62]. Tart cherry enriched in cyan-3-glc also altered the activity of PPARs in the Zucker fatty rat. Tart cherry diet increases the activity of PPAR-α and PPAR-γ as well as decreases the pro-inflammatory cytokine mRNA expression and NF-κB activity in retroperitoneal fat. Therefore, the effects of anthocyanins on obesity-related disease may be related with anti-inflammatory effects.

One study compared the prevention of obesity between whole-berry supplement and purified berry anthocyanin supplement in high fat diet-induced obese male C57BL/6J mice. In the study, purified anthocyanin showed decrease in serum cholesterol and TG level and serum leptin level. However, it was not shown in whole-berry supplement [63]. The similar results were observed from other berries including strawberry, black raspberry, and Concord grape [64]. These findings suggest that the varying amounts of berries consumed might be the reason of the discrepancies between the studies.

9.5 CONCLUSION

Oxidative stress and inflammation are not independent processes and play an important role in the development of various obesity-related chronic diseases. Anthocyanins, particularly those found in berries, have both antioxidant and anti-inflammatory effects that may reduce the risk of these diseases. Different berries exhibit variation in anthocyanin composition, which might account for the distinct antioxidant and anti-inflammatory effects of different berries.

REFERENCES

1. Hojgaard B, Olsen KR, Sogaard J, Gyrd-Hansen D, Sorensen TI. 2009. Obesity related health care costs assessed from BMI or waist circumference—Secondary publication. *Ugeskr Laeger.* 171:3068–3071.
2. Chandramohan G, Kalantar-Zadeh K, Kermah D, Go SC, Vaziri ND, Norris KC. 2012. Relationship between obesity and pulse pressure in children: Results of the National Health and Nutrition Survey (NHANES) 1988–1994. *J Am Soc Hypertens.* 6:277–283.
3. Maher CA, Mire E, Harrington DM, Staiano AE, Katzmarzyk PT. 2013. The independent and combined associations of physical activity and sedentary behavior with obesity in adults: NHANES 2003–06. *Obesity (Silver Spring).* 21:E730–E737.
4. Voelker R. 2012. Escalating obesity rates pose health, budget threats. *JAMA.* 308:1514.
5. Magnusson P, Torp-Pedersen CT, Backer V, Beyer N, Andersen LB, Hansen IL, Dela F, Astrup AV, Pedersen BK, Tjonneland AM, et al. 2004. Physical activity and chronic disease II. Type 2 diabetes, obesity and cancer. *Ugeskr Laeger.* 166:1547–1551.
6. Kahn BB, Flier JS. 2000. Obesity and insulin resistance. *J Clin Invest.* 106:473–481.
7. Hubert HB, Feinleib M, McNamara PM, Castelli WP. 1983. Obesity as an independent risk factor for cardiovascular disease: A 26-year follow-up of participants in the Framingham Heart Study. *Circulation.* 67:968–977.
8. Calabro P, Golia E, Maddaloni V, Malvezzi M, Casillo B, Marotta C, Calabro R, Golino P. 2009. Adipose tissue-mediated inflammation: The missing link between obesity and cardiovascular disease? *Intern Emerg Med.* 4:25–34.
9. He J, Giusti MM. 2010. Anthocyanins: Natural colorants with health-promoting properties. *Annu Rev Food Sci Technol.* 1:163–187.
10. Kahkonen MP, Heinonen M. 2003. Antioxidant activity of anthocyanins and their aglycons. *J Agric Food Chem.* 51:628–633.
11. Egger G, Dixon J. 2010. Inflammatory effects of nutritional stimuli: Further support for the need for a big picture approach to tackling obesity and chronic disease. *Obes Rev.* 11:137–149.
12. Fernandez-Sanchez A, Madrigal-Santillan E, Bautista M, Esquivel-Soto J, Morales-Gonzalez A, Esquivel-Chirino C, Durante-Montiel I, Sanchez-Rivera G, Valadez-Vega C, Morales-Gonzalez JA. 2011. Inflammation, oxidative stress, and obesity. *Int J Mol Sci.* 12:3117–3132.
13. Dandona P, Aljada A, Bandyopadhyay A. 2004. Inflammation: The link between insulin resistance, obesity and diabetes. *Trends Immunol.* 25:4–7.
14. Galassetti P. 2012. Inflammation and oxidative stress in obesity, metabolic syndrome, and diabetes. *Exp Diabetes Res.* 2012:943706.
15. Morgan MJ, Liu ZG. 2011. Crosstalk of reactive oxygen species and NF-kappaB signaling. *Cell Res.* 21:103–115.
16. Xu H, Barnes GT, Yang Q, Tan G, Yang D, Chou CJ, Sole J, Nichols A, Ross JS, Tartaglia LA, Chen H. 2003. Chronic inflammation in fat plays a crucial role in the development of obesity-related insulin resistance. *J Clin Invest.* 112:1821–1830.
17. Gustafson B. 2010 Adipose tissue, inflammation and atherosclerosis. *J Atheroscler Thromb.* 17:332–341.
18. Hammond WG. 1995 Obesity and cell transplantation. *Nutrition.* 11:48–49.
19. Carocho M, Ferreira IC. 2013. A review on antioxidants, prooxidants and related controversy: Natural and synthetic compounds, screening and analysis methodologies and future perspectives. *Food Chem Toxicol.* 51:15–25.
20. Ishii T, Itoh K, Yamamoto M. 2002. Roles of Nrf2 in activation of antioxidant enzyme genes via antioxidant responsive elements. *Methods Enzymol.* 348:182–190.
21. Kim JK, Jang HD. 2014. Nrf2-mediated HO-1 induction coupled with the ERK signaling pathway contributes to indirect antioxidant capacity of caffeic acid phenethyl ester in HepG2 cells. *Int J Mol Sci.* 15:12149–12165.
22. Agoroaei L, Mircea C, Butnaru E, Ilicenco D, Proca M. 2003. Super-oxide dismutase and catalase in smokers. *Rev Med Chir Soc Med Nat Iasi.* 107:747–751.
23. Soldatov AA, Gostiukhina OL, Golovina IV. 2007. Antioxidant enzyme complex of tissues of the bivalve *Mytilus galloprovincialis* Lam. under normal and oxidative-stress conditions: A review. *Prikl Biokhim Mikrobiol.* 43:621–628.
24. Araujo JA, Zhang M, Yin F. 2012. Heme oxygenase-1, oxidation, inflammation, and atherosclerosis. *Front Pharmacol.* 3:119.
25. Yang CM, Huang SM, Liu CL, Hu ML. 2012. Apo-8'-lycopenal induces expression of HO-1 and NQO-1 via the ERK/p38-Nrf2-ARE pathway in human HepG2 cells. *J Agric Food Chem.* 60:1576–1585.

26. Dinkova-Kostova AT, Talalay P. 2010. NAD(P)H:quinone acceptor oxidoreductase 1 (NQO1), a multifunctional antioxidant enzyme and exceptionally versatile cytoprotector. *Arch Biochem Biophys.* 501:116–123.
27. Liu Y, Qi W, Richardson A, Van Remmen H, Ikeno Y, Salmon AB. 2013. Oxidative damage associated with obesity is prevented by overexpression of CuZn- or Mn-superoxide dismutase. *Biochem Biophys Res Commun.* 438:78–83.
28. Savini I, Catani MV, Evangelista D, Gasperi V, Avigliano L. 2013. Obesity-associated oxidative stress: Strategies finalized to improve redox state. *Int J Mol Sci.* 14:10497–10538.
29. Holt EM, Steffen LM, Moran A, Basu S, Steinberger J, Ross JA, Hong CP, Sinaiko AR. 2009. Fruit and vegetable consumption and its relation to markers of inflammation and oxidative stress in adolescents. *J Am Diet Assoc.* 109:414–421.
30. Scalbert A, Manach C, Morand C, Remesy C, Jimenez L. 2005. Dietary polyphenols and the prevention of diseases. *Crit Rev Food Sci Nutr.* 45:287–306.
31. Wang Y, Yang M, Lee SG, Davis CG, Koo SI, Fernandez ML, Volek JS, Chun OK. 2014. Diets high in total antioxidant capacity improve risk biomarkers of cardiovascular disease: A 9-month observational study among overweight/obese postmenopausal women. *Eur J Nutr.* 53:1363–1369.
32. Kaplan O, Meric M, Acar Z, Kale A, Demircan S, Yilmaz O, Demircan G, Yilmaz Miroglu Y. 2013. The effect of exercise and antioxidant enzyme levels in syndrome X and coronary slow flow phenomenon: An observational study. *Anadolu Kardiyol Derg.* 13:641–646.
33. Ness AR, Powles JW. 1997. Fruit and vegetables, and cardiovascular disease: A review. *Int J Epidemiol.* 26:1–13.
34. Bazzano LA, He J, Ogden LG, Loria CM, Vupputuri S, Myers L, Whelton PK. 2002. Fruit and vegetable intake and risk of cardiovascular disease in US adults: The first National Health and Nutrition Examination Survey Epidemiologic Follow-up Study. *Am J Clin Nutr.* 76:93–99.
35. Zafra-Stone S, Yasmin T, Bagchi M, Chatterjee A, Vinson JA, Bagchi D. 2007. Berry anthocyanins as novel antioxidants in human health and disease prevention. *Mol Nutr Food Res.* 51:675–683.
36. Marja P K, Johanna H, Velimatti O, Marina H. 2003. Berry anthocyanins: Isolation, identification and antioxidant activities. *J Sci Food Agric.* 83:1403–1411.
37. Chun OK, Chung SJ, Song WO. 2007. Estimated dietary flavonoid intake and major food sources of U.S. adults. *J Nutr.* 137:1244–1252.
38. Wu X, Beecher GR, Holden JM, Haytowitz DB, Gebhardt SE, Prior RL. 2006. Concentrations of anthocyanins in common foods in the United States and estimation of normal consumption. *J Agric Food Chem.* 54:4069–4075.
39. Wu X, Prior RL. 2005. Systematic identification and characterization of anthocyanins by HPLC-ESI-MS/MS in common foods in the United States: Fruits and berries. *J Agric Food Chem.* 53:2589–2599.
40. Seyoum A, Asres K, El-Fiky FK. 2006. Structure-radical scavenging activity relationships of flavonoids. *Phytochemistry.* 67:2058–2070.
41. Dudonne S, Vitrac X, Coutiere P, Woillez M, Merillon JM. 2009. Comparative study of antioxidant properties and total phenolic content of 30 plant extracts of industrial interest using DPPH, ABTS, FRAP, SOD, and ORAC assays. *J Agric Food Chem.* 57:1768–1774.
42. Benzie IF, Strain JJ. 1996. The ferric reducing ability of plasma (FRAP) as a measure of "antioxidant power": The FRAP assay. *Anal Biochem.* 239:70–76.
43. Rice-Evans CA, Miller NJ, Paganga G. 1996. Structure-antioxidant activity relationships of flavonoids and phenolic acids. *Free Rad Biol Med.* 20:933–956.
44. Chang H-J, Choi EH, Chun HS. 2008. Quantitative structure-activity relationship (QSAR) of antioxidative anthocyanidins and their glycosides. *Food Sci Biotechnol.* 17:501–507.
45. Wang Y, Chen X, Zhang Y, Chen X. 2012. Antioxidant activities and major anthocyanins of Myrobalan plum (*Prunus cerasifera* Ehrh.). *J Food Sci.* 77:C388–C393.
46. Wang H, Cao G, Prior RL. 1997. Oxygen radical absorbing capacity of anthocyanins. *J Agric Food Chem.* 45:304–309.
47. García-Alonso M, Rimbach G, Rivas-Gonzalo JC, Pascual-Teresa Sd. 2004. Antioxidant and cellular activities of anthocyanins and their corresponding vitisins-A studies in platelets, monocytes, and human endothelial cells. *J Agric Food Chem.* 52:3378–3384.
48. Pergola C, Rossi A, Dugo P, Cuzzocrea S, Sautebin L. 2006. Inhibition of nitric oxide biosynthesis by anthocyanin fraction of blackberry extract. *Nitric Oxide.* 15:30–39.
49. Wang Q, Xia M, Liu C, Guo H, Ye Q, Hu Y, Zhang Y, Hou M, Zhu H, Ma J, Ling W. 2008. Cyanidin-3-O-beta-glucoside inhibits iNOS and COX-2 expression by inducing liver X receptor alpha activation in THP-1 macrophages. *Life Sci.* 83:176–184.

50. Kaume L, Gilbert WC, Brownmiller C, Howard LR, Devareddy L. 2012. Cyanidin 3-O-β-d-glucoside-rich blackberries modulate hepatic gene expression, and anti-obesity effects in ovariectomized rats. *J Func Foods.* 4:480–488.
51. Cheng A, Yan H, Han C, Wang W, Tian Y, Chen X. 2014. Polyphenols from blueberries modulate inflammation cytokines in LPS-induced RAW264.7 macrophages. *Int J Biol Macromol.* 69:382–387.
52. Huang WY, Liu YM, Wang J, Wang XN, Li CY. 2014. Anti-inflammatory effect of the blueberry anthocyanins malvidin-3-glucoside and malvidin-3-galactoside in endothelial cells. *Molecules.* 19:12827–12841.
53. Vendrame S, Daugherty A, Kristo AS, Riso P, Klimis-Zacas D. 2013. Wild blueberry (*Vaccinium angustifolium*) consumption improves inflammatory status in the obese Zucker rat model of the metabolic syndrome. *J Nutr Biochem.* 24:1508–1512.
54. Riso P, Klimis-Zacas D, Del Bo C, Martini D, Campolo J, Vendrame S, Moller P, Loft S, De Maria R, Porrini M. 2013. Effect of a wild blueberry (*Vaccinium angustifolium*) drink intervention on markers of oxidative stress, inflammation and endothelial function in humans with cardiovascular risk factors. *Eur J Nutr.* 52:949–961.
55. Hou DX, Yanagita T, Uto T, Masuzaki S, Fujii M. 2005. Anthocyanidins inhibit cyclooxygenase-2 expression in LPS-evoked macrophages: Structure-activity relationship and molecular mechanisms involved. *Biochem Pharmacol.* 70:417–425.
56. Guo H, Xia M, Zou T, Ling W, Zhong R, Zhang W. 2012. Cyanidin 3-glucoside attenuates obesity-associated insulin resistance and hepatic steatosis in high-fat diet-fed and db/db mice via the transcription factor FoxO1. *J Nutr Biochem.* 23:349–360.
57. Wei X, Wang D, Yang Y, Xia M, Li D, Li G, Zhu Y, Xiao Y, Ling W. 2011. Cyanidin-3-O-beta-glucoside improves obesity and triglyceride metabolism in KK-Ay mice by regulating lipoprotein lipase activity. *J Sci Food Agric.* 91:1006–1013.
58. Rojo LE, Ribnicky D, Logendra S, Poulev A, Rojas-Silva P, Kuhn P, Dorn R, Grace MH, Lila MA, Raskin I. 2012. In vitro and in vivo anti-diabetic effects of anthocyanins from Maqui Berry (*Aristotelia chilensis*). *Food Chem.* 131:387–396.
59. Hidalgo J, Flores C, Hidalgo MA, Perez M, Yanez A, Quinones L, Caceres DD, Burgos RA. 2014. Delphinol(R) standardized maqui berry extract reduces postprandial blood glucose increase in individuals with impaired glucose regulation by novel mechanism of sodium glucose cotransporter inhibition. *Panminerva Med.* 56:1–7.
60. Lehtonen HM, Suomela JP, Tahvonen R, Yang B, Venojarvi M, Viikari J, Kallio H. 2011. Different berries and berry fractions have various but slightly positive effects on the associated variables of metabolic diseases on overweight and obese women. *Eur J Clin Nutr.* 65:394–401.
61. Torronen R, Sarkkinen E, Tapola N, Hautaniemi E, Kilpi K, Niskanen L. 2010. Berries modify the postprandial plasma glucose response to sucrose in healthy subjects. *Br J Nutr.* 103:1094–1097.
62. Kersten S. 2008. Peroxisome proliferator activated receptors and lipoprotein metabolism. *PPAR Res.* 2008:132960.
63. Prior RL, Wu X, Gu L, Hager TJ, Hager A, Howard LR. 2008. Whole berries versus berry anthocyanins: Interactions with dietary fat levels in the C57BL/6J mouse model of obesity. *J Agric Food Chem.* 56:647–653.
64. Prior RL, Wu X, Gu L, Hager T, Hager A, Wilkes S, Howard L. 2009. Purified berry anthocyanins but not whole berries normalize lipid parameters in mice fed an obesogenic high fat diet. *Mol Nutr Food Res.* 53:1406–1418.

Section III

Cardiovascular Health

10 Nutrition and Cardiovascular Health
A Review

Mash Hamid, Clare Stradling, Shahrad Taheri, and G. Neil Thomas

CONTENTS

10.1 INTRODUCTION

Atherosclerosis, which begins early in life, is a disease that subsequently leads to cardiovascular disease (CVD) including coronary heart disease (CHD) and peripheral and cerebrovascular disease. CVD is one of the leading causes of mortality worldwide. According to the World Health Organisation, 17.3 million individuals died of CVD in 2008, and it is estimated that within the next 15 years, nearly 30 million lives will be lost to CVD (World Health Organisation 2011). Various factors such as lifestyle, smoking, alcohol, family history of CVD, environment, and diet have been suggested to be among the contributors of CVD. Diet is a major modifiable risk factor for the development of CVD.

Epidemiological studies in the past have shown reduced risk of CVD with food groups such as whole grain (Mellen et al. 2008), fruit and vegetables (Oude Griep et al. 2010), and nuts (Kelly and Sabate 2006). Recently, dietary pattern analysis has shown an effect on CVD beyond that of individual food groups (Jacques and Tucker 2001). Several investigations have demonstrated protective effects of plant-based dietary patterns such as the Dietary Approach to Stop Hypertension (DASH) (Fung et al. 2008) and the Mediterranean diet on CVD. There is also evidence that distinct dietary patterns such as the very-low-carbohydrate diet (VLCD) also offer cardiovascular benefits (Santos et al. 2012). Dietary recommendations based on dietary pattern analysis have become part of the guidelines for CVD prevention. In the United Kingdom, the dietetic guidelines recommend following plant-based diets similar to the Mediterranean (Mead et al. 2006). These recommendations are also in agreement with the UK guidelines for the prevention of myocardial infarction (MI) (Cooper et al. 2007).

The aim of this chapter is to review the evidence in relation to most popular dietary patterns focusing on the DASH, Mediterranean, and VLCD. A comprehensive review of all studies assessing these dietary factors is beyond the scope of this chapter; therefore, systematic reviews and meta-analyses have been reviewed when applicable.

10.2 RATIONALE FOR DIETARY PATTERN ANALYSIS

The limitation of single food item and/or individual food group analyses is that humans eat a diet comprising combinations of several food groups. For example consumers of fruits and vegetables are more likely to have a diet with whole grain and nuts (Hu et al. 2000), whereas consumers of sugary foods are more likely to have high-fat foods (Nettleton et al. 2009). Likewise, single food item analyses fail to identify the health benefits of food combinations (Jacques and Tucker 2001). Another limitation of single food analyses is that they are unable to produce cumulative effects. For instance, increasing vegetable and fruit intake together with sodium restriction is more efficient in lowering blood pressure than either alone as demonstrated in the DASH diet trial (Sacks et al. 2001). Dietary patterns overcome these limitations and therefore have been widely used to determine the relationship with chronic disease (Hu et al. 2000).

10.3 CHARACTERIZING DIETARY PATTERNS

Dietary patterns rely on statistical methods to be characterized because they cannot be measured directly. They are characterized using empirical (a posteriori) and theoretical (a priori) methods. A posteriori methods include data-driven methods such as principal component factor analysis (PCFA) and cluster analysis (Michels and Schulze 2005). The PCFA relies on nutritional data from a population under study to identify dietary patterns based on correlations between food items and/or food groups. The correlated groups of food groups are then allocated a name, and a summary score is used in correlation and regression analysis (Hu 2000). For example the Health Professionals Follow-Up study used PCFA and identified the *prudent diet*, which was found to be inversely associated with CHD (relative risk (RR) 0.70, 95% confidence interval 0.56–0.86) (Hu et al. 2000). The limitation of a posteriori method is that they may not identify ideal dietary patterns (Hu 2002). An alternative approach to the PCFA is to develop a diet index score based on preexisting dietary patterns or prespecified nutritional guidelines (Jacques and Tucker 2001).

Theoretically defined or a priori dietary patterns assign a score or index to selection of food items or groups that are deemed beneficial for health. The composite index score is then used as a single variable in statistical analyses (Hu 2002). Epidemiological studies that have assessed whether dietary indices predict CVD are discussed under the DASH and Mediterranean sections. The limitation of diet index score is that they are as good as only the guidelines they were constructed on (Waijers et al. 2007). Similarly, arbitrary decisions are made in selecting the components, scoring method, and the cutoff points, which can influence the strength of associations. Furthermore, multiple lifestyle factors affect health and life span, and they cannot be fully accounted for when assessing diet. The advantage of diet index scores is that they can be useful in assessing adherence to nutritional guidelines and whether they are efficient in lowering the risk of CVD and mortality. For instance, the Healthy Eating Index (HEI) score was one of the earliest diet scores constructed to assess adherence to dietary guidelines developed by the American and Food Guide Pyramid. It consisted of 10 components, and the Health Professionals Study found the score to be associated with a 28% (RR 0.72, 95%CI 0.60–0.88) modest reduction of CVD after adjusting for potential confounders (McCullough et al. 2000). To improve the predicted risk more accurately, an alternative HEI (AHEI) score was subsequently developed, which removed potatoes from the vegetable component and made some distinctions between meats and fats (McCullough et al. 2002). In a larger study, the AHEI score showed a stronger association with CVD (RR 0.61, 95%CI 0.49–0.75) after adjusting for potential confounders.

10.4 DIETARY APPROACH TO STOP HYPERTENSION

A clinical trial in the 1980s showed that a vegetarian diet lowered blood pressure (Rouse et al. 1983). Reflecting this plant-based diet, the National Heart, Lung, and Blood Institute designed the DASH diet by incorporating food groups that have been shown to lower blood pressure. The DASH diet consisted of whole grain, fruit, vegetables, nuts, legumes, and low-fat dairy, and recommended limiting the consumption of meat and sweetened drinks. A clinical trial was then carried out to assess the effect of the diet on blood pressure.

The DASH diet trial recruited 459 individuals with mild hypertension and randomized them into three diet groups: (1) typical American diet, (2) fruit and vegetables, and (3) DASH combination diet for 8 weeks (Appel et al. 1997). All diets provided 3000 mg sodium/day, and subjects were provided with prepared meals during the intervention period. At the end of the trial, reduction in systolic blood pressure (–5.5 mmHg, 95%CI –7.4 to –3.7) was greater for the DASH compared to the fruit and vegetable group, which lowered systolic blood pressure by –2.8 mmHg (95%CI –4.7 to –0.9) compared to the control group. The reduction in blood pressure seen in the DASH diet group suggests that meat reduction in conjunction with increased intake of low-fat dairy with fruit and vegetables provides benefits beyond that of fruit and vegetable consumption alone in lowering blood pressure–related CVD. Besides improvement in blood pressure, the DASH diet also lowered total cholesterol (–0.35 mmol/L, 95%CI –0.49 to –0.22), low-density lipoprotein (LDL) cholesterol (–0.28 mmol/L, 95%CI –0.40 to –0.16), and high-density lipoprotein (HDL) cholesterol (–0.09 mmol/L, 95%CI –0.13 to –0.06) compared to the fruit and vegetable and control diets. The authors estimated the resulting changes in 10-year CHD risk using the Framingham equation and detected an 18% (RR 0.82, 95%CI 0.75–0.90) reduction in estimated CHD risk at week 8 compared to baseline values for individuals who were assigned to the DASH diet when compared to the control group (Chen et al. 2010). Comparison with the fruit and vegetable group, an 11% (RR 0.89, 95%CI 0.81–0.97) reduction in CHD risk was seen for the DASH diet group. This suggests that the reduction in HDL cholesterol is compensated for by the concomitant reductions in blood pressure and LDL cholesterol.

A follow-up DASH–sodium trial was performed to assess the effects of sodium reduction together with the DASH diet on blood pressure since sodium restriction was not part of the first trial. It recruited 412 adults and allocated the subjects to three levels of sodium (high 150 mmol/day, intermediate 100 mmol/day, and low 50 mmol/day) for 30 days each in a random order in this randomized crossover trial. The results showed a reduction in blood pressure with the DASH–sodium diet at each sodium level (–1.3 mmHg, 95%CI –2.6 to 0.0 and –1.7 mmHg, 95%CI –3.0 to –0.4) and the control diet (–2.1 mmHg, 95%CI –3.4 to –0.8 and –4.6 mmHg, 95%CI –5.9 to –3.2). The DASH–sodium group showed an additional reduction of –5.6 and –2.2 mmHg showing greater benefits with the DASH diet (Sacks et al. 2001). This suggests that a significant reduction in blood pressure is achievable, equivalent to that of antihypertensive medication when the DASH diet is used together with sodium restriction. Fifty-six subjects from the trial were observed after 12 months. The authors noted that subjects from the DASH group consumed more fruit and vegetables and had a slight increase in sodium intake compared to the control group but were able to sustain their blood pressure reduction (Ard et al. 2004).

The earlier-mentioned randomized controlled trials (RCTs) were short-term trials and were performed in healthy subjects. To address the limitations of short-term RCTs, cohorts have been able to explore the long-term relationship between adherence to a DASH-style diet and CVD risk. Using the a priori method, the Nurses' Health Study of 88,517 female subjects developed a DASH-style diet score based on eight food components and one nutrient component (whole grain, fruits, vegetables, nuts, legumes, low-fat dairy, reduced intake of red meat, sugary beverages, and sodium). A food frequency questionnaire that was administered seven times during the 24-year follow-up was used to collect dietary data. After adjusting for potential confounders, females in the highest quintile of DASH-style diet had a 24% (RR 0.76, 95%CI 0.67–0.85) lower risk of CHD. The DASH-style diet was also associated with a 22% (RR 0.78, 95%CI 0.67–0.90) lower risk of nonfatal CHD and a 29% (RR 0.71, 95%CI 0.58–0.89) lower risk of fatal CHD (Fung et al. 2008). Subsequently, the Women's Health Study applied the same DASH-style diet score to their study and assessed the association with CVD and fatal CHD in 34,827 subjects. The multivariable model that adjusted for age, energy intake, and randomization status showed that the DASH diet score was inversely associated with CVD risk (hazard ratio (HR) 0.64, 95%CI 0.53–0.78) and fatal CHD (HR 0.59, 95%CI 0.44–0.80).

Further adjustment for physical activity, smoking, alcohol, education, hormone therapy, and post-menopausal status attenuated the association for both CVD (HR 0.88, 95%CI 0.72–1.07) and fatal CHD (HR 0.90, 95%CI 0.65–1.24) (Fitzgerald et al. 2012). These results are consistent with that of the Iowa Women's Health Study, which observed an inverse association (HR 0.67, 95%CI 0.52–0.86) with CHD death after adjusting for age and energy. Adjusting for other confounders attenuated (HR 0.86, 95%CI 0.67–1.12) the relationship (Folsom et al. 2007). A possible explanation of diluted effects of the Fitzgerald et al. (2012) and Folsom et al. (2007) cohorts could be differences in CHD events, number of subjects, and follow-up duration when comparing to Fung et al. (2008). The DASH scores in both studies were also different. The Fung score was designed to assess adherence to the overall pattern (Fung et al. 2008), whereas the Folsom score allocated points for selected food groups at 2000 cal (Folsom et al. 2007). A recent systematic review that pooled the results from these cohorts found that the DASH-style diet lowered the risk of CHD by 21% (RR 0.79, 95%CI 0.71–0.88) and for CVD by 20% (RR 0.80, 95%CI 0.74–0.86) (Salehi-Abargouei et al. 2013).

The DASH diet has been shown to lower blood pressure and cholesterol in clinical trials and is a suitable alternative to antihypertensive medication. Very few studies have assessed the effects of the DASH diet on CVD under free-living conditions. The limited data from observational studies indicate that DASH does reduce the risk of CVD, but the evidence is weak.

10.5 MEDITERRANEAN DIET

The Mediterranean diet was designed in the 1960s when the Seven Countries Study (Keys 1997) suggested that this dietary pattern was the reason for the lower CVD rates and increased longevity among inhabitants in these olive-growing regions. Consistent with the principles of the DASH diet, the Mediterranean diet also emphasizes increased intake of whole grain, fruits, vegetables, nuts, legume, olive oil, moderate intake of dairy, poultry, fish, alcohol, and low intake of red meat. The Mediterranean diet encompasses a lifestyle that encourages engaging in physical activity, obtaining optimal vitamin D levels through exposure to sun, and having siestas.

The first Mediterranean diet score (MDS) was developed by Trichopoulou et al. (1995), who based it on the diet of older Greek adults and showed a link with survival. The score included eight components, and a positive score was given for a higher-than-median intake of fruit and nuts, vegetables, legumes, cereal, and dairy. A positive score was also given for lower-than-median intake of meat, alcohol, and saturated fat. The final score ranged between 0 and 8 to assess adherence to the diet. The research team then used the MDS in the Greek European Prospective Study into Cancer and Nutrition (EPIC) that had a 44-month follow-up period and 22,043 subjects. A two-point increase in MDS was associated with a 33% (HR 0.67, 95%CI 0.47–0.94) reduction in CHD mortality (Trichopoulou et al. 2003). The Greek EPIC study later published gender-stratified results after a median follow-up period of 10 years. Again, a two-point increase in MDS reduced cardiovascular mortality by 19% (HR 0.81, 95%CI 0.67–0.99) in men and by 25% (HR 0.75, 95%CI 0.57–0.98) in women. Similar trend was observed for CHD incidence but yielded less precision in the results because of wider confidence intervals (Dilis et al. 2012).

Several meta-analyses of cohort studies have also produced similar results (Sofi et al. 2008, 2010, 2014). A meta-analysis of eight cohort studies involving 514,816 individuals with study duration from 3 to 18 years assessed the association between the Mediterranean diet and cardiovascular mortality in primary prevention setting. The two-point increase in the MDS reduced the risk of cardiovascular mortality by 9% (RR 0.91, 95%CI 0.87–0.95) (Sofi et al. 2008). The same research group later updated the study by adding 10 more cohorts to the analyses involving 2,190,627 individuals. A 10% (RR 0.90, 95%CI 0.87–0.93) reduced risk of cardiovascular mortality was observed with a two-point increase in the MDS (Sofi et al. 2010). Further inclusion of 18 cohort studies showed a 10% (RR 0.90, 95%CI 0.87–0.92) reduced risk of CVD with a two-point increase in the MDS in a recent meta-analysis (Sofi et al. 2014).

RCTs have played an important role in the acquisition of knowledge in this field. RCTs have slightly modified the diet by (1) allowing moderate fat intake, (2) replacing beef and lamb with chicken and fish, and (3) adding healthy fats to the diet such as nuts and olive oil. A meta-analysis of six RCTs that compared the Mediterranean diet to the low-fat diet showed improvements in wide range of cardiovascular risk factors in subjects allocated to the Mediterranean diet (Nordmann et al. 2011). After 2 years of follow-up, subjects assigned to the Mediterranean diet lost more weight (weighted mean difference (WMD) −2.2 kg, 95%CI −3.9 to −0.6), had a reduced waist circumference (WMD −0.9 cm, 95%CI −2.0 to −0.2), and lower fasting glucose (WMD −0.21 mmol/L, 95%CI −0.39 to −0.03), systolic blood pressure (WMD −1.7 mmHg, 95%CI −3.4 to −0.1), and total cholesterol (WMD −0.19 mmol/L, 95%CI −0.26 to −0.11). The Mediterranean diet also reduced high-sensitivity C-reactive protein (WMD −9.52 nmol/L, 95%CI −14.29 to −4.76), an inflammatory marker associated with increased risk of CVD. Significant heterogeneity was present between the trials because of imbalances in interventions where greater support was given to the Mediterranean diet group. The effects of the Mediterranean diet on cardiovascular risk factors were also assessed by another meta-analysis, but the results of the analyses are unreliable because of inappropriate pooling of the studies and significant heterogeneity between the trials (Kastorini et al. 2011).

Recent RCTs have also enhanced the understanding of the overall benefits of the Mediterranean diet. The Primary Prevention of Cardiovascular Disease with a Mediterranean Diet trial randomized 7447 Spanish adults at high cardiovascular risk to one of three groups: (1) Mediterranean diet with provision of olive oil, (2) Mediterranean diet with provision of nuts, and (3) low-fat diet, during a median follow-up of 4.8 years. This study was stopped because of the primary endpoint crossing the stopping boundary during the interim analysis. The trial results demonstrated that the Mediterranean diet with provision of olive oil reduced the risk of cardiovascular events by 30% (HR 0.70, 95%CI 0.54–0.92), and the Mediterranean diet with provision of nuts reduced the risk by 28% (HR 0.72, 95%CI 0.54–0.96) compared to the low-fat diet (Estruch et al. 2013).

Most Mediterranean diet studies have been performed in healthy individuals and have shown evidence for primary prevention, but little is known about the effects of the diet in individuals with preexisting CVD. The Heart Institute of Spokane Diet Intervention and Evaluation Trial randomized 101 adults with MI to the Mediterranean-style diet or a low-fat diet and followed them up for a median period of 46 months in a case–control analysis. After adjusting for obesity, LDL cholesterol, smoking, and medication, the Mediterranean diet group experienced fewer cardiovascular events (Odds Ratio [OR] 0.28, 95%CI 0.13–0.63) (Tuttle et al. 2008). Other RCTs performed in individuals with existing CVD also have not been without problems. For instance, the Lyon Diet Heart Study reported a reduction in MI after 27 months, but the Data Monitoring Committee overestimated the net health benefits of the trial and stopped it early. This trial also did not perform intention-to-treat analysis (de Lorgeril et al. 1999).

There have been some concerns regarding the high-fat content of the Mediterranean diet, which may contribute to weight gain. The meta-analysis by Nordmann et al. (2011) discussed earlier showed reductions in waist circumference and body weight with the diet, which suggests that weight gain is unlikely. This has been supported by a meta-analysis of 16 RCTs, which showed a mean difference of −1.75 kg (95%CI −2.86 to −0.64) between the groups. The results also showed enhanced weight loss (mean difference −2.69 kg, 95%CI −3.99 to −1.38) with the Mediterranean diet with study duration lasting over 6 months. Further analyses showed that weight loss was greater when the Mediterranean diet was combined with calorie restriction (mean difference −3.88 kg, 95%CI −6.54 to −1.21) and increased exercise (mean difference −4.01 kg, 95%CI −5.79 to 2.23) (Esposito et al. 2011). This suggests that the Mediterranean diet in conjunction with calorie restriction and physical activity is an important tool for weight loss and cardiovascular outcomes.

A review of the literature suggests that the Mediterranean diet reduces cardiovascular mortality, and several RCTs including meta-analysis have demonstrated its benefits on the majority of cardiovascular risk factors. Most clinical trials have used the low-fat diet as a comparator.

10.6 VERY-LOW-CARBOHYDRATE DIET (VLCD)

A VLCD program is frequently used for weight loss in clinical trials (Gardner et al. 2007; Shai et al. 2008). VLCD recommended between 20 and 50 g of carbohydrates (CHO) per day, roughly 20% of daily energy from CHO (Westman et al. 2007). VLCD, which is termed the ketogenic diet, allows ad libitum intake of protein and fats. A popular example of the VLCD is the Atkins diet.

On this diet, energy is primarily obtained from ketones and fats (Last and Wilson 2006; Westman et al. 2007; Wylie-Rosett and Davis 2009). A VLCD results in ketosis. Ketosis occurs when the body starts burning fat instead of CHO for fuel (Dashti et al. 2004). Weight loss in the early phase of the VLCD is due to the diuretic effects of the diet as glycogen releases bound water through urine (Adam-Perrot et al. 2006; Last and Wilson 2006). Another reason for weight loss on the VLCD is calorie restriction because the food choices are limited to ensure that CHO does not exceed above the maximum requirements (Adam-Perrot et al. 2006).

Clinical trials have implemented the VLCD to study the extent to which the diet improves cardiovascular risk factors. An earlier meta-analysis of five RCTs that involved 447 obese subjects aged 42–49 years compared VLCD to the low-fat diets (Nordmann et al. 2006). At 6 months, the VLCD reduced the weight by −3.3 kg (95%CI −5.3 to −1.4). Weight loss led to no improvements in diastolic blood pressure (WMD −1.8 mmHg, 95%CI −3.7 to 0.1), systolic blood pressure (WMD 2.4 mmHg, 95%CI −4.9 to 0.1), LDL cholesterol (WMD 0.14 mmol/L, 95%CI 0.03–0.26), and triglycerides (WMD −0.25 mmol/L, 95%CI − 0.43 to −0.06), but increased HDL cholesterol (WMD 0.12 mmol/L, 95%CI 0.04–0.21). Weight loss was no longer maintained at 12 months. Since this has been carried out, several RCTs have emerged that have advanced the knowledge in the field.

In a recent systematic review and meta-analysis by Santos et al. (2012), the long-term effects of VLCD have been assessed. This review evaluated 23 RCTs lasting 3–24 months involving 1141 obese adults. They performed the analyses within the VLCD group and compared baseline data to four follow-up periods: (1) less than 6 months, (2) 6–11 months, (3) 12–23 months, and (4) post 24 months. The VLCD resulted in significant weight loss (−6.82 kg, 95%CI −7.03 to −6.61: eight RCTs) at 6 months. The effects were maintained at 23 months, but at 24 months, there was a slight rebound in weight (−4.65 kg, 95%CI −5.37 to −3.93: four RCTs). Figure 10.1 illustrates average weight loss with VLCD over 24 months. Most studies showed improvements in blood pressure, HDL cholesterol, waist circumference, glycemia, and triglycerides at 6 and 12 months. Improvements in LDL cholesterol were not observed at 6 months, but between 12 and 23 months, there was a mean

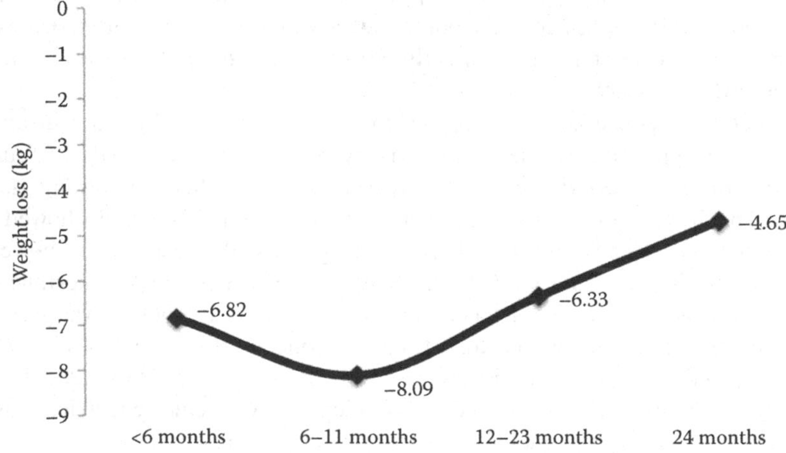

FIGURE 10.1 Weight loss with very-low-carbohydrate diet over 24 months.

reduction of −0.07 mmol/L (95%CI −0.13 to −0.10: six RCTs) and of −0.08 mmol/L (95%CI −0.16 to −0.10: two RCTs) post 24 months. This finding shows that weight loss maintenance can eventually lower LDL cholesterol levels.

The criticism of the VLCD is an increase in LDL cholesterol because of a higher saturated fat intake (Brinkworth et al. 2009; Crowe 2005). Prolonged saturated fat intake causes hyperlipidemia, which elevates the risk of CVD (Ebbert and Jensen 2013). An RCT of VLCD that prescribed a higher saturated fat showed that after 12 months, half of the study subjects experienced a 10% increase in LDL cholesterol (Brinkworth et al. 2009). A strategy to lower LDL cholesterol–induced CVD risk in patients with hyperglycemia was tested by Tay et al. (2014). They substituted saturated fats with unsaturated fat/low saturated fat and found reduction in LDL cholesterol at the end of the trial. This suggests that substituting unhealthy fats for healthy fats does not increase LDL cholesterol. The study also showed that VLCD reduced fasting glucose and led to reduced dosages of anti-glycemic medication suggesting that lowering saturated fat in VLCD at least in the short term is an effective therapy for hyperglycemia.

Nutritional deficiencies on VLCD are common because foods purported to lower CVD risk such as fruits, vegetables, nuts, and whole grains are reduced (Floegel and Pischon 2012). Lack of micronutrients such as magnesium and folic acid can result in nutritional deficiencies. A post hoc analysis of the “A TO Z” study comparing VLCD to three diet programs in obese women showed that subjects allocated to the VLCD had the lowest magnesium and folic acid levels (Gardner et al. 2010). Magnesium has been shown to lower the risk of CVD (Del Gobbo et al. 2013), and low folic acid levels can impair brachial artery flow-mediated dilation (Woo et al. 2002). This was shown in a 12-month RCT that compared VLCD to a low-fat diet where comparison with baseline value showed that VLCD group had their plasma folate reduced by −4.2 nmol/L (Hashimoto et al. 1998). The endothelial function appears to be affected by VLCD, but whether it adversely affects cardiovascular endpoints has not been evaluated (Wycherley et al. 2010).

In addition to the nutritional deficiencies discussed earlier, the adverse effects of VLCD have been addressed by few trials (Westman et al. 2002; Yancy et al. 2004). An RCT of 120 obese adults comparing VLCD to the low-fat found that the VLCD group experienced more side effects than the low-fat diet group. These included constipation (68% vs. 35%), headaches (60% vs. 40%), halitosis (38% vs. 8%), muscle cramps (35% vs. 7%), fatigue (25% vs. 8%), diarrhea (23% vs. 7%), and rash (13% vs. 0%) (Yancy et al. 2004). High attrition rates detected in the VLCD studies could be the result of these adverse effects (Westman et al. 2002; Yancy et al. 2004). Nutritional deficiencies and the adverse effects on VLCD have been questioned. A systematic review of 94 studies of different study designs (24 RCTs, 19 crossover trials, 25 pre–post studies, 17 trial with control or comparison groups, and 9 sequential study design) with a duration lasting 4–12 months showed that very few studies had data on surrogated markers such as systolic blood pressure (four studies), LDL cholesterol (seven studies), HDL cholesterol (nine studies), and fasting insulin (five studies). The data over 3 months were limited to five studies, and the diet was not adequately evaluated for longer than this period. However, the diet showed no adverse effects on serum lipids and fasting glucose. No information on the side effects was available, and the lack of long-term data limited the understanding of the safety of VLCD (Bravata et al. 2003).

VLCD appear to be effective for weight loss at 6 months, with weight loss mediating the cardiovascular benefits, which can be observed in the longer-term studies of up to 2 years. However, with weight regain, which is observed at 24 months, these benefits are reduced. The diet's high saturated fat content and the increase in LDL cholesterol have been a concern, but short-term trials have addressed this by replacing saturated fat with unsaturated fats. This strategy appears to be promising, but the long-term effects are warranted. VLCD also restricts healthy foods, which increases the risk of nutritional deficiencies, thus questioning their safety. The majority of VLCD trials are of short duration making it impossible to address their safety.

10.7 SUMMARY

Dietary pattern analyses have strengthened our understanding of the role of diet in the prevention of CVD. A small number of clinical trials have shown that the DASH diet pattern has a beneficial effect on blood pressure and cholesterol and, with partial support from large epidemiological studies, suggest that the DASH diet pattern may potentially reduce the CVD risk. This evidence for primary prevention of CVD is stronger with the Mediterranean diet pattern as demonstrated by both RCTs and epidemiological studies. Overlapping of food groups in both diets shows an emphasis toward plant-based diets. In contrast, improvements in cardiovascular risk factors with VLCD appear to be through weight loss. The long-term effect of VLCD on cardiovascular mortality is unknown, and their safety has not been adequately assessed.

REFERENCES

Adam-Perrot, A., P. Clifton, and F. Brouns. 2006. Low-carbohydrate diets: Nutritional and physiological aspects. *Obesity Reviews* 7(1): 49–58.

Appel, L. J., T. J. Moore, E. Obarzanek, W. M. Vollmer, L. P. Svetkey, F. M. Sacks, G. A. Brayet al. 1997. A clinical trial of the effects of dietary patterns on blood pressure. DASH collaborative research group. *New England Journal of Medicine* 336(16): 1117–1124.

Ard, J. D., C. J. Coffman, P. H. Lin, and L. P. Svetkey. 2004. One-year follow-up study of blood pressure and dietary patterns in dietary approaches to stop hypertension (DASH)-sodium participants. *American Journal of Hypertension* 17: 1156–1162.

Bravata, D. M., L. Sanders, J. Huang, H. M. Krumholz, I. Olkin, C. D. Gardner, and D. M. Bravata. 2003. Efficacy and safety of low-carbohydrate diets: A systematic review. *Journal of the American Medical Association* 289: 1837–1850.

Brinkworth, G. D., M. Noakes, J. D. Buckley, J. B. Keogh, and P. M. Clifton. 2009. Long-term effects of a very-low-carbohydrate weight loss diet compared with an isocaloric low-fat diet after 12 mo. *American Journal of Clinical Nutrition* 90: 23–32.

Chen, S. T., N. M. Maruthur, and L. J. Appel. 2010. The effect of dietary patterns on estimated coronary heart disease risk: Results from the Dietary Approaches to Stop Hypertension (DASH) Trial. *Circulation. Cardiovascular Quality and Outcomes* 3: 484–489.

Cooper, A., J. Skinner, G. Nherera, G. Feder, G. Ritchie, M. Kathoria, N. Turnbull et al. 2007. *Clinical Guidelines and Evidence Review for Post Myocardial Infarction: Secondary Prevention in Primary and Secondary Care for Patients Following a Myocardial Infarction.* National Collaborating Centre for Primary Care and Royal College of General Practitioners: London, U.K.

Crowe, T. C. 2005. Safety of low-carbohydrate diets. *Obesity Reviews* 6: 235–245.

Dashti, H. M., T. C. Mathew, T. Hussein, S. K. Afsar, A. Behbahani, M. A. Khoursheed, H. M. Al-Sayer, Y. Y. Bo-Abbas, and N. S. Al-Zaid. 2004. Long-term effects of a ketogenic diet in obese patients. *Experimental and Clinical Cardiology* 9: 200–205.

de Lorgeril, M., P. Salen, J. L. Martin, I. Monjaud, J. Delaye, and N. Mamelle. 1999. Mediterranean diet, traditional risk factors, and the rate of cardiovascular complications after myocardial infarction: Final report of the Lyon Diet Heart Study. *Circulation* 99: 779–785.

Del Gobbo, L. C., F. Imamura, J. H. Wu, M. C. de Oliveira Otto, S. E. Chiuve, and D. Mozaffarian. 2013. Circulating and dietary magnesium and risk of cardiovascular disease: A systematic review and meta-analysis of prospective studies. *American Journal of Clinical Nutrition* 98: 160–173.

Dilis, V., M. Katsoulis, P. Lagiou, D. Trichopoulos, A. Naska, and A. Trichopoulou. 2012. Mediterranean diet and CHD: The Greek European Prospective Investigation into Cancer and Nutrition Cohort. *British Journal of Nutrition* 108: 699–709.

Ebbert, J. O. and M. D. Jensen. 2013. Fat depots, free fatty acids, and dyslipidemia. *Nutrients* 5: 498–508.

Esposito, K., C. M. Kastorini, D. B. Panagiotakos, and D. Giugliano. 2011. Mediterranean diet and weight loss: Meta-analysis of randomized controlled trials. *Metabolic Syndrome and Related Disorders* 9: 1–12.

Estruch, R., E. Ros, J. Salas-Salvado, M. I. Covas, D. Corella, F. Aros, E. Gomez-Gracia et al. 2013. Primary prevention of cardiovascular disease with a Mediterranean diet. *New England Journal of Medicine* 368: 1279–1290.

Fitzgerald, K. C., S. E. Chiuve, J. E. Buring, P. M. Ridker, and R. J. Glynn. 2012. Comparison of associations of adherence to a Dietary Approaches to Stop Hypertension (DASH)-style diet with risks of cardiovascular disease and venous thromboembolism. *Journal of Thrombosis and Haemostasis* 10: 189–198.

Floegel, A. and T. Pischon. 2012. Low carbohydrate-high protein diets. *British Medical Journal* 344: e3801.

Folsom, A. R., E. D. Parker, and L. J. Harnack. 2007. Degree of concordance with DASH diet guidelines and incidence of hypertension and fatal cardiovascular disease. *American Journal of Hypertension* 20: 225–232.

Fung, T. T., S. E. Chiuve, M. L. McCullough, K. M. Rexrode, G. Logroscino, and F. B. Hu. 2008. Adherence to a DASH-Style diet and risk of coronary heart disease and stroke in women. *Archives of Internal Medicine* 168: 713–720.

Gardner, C. D., A. Kiazand, S. Alhassan, S. Kim, R. S. Stafford, R. R. Balise, H. C. Kraemer, and A. C. King. 2007. Comparison of the Atkins, Zone, Ornish, and LEARN diets for change in weight and related risk factors among overweight premenopausal women: The A TO Z weight loss study: A randomized trial. *Journal of the American Medical Association* 297: 969–977.

Gardner, C. D., S. Kim, A. Bersamin, M. Dopler-Nelson, J. Otten, B. Oelrich, and R. Cherin. 2010. Micronutrient quality of weight-loss diets that focus on macronutrients: Results from the A TO Z study. *American Journal of Clinical Nutrition* 92: 304–312.

Hashimoto, M., M. Akishita, M. Eto, K. Kozaki, J. Ako, N. Sugimoto, M. Yoshizumi, K. Toba, and Y. Ouchi. 1998. The impairment of flow-mediated vasodilatation in obese men with visceral fat accumulation. *International Journal of Obesity and Related Metabolic Disorders* 22: 477–484.

Hu, F. B. 2002. Dietary pattern analysis: A new direction in nutritional epidemiology. *Current Opinion in Lipidology* 13: 3–9.

Hu, F. B., E. B. Rimm, M. J. Stampfer, A. Ascherio, D. Spiegelman, and W. C. Willett. 2000. Prospective study of major dietary patterns and risk of coronary heart disease in Men. *American Journal of Clinical Nutrition* 72: 912–921.

Jacques, P. F. and K. L. Tucker. 2001. Are dietary patterns useful for understanding the role of diet in chronic disease? *American Journal of Clinical Nutrition* 73: 1–2.

Kastorini, C. M., H. J. Milionis, K. Esposito, D. Giugliano, J. A. Goudevenos, and D. B. Panagiotakos. 2011. The effect of Mediterranean diet on metabolic syndrome and its components: A meta-analysis of 50 studies and 534,906 individuals. *Journal of the American College of Cardiology* 57: 1299–1313.

Kelly, J. H., Jr., and J. Sabate. 2006. Nuts and coronary heart disease: An epidemiological perspective. *British Journal of Nutrition* 96: S61–S67.

Keys, A.1997. Coronary heart disease in seven countries. 1970. *Nutrition* 13: 250–252; discussion 249, 253.

Last, A. R. and S. A. Wilson. 2006. Low-carbohydrate diets. *American Family Physician* 73: 1942–1948.

McCullough, M. L., D. Feskanich, E. B. Rimm, E. L. Giovannucci, A. Ascherio, J. N. Variyam, D. Spiegelman, M. J. Stampfer, and W. C. Willett. 2000. Adherence to the dietary guidelines for Americans and risk of major chronic disease in men. *American Journal of Clinical Nutrition* 72: 1223–1231.

McCullough, M. L., D. Feskanich, M. J. Stampfer, E. L. Giovannucci, E. B. Rimm, F. B. Hu, D. Spiegelman, D. J. Hunter, G. A. Colditz, and W. C. Willett. 2002. Diet quality and major chronic disease risk in men and women: Moving toward improved dietary guidance. *American Journal of Clinical Nutrition* 76: 1261–1271.

Mead, A., G. Atkinson, D. Albin, D. Alphey, S. Baic, O. Boyd, L. Cadigan et al. 2006. Dietetic guidelines on food and nutrition in the secondary prevention of cardiovascular disease—Evidence from systematic reviews of randomized controlled trials. *Journal of Human Nutrition and Dietetics* 19: 401–419.

Mellen, P. B., T. F. Walsh, and D. M. Herrington. 2008. Whole grain intake and cardiovascular disease: A meta-analysis. *Nutrition, Metabolism, and Cardiovascular Diseases* 18: 283–290.

Michels, K. B. and M. B. Schulze. 2005. Can dietary patterns help us detect diet-disease associations? *Nutrition Research Reviews* 18: 241–248.

Nettleton, J. A., J. F. Polak, R. Tracy, G. L. Burke, and D. R. Jacobs Jr. 2008. Dietary patterns and incident cardiovascular disease in the multi-ethnic study of atherosclerosis. *American Journal of Clinical Nutrition* 90: 647–654.

Nordmann, A. J., A. Nordmann, M. Briel, U. Keller, W. S. Yancy Jr., B. J. Brehm, and H. C. Bucher. 2006. Effects of low-carbohydrate vs low-fat diets on weight loss and cardiovascular risk factors: A meta-analysis of randomized controlled trials. *Archives of Internal Medicine* 166: 285–293.

Nordmann, A. J., K. Suter-Zimmermann, H. C. Bucher, I. Shai, K. R. Tuttle, R. Estruch, and M. Briel. 2011. Meta-analysis comparing Mediterranean to low-fat diets for modification of cardiovascular risk factors. *American Journal of Medicine* 124: 841–851.e2.

Oude Griep, L. M., J. M. Geleijnse, D. Kromhout, M. C. Ocke, and W. M. Verschuren. 2010. Raw and processed fruit and vegetable consumption and 10-year coronary heart disease incidence in a population-based cohort study in the Netherlands. *PLoS ONE* 5(10): e13609.

Rouse, I. L., L. J. Beilin, B. K. Armstrong, and R. Vandongen. 1983. Blood-pressure-lowering effect of a vegetarian diet: Controlled trial in normotensive subjects. *Lancet* 1: 5–10.

Sacks, F. M., L. P. Svetkey, W. M. Vollmer, L. J. Appel, G. A. Bray, D. Harsha, E. Obarzanek et al. 2001. Effects on blood pressure of reduced dietary sodium and the Dietary Approaches to Stop Hypertension (DASH) diet. DASH-sodium collaborative research group. *New England Journal of Medicine* 344: 3–10.

Salehi-Abargouei, A., Z. Maghsoudi, F. Shirani, and L. Azadbakht. 2013. Effects of Dietary Approaches to Stop Hypertension (DASH)-style diet on fatal or nonfatal cardiovascular diseases-incidence: A systematic review and meta-analysis of observational prospective studies. *Nutrition* 29: 611–618.

Santos, F. L., S. S. Esteves, A. da Costa Pereira, W. S. Yancy Jr., and J. P. Nunes. 2012. Systematic review and meta-analysis of clinical trials of the effects of low carbohydrate diets on cardiovascular risk factors. *Obesity Reviews* 13: 1048–1066.

Shai, I., D. Schwarzfuchs, Y. Henkin, D. R. Shahar, S. Witkow, I. Greenberg, R. Golan et al. 2008. Weight loss with a low-carbohydrate, Mediterranean, or low-fat diet. *New England Journal of Medicine* 359: 229–241.

Sofi, F., R. Abbate, G. F. Gensini, and A. Casini. 2010. Accruing evidence on benefits of adherence to the Mediterranean diet on health: An updated systematic review and meta-analysis. *American Journal of Clinical Nutrition* 92: 1189–1196.

Sofi, F., F. Cesari, R. Abbate, G. F. Gensini, and A. Casini. 2008. Adherence to Mediterranean diet and health status: Meta-analysis. *British Medical Journal* 337: a1344.

Sofi, F., C. Macchi, R. Abbate, G. F. Gensini, and A. Casini. 2014. Mediterranean diet and health status: An updated meta-analysis and a proposal for a literature-based adherence score. *Public Health Nutrition* 17: 2769–2782.

Tay, J., N. D. Luscombe-Marsh, C. H. Thompson, M. Noakes, J. D. Buckley, G. A. Wittert, W. S. Yancy Jr., and G. D. Brinkworth. 2014. A very low carbohydrate, low saturated fat diet for type 2 diabetes management: A randomized trial. *Diabetes Care* 37: 2909–2918.

Trichopoulou, A., T. Costacou, C. Bamia, and D. Trichopoulos. 2003. Adherence to a Mediterranean diet and survival in a Greek population. *New England Journal of Medicine* 348: 2599–2608.

Trichopoulou, A., A. Kouris-Blazos, M. L. Wahlqvist, C. Gnardellis, P. Lagiou, E. Polychronopoulos, T. Vassilakou, L. Lipworth, and D. Trichopoulos. 1995. Diet and overall survival in elderly people. *British Medical Journal* 311: 1457–1460.

Tuttle, K. R., L. A. Shuler, D. P. Packard, J. E. Milton, K. B. Daratha, D. M. Bibus, and R. A. Short. 2008. Comparison of low-fat versus Mediterranean-style dietary intervention after first myocardial infarction (from the Heart Institute of Spokane Diet Intervention and Evaluation Trial). *American Journal of Cardiology* 101: 1523–1530.

Waijers, P. M., E. J. Feskens, and M. C.Ocke. 2007. A critical review of predefined diet quality scores. *British Journal of Nutrition* 97: 219–231.

Westman, E. C., W. S. Yancy, J. S. Edman, K. F. Tomlin, and C. E. Perkins. 2002. Effect of a 6-month adherence to a very low carbohydrate program. *American Journal of Medicine* 113: 30–36.

Westman, E. C., R. D. Feinman, J. C. Mavropoulos, M. C. Vernon, J. S. Volek, J. A. Wortman, W. S. Yancy, and S. D. Phinney. 2007. Low-carbohydrate nutrition and metabolism. *American Journal of Clinical Nutrition* 86: 276–284.

Woo, K. S., P. Chook, L. L. Chan, A. S. Cheung, W. H. Fung, Mu Qiao, Y. I. Lolin et al. 2002. Long-term improvement in homocysteine levels and arterial endothelial function after 1-year folic acid supplementation. *The American Journal of Medicine* 112: 535–539.

World Health Organisation. 2011. *Cardiovascular Diseases (CVDs)*. World Health Organisation Media Centre, Geneva, Switzerland.

Wycherley, T. P., G. D. Brinkworth, J. B. Keogh, M. Noakes, J. D. Buckley, and P. M. Clifton. 2010. Long-term effects of weight loss with a very low carbohydrate and low fat diet on vascular function in overweight and obese patients. *Journal of Internal Medicine* 267: 452–461.

Wylie-Rosett, J. and N. J. Davis. 2009. Low-carbohydrate diets: An update on current research. *Current Diabetes Reports* 9: 396–404.

Yancy, W. S. Jr., M. K. Olsen, J. R. Guyton, R. P. Bakst, and E. C. Westman. 2004. A low-carbohydrate, ketogenic diet versus a low-fat diet to treat obesity and hyperlipidemia: A randomized, controlled trial. *Annals of Internal Medicine*140: 769–777.

Section IV

Arthritis, Inflammation, and Joint Disorders

11 Review on the Efficacy of Probiotics in the Treatment of Rheumatic Diseases

Elnaz Vaghef-Mehrabany and Leila Vaghef-Mehrabany

CONTENTS

11.1 INTRODUCTION

Rheumatic diseases, representing more than a hundred distinct musculoskeletal diseases and syndromes, are a major health concern and the principal cause of physical disability worldwide, imposing remarkable economic burden on the governments. It is estimated that 20% of the population is affected by rheumatic diseases, with older adults and women suffering the most. Pain and stiffness are the commonest symptoms of rheumatic diseases; many extra-articular features including fever, fatigue, weakness, and eye and pulmonary symptoms may also accompany the musculoskeletal discomforts (Kavanaugh 2007, Klippel et al. 2008, Arend and Lawry 2008, Kool 2011). Most therapies for these patients are not disease specific and result in many undesirable health consequences; gastrointestinal complications and nephrotoxicity follow long-term use of nonsteroidal anti-inflammatory drugs (NSAIDs); osteoporosis, adrenal insufficiency, cataract, skin atrophy, peptic ulcers, and infection are some of the well-known adverse effects for glucocorticoids; and liver toxicity and suppressed immune system, which predispose the patient to infections and malignancies, are documented side effects of disease-modifying antirheumatic drugs (DMARDs; Grove et al. 2001, Quan et al. 2008). Thus, it is a necessity to investigate new drugs and nutritional supplements for more efficient control of these debilitating disorders.

In 2002, FAO/WHO defined probiotics as "live microorganisms which, when administered in adequate amounts, confer a health benefit on the host" (Anonymous 2002). It is believed that a probiotic product should contain $\geq 10^6$–10^8 colony-forming units (CFU)/g or $\geq 10^8$–10^{10} CFU/day of viable cells; however, no precise cell count has been established to guarantee a particular health effect thus far (Champagne et al. 2011). Probiotics have been reported to help patients with a variety of disorders including gastrointestinal discomforts (Briand et al. 2006, Mcfarland 2006, Allen et al. 2010, Chitapanarux et al. 2010), lactose maldigestion (Mustapha et al. 1997), obesity, hyperlipidemia, and hypertension (Pickup 2004, Lye et al. 2009, Ley 2010, Musso et al. 2010). Regulation of immune system function is among the most documented benefits of probiotic bacteria. Anticarcinogenic and antidiabetic effects of probiotics are proposed to be chiefly due to their immunoregulatory properties (Commane et al. 2005).

Human immune system is made up of two major arms: innate and adaptive immune system, each involving particular cells and molecules (Janeway et al. 2001, Haddad et al. 2005, Gill et al. 2009). A proper cooperation between innate and adaptive immune responses is crucial for the protection of the body against pathogenic microbes (bacteria, viruses, and parasites), autoimmunities, immunodeficiencies, and metabolic diseases. Gut-associated lymphoid tissue is the largest lymphoid tissue of the human body. It is primarily exposed to microbial antigens during the initial intestinal colonization, which begins at birth. The mode of birth and feeding, hygiene levels, and medication use influence the type of organisms colonizing the gut. Development of a functional and balanced immune system rests upon the stimuli provided by the commensal bacteria colonized in the intestines (Borchers et al. 2009).

Results of *in vitro* and *in vivo* studies have revealed that probiotics influence both local and systemic immune responses (Delcenserie et al. 2008). Both viable and nonviable probiotic bacteria affect immune system functions. This suggests that metabolic and secreted factors as well as structural or other cellular components may mediate some of the immunomodulatory activities of probiotics. Based on *in vitro* investigations, different probiotics influence immune responses in a strain-specific manner; some probiotics increase T-helper 1 (Th1) cytokines, which makes them good candidates for investigation and probable application in those suffering from immunodeficiencies as in acquired immune deficiency syndrome, and others increase T-helper 2 (Th2) cytokines, which allows them to be studied and, in case of confirmed benefits, administered to patients with autoimmunities like rheumatoid arthritis (RA), inflammatory bowel disease, or allergies. Variations in structure or secreted mediators may explain the specific effects of different probiotic strains on cytokine production patterns. Despite this, results of animal and human studies do not yet support one precise immune-regulatory effect for each probiotic strain. It is assumed that the interaction between the host's intestinal microbiota (which is unique to each person) and the administered probiotic bacteria affects the net influence of the probiotic therapy. Considering an appropriate dosage is also crucial to come up with the results expected (Weng and Walker 2006, Borchers et al. 2009). In a clinical trial by Gill et al. (2001), administration of lower doses was more effective than high doses in immune-related conditions.

Since a number of observational studies have shown gut microbiota alterations in some rheumatic diseases and have suggested a contributory role of these changes in the development or progression of the disease and due to the immune-regulatory effects of probiotics, great interest has aroused as to whether or not probiotics can be safely prescribed as complementary drugs or supplements to rheumatic patients. Only a limited number of *in vitro* and *in vivo* studies have been conducted in an attempt to tackle this question. Details on the results of the relevant studies are presented in the upcoming sections.

11.2 PROBIOTICS IN SYSTEMIC RHEUMATIC DISEASES

11.2.1 Rheumatoid Arthritis

RA is an autoimmune disease with a prevalence of 0.5%–1.0% of adults worldwide. Progressive joint disorder, great tenderness, and functional disability are the chief characteristics of RA. RA is of unknown etiology and primarily affects synovial tissues (O'Dell 2008, Zyrianova 2011). Genetic factors have been proposed to contribute to 50%–60% of RA risk (Tobon et al. 2010,

Firestein 2012). Several environmental factors including smoking, some specific bacteria and viruses (*Mycobacterium*, *Streptococcus*, *Mycoplasma*, *Escherichia coli*, *Helicobacter pylori*, *Rubella*, *Epstein–Barr* virus, and *Parvovirus*), and dietary factors may trigger the development of RA in genetically susceptible subjects (O'Dell 2008, Hagen et al. 2009, Tobon et al. 2010). NSAIDs, corticosteroids, and DMARDs (both synthetic and biologic) are the main therapies for RA (O'Dell 2004).

11.2.1.1 Gut Microbiota and Rheumatoid Arthritis

A number of human studies have reported that gut microbiota is altered in RA patients (McCulloch et al. 1993, Eerola et al. 1994, Malin et al. 1996, Peltonen et al. 1997). A higher carriage rate of *Clostridium perfringens* has been found in those suffering from RA (Shinebaum et al. 1987). It was in the late 1970s when, for the first time, germ-free rats were shown to be greatly susceptible to the development of RA, while those raised under conventional conditions had mild disease and a lower incidence in an adjuvant-induced arthritis model. The use of *gnotobiotic* animals (germ-free mice colonized with certain microbiota at specific stages of their life) also proposed a role of intestinal microbial communities in RA development (Scher and Abramson 2011). Bowel inflammation has been found to be complicated by joint inflammation in about 20% of the patients suffering from Crohn's disease and ulcerative colitis. Moreover, joint inflammation is provoked by bowel infection caused by enteropathogens such as *Salmonella* and *Yersinia* in these patients. Altered bowel anatomy, autoimmunity due to molecular mimicry, altered bowel permeability, and toxin-mediated synovitis are the possible mechanisms through which intestinal bacteria may have an impact on the initiation or propagation of the disease (Saarela et al. 2002).

11.2.1.2 Probiotics in the Treatment of Rheumatoid Arthritis

The effect of probiotic administration, in either prevention or the treatment of RA, has been investigated in a limited number of animal and human studies. The results are summarized in the following text.

11.2.1.2.1 Animal Studies

In a study conducted by Kato et al. (1998), mice to which collagen type II (CII) was injected (for experimental induction of RA) were given either an oral suspension of *L. casei* Shirota preparation (2×10^{11} CFU/g) or distilled water. The probiotic group showed a reduced incidence and development of RA; the level of serum antibody against CII was lesser in the treatment group as well. Moreover, the CII-specific IgG2a and IgG2b antibodies in serum were down-regulated, and the delayed-type hypersensitivity response was inhibited in the probiotic-receiving mice. Orally administered *L. casei* suppressed the CII-specific secretion of interferon-γ (IFN-γ) from splenocytes ex vivo.

Lewis rats injected bovine tropomyosin or complete Freund's adjuvant to induce tropomyosin arthritis or adjuvant arthritis (AA), respectively, were shown to have reduced arthritis clinical scores when administered with any commercial yogurt (fermented with 10^{11} CFU/L *L. bulgaricus*), live or killed LGG (10^8 CFU suspended in 1 mL sterile water), compared to the group who were fed milk (Baharav et al. 2004).

In another study, in which CII was used for RA induction, rats were treated with one of the following: (1) *L. casei* (2×10^{10} CFU, 500 mg/kg); (2) CII/Glu (type II collagen, 250 mg/kg; glucosamine (Gln), 250 mg/kg); (3) mixture (*L. casei*, 2×10^{10} CFU, 500 mg/kg; CII, 250 mg/kg; Gln, 250 mg/kg); (4) MTX (methotrexate, 300 μg/kg; two times per week); (5) control (1 mL PBS). Coadministration of *L. casei* with CII more effectively suppressed clinical symptoms, paw swelling, lymphocyte infiltration, and destruction of cartilage tissues of experimental arthritis than other treatments. This enhanced therapeutic efficacy was associated with an increase in anti-inflammatory cytokines (IL-10 and TGF-β) and decreased pro-inflammatory cytokines (IL-1β, IL-2, IL-6, IL-12, IL-17, IFN-γ, and TNF-α).

Coadministration of *L. casei* and CII suppressed CII-reactive T cell proliferation and the levels of Th1-type IgG2a and IgG2b effectively and up-regulated Foxp3 expression levels and the population of Foxp3$^+$ CD4$^+$ T cells (So et al. 2008a).

In another study conducted by the same team, oral administration of 5 × 10^9 CFU/day *L. casei* suppressed collagen-induced arthritis and reduced paw swelling, lymphocyte infiltration, and destruction of cartilage tissue in Lewis rats. *L. casei* administration reduced CII-reactive pro-inflammatory molecules (IL-1β, IL-2, IL-6, IL-12, IL-17, IFN-γ, tumor necrosis factor-α [TNF-α], and cyclooxygenase-2 [COX-2]) produced by CD4$^+$ T cells. *L. casei* administration also reduced the translocation of nuclear factor-κB (NF-κB) into nucleus and CII-reactive Th1-type IgG2a and IgG2b and increased immune-regulatory IL-10 levels (So et al. 2008b).

E. coli strain O83 (Colinfant), when administered in combination with methotrexate, significantly inhibited both inflammation and destructive arthritis-associated changes; the effects were not significantly different from those with methotrexate alone. The combination treatment inhibited both the hind paw swelling and arthrogram score remarkably, though not significantly greater than methotrexate alone. Treatment with the probiotic alone had no effect on AA in rats (Rovensky et al. 2009).

Amdekar et al. (2011) found that feeding Wistar rats with 2 × 10^8 CFU/mL *L. casei* ATCC334 in 500 μL distilled water led to normal histopathology without any synovial infiltration, pannus formation, and cartilage and bone destruction. Arthritis score was also lower for the group treated with *L. casei*. Oral administration of *L. casei* significantly decreased the pro-inflammatory cytokines as well.

11.2.1.2.2 Human Studies

To assess the effects of LGG on RA, 21 patients were recruited to receive either two probiotic capsules each containing ≥5 × 10^9 CFU of LGG or placebo capsules each day for a 12-month period. The results indicated that the mean number of tender and swollen joints had a greater decrease in the probiotic group than the placebo. Also, RA activity, according to global assessments, reduced more remarkably in the LGG group. However, none of these differences were significant. Serum IL-1β increased slightly in the probiotic group, but no differences were detected in the serum levels of IL-6, TNF-α, myeloperoxidase, IL-10, or IL-12. Although the probiotic supplementation showed no particular advantage for the RA patients, the authors reported that more subjects in the probiotic group reported subjective well-being (Hatakka et al. 2003).

Mandel et al. (2010) supplemented 45 RA patients with a daily probiotic caplet containing 2 × 10^9 CFU *Bacillus coagulans* GBI-30, green tea extract, methylsulfonylmethane, and vitamins and minerals (including vitamins A, B, C, D, E, folic acid, and selenium) or a matching placebo that contained microcrystalline cellulose for 60 days. Subjects in the probiotic group experienced improvement in their pain level according to the results obtained from Patient Pain Assessment score and Pain Scale. Compared to placebo, *B. coagulans* GBI-30 treatment resulted in greater improvement in self-assessed disability as assessed by Patient Global Assessment, reduction in C-reactive protein (CRP), as well as increased ability to walk 2 mi, reach, and participate in daily activities. No treatment-related adverse events were reported throughout this study. The effect of probiotic therapy on serum cytokines level was not assessed.

In another clinical trial conducted by Pineda et al. (2011), 29 patients were administered a daily probiotic capsule containing 2 × 10^9 CFU of *L. rhamnosus* GR-1 and *L. reuteri* RC-14 or a placebo containing the same inactive agents as the probiotic capsules (dextrose, potato starch, microcrystalline cellulose, and magnesium stearate). After 3 months of intervention, a significant improvement in the Health Assessment Questionnaire score was observed in the probiotic group. However, no significant between-group changes were reported. Twenty percent of the patients in the probiotic group and seven percent of those in the placebo group achieved an American College of Rheumatology 20 response; the difference between the two groups was insignificant though. The changes in the cytokine levels favored the placebo group over the probiotic.

In a recently performed study, the effects of probiotic supplementation were evaluated on disease symptoms, European league against rheumatism (EULAR) response, inflammatory biomarkers, and oxidative stress indices in women with RA. In a randomized, double-blind, placebo-controlled clinical trial, 46 RA patients were assigned into two groups: patients in the probiotic group received a daily capsule containing 10^8 (CFU) of *L. casei* 01 and those in the placebo group took identical capsules containing maltodextrin for 8 weeks. Serum high-sensitivity CRP (hs-CRP), tender and swollen joint counts, and disease activity score 28 decreased significantly only in the probiotic group, while global health score significantly decreased in both groups by the end of the study. The between-group differences were significant for all these parameters at the end of the study ($P < 0.05$). Regarding the EULAR criteria, a significant difference was found between the groups ($P < 0.01$). In the probiotic group, a significant reduction in serum levels of TNF-α and IL-12 and an increase in serum IL-10 were observed ($P < 0.05$). Also, a significant difference was found between the two groups for TNF-α, IL-6, IL-12, and IL-10 at the end of the study ($P < 0.05$). Superoxide dismutase activity decreased in the probiotic group and glutathione peroxidase activity decreased in both groups ($P < 0.05$). Although serum malondialdehyde was lower in the probiotic group and total antioxidant capacity was higher in the probiotic group as compared to the placebo by the end of the study course, no significant difference was observed between the groups for any of the measured indices ($P > 0.05$) (Vaghef-Mehrabany et al. 2014, 2015).

11.2.2 Gout

Gout is the commonest form of inflammatory arthritis that results from immunological responses to microcrystals of monosodium urate (MSU) deposited in and around the joints; deposition of MSU occurs when physiological saturation threshold for uric acid is exceeded in body fluids. Metatarsophalangeal joints are most affected by the disease; however, tarsal joints, ankles, knees, and wrists may be influenced as well (Suresh 2005, Roddy and Doherty 2010). Global prevalence of gout has been increasing since the last decades and was estimated to be 0.08% in 2010 (Smith et al. 2014). Physical manifestations of gout include redness, swelling, heat, tenderness, and global loss of movement (Suresh 2005). Hyperuricemia, genetic factors, dietary factors, alcohol consumption, metabolic syndrome, diuretic use, renal diseases, and osteoarthritis (OA) are among the most well-known risk factors for gout (Roddy and Doherty 2010). Aside from NSAIDs and corticosteroids, colchicine is a drug particularly administered to gout patients (Suresh 2005).

No animal studies or clinical trials have evaluated probiotic supplementation effects in gout disease thus far. However, considering the results of an animal study by Savcheniuk et al. (2014) might be relevant in this regard. In this study, monosodium glutamate (MSG) was used to induce obesity in newborn rats. MSG is found abundantly in natural foods and is applied as a food additive in industrially produced canned or semifinished products. Obesogenic properties of MSG have been investigated in many studies (Dolnikoff et al. 1988, Marmo et al. 1994, Hirata et al. 1997). It is noteworthy that MSG results in hyperuricemia and is discouraged for those suffering from gout. Following an altered glutamate catabolism in the body, liver overutilizes glutamine and overproduces uric acid (Pagliara and Goodman 1969, Gutman 1973). Savcheniuk et al. (2014) found that feeding the study rats with a probiotic mixture (*L. casei* IMVB-7280, *B. animalis* VKL, *B. animalis* VKB) at the dose of 5×10^9 CFU/kg (50 mg/kg) intragastrically could prevent obesity and lipid metabolism disorders in adulthood. With regard to the strong association between obesity and hyperuricemia (Li-Ying et al. 2007, Baldwin et al. 2011) and the causal role suggested by some studies for hyperuricemia in the incidence of obesity and metabolic syndrome (Masuo et al. 2003, Nakagawa et al. 2005), it is probable that probiotics have prevented extreme weight gain in the MSG-injected rats through prohibiting hyperuricemia. Unfortunately, serum uric acid levels were not evaluated in this study; thus, it is yet too soon to draw a definite conclusion about the probable benefits of probiotics for hyperuricemia and gout.

11.2.3 Sjögren's Syndrome

Sjögren's syndrome (SS) is a chronic autoimmune disease characterized by the malfunction of exocrine glands such as salivary and lacrimal glands. The estimated prevalence of SS is 0.5% among adults, when classified according to the American–European Consensus Criteria (Groom et al. 2002, Vitali et al. 2002, Bowman et al. 2004, Theander and Jacobsson 2005). The main symptoms of SS are dry mouth (xerostomia) and eyes (keratoconjunctivitis sicca), and lymphoproliferative malignancy is the most devastating consequence of the disease (Theander et al. 2006). The etiology of this inflammatory disorder remains unclear; genetic, hormonal, environmental (mainly infections), and other factors (such as birth weight) contribute to its pathogenesis (Delaleu et al. 2005, Jonsson et al. 2005, Mostafavi et al. 2005). Eye dryness is not efficiently alleviated by systemic treatments in SS patients; artificial tears may help with this problem (Bell et al. 1999).

Considering the antibacterial functions of saliva, xerostomia in SS can result in many oral difficulties including various infections (Mathews et al. 2008). Normal microbiota can protect oral cavity against pathogenic bacteria. Probiotics have been suggested to be efficacious in combating oral diseases by two means: fighting with the pathogens and reducing inflammation and tissue damages. By aggregating, competing for adhesion sides, nutrients, and growth factors, and producing antimicrobial agents like acids, probiotics eliminate the pathogenic bacteria off the mouth. Probiotics reduce inflammation in the mouth through enhancing production of IgA and defensins, decreasing MMP production, and decreasing pro-inflammatory cytokine release by the pathogens (Haukioja 2010). Although no clinical trials have investigated the probable positive effects of probiotic supplementation in SS patients, it is apparent that aside from systemic immune-regulatory effects of probiotics on the overall process of the disease, a local anti-infection effect can be expected for these useful microorganisms in the mouth. Developing probiotic chewing tablets or mouthwashes may be most beneficial if the latter is aimed.

11.2.4 Fibromyalgia

Fibromyalgia (FM) is a chronic musculoskeletal hypersensitivity with unknown etiology that affects approximately 2% of people in communities (Wolfe et al. 1995, Garcia-Campayo et al. 2008). The main symptoms of FM include benign widespread pain, muscle tenderness, sleep disturbances, fatigue, morning stiffness, and depressed mood (Mas et al. 2008, Garcia-Campayo et al. 2008). Abnormal pain processing in the central nervous system is believed to play a major role in the pathophysiology of FM; dysfunction in peripheral tissues may contribute to the disease to some extent as well (Abeles et al. 2007). Many pharmacologic and nonpharmacologic treatments are available for FM patients: NSAIDs, tricyclic antidepressants, other antidepressants including selective serotonin reuptake inhibitors, cyclobenzaprine, *S*-adenosylmethionine (SAM-e), and 5-hydroxytryptophan. These therapies only modestly alleviate the symptoms in a minority of patients (Tofferi et al. 2004). FM has overlapping symptoms with chronic fatigue syndrome (CFS), and patients with CFS usually fit the criteria for FM and vice versa; however, these diseases are not the same (Gantz and Coldsmith 2001).

Gut microbiota has a strong link with somatic hypersensitivity; 30%–75% of those with FM exert also inflammatory bowel syndrome (IBS) manifestations, and IBS patients generally report somatic hypersensitivity (Whitehead et al. 2002). Small intestine bacterial overgrowth (SIBO) is a common characteristic of both conditions and may contribute to the induction of hypersensitivity in the two diseases (Pimentel et al. 2004). Animal studies have shown that bacterial toxins can cause local inflammation and hypersensitivity, probably through increased production of prostaglandins and reduced nitrous oxide production (Kanaan et al. 1996, Tunctan et al. 2006). Also, lipopolysaccharides (LPS), a component of the outer layer of gram-negative bacteria, induced hypersensitivity in rats (Coelho et al. 2000). Probiotics may be helpful in treating SIBO and clearing the gut from the toxins and LPS of putrefactive gram-negative bacteria.

The results of a study in 121 patients with encephalomyelitis (ME)/CFS or CF found a significant positive correlation between IgA response to commensal bacterial LPS and inflammatory cytokines. In addition, higher inflammatory cytokine levels are significantly related to disease symptoms including fatigue and sadness. The study concluded that the disease activity in patients might be a result of increased translocation of commensal bacteria (Maes et al. 2012).

Two months of probiotic supplementation (24 million CFU of *L. casei* Shirota) in CFS patients significantly increased *lactobacilli* and *bifidobacteria* counts in stool samples and decreased anxiety symptoms (Rao et al. 2009). Whether colonization of gut with gram probiotic bacteria can help with the symptoms of FM is yet to be investigated.

11.2.5 Systemic Lupus Erythematosus

Systemic lupus erythematosus (SLE) is an inflammatory and multisystemic autoimmune disease resulting from immune-system-mediated tissue destruction (Danchenko et al. 2006). The prevalence of SLE is estimated to be 124/100,000 of Americans. Since all aspects of immune system are affected by SLE, the manifestations of the disease are so similar to those of microbial infections. Musculoskeletal, renal, cardiovascular, pulmonary, nervous, gastrointestinal, and hematologic systems as well as the skin are involved in SLE (Crow 2008). Genetic susceptibility along with environmental factors consisting of infections, hormones, smoking, alcohol consumption and contaminants, dietary factors like saturated fatty acids, and some drugs play a role in the pathogenesis of SLE (Cuchacovich and Gedalia 2009). Immune-suppressive agents, purine synthesis inhibitors, and methotrexate are some of the commonly prescribed treatments for SLE patients (Crow 2008).

Polyclonal B-cell activation, which results in increased production of antibodies, precedes SLE development in animal models. On the other hand, bacterial products like LPS might be effective in polyclonal B-cell activation (Klinman 1989, 1990). Measuring the resistance of gut to colonization of pathogenic bacteria in SLE patients in comparison with healthy individuals revealed that colonization resistance was significantly lower in the patients, which may lead to higher bacterial translocation across the gut in these subjects; some of these bacteria may serve as polyclonal B-cell activators (Apperloo-renkemal et al. 1994). Thus, a link between gut microbiota alterations and SLE initiation or propagation is most probable (Zhang and Reichlin 2008, Al-Salami et al. 2012). Some animal studies have come up with promising results regarding the effects of probiotics in treating SLE. Intraperitoneal injection of heat-killed *L. casei* prolonged life span in MRL/lpr mice, which develop an autoimmune disease similar to human SLE (Mike et al. 1999). Also, feeding probiotics to (NZB×NZW) F1 (BWF1) lupus-prone mice postponed lupus onset, decreased disease severity, and increased survival; increased percentage of CD4+Foxp3+ regulatory cells and IL-10 production was associated with the protection observed (Alard et al. 2009).

Well-designed clinical trials are warranted to confirm the results obtained from animal studies. Only then can probiotics be claimed efficient supplements in managing SLE.

11.2.6 Scleroderma (Systemic Sclerosis)

Systemic sclerosis (SSc) is a rare immune-mediated multisystem disease characterized by widespread vascular damage and progressive fibrosis of the skin and visceral organs (Kowal-Bielecka et al. 2013). The prevalence of scleroderma ranges from 7/million to 489/million with significant geographical differences (Bonifazi et al. 2013). The most common clinical manifestations of the disease are Reynaud's phenomenon (episodic color changes of the skin caused by cold exposure or anxiety), cutaneous fibrosis, gastrointestinal disorders, dyspnea, cardiac diseases, proteinuria, and musculoskeletal symptoms. Factors contributing to SSc development include autoimmune, genetic, hormonal, and environmental issues (Wigley 2008). Since universal disease-modifying therapies are inefficient in treating SSc, organ-targeted therapy is used to manage the disease. Treatment of SSc-related vascular disease, immunosuppressive therapy, stem cell transplantation, biological therapies, and kinase receptor inhibitors are some of the most recently used strategies used to treat SSc (Kowal-Bielecka et al. 2013).

Although there is no evidence on the probable role of gut microbiota changes in the pathogenesis of SSc, studies suggest that this inflammatory diseases is followed by SIBO (Madrid et al. 2002, Marie et al. 2009), which may be responsible for some gastrointestinal symptoms of SSc patients including dysphagia (Singh and Toskes 2003). Probiotics have been shown to be beneficial in the case of SIBO in animal studies. The probable mechanisms include barrier-enhancing, antibacterial, immune-modulating, and anti-inflammatory effects. However, these benefits need to be investigated and confirmed in human studies (Quigley and Quera 2006). The results of a study in which 22 patients with SIBO and chronic diarrhea were supplemented with two *lactobacilli* strains proposed that only prolonged courses of probiotic use may be beneficial in the treatment of SIBO (Gaon et al. 2002).

Gastrointestinal manifestations of SSc particularly its motility abnormalities are believed to result from autonomic nerve dysfunction (Cerinic et al. 1996, Straub et al. 1996, Lock et al. 1998, Malandrini et al. 2000, Iovino et al. 2001). To manage incontinence of stool, a common condition due to bowel and sphincter's dysfunction, it is essential that constipation–diarrhea cycle be prohibited; probiotic administration may help with this issue (Shah and Wigley 2013). Moreover, in a clinical trial carried out in SSc patients, reflux and bloating/distention were revealed to decrease significantly after 2 months of probiotic supplementation (Frech et al. 2011). To encourage regular use of probiotics to SSc patients, the current evidence needs to be strengthened by further clinical trials.

11.3 PROBIOTICS IN NONSYSTEMIC RHEUMATIC DISEASES

11.3.1 Osteoarthritis

OA, a progressive rheumatic disease with high prevalence, is the major cause of disability in the elderly people (Peat et al. 2001, Srikanth et al. 2005). About 15% of the world's adult population suffers joint pain and disability resulting from OA (Felson 1995). In the United States, approximately 6% of adults 30 years of age or older are affected by symptomatic disease in the knee; symptomatic hip OA occurs in nearly 3% (Felson and Zhang 1998). The chief symptoms of OA are joint pain, stiffness, and limitation of movement. This rheumatic disease develops slowly but can eventually lead to joint failure. The major risk factors of OA include age, gender, ethnicity and race, nutritional factors, osteoporosis, smoking, obesity and metabolic diseases, sarcopenia, and local mechanical risk factors (Cooper et al. 2013). Aside from drug therapies including non-opioid analgesics, NSAIDs, topical analgesics, opioid analgesics, and intra-articular steroid injection, physiotherapy and antidepressants as well as patient education are used to treat OA. Herbal medicine is also getting popular among the OA patients and has been shown to be safe and usually effective in alleviating the symptoms (Long et al. 2001).

Although inflammation is usually assumed to follow OA than precede its occurrence, some researchers suggest that inflammation may have a contributory role. Obesity, a major risk factor for OA, and its association with inflammation may help explain this. Population studies have revealed that OA risk rises by 9%–13% for each kilogram of body mass increase (Hart and Spector 1993), and a 5 kg body weight decrease reduces OA incidence by 50% (Felson et al. 1992). Obesity is also associated with OA progression, especially in those who gained weight after being diagnosed with the disease (Cooper et al. 2000). Obesity, being interrelated with compromised gut mucosa, translocation of microbiota, and increased serum LPS, has been demonstrated to result in metabolic endotoxemia and chronic low-grade inflammation (Ley et al. 2005, Brun et al. 2007, Cani et al. 2007, Lira et al. 2010, Sun et al. 2010). On the other hand, inflammatory mediators have been shown to disrupt articular cartilage in some *in vitro* studies (Attur et al. 1998, Distel et al. 2009). Endotoxins may trigger OA by the activation of macrophages in the synovial fluid, via toll-like receptor-4 (TLR-4) (Metcalfe et al. 2012).

An animal study investigated the effects of *L. casei* supplementation on pathological and inflammatory responses of OA rats. OA was induced by monosodium iodoacetate (MIA) injection in the animals. *L. casei* alone or together with CII and Gln was orally administered to the rats, beginning from 14 days prior to MIA injection and was continued for 8 weeks. Coadministration of *L. casei* with CII/Gln significantly decreased pain, cartilage destruction, and lymphocyte infiltration. Moreover, expression of several pro-inflammatory cytokines (IL-1β, IL-2, IL-6, IL-12, IL-17, TNF-α, and IFN-γ) and metalloproteinases (MMP1, MMP3, and MMP13) was reduced while anti-inflammatory cytokine (IL-4 and IL-10) levels were increased by the treatment. The effects observed for *L. casei* in combination with CII/Gln were significantly greater than *L. casei* or Gln alone (So et al. 2011). In a nonblind clinical trial conducted by Coulson et al. (2013), green-lipped mussel (GLM) and glucosamine sulfate (GS) caused a moderate decrease in *Clostridium* and *Staphylococcus* species and increase in *Lactobacillus*, *Streptococcus*, and *Eubacterium* species in the gastrointestinal tract of OA patients. The authors suggested that nutritional supplements like GLM and GS may regulate some of the metabolic and immunological activities of the gut microbiota (Coulson et al. 2013); this may be in part responsible for the therapeutic effects of these supplements (Laverty et al. 2005).

Due to their antiobesity effects reported by many studies (Kadooka et al. 2010, Chang et al. 2011, Jung et al. 2013, Sharafedtinov et al. 2013) and anti-inflammatory properties, probiotics may be profitable for OA patients. Animal studies and clinical studies directly performed in OA patients are required to draw definite conclusion though.

11.3.2 Bursitis and Tendonitis

Bursitis is the inflammation of bursae of synovial fluid in the body. Trauma, autoimmune disorders, infections, and iatrogenic etiologies can all lead to bursitis. The major symptoms are local warmth and erythema, joint pain, and stiffness. Ice, elevation, physiotherapy, anti-inflammatory drugs, and pain-relieving medications are used to treat noninfectious bursitis; antibiotic therapy is also applied in the case of infectious bursitis (Vigorita and Ghelman 1999).

Tendinitis (also tendonitis), meaning inflammation of a tendon, is accompanied with inflammatory symptoms including pain and redness; these symptoms are proportional to vascular disruption, hematoma, or atrophy-related cell necrosis. Repetitive use of the joints in endurance activities and abnormal stresses and loads on soft tissues are two of the main contributing factors to tendon overuse injuries (Giffin and Stanish 1993). Treatment of tendonitis includes the use of NSAIDs, rest, and gradual return to exercise (Wilson and Best 2005).

There is no evidence on probable alterations of gut microbiota in bursitis or tendonitis patients; no animal studies and clinical trials have been conducted to investigate the effects of probiotic supplementation in these two conditions either. Although inflammation occurs as a secondary event and affects only the injured areas of the body, it may be possible that probiotics reduce pain by affecting immune responses systemically.

11.4 CONCLUSION AND FUTURE TRENDS

Gut microbiota has been shown to be altered in some rheumatic diseases, particularly systemic ones. These microbial changes may be either the cause or the consequence of the disease; a few studies have suggested a contributory role of these changes in the pathogenesis of a number of rheumatic diseases. Probiotics have exerted favorable results in some clinical trials; these positive effects are largely attributed to their immune-regulatory properties.

With regard to the relatively small number of studies performed in this field, it is yet too soon to consider probiotics as adjunct therapy in the treatment of all rheumatic diseases. However, due to beneficial effects of probiotics in the improvement of some metabolic abnormalities, which may follow many of the rheumatic diseases and the common therapies used by them, it may be wise to recommend the patients to consume probiotic foods, to increase their overall health (Homayouni-Rad et al. 2015).

It is suggested that future studies aim toward the identification of possible gut microbiota changes of rheumatic patients in comparison to healthy subjects, selection of efficient probiotic strains based on evidence, and investigation of their effects in different dosages and vehicles (foods vs. supplements), in various rheumatic diseases.

REFERENCES

Abeles, A.M., Pillinger, M.H., Solitar, B.M., and Abeles, M. 2007. Narrative review: The pathophysiology of fibromyalgia. *Annals of Internal Medicine* 146:726–734.

Alard, P., Parnell, S., Manirarora, J., Kosiewicz, M., and Atay, S. 2009. Probiotics control lupus progression via induction of regulatory cells and IL-10 production. *The Journal of Immunology* 182: 50.30 (Meeting Abstract Supplement).

Allen, S.J., Martinez, E.G., Gregorio, G.V., and Dans, L.F. 2010. Probiotics for treating acute infectious diarrhea. *The Cochrane Library* 11:1–124.

Al-Salami, H., Caccetta, R., Golocorbin-Kon, S., and Mikov, M. 2012. Probiotics applications in autoimmune diseases. In: Rigobelo, E.C. (ed.), *Probiotics*, pp. 325–366. Rijeka, Croatia: Intech.

Amdekar, S., Singh, V., Singh, R., Sharma, P., Keshav, P., and Kumar, A. 2011. *Lactobacillus casei* reduces the inflammatory joint damage associated with collagen-induced arthritis (CIA) by reducing the pro-inflammatory cytokines. *Journal of Clinical Immunology* 31(2):147–154.

Anonymous. 2002. Guidelines for the evaluation of probiotics in food. Food and Agriculture Organization of the United Nations and World Health Organization Expert Consultation Report. pp. 1–11. http://www.who.int/foodsafety/publications/fs_management/probiotics2/en (accessed January 05, 2012).

Apperloo-renkemal, H.Z., Bootsma, H., Mulder, B.I., Kallenberg, C.G., and Van Der Waajj, D. 1994. Host-microflora interaction in systemic lupus erythematosus (SLE): Colonization resistance of the indigenous bacteria of the intestinal tract. *Epidemiology and Infection* 112:367–373.

Arend, W.P. and Lawry, G.V. 2008. Rheumatic disease. In: Goldman, L. and Ausiello, D. (eds.), *Cecil Medicine*, pp. 1963–1975. Philadelphia, PA: Saunders.

Attur, M.G., Patel, I.R., Patel, R.N., Abramson, S.B., and Amin, A.R. 1998. Autocrine production of IL-1β by human osteoarthritis-affected cartilage and differential regulation of endogenous nitric oxide, IL-6, prostaglandin E2, and IL-8. *Proceedings of the Association of American Physicians* 110:65–72.

Baharav, E., Mor, F., Halpern, M., and Winberger, A. 2004. *Lactobacillus GG* bacteria ameliorate arthritis in lewis rats. *The Journal of Nutrition* 134(8):1964–1969.

Baldwin, W., McRae, S., Marek, G., Wymer, D., Pannu, V., Baylis, C. et al. 2011. Hyperuricemia as a mediator of the proinflammatory endocrine imbalance in the adipose tissue in a murine model of the metabolic syndrome. *Diabetes* 60:1258–1269.

Bell, M., Askari, A., Bookman, A., Frydrych, S., Lamont, J., McComb, J. et al. 1999. Sjögren's syndrome: A critical review of clinical management. *The Journal of Rheumatology* 26:2051–2061.

Bonifazi, M., Tramacere, I., Pomponio, G., Gabrielli, B., Avvedimento, E.V., La Vecchia, C. et al. 2013. Systemic sclerosis (scleroderma) and cancer risk: Systematic review and meta-analysis of observational studies. *Rheumatology* 52:143–154.

Borchers, A.T., Selmi, C., Meyers, F.J., Keen, C.L., and Gershwin, M.E. 2009. Probiotics and immunity. *Journal of Gastroenterology* 44(1):26–46.

Bowman, S.J., Ibrahim, G.H, Holmes, G., Hamburger, J., and Ainsworth, J.R. 2004. Estimating the prevalence among Caucasian women of primary Sjögren's syndrome in two general practices in Birmingham, UK. *Scandinavian Journal of Rheumatology* 33:39–43.

Briand, V., Buffet, P., Genty, S., Lacombe, K., Godineau, N., Salomon, J. et al. 2006. Absence of efficacy of nonviable *Lactobacillus acidophilus* for the prevention of traveler's diarrhea: A randomized, double-blind, controlled study. *Clinical Infectious Diseases* 43(9):1170–1175.

Brun, P., Castagliuolo, I., Di Leo, V., Buda, A., Pinzani, M., Palu, G. et al. 2007. Increased intestinal permeability in obese mice: New evidence in the pathogenesis of nonalcoholic steatohepatitis. *The American Journal of Physiology-Gastrointestinal and Liver Physiology* 292: 518–525.

Cani, P.D., Amar, J., Iglesias, M.A., Poggi, M., Knauf, C., Bastelica, D. et al. 2007. Metabolic endotoxemia initiates obesity and insulin resistance. *Diabetes* 56:1761–1772.

Cerinic, M.M., Generini, S., Pignone, A., and Casale, R. 1996. The nervous system in systemic sclerosis (scleroderma): Clinical features and pathogenetic mechanisms. *Rheumatic Disease Clinics of North America* 22:879–892.

Champagne, C.P., Ross, R.P., Saarela, M., Hansen, K.F., and Charalampopoulos, D. 2011. Recommendations for the viability assessment of probiotics as concentrated cultures and in food matrices. *International Journal of Food Microbiology* 149(3):185–193.

Chang, B.J., Park, S.U., Jang, Y.S., Ko, S.H., Joo, N.M., Kim, S.I. et al. 2011. Effect of functional yogurt NY-YP901 in improving the trait of metabolic syndrome. *European Journal of Clinical Nutrition* 65:1250–1255.

Chitapanarux, I., Chitapanarux, T., Traisathit, P., Kudumpee, S., Tharavichitkul, E., and Lorvidhaya, V. 2010. Randomized controlled trial of live *Lactobacillus acidophilus* plus *Bifidobacterium bifidum* in prophylaxis of diarrhea during radiotherapy in cervical cancer patients. *Radiation Oncology* 5:31–36.

Coelho, A.M., Fioramonti, J., and Bueno, L. 2000. Systemic lipopolysaccharide influences rectal hypersensitivity in rats: Role of mast cells, cytokines, and vagus nerve. *American Journal of Physiology-Gastrointestinal and Liver Physiology* 279:781–790.

Commane, D., Hughes, R., Shortt, C., and Rowland, I. 2005. The potential mechanisms involved in the anticarcinogenic action of probiotics. *Mutation Research* 591(1–2):276–289.

Cooper, C., Denni son, E., Edwards, M., and Litwic, A. 2013. Epidemiology of osteoarthritis. *Medicographia* 35:145–151.

Cooper, C., Snow, S., McAlindon, T.E., Kellingray, S.,Stuart, B., Coggon, D. et al. 2000. Risk factors for the incidence and progression of radiographic knee osteoarthritis. *Arthritis and Rheumatism* 43:995–1000.

Coulson, S., Butt, H., Vecchio, P., Gramotnev, H., and Vitetta, L. 2013. Green-lipped mussel extract (*Perna canaliculus*) and glucosamine sulphate in patients with knee osteoarthritis: Therapeutic efficacy and effects on gastrointestinal microbiota profiles. *Inflammopharmacology* 21(1):79–90.

Crow, M.K. 2008. Systemic lupus erythematosus. In: Goldman, L. and Ausiello, D. (eds.), *Cecil Medicine*, pp. 2022–2032. Philadelphia, PA: Saunders.

Cuchacovich, R. and Gedalia, A. 2009. Pathophysiology and clinical spectrum of infections in systemic lupus erythematosus. *Rheumatic Diseases Clinics of North America*. 35(1):75–93.

Danchenko, N., Satia, J.A., and Anthony, M.S. 2006. Epidemiology of systemic lupus erythematosus: A comparison of worldwide disease burden. *Lupus* 15:308–318.

Delaleu, N., Jonsson, R., and Koller, M.M. 2005. Sjögren's syndrome. *European Journal of Oral Sciences* 113:101–113.

Delcenserie, V., Martel, D., Lamoureux, M., Amiot, J., Boutin, Y., and Roy, D. 2008. Immunomodulatory effects of probiotics in the intestinal tract. *Current Issues in Molecular Biology* 10:37–54.

Distel, E., Cadoudal, T., Durant, S., Poignard, A., Chevalier, X., and Benelli, C. 2009. The infrapatellar fat pad in knee osteoarthritis: An important source of interleukin-6 and its soluble receptor. *Arthritis and Rheumatism* 60:3374–3377.

Dolnikoff, M.S., Kater, C.E., Egami, M., Andrade, I.S., and Marmo, M.R. 1988. Neonatal treatment with monosodium glutamate increases plasma corticosterone in the rat. *Neuroendocrinology* 48:645–649.

Eerola, E., Mottonen, T., Hannonen, P., Luukkainen, R., Kantola, I., Vuori, K. et al. 1994. Intestinal flora in early rheumatoid arthritis. *British Journal of Rheumatology* 33(11):1030–1038.

Felson, D.T. 1995. The epidemiology of osteoarthritis: Prevalence and risk factors. In: Kuettner, K.E. and Goldberg, V.M. (eds.), *Osteoarthritis Disorders*, pp. 13–24. Rosemont, IL: American Academy of Orthopaedic Surgeons.

Felson, D.T. and Zhang, Y. 1998. An update on the epidemiology of knee and hip osteoarthritis with a view to prevention. *Arthritis and Rheumatism* 41:1343–1355.

Felson, D.T., Zhang, Y., Anthony, J.M., Naimark, A., and Anderson, J.J. 1992. Weight loss reduces the risk for symptomatic knee osteoarthritis in women. The Framingham Study. *Annals of Internal Medicine* 116:535–539.

Firestein, G.S. 2012. Etiology and pathogenesis of rheumatoid arthritis. In: Firestein, G.S., Budd, R., Gabriel, S., McInnes, I., and O'Dell, J. (eds.), *Kelley's Textbook of Rheumatology*, p. 1035. St. Louis, MO: Saunders.

Frech, T.M., Khanna, D., Maranian, P., Frech, E.J., Sawitzke, A.D., and Murtaugh, M.A. 2011. Probiotics for the treatment of systemic sclerosis-associated gastrointestinal bloating/distention. *Clinical and Experimental Rheumatology* 29 (Suppl.65):S22–S25.

Gantz, N.M. and Coldsmith, E.E. 2001. Chronic fatigue syndrome and fibromyalgia resources on the World Wide Web: A descriptive journey. *Clinical Infectious Diseases* 32:938–948.

Gaon, D., Garmendia, C., Murrielo, No., deCuccoGames, A., Cerchio, A., Quintas, R. et al. 2002. Effect of *Lactobacillus* strains (*L. casei* and *L. acidophilus* strains cereal) on bacterial overgrowth related chronic diarrhea. *Medicina (B Aires)* 62:159–163.

Garcia-Campayo, J., Magdalena, J., Magallón, R., Fernández-García, F., Salas, M., and Andrés, E. 2008. A meta-analysis of the efficacy of fibromyalgia treatment according to level of care. *Arthritis Research & Therapy* 10(4):81–96.

Giffin, J.R. and Stanish, N.D. 1993. Overuse tendonitis and rehabilitation. *Canadian Family Physician* 39:1762–1769.

Gill, H.S., Grover, S., Batish, V.K., and Gill, P. 2009. Immunological effects of probiotics and their significance to human health. In: Charalampopoulos, D. and Rastall, R.A. (eds.), *Prebiotics and Probiotics Science and Technology*, pp. 901–948. Berlin, Germany: Springer.

Gill, H.S., Rutherfurd, K.J., Cross, M.L., and Gopal, P.K. 2001. Enhancement of immunity in the elderly by dietary supplementation with the probiotic *Bifidobacterium lactis* HN019. *The American Journal of Clinical Nutrition* 74(5):833–839.

Groom, J., Kalled, S.L., Cutler, A.H., Olson, C., Woodcock, S.A., Schneider, P. et al. 2002. Association of BAFF/BLyS overexpression and altered B cell differentiation with Sjögren's syndrome. *The Journal of Clinical Investigation* 109:59–68.

Grove, M.L., Hassell, A.B., Hay, E.M., and Shadforth, M.F. 2001. Adverse reactions to disease-modifying anti-rheumatic drugs in clinical practice. *Quarterly Journal of Medicine* 94:309–319.

Gutman, A.B. 1973. The past four decades of progress in the knowledge of gout, with an assessment of the present status. *Arthritis and Rheumatism* 16(4):431–445.

Haddad, P.S., Azar, G.A., Groom, S., and Boivin, M. 2005. Natural health products, modulation of immune function and prevention of chronic diseases. *Evidence-Based Complementary and Alternative Medicine* 2(4):513–520.

Hagen, K.B., Byfuglien, M.G., Falzon, L., Olsen, S.U., and Smedslund, G. 2009. Dietary interventions for rheumatoid arthritis. *Cochrane Database Systematic Reviews* 1, CD006400.

Hart, D.J. and Spector, T.D. 1993. The relationship of obesity, fat distribution and osteoarthritis in women in the general population: The Chingford study. *The Journal of Rheumatology* 20:331–335.

Hatakka, K., Martio, J., Korpela, M., Poussa, T., Laasanen, T., Saxelin, M. et al. 2003. Effects of probiotic therapy on the activity and activation of mild rheumatoid arthritis—A pilot study. *Scandinavian Journal of Rheumatology* 32(4):211–215.

Haukioja, A. 2010. Probiotics and oral health. *European Journal of Dentistry* 4:348–355.

Hirata, A.E., Andrade, I.S., Vaskevicius, P., and Dolnikoff, M.S. 1997. Monosodium glutamate (MSG)-obese rats develop glucose intolerance and insulin resistance to peripheral glucose uptake. *Brazilian Journal of Medical and Biological Research* 30(5):671–674.

Homayouni-Rad, A., Vaghef-Mehrabany, E., Alipoor, B., and Vaghef-Mehrabany, L. 2015. The comparison of food and supplement as probiotic delivery vehicles. *Critical Reviews in Food Science and Nutrition*. DOI:10.1080/10408398.2012.733894.

Iovino, P., Valentini, G., Ciacci, C., De Luca, A., Tremolaterra, F., Sabbatini, F. et al. 2001. Proximal stomach function in systemic sclerosis: Relationship with autonomic nerve function. *Digestive Diseases and Sciences* 46:723–730.

Janeway, C.A., Travers, J.P., Walport, M., and Shlomchik, M.J. 2001 *Immunobiology, The Immune System in Health and Disease*, pp. 37–99. New York: Garland Science.

Jonsson, R., Bowman, S., and Gordon, T. 2005. Sjögren's syndrome. In: Koopman, W. and Moreland, L. (eds.), *Arthritis and Allied Conditions—A Textbook of Rheumatology*, pp. 1681–1705. Philadelphia, PA: Lippincott Williams & Wilkins.

Jung, S.P., Lee, K.M., Kang, J.H., Yun, S.I., Park, H.O., Moon, Y. et al. 2013. Effect of *Lactobacillus gasseri* BNR17 on overweight and obese adults: A randomized, double-blind clinical trial original article. *Korean Journal of Family Medicine* 34:80–39.

Kadooka, Y., Sato, M., Imaizumi, K., Ogawa, A., Ikuyama, K., Akai, Y. et al. 2010. Regulation of abdominal adiposity by probiotics (*lactobacillus gasseri* SBT2055) in adults with obese tendencies in a randomized controlled trial. *European Journal of Clinical Nutrition* 64:636–643.

Kanaan, S., Saade, N., Haddad, J., Abdelnoor, A.M., Atweh, S.F., Jabbur, S.J. et al. 1996. Endotoxin-induced local inflammation and hyperalgesia in rats and mice: A new model for inflammatory pain. *Pain* 66(2–3):373–379.

Kato, I., Endo-Tanaka, K., and Yokokura, T. 1998. Suppressive effects of the oral administration of *Lactobacillus casei* on type II collagen-induced arthritis in DBA/1 mice. *Life Sciences* 63(8):635–644.

Kavanaugh, A. 2007. Rheumatic diseases in the elderly: A "Perfect storm". *Rheumatic Disease Clinics of North America* 33(1):xi–xiii.

Klinman, D.M. 1989. Regulation of B cell activation in autoimmune mice. *Clinical Immunology and Immunopathology* 53:825–834.

Klinman, D.M. 1990. Polyclonal B cell activation in lupus-prone mice precedes and predicts the development of autoimmune disease. *The Journal of Clinical Investigation* 86:1249–1254.

Klippel, J.H., Stone, J.H., Crofford, L.J., and White, P.H. 2008. *Primer on the Rheumatic Diseases*. New York: Springer.

Kool, M. 2011. Understanding lack of understanding; Invalidation in rheumatic diseases. PhD disseration, de Universiteit Utrecht, Utrecht, the Netherlands.

Kowal-Bielecka, O., Bielecki, M., and Kowal, K. 2013. Recent advances in the diagnosis and treatment of systemic sclerosis. *Polskie Archiwum Medycyny Wewnętrznej* 123(1–2):51–58.

Laverty, S., Sandy, J., Celeste, C., Vachon, P., Marier, J., and Plaas, A. 2005. Synovial fluid levels and serum pharmacokinetics in a large animal model following treatment with oral glucosamine at clinically relevant doses. *Arthritis and Rheumatism* 52:181–191.

Ley, R.E. 2010. Obesity and the human microbiome. *Current Opinion in Gastroenterology* 26(1):5–11.

Ley, R.E., Backhed, F., Turnbaugh, P., Lozupone, C.A., Knight, R.D., and Gordon, J.I. 2005. Obesity alters gut microbial ecology. *Proceedings of the National Academy of Sciences of the United States of America* 102:11070–11075.

Lira, F.S., Rosa, J.C., Pimentel, G.D., Souza, H.A., Caperuto, E.C., Carnevali, L.C. Jr. et al. 2010. Endotoxin levels correlate positively with a sedentary lifestyle and negatively with highly trained subjects. *Lipids in Health and Disease* 9:82.

Li-Ying, C., Wen-hua, Z., Zhou-wen, Z., Hong-lei, D., Jing-jing, R., Jian-hua, C. et al. 2007. Relationship between hyperuricemia and metabolic syndrome. *Journal of Zhejiang University Science B* 8(8):593–598.

Lock, G., Straub, R.H., Zeuner, M., Antoniou, E., Holstege, A., Scholmerich, J. et al. 1998. Association of autonomic nervous dysfunction and esophageal dysmotility in systemic sclerosis. *The Journal of Rheumatology* 25:1330–1335.

Long, L., Soeken, K., and Ernst, E. 2001. Herbal medicine for the treatment of osteoarthritis: A systemic review. *Rheumatology* 40:779–793.

Lye, H.S., Kuan, C.Y., Ewe, J.A., Fung, W.Y., and Liong, M.T. 2009. The improvement of hypertension by probiotics: Effects on cholesterol, diabetes, renin and phytoestrogens. *International Journal of Dairy Sciences* 10(9):3755–3775.

Madrid, A.M., Soto, L., Defilippi, C., Cuchacovich, M., Defilippi, C.L., and Henriquez, A. 2002. Gastrointestinal motor involvement in scleroderma and its clinical correlation. *Acta Gastroenterol Latinoam* 13:381.

Maes, M., Twisk, F.N.M., Kubera, M., Ringel, K., Leunis, J.C., and Geffard, M. 2012. Increased IgA responses to the LPS of commensal bacteria is associated with inflammation and activation of cell-mediated immunity in chronic fatigue syndrome. *Journal of Affective Disorders* 136:909–917.

Malandrini, A., Selvi, E., Villanova, M., Berti, G., Sabadini, L., Salvadori, C. et al. 2000. Autonomic nervous system and smooth muscle cell involvement in systemic sclerosis: Ultrastructural study of 3 cases. *The Journal of Rheumatology* 27:1203–1206.

Malin, M., Verronen, P., Mykkänen, H., Salininen, S., and Isolauri, E. 1996. Increased bacterial urease activity in faeces in juvenile chronic arthritis: Evidence of altered intestinal microflora? *British Journal of Rheumatology* 35(7):689–694.

Mandel, D.R., Eichas, K., and Holmes, J. 2010. *Bacillus coagulans*: A viable adjunct therapy for relieving symptoms of rheumatoid arthritis according to a randomized, controlled trial. *Complementary and Alternative Medicine* 10:1–7.

Marie, I., Ducrotte, P., Denis, P., Menard, J.F.O., and Levesque, H. 2009. Small intestinal bacterial overgrowth in systemic sclerosis. *Rheumatology* 48:1314–1319.

Marmo, M.R., Dolnikoff, M.S., Kettelhut, I.C., Matsuchita, D.M., Hell, N.S., and Lima, F.B. 1994. Neonatal monosodium glutamate treatment increases epididymal adipose tissue sensitivity to insulin in three-month old rats. *Brazilian Journal of Medical and Biological Research* 27:1249–1253.

Mas, A.J., Carmona, L., Valverde, M., Ribas, B., and the EPISER Study Group. 2008. Prevalence and impact of fibromyalgia on function and quality of life in individuals from the general population: Results from a nationwide study in Spain. *Clinical and Experimental Rheumatology* 26:519–526.

Masuo, K., Kawaguchi, H., Mikami, H., Ogihara, T., and Tuck, M.L. 2003. Serum uric acid and plasma norepinephrine concentrations predict subsequent weight gain and blood pressure elevation. *Hypertension* 42:474–480.

Mathews, S.A., Kurien, B.T., and Scofield, R.H. 2008. Oral manifestations of Sjögren's syndrome. *Journal of Dental Research* 87(4):308–318.

McCulloch, J., Lydyard, P.M., and Rook, J.A.W. 1993. Rheumatoid arthritis: How well do the theories fit the evidence? *Clinical and Experimental Immunology* 92(1):1–6.

Mcfarland, L.V. 2006. Meta-analysis of probiotics for the prevention of antibiotic associated diarrhea and the treatment of *Clostridium difficile* disease. *The American Journal of Gastroenterology* 101(4):812–822.

Metcalfe, D., Harte, A.L., Aletrari, M.O., Al Daghri, N.M., Al Disi, D., Tripathi, G. et al. 2012. Does endotoxaemia contribute to osteoarthritis in obese patients? *Clinical Science* 123:627–634.

Mike, A., Nagaoka, N., Tagami, Y., Miyashita, M., Shimada, S., Uchida, K. et al. 1999. Prevention of B220+ T cell expansion and prolongation of lifespan induced by *Lactobacillus casei* in MRL/lpr mice. *Clinical and Experimental Immunology* 117:368–375.

Mostafavi, B., Akyuz, S., Jacobsson, M.E., Nilsen, L.V., Theander, E., and Jacobsson, L.H. 2005. Perinatal characteristics and risk of developing primary Sjögren's syndrome: A case-control study. *The Journal of Rheumatology* 32:665–668.

Musso, G., Gambino, R., and Cassader, M. 2010. Obesity, diabetes and gut microbiota: The hygiene hypothesis expanded? *Diabetes Care* 33(10):2277–2284.

Mustapha, A., Jiang, T., and Savaiano, D.A. 1997. Improvement of lactose digestion by humans following ingestion of unfermented acidophilus milk: Influence of bile sensitivity, lactose transport and acid tolerance of *Lactobacillus acidophilus*. *Journal of Dairy Science* 80(8):1537–1545.

Nakagawa, T., Tuttle, K.R., Short, R.A., and Johnson, R.J. 2005. Hypothesis: Fructose-induced hyperuricemia as a causal mechanism for the epidemic of the metabolic syndrome. *Nature Reviews Nephrology* 1:80–86.

O'Dell, J.R. 2004. Therapeutic strategies for rheumatoid arthritis. *The New England Journal of Medicine* 350(25):2591–2602.

O'Dell, J.R. 2008. Rheumatoid arthritis. In: Goldman, L. and Ausiello, D. (eds.), *Cecil Medicine*, pp. 2003–2011. Philadelphia, PA: Saunders.

Pagliara, A.S. and Goodman, A.D. 1969. Elevation of plasma glutamate in gout: Its possible role in the pathogenesis of hyperuricemia. *The New England Journal of Medicine* 281:767–770.

Peat, G., McCarney, R., and Croft, P. 2001. Knee pain and osteoarthritis in older adults: A review of community burden and current use of primary health care. *Annals of the Rheumatic Diseases* 60:91–97.

Peltonen, R., Nenonen, M., Helve, T., Hanninen, O., Toivanen, P., and Eerola, E. 1997. Faecal microbial flora and disease activity in rheumatoid arthritis during a vegan diet. *British Journal of Rheumatology* 36(1):64–68.

Pickup, J.C. 2004. Inflammation and activated innate immunity in the pathogenesis of type 2 diabetes. *Diabetes Care* 27(3):813–823.

Pimentel, M., Wallace, D., Hallegua, D., Chow, E., Kong, Y., Park, S. et al. 2004. A link between irritable bowel syndrome and fibromyalgia may be related to findings on lactulose breath testing. *Annals of the Rheumatic Diseases* 63(4):450–452.

Pineda, M.A., Thompson, S.F., Summers, K., Leon, F., Pope, J., and Reid, G. 2011. A randomized, double-blinded, placebo-controlled pilot study of probiotics in active rheumatoid arthritis. *Medical Science Monitor* 17(6):347–354.

Quan, L.D., Thiele, G.M., Tian, J., and Wang, D. 2008. The development of novel therapies for rheumatoid arthritis. *Expert Opinion on Therapeutic Patents* 18(7):723–738.

Quigley, E.M.M. and Quera, R. 2006. Small intestinal bacterial overgrowth: Roles of antibiotics, prebiotics, and probiotics. *Gastroenterology* 130:S78–S90.

Rao, A.V., Bested, A.C., Beaulne, T.M., Katzman, M.A., Iorio, C., Berardi, J.M. et al. 2009. A randomized, double-blind, placebo-controlled pilot study of a probiotic in emotional symptoms of chronic fatigue syndrome. *Gut Pathogens* 1:6–12.

Roddy, E. and Doherty, M. 2010. Epidemiology of gout. *Arthritis Research & Therapy* 12:223–234.

Rovensky, J., Stancikova, J., Svik, K., Uteseny, J., Bauerova, J., and Jurcovocova, J. 2009. Treatment of adjuvant-induced arthritis with the combination of methotrexate and probiotic bacteria *Escherichia coli* O83 (Colinfant®). *Folia Microbiology* 54(4):359–363.

Saarela, M., Lahteenmaki, L., Crittenden, R., Salminen, S., and Mattila-Sandholm, T. 2002. Gut bacteria and health foods—The European perspective. *International Journal of Food Microbiology* 78(1–2):99–117.

Savcheniuk, O.A., Virchenkol, O.V., Falalyeyeva, T.M., Beregova, T.V., Babenko, L.P., Lazarenko, L.M. et al. 2014. The efficacy of probiotics for monosodium glutamate-induced obesity: Dietology concerns and opportunities for prevention. *The EPMA Journal* 5(1):2. DOI:10.1186/1878-5085-5-2.

Scher, J.U. and Abramson, S.B. 2011. The microbiome and rheumatoid arthritis. *Nature Reviews Rheumatology* 7(10):569–578.

Shah, A.A. and Wigley, F.M. 2013. *My approach to the treatment of scleroderma. Mayo Clinic Proceedings* 88(4):377–393.

Sharafedtinov, K.K., Plotnikova, O.A., Alexeeva, R.I., Sentsova, T.B., Songisepp, E., Stsepetova, J. et al. 2013. Hypocaloric diet supplemented with probiotic cheese improves body mass index and blood pressure indices of obese hypertensive patients—A randomized double-blind placebo-controlled pilot study. *Nutrition Journal* 12:138–148.

Shinebaum, R., Neumann, V.C., Cooke, E.M., and Wright, V. 1987. Comparison of faecal flora in patients with rheumatoid arthritis and controls. *British Journal of Rheumatology* 26(5):329–333.

Singh, V.V. and Toskes, P.P. 2003. Small bowel bacterial overgrowth: Presentation, diagnosis, and treatment. *Current Gastroenterology Reports* 5:365–372.

Smith, E., Hoy, D., Cross, M., Merriman, T.R., Vos, T., Buchbinder, R. et al. 2014. The global burden of gout: Estimates from the Global Burden of Disease 2010 study. *Annals of the Rheumatic Diseases* 73(8):1462–1469.

So, J.S., Kwon, H.K., Lee, C.G., Yi, H.J., Park, J.A., Lim, S.Y. et al. 2008b. *Lactobacillus casei* suppresses experimental arthritis by down-regulating T helper 1effector functions. *Molecular Immunology* 45(9):2690–2699.

So, J.S., Lee, C.G., Kwon, H.K., Yi, H.J., Chae, C.S., Park, J.A. et al. 2008a. *Lactobacillus casei* potentiates induction of oral tolerance in experimental arthritis. *Molecular Immunology* 46(1):172–180.

So, J.S., Song, M.K., Kwon, H.K., Lee, C.G., Chae, C.S., Sahoo, A. et al. 2011. *Lactobacillus casei* enhances type II collagen/glucosamine-mediated suppression of inflammatory responses in experimental osteoarthritis. *Life Sciences* 88:358–366.

Srikanth, V.K., Fryer, J.L., Zhai, G., Winzenberg, T.M., Hosmer, D., and Jones, G. 2005. A meta-analysis of sex differences prevalence, incidence and severity of osteoarthritis. *Osteoarthritis and Cartilage* 13:769–781.

Straub, R.H., Zeuner, M., Lock, G., Rath, H., Hein, R., Scholmerich, J. et al. 1996. Autonomic and sensorimotor neuropathy in patients with systemic lupus erythematosus and systemic sclerosis. *The Journal of Rheumatology* 23:87–92.

Sun, Y., Sun, J., Wang, X., You, W., and Yang, M. 2010. Variants in the fat mass and obesity associated (FTO) gene are associated with obesity and C-reactive protein levels in Chinese Han populations. *Clinical and Investigative Medicine* 33:405–412.

Suresh, E. 2005. Diagnosis and management of gout: A rational approach. *Postgraduate Medical Journal* 81:572–579.

Theander, E., Henriksson, G., Ljungberg, O., Mandl, T., Manthorpe, R., and Jacobsson, L.T.H. 2006. Lymphoma and other malignancies in primary Sjögren's syndrome: A cohort study on cancer incidence and lymphoma predictors. *Annals of Rheumatic Diseases* 65:796–803.

Theander, E. and Jacobsson, L. 2005. Reply: Prevalence of primary SS. *Arthritis and Rheumatology* 52:369–370.

Tobon, G.J., Youinou, P., and Saraux, A. 2010. The environment, geo-epidemiology, and autoimmune disease: Rheumatoid arthritis. *Journal of Autoimmunity* 35(1):10–14.

Tofferi, J.K., Jackson, J.L., and O'malley, P.G. 2004. Treatment of fibromyalgia with cyclobenzaprine: A meta-analysis. *Arthritis & Rheumatism* 51(1):9–13.

Tunctan, B., Ozveren, E., Korkmaz, B., Buharalioglu, C.K., Tamer, L., Degirmenci, U. et al. 2006. Nitric oxide reverses endotoxin induced inflammatory hyperalgesia via inhibition of prostacyclin production in mice. *Pharmacological Research* 53(2):177–192.

Vaghef-Mehrabany, E., Alipour, B., Homayouni-Rad, A., Sharif, S.K., Asghari-Jafarabadi, M., and Zavvari, S. 2014a. Probiotic supplementation improves inflammatory status in patients with rheumatoid arthritis. *Nutrition* 30:430–435.

Vaghef-Mehrabany, E., Homayouni-Rad, A, Alipour, B., Sharif, S.K., Vaghef-Mehrabany, L., and Alipour-Ajiry, S. 2015. Effects of probiotic supplementation on oxidative stress indices in rheumatoid arthritis women: A randomized double-blind clinical trial. *Journal of the American College of Nutrition*. 9:1–9.

Vigorita, V.J. and Ghelman, B. 1999. *Orthopaedic Pathology*. Philadelphia, PA: Lippincott Williams & Wilkins.

Vitali, C., Bombardieri, S., Jonsson, R., Moutsopoulos, H.M., Alexander, E.L., Carsons, S.E. et al. 2002. Classification criteria for Sjögren's syndrome: A revised version of the European criteria proposed by the American-European Consensus Group. *Annals of Rheumatic Diseases* 61:554–558.

Weng, M. and Walker, W.A. 2006. Bacterial colonization, probiotics and clinical disease. *Journal of Pediatrics* 149(5):S107–S114.

Whitehead, W., Palsson, O., and Jones, K. 2002. Systematic review of the comorbidity of irritable bowel syndrome with other disorders: What are the causes and implications? *Gastroenterology* 122:1140–1156.

Wigley, F.M. 2008. Scleroderma (Systemic sclerosis). In: Goldman, L. and Ausiello, D. *Cecil Medicine*, pp. 2035–2039. Philadelphia, PA: Saunders.

Wilson, J.J. and Best, T.M. 2005. Common overuse tendon problems: A review and recommendations for treatment. *American Family Physician* 72:811–818.

Wolfe, F., Ross, K., Anderson, J., and Russell, I.J. 1995. The prevalence and characteristics of fibromyalgia in the general population. *Arthritis and Rheumatism* 38:19–28.

Zhang, W. and Reichlin, M. 2008. A possible link between infection with burkholderia bacteria and systemic lupus erythematosus based on epitope mimicry. *Clinical and Developmental Immunology* 2008:1–7.

Zyrianova, Y. 2011. Rheumatoid arthritis: A historical and biopsychosocial perspective. In: Lemmey, A.B. (ed.), *Rheumatoid Arthritis-Etiology, Consequences and Co-Morbidities*, p. 189. Rijeka, Croatia: InTech.

12 Phytochemicals as Anti-Inflammatory Agents

Kartick C. Pramanik and Atreyi Maiti

CONTENTS

12.1 INTRODUCTION

Inflammation is defined as a complex biological response of vascular tissues to harmful stimuli, such as pathogens, damage cells, or irritants characterized by local redness, swelling, joint pain, heat, and loss of joint function [1]. A large number of chemical mediators such as kinins, eicosanoids, complement proteins, histamine, and monokines regulate these inflammatory manifestations. Inflammation is either acute or chronic. Acute inflammation may be associated with an initial response of the body to harmful stimuli, and failure of acute inflammation to resolve may predispose to autoimmunity, chronic dysplastic inflammation, and excessive tissue damage. Chronic inflammation is an inflammatory response that is out of proportion, resulting in damage to the body. Prostaglandins (PGs), prostacyclins, and thromboxanes play a key role in the generation of the inflammatory response, pain, and platelet aggregation, and they are generated by the action of cyclooxygenase (COX) isoenzyme. Chronic inflammation causes many advanced aged diseases such as heart attack, Alzheimer's disease, and cancer [2]. Nonsteroidal anti-inflammatory drugs (NSAIDs) are the most commonly used drugs to prevent and treat inflammation and/or postoperative pain [3]. These drugs block PG production by attenuating COX-1 and COX-2 enzyme activity. The long-term use of steroidal anti-inflammatory drugs (SAIDs) and NSAIDs causes adverse side effects and also damages the human biological systems such as the digestive (specifically the liver and gastrointestinal tract), renal, and cardiovascular systems [4–6]. Therefore, there is an urgent need to develop new, safe, potent, nontoxic anti-inflammatory drugs.

Nature has provided many things for mankind over the years, including the tools for the first attempt at therapeutic intervention. From the ancient time, plants have provided a large variety of potent drugs to alleviate suffering from various diseases, which is also a rich source of effective and safe medicines. Since the past decade, worldwide use of medicinal plants has become important in primary health-care needs, especially in developing countries. Plant and plant-derived chemicals, known as phytochemicals, have provided tremendous support in the traditional health-care system, and they have been used as a source of new potential drugs to prevent various kinds of diseases in modern pharmaceutical industries. According to the World Health Organization (WHO), about 80% of the world's population relies mainly on plant-based drugs. In recent years, investigators have paid great attention to the potent phytochemicals to develop modern medicine as they are easily available, less expensive, and have no side effects. Phytochemicals are more important to treat inflammation, and there is an increasing awareness to develop a phytochemical acting as an anti-inflammatory agent. In the United States, a modification of traditional medicine is termed as complementary and alternative medicine (CAM) and defined as a group of diverse medical and health-care system, practices, and products that are not presently considered to be a part of conventional medicine (NCCAM website, 2005). It was also reported that 158 million people of the American adult population use complementary medicine and about $17 billion were spent on traditional remedies in 2000 (NCCAM website, 2005). It has been shown that some of the phytochemicals are abundant in fruits, vegetables, and in spices, teas, cocoa, or red wine. These have been used for centuries as antioxidant and anti-inflammatory agents. The focus of this chapter is to summarize some of the potent anti-inflammatory phytochemicals and their possible mechanism of action through which they can inhibit inflammatory signals.

12.2 PHYTOCHEMICALS AND THEIR CLASSIFICATION

Phytochemical is derived from the Greek word "phyto," which means plant. Phytochemicals are defined as a bioactive plant chemical in fruits, vegetables, grain, and other plant foods that protect plants against bacteria, viruses, and fungi, and consumption of large amount of brightly colored fruits and vegetables (yellow, orange, red, green, white, blue, purple), whole grain/cereals, and beans has been linked to reduce the risk of major chronic diseases. A large number (>5000) of individual phytochemicals have been identified, but a large percentage still remain undiscovered. It is an urgent need to identify them before we can fully understand the health beneficial effect in whole food [7]. There is a promising report from the National Academy of Sciences on diet and health

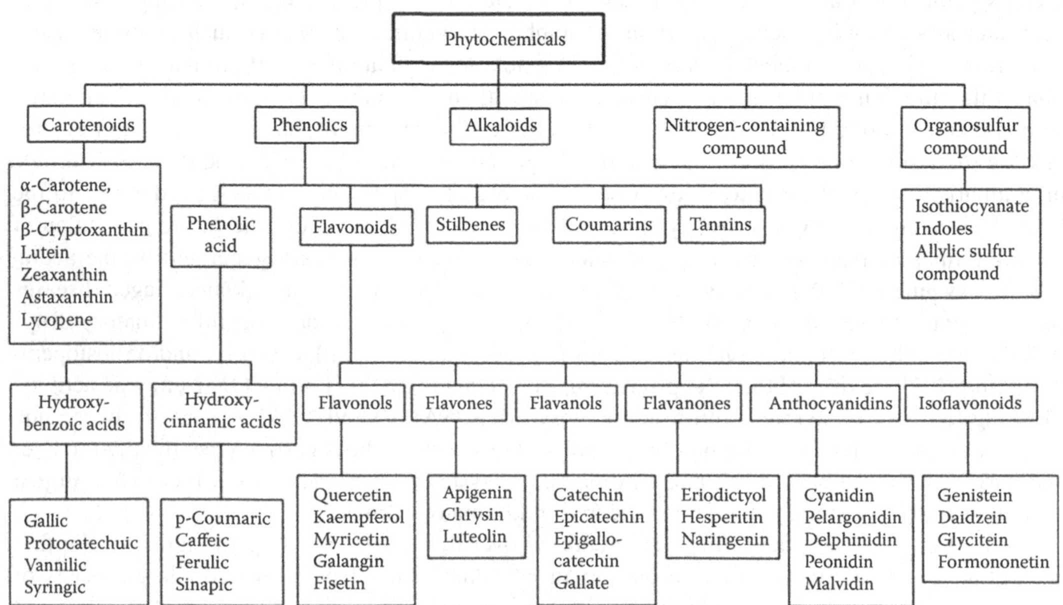

FIGURE 12.1 Classification of phytochemicals.

that recommended consuming five or more servings of fruits and vegetables daily for reducing the risk of both cancer and heart disease. However, there is a new light from the convincing evidences that the beneficial effect of phytochemical in fruits and vegetables is even greater than is currently understood [8]. Phytochemicals can be classified as given later (Figure 12.1). Interestingly, most studies of phytochemicals are the phenolic and carotenoid groups.

12.3 CELL SIGNALING PATHWAY ASSOCIATED WITH INFLAMMATION

In the past decade, there is an increased interest on the cellular and molecular mechanism involved in inflammatory process and this opened a new era to the discovery of many targets for the development of new drugs to treat chronic inflammation [9]. The inflammatory process itself is not considered a disease, but failure to resolve it in a timely fashion resulted in tissue damage and modulation of cell signaling pathways [10]. Inflammation is associated with the release of a great number of inflammatory mediators including kinins, platelet-activating factor (PAF), PGs, leukotrienes (LTs), amines, purines, cytokines, chemokines, and other adhesion molecules. These mediators lead to the local release of other mediators from leukocytes to the site of inflammation [11].

Inflammatory pathway can be classified into arachidonic acid (AA)-dependent and AA-independent pathways [12]. It has been discovered that COX, lipooxygenase (LOX), and phospholipase A2 (PLA2) involved in AA-dependent pathway and nitric oxide synthase (NOS), NF-κB, peroxisome proliferator activated receptors (PPAR), and NSAID-activated gene-1 (NAG) belong to AA-independent pathway (Figure 12.2). The metabolism of AA is either via COX pathway–resulted production of PGs or thromboxane A2 or via LOX pathway–resulted production of hydroperoxye-icosatetraenoic acid (HETES) and LTs. Products from both pathways have been shown to be key players in the process of inflammation [13–15].

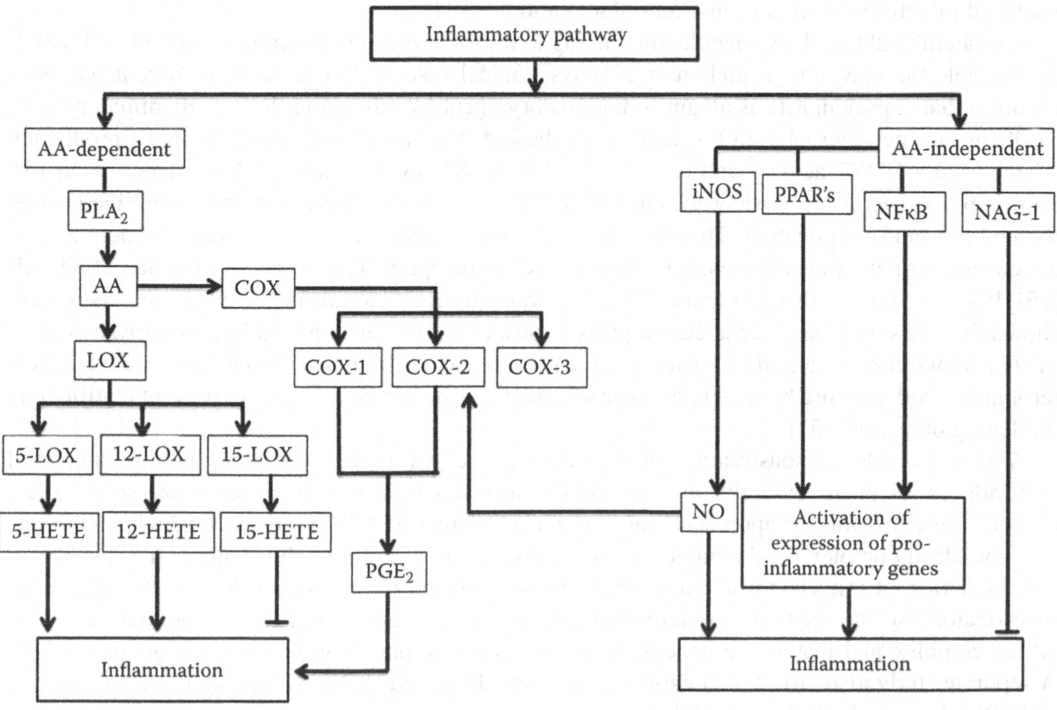

FIGURE 12.2 Inflammatory pathways in inflammation.

12.4 PHYTOCHEMICALS AND THEIR EFFECT ON INFLAMMATION

Despite the immense valuable research on different phytochemicals on inflammation, some of them entered in clinical trial. In this chapter, we will focus our attention on selective representative molecules and their mechanism as anti-inflammatory agent like capsaicin, curcumin, catechin, resveratrol, quercetin, genistein, indole-3-carbinol, lycopene, apigenin, and luteolin.

12.4.1 CAPSAICIN

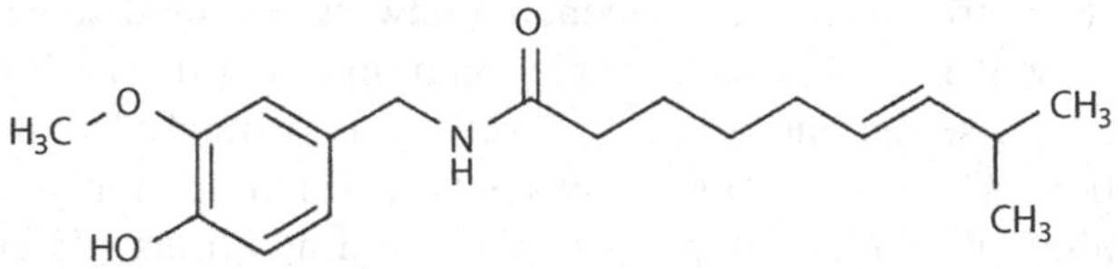

Capsaicin

Capsaicin is an active and pungent component in hot red and chili peppers. It has been widely used as spice or as food additive mostly in South Asian and Latin American countries [16–18]. In addition, it has been used as a folk medicine for stimulating circulation, aiding digestion, and relieving topical pain. Capsaicin is a potent anti-inflammatory agent and has been known a fighter for chronic and subchronic inflammation [19,20]. A study has reported that capsaicin inhibits carrageenan-induced paw inflammation and adjuvant-induced arthritis in rats and ethanol-induced inflammation [21–24]. Numerous investigators reported that capsaicin is used to treat pain and inflammation and may also have potential in treating a number of diseases such as rheumatoid arthritis, diabetic neuropathy, cluster of headache, and herpes zoster [25–28]. Besides anti-inflammatory activity, capsaicin is also used as an anticancer, antiobesity, and antioxidant agent [29–31]. Studies have shown that capsaicin also improves digestion by increasing digestive fluid in the stomach and preventing bacterial infection that could cause an inflammation [32,33].

Capsaicin could work by specifically binding to transient receptor potential vanilloid 1 (TRPV1) by multiple noxious stimuli and show its physiological response in sensory neuron. It has been reported that capsaicin acts as an anti-inflammatory agent by repressing the proinflammatory gene iNOS in murine macrophase [34]. Kim et al. showed that capsaicin can inhibit PGE_2 production by repressing COX2 activity and can also inhibit NF-KB by attenuating I-KBα degradation further. Capsaicin activates PPAR-γ, which can inhibit tumor necrosis factor-α (TNF-α) production and thereby prevent inflammation. Therefore, from the above evidence it is clear that capsaicin acts as an anti-inflammatory agent by the activation of nuclear receptor PPAR-γ and inactivation of NF-KB [35]. It is well known that substance P is a key transmitter of pain to the brain. Researchers have shown that consumption of capsaicin suppresses substance P production [17]. Interestingly, capsaicin may prevent diarrhea caused by bacterial infection [36]. Apart from this, it may lower blood cholesterol and blood pressure by stimulating cardiovascular system and also help to prevent clotting and hardening of arteries [37].

A recent study demonstrated that capsaicin decreases mitochondrial membrane potential and induces apoptosis by activating caspase cascade and thereby can prevent pancreatic cancer [38]. Capsaicin-mediated apoptosis was through mitochondrial ROS generation, which inhibits mitochondrial complex I and complex III activities, disruption of mitochondrial membrane potential, oxidation of mitochondrial cardiolipin, and misbalance of antioxidant levels [39]. The same investigator also showed that capsaicin-mediated oxidative stress dissociates the interaction of Trx/ASK1 complex and may cause pancreatic tumor growth suppression by inducing apoptosis [40]. A separate study also proved that capsaicin activates JNK and FOXO-1, leading to the acetylation of FOXO-1 through CBP and SirT-1. In addition, acetylated FOXO1 induced apoptosis in pancreatic cancer cells through BIM activation in vitro and in vivo [41]. A further study also proved that capsaicin can prevent adipogenesis and obesity by activating vanilloid receptor 1 (VR-1), which promotes a calcium influx [42]. Capsaicin-mediated suppression of obesity-induced inflammation was associated with decrease in fasting glucose, insulin, and triglyceride levels and suppression of interleukin (IL)-6 and MCP-1 expression and secretion from obese adipose tissue. Nowadays, various pharmaceutical formulation of capsaicin is available over the counter for the treatment of peripheral neuropathies and chronic musculoskeletal pain. Therefore, the evidence suggested that capsaicin might be regarded as an important phytochemical used as anti-inflammatory and anticancer agents.

12.4.2 Curcumin

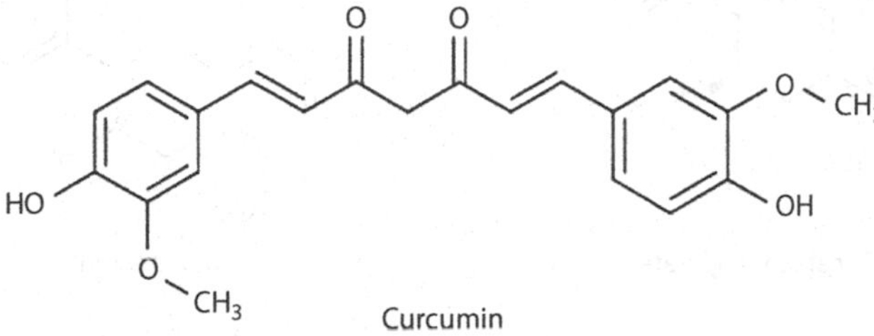

Curcumin

Curcumin, a natural compound present in turmeric (*Curcuma longa*), is used as a yellow spice in Indian food and has been acting as an anti-inflammatory agent for centuries in Indian Ayurvedic medicine. There are three curcuminoids extracted from turmeric: curcumin, demethoxycurcumin, and bismethoxycurcumin. Curcumin is a major active constituent that is responsible for the yellow pigment. In the past few decades, several investigators have shown immense interest in curcumin for its various purposes to cure different diseases. Several reports have shown that curcumin exhibits anti-inflammatory, anticancer, and antioxidant properties [43,44]. This chapter considered curcumin as an anti-inflammatory agent. The effect of curcumin on cancer from an anti-inflammatory perspective has also been discussed.

Curcumin acts as an anti-inflammatory agent by interacting with various molecular targets. Its anti-inflammatory activity is mediated through the inhibition of induction of COX-2, LOX, and nitric oxide synthase (iNOS). In addition, it also inhibits the production of the inflammatory cytokines, such as TNF-α, ILs, and activates transcription factors like NF-KB and AP-1 [45,46]. Expanding bodies of evidence demonstrated that curcumin attributes its anti-inflammatory property by inhibiting COX-2 enzyme activity and thereby suppresses PGs synthesis [47]. It has also been shown that curcumin significantly inhibits PLA2, COX-2, and LOX activities and modifies PGE_2 levels in clonic mucosa and tumor [48]. Reports also suggested that obesity-induced inflammatory response in obese mice was attenuated by curcumin by inhibiting the release of MCP-1 and TNF-α [49]. NF-KB is a known transcription factor that regulates inflammation, cellular proliferation, and tumorigenesis. Several lines of evidence suggested that curcumin mediated the suppression of upstream transcriptional factor NF-KB by blocking the phosphorylation of inhibitory factor I-kappa B kinase (IKB), which in turn inhibits COX-2 and iNOS activity and thereby prevents inflammatory signal and tumorigenesis [50,51]. Curcumin also inhibits cytokine production by down-regulating protein kinase C (PKC). Apart from the cell line data, several investigators have shown animal studies on curcumin as an anti-inflammatory agent [52]. It is noteworthy that tetrahydrocurcumin, one of the strong metabolites of curcumin, exhibits stronger antioxidant and anti-inflammatory activity than curcumin.

It is well known that proinflammatory states are well linked with the tumor promotion [53,54]. Several evidences suggested that curcumin acts as a strong anti-inflammatory agent that is anticipated to have chemopreventive activity. Several lines of studies have shown that curcumin inhibits carcinogenesis in a number of cancer types including pancreatic, gastric, prostate, breast, hepatic and colorectal, and oral cancers and leukemia [55]. It has also been shown that the entire anti-inflammatory pathway has been implicated in the anticarcinogenic potential of curcumin [47,51,56,57].

Therefore, a number of evidences have proved that curcumin acts as an anti-inflammatory agent *in vitro* and *in vivo* but still a lot needs to be proved in human clinical trial to strongly establish curcumin as an anti-inflammatory agent.

12.4.3 Catechins

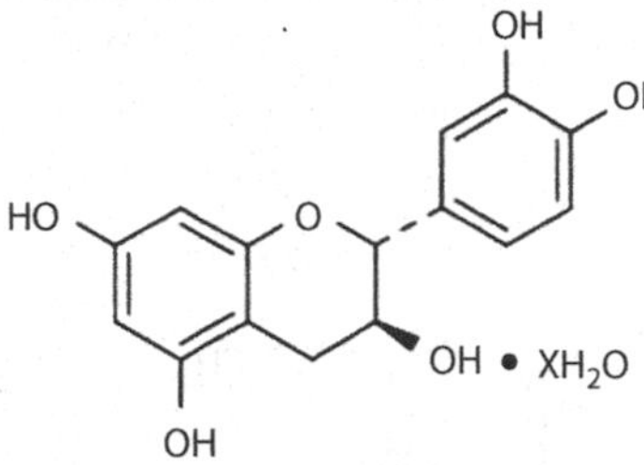

(+)- catechin hydrate

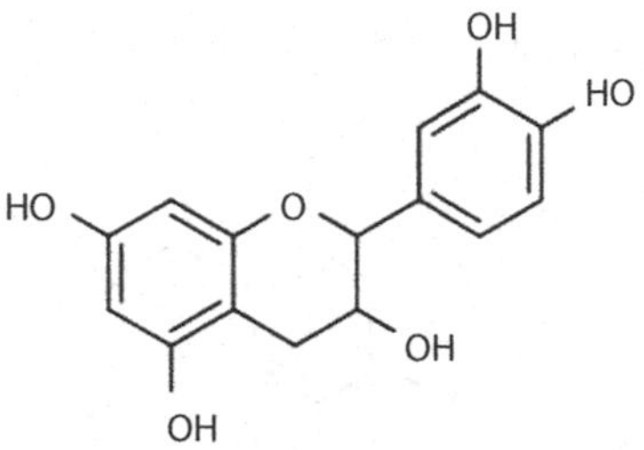

DL-catechin

Catechins are the main bioactive components of tea polyphenols and show many biological functions including anti-inflammatory, antioxidant, and anticancer effects. At present, there are eight catechins isolated from green tea, out of which the major tea catechins are epigallocatechin-3 gallate (EGCG), epigallocatechin (EGC), and epicatechin-3 gallate (ECG). EGCG is the most widely used catechin and is thought to be responsible for a majority of biological effects of green tea, especially for anti-inflammatory effect. A line of evidence suggested that the anti-inflammatory effect of catechins is due to their scavenging of NO and inhibition of NO synthase activity and EGCG being the most effective on that [58–63]. NO produced from neuronal NOS (nNOS) is inhibited by EGCG and oligomeric proanthocyanidins in BL21 (DE3) *Escherichia coli* cells [64]. Reports suggested that EGCG inhibited nNOS production induced by lipopolysaccharide (LPS) and interferon-γ (IFN-γ) in peritoneal cells. In addition, EGCG also inhibits iNOS mRNA and activity induced by LPS, IFN-γ, TNF-α, and IL-1 in vitro and thereby prevent inflammation [60,65,66]. The mechanism behind this anti-inflammatory effect was EGCG preventing IKB degradation, which in turn inhibits NF-KB from binding to the promoter of iNOS gene [66]. Catechins can bind to the promoter region of endothelial NOS (eNOS) containing antioxidant response element and activate eNOS. On the other hand, a contradictory report demonstrated that ECG develops the quality of wound by inducing proinflammatory enzymes like iNOS and COX-2 [67]. This discrimination needs to be clarified by further investigation. EGCG also showed its anti-inflammatory activity by inducing eNOS to produce NO, which in turn increased the phosphorylation of PI3K and AKT and causes vasorelaxation [68]. Importantly, EGCG specifically inhibited proteasome *in vitro* and *in vivo* and this phenomenon may be causative for its anti-inflammatory activity [69]. Furthermore, EGCG also prevented the induction of vascular adhesion molecules-1 by TNF-α and IL-1, which in turn reduced monocyte adhesion [70]. Catechins also inhibits proinflammatory cytokine IL-1 induced by polymorphonuclear leukocytes exposed to LPS [71].

A line of evidence suggested that catechins exhibit its anti-inflammatory activity in animal models by suppressing the oxidative stress and proinflammatory cytokine and increasing catalase and superoxide dismutase and decreasing iNOS and TNF-α and NF-KB expression [72,73]. Of note, topical application of EGCG on rat also prevents UVB-induced inflammation by inhibiting immunosuppression, infiltration of cluster of differentiation (CD) 11b+ leukocytes, and depletion of antigen-presenting cells such as macrophages and dendritic cells [74]. Most of the time inflammation brings arthritis disease. Importantly, catechins prevent arthritis-induced cartilage degradation by preventing the breakdown of proteoglycan and type II collagen [75]. Interestingly, reports also suggested that the daily intake of six to eight cups of green tea, which is approximately 800 mg of catechin, may counteract oxidative stress and inflammation and trigger obesity, indicating that drinking green tea may be a useful prophylactic against inflammation and obesity [76] and that catechin might be a promising anti-inflammatory agent in the near future.

12.4.4 Resveratrol

OH OH

HO

Resveratrol

Resveratrol (*trans*-3, 5, 4′-trihydroxystilbene) is a polyphenolic phytoalexin synthesized in response to microbial attack in various plants, including grapes, berries, peanuts, and Japanese knotweed [77–80]. The concentration of resveratrol varies from 50 to 100 μg/g in fresh grape skin and from 0.1 to 14 mg/L in red wine [81,82]. One Spanish study suggested that it is also found in white and rose wine and the concentration varies from 0.011 to 0.547 and 0.07 to 1.06 mg/L, respectively [83]. Resveratrol exists in two isoform, *trans* and *cis*, and it is noteworthy that *trans*-isomer is more stable than *cis*-isomer [84].

An expanding body of evidence suggested that resveratrol is a potent anti-inflammatory agent. In this chapter, we discussed how resveratrol exhibits its anti-inflammatory properties. Recent studies showed that resveratrol can inhibit TNF-α-induced vascular leakage in mouse liver perfusion model [85] and can also inhibit IL-8 and granulocytes-macrophage colony by stimulating factor-induced inflammation in A549 cells. Another study showed that resveratrol can inhibit the release of TNF-α in bone marrow–derived mouse mast cells [85] and thereby prevents inflammation. Recruits effector of inflammatory response identifies neutrophils due to which it plays an important role in the first stage of inflammation. Studies proved that resveratrol could inhibit all physiological phases of inflammatory response induced by neutrophils [82,86]. A study also showed that TNF-α regulates the expression of some adhesion molecules and cytokines on endothelial cells and the same study evaluated that resveratrol can inhibit the expression of adhesion molecules like vascular cell adhesion molecules-1 (VCAM-1) and intercellular adhesion molecules-1 (ICAM-1) and neutrophil adhesion induced by TNF-α in human umbilical vein endothelial cells [87]. A recent study showed that resveratrol attenuates carrageenan-induced paw edema through the inhibition of COX-2 [88]. It can also inhibit inflammation by inhibiting the expression of iNOS and COX-2 in cytokine-stimulated human primary airway epithelial cells [89]. An interesting study discriminated the action of resveratrol between the COX isoform, and it was suggested that resveratrol led the elimination of PGs synthesis via COX-1 not COX-2 [90]. Therefore, the anti-inflammatory activity of resveratrol may be explained by the inhibition of both isoenzymes. A study also suggested that resveratrol significantly reduces the colon injury and neutrophil infiltration by decreasing the expression of COX-2 [91]. Resveratrol also acts as an anti-inflammatory agent by suppressing the secretion of TNF-α and nitric oxide in LPS-stimulated rat cortical microglia and N9 microglial cells [92]. In addition, resveratrol incubation (10–40 μM) attenuates the release of inflammatory cytokines (TNF-α, IL-1β, IL-6, and MIP-1α) from C5a-stimulated human and mouse neutrophils [93]. Extensive research in the last few years brings the light on the effect of resveratrol on regulation of transcription factor, which regulates the expression of inflammatory mediators. These transcription factors include NF-KB, AP-1, C/EBP, and fos/jun. Resveratrol may interfere with the activation of all of these transcription factors [82]. Existing reports also suggested that NF-KB activation is the key cause of inflammation and suppression of the nuclear transcription factor attenuates inflammation. Resveratrol inhibits NF-KB activation by inhibiting I-KB kinase [94].

PGs synthesis may also stimulate tumor cell growth, and it may direct the correlation of inflammation and cancer [95–98]. An impressive body of evidence suggested that resveratrol inhibits cancer by interfering in the cellular proliferation and growth, apoptosis, inflammation, invasion, angiogenesis, and metastasis [99,100], and thereby can exhibit its chemopreventive agent. The most interesting properties are that the anticancer effect of resveratrol also has reflected on strong anti-inflammatory and antioxidant properties.

12.4.5 Quercetin

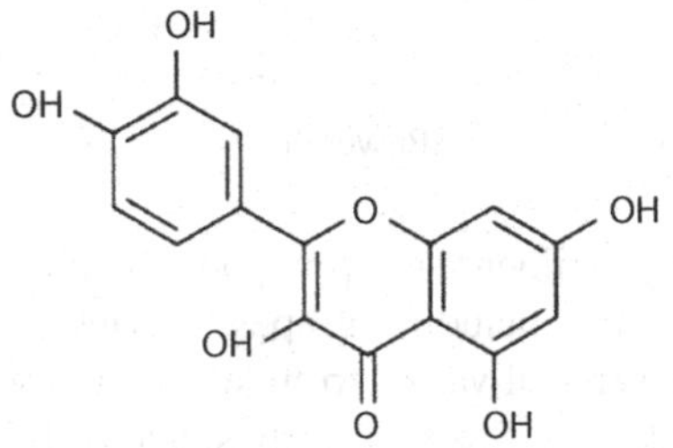

Quercetin

Quercetin (3,3′,4′,5–7-pentahydroxyflavone) is one of the important dietary flavonoids present in multiple green vegetables, citrus fruits, tea, berries, onions, parsley, and red grape wines and has been extensively studied for its beneficial heath effect [101]. Quercetin mainly exists in glycosylated form such as quercitrin or rutoside [102].

The anti-inflammatory property of quercetin has been shown by many investigators [103,104]. For instance, it has been reported that quercetin inhibits TNF-α-induced inflammation by inhibiting NF-KB signaling in hepatic cells [105]. This flavonoid also has the capability to inhibit LPS-induced TNF-α production in macrophages [106] and IL-8 production in lung cancer cells [107]. It was also reported that quercetin attenuates mRNA levels of TNF-α and IL-1α induced by LPS in glial cells [108]. Noh et al. reported that quercetin acts as an anti-inflammatory agent by inhibiting MIP-1α-induced inflammation in macrophages. The mechanism behind this was that quercetin down-regulates CCR1/CCR5 and inhibits the activation of c-Jun N-terminal kinase, $_{\mathrm{p}}$38 MAPK and I-KB kinase, and I-KBα degradation [109]. Endale et al. evaluated quercetin anti-inflammatory activity by inhibiting LPS-induced NO, iNOS, COX-2, TNF-α, IL-1β, IL-6, and PGE-2 production in macrophages [110]. Another separate study reported that the anti-inflammatory action of quercetin by inhibiting IL-1β induced the production of MMPs, COX-2, and PGE-2 in rheumatoid synovial fibroblast [111]. In addition, quercetin also attenuated the TNF-α-induced expression of inflammatory genes such as IL-1β, IL-6, and IL-8 in human adipocytes and thereby exhibited its anti-inflammatory activity [112]. An interesting report by Stewart et al. demonstrated that quercetin supplementation (0.8%) in high-fat diet decreased the inflammatory markers like INF-γ, IL-1α, and IL-4 [113]. The overall evidence may explain the anti-inflammatory effect of quercetin by interplay between oxidative stress and inflammation. Because the induction of oxidative stress promoted inflammatory process by the activation of transcription factor such as NF-KB and AP-1, which in turn produces cytokines like TNF-α [114,115]. And quercetin mitigated inflammation by inhibiting this cytokine production.

However, the properties of quercetin are not limited as an anti-inflammatory agent, but this phytochemical is also known as an anticancer agent. This anti-inflammatory effect of quercetin is also anticipated in anticancer effect. An expanding body of evidence suggested that the anticancer effect of quercetin was induced by cell death or cell cycle arrest and that too was mediated through the suppression of oncogenes such as Mcl-1, MEK, PI3K, RAS, and induction of tumor suppressor genes like P53 and P21. Unfortunately, no clinical trials data have yet been published where quercetin could be proved as an anticancer agent. Therefore, evidences suggested that the use of quercetin could inhibit inflammation and cancer and that quercetin would be a promising anti-inflammatory agent in human health care.

12.4.6 Genistein

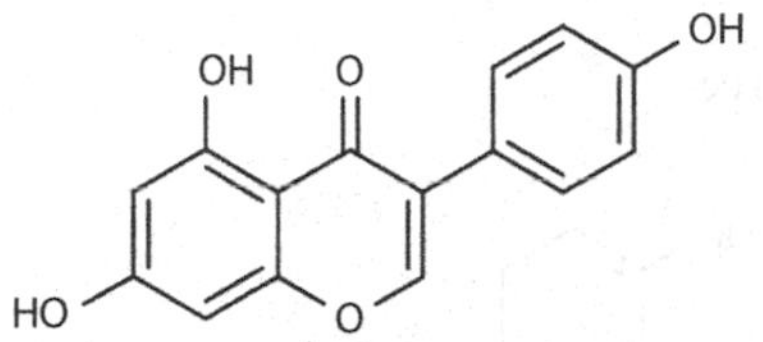

Genistein

Genistein (4′,5,7-trihydroxyisoflavone) is a phytoestrogen found in soy bean and soy-enriched product. It has been reported that the daily intake concentration of isoflavones varies from 25 to 30 mg in the Japanese diet and even reaches up to 100 mg in 10% of Asian diet [116]. In the United States, concentration of isoflavones varies from 0.15 to 3 mg [117,118]. This difference in genistein concentration leads to different outcomes in respect of variety of clinical contexts such as cholesterol regulation, osteoporosis, and cancer from the Asian to Western society. In this chapter, we have attempted to summarize the anti-inflammatory effect of genistein.

The anti-inflammatory effect of this phytochemical is due to the inhibition of LPS-induced TNF-α and IL-6 production in mouse macrophages [1]. It has also been reported that genistein blocks the secretion of TNF-α and IL-1β in phytohemagglutinin-stimulated macrophages and thereby acts as an anti-inflammatory agent [119]. Liang et al. reported that the anti-inflammatory effect of genistein due to suppression of LPS-induced expression of COX-2 and iNOS by mouse macrophages [120]. Relic et al. reported its anti-inflammatory properties in adipocytes. In addition, it also down-regulates leptin production [121]. Several reports have demonstrated that genistein is especially use as a small molecule inhibitor in breast and prostate cancer [122,123]. And this effect has been more anticipated in Asian countries where people take more genistein.

12.4.7 Indole-3-Carbinol and Lycopene

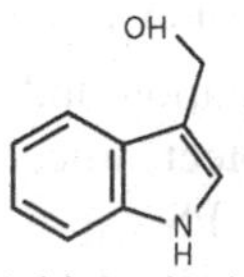

Indole-3-carbinol

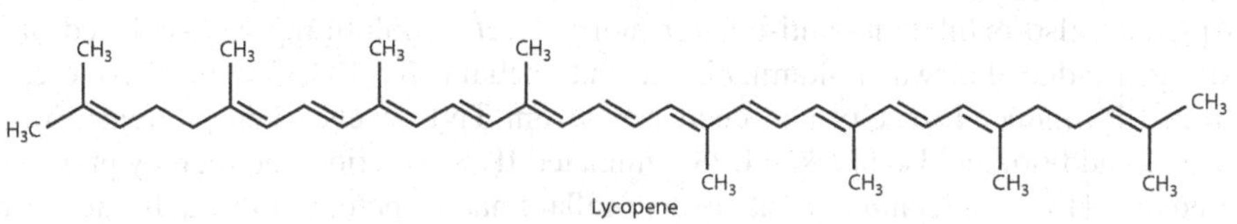

Lycopene

Indole-3-carbinol (13C) is a glucobrassicin derivative found in cruciferous vegetable such as broccoli, cabbage, cauliflower, bok choy, Brussels sprouts, mustard green, and kale. The anti-inflammatory activity of this cruciferous vegetable has been shown by a number of investigators. For instance, 13C acts as an anti-inflammatory agent by inhibiting the production of proinflammatory mediators such as TNF-α, IL-1β, IL-6, IL-12, and NO induced by LPS in dendritic cells [124]. In addition, it also suppresses proinflammatory mediators such as IL-6, IL-1β, TNF-α, IL-10, iNOS, and NO in macrophages [125–127]. Apart from this report, 13C showed its anti-inflammatory effect by the inhibition of NF-KB and nuclear factor of kappa light polypeptide gene enhancer in B-cell inhibitor alpha (I-KB-α) kinase activation [128].

Lycopene is a naturally occurring carotenoid compound found in tomato, papaya, pink grapefruit, pink guava, and watermelon. Lycopene is widely used as an anti-inflammatory agent. It has been shown that lycopene attenuates proinflammatory mediator TNF-α secretion induced by LPS in macrophages [129]. Simone et al. also demonstrated that lycopene can inhibit NF-KB-mediated IL-8 expression in cigarette smoke–stimulated macrophages [130]. Lycopene also showed its anti-inflammatory effect by inhibiting proinflammatory cytokines such as MCP-1, IL-6 in HUVECs cells, and so on [131].

12.4.8 Apigenin and Luteolin

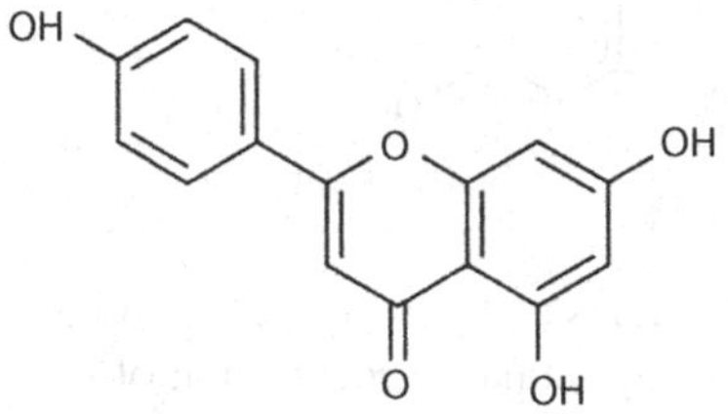

Apigenin

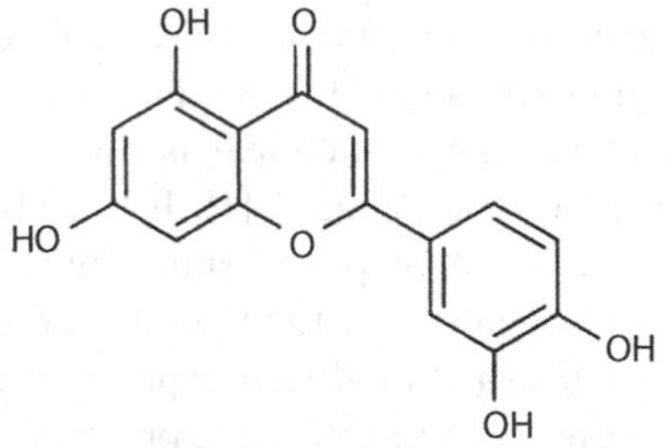

Luteolin

Apigenin (4′,5,7-trihydroxyflavone) is a natural flavonoid found in parsley and celery and abundantly present in common fruits and vegetables. During the last decade, researchers have taken great interest in apigenin because of its low intrinsic toxicity and high anti-inflammatory effect. An expanding body of evidence reported that apigenin has a strong anti-inflammatory effect. For instance, Kowalski et al. and Nicholas et al. demonstrated that apigenin inhibits the expression of TNF-α and IL-1β in LPS-stimulated mouse macrophages and human monocytes [132,133]. Apigenin also exhibits its anti-inflammatory effect by inhibiting LPS-induced inflammation and allergen-induced airway inflammation in endothelial cells [134,135]. Furthermore, it protects mice from LPS-induced toxicity and decreases serum TNF levels when pretreated before LPS exposure. In addition, it also blocked LPS-stimulated IL-8 secretion and thereby prevents inflammatory mediator [133]. Apigenin exhibits its anti-inflammatory potential through interacting with several intracellular signaling pathways, such as NF-KB, MAPK/ERK, and JNK pathway [133,136]. For example apigenin inhibits proinflammatory mediator induced by LPS in mouse macrophages and also suppressed inflammatory response through the inactivation of NF-KB [120,133]. Moreover, Gerritsen et al. showed that apigenin can exhibit its anti-inflammatory effect by attenuating neutrophil and lymphocyte adhesion in endothelial cells, and Lee et al. showed that apigenin can prevent monocyte adhesion in HUVECs cells. The mechanism behind both the experiments was that apigenin regulates the expression of ICAM and VCAM [137,138].

Luteolin (3′,4′,5,7-tetrahydroxyflavone) is a flavone found in edible plants and various fruits and vegetables. This common flavone exhibits its beneficial effect including anti-inflammatory, antioxidant, and antiproliferative function. Here, we discussed its anti-inflammatory effect. Park et al. and Xagorari et al. showed that luteolin show its anti-inflammatory effect by inhibiting the LPS-induced release of TNF-α, IL-6, and NO by macrophages [139,140]. It also inhibited LPS-induced secretion of proinflammatory mediator such as INF-γ, COX-2, IL-6, and iNOS in alveolar macrophage and peripheral macrophage in RAW 264.7 cell lines. The mechanism behind this anti-inflammatory effect was that luteolin suppresses NF-KB activation and I-KB degradation and AP-1 activation in LPS-stimulated macrophage [141]. Moreover, luteolin blocks COX-2 expression and also inhibits carrageenan-induced paw edema in rat and thereby exhibits its anti-inflammatory effect [142].

12.5 CONCLUSION

The chapter emphasized the anti-inflammatory effect of most common and important dietary phytochemicals, including capsaicin, curcumin, catechin, resveratrol, quercetin, genistein, indole-3-carbinol, lycopene, apigenin, and luteolin that are able to interfere at several points of cellular inflammatory pathways. This chapter especially highlighted the dietary phytochemicals as anti-inflammatory weapons. For many decades, SAIDs and NSAIDs have been used to treat acute inflammation, but they were also clinically unsuccessful because of their unexpected side effects. Recently, considerable attention has been devoted to develop naturally potent therapeutic agents that can treat inflammation. Therefore, phytochemicals, which are safe and cheap, have attracted attention all over the world to treat inflammation. Inflammation is associated to develop several chronic diseases including diabetes, obesity, arteriosclerosis, neurodegenerative disease, and even cancer. Many scientists have shown the beneficial effect of these phytochemicals to treat other diseases. Thus, to develop a safe anti-inflammatory effect, phytochemicals may be useful to treat such kinds of disease, especially cancer. Here, we also emphasized the possible effect of phytochemicals in the prevention and treatment of cancer on the basis of their anti-inflammatory perspective. Out of the mentioned phytochemicals, the phenolic and carotenoid group has a strong anti-inflammatory effect. They act through either inhibition of proinflammatory mediators such as TNF-α, IL-1β, IL-6, IL-8, IL-10, IL-12, iNOS, COX-2, and NO production or inhibition of NF-KB, MAPK/ERK, and JNK pathway induced by either LPS or external stimulators. A number of investigators have proved most of the phytochemical's anti-inflammatory efficacy in vitro and in vivo as a preclinical condition, but the beneficial effect of these dietary phytochemicals in humans is still in vague. However, in the present scenario, scientists are more interested in the synthetic analogue of dietary phytochemicals because most of the phytochemicals have limitation of poor potency and bioavailability and the synthetic analogue could be the solution of these limitations. Taken together, this chapter provides new insights into the anti-inflammatory effects of important phytochemicals, which could be promising natural anti-inflammatory agents in the near future.

REFERENCES

1. Calixto, J.B., Campos, M.M., Otuki, M.F., and Santos, A.R. (2004) Anti-inflammatory compounds of plant origin. Part II. Modulation of pro-inflammatory cytokines, chemokines and adhesion molecules. *Planta Med*, **70**, 93–103.
2. Banerjee, S., Zhang, Y., Wang, Z., Che, M., Chiao, P.J., Abbruzzese, J.L., and Sarkar, F.H. (2007) In vitro and in vivo molecular evidence of genistein action in augmenting the efficacy of cisplatin in pancreatic cancer. *Int J Cancer*, **120**, 906–917.
3. Luna, S.P., Basilio, A.C., Steagall, P.V., Machado, L.P., Moutinho, F.Q., Takahira, R.K., and Brandao, C.V. (2007) Evaluation of adverse effects of long-term oral administration of carprofen, etodolac, flunixin meglumine, ketoprofen, and meloxicam in dogs. *Am J Vet Res*, **68**, 258–264.

4. Rao, C.V., Reddy, B.S., Steele, V.E., Wang, C.X., Liu, X., Ouyang, N., Patlolla, J.M., Simi, B., Kopelovich, L., and Rigas, B. (2006) Nitric oxide-releasing aspirin and indomethacin are potent inhibitors against colon cancer in azoxymethane-treated rats: Effects on molecular targets. *Mol Cancer Ther*, **5**, 1530–1538.
5. Shukla, S., Mishra, A., Fu, P., MacLennan, G.T., Resnick, M.I., and Gupta, S. (2005) Up-regulation of insulin-like growth factor binding protein-3 by apigenin leads to growth inhibition and apoptosis of 22Rv1 xenograft in athymic nude mice. *FASEB J*, **19**, 2042–2044.
6. Tyagi, A., Agarwal, R., and Agarwal, C. (2003) Grape seed extract inhibits EGF-induced and constitutively active mitogenic signaling but activates JNK in human prostate carcinoma DU145 cells: Possible role in antiproliferation and apoptosis. *Oncogene*, **22**, 1302–1316.
7. Liu, R.H. (2003) Health benefits of fruit and vegetables are from additive and synergistic combinations of phytochemicals. *Am J Clin Nutr*, **78**, 517S–520S.
8. Ames, B.N. and Gold, L.S. (1991) Endogenous mutagens and the causes of aging and cancer. *Mutat Res*, **250**, 3–16.
9. Calixto, J.B., Otuki, M.F., and Santos, A.R. (2003) Anti-inflammatory compounds of plant origin. Part I. Action on arachidonic acid pathway, nitric oxide and nuclear factor kappa B (NF-kappaB). *Planta Med*, **69**, 973–983.
10. Serhan, C.N. and Savill, J. (2005) Resolution of inflammation: The beginning programs the end. *Nat Immunol*, **6**, 1191–1197.
11. Kim, Y.S., Young, M.R., Bobe, G., Colburn, N.H., and Milner, J.A. (2009) Bioactive food components, inflammatory targets, and cancer prevention. *Cancer Prev Res (Phila)*, **2**, 200–208.
12. Yoon, J.H. and Baek, S.J. (2005) Molecular targets of dietary polyphenols with anti-inflammatory properties. *Yonsei Med J*, **46**, 585–596.
13. Claria, J. and Romano, M. (2005) Pharmacological intervention of cyclooxygenase-2 and 5-lipoxygenase pathways. Impact on inflammation and cancer. *Curr Pharm Des*, **11**, 3431–3447.
14. Conrad, D.J. (1999) The arachidonate 12/15 lipoxygenases. A review of tissue expression and biologic function. *Clin Rev Allergy Immunol*, **17**, 71–89.
15. Moore, T.L. and Weiss, T.D. (1985) Mediators of inflammation. *Semin Arthritis Rheum*, **14**, 247–262.
16. Govindarajan, V.S. and Sathyanarayana, M.N. (1991) Capsicum—Production, technology, chemistry, and quality. Part V. Impact on physiology, pharmacology, nutrition, and metabolism; structure, pungency, pain, and desensitization sequences. *Crit Rev Food Sci Nutr*, **29**, 435–474.
17. Lopez-Carrillo, L., Hernandez Avila, M., and Dubrow, R. (1994) Chili pepper consumption and gastric cancer in Mexico: A case-control study. *Am J Epidemiol*, **139**, 263–271.
18. Monsereenusorn, Y. (1983) Subchronic toxicity studies of capsaicin and capsicum in rats. *Res Commun Chem Pathol Pharmacol*, **41**, 95–110.
19. Castellani, M.L., Bhattacharya, K., Tagen, M., Kempuraj, D., Perrella, A., De Lutiis, M., Boucher, W., Conti, P., Theoharides, T.C., Cerulli, G., Salini, V., and Neri, G. (2007) Anti-chemokine therapy for inflammatory diseases. *Int J Immunopathol Pharmacol*, **20**, 447–453.
20. Sbarsi, I., Falcone, C., Boiocchi, C., Campo, I., Zorzetto, M., De Silvestri, A., and Cuccia, M. (2007) Inflammation and atherosclerosis: The role of TNF and TNF receptors polymorphisms in coronary artery disease. *Int J Immunopathol Pharmacol*, **20**, 145–154.
21. Gonzalez, G.G., Garcia de la Rubia, P., Gallar, J., and Belmonte, C. (1993) Reduction of capsaicin-induced ocular pain and neurogenic inflammation by calcium antagonists. *Invest Ophthalmol Vis Sci*, **34**, 3329–3335.
22. Joe, B., Rao, U.J., and Lokesh, B.R. (1997) Presence of an acidic glycoprotein in the serum of arthritic rats: Modulation by capsaicin and curcumin. *Mol Cell Biochem*, **169**, 125–134.
23. Nagahisa, A., Kanai, Y., Suga, O., Taniguchi, K., Tsuchiya, M., Lowe, J.A. 3rd, and Hess, H.J. (1992) Antiinflammatory and analgesic activity of a non-peptide substance P receptor antagonist. *Eur J Pharmacol*, **217**, 191–195.
24. Park, J.S., Choi, M.A., Kim, B.S., Han, I.S., Kurata, T., and Yu, R. (2000) Capsaicin protects against ethanol-induced oxidative injury in the gastric mucosa of rats. *Life Sci*, **67**, 3087–3093.
25. Holzer, P. (1991) Capsaicin: Cellular targets, mechanisms of action, and selectivity for thin sensory neurons. *Pharmacol Rev*, **43**, 143–201.
26. Matucci Cerinic, M., McCarthy, G., Lombardi, A., Pignone, A., and Partsch, G. (1995) Neurogenic influences in arthritis: Potential modification by capsaicin. *J Rheumatol*, **22**, 1447–1449.
27. Sicuteri, F., Fusco, B.M., Marabini, S., Campagnolo, V., Maggi, C.A., Geppetti, P., and Fanciullacci, M. (1989) Beneficial effect of capsaicin application to the nasal mucosa in cluster headache. *Clin J Pain*, **5**, 49–53.

28. Watson, C.P., Evans, R.J., and Watt, V.R. (1988) Post-herpetic neuralgia and topical capsaicin. *Pain*, **33**, 333–340.
29. Alvarez-Parrilla, E., de la Rosa, L.A., Amarowicz, R., and Shahidi, F. (2011) Antioxidant activity of fresh and processed Jalapeno and Serrano peppers. *J Agric Food Chem*, **59**, 163–173.
30. Kang, J.H., Kim, C.S., Han, I.S., Kawada, T., and Yu, R. (2007) Capsaicin, a spicy component of hot peppers, modulates adipokine gene expression and protein release from obese-mouse adipose tissues and isolated adipocytes, and suppresses the inflammatory responses of adipose tissue macrophages. *FEBS Lett*, **581**, 4389–4396.
31. Yoshitani, S.I., Tanaka, T., Kohno, H., and Takashima, S. (2001) Chemoprevention of azoxymethane-induced rat colon carcinogenesis by dietary capsaicin and rotenone. *Int J Oncol*, **19**, 929–939.
32. Di Bonaventura, G., Piccolomini, R., Pompilio, A., Zappacosta, R., Piccolomini, M., and Neri, M. (2007) Serum and mucosal cytokine profiles in patients with active *Helicobacter pylori* and ischemic heart disease: Is there a relationship? *Int J Immunopathol Pharmacol*, **20**, 163–172.
33. Montagna, M., Avanzini, M.A., Visai, L., Locatelli, F., Montillo, M., Morra, E., and Regazzi, M.B. (2007) A new sensitive enzyme-linked immunosorbent assay (ELISA) for Alemtuzumab determination: Development, validation and application. *Int J Immunopathol Pharmacol*, **20**, 363–371.
34. Kim, C.S., Kawada, T., Kim, B.S., Han, I.S., Choe, S.Y., Kurata, T., and Yu, R. (2003) Capsaicin exhibits anti-inflammatory property by inhibiting IkB-a degradation in LPS-stimulated peritoneal macrophages. *Cell Signal*, **15**, 299–306.
35. Park, J.Y., Kawada, T., Han, I.S., Kim, B.S., Goto, T., Takahashi, N., Fushiki, T., Kurata, T., and Yu, R. (2004) Capsaicin inhibits the production of tumor necrosis factor alpha by LPS-stimulated murine macrophages, RAW 264.7: A PPARgamma ligand-like action as a novel mechanism. *FEBS Lett*, **572**, 266–270.
36. Banche, G., Allizond, V., Mandras, N., Garzaro, M., Cavallo, G.P., Baldi, C., Scutera, S. et al. (2007) Improvement of clinical response in allergic rhinitis patients treated with an oral immunostimulating bacterial lysate: In vivo immunological effects. *Int J Immunopathol Pharmacol*, **20**, 129–138.
37. Pyun, B.J., Choi, S., Lee, Y., Kim, T.W., Min, J.K., Kim, Y., Kim, B.D., Kim, J.H., Kim, T.Y., Kim, Y.M., and Kwon, Y.G. (2008) Capsiate, a nonpungent capsaicin-like compound, inhibits angiogenesis and vascular permeability via a direct inhibition of Src kinase activity. *Cancer Res*, **68**, 227–235.
38. Zhang, R., Humphreys, I., Sahu, R.P., Shi, Y., and Srivastava, S.K. (2008) In vitro and in vivo induction of apoptosis by capsaicin in pancreatic cancer cells is mediated through ROS generation and mitochondrial death pathway. *Apoptosis*, **13**, 1465–1478.
39. Pramanik, K.C., Boreddy, S.R., and Srivastava, S.K. (2011) Role of mitochondrial electron transport chain complexes in capsaicin mediated oxidative stress leading to apoptosis in pancreatic cancer cells. *PLoS One*, **6**, e20151.
40. Pramanik, K.C. and Srivastava, S.K. (2012) Apoptosis signal-regulating kinase 1-thioredoxin complex dissociation by capsaicin causes pancreatic tumor growth suppression by inducing apoptosis. *Antioxid Redox Signal*, **17**, 1417–1432.
41. Pramanik, K.C., Fofaria, N.M., Gupta, P., and Srivastava, S.K. (2014) CBP-mediated FOXO-1 acetylation inhibits pancreatic tumor growth by targeting SirT. *Mol Cancer Ther*, **13**, 687–698.
42. Zhang, L.L., Yan Liu, D., Ma, L.Q., Luo, Z.D., Cao, T.B., Zhong, J., Yan, Z.C. et al (2007) Activation of transient receptor potential vanilloid type-1 channel prevents adipogenesis and obesity. *Circ Res*, **100**, 1063–1070.
43. Mukhopadhyay, A., Basu, N., Ghatak, N., and Gujral, P.K. (1982) Anti-inflammatory and irritant activities of curcumin analogues in rats. *Agents Actions*, **12**, 508–515.
44. Reddy, A.C. and Lokesh, B.R. (1994) Effect of dietary turmeric (*Curcuma longa*) on iron-induced lipid peroxidation in the rat liver. *Food Chem Toxicol*, **32**, 279–283.
45. Abe, Y., Hashimoto, S., and Horie, T. (1999) Curcumin inhibition of inflammatory cytokine production by human peripheral blood monocytes and alveolar macrophages. *Pharmacol Res*, **39**, 41–47.
46. Goel, A., Kunnumakkara, A.B., and Aggarwal, B.B. (2008) Curcumin as "Curecumin": From kitchen to clinic. *Biochem Pharmacol*, **75**, 787–809.
47. Huang, M.T., Lysz, T., Ferraro, T., Abidi, T.F., Laskin, J.D., and Conney, A.H. (1991) Inhibitory effects of curcumin on in vitro lipoxygenase and cyclooxygenase activities in mouse epidermis. *Cancer Res*, **51**, 813–819.
48. Kawamori, T., Rao, C.V., Seibert, K., and Reddy, B.S. (1998) Chemopreventive activity of celecoxib, a specific cyclooxygenase-2 inhibitor, against colon carcinogenesis. *Cancer Res*, **58**, 409–412.

49. Woo, H.M., Kang, J.H., Kawada, T., Yoo, H., Sung, M.K., and Yu, R. (2007) Active spice-derived components can inhibit inflammatory responses of adipose tissue in obesity by suppressing inflammatory actions of macrophages and release of monocyte chemoattractant protein-1 from adipocytes. *Life Sci*, **80**, 926–931.
50. Jobin, C., Bradham, C.A., Russo, M.P., Juma, B., Narula, A.S., Brenner, D.A., and Sartor, R.B. (1999) Curcumin blocks cytokine-mediated NF-kappa B activation and proinflammatory gene expression by inhibiting inhibitory factor I-kappa B kinase activity. *J Immunol*, **163**, 3474–3483.
51. Surh, Y.J., Chun, K.S., Cha, H.H., Han, S.S., Keum, Y.S., Park, K.K., and Lee, S.S. (2001) Molecular mechanisms underlying chemopreventive activities of anti-inflammatory phytochemicals: Down-regulation of COX-2 and iNOS through suppression of NF-kappa B activation. *Mutat Res*, **480–481**, 243–268.
52. Srimal, R.C. and Dhawan, B.N. (1973) Pharmacology of diferuloylmethane (curcumin), a non-steroidal anti-inflammatory agent. *J Pharm Pharmacol*, **25**, 447–452.
53. Bennett, A. (1986) The production of prostanoids in human cancers, and their implications for tumor progression. *Prog Lipid Res*, **25**, 539–542.
54. Qiao, L., Kozoni, V., Tsioulias, G.J., Koutsos, M.I., Hanif, R., Shiff, S.J., and Rigas, B. (1995) Selected eicosanoids increase the proliferation rate of human colon carcinoma cell lines and mouse colonocytes in vivo. *Biochim Biophys Acta*, **1258**, 215–223.
55. Aggarwal, B.B., Kumar, A., and Bharti, A.C. (2003) Anticancer potential of curcumin: Preclinical and clinical studies. *Anticancer Res*, **23**, 363–398.
56. Cho, J.W., Lee, K.S., and Kim, C.W. (2007) Curcumin attenuates the expression of IL-1beta, IL-6, and TNF-alpha as well as cyclin E in TNF-alpha-treated HaCaT cells; NF-kappaB and MAPKs as potential upstream targets. *Int J Mol Med*, **19**, 469–474.
57. Liu, J.Y., Lin, S.J., and Lin, J.K. (1993) Inhibitory effects of curcumin on protein kinase C activity induced by 12-O-tetradecanoyl-phorbol-13-acetate in NIH 3T3 cells. *Carcinogenesis*, **14**, 857–861.
58. Chan, M.M., Ho, C.T., and Huang, H.I. (1995) Effects of three dietary phytochemicals from tea, rosemary and turmeric on inflammation-induced nitrite production. *Cancer Lett*, **96**, 23–29.
59. Nagai, K., Jiang, M.H., Hada, J., Nagata, T., Yajima, Y., Yamamoto, S., and Nishizaki, T. (2002) (-)-Epigallocatechin gallate protects against NO stress-induced neuronal damage after ischemia by acting as an anti-oxidant. *Brain Res*, **956**, 319–322.
60. Paquay, J.B., Haenen, G.R., Stender, G., Wiseman, S.A., Tijburg, L.B., and Bast, A. (2000) Protection against nitric oxide toxicity by tea. *J Agric Food Chem*, **48**, 5768–5772.
61. Sutherland, B.A., Shaw, O.M., Clarkson, A.N., Jackson, D.N., Sammut, I.A., and Appleton, I. (2005) Neuroprotective effects of (-)-epigallocatechin gallate following hypoxia-ischemia-induced brain damage: Novel mechanisms of action. *FASEB J*, **19**, 258–260.
62. Suzuki, M., Tabuchi, M., Ikeda, M., Umegaki, K., and Tomita, T. (2004) Protective effects of green tea catechins on cerebral ischemic damage. *Med Sci Monit*, **10**, BR166–BR174.
63. Tedeschi, E., Menegazzi, M., Yao, Y., Suzuki, H., Forstermann, U., and Kleinert, H. (2004) Green tea inhibits human inducible nitric-oxide synthase expression by down-regulating signal transducer and activator of transcription-1alpha activation. *Mol Pharmacol*, **65**, 111–120.
64. Stevens, J.F., Miranda, C.L., Wolthers, K.R., Schimerlik, M., Deinzer, M.L., and Buhler, D.R. (2002) Identification and in vitro biological activities of hop proanthocyanidins: Inhibition of nNOS activity and scavenging of reactive nitrogen species. *J Agric Food Chem*, **50**, 3435–3443.
65. Chan, M.M., Fong, D., Ho, C.T., and Huang, H.I. (1997) Inhibition of inducible nitric oxide synthase gene expression and enzyme activity by epigallocatechin gallate, a natural product from green tea. *Biochem Pharmacol*, **54**, 1281–1286.
66. Lin, Y.L. and Lin, J.K. (1997) (-)-Epigallocatechin-3-gallate blocks the induction of nitric oxide synthase by down-regulating lipopolysaccharide-induced activity of transcription factor nuclear factor-kappaB. *Mol Pharmacol*, **52**, 465–472.
67. Frank, S., Stallmeyer, B., Kampfer, H., Kolb, N., and Pfeilschifter, J. (1999) Nitric oxide triggers enhanced induction of vascular endothelial growth factor expression in cultured keratinocytes (HaCaT) and during cutaneous wound repair. *FASEB J*, **13**, 2002–2014.
68. Lorenz, M., Wessler, S., Follmann, E., Michaelis, W., Dusterhoft, T., Baumann, G., Stangl, K., and Stangl, V. (2004) A constituent of green tea, epigallocatechin-3-gallate, activates endothelial nitric oxide synthase by a phosphatidylinositol-3-OH-kinase-, cAMP-dependent protein kinase-, and Akt-dependent pathway and leads to endothelial-dependent vasorelaxation. *J Biol Chem*, **279**, 6190–6195.
69. Nam, S., Smith, D.M., and Dou, Q.P. (2001) Ester bond-containing tea polyphenols potently inhibit proteasome activity in vitro and in vivo. *J Biol Chem*, **276**, 13322–13330.

70. Ludwig, A., Lorenz, M., Grimbo, N., Steinle, F., Meiners, S., Bartsch, C., Stangl, K., Baumann, G., and Stangl, V. (2004) The tea flavonoid epigallocatechin-3-gallate reduces cytokine-induced VCAM-1 expression and monocyte adhesion to endothelial cells. *Biochem Biophys Res Commun*, **316**, 659–665.
71. Crouvezier, S., Powell, B., Keir, D., and Yaqoob, P. (2001) The effects of phenolic components of tea on the production of pro- and anti-inflammatory cytokines by human leukocytes in vitro. *Cytokine*, **13**, 280–286.
72. Abd El-Aziz, T.A., Mohamed, R.H., Pasha, H.F., and Abdel-Aziz, H.R. (2012) Catechin protects against oxidative stress and inflammatory-mediated cardiotoxicity in adriamycin-treated rats. *Clin Exp Med*, **12**, 233–240.
73. Suzuki, J., Ogawa, M., Futamatsu, H., Kosuge, H., Sagesaka, Y.M., and Isobe, M. (2007) Tea catechins improve left ventricular dysfunction, suppress myocardial inflammation and fibrosis, and alter cytokine expression in rat autoimmune myocarditis. *Eur J Heart Fail*, **9**, 152–159.
74. Katiyar, S.K. and Mukhtar, H. (2001) Green tea polyphenol (-)-epigallocatechin-3-gallate treatment to mouse skin prevents UVB-induced infiltration of leukocytes, depletion of antigen-presenting cells, and oxidative stress. *J Leukoc Biol*, **69**, 719–726.
75. Adcocks, C., Collin, P., and Buttle, D.J. (2002) Catechins from green tea (*Camellia sinensis*) inhibit bovine and human cartilage proteoglycan and type II collagen degradation in vitro. *J Nutr*, **132**, 341–346.
76. Khokhar, S. and Magnusdottir, S.G. (2002) Total phenol, catechin, and caffeine contents of teas commonly consumed in the United kingdom. *J Agric Food Chem*, **50**, 565–570.
77. Burns, J., Yokota, T., Ashihara, H., Lean, M.E., and Crozier, A. (2002) Plant foods and herbal sources of resveratrol. *J Agric Food Chem*, **50**, 3337–3340.
78. Delmas, D., Lancon, A., Colin, D., Jannin, B., and Latruffe, N. (2006) Resveratrol as a chemopreventive agent: A promising molecule for fighting cancer. *Curr Drug Targets*, **7**, 423–442.
79. Ibern-Gomez, M., Roig-Perez, S., Lamuela-Raventos, R.M., and de la Torre-Boronat, M.C. (2000) Resveratrol and piceid levels in natural and blended peanut butters. *J Agric Food Chem*, **48**, 6352–6354.
80. Ignatowicz, E. and Baer-Dubowska, W. (2001) Resveratrol, a natural chemopreventive agent against degenerative diseases. *Pol J Pharmacol*, **53**, 557–569.
81. Mark, L., Nikfardjam, M.S., Avar, P., and Ohmacht, R. (2005) A validated HPLC method for the quantitative analysis of trans-resveratrol and trans-piceid in Hungarian wines. *J Chromatogr Sci*, **43**, 445–449.
82. Pervaiz, S. (2003) Resveratrol: From grapevines to mammalian biology. *FASEB J*, **17**, 1975–1985.
83. Martinez-Ortega, M.V., Carcia-Parrilla, M.C., and Troncoso, A.M. (2000) Resveratrol content in wines and musts from the south of Spain. *Nahrung*, **44**, 253–256.
84. Shakibaei, M., Harikumar, K.B., and Aggarwal, B.B. (2009) Resveratrol addiction: To die or not to die. *Mol Nutr Food Res*, **53**, 115–128.
85. Baolin, L., Inami, Y., Tanaka, H., Inagaki, N., Iinuma, M., and Nagai, H. (2004) Resveratrol inhibits the release of mediators from bone marrow-derived mouse mast cells in vitro. *Planta Med*, **70**, 305–309.
86. Cavallaro, A., Ainis, T., Bottari, C., and Fimiani, V. (2003) Effect of resveratrol on some activities of isolated and in whole blood human neutrophils. *Physiol Res*, **52**, 555–562.
87. Ferrero, M.E., Bertelli, A.A., Pellegatta, F., Fulgenzi, A., Corsi, M.M., and Bertelli, A. (1998) Phytoalexin resveratrol (3–4′-5-trihydroxystilbene) modulates granulocyte and monocyte endothelial adhesion. *Transplant Proc*, **30**, 4191–4193.
88. Jang, M., Cai, L., Udeani, G.O., Slowing, K.V., Thomas, C.F., Beecher, C.W., Fong, H.H. et al. (1997) Cancer chemopreventive activity of resveratrol, a natural product derived from grapes. *Science*, **275**, 218–220.
89. Donnelly, L.E., Newton, R., Kennedy, G.E., Fenwick, P.S., Leung, R.H., Ito, K., Russell, R.E., and Barnes, P.J. (2004) Anti-inflammatory effects of resveratrol in lung epithelial cells: Molecular mechanisms. *Am J Physiol Lung Cell Mol Physiol*, **287**, L774–L783.
90. Szewczuk, L.M., Forti, L., Stivala, L.A., and Penning, T.M. (2004) Resveratrol is a peroxidase-mediated inactivator of COX-1 but not COX-2: A mechanistic approach to the design of COX-1 selective agents. *J Biol Chem*, **279**, 22727–22737.
91. Martin, A.R., Villegas, I., La Casa, C., and de la Lastra, C.A. (2004) Resveratrol, a polyphenol found in grapes, suppresses oxidative damage and stimulates apoptosis during early colonic inflammation in rats. *Biochem Pharmacol*, **67**, 1399–1410.
92. Bi, X.L., Yang, J.Y., Dong, Y.X., Wang, J.M., Cui, Y.H., Ikeshima, T., Zhao, Y.Q., and Wu, C.F. (2005) Resveratrol inhibits nitric oxide and TNF-alpha production by lipopolysaccharide-activated microglia. *Int Immunopharmacol*, **5**, 185–193.
93. Issuree, P.D., Pushparaj, P.N., Pervaiz, S., and Melendez, A.J. (2009) Resveratrol attenuates C5a-induced inflammatory responses in vitro and in vivo by inhibiting phospholipase D and sphingosine kinase activities. *FASEB J*, **23**, 2412–2424.

94. Holmes-McNary, M. and Baldwin, A.S. Jr. (2000) Chemopreventive properties of trans-resveratrol are associated with inhibition of activation of the IkappaB kinase. *Cancer Res*, **60**, 3477–3483.
95. Goodwin, J.S. and Ceuppens, J. (1983) Regulation of the immune response by prostaglandins. *J Clin Immunol*, **3**, 295–315.
96. Gupta, R.A., Tejada, L.V., Tong, B.J., Das, S.K., Morrow, J.D., Dey, S.K., and DuBois, R.N. (2003) Cyclooxygenase-1 is overexpressed and promotes angiogenic growth factor production in ovarian cancer. *Cancer Res*, **63**, 906–911.
97. Tsujii, M. and DuBois, R.N. (1995) Alterations in cellular adhesion and apoptosis in epithelial cells overexpressing prostaglandin endoperoxide synthase 2. *Cell*, **83**, 493–501.
98. Tsujii, M., Kawano, S., Tsuji, S., Sawaoka, H., Hori, M., and DuBois, R.N. (1998) Cyclooxygenase regulates angiogenesis induced by colon cancer cells. *Cell*, **93**, 705–716.
99. Athar, M., Back, J.H., Kopelovich, L., Bickers, D.R., and Kim, A.L. (2009) Multiple molecular targets of resveratrol: Anti-carcinogenic mechanisms. *Arch Biochem Biophys*, **486**, 95–102.
100. Pirola, L. and Frojdo, S. (2008) Resveratrol: One molecule, many targets. *IUBMB Life*, **60**, 323–332.
101. Miean, K.H. and Mohamed, S. (2001) Flavonoid (myricetin, quercetin, kaempferol, luteolin, and apigenin) content of edible tropical plants. *J Agric Food Chem*, **49**, 3106–3112.
102. Hertog, M.G., Feskens, E.J., Hollman, P.C., Katan, M.B., and Kromhout, D. (1993) Dietary antioxidant flavonoids and risk of coronary heart disease: The Zutphen Elderly Study. *Lancet*, **342**, 1007–1011.
103. Orsolic, N., Knezevic, A.H., Sver, L., Terzic, S., and Basic, I. (2004) Immunomodulatory and antimetastatic action of propolis and related polyphenolic compounds. *J Ethnopharmacol*, **94**, 307–315.
104. Read, M.A. (1995) Flavonoids: Naturally occurring anti-inflammatory agents. *Am J Pathol*, **147**, 235–237.
105. Granado-Serrano, A.B., Martin, M.A., Bravo, L., Goya, L., and Ramos, S. (2012) Quercetin attenuates TNF-induced inflammation in hepatic cells by inhibiting the NF-kappaB pathway. *Nutr Cancer*, **64**, 588–598.
106. Manjeet, K.R. and Ghosh, B. (1999) Quercetin inhibits LPS-induced nitric oxide and tumor necrosis factor-alpha production in murine macrophages. *Int J Immunopharmacol*, **21**, 435–443.
107. Geraets, L., Moonen, H.J., Brauers, K., Wouters, E.F., Bast, A., and Hageman, G.J. (2007) Dietary flavones and flavonoles are inhibitors of poly(ADP-ribose)polymerase-1 in pulmonary epithelial cells. *J Nutr*, **137**, 2190–2195.
108. Bureau, G., Longpre, F., and Martinoli, M.G. (2008) Resveratrol and quercetin, two natural polyphenols, reduce apoptotic neuronal cell death induced by neuroinflammation. *J Neurosci Res*, **86**, 403–410.
109. Noh, H.J., Kim, C.S., Kang, J.H., Park, J.Y., Choe, S.Y., Hong, S.M., Yoo, H., Park, T., and Yu, R. (2014) Quercetin suppresses MIP-1alpha-induced adipose inflammation by downregulating its receptors CCR1/CCR5 and inhibiting inflammatory signaling. *J Med Food*, **17**, 550–557.
110. Endale, M., Park, S.C., Kim, S., Kim, S.H., Yang, Y., Cho, J.Y., and Rhee, M.H. (2013) Quercetin disrupts tyrosine-phosphorylated phosphatidylinositol 3-kinase and myeloid differentiation factor-88 association, and inhibits MAPK/AP-1 and IKK/NF-kappaB-induced inflammatory mediators production in RAW 264.7 cells. *Immunobiology*, **218**, 1452–1467.
111. Sung, M.S., Lee, E.G., Jeon, H.S., Chae, H.J., Park, S.J., Lee, Y.C., and Yoo, W.H. (2012) Quercetin inhibits IL-1beta-induced proliferation and production of MMPs, COX-2, and PGE2 by rheumatoid synovial fibroblast. *Inflammation*, **35**, 1585–1594.
112. Chuang, C.C., Martinez, K., Xie, G., Kennedy, A., Bumrungpert, A., Overman, A., Jia, W., and McIntosh, M.K. (2010) Quercetin is equally or more effective than resveratrol in attenuating tumor necrosis factor-{alpha}-mediated inflammation and insulin resistance in primary human adipocytes. *Am J Clin Nutr*, **92**, 1511–1521.
113. Stewart, L.K., Soileau, J.L., Ribnicky, D., Wang, Z.Q., Raskin, I., Poulev, A., Majewski, M., Cefalu, W.T., and Gettys, T.W. (2008) Quercetin transiently increases energy expenditure but persistently decreases circulating markers of inflammation in C57BL/6J mice fed a high-fat diet. *Metabolism*, **57**, S39–S46.
114. MacNee, W. (2001) Oxidative stress and lung inflammation in airways disease. *Eur J Pharmacol*, **429**, 195–207.
115. Rahman, I. (2002) Oxidative stress, transcription factors and chromatin remodelling in lung inflammation. *Biochem Pharmacol*, **64**, 935–942.
116. Messina, M., Nagata, C., and Wu, A.H. (2006) Estimated Asian adult soy protein and isoflavone intakes. *Nutr Cancer*, **55**, 1–12.
117. de Kleijn, M.J., van der Schouw, Y.T., Wilson, P.W., Adlercreutz, H., Mazur, W., Grobbee, D.E., and Jacques, P.F. (2001) Intake of dietary phytoestrogens is low in postmenopausal women in the United States: The Framingham study(1–4). *J Nutr*, **131**, 1826–1832.

118. Horn-Ross, P.L., John, E.M., Lee, M., Stewart, S.L., Koo, J., Sakoda, L.C., Shiau, A.C., Goldstein, J., Davis, P., and Perez-Stable, E.J. (2001) Phytoestrogen consumption and breast cancer risk in a multiethnic population: The Bay Area Breast Cancer Study. *Am J Epidemiol*, **154**, 434–441.
119. Kesherwani, V. and Sodhi, A. (2007) Involvement of tyrosine kinases and MAP kinases in the production of TNF-alpha and IL-1beta by macrophages in vitro on treatment with phytohemagglutinin. *J Interferon Cytokine Res*, **27**, 497–505.
120. Liang, Y.C., Huang, Y.T., Tsai, S.H., Lin-Shiau, S.Y., Chen, C.F., and Lin, J.K. (1999) Suppression of inducible cyclooxygenase and inducible nitric oxide synthase by apigenin and related flavonoids in mouse macrophages. *Carcinogenesis*, **20**, 1945–1952.
121. Relic, B., Zeddou, M., Desoroux, A., Beguin, Y., de Seny, D., and Malaise, M.G. (2009) Genistein induces adipogenesis but inhibits leptin induction in human synovial fibroblasts. *Lab Invest*, **89**, 811–822.
122. Farina, H.G., Pomies, M., Alonso, D.F., and Gomez, D.E. (2006) Antitumor and antiangiogenic activity of soy isoflavone genistein in mouse models of melanoma and breast cancer. *Oncol Rep*, **16**, 885–891.
123. Lakshman, M., Xu, L., Ananthanarayanan, V., Cooper, J., Takimoto, C.H., Helenowski, I., Pelling, J.C., and Bergan, R.C. (2008) Dietary genistein inhibits metastasis of human prostate cancer in mice. *Cancer Res*, **68**, 2024–2032.
124. Benson, J.M. and Shepherd, D.M. (2011) Dietary ligands of the aryl hydrocarbon receptor induce anti-inflammatory and immunoregulatory effects on murine dendritic cells. *Toxicol Sci*, **124**, 327–338.
125. Chen, Y.H., Dai, H.J., and Chang, H.P. (2003) Suppression of inducible nitric oxide production by indole and isothiocyanate derivatives from Brassica plants in stimulated macrophages. *Planta Med*, **69**, 696–700.
126. Jiang, J., Kang, T.B., Shim do, W., Oh, N.H., Kim, T.J., and Lee, K.H. (2013) Indole-3-carbinol inhibits LPS-induced inflammatory response by blocking TRIF-dependent signaling pathway in macrophages. *Food Chem Toxicol*, **57**, 256–261.
127. Tsai, J.T., Liu, H.C., and Chen, Y.H. (2010) Suppression of inflammatory mediators by cruciferous vegetable-derived indole-3-carbinol and phenylethyl isothiocyanate in lipopolysaccharide-activated macrophages. *Mediators Inflamm*, **2010**, 293642.
128. Takada, Y., Andreeff, M., and Aggarwal, B.B. (2005) Indole-3-carbinol suppresses NF-kappaB and IkappaBalpha kinase activation, causing inhibition of expression of NF-kappaB-regulated antiapoptotic and metastatic gene products and enhancement of apoptosis in myeloid and leukemia cells. *Blood*, **106**, 641–649.
129. Marcotorchino, J., Romier, B., Gouranton, E., Riollet, C., Gleize, B., Malezet-Desmoulins, C., and Landrier, J.F. (2012) Lycopene attenuates LPS-induced TNF-alpha secretion in macrophages and inflammatory markers in adipocytes exposed to macrophage-conditioned media. *Mol Nutr Food Res*, **56**, 725–732.
130. Simone, R.E., Russo, M., Catalano, A., Monego, G., Froehlich, K., Boehm, V., and Palozza, P. (2011) Lycopene inhibits NF-kB-mediated IL-8 expression and changes redox and PPARgamma signalling in cigarette smoke-stimulated macrophages. *PLoS One*, **6**, e19652.
131. Wang, Y., Gao, Y., Yu, W., Jiang, Z., Qu, J., and Li, K. (2013) Lycopene protects against LPS-induced proinflammatory cytokine cascade in HUVECs. *Pharmazie*, **68**, 681–684.
132. Kowalski, J., Samojedny, A., Paul, M., Pietsz, G., and Wilczok, T. (2005) Effect of apigenin, kaempferol and resveratrol on the expression of interleukin-1beta and tumor necrosis factor-alpha genes in J774.2 macrophages. *Pharmacol Rep*, **57**, 390–394.
133. Nicholas, C., Batra, S., Vargo, M.A., Voss, O.H., Gavrilin, M.A., Wewers, M.D., Guttridge, D.C., Grotewold, E., and Doseff, A.I. (2007) Apigenin blocks lipopolysaccharide-induced lethality in vivo and proinflammatory cytokines expression by inactivating NF-kappaB through the suppression of p65 phosphorylation. *J Immunol*, **179**, 7121–7127.
134. Duarte, S., Arango, D., Parihar, A., Hamel, P., Yasmeen, R., and Doseff, A.I. (2013) Apigenin protects endothelial cells from lipopolysaccharide (LPS)-induced inflammation by decreasing caspase-3 activation and modulating mitochondrial function. *Int J Mol Sci*, **14**, 17664–17679.
135. Li, R.R., Pang, L.L., Du, Q., Shi, Y., Dai, W.J., and Yin, K.S. (2010) Apigenin inhibits allergen-induced airway inflammation and switches immune response in a murine model of asthma. *Immunopharmacol Immunotoxicol*, **32**, 364–370.
136. Wang, J., Liao, Y., Fan, J., Ye, T., Sun, X., and Dong, S. (2012) Apigenin inhibits the expression of IL-6, IL-8, and ICAM-1 in DEHP-stimulated human umbilical vein endothelial cells and in vivo. *Inflammation*, **35**, 1466–1476.
137. Gerritsen, M.E., Carley, W.W., Ranges, G.E., Shen, C.P., Phan, S.A., Ligon, G.F., and Perry, C.A. (1995) Flavonoids inhibit cytokine-induced endothelial cell adhesion protein gene expression. *Am J Pathol*, **147**, 278–292.

138. Lee, J.H., Zhou, H.Y., Cho, S.Y., Kim, Y.S., Lee, Y.S., and Jeong, C.S. (2007) Anti-inflammatory mechanisms of apigenin: Inhibition of cyclooxygenase-2 expression, adhesion of monocytes to human umbilical vein endothelial cells, and expression of cellular adhesion molecules. *Arch Pharm Res*, **30**, 1318–1327.
139. Park, E., Kum, S., Wang, C., Park, S.Y., Kim, B.S., and Schuller-Levis, G. (2005) Anti-inflammatory activity of herbal medicines: Inhibition of nitric oxide production and tumor necrosis factor-alpha secretion in an activated macrophage-like cell line. *Am J Chin Med*, **33**, 415–424.
140. Xagorari, A., Papapetropoulos, A., Mauromatis, A., Economou, M., Fotsis, T., and Roussos, C. (2001) Luteolin inhibits an endotoxin-stimulated phosphorylation cascade and proinflammatory cytokine production in macrophages. *J Pharmacol Exp Ther*, **296**, 181–187.
141. Chen, C.Y., Peng, W.H., Tsai, K.D., and Hsu, S.L. (2007) Luteolin suppresses inflammation-associated gene expression by blocking NF-kappaB and AP-1 activation pathway in mouse alveolar macrophages. *Life Sci*, **81**, 1602–1614.
142. Ziyan, L., Yongmei, Z., Nan, Z., Ning, T., and Baolin, L. (2007) Evaluation of the anti-inflammatory activity of luteolin in experimental animal models. *Planta Med*, **73**, 221–226.

Section V

Brain Functions

13 ω-3 PUFA, Advancing Age, and Brain Function

A Review

Isabelle Denis and Gaëlle Champeil-Potokar

CONTENTS

13.1 INTRODUCTION

Over the past four decades or so, studies published on the way omega-3 polyunsaturated fatty acids (ω-3 PUFAs) influence human health have gradually revealed the need for these specific PUFAs, quite separately from the need for the other essential PUFA, omega-6 fatty acids. It was found that a lack of dietary ω-3 PUFA, which is rare in humans (clinical cases of parenteral nutrition), is associated with neurological symptoms (Holman et al. 1982). This resulted in questions being raised about the role of ω-3 PUFA in brain physiology (Bourre et al. 1984). These findings have triggered considerable interest among scientists, the food industry, the media, and the general population. ω-3 PUFAs are claimed to help improve memory, alleviate mood disorders, and protect the brain against aging. The fad for a nutritional fountain of youth is, in fact, based on a great deal of experimental and epidemiological data. While these data have enhanced our understanding of the role of fatty acid (FA) in brain physiology, we still cannot say definitely that dietary ω-3 PUFA can optimize the resistance of the human brain to aging.

This chapter is designed to provide an up-to-date account of the scientific findings resulting from experimental and observational studies showing the potential capacity of dietary FA to slow brain aging. The first part examines why dietary ω-3 PUFAs are important for the brain and how diet and aging influence the lipid content of the brain. The second part covers the many observational and interventional studies on humans that, unfortunately, still provide no firm evidence that dietary ω-3 PUFA can prevent brain aging because of the many biases and confounders that complicate this work. Part 3 summarizes the main alterations in the brain that result from aging and looks at how ω-3 PUFAs influence these alterations, using data from experimental studies reported during the last 20 years. The last part focuses on the alterations of neurotransmission in the hippocampus associated with cognitive decline, the role of the endogenous repairing processes, and their impairment associated with low-grade inflammation and oxidative damage occurring in the aging brain.

13.2 DIETARY ω-3 PUFA AND THE BRAIN

13.2.1 ω-3 PUFA in the Brain: Type, Structure, and Abundance

The brain is one of the fattest tissues in the body, with lipids accounting for about half of its dry weight. The lipid status of the brain is qualitatively unique in that half of its constitutive fatty acids are PUFA, of which half are ω-3 PUFA (Agranoff and Hajra 1993, Bourre et al. 1995). This is related to the importance and specificity of the neuronal and glial cell membranes. The cell membrane bilayer contains a variety of phospholipids, each of which is made up of a polar phosphoglycerol head and two fatty acid tails. Nearly all the phospholipid units in the brain contain one PUFA, located in the sn2 position. These are mainly equal amounts of either arachidonic acid (AA) or docosahexaenoic acid (DHA). These brain membrane phospholipids contain much higher PUFA concentrations than do other tissues. This strongly suggests that their supply is important for neurophysiological processes. DHA is the main long-chain PUFA (LC-PUFA) derived from the ω-3 PUFA series while AA is the main PUFA of the ω-6 PUFA series. These series differ in the position of the first double bond on the fatty acids carbon chain: it is on the third carbon from the methyl terminal end in the ω-3 PUFA and on the sixth carbon in the ω-6 PUFA. The precursor of the ω-3 PUFA series is α-linolenic acid (ALA), which has 18 carbon atoms and 3 double bonds (18:3 n-3), and the precursor of the ω-6 PUFA series is linoleic acid (LA) with 18 carbons and 2 double bonds (18:2 n-6). Mammals cannot synthesize these precursors de novo; they must be supplied by the diet. Nevertheless, they can be elongated and further desaturated by a battery of enzymes, the elongases and desaturases, which are the same for the two series (Figure 13.1). These enzymatic reactions give rise to several longer PUFA, the main ones being AA (20:4 n-6) for the ω-6 PUFA series and DHA (22:6 n-3) and eicosapentaenoic acid (EPA: 20:5 n-3) for the ω-3 PUFA series. The major PUFA in the brain membrane phospholipids are AA and DHA; AA accounts for 37% of the total brain PUFA and DHA for 48%. Analyses of rodent brains indicate that all the other PUFA together account for no more than 15% of the total PUFA (Champeil-Potokar et al. 2006, Latour et al. 2013). The FA composition of human brains is quite similar, although it is less well documented than that of rats and mice.

The abundance of PUFA varies from one class of phospholipid to another: it is 13% of the total FA in phosphatidylcholine (PC), the main class (40% of total phospholipids), and 35%–45% in phosphatidylinositol (PI), phosphatidylserine (PS), and phosphatidylethanolamine (PE) (3.5%, 12%, and 36% of total phospholipids, respectively) (Agranoff and Hajra 1993, Ximenes da Silva et al. 2002, Champeil-Potokar et al. 2004, 2006). These differences between phospholipid classes may account for specific roles of PUFA in distinct cell processes. For instance, the high concentration of PUFA in PE may be related to the segregation of lipid rafts within the membrane thus favoring the combined regulation of proteins assigned to one function (Stillwell and Wassall 2003).

In addition to the great variation in the PUFA content of phospholipid classes, the relative amounts of individual PUFA in each class also vary to a smaller degree. Furthermore, the relative amount of

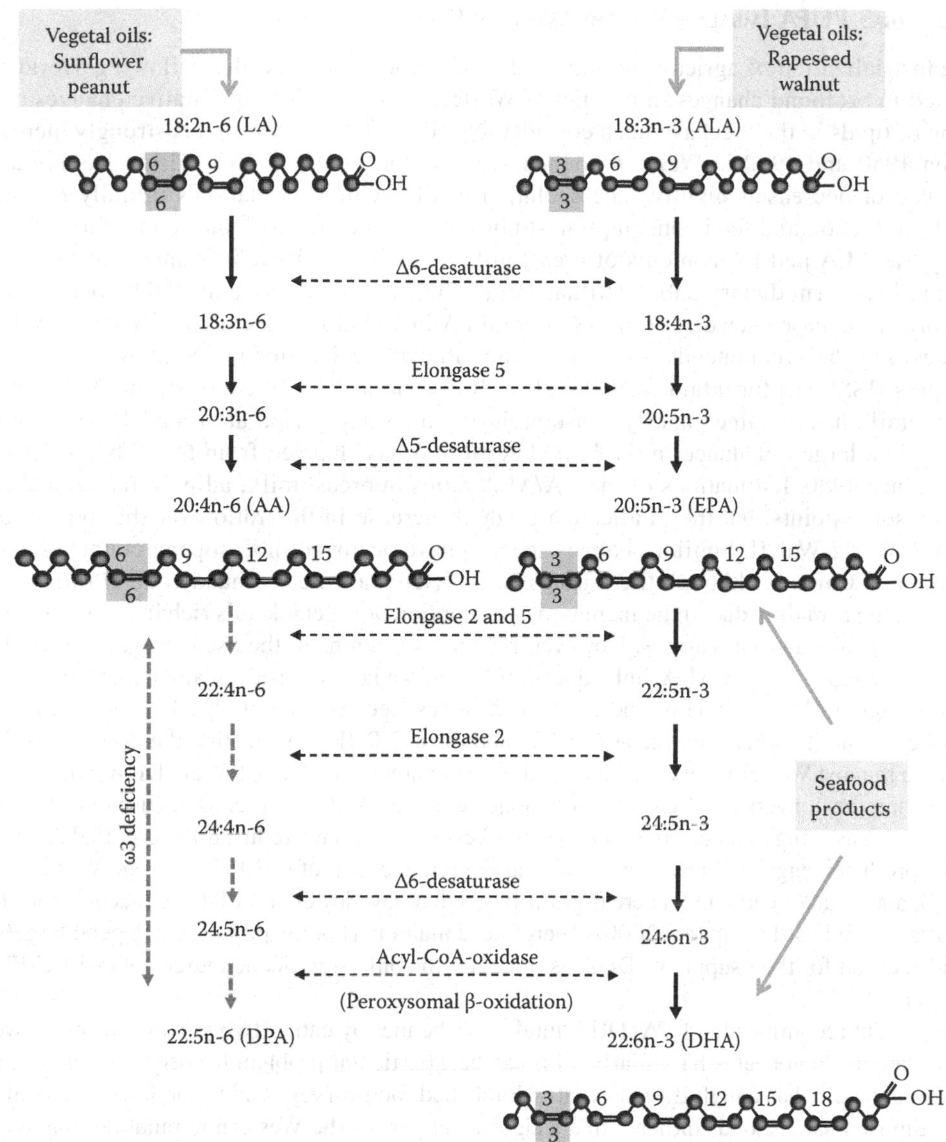

FIGURE 13.1 ω-6 and ω-3 PUFA metabolism via the elongation–desaturation pathway: The mammalian bioconversion pathways produce ω-6 (or n-6) and ω-3 (or n-3) long-chain polyunsaturated fatty acids (LC-PUFAs) from their vegetal precursors (linoleic acid [LA] and linolenic acid [ALA]) by sequential steps of desaturation and elongation. They mainly take place in the liver, which is the major LC-PUFA provider for all the tissues of the organism, including brain. The involved enzymes (elongases and desaturases) are the same for the ω-6 and ω-3 series. The production of ω-3 LC-PUFA (eicosapentaenoic acid [EPA] and docosahexaenoic acid [DHA]) is, therefore, in competition with that of arachidonic acid (AA), the main ω-6 LC-PUFA.

each PUFA in each class varies slightly from one region of the brain to another. For instance, there is more DHA in the PE in the cortex (23% of total FA) of the brains of adult rats than in the PE of the hippocampus (20% of total FA); it is even less abundant in some hypothalamic nuclei (18% of total FA), in striatum (16% of total FA), and in the pineal gland (13% of total FA) (Ximenes da Silva et al. 2002, Lavialle et al. 2008).

But, despite these variations, the impact of diet or age on the PUFA composition of each class of phospholipid and region is very similar.

13.2.2 ω-3 PUFA Imbalance in the Western Diet

The industrialization of agriculture and food production in the decades following World War II has led to profound changes in the diet of Western countries. The qualitative changes of the fraction of lipids in the diet have been considerable. The intake of ω-6 PUFA strongly increased between 1950 and 1990 in Western countries, while the intake of ω-3 PUFAs has remained unchanged or decreased slightly. The evolution of PUFA intakes that was initially measured in food production and food consumption studies has been confirmed and refined in studies on the way the ALA and LA contents of breast milk and adipose tissue in women have changed, reflecting long-term dietary habits (Ailhaud et al. 2006). The LA content of the breast milk of U.S. women increased steadily from 6% of total FA in 1945 to a plateau of 15%–16% by 1990, far exceeding the recommendation of the International Society for the Study of Fatty Acids and Lipids (ISSFAL) for infant formulas (LA: 10% of total FA). In contrast, the ALA content of breast milk has remained nearly constant during the same period at around 1% of total FA, resulting in a large imbalance in the LA/ALA ratio; it has changed from 6 to 8 before 1970 to over 15 since 1980. Estimations of the LA/ALA ratios in breast milk, adipose tissue, and food differ on some points, but they indicate a gradual increase in this ratio over the four decades following World War II. Similar changes seem to have occurred in European countries and in Australia and Canada, although the timings have differed a little (Ailhaud et al. 2006).

The change is mainly due to the increased consumption of vegetable oils rich in LA such as corn and sunflower oils and margarines. However, regional variations in the use of vegetable oils have led to less pronounced LA/ALA imbalances in Scandinavian countries, Canada, and the United Kingdom, than in France, Spain, and the United States (see Ailhaud et al. 2006 for details). The metabolic competition between the ω-6 PUFA and the ω-3 PUFA means that the current LA/ALA imbalance in most Western diets can hamper the conversion of ALA to EPA and DHA, which is less efficient than the conversion of LA to AA (Choque et al. 2014). In parallel to the use of ω-6 PUFA-rich oils for seasoning and cooking, changes in livestock feed have reduced the ω-3 PUFA content of dairy products, eggs, and meat, exacerbating the relative lack of ω-3 PUFA in the Western diet. The milk and meat of cattle fed a cereal-grain-based diet have lower ω-3 PUFA concentrations than those of grass-fed cattle (Sanders 2000). Therefore, a major part of the population depend largely on fish and seafood for their supply of DHA as these are the only significant sources of ω-3 LC-PUFA in the diet.

The present recommended EPA+DHA intake can be met by eating two portions of fish a week, but most people do not eat fish regularly. This can be a particular problem for people living in countries where the diet has a high LA/ALA ratio. Published food surveys and tissue fatty acid analyses (milk, adipose tissue, blood) indicate that a significant part of the Western population may not eat sufficient fish and so cannot restore the unbalanced dietary LA/ALA ratio (Vyncke et al. 2012, Sioen et al. 2013). This can lead to a deficit in DHA in Western populations due to a combination of poor dietary supply and low synthesis from ALA.

The recent national and international dietary surveys indicate that the LA/ALA ratio tends to decrease since 2000s and that the ALA intakes were adequate in many countries in 2010 (Micha et al. 2014). The LA/ALA ratio has been recently evaluated to be around 8–10 in several Western countries (Harika et al. 2011, Vyncke et al. 2012, Sioen et al. 2013). However, Micha et al. (2014), evaluating fat consumption in 266 countries in 2010, also point for some large regional discrepancies in the fish and seafood consumption, estimating that 80% of the world's population have mean ω-3 LC-PUFA intakes below 250 mg/day (while the World Health Organization [WHO] recommendations for ω-3 LC-PUFA are 300–500 mg/day). This study also estimates to 44% only the part of the world's population consuming more than 1.1 g ALA/day (current WHO recommendation for ALA is 2 g/day) while more than half the global population have elevated ω-6 PUFA intakes (more than 5% of total energy intake with large regional discrepancies ranging from 1.2% to 12.5% of energy intakes).

13.2.3 Influence of the Diet on Brain Lipid Composition

The influence of PUFA dietary intake on the brain lipid composition of various animals has been studied for decades. Despite the multiplicity of models and study protocols used, the results are particularly robust and convergent. They show that the ω-6/ω-3 PUFA ratio in the diet strongly determines the ratio in the brain. Thus, the amount of DHA in the brain membranes is low when this ratio is high and increases progressively when the ratio decreases, to reach a plateau when the dietary LA/ALA ratio is around 4. This ratio of 4 is, therefore, considered to be the reference ration for a balanced PUFA intake, leading to a physiologically optimal incorporation of DHA into brain membranes.

The amount of DHA in the brains of rats fed a diet containing vegetal oils (a mixture of sunflower and rapeseed oil) providing a LA/ALA ratio of 4 is around 25% of the total FA in PE, while that of AA is around 15% (Champeil-Potokar et al. 2006, Hennebelle et al. 2012, Latour et al. 2013). Supplementing this diet with a high concentration of fish oil, a direct source of EPA and DHA, results in only a small increase in the amount of the DHA incorporated in cortical PE, from 25% to 27% of total FA in our rat model, and this is offset by an equivalent decrease in AA (Hennebelle et al. 2012). Therefore, the maximal amount of DHA in the mammalian brain seems to be around 25%–30% of the total FA, in the richer PUFA containing phospholipid classes (PE and PS). The very limited amount of EPA in brain membranes (usually less than 0.5% of total fatty acids) may double in animals fed a diet rich in fish oil (Hennebelle et al. 2012), but it generally remains below 1%–2% of the total FA content (Bourre et al. 1992, Cutuli et al. 2014).

Depriving the diet of ω-3 PUFA strongly reduces the amount of DHA in the brain. The extent depends on the duration of the deprivation and the age of the animal. The perinatal period is the crucial time for the accretion of DHA in brain membranes, as this is when myelination and synaptogenesis occur; these processes are particularly intense during the last 3 months of gestation and the neonatal period. As much as 1 g of DHA is incorporated into the brain membranes of humans during the first 6 months of life, which is nearly half of the total amount of DHA incorporated into the whole body (Cunnane et al. 2000). These authors compared infants given ω-3 PUFA-poor formula and those fed on breast milk, which provided at least 60 mg DHA/day. They found that a lack of ω-3 PUFA during this period can halve the amount of DHA incorporated into the brain. They also found that the other organs of the formula-fed infants were more severely depleted in DHA than was the brain, indicating that DHA was preferentially incorporated into brain membranes (Cunnane et al. 2000).

Studies on rat models indicate that a lack of dietary ω-3 PUFA during gestation results in a 50% lower brain DHA in the offspring at birth and adult age, if maintained under an ω-3 PUFA-deficient diet (Ximenes da Silva et al. 2002, Pifferi et al. 2005, Hennebelle et al. 2012, Latour et al. 2013). When two generations of rats are fed a diet lacking ω-3 PUFA, the brains of the second generation can lack up to 80% of their normal DHA content (Aïd et al. 2003, 2005, Mathieu et al. 2008). The decreased brain DHA is offset by an equivalent increase in the ω-6 PUFA, docosapentaenoic acid (DPA, 22:5 n-6). This ω-6 PUFA, which has one unsaturated bond less than DHA, is not usually present in cell membranes. It is synthesized from LA when ALA is lacking and is therefore characteristic of an ω-3 PUFA deficiency. The amplitude of the decrease in DHA in rats fed an ω-3 PUFA-deficient diet is usually the same in the different classes of membrane phospholipids, but it can differ slightly between brain regions (Ximenes da Silva et al. 2002).

While the perinatal period is particularly sensitive to ω-3 PUFA deprivation, adults also require an adequate dietary supply because there is a regular turnover of membrane phospholipids in the brain. This leads to a renewal of 5%–8% of AA and DHA each day in adult rats (Rapoport 2003) and to a turnover of 18 mg AA and 4.6 mg DHA each day in the human brain (Rapoport et al. 2007). Both AA and DHA are continuously released from membrane phospholipids by phospholipase A2 (PLA2) that is activated in response to many signals. The released PUFA can be converted to signaling molecules (notably eicosanoids and docosanoids) by enzymatic or nonenzymatic oxygenation, metabolized via the β-oxidation pathway to energy-producing substrates, re-esterified back to membrane phospholipids; they can even diffuse back into the blood plasma. The studies from Rapoport's laboratory using radiolabeled PUFA and positron emission tomography (PET) imaging have shown that the rate of this turnover is greatly reduced in animals fed a diet lacking ω-3 PUFA. This allows the brain to save the precious DHA. Brain DHA turnover is four times lower in adult rats fed a diet lacking ω-3 PUFA than in rats fed a balanced diet (DeMar et al. 2004). DHA turnover is reduced mainly by the inhibition of the calcium-independent isoform of PLA2, iPLA2 (Rao et al. 2007).

Therefore, a lack of ω-3 PUFA has two major consequences for brain physiology: the DHA in cell membrane phospholipids is replaced by ω-6 DPA and the turnover of DHA is slowed down by inhibiting specific PLA2 signaling pathways. The first change may alter the dynamics and flexibility of the membrane bilayer (Stillwell and Wassall 2003), while the second may alter the ratio of the active metabolites resulting from the oxygenation of AA and DHA, which in turn may upset the balance between proinflammatory and anti-inflammatory pathways (Bazan 2007).

The very low rate at which ALA is converted to DHA in humans (<1%) (Burdge 2004 (review), Goyens et al. 2005, Hussein et al. 2005) combined with the excessively high LA/ALA ratio and the lack of DHA in the current Western diet are likely, together, to endanger the optimal accretion of DHA in the brain. While the total deprivation of ω-3 PUFA that can be obtained in experimental animals is more dramatic than anything experienced by humans, a significant part of the population may have brains that are exposed to membrane and signaling disturbances because of the suboptimal accretion of DHA.

13.2.4 Aging and the Brain Lipid Composition

The influence of aging on the fatty acid content of brain membranes is less clear than that of the diet. The pioneering studies on aged rodents all showed a decrease in brain LC-PUFA with aging, but did not agree on the period or the amplitude of the decrease, the specific PUFA concerned, AA and/or DHA, or the brain region(s) involved (Delion et al. 1997, Giusto et al. 2002, Ledesma et al. 2012). We have recently shown that the brains of old rats fed a diet containing adequate ALA have from 15% to 47% less DHA in their cortical membrane phospholipids than do the brains of young rats and that this loss is offset by an increase in monounsaturated fatty acids (MUFAs); the amounts of AA in young and old rats remain similar (Latour et al. 2013, Roy et al. 2013). We found that the sum of DHA+ω-6DPA in old ω-3 PUFA-deprived rats was also 15% lower than in young ω-3 PUFA-deprived rats (Latour et al. 2013). This suggests a specific alteration in the enzymes responsible for renewing the DHA site on the phospholipid molecules with aging. The LC-acyl-CoA synthetases responsible for the reincorporation of PUFA into phospholipids seem to be specific for individual PUFA (Chen et al. 2008), the one specific for DHA and ω-6DPA may be particularly sensitive to aging.

Data on the human brain are still scarce, but they suggest that the brain membranes of the elderly contain less than normal amounts of DHA and AA (McNamara et al. 2008). Paradoxically, the plasma concentrations of ω-3 PUFA are likely to be increased in older people, as shown repeatedly and recently reviewed by Hennebelle et al. (2014). Cunnane's group used carbon-13 tracers to show that the age-related increases in plasma DHA and EPA are independent of the dietary intakes and may result from changes in DHA homeostasis. The transit of PUFA through the plasma, their retro-conversion, and β-oxidation may all be altered with age (Hennebelle et al. 2014). A recent study on the age-related increase in plasma ω-3 PUFA in elderly Japanese also found that the change was independent of dietary ω-3 PUFA. These subjects ate much more fish than do Western populations (Otsuka et al. 2013). This suggests that a high LC-ω-3 PUFA intake cannot prevent age-related changes in DHA metabolism. However, the plasma AA decreased with age in these Japanese high-fish consumers, which does not occur in Western seniors, and may contribute to the anti-inflammatory properties of fish consumption. We recently found that prolonged feeding of old rats a diet supplemented with fish oil prevented the small age-related decrease in brain DHA that normally occurs in these animals, which agrees well with the concept of a fish-rich diet being beneficial for the elderly (Latour et al., in preparation).

The increased plasma DHA concentration observed in aged human populations may be associated with a decreased DHA concentration in brain membranes resulting from an increase in its turnover and the reduced activity of enzymes like LC-acyl-CoA synthetase that catalyze the reincorporation of DHA into brain cell membranes. The increased DHA turnover in older people is also suggested by the increased PLA2 activity and low-grade inflammatory status of the brain associated with aging. This was recently confirmed by the observation that elderly people with mild cognitive impairment and late-onset Alzheimer's disease (AD) showed a gradual increase in PLA2 activity, glycerophospholipid breakdown, and inflammatory lipids in their cerebrospinal fluid (CSF) while cognitively healthy elderly people did not (Fonteh et al. 2013). However, supplementing the diet of AD patients with ω-3 PUFA for 6 months seems to increase the DHA concentration in their CSF in a way that is inversely correlated with inflammatory markers (Freund-Levi et al. 2014).

There is no clear evidence showing how the dietary intake of ω-3 PUFA changes with age; it seems to depend on cultural, economic, age, and health factors. Some recent food survey studies suggest that the ω-3 PUFA intakes of adolescents and young adults are lower than that of older adults (Gonzales-Rodriguez et al. 2013 [Spain], Sioen et al. 2013 [Belgium]), with a positive correlation between age and the consumption of healthy food such as fish, vegetables, fruit, and oils (Meyer et al. 2003 [*Australia*], Gonzales-Rodriguez et al. 2013). This may well be true for younger elderly people but older elderly and community-dwelling elderly people frequently have low ω-3 PUFA intakes (Hennebelle et al. 2014).

13.3 DIETARY ω-3 PUFA AND BRAIN AGING IN HUMANS: A HARD-TO-ESTABLISH LINK

The increased longevity of people living in most parts of the world has led to growing concern about aging. Brain aging is characterized by cognitive disabilities and an increased susceptibility to neurodegenerative disease including AD and various age-related dementias. The increasing socioeconomic burden resulting from cognitive impairment and the associated loss of autonomy in the elderly makes it essential to look for preventive strategies. Research carried out over the past few decades on the possible influence of ω-3 PUFA on brain physiology and cognitive performance has led to the popular idea that these nutrients could be the Holy Grail for slowing down brain aging. However, the findings of the dozens of observational and interventional studies done on humans so far have not resolved the question of whether dietary ω-3 PUFAs are of any real benefit in preventing brain aging (for a recent update, see Denis et al. 2015). The following section summarizes the main findings and problems of the studies linking ω-3 PUFA and normal or pathological brain aging.

13.3.1 Human Studies on "ω-3 PUFA and Brain Aging": A Brief History

The first indications that ω-3 PUFA can help the brain to cope with age-related damage came from epidemiological studies linking high ω-3 PUFA dietary intakes or fish consumption with a lower risk of AD. However, subsequent studies have failed to confirm this correlation (for review, see Cunnane et al. 2009). The influence of ω-3 PUFA dietary intake on the cognitive decline that characterizes normal brain aging has now been evaluated in observational and interventional (randomized placebo controlled) studies with more consistent findings. Two meta-analyses of the published data (including observational studies and clinical trials) concluded that ω-3 PUFA help slow down cognitive decline in old dementia-free people (Fotuhi et al. 2009, Mazereeuw et al. 2012).

Recent developments in human brain imaging (magnetic resonance imaging [MRI]) have made it possible to evaluate the effects of ω-3 PUFA on brain aging by measuring physiological traits in addition to cognitive changes. The main age-related changes in the brain characterized by MRI are a decrease in gray matter volume, reflecting synaptic and cell loss, and alterations in the quality of white matter, generally referred as white matter hyper-intensities, reflecting vascular and myelin damage. About 10 studies published in the last 2 years provide some MRI evaluation of brain aging in relation to ω-3 PUFA status. They all show an inverse relation between ω-3 PUFA intake, or the ω-3 PUFA status measured in blood (DHA+EPA concentration in plasma or erythrocyte membranes), and some age-associated alteration measured in the brain by MRI (Denis et al. 2015). For instance, Pottalla et al. (2014) found that elevated red blood cell DHA+EPA was associated with a greater total brain or hippocampus volume, while their previous study on the same cohort of elderly American women found no association between the ω-3 PUFA status and age-related cognitive decline (Ammann et al. 2013). Studies published in the last 2 years have shown a positive correlation between ω-3 PUFA status and a greater gray matter volume and/or a better grade of white matter in elderly subjects. However, the findings remain fragile as they vary from one study to another. Some found that the influence of ω-3 PUFA was restricted to specific regions of the brain (Samieri et al. 2012) and to white or gray matter only. Thus, Virtanen et al. (2013) found no association between the plasma DHA concentration and brain atrophy in a cohort of elderly American subjects, in contrast to the findings of Pottala's study or Titova et al. (2013) working on elderly Swedish people.

The promising results of one recent interventional study found that feeding 65 early elderly subjects (50–75 years old) a diet with a DHA+EPA supplement of 2.2 g/day for 26 weeks reduced loss of gray matter and improved white matter intensity in their brains (Witte et al. 2014).

13.3.2 Main Pitfalls of Human Studies

Although most of the findings of recent human studies indicated that dietary ω-3 PUFA supplements have a positive influence on MRI-measured brain changes associated with aging, it is important to understand the limitations of these studies. The major one is the close association between an adequate ω-3 PUFA status (generally due to a high fish intake) and an overall healthy diet (low sugar, low saturated fat, highly diversified, and well balanced), which is itself closely associated with a high socioeconomic status, a global healthy way of life (physical activity, social interactions) and better cognitive scores. These features are strongly predictive of a slower cognitive decline (Bennett et al. 2014). Therefore, the very role of ω-3 PUFA can hardly be individualized among these many confounders. The French Three-Cities study and the Cardiovascular Health Study analyses demonstrated the association between a high ω-3 PUFA status and a healthy diet and lifestyle (Barberger-Gateau et al. 2002, Virtanen et al. 2013). Another analysis of the same cohort found that fish consumption was correlated with a greater gray matter volume, while ω-3 PUFA status was not, suggesting that lifestyle had more influence than biological factors (Raji et al. 2014).

Another caveat is the difficulty of estimating ω-3 PUFA status or intake over the long term. Most of the referenced studies are based on a single report of ω-3 PUFA status/intake, which is often separated by some years from the time of MRI or cognitive evaluation (Pottala et al. 2014). Determining the ω-3 PUFA status or intake is itself difficult. The plasma ω-3 PUFA status was not correlated with the ω-3 PUFA intake in some studies, highlighting the inaccuracy of food recording or plasma sample analyses/conservation in large cohorts (Titova et al. 2013). The dissociation between dietary intake and plasma ω-3 LC-PUFA may also result from an altered turnover in elderly people (as mentioned in Section 13.2.4).

Furthermore, there is still disagreement about the cognitive aging stage that is sensitive to ω-3 PUFA: most recent studies obtained their correlations in cognitively healthy seniors, whereas previous positive results were restricted to patients with mild cognitive impairment (Mazereeuw et al. 2012). It now appears quite clear that ω-3 PUFA has no benefit for patients with established dementia (Cunnane et al. 2009), and most of the recent studies excluded them. There are probably also subgroup effects due to genetic differences, since carriers of apolipoprotein Eε4 (ApoEε4) alleles, representing about 15% of the general population and more prone to cognitive decline or dementia, seem to be insensitive to ω-3 PUFA (Cunnane et al. 2009).

To date, while the evidence from human studies that ω-3 PUFAs have a neuroprotective effect accumulates slowly, the many caveats of these studies need to be offset by experimental investigations in order to progress in our understanding of the impact of ω-3 PUFA on brain aging.

13.4 BRAIN AGING: HOW CAN ω-3 PUFA HELP? MECHANISMS REVEALED BY EXPERIMENTAL STUDIES

The link between ω-3 PUFA and brain aging or neurodegenerative disease has been extensively investigated in animal models, mainly rodents. Despite the inconsistent results of human studies, the vast majority of these experiments have produced positive results showing that ω-3 PUFAs protect the brain against cognitive decline and the neurophysiological damage associated with aging. However, as with human studies, the reliability of these experimental studies is open to question and the many caveats mean that it is not yet possible to conclude that dietary ω-3 PUFA have specific antiaging actions, or to explain precisely how they act. One difficulty is that the great variation in the dietary manipulations performed in different studies makes it difficult to compare their findings. We must also distinguish between ω-3 PUFA deficiencies in adults and in the first or successive generations and between the details of the ω-3 PUFA supplementation, their duration, and composition (mostly EPA or mostly DHA). Another difficulty is the huge diversity of the age-related changes in brain processes, either cognitive or physiological, and the relative frailty of knowledge in this rapidly expanding domain of research. Explorations of brain aging are further complicated by the fact that variations between individual old animals (as in elderly humans) are much greater than between young ones. Cognitive impairment due to aging has been correlated with changes in neurotransmission, loss of dendritic spines and synapses, vascular and metabolic disturbances, neuroinflammation including changes in glial phenotype, intracellular alterations including oxidative stress, mitochondrial and calcium signaling modifications. This section examines the link between the ω-3 PUFA status and the main manifestations of age-related brain damage.

13.4.1 ω-3 PUFA and Cognitive Decline

Experimental studies on young adult rodents carried out over the past 20 years have shown that a lack of ω-3 PUFA is associated with impaired learning capacities. The cognitive deficit has been demonstrated using a wide range of behavioral tests, evaluating learning capacities on the basis of spatial memorization, sensory discrimination, and avoidance tasks (McCann and Ames 2005). They suggest that the cognitive impact of a lack of dietary ω-3 PUFA is not specific to one type of memory, although most of the tests evaluated hippocampus-dependent learning. The wide range of tests used also makes unlikely that the cognitive deficit is linked to a sensory or physical deficit. Nevertheless, the influence of ω-3 PUFA on emotional behavior, also shown in rodents, can interfere with all the cognitive tests used; ω-3 PUFA deficiency has been particularly associated with increased anxiety and hyperactivity (Fedorova and Salem 2006, Lavialle et al. 2010).

Much less work has been done on the impact of ω-3 PUFA on cognitive decline in aged rodents. The studies have used a range of learning tests, most of them testing hippocampal memorization (Y maze, Moris water maze, avoidance tests, object recognition). Some studies have found that the learning capacities of first-generation ω-3 PUFA-deficient old mice (Umezawa et al. 1995, Carrie et al. 2002) and old ω-3 PUFA-deficient rats (Yamamoto et al. 1991) are inferior to those of ω-3 PUFA-replete old animals, while others have found them to be unchanged (Moranis et al. 2011). Short-term supplementation with ω-3 LC-PUFA can restore the spatial learning ability of old rats (Gamoh et al. 2001 [several weeks on a DHA supplement], Kelly et al. 2011 [2 months on an EPA supplement]), and of old mice (Labrousse et al. 2012 [2 months on a fish oil supplement]). An ω-3 LC-PUFA dietary supplement also improved the cognitive capacity when tested in rodent models of AD (Calon et al. 2004, Hashimoto et al. 2005 [several weeks on a DHA supplement]), although, again, there are contradictory results (Barcelo-Coblijn et al. 2003, Arendash et al. 2007 [after weeks or months on a fish oil supplement]). However, the Morris water maze was used to show that ω-3 LC-PUFA supplementation had no beneficial effect, and this test is not well adapted to old animals with a physical impairment and an enhanced anxiety for swimming. A recent study using a 2-month ω-3 LC-PUFA supplementation showed that treatment improved spatial learning, object recognition, and aversive response retention in old mice (Cutuli et al. 2014). The interesting point in this study is that the ω-3 LC-PUFA supplementation did not alter the anxiety level of the mice, supporting the specificity of the cognitive effect. Overall most of the reported cognitive deficits alleviated by ω-3 PUFA in experimental studies depend on hippocampal function. Other aspects of cognition may also be concerned, but they have not been tested.

13.4.2 ω-3 PUFA and Neurotransmission (Figure 13.2)

The hippocampus seems to be one of the first and most severely altered areas of the humans and animal brains during aging. However, the real extent of normal aging-related damage has not yet been clearly established; the literature contains many contradictory observations. The hippocampal volume, number of neurons, and dendritic arborization may all remain relatively intact during aging, while there may be more subtle changes that account for the cognitive deficits, like place strategy in spatial learning tasks that is clearly affected by aging (Samson and Barnes 2013). In particular, there are many changes in glutamatergic neurotransmission and the associated synaptic plasticity in the aging hippocampus.

The main neuronal pathways in the hippocampus rely on glutamatergic transmission involving the release of glutamate from the pre-synaptic neuron, which is then bound to specific ionotropic receptors (2-amino-3-propionic acid [AMPA] and N-methyl-D-aspartate [NMDA] receptors) on the postsynaptic neuron, triggering excitatory postsynaptic potentials (EPSP). The astrocyte, the third cell partner in the synapse, acts in many ways to modulate the system by scavenging glutamate, releasing regulatory molecules (gliotransmitters), and regulating the extra-synaptic volume (Nedergaard and Verkhratsky 2012). The efficacy of neurotransmission (synaptic efficiency) can be durably potentiated (long-term potentiation [LTP]) or depressed (long-term depression [LTD]), mainly by activating NMDA and calcium-dependent cascades of phosphorylation or de-phosphorylation in order to modulate the amount of AMPA receptors at the postsynaptic membrane. The astrocytes also participate in these modulations of synaptic efficiency (Todd et al. 2006).

Experiments on rodents have shown that the age-related alterations in these processes of synaptic plasticity are clearly correlated with defects in spatial memory (Samson and Barnes 2013). Studies conducted in the laboratory of M. Lynch have shown that the improved spatial learning in the Morris water maze produced by ω-3 LC-PUFA supplementation in aged rats is associated with a restoration of LTP in the hippocampus. In this model, ω-3 LC-PUFA supplementation was sufficient to offset the age-related decrease in brain DHA (Martin et al. 2002, Lynch et al. 2007, Kelly et al. 2011). However, both this group and another reported a similar restoration of LTP when aged rats were given a supplementation containing AA and ϒ-linolenic acid, which suggests that both ω-6 and ω-3 LC-PUFA help preserve synaptic plasticity during aging (McGahon et al. 1999, Kotani et al. 2003). In a mice model of aging and neuroinflammation, 4 months of ω-3 PUFA supplied diet at the adult age restored LTP in the dentate gyrus of the hippocampus as compared to mice receiving an ω-3 PUFA-deficient diet (Crupi et al. 2012). Others have shown that a ω-3 PUFA deficiency also impairs LTP in the hippocampus of young mice and is associated with a decrease in the amount of postsynaptic NMDA receptors (Cao et al. 2009).

The numbers of some specific subunits of AMPA and NMDA receptors seem to decrease with aging, which may contribute to the impairment of synaptic plasticity in old animals. A 3-month

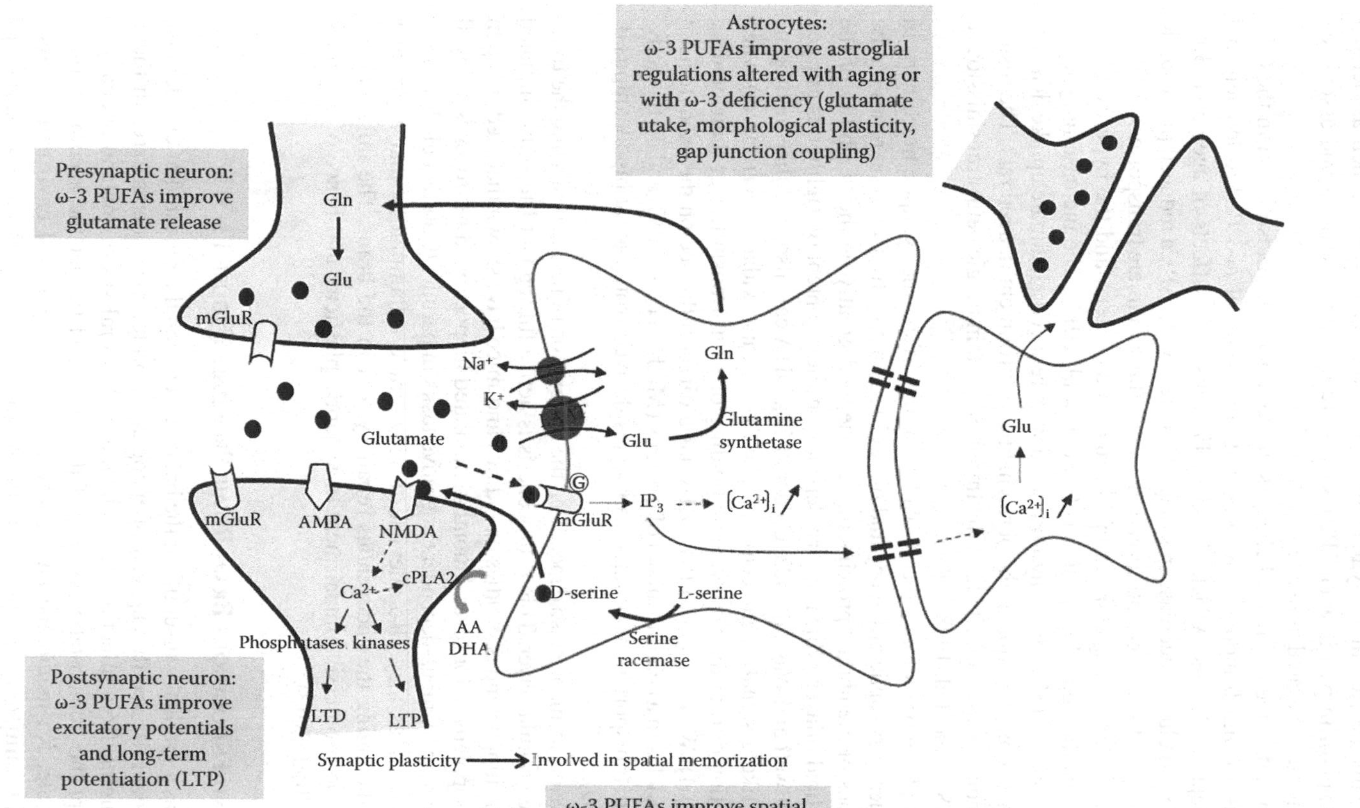

FIGURE 13.2 **(See color insert.)** ω-3 PUFA implication in the synaptic activity and regulation: Glutamatergic neurotransmission relies on a finely regulated cross-talk between the presynaptic and postsynaptic neurons and the astrocytes. Notably, the presynaptic release of glutamate (Glu) is controlled by the feedback activation of metabotropic receptors (mGluR), its postsynaptic binding on ionotropic receptors (AMPA and NMDA) is modified by gliotransmitters (such as D-serine), its concentration in the synaptic cleft depends on the astroglial glutamate uptake activity, and its extrasynaptic leakage varies according to the extent of the astroglial sheath around the synapse. The changes in synaptic efficiency, called long-term potentiation (LTP) and long-term depression (LTD), are considered to sustain memory formation and are notably involved in spatial learning. Several of these mechanisms are affected directly by DHA or by the ω-3 PUFA status of brain cell membranes Gln (Glutamine).

dietary fish oil supplement can restore the numbers of NMDA and AMPA receptor NR2B and GLUR2 subunits in old rats (Dyall et al. 2007). Similarly, ω-3 PUFA influences the synthesis of several proteins involved in glutamatergic synaptic signaling in young rodents (for review, see Su 2010, Denis et al. 2013). This increase in the synthesis of synaptic receptors and/or their associated signaling proteins may explain in part how ω-3 PUFAs restore synaptic plasticity and associated cognitive abilities that have deteriorated with age.

We have recently shown that the age-related changes in glutamatergic transmission in the CA1 area of the hippocampus are much more severe in a first generation of ω-3 PUFA-deficient old rats than in ω-3 PUFA-replete old rats. A lack of ω-3 PUFA makes the effects of age about 30% more severe. These changes include a decrease in synaptic efficiency (EPSP), a reduced presynaptic release of glutamate linked to a lower concentration of the vesicular glutamate transporters (VGlut-1 and VGlut-2), a decrease in astroglial glutamate uptake and transporters, and the hypertrophy of astrocytes that characterizes the aging hippocampus (Latour et al. 2013). The increase in synaptic astroglial coverage due to astrocyte hypertrophy, combined with reduced glutamate uptake, leads to a greater ambient glutamate concentration in the perisynaptic environment in aged rats. The resulting changes in synaptic homeostasis contribute to the impaired glutamatergic neurotransmission in the aging hippocampus (Sykova et al. 1998, 2002).

The ω-3 PUFA status of the brain (or of the whole body) may affect the synaptic machinery in several ways and so influence synaptic efficiency and plasticity. Synaptic transmission relies on the movement and interactions of membrane proteins that can depend greatly on the flexibility of the molecules that form the lipid bilayer, which in turn depends on their content of highly unsaturated fatty acids like DHA (Stillwell and Wassall 2003, Calder 2012). DHA can also modulate membrane proteins directly, acting like a signaling molecule (in itself or via its oxidative derivatives) when released by PLA2 activation during the postsynaptic binding of neurotransmitter or their binding to astroglia (Lee et al. 2011). We have shown that DHA has a direct influence on the exocytosis of neurotransmitter from vesicles in a cell line model of neurons (Mathieu et al. 2010) and on the activity of astroglial glutamate transporters in cultured astrocytes derived from the rat hippocampus or cortex (Grintal et al. 2009).

Hippocampal cognitive performance also depends on the integration of new neurons into the functional network within the granular layer. This neurogenesis is active throughout life and is initiated in the dentate gyrus of the hippocampus. Studies on old rats and mice have shown that feeding them a dietary ω-3 LC-PUFA supplement for several months stimulated hippocampal neurogenesis (Dyall et al. 2010) and improved hippocampus-dependent cognitive tasks in parallel (Cutuli et al. 2014).

An optimal ω-3 PUFA status may also alleviate the low-grade inflammation that aggravates aging by soliciting and damaging the endogenous repair system in the brain. The inflammation therefore contributes to the progressive impairment of synaptic plasticity and hence of cognitive decline (Norden and Godbout 2013).

13.4.3 ω-3 PUFA and Endogenous Brain Repair Processes (Figure 13.3)

Aging may be regarded as a gradual worsening of the balance between the repeated micro-damage events that occur throughout life and the capacity of endogenous protective systems to repair them. All sorts of stresses, ranging from infections, to ischemia, behavioral stress, metabolic changes, and free radicals, disrupt the homeostatic systems of the brain and trigger the accumulation of toxic molecules (glutamate, K^+, membrane fatty acids, etc.) in the neuronal environment. Such disruption is considered to initiate and/or propagate the brain damage associated with aging and neurological disorders (Matute et al. 2006, Yi and Hazell 2006, Sheldon and Robinson 2007). The brain responds to disrupted homeostasis by activating microglial cells; these in turn activate astrocytes by releasing proinflammatory cytokines such as IL-6, IL-1β, and TNF-α. Microglia are pivotal cells in the immune surveillance in the brain and also propagate peripheral inflammatory signals to the brain. Activated astrocytes can become more protective by taking up glutamate and

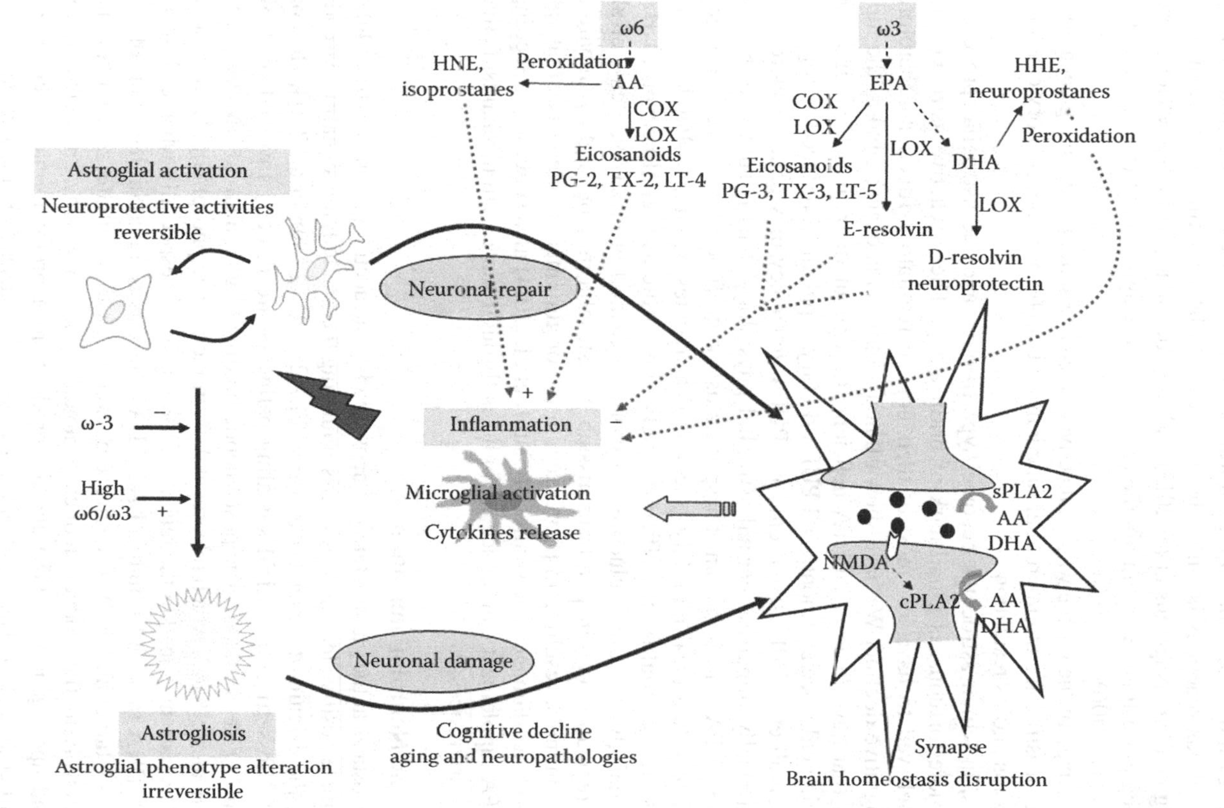

FIGURE 13.3 **(See color insert.)** Glial activation—an endogenous brain repair system: Changes in the homeostasis of the neuronal/synaptic environment (such as increased glutamate release) activate microglia, the immune cells of the brain, which in turn activate the astrocytes. Reversibly activated astrocytes reinforce their neuroprotective activities to restore the homeostasis. During aging, astrocyte activation turns to an irreversible alteration of the astrocyte phenotype called astrogliosis, resulting in impaired synaptic regulations. The underlying signaling pathways involve oxygenated derivatives of LC-PUFA, thought to be proinflammatory when derived from the ω-6 series and anti-inflammatory when derived from the ω-3 series. An adequate ω-3 PUFA dietary intake providing sufficient DHA to the brain may, therefore, limit the glial activation and slow down the age-induced brain damages.

releasing neurotrophic/growth factors like brain-derived neurotrophic factor (BDNF), leading to enhanced synaptic regulation and neuron repair. Astrocytes become irreversibly activated when the insults are too intense or too frequent, and the astrocyte phenotype is altered by the process of astrogliosis (Cotrina and Nedergaard 2002, Sofroniew and Vinters 2010). This further disrupts homeostasis, aggravates the damage to neurons, and progressively exacerbates the dysfunction associated with neurological disorders and aging (Morale et al. 2006). The switch in glial activity from repairing to deleterious reactions is currently considered to be a continuum of changes in response to a changing context (Nagelhus et al. 2013) and may be an accessible target for therapeutic/preventive strategies designed to maintain the function of the aging brain (Sun et al. 2004, Heneka 2006, Morale et al. 2006).

The ω-3 PUFA status may influence the way glial activation changes and its repairing capacities in several ways, acting on astroglial and microglial functions and on the proinflammatory cascades involved in glial activation and its resolution.

Diffuse astrogliosis, in which astrocytes become hypertrophic, and the astroglial processes become thicker and more tortuous, is a hallmark of brain aging. These reactive astrocytes in the aging brain are believed to have lost most of their normal regulatory functions, therefore contributing to the cognitive decline. We have shown that astrogliosis is exacerbated in the hippocampus of old rats that have been ω-3 PUFA deficient throughout their lives (Latour et al. 2013). Conversely, giving old mice a 2-month ω-3 PUFA dietary supplement reduced astrogliosis in the hippocampus (Cutuli et al. 2014). A chronic ω-3 PUFA deficiency may enhance astrogliosis during aging by gradually impairing normal astroglial physiology. This is suggested by our work showing that ω-3 PUFAs are important for specific astrocyte functions: DHA favors gap junction coupling and morphological plasticity in cultured astrocytes (Champeil-Potokar et al. 2006), both properties are essential for the efficient functioning of the astroglial network; DHA also modulates astroglial glutamate and glucose transporters (Grintal et al. 2009, Denis et al. 2013). Therefore, the regulation of synaptic transmission by astroglia may be slightly impaired in ω-3 PUFA-deficient animals, resulting in poorer regulation of glutamate homeostasis that can lead to enhanced age-related damage. The studies of Cutuli et al. (2014) also suggest that feeding old animals a ω-3 PUFA supplement can reduce astrogliosis through short-term mechanisms that attenuate proinflammatory processes.

13.4.3.1 ω-3 PUFA and Neuroinflammation

The disruption of homeostasis at the glutamatergic synapse leads to an accumulation of extracellular glutamate that may initiate positive feedback by over-stimulating the arachidonic signaling cascade initiated by activating the calcium-dependent isoform of PLA2, cPLA2 (Sun et al. 2004, Haydon and Carmignoto 2006, Bossetti 2007). Lipid signaling pathways are directly involved in these mechanisms (Phillis and O'Regan 2004). The postsynaptic binding of glutamate to NMDA and to astroglial receptors activates cPLA2, which releases AA from membrane phospholipids (Ramadan et al. 2010). Excess glutamate may lead to the release of too much AA, especially when cell membranes have a high AA/DHA ratio and a high cPLA2/iPLA2 ratio, as is found in the brains of ω-3 PUFA-deficient animals (Rao et al. 2007). The release of excess AA then initiates a proinflammatory cascade of events involving the production of eicosanoids via the activation of inducible cyclooxygenase (COX2) and lipoxygenases (LOX) and the production of proinflammatory cytokines (Bazan 2007, Farooqui et al. 2007). The onset of the AA signaling cascade is moderated by ω-3 PUFA, which inhibits the synthesis of proinflammatory isoforms (cytoplasmic [cPLA2] and secretory [sPLA2]) of PLA2 and cyclooxygenase (COX2) and reduces the production of eicosanoids. This capacity of ω-3 PUFA to counteract the influence of the AA signaling cascade has been described in peripheral tissues (Calder 2013) and in the brain (Rao et al. 2007, Rapoport 2008).

Low-grade inflammation is a hallmark of aging characterized by elevated concentrations of inflammatory cytokines in the blood and in the brain, where they are produced by microglia and astrocytes (Norden and Godbout 2013, Joffre et al. 2014). The anti-inflammatory properties of ω-3

PUFA may be a major feature of their protection of the brain against aging (Calder 2011, 2013). A chronic ω-3 PUFA deficiency enhances the LPS-induced increase in IL-6 concentrations in the plasma and hippocampus of mice (Mingam et al. 2008), while a dietary ω-3 LC-PUFA supplement reduces cytokine production and microglial activation associated with aging in several rodent models (Lynch et al. 2007, Kelly et al. 2011, Labrousse et al. 2012). Recent *in vitro* studies have shown that DHA and EPA dampen the development of the proinflammatory M1 phenotype of microglia and favor their repairing phenotype (phagocytosis of β-amyloid) (Hjorth et al. 2013). The anti-inflammatory action of DHA involves the down-regulation of nuclear factor-κB in microglia, and the enzymatic production of oxygenated derivatives, via the activities of COX and LOX, called resolvins and neuroprotectins, which actively participate to the resolution of the inflammatory process (Calder 2011, Orr et al. 2013). In a model of brain acute ischemia, DHA has been shown to temper microglial activation and the inflammation-associated brain injuries while promoting the survival of neurons and astroglia (Eady et al. 2014).

13.4.3.2 ω-3 PUFA and Oxidative Damage

Mitochondrial-based oxidative phosphorylation is very active in brain cells that are huge oxygen consumers. The production of large amounts of free radicals, combined with a progressive decline in antioxidant defense systems, is thought to play a major role in brain aging. The high PUFA content of brain cell membranes also contributes to the specific vulnerability of the brain to oxidative damages. PUFAs are targets of reactive oxygen species (ROS) and their oxidation leads to peroxidation derivatives such as 4-hydroxy-nonenal (HNE) from ω-6 PUFA, and 4-hydroxy-hexenal (4-HHE) from ω-3 PUFA. These aldehydes and their protein adducts are used to quantify oxidative stress and lipid peroxidation in blood, tissues, and cells. They are clearly associated with oxidative damage by increasing ROS, protein, and phospholipid adducts, by altering DNA and by decreasing antioxidative defenses (glutathione) (Long et al. 2010). While the effects of HNE have been studied for longer than those of HHE, both compounds are cytotoxic and induce apoptosis in many cellular models including neurons. They also activate signaling pathways such as NFκB, extracellular signal–regulated kinase (ERK), or mitogen-activated protein (MAP) kinase pathways. HHE activity seems to differ from that of HNE, at least to a certain extent. Each compound has different protein targets for adduct formation and HHE alters cell signaling pathways at a lower concentration than does HNE (Long et al. 2010). HHE is much more abundant than HNE in DHA-rich tissues such as the brain (Long et al. 2010).

These observations suggest that dietary ω-3 and ω-6 PUFA are pro-oxidative, triggering proinflammatory processes. Paradoxically, measurements of changes in peroxidation and inflammation markers in response to the dietary supply of ω-3 LC-PUFA have not shown that they increase. Instead, the index of oxidative stress and inflammation status was found to decrease. The dose–response study of Calzada et al. (2010) showed that 200–800 mg/day DHA increased the plasma antioxidant status of early aging human subjects and that only higher DHA intakes (800–1600 mg/day) increased the concentration of circulating HHE, without altering the plasma oxidative status of the subjects. HHE may have a paradoxically antioxidant action by stimulating the heme-oxygenase-1 (HO-1), a protective enzyme whose activity is induced by cellular oxidative stress (Ishikado et al. 2013, Nakagawa et al. 2014). Nonenzymatic oxygenation of DHA also produces neuroprostanes that may play a key role in the anti-inflammatory effects of dietary ω-3 LC-PUFA (Musiek et al. 2008, Gladine et al. 2014).

A recent study on adult Korean subjects also showed an inverse correlation between the ω-3 LC-PUFA concentration in blood erythrocytes, which is a good index of ω-3 PUFA dietary intake, and the circulating markers of inflammation and oxidative stress (Baek and Park 2013). Others have shown that a dietary ω-3 LC-PUFA supplement improves the hippocampus antioxidant status of aged rats (Jiang et al. 2013), as well as in a rat model of metabolic syndrome (Maruyama et al. 2014).

Last, a dietary ω-3 LC-PUFA supplement was found to protect mitochondrial function from age-related changes in rodent models of aging and AD (Eckert et al. 2013).

Overall, the current state of knowledge indicates that dietary ω-3 LC-PUFAs promote the anti-oxidative and anti-inflammatory status of animals, including humans, despite their highly peroxidative nature. However, a diet poor in ω-3 PUFA and rich in ω-6 PUFA, like those of many Western and emerging countries, seems to increase peroxidative markers and favor low-grade inflammation in both the body and the brain. These global effects probably result from the production of enzyme-catalyzed (resolvins, protectins) and nonenzyme-catalyzed (HHE, neuroprostanes) derivatives of ω-3 LC-PUFA. These may trigger more beneficial cellular signaling than those associated with ω-6 PUFA derivatives. However, we need to know more about the biological activities of PUFA derivatives before we can clearly understand the impact of ω-3 PUFA and ω-6 PUFA on oxidative stress in tissues, including the brain.

13.4.3.3 ω-3 PUFA and Cerebral Circulation

The beneficial effects of ω-3 PUFA on the cardiovascular system have been studied for decades and are now well documented. A diet rich in ω-3 PUFA reduces the risk for cardiovascular disease by acting on many mechanisms, notably by lowering platelet aggregation, dampening the oxidation of plasma low-density lipoproteins (LDL), reducing the concentration of circulating triglycerides, and limiting the inflammatory signaling in artery walls (Chang and Deckelbaum 2013). Vascular disorders contribute to brain aging and neurodegenerative disease, and the beneficial action of ω-3 PUFA for the general and brain vascular system probably contributes to prevent damage to neurons and synaptic impairment. Several studies on animal models, including aged animals, have shown that ω-3 LC-PUFA dietary supplements increase regional cerebral blood flow (Haast and Kiliaan 2014), and fish oil supplements increase the oxyhemoglobin content of the cortex of elderly human subjects performing cognitive tasks (Konagai et al. 2013). ω-3 PUFA may act on cerebral blood flow through vasodilating mechanisms involving nitric oxide synthase and TREK-1 channels (Haast and Kiliaan 2014). An increase in blood flow will help the aging brain maintain sufficient supplies of oxygen and energy substrates to the neurons. The brains of adult rats that are ω-3 PUFA deficient use less-than-normal amounts of glucose and the concentrations of the glucose transporter GLUT1 on the endothelial cells of brain vessels and the astrocytes are subnormal (Ximenes da Silva et al. 2002, Pifferi et al. 2005). Astrocytes are part of the blood–brain barrier and play a crucial role in adapting blood flow to neuron activity. The beneficial effects of ω-3 PUFA on astroglial function described earlier may also help these cells maintain an adequate blood flow.

13.5 CONCLUSION

The decade-long imbalance between ω-6 and ω-3 PUFA that has persisted in Western diets seems likely to endanger brain and cognitive functions as people get older. The high ω-6/ω-3 PUFA ratio in the diet may decrease the incorporation of DHA into membranes of brain cells, including neurons, astrocytes and microglia, and hamper DHA signaling, while simultaneously increasing AA signaling in both brain cells and peripheral tissues. The above-normal ω-6 PUFA signaling favors the low-grade inflammatory status associated with aging, while the data cited earlier all point to DHA being involved in numerous aspects of cerebral function.

There is an increasing body of evidence documenting the beneficial effect of an adequate ω-3 PUFA intake on brain aging in humans. However, there are many caveats about ω-3 PUFA and human studies, including lifestyle confounders and variations in the determinants (evaluation and stage of cognitive decline and nutritional status).

Experimental studies on rodents and on cellular models continue to add to our understanding of how ω-3 PUFAs act in brain cells. The most advanced leads are those involving DHA in synapse regulation and neuroinflammation, which are a great challenge to the aging brain. There are now sufficient data indicating that the amount of DHA in membranes influences several steps of synaptic transmission, notably at the glutamatergic synapses in the hippocampus. These steps are neurotransmitter release, postsynaptic transmitter reception, and regulation by astrocytes.

DHA may also temper the exacerbation of the glial reaction and the resulting proinflammatory events that accelerate brain aging through its effects on astroglia and the way it antagonizes AA in the PLA2/COX signaling pathway. The few published studies on the role of DHA in neurogenesis in the adult hippocampus suggest that DHA also promotes the supply of newly formed neurons to support the memory throughout life. The emerging and expanding research on the specific roles of the enzymatic and nonenzymatic derivatives of DHA and EPA as distinct from those derived from AA promise to help our understanding of how dietary ω-3 PUFAs enable the brain to cope with aging. These compounds may be particularly important for limiting oxidative stress and low-grade inflammation and for coupling cerebral blood flow and neuron activity.

Investigation into the beneficial impact of dietary ω-3 PUFA on brain processes still continues. It is now clear that we need to rebalance the ω-3 PUFA content of our Western diet in order to preserve cognitive function in older people.

ACKNOWLEDGMENT

The authors thank Dr. Owen Parkes for editing the English manuscript.

REFERENCES

Agranoff BW, Hajra AK. 1993. Lipids. In *Basic Neurochemistry*, ed. Siegel G et al. New-York: Raven Press.

Aid S, Vancassel S, Poumes-Ballihaut C, Chalon S, Guesnet P, Lavialle M. 2003. Effect of a diet-induced n-3 PUFA depletion on cholinergic parameters in the rat hippocampus. *Journal of Lipid Research* 44(8):1545–1551.

Aid S, Vancassel S, Linard A, Lavialle M, Guesnet P. 2005. Dietary docosahexaenoic acid 22:6(n-3) as a phospholipid or a triglyceride enhances the potassium chloride-evoked release of acetylcholine in rat hippocampus. *Journal of Nutrition* 135(5):1008–1013.

Ailhaud G, Massiera F, Weill P, Legrand P, Alessandri JM, Guesnet P. 2006. Temporal changes in dietary fats: Role of n-6 polyunsaturated fatty acids in excessive adipose tissue development and relationship to obesity. *Progress in Lipid Research* 45(3):203–236.

Ammann EM, Pottala JV, Harris WS, Espeland MA, Wallace R, Denburg NL, Carnahan RM, Robinson JG. 2013. Omega-3 fatty acids and domain-specific cognitive aging: Secondary analyses of data from WHISCA. *Neurology* 81(17):1484–1491.

Arendash GW, Jensen MT, Salem N, Hussein N, Cracchiolo J, Dickson A, Leighty R, Potter H. 2007. A diet high in omega-3 fatty acids does not improve or protect cognitive performance in Alzheimer's transgenic mice. *Neuroscience* 149(2):286–302.

Baek D, Park Y. 2013. Association between erythrocyte n-3 polyunsaturated fatty acids and biomarkers of inflammation and oxidative stress in patients with and without depression. *Prostaglandins Leukotrienes and Essential Fatty Acids* 89(5):291–296.

Barberger-Gateau P, Letenneur L, Deschamps V, Peres K, Dartigues J-F, Renaud S. 2002. Fish, meat, and risk of dementia: Cohort study. *BMJ* (Clinical research ed) 325(7370):932–933.

Barcelo-Coblijn G, Hogyes E, Kitajka K, Puskas LG, Zvara A, Hackler L, Nyakas C, Penke Z, Farkas T. 2003. Modification by docosahexaenoic acid of age-induced alterations in gene expression and molecular composition of rat brain phospholipids. *Proceedings of the National Academy of Sciences of the United States of America* 100(20):11321–11326.

Bazan NG. 2007. Omega-3 fatty acids, pro-inflammatory signaling and neuroprotection. *Current Opinion in Clinical Nutrition and Metabolic Care* 10(2):136–141.

Bennett DA, Arnold SE, Valenzuela MJ, Brayne C, Schneider JA. 2014. Cognitive and social lifestyle: Links with neuropathology and cognition in late life. *Acta Neuropathologica* 127(1):137–150.

Bossetti F. 2007. Arachidonic acid metabolism in brain physiology and pathology: Lessons from genetically altered mouse models. *Journal of Neurochemistry* 102:577–586.

Bourre JM, Pascal G, Durand G, Masson M, Dumont O, Piciotti M. 1984. Alteration in the fatty acid composition of rat brain cells (neurons, astrocytes and oligodendrocytes) and of subcellular fractions (myelin and synaptosomes) induced by a diet devoid of n-3 fatty acids. *Journal of Neurochemistry* 43(2):342–348.

Bourre JM, Bonneil M, Chaudière J, Clément M, Dumont O, Durand G, Lafont H, Nalbone G, Pascal G, Piciotti M. 1992. Structural and functional importance of dietary polyunsaturated fatty acids in the nervous system. *Advances in Experimental Medicine and Biology* 318:211–229.

Bourre JM, Dumont O, Clement M, Durand G. 1995. Fatty acids of the alpha-linolenic family and the structures and functions of the brain – Their nature, role, origin and dietary importance – Animal model. *Ocl-Oleagineux Corps Gras Lipides* 2(4):254–263.

Burdge G. 2004. Alpha-linolenic acid metabolism in men and women: nutritional and biological implications. *Current Opinion in Clinical Nutrition and Metabolism Care* 7(2):137–144.

Calder PC. 2011. Fatty acids and inflammation: The cutting edge between food and pharma. *European Journal of Pharmacology* 668:S50–S58.

Calder PC. 2012. Mechanisms of action of (n-3) fatty acids. *The Journal of Nutrition* 142(3):592S–599S.

Calder PC. 2013. Omega-3 polyunsaturated fatty acids and inflammatory processes: Nutrition or pharmacology? *British Journal of Clinical Pharmacology* 75(3):645–662.

Calon F, Lim GP, Yang FS, Morihara T, Teter B, Ubeda O, Rostaing P, Triller A, Salem N, Ashe KH, Frautschy SA, Cole GM. 2004. Docosahexaenoic acid protects from dendritic pathology in an Alzheimer's disease mouse model. *Neuron* 43(5):633–645.

Calzada C, Colas R, Guillot N, Guichardant M, Laville M, Vericel E, Lagarde M. 2010. Subgram daily supplementation with docosahexaenoic acid protects low-density lipoproteins from oxidation in healthy men. *Atherosclerosis* 208(2):467–472.

Cao DH, Kevala K, Kim J, Moon HS, Jun SB, Lovinger D, Kim HY. 2009. Docosahexaenoic acid promotes hippocampal neuronal development and synaptic function. *Journal of Neurochemistry* 111(2):510–521.

Carrie I, Smirnova M, Clement M, De Javel D, Frances H, Bourre JM. 2002. Docosahexaenoic acid-rich phospholipid supplementation: Effect on behavior, learning ability, and retinal function in control and n-3 polyunsaturated fatty acid deficient old mice. *Nutritional Neuroscience* 5(1):43–52.

Champeil-Potokar G, Denis I, Goustard-Langelier B, Alessandri JM, Guesnet P, Lavialle M. 2004. Astrocytes in culture require docosahexaenoic acid to restore the n-3/n-6 polyunsaturated fatty acid balance in their membrane phospholipids. *Journal of Neuroscience Research* 75(1):96–106.

Champeil-Potokar G, Chaumontet C, Guesnet P, Lavialle M, Denis I. 2006. Docosahexaenoic acid (22:6 n-3) enrichment of membrane phospholipids increases gap junction coupling capacity in cultured astrocytes. *European Journal of Neuroscience* 24(11):3084–3090.

Chang CL, Deckelbaum RJ. 2013. Omega-3 fatty acids: Mechanisms underlying "protective effects" in atherosclerosis. *Current Opinion in Lipidology* 24(4):345–350.

Chen CT, Green JT, Orr SK, Bazinet RP. 2008. Regulation of brain polyunsaturated fatty acid uptake and turnover. *Prostaglandins Leukotrienes and Essential Fatty Acids* 79(3–5):85–91.

Choque B, Catheline D, Rioux V, Legrand P. 2014. Linoleic acid: Between doubts and certainties. *Biochimie* 96C:14–21.

Cotrina ML, Nedergaard M. 2002. Astrocytes in the aging brain. *Journal of Neuroscience Research* 67(1):1–10.

Crupi R, Cambiaghi M, Deckelbaum R, Hansen I, Mindes J, Spina E, Battaglia F. 2012. n-3 fatty acids prevent impairment of neurogenesis and synaptic plasticity in B-cell activating factor (BAFF) transgenic mice. *Preventive Medicine* 54:S103–S108.

Cunnane SC, Francescutti V, Brenna JT, Crawford MA. 2000. Breasts-fed infants achieve a higher rate of brain and whole body docosahexaenoate accumulation than formula-fed infants not consuming dietary docosahexaenoate. *Lipids* 35(1):105–111.

Cunnane SC, Plourde M, Pifferi F, Begin M, Feart C, Barberger-Gateau P. 2009. Fish, docosahexaenoic acid and Alzheimer's disease. *Progress in Lipid Research* 48(5):239–256.

Cutuli D, De Bartolo P, Caporali P, Laricchiuta D, Foti F, Ronci M, Rossi C, et al. 2014. n-3 polyunsaturated fatty acids supplementation enhances hippocampal functionality in aged mice. *Frontiers in Aging Neuroscience* 6.

Delion S, Chalon S, Guilloteau D, Lejeune B, Besnard JC, Durand G. 1997. Age-related changes in phospholipid fatty acid composition and monoaminergic neurotransmission in the hippocampus of rats fed a balanced or an n-3 polyunsaturated fatty acid-deficient diet. *Journal of Lipid Research* 38(4):680–689.

DeMar JC, Ma KZ, Bell JM, Rapoport SI. 2004. Half-lives of docosahexaenoic acid in rat brain phospholipids are prolonged by 15 weeks of nutritional deprivation of n-3 polyunsaturated fatty acids. *Journal of Neurochemistry* 91(5):1125–1137.

Denis I, Potier B, Vancassel S, Heberden C, Lavialle M. 2013. Omega-3 fatty acids and brain resistance to ageing and stress: Body of evidence and possible mechanisms. *Ageing Research Reviews* 12(2):579–594.

Denis I, Potier B, Heberden C, Vancassel S. 2015. ω-3 polyunsaturated fatty acids and brain aging. *Current Opinion in Clinical Nutrition and Metabolic Care.* 18(2):139–146.

Dyall SC, Michael GJ, Whelpton R, Scott AG, Michael-Titus AT. 2007. Dietary enrichment with omega-3 polyunsaturated fatty acids reverses age-related decreases in the GluR2 and NR2B glutamate receptor subunits in rat forebrain. *Neurobiology of Aging* 28(3):424–439.

Dyall SC, Michael GJ, Michael-Titus AT. 2010. Omega-3 fatty acids reverse age-related decreases in nuclear receptors and increase neurogenesis in old rats. *Journal of Neuroscience Research* 88(10):2091–2102.

Eady TN, Khoutorova L, Obenaus A, Mohd-Yusof A, Bazan NG, Belayev L. 2014. Docosahexaenoic acid complexed to albumin provides neuroprotection after experimental stroke in aged rats. *Neurobiology of Disease* 62:1–7.

Eckert GP, Lipka U, Muller WE. 2013. Omega-3 fatty acids in neurodegenerative diseases: Focus on mitochondria. *Prostaglandins Leukotrienes and Essential Fatty Acids* 88(1):105–114.

Farooqui AA, Horrocks LA, Farooqui T. 2007. Modulation of inflammation in brain: A matter of fat. *Journal of Neurochemistry* 101(3):577–599.

Fedorova I, Salem N. 2006. Omega-3 fatty acids and rodent behavior. *Prostaglandins Leukotrienes and Essential Fatty Acids* 75(4–5):271–289.

Fonteh AN, Chiang J, Cipolla M et al. 2013. Alterations in cerebrospinal fluid glycerophospholipids and phospholipase A2 activity in Alzheimer's disease. *Journal of Lipid Research* 54(10):2884–2897.

Fotuhi M, Mohassel P, Yaffe K. 2009. Fish consumption, long-chain omega-3 fatty acids and risk of cognitive decline or Alzheimer disease: A complex association. *Nature Clinical Practice Neurology* 5(3):140–152.

Freund-Levi Y, Vedin I, Hjorth E, Basun H, Irving GF, Schultzberg M, Eriksdotter M, Palmblad J, Vessby B, Wahlund LO, Cederholm T, Basu S. 2014. Effects of supplementation with omega-3 fatty acids on oxidative stress and inflammation in patients with Alzheimer's disease: The OmegAD Study. *Journal of Alzheimers Disease* 42(3):823–831.

Gamoh S, Hashimoto M, Hossain S, Masumura S. 2001. Chronic administration of docosahexaenoic acid improves the performance of radial arm maze task in aged rats. *Clinical and Experimental Pharmacology and Physiology* 28(4):266–270.

Giusto NM, Salvador GA, Castagnet PI, Pasquare SJ, de Boschero MGI. 2002. Age-associated changes in central nervous system glycerolipid composition and metabolism. *Neurochemical Research* 27(11):1513–1523.

Gladine C, Newman JW, Durand T, Pedersen TL, Galano J-M, Demougeot C, Berdeaux O, Pujos-Guillot E, Mazur A, Comte B. 2014. Lipid profiling following intake of the omega 3 fatty acid DHA identifies the peroxidized metabolites F-4-neuroprostanes as the best predictors of atherosclerosis prevention. *PLoS One* 9(2):e89393.

Gonzalez-Rodriguez LG, Aparicio A, Lopez-Sobaler AM, Ortega RM. 2013. Omega 3 and omega 6 fatty acids intake and dietary sources in a representative sample of Spanish adults. *International Journal for Vitamin and Nutrition Research Internationale Zeitschrift fur Vitamin- und Ernahrungsforschung Journal international de vitaminologie et de nutrition* 83(1):36–47.

Goyens PL, Spilker ME, Zock PL, Katan MB, Mensink RP. 2005. Compartmental modeling to quantify alpha-linolenic acid conversion after longer-term intake of multiple tracer boluses. *Journal of Lipid Research* 46:1474–1483.

Grintal B, Champeil-Potokar G, Lavialle M, Vancassel S, Breton S, Denis I. 2009. Inhibition of astroglial glutamate transport by polyunsaturated fatty acids: Evidence for a signalling role of docosahexaenoic acid. *Neurochemistry International* 54(8):535–543.

Haast RAM, Kiliaan AJ. 2014. Impact of fatty acids on brain circulation, structure and function. *Prostaglandins, Leukotrienes and Essential Fatty Acids* 92:3–14.

Hashimoto M, Tanabe Y, Fujii Y, Kikuta T, Shibata H, Shido O. 2005. Chronic administration of docosahexaenoic acid ameliorates the impairment of spatial cognition learning ability in amyloid beta-infused rats. *Journal of Nutrition* 135(3):549–555.

Haydon PG, Carmignoto G. 2006. Astrocyte control of synaptic transmission and neurovascular coupling. *Physiological Reviews* 86(3):1009–1031.

Heneka MT. 2006. Inflammation in Alzheimer's disease. *Clinical Neuroscience Research* 6(5):247–260.

Hennebelle M, Balasse L, Latour A, Champeil-Potokar G, Denis S, Lavialle M, Gisquet-Verrier P, Denis I, Vancassel S. 2012. Influence of omega-3 fatty acid status on the way rats adapt to chronic restraint stress. *PLoS One* 7(7):e42142.

Hennebelle M, Champeil-Potokar G, Lavialle M, Vancassel S, Denis I. 2014. Omega-3 polyunsaturated fatty acids and chronic stress-induced modulations of glutamatergic neurotransmission in the hippocampus. *Nutrition Reviews* 72(2):99–112.

Hjorth E, Zhu M, Toro VC, Vedin I, Palmblad J, Cederholm T, Freund-Levi Y et al. 2013. Omega-3 fatty acids enhance phagocytosis of Alzheimer's disease-related amyloid-beta(42) by human microglia and decrease inflammatory markers. *Journal of Alzheimers Disease* 35(4):697–713.

Holman RT, Johnson SB, Hatch TF. 1982. Human linolenic acid deficiency - Reply. *American Journal of Clinical Nutrition* 36(6):1254–1255.

Hussein N, Ah-Sing E, Wilkinson P, Leach C, Griffin BA, Millward DJ. 2005. Long-chain conversion of C-13 linoleic acid and alpha-linolenic acid in response to marked changes in their dietary intake in men. *Journal of Lipid Research* 46(2):269–280.

Ishikado A, Morino K, Nishio Y, Nakagawa F, Mukose A, Sono Y, Yoshioka N et al. 2013. 4-Hydroxy hexenal derived from docosahexaenoic acid protects endothelial cells via Nrf2 activation. *PLoS One* 8(7):e69415 [69413pp.]–e69415 [69413pp.].

Jiang L-H, Yan S, Wang J, Liang Q-y. 2013. Oral administration of docosahexaenoic acid activates the GDNF-MAPK-CERB pathway in hippocampus of natural aged rat. *Pharmaceutical Biology* 51(9):1188–1195.

Joffre C, Nadjar A, Lebbadi M, Calon F, Laye S. 2014. n-3 LCPUFA improves cognition: The young, the old and the sick. *Prostaglandins Leukotrienes and Essential Fatty Acids* 91(1–2):1–20.

Kelly L, Grehan B, Della Chiesa A, O'Mara SM, Downer E, Sahyoun G, Massey KA, Nicolaou A, Lynch MA. 2011. The polyunsaturated fatty acids, EPA and DPA exert a protective effect in the hippocampus of the aged rat. *Neurobiology of Aging* 32(12):2318.

Konagai C, Yanagimoto K, Hayamizu K, Han L, Tsuji T, Koga Y. 2013. Effects of krill oil containing n-3 polyunsaturated fatty acids in phospholipid form on human brain function: A randomized controlled trial in healthy elderly volunteers. *Clinical Interventions in Aging* 8:1247–1257.

Kotani S, Nakazawa H, Tokimasa T, Akimoto K, Kawashima H, Toyoda-Ono Y, Kiso Y, Okaichi H, Sakakibara M. 2003. Synaptic plasticity preserved with arachidonic acid diet in aged rats. *Neuroscience Research* 46(4):453–461.

Labrousse VF, Nadjar A, Joffre C, Costes L, Aubert A, Gregoire S, Bretillon L, Laye S. 2012. Short-term long chain omega3 diet protects from neuroinflammatory processes and memory impairment in aged mice. *PLos One* 7(5):e36861.

Latour A, Grintal B, Champeil-Potokar G, Hennebelle M, Lavialle M, Dutar P, Potier B, Billard JM, Vancassel S, Denis I. 2013. Omega-3 fatty acids deficiency aggravates glutamatergic synapse and astroglial aging in the rat hippocampal CA1. *Aging Cell* 12(1):76–84.

Lavialle M, Champeil-Potokar G, Alessandri JM, Balasse L, Guesnet P, Papillon C, Pevet P, Vancassel S, Vivien-Roels B, Denis I. 2008. An (n-3) polyunsaturated fatty acid-deficient diet disturbs daily locomotor activity, melatonin rhythm, and striatal dopamine in Syrian hamsters. *Journal of Nutrition* 138(9):1719–1724.

Lavialle M, Denis I, Guesnet P, Vancassel S. 2010. Involvement of omega-3 fatty acids in emotional responses and hyperactive symptoms. *Journal of Nutritional Biochemistry* 21(10):899–905.

Ledesma MD, Martin MG, Dotti CG. 2012. Lipid changes in the aged brain: Effect on synaptic function and neuronal survival. *Progress in Lipid Research* 51(1):23–35.

Lee JCM, Simonyi A, Sun AY, Sun GY. 2011. Phospholipases A2 and neural membrane dynamics: Implications for Alzheimer's disease. *Journal of Neurochemistry* 116(5):813–819.

Long EK, Rosenberger TA, Picklo MJ Sr. 2010. Ethanol withdrawal increases glutathione adducts of 4-hydroxy-2-hexenal but not 4-hydroxyl-2-nonenal in the rat cerebral cortex. *Free Radical Biology and Medicine* 48(3):384–390.

Lynch AM, Loane DJ, Minogue AM, Clarke RM, Kilroy D, Nally RE, Roche OJ, O'Connell F, Lynch MA. 2007. Eicosapentaenoic acid confers neuroprotection in the amyloid-beta challenged aged hippocampus. *Neurobiology of Aging* 28(6):845–855.

Martin DS, Spencer P, Horrobin DF, Lynch MA. 2002. Long-term potentiation in aged rats is restored when the age-related decrease in polyunsaturated fatty acid concentration is reversed. *Prostaglandins Leukotrienes and Essential Fatty Acids* 67:121–130.

Maruyama H, Takahashi M, Sekimoto T, Shimada T, Yokosuka O. 2014. Linoleate appears to protect against palmitate-induced inflammation in Huh7 cells. *Lipids in Health and Disease* 13:78.

Mathieu G, Denis S, Lavialle M, Vancassel S. 2008. Synergistic effects of stress and omega-3 fatty acid deprivation on emotional response and brain lipid composition in adult rats. *Prostaglandins Leukotrienes and Essential Fatty Acids* 78(6):391–401.

Mathieu G, Denis S, Langelier B, Denis I, Lavialle M, Vancassel S. 2010. DHA enhances the noradrenaline release by SH-SY5Y cells (vol. 56, p. 94, 2010). *Neurochemistry International* 57(6):690–690.

Matute C, Domercq M, Sanchez-Gomez MV. 2006. Glutamate-mediated glial injury: Mechanisms and clinical importance (vol. 53, p. 212, 2006). *Glia* 53(6):675–675.

Mazereeuw G, Lanctot KL, Chau SA, Swardfager W, Herrmann N. 2012. Effects of omega-3 fatty acids on cognitive performance: A meta-analysis. *Neurobiology of Aging* 33(7):1482.e1417–e1429.

McCann JC, Ames BN. 2005. Is docosahexaenoic acid, an n-3 long-chain polyunsaturated fatty acid, required for development of normal brain function? An overview of evidence from cognitive and behavioral tests in humans and animals. *American Journal of Clinical Nutrition* 82(2):281–295.

McGahon BM, Murray CA, Horrobin DF, Lynch MA. 1999. Age-related changes in oxidative mechanisms and LTP are reversed by dietary manipulation. *Neurobiology of Aging* 20(6):643–653.

McNamara RK, Liu Y, Jandacek R, Rider T, Tso P. 2008. The aging human orbitofrontal cortex: Decreasing polyunsaturated fatty acid composition and associated increases in lipogenic gene expression and stearoyl-CoA desaturase activity. *Prostaglandins, Leukotrienes, and Essential Fatty Acids* 78(4–5):293–304.

Meyer BJ, Mann NJ, Lewis JL, Milligan GC, Sinclair AJ, Howe PRC. 2003. Dietary intakes and food sources of omega-6 and omega-3 polyunsaturated fatty acids. *Lipids* 38(4):391–398.

Micha R, Khatibzadeh S, Shi P, Fahimi S, Lim S, Andrews KG, Engell RE, Powles J, Ezzati M, Mozaffarian D, Global Burden of Diseases Nutrition and Chronic Diseases Expert Group NutriCo DE. 2014. Global, regional, and national consumption levels of dietary fats and oils in 1990 and 2010: A systematic analysis including 266 country-specific nutrition surveys. *BMJ* (Clinical research ed) 348:g2272.

Mingam R, Moranis A, Bluthe R-M, De Smedt-Peyrusse V, Kelley KW, Guesnet P, Lavialle M, Dantzer R, Laye S. 2008. Uncoupling of interleukin-6 from its signalling pathway by dietary n-3-polyunsaturated fatty acid deprivation alters sickness behaviour in mice. *European Journal of Neuroscience* 28(9):1877–1886.

Morale MC, Serra PA, L'Episcopo F, Tirolo C, Caniglia S, Testa N, Gennuso F et al. 2006. Estrogen, neuroinflammation and neuroprotection in Parkinson's disease: Glia dictates resistance versus vulnerability to neurodegeneration. *Neuroscience* 138(3):869–878.

Moranis A, Delpech JC, De Smedt-Peyrusse V, Aubert A, Guesnet P, Lavialle M, Joffre C, Laye S. 2011. Long term adequate n-3 polyunsaturated fatty acid diet protects from depressive-like behavior but not from working memory disruption and brain cytokine expression in aged mice. *Brain, Behavior, and Immunity* 26:721–731.

Musiek ES, Brooks JD, Joo M, Brunoldi E, Porta A, Zanoni G, Vidari G et al. 2008. Electrophilic cyclopentenone neuroprostanes are anti-inflammatory mediators formed from the peroxidation of the omega-3 polyunsaturated fatty acid docosahexaenoic acid. *The Journal of Biological Chemistry* 283(29):19927–19935.

Nagelhus EA, Amiry-Moghaddam M, Bergersen LH, Bjaalie JG, Eriksson J, Gundersen V, Leergaard TB et al. 2013. The glia doctrine: Addressing the role of glial cells in healthy brain ageing. *Mechanisms of Ageing and Development* 134(10):449–459.

Nakagawa F, Morino K, Ugi S, Ishikado A, Kondo K, Sato D, Konno S et al. 2014. 4-Hydroxy hexenal derived from dietary n-3 polyunsaturated fatty acids induces anti-oxidative enzyme heme oxygenase-1 in multiple organs. *Biochemical and Biophysical Research Communications* 443(3):991–996.

Nedergaard M, Verkhratsky A. 2012. Artifact versus reality-How astrocytes contribute to synaptic events. *Glia* 60(7):1013–1023.

Norden DM, Godbout JP. 2013. Review: Microglia of the aged brain: Primed to be activated and resistant to regulation. *Neuropathology and Applied Neurobiology* 39(1):19–34.

Orr SK, Palumbo S, Bosetti F, Mount HT, Kang JX, Greenwood CE, Ma DWL, Serhan CN, Bazinet RP. 2013. Unesterified docosahexaenoic acid is protective in neuroinflammation. *Journal of Neurochemistry* 127(3):378–393.

Otsuka R, Kato Y, Imai T, Ando F, Shimokata H. 2013. Higher serum EPA or DHA, and lower ARA compositions with age independent fatty acid intake in Japanese aged 40 to 79. *Lipids* 48(7):719–727.

Phillis JW, O'Regan MH. 2004. A potentially critical role of phospholipases in central nervous system ischemic, traumatic, and neurodegenerative disorders. *Brain Research Reviews* 44(1):13–47.

Pifferi F, Roux F, Langelier B, Alessandri JM, Vancassel S, Jouin M, Lavialle M, Guesnet P. 2005. (n-3) polyunsaturated fatty acid deficiency reduces the expression of both isoforms of the brain glucose transporter GLUT1 in rats. *Journal of Nutrition* 135(9):2241–2246.

Pottala JV, Yaffe K, Robinson JG, Espeland MA, Wallace R, Harris WS. 2014. Higher RBC EPA + DHA corresponds with larger total brain and hippocampal volumes: WHIMS-MRI study. *Neurology* 82(5):435–442.

Raji CA, Erickson KI, Lopez OL, Kuller LH, Gach HM, Thompson PM, Riverol M, Becker JT. 2014. Regular fish consumption and age-related brain gray matter loss. *American Journal of Preventive Medicine* 47(4):444–451.

Ramadan E, Rosa AO, Chang L, Chen M, Rapoport SI, Basselin M. 2010. Extracellular-derived calcium does not initiate in vivo neurotransmission involving docosahexaenoic acid. *Journal of Lipid Research* 51(8):2334–2340.

Rao JS, Ertley RN, Demar JC, Rapoport SI, Bazinet RP, Lee HJ. 2007. Dietary n-3 PUFA deprivation alters expression of enzymes of the arachidonic and docosahexaenoic acid cascades in rat frontal cortex. *Molecular Psychiatry* 12(2):151–157.

Rapoport SI. 2003. In vivo approaches to quantifying and imaging brain arachidonic and docosahexaenoic acid metabolism. *Journal of Pediatrics* 143(4):S26–S34.

Rapoport SI. 2008. Arachidonic acid and the brain. *Journal of Nutrition* 138(12):2515–2520.

Rapoport SI, Rao JS, Igarashi M. 2007. Brain metabolism of nutritionally essential polyunsaturated fatty acids depends on both the diet and the liver. *Prostaglandins, Leukotrienes and Essential Fatty Acids* 77:251–261.

Roy M, Hennebelle M, St-Pierre V, Courchesne-Loyer A, Fortier M, Bouzier-Sore AK, Gallis JL, Beauvieux MC, Cunnane SC. 2013. Long-term calorie restriction has minimal impact on brain metabolite and fatty acid profiles in aged rats on a Western-style diet. *Neurochemistry International* 63(5):450–457.

Samieri C, Maillard P, Crivello F, Proust-Lima C, Peuchant E, Helmer C, Amieva H et al. 2012. Plasma long-chain omega-3 fatty acids and atrophy of the medial temporal lobe. *Neurology* 79(7):642–650.

Samson RD, Barnes CA. 2013. Impact of aging brain circuits on cognition. *European Journal of Neuroscience* 37(12):1903–1915.

Sanders TAB. 2000. Polyunsaturated fatty acids in the food chain in Europe. *American Journal of Clinical Nutrition* 71:176S–178S.

Sheldon AL, Robinson MB. 2007. The role of glutamate transporters in neurodegenerative diseases and potential opportunities for intervention. *Neurochemistry International* 51(6–7):333–355.

Sioen I, Vyncke K, De Maeyer M, Gerichhausen M, De Henauw S. 2013. Dietary intake and food sources of total and individual polyunsaturated fatty acids in the Belgian population over 15 years old. *Lipids* 48(7):729–738.

Sofroniew MV, Vinters HV. 2010. Astrocytes: Biology and pathology. *Acta Neuropathologica* 119(1):7–35.

Sprecher H, Luthria DL, Mohammed BS, Baykousheva SP. 1995. Reevaluation of the pathways for the biosynthesis of polyunsaturated fatty acids. *Journal of Lipid Research* 36:2471–2477.

Stillwell W, Wassall SR. 2003. Docosahexaenoic acid: Membrane properties of a unique fatty acid. *Chemistry and Physics of Lipids* 126(1):1–27.

Su HM. 2010. Mechanisms of n-3 fatty acid-mediated development and maintenance of learning memory performance. *Journal of Nutritional Biochemistry* 21(5):364–373.

Sun GY, Xu JF, Jensen MD, Simonyi A. 2004. Phospholipase A(2) in the central nervous system: Implications for neurodegenerative diseases. *Journal of Lipid Research* 45(2):205–213.

Sykova E, Mazel T, Simonova Z. 1998. Diffusion constraints and neuron-glia interaction during aging. *Experimental Gerontology* 33(7–8):837–851.

Sykova E, Mazel T, Hasenohrl RU, Harvey AR, Simonova Z, Mulders W, Huston JP. 2002. Learning deficits in aged rats related to decrease in extracellular volume and loss of diffusion anisotropy in hippocampus. *Hippocampus* 12(2):269–279.

Titova OE, Sjogren P, Brooks SJ, Kullberg J, Ax E, Kilander L, Riserus U et al. 2013. Dietary intake of eicosapentaenoic and docosahexaenoic acids is linked to gray matter volume and cognitive function in elderly. *Age* (Dordrecht, Netherlands) 35(4):1495–1505.

Todd KJ, Serrano A, Lacaille JC, Robitaille R. 2006. Glial cells in synaptic plasticity. *Journal of Physiology-Paris* 99(2–3):75–83.

Umezawa M, Ohta A, Tojo H, Yagi H, Hosokawa M, Takeda T. 1995. Dietary alpha-linolenate/linoleate balance influences learning and memory in the senescence-accelerated mouse (SAM). *Brain Research* 669(2):225–233.

Virtanen JK, Siscovick DS, Lemaitre RN, Longstreth WT, Spiegelman D, Rimm EB, King IB, Mozaffarian D. 2013. Circulating omega-3 polyunsaturated fatty acids and subclinical brain abnormalities on MRI in older adults: The Cardiovascular Health Study. *Journal of the American Heart Association* 2(5):e000305.

Vyncke KE, Libuda L, De Vriendt T, Moreno LA, Van Winckel M, Manios Y, Gottrand F et al. 2012. Dietary fatty acid intake, its food sources and determinants in European adolescents: The HELENA (Healthy Lifestyle in Europe by Nutrition in Adolescence) Study. *The British Journal of Nutrition* 108(12):2261–2273.

Witte AV, Kerti L, Hermannstadter HM, Fiebach JB, Schreiber SJ, Schuchardt JP, Hahn A, Floel A. 2014. Long-chain omega-3 Fatty acids improve brain function and structure in older adults. *Cerebral Cortex* (New York: 1991) 24(11):3059–3068.

Ximenes da Silva A, Lavialle F, Gendrot G, Guesnet P, Alessandri J-M, Lavialle M. 2002. Glucose transport and utilization are altered in the brain of rats deficient in n-3 polyunsaturated fatty acids. *Journal of Neurochemistry* 81(6):1328–1337.

Yamamoto N, Okaniwa Y, Mori S, Nomura M, Okuyama H. 1991. Effects of a high-linoleate and a high-alpha-linolenate diet on the learning ability of aged rats. Evidence against an autoxidation-related lipid peroxide theory of aging. *Journal of Gerontology* 46:B17–B22.

Yi JH, Hazell AS. 2006. Excitotoxic mechanisms and the role of astrocytic glutamate transporters in traumatic brain injury. *Neurochemistry International* 48(5):394–403.

14 Stress, Parkinson's, and Alzheimer's Disease
Role of Dietary Supplements

Raj K. Keservani, Rajesh K. Kesharwani, Anil K. Sharma, and Mohd Fasih Ahmad

CONTENTS

14.1 INTRODUCTION

As per the U.S. Food and Drug Administration (FDA), dietary supplements are products that are not pharmaceutical drugs, food additives like spices or preservatives, or conventional food, and which also complies with any of these criteria: (1) The product is supposed to add nutrition to a person's diet, despite it not being utilized as a meal substitute. (2) The product is or contains a vitamin, dietary element, herb used for herbalism or botanical used as a medicinal plant, amino acid, any substance that adds to other food eaten, or any concentrate, metabolite, ingredient, extract, or a combination of these things. (3) The product is labeled as a dietary supplement (IMNRC 2004).

A dietary supplement is believed to supply nutrients that may otherwise not be consumed in sufficient quantities. Supplements as generally apprehended may be comprised of vitamins, minerals, fiber, fatty acids, or amino acids, besides other substances. U.S. authorities describe dietary supplements as foods, whereas in other parts of the world, these may be categorized as drugs or other products. There are over 50,000 dietary supplements in the market (Grace 2013, Park 2011).

Stress is the way in which human beings react both physically and mentally to changes, events, and situations in their lives. People experience stress in different ways and for different reasons. The reaction is based on your perception of an event or situation. If you view a situation negatively, you will likely feel distressed overwhelmed, oppressed, or out of control. Distress is the more familiar form of stress. The other form, eustress, results from a "positive" view of an event or situation, which is why it is also called "good stress" (Ayala 2008).

The basic concept that explained the physiology of the stress response, specifically the immediate, intermediate, and prolonged effects on the body is involvement of different systems. Three systems are directly involved with the physiology of stress: the nervous system, the endocrine system, and the immune system (George 2006).

Parkinson's disease (PD) is a progressive disorder in neurology, which results from degeneration of cells in the portion of the brain producing dopamine neurotransmitter (chemical messenger). It is manifested through the loss of motor control, for example slowness of movement, rigidity, tremor, and balance problems, and nonmovement-type symptoms may include constipation, low mood, fatigue, sleep, and memory problems (Tripathi 2009).

Traditionally, treatment may involve drugs, which is primarily focused at enhancing dopamine activity. Since dopamine is synthesized in the body from amino acids, which are the structural and functional units of protein, diet may play a vital role in ensuring that the appropriate nutrients are available to reinforce the body's ability to produce dopamine. Maneuvering nutritional status and considering comorbidities—viz constipation, depression, fatigue, and insomnia—is also an area that may be improved through diet (Corell et al. 1998, Thiruchevlvam et al. 2000).

Major dietary determinants discussed later include reduction in toxic load, homocysteine with folic acid, vitamins B12 and B6, zinc, and tri-methyl-glycine (TMG) and increase in omega-3 fats, vitamin D, and magnesium (Postuma et al. 2006, Paus et al. 2007, Silva et al. 2008).

Alzheimer's disease (AD) is a progressive neurodegenerative disorder that affects geriatric individuals and is the paramount cause of dementia. It can develop to an entirely vegetative condition. Atrophy of cortical and subcortical areas is linked with the deposition of α-amyloid protein in the form of senile plaques and formation of neurofibrillary tangles. There is significant cholinergic deficiency in the brain, though other neurotransmitter systems are affected too (Tripathi 2009).

Many fruits and vegetables are good sources of antioxidants, including vitamins A, B (riboflavin), C, and E, which are present at low concentrations in some PD patients. Several studies have reported reduction in peroxidase (Ambani et al. 1975), glutathione-peroxidase activities (Kish et al. 1985), and glutathione (Riederer et al. 1989) in the substantia nigra (SN) of PD patients postmortem; this phenomenon suggests that metabolic failure in antioxidant mechanisms and chemical processes may result in lipid peroxidation and Parkinsonian characteristics (Uttara et al. 2009).

Although the antioxidant potential of some fruits and vegetables is visible in numerous studies, a recent investigation rang alarm about the antioxidant properties of pomegranate. In contrast to the earlier reports, regarding neuroprotective effects seen in AD (Hartman et al. 2006), pomegranate juice worsened oxidative stress and neurodegeneration in a rotenone model of PD (Tapias et al. 2013).

14.2 ROLE OF DIETARY SUPPLEMENTS ON STRESS

The effect of stress on health is quite dangerous and may jeopardize functioning of every major system in our body. Improper measures to handle stress can lead to conditions such as heart disease, headaches, weight gain, and cancer. The right nutrition can reduce the problems that stress may cause to our body and effectively repair any damage that has been done in the past. A balanced diet also conditions our body for stress that may be thrust upon our body in the future. The following rules may provide assistance in maintaining the body's innate defenses up and render the body more resistant toward stress.

- Good nutrition
- Good diet plan
- Avoiding certain foods
- Increasing "immune system–enhancing" nutrients
- Psychologically counteracting stress

Stress is quite common in a person's life nowadays and may occur more than once. However, as inevitable as stress can sometimes be, it is a choice. You may either allow the stress to cause suffering to your body or you may opt to do something about it. When stress takes place, including an adequately balanced diet plan to your routine will help you conquer any challenges offered by stress that you may come across.

We all are familiar with indispensability of a good nutritional plan for healthy body. Another effective characteristic of healthy nutrition is the perks it offers while dealing with stress. It is suggested that you should supply your body with all vital nutrients while facing stress. Failing to do so will be troublesome for your body, and you will not be able to combat against stress in an effective way.

A broad category of foods is needed in order to stay healthy; that is why there is no single food available that contains all the required nutrients. So you should have a selection of foods. Nutrients that you require include minerals, vitamins, proteins, good fatty acids, and energy derived from foods containing carbohydrates, protein, and fats. Consumption of your required nutrients (typically between 40 and 60 nutrients) per day is key to a healthy, sound body. There are a variety of foods that you need to keep a distance from. Sugar is one of the prime and common foods you need to disrespect. The food itself contains no vital nutrients that we require. Sugar also provides the person a huge burst of energy for a shorter span only. When this "extreme" runs out, the person will suffer a massive comedown from this and suffer a longer "low" period.

Next are alcohol and coffee; we must now consider B vitamins in your body. B vitamins are required for handling stress since they are utilized to boost your metabolism. Substances such as alcohol and caffeine will deplete these resources and influence the dynamics of your brain. Caffeine may be the culprit behind inducing the first stage of stress. When consumed under stress, the body makes use of reserve B vitamins so that you have no resources left to deal with the menace. Caffeine is also responsible for rendering people hyperactive and nervous. Due to this, the person's sleeping cycle is affected remarkably. If you have problem while checking your stress and always feel fatigue, it is imperative here that you review your diet to look if you are lacking any nutrients. If the problem is due to a deficiency in the nutritional part, then you need to find a solution to this problem. This may be readily corrected by changing your food habits to make up for the nutrients that you are lacking. Another option is to consume nutrient supplements. When the body is stressed, it is evident that the body utilizes its stores until it is depleted. The following are the main nutrients that the body will use up:

- *B vitamins*: These help the body to cope with stress (build your metabolism) and control the whole nervous system.
- *Proteins*: Assist in growth and tissue repair.
- *A vitamins*: Essential for normal vision.
- *C vitamins*: Protection of the immune system (antioxidants, diabetes protection, etc.). Lowers the amount of cortisol in your body.
- *Magnesium*: Needed for a variety of tasks such as muscle relaxation, fatty acid formation, making new cells, and heartbeat regulation.

In order to consume the following nutrients, a person should have some kind of food habit in order to consume the following nutrients. Going by a strict scheme will prepare the body to cope up stress and other ailments that are inflicted on the body. Balanced diet is one of the most important variables in the reduction of stress. With a balanced diet and a correct nutritional strategy, your body will be ready to face challenging circumstances where stress is thrust upon the body. While under stress, it is necessary for the body to use all vital nutrients in order to cope and function effectively. You can have these nutrients from a broad variety of foods (Figure 14.1).

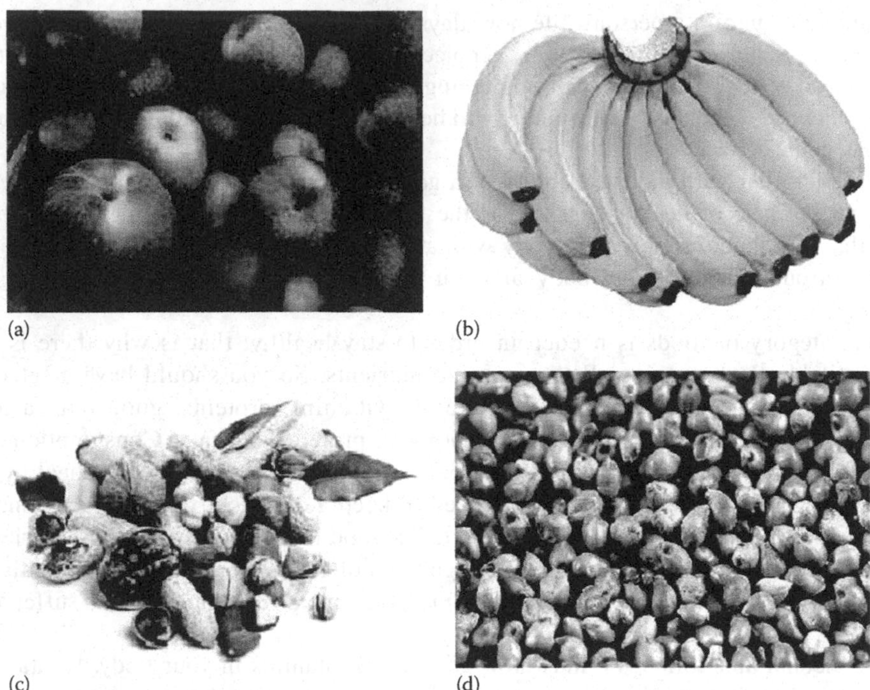

FIGURE 14.1 Structure of dietary supplements used in prevention of stress: (a) apple, (b) banana, (c) nuts, (d) protein-rich seeds.

- *B vitamins*: There are many B vitamin types, each as important as its counterpart. B vitamins can be found in foods such as seaweed and raw foods.
- *Proteins and iron*: Meats, eggs, seeds, nuts, etc.
- *A vitamins*: Cheese, eggs, fish with oil, milk, etc.
- *C vitamins*: Fruits (apple, banana, orange, etc.).
- *Magnesium*: Green leaved vegetables (e.g. cabbage), fish, and meat and dairy products.

Magnesium (Keservani et al. 2010a) is the key element that ought to be consumed on a regular basis. Besides, magnesium deficiencies are also associated with stress personality problems such as uneasiness and anxiety. If you are undergoing a surge of stress for a long span, then it is suggested that you consume plentiful of calcium-rich foods. This is available in foods such as milk and cheese.

14.3 SIGNIFICANCE OF NUTRITION IN PARKINSON'S DISEASE

PD affects health in a variety of ways. It may slow down the gastrointestinal tract, resulting in constipation, slowed stomach emptying, and difficulty in swallowing; it can progress to loss to perceive smell and taste. Drugs used to treat PD may cause nausea and low appetite. And, one of the most important drugs, levodopa, should compete with protein for absorption through the small intestine. Persons with PD are at enhanced danger for malnutrition; yet, with focus to diet, you will experience better, keep away nutrition-linked diseases, and ward off hospitalization. A stay in the hospital may be expensive, traumatic, and painful, but for those with PD, there are extra concerns (Holden 2005).

- Some hospital staff people are not used to the special drugs used for PD.
- Dosing of medications can be difficult for staff, which may already have complicated regimens in place.

By abiding good nutrition practices, you will feel better, and there are much more chances to be healthy and avoid the hospital visits.

14.3.1 Optimal Nutrition for People Afflicted by Parkinson's Disease

PD influences every individual in a different manner, few factors that may change your dietary requirements include your age, your gender, past record of any other diagnosed conditions—viz high blood pressure, food allergies, diabetes, etc. Besides, drugs commonly used may have numerous side effects that may affect the nutritional health of the patient. This comprises of drugs for heart disease, blood pressure, and other conditions, and PD medications; it further covers many over-the-counter medications.

We will also discuss in the following some of the most common issues, few of which may be serious enough over time to necessitate hospitalization (Holden 2005).

14.3.1.1 Bone Thinning

Regarding bone thinning, people consume foods that supply the bone-strengthening nutrients: in particular, calcium, magnesium, and vitamins D and K. Further regular exposure to sunlight (which provides vitamin D, a bone-strengthening vitamin) and weight-bearing exercise, such as walking, are needed. Nutrients, sunlight, and weight-bearing exercise will help in keeping the bones strong, preventing fractures and hospitalization.

Osteoporosis is serious. It can lead to fractures of the hip, spine, or wrist and influences many women over the age of 60. Osteoporosis is a disease that results in weakened bones. Calcium is replaced from bones, leaving small apertures. The preliminary stage of such bone thinning is known as osteopenia; when it advances too far, it is termed osteoporosis.

14.3.1.2 Dehydration

PD medicaments may pose the danger of dehydration. Most people with PD do not understand the vital role of water to stay healthy. Dehydration may result in confusion, weakness, balance problems, respiratory failure, kidney failure, and eventually death. Water helps in the lubrication of our joints and acts as a shock absorber within the eyes and the spinal cord. And, when the digestive system converts the food into fuel to be used by the body, a number of toxins and wastes are produced. Water is the driving force that excretes these wastes out of the body in the form of breath, urine, and fecal matter. Truly, water is miraculous.

Bladder and urinary tract infections are quite common with progressing age and people with PD. The thirst sensation is slowed down as we age, so we do not feel thirsty even when we require fluids. Older adults are, in general, in a state of mild and prolonged dehydration. This allows bacterial growth and bacteria thrive in the bladder and urinary tract, causing infection.

A large glass of cranberry juice regularly, with at least four (preferably eight) glasses of water, in addition to any juices or other beverages usually taken up, is a good approach. Cranberry juice may help in the prevention and cure of infections in many cases, along with drugs.

Some people observe that they often perceive thirst and sometimes have dry mouth, thick or sticky saliva, and dry eyes. This may be attributed to anti-Parkinson medicaments; the anti-cholinergic drugs Artane or Cogentin used to treat tremor are, in particular, known to cause such symptoms. Dry mouth may also a result of difficulty in swallowing, sleeping with the mouth open, or breathing through the mouth while staying awake. Ensure you are drinking plenty of fluids to combat dry mouth.

14.3.1.3 Bowel Impaction

PD can reduce the movement of the colon, leading to constipation. This renders it significant to include enough fiber in the daily menu. Fiber, along with water, maintains the smooth functioning of our bowels. Insoluble fiber works hand in hand with water. Every bit of fiber imbibes water like a tiny sponge and swells up to many times its original size. All these small water-soaked sponges add bulk to the stool, impart it softness, and make it easy to pass. They also improve the tone of the muscles of the intestine so they stay strong and healthy. More frequent bowel movements are generally the outcome. This not only helps to ward off constipation but it can prevent or ease hemorrhoids as well. These happen when we strain to pass the stool. Fiber can also minimize the risk of colon and rectal cancers. The task of the large intestine, or colon, is to keep enough water in the stool to keep it soft. If not handled properly, constipation may lead to a mass of dry, hard feces, which is hard to pass off normally. This is termed as bowel impaction. People with bowel impaction may need hospitalization, sometimes even surgery (Holden 2005).

14.3.1.4 Weight Loss

People with PD lose weight, at some point in life a crucial amount of weight, ignorantly. There are several possible reasons for this: depression may cause poor appetite and willingness to eat; chewing or swallowing difficulties may render it difficult to eat at a normal rate; it can take hours to finish a meal as some have difficulty in maneuvering a fork and knife; or tremor and dyskinesia burn up additional calories. In other cases, people with PD apprise that their appetites are nice, they enjoy taking meals, and yet they still lose weight in a strange manner.

When we lose weight, precious muscle mass is lost, too. Muscle wasting leads to difficulty in walking, keeping appropriate balance, and performing the routine activities of daily life. Furthermore, the body has shortage of nutrients, like vitamins and minerals. This wastage may lead to behavior change, altered mental function, compromised immune system, weakened bones, and other undesirable situations.

In addition to these variants, we require regular meals to keep our energy. People with PD generally feel fatigue because of disease or drugs used to treat PD; deficiency of glucose may make this tiredness worst, too. Food provides a steady stream of blood glucose, which our body's cells utilize for nourishment, energy, and work. Without this glucose, we may feel tired, listless, and apathetic. To attain weight, consumption of cooked vegetables, vegetable juices, and vegetable soups may be better alternatives. Pureed soups can be shipped from a mug, obviating the need for a spoon (Holden 2005).

14.3.2 Role of Dietary Supplements in Parkinson's Disease

A routine menu comprised of whole grains, enriched with vegetables and fruits, calcium-rich foods, and smaller parts of high-protein foods, is the best feasible option for people with PD. The whole grains have the fiber that helps regulate the constipation that generally occurs in PD, as well as helping in the management of blood sugar, blood pressure, cholesterol, and heart disease. Vegetables and fruits are rich in antioxidants, phytochemicals (Keservani and Sharma 2014), minerals (Keservani et al. 2010a), and vitamins (Keservani et al. 2010b) that nourish and strengthen the muscles, nervous system, and organs of the body. Calcium is important in particular, as it helps to maintain the bones strong, preventing fractures. And protein makes the muscular system healthy; strong, toned muscles help sustain balance and strength (Holden 2005).

Nutrition has a significant role both potentially in reducing the risk for PD and in the therapeutic help and treatment of PD at all stages. Few of dietary supplements which are mentioned in the following sections are used in the management of the PD (Table 14.1, Figure 14.2).

14.4 ROLE OF SUPPLEMENTS IN ALZHEIMER'S DISEASE

The one, outstanding nutritional discovery is that your risk of developing Alzheimer's is closely linked to your level of toxic amino acid homocysteine, which can be determined from a pinprick of blood on a domestic test kit. The lower is your level throughout life, the smaller your tendencies of

TABLE 14.1
Beneficial Nutrients and Their Food Source for PD

Nutrients	Recommended Daily Dose	Food Sources
Folate (folic acid)	400 μg	Enriched products (grains, cereals, and breads), dark leafy vegetables, dried peas, beans, lentils, and orange juice.
Vitamin B6	10–15 mg	Avocados, bananas, potatoes, fish, poultry, and meat.
Vitamin B12	2.4 μg	Liver, eggs, fish, milk, and meats.
Vitamin D	10–15 μg or 400–600 IU	Fatty fish (such as tuna, salmon, and mackerel), fortified milk products, and cereals.
Vitamin E (alpha tocopherol)	15 mg	Vegetable oils, whole grains, nuts, fruits, vegetables, and meats.
Calcium	1000–1200 mg	Milk, yogurt, cheese, calcium-set tofu, broccoli, kale, and Chinese cabbage.
Fiber	30–35 g	*Soluble fiber sources*: Fresh fruits/vegetables, whole grains (brown rice, barely oat bran), peas, beans, and lentils.
Fluid	1 mL/calorie; usually about 6–8 cups/day	Fluid can come from water, juice, tea, and sodas. Remember that water is calorie-free.

developing serious memory recession. Homocysteine is a neurotoxin able to cause straightforward damage to the medial temporal lobe, which is the part of the brain that rapidly degenerates in AD. Homocysteine is readily lowered with economic B vitamins.

One of such important studies, published in 2002 in the *New England Journal of Medicine*, listed the health of 1092 elderly people without dementia and measured their homocysteine levels (Seshadri et al. 2002). After 8 years, 111 were identified with dementia, 83 of whom were assigned the diagnosis of Alzheimer's. Those with elevated blood homocysteine levels (above 14 units) were at about double the risk of Alzheimer's. There is also proof that even before a decline in mental function begins to emerge in so-called healthy elderly individuals, high homocysteine forecasts physical degeneration in certain portions of the brain.

In Scotland, researchers have observed that reduction in mental performance in old age is quite linked with high homocysteine and low levels of vitamins B12 and folic acid. In a feedback from participants in the Scottish Mental Surveys of 1932 and 1947, which surveyed childhood intelligence, they observed that the most mentally active had the highest levels of B vitamins and lowest concentration of homocysteine; high homocysteine was linked with a 7%–8% decrease in mental activity (Sachdev et al. 2002).

Another Californian study of the same pattern advised 579 men and women aged 60 years and over to record their diet and the supplements they consumed (Duthie et al. 2002). Nine years later, 57 of them had Alzheimer's. Those with the highest folate consumption lowered their risk of progressing Alzheimer's by 55%.

A research group headed by Dr Teodoro Bottiglieri at the Baylor University Metabolic Disease Center in Dallas, Texas, recommended that the low concentration of folic acid (which leads to high homocysteine) can lead to brain damage that kicks up dementia and Alzheimer's. Their research has observed that one-third of those with both dementia and homocysteine levels above 14 units were lacking folic acid (Bottiglieri et al. 2001).

Both high homocysteine levels and low folic acid and B12 levels in blood correlate very well with increasing risk for Alzheimer's according to a systematic review (Van and Van Gool 2009). Another review, in 2008, concludes that of "Seventy-seven cross-sectional studies on more than 34,000 subjects and 33 prospective studies on more than 12,000 subjects have shown associations between cognitive deficit or dementia and homocysteine and/or B vitamins" (Smith 2008). Homocysteine levels also predict and correlate with the rate of cognitive decline (Oulhaj et al. 2010) as does B12 status

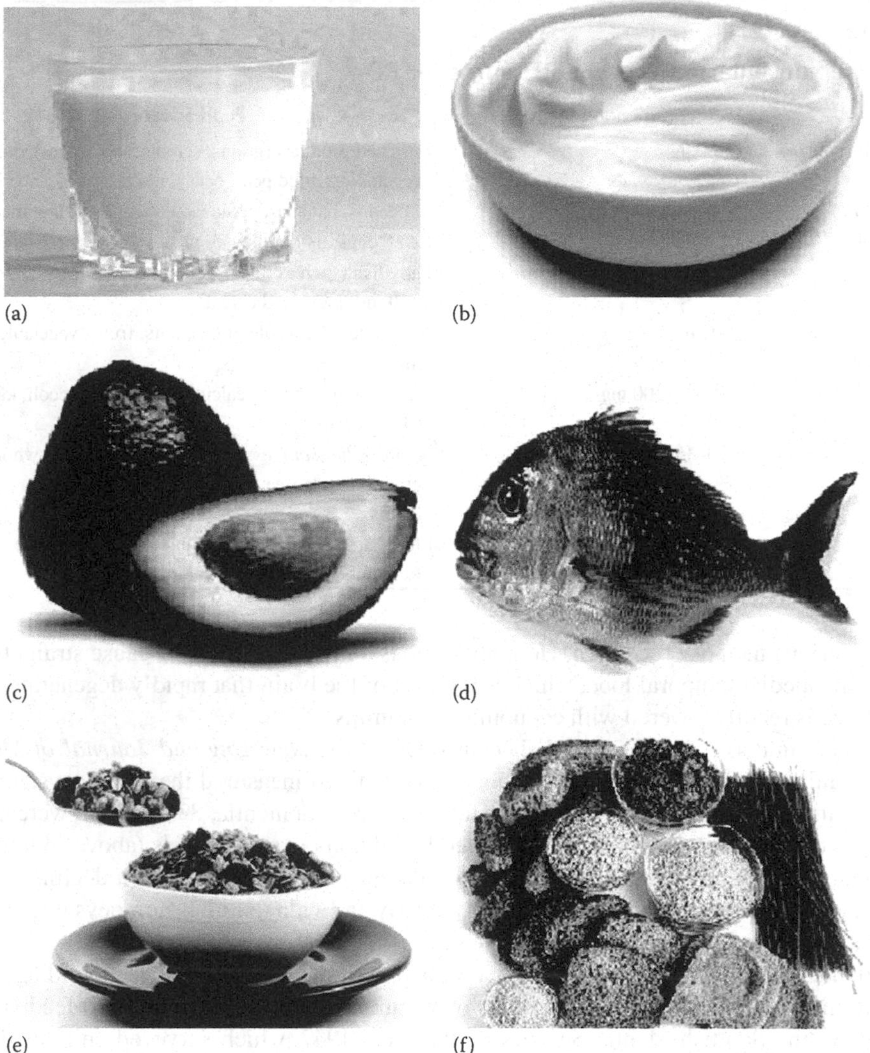

FIGURE 14.2 Beneficial dietary supplements used in the prevention of Parkinson's disease: (a) milk, (b) yogurt, (c) avocado, (d) fish, (e) fortified cereals, (f) fibre.

(Smith and Refsum 2009). There is, therefore, ample evidence to propose that lowering homocysteine by giving appropriate supplemental levels of homocysteine lowering nutrients, including B6, B12, and folic acid, would reduce risk (Tangney et al. 2009). The main question being at what point in the process is cognitive decline reversible and what dosage of nutrients confers maximum protection?

But why should homocysteine and a deficiency of these B vitamins predict cognitive tapering? The cause for this relation can be that the body requires B vitamins to change the toxic and brain-damaging homocysteine into two very handy chemicals called glutathione—an antioxidant—and the amino acid called SAMe. SAMe is essential for "methylation," which is a prime chemical activity occurring millions of times every second, which maintains the brain's chemistry in order. Therefore, the theory has sense but does supplementing with vitamins control, or in fact reverse memory loss? A study in Holland provided 818 people aged between 50 and 75 years either a vitamin having 800 μg of folic acid once a day—approximately three times the RDA and the equivalent of 2.5 lb of strawberries—or a placebo pill (Durga et al. 2007). Three years later, supplement consumers had scores on memory tests at par with people 5.5 years younger. While testing cognitive speed, the folic acid supported takers to perform as good as people 1.9 years younger.

Professor David Smith and his associates at the Optima Project at the University of Oxford studied the influences of administering B vitamins against dummy pills to those with mild cognitive impairment, mapping brain shrinkage with an MRI scan, and cognitive function (Smith et al. 2010). In this study, homocysteine levels above 9.5 mmol/L was associated with accelerated brain shrinkage and cognitive deficiency. Those given folic acid (0.8 mg/day), vitamin B12 (0.5 mg/day), and vitamin B6 (20 mg/day) had a significant reduction in the propensity of brain shrinkage. The rate of atrophy in subjects with homocysteine above 13 mmol/L was 53% low in the active treatment group. A higher rate of atrophy was linked with a lower ultimate cognitive test scores.

A study from the University of California provided homocysteine-lowering B vitamins to those already having mild-to-moderate Alzheimer's (Aisen et al. 2008). The selection of patients was not based on homocysteine levels (average homocysteine was 9.1 mmol/L at baseline), and brain scans were not carried out; therefore, it was not as credible as the past University of Oxford study. The patients were given folic acid (5 mg/day), B12 (1 mg/day), and B6 (25 mg/day for 18 months). No significant difference was observed in the rate of cognitive damage in those on the supplements against dummy pills. But when the patients were segregated as those with high and low cognitive test scores at the beginning, those who were suffering from milder Alzheimer's did remarkably respond; those consuming B vitamins hardly got morbid over 15 months, while those on the dummy exhibited a steady decrease. The average fall in homocysteine over the 18 months was from 9.1 to 6.8 μmol/L.

To date, the proofs recommend that, if patients with high homocysteine are supplemented by 1000 μg of folic acid, 20 mg of B6, and 500 μg of B12, this may lead to a control of age-related memory loss and brain shrinkage and may even support those in the preliminary stages of AD.

These values of nutrients are a far cry from the RDA concentration, in particular for vitamin B12. The lowest oral dose of vitamin B12 i.e.-500 μg, is 250 times higher than RDA (2.5 μg) which is even more than having received a well balanced food.

Such high quantities are exploited for the simple cause that they work. "The lowest dose of oral cyanocobalamin (B12) required to keep in check mild vitamin B12 deficiency in older people is more than 200 times the recommended dietary allowance," findings from a paper by scientist at the University of Wageningen in Holland, one of the top B12 research centers around the globe (Eussen et al. 2005). It is definitely meaningful to test your homocysteine values and if it is over 9 mmol/L, try to ensure an optimal consumption of B6, B12, and folic acid. There are other nutrients that paves way to lower homocysteine significantly: zinc, TMG (1000–2000 mg), and *N*-acetyl cysteine (NAC: 500–1000 mg). There is also proof that methyl B12 may be a more active form of this vitamin. The simplest way to attain an optimal consumption of all these nutrients is by having a homocysteine-lowering supplement containing all these nutrients in such doses.

14.4.1 Diet and Supplements for Alzheimer's Disease

The brain is a flesh and blood organ which the appropriate fuel to work well. Developing a better memory, controlling Alzheimer's and memory loss, and addressing the causes of AD, all depend on your lifestyle. The diet plays key role in maintaining good health of brain. And with the apt Alzheimer's diet, you may in fact affect the health of your genes. That is the right approach and it begins with the foods you consume daily (Oken et al. 1998, Feart et al. 2010).

14.4.1.1 Alzheimer's Prevention Diet

One of the best choices you may provide input to your brain in order to have better memory is via abstaining from a diet rich in trans-fat and saturated fat. These fats, like those coming from animal products (especially red meats), may lead to inflammation and generate free radicals. As you might be aware, free radicals are the by-products of your metabolism, but in higher amounts, they may destroy and even can cause death of your vital brain cells.

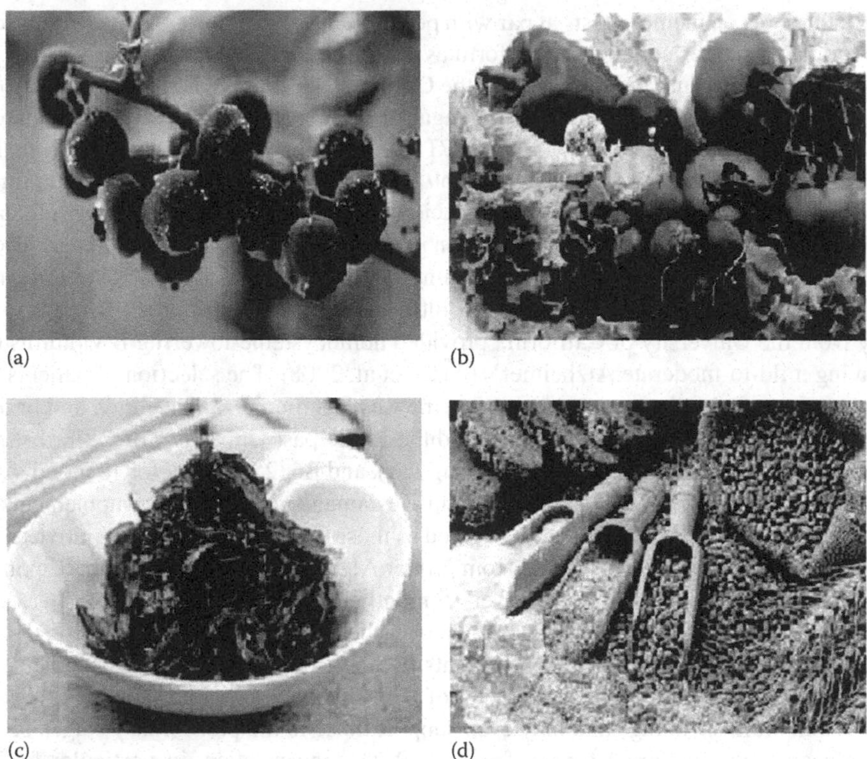

FIGURE 14.3 Structure of some dietary supplements for Alzheimer's disease: (a) blueberries, (b) fresh vegetables, (c) seaweeds, (d) whole grains.

Consuming foods that are rich in antioxidants such as vitamins C and E is a marvelous natural way to get rid of free radicals from your body. Similarly, scientists trust that eating of fruits and vegetables, taking fish high in omega-3 oils (Kalmijn et al. 1997, Conquer et al. 2000, Swanson et al. 2012), and vegetarian protein alternatives (such as soy) are natural defense against memory loss.

Besides revising Alzheimer's diet, search more about the best vitamins and nutrients to help your memory and stay away from AD early symptoms.

The ideal prevention diet (Figure 14.3) is given as follows:

- *20% good fats.* Items in this group include extra virgin olive oil, avocado, and flax seed oil.
- *40% lean proteins.* Include fish, chicken, turkey, and soy on a daily basis.
- *40% complex carbohydrates.* Discover the rewards of a spectrum of fresh vegetables, whole grains, legumes, and fresh fruits.
- *Superfoods for the brain—as much as you want!* These superfoods, including blueberries, spinach, and seaweed, have fabulous antioxidant properties, preventing causes of Alzheimer's.

14.4.1.2 Vitamins and Other Memory-Specific Nutrients for Alzheimer's

If you are concerned about the control of Alzheimer's and correcting memory loss, you should for sure consume a potent multiple vitamin and mineral capsule. Ensure the vitamin formula you opted has folic acid and vitamin C. Folic acid minimizes homocysteine levels as high homocysteine values may land you at jeopardy for heart disease as well as memory loss. Vitamin C (Keservani et al. 2010a) has been known to alleviate your risk of AD by 20% when coadministered with vitamin E. To avail benefit up to a maximum extent, you should consume a dose of 2000 mg of vitamin C every day.

When you prepare a balanced diet that keeps your overall health in good shape, you are not only doing good for your body, but you are also strengthening and improving your memory as well.

Have a look upon the following memory-specific nutrients in your daily vitamin schedule (Chen and Tappel 1995, Nagamatsu et al. 1995, Oyama et al. 1996):

- Coenzyme Q10
- Alpha lipoic acid
- *Ginkgo biloba*
- Phosphatidylserine
- DHA (an omega-3 oil)
- Acetyl-L-carnitine

Two additional nutrients are suggested only for people who have moderate-to-severe memory loss (Nagamatsu et al. 1995, Szatmari and Whitehouse 2003, Li et al. 2008):

- Huperzine-A
- Vinpocetine

14.5 CONCLUSIONS

The body, under stress, demands foods that are rich in sugars and fats. These foods provide no benefits for you except supply a prima facie transient burst of energy. This energy explosion will deplete fast, followed by an extended period of tiredness. Therefore, a well-balanced diet is required to replenish foods that are in demand during stressful circumstances. A latest research investigation observed that age-linked downfall could begin as early as 45 despite promising strength of these nutrients in PD. A budding body of proof recommends that nutrition can play a key role in PD. Epidemiological and biochemical studies have recently recognized potential components in some food classes that can elicit neuroprotection in PD. The good news is that a plenty of encouraging research avenues heralds that risk of dementia and Alzheimer's could be lowered in the early stages by a comprehensive optimum nutrition strategy. The most robust evidence to date pertains to elevated homocysteine levels, which both assess risk and may lead to the kind of brain damage observed in Alzheimer's, caused by the deficiency of B vitamins, particularly B12, which is very poorly absorbed with age.

REFERENCES

Aisen, P.S., L.S. Schneider, M. Sano, R. Diaz-Arrastia et al. 2008. High-dose B vitamin supplementation and cognitive decline in Alzheimer disease. *JAMA*. 300(15):1774–1783.

Ambani, L.M., W.M.H. Van, S. Murphy. 1975. Brain peroxidase and catalase in Parkinson disease. *Arch. Neurol.* 32:114–118.

Ayala, S. 2008. *Stress. Health Tips from Army Medicine*. Madigan Army Medical Center, Fort Lewis, WA. Retrieved June 13, 2008 from http://www.armymedicine.army.mil/hc/health tips/08/stress.cfm (accessed on July 12, 2014).

Bottiglieri, T. et al. 2001. Plasma total homocysteine levels and the C677T mutation in the methylenetetrahydrofolate reductase (MTHFR) gene: A study in an Italian population with dementia. *Mech. Age. Develop.* 122(16):2013–2023.

Chen, H., A.L. Tappel. 1995. Vitamin E, selenium, trolox C, ascorbic acid palmitate, acetylcysteine, coenzyme Q, b-carotene, canthaxanthin, and (+)-catechin protect against oxidative damage to kidney, heart, lung and spleen. *Free Radic Res.* 22:177–186.

Conquer, J.A., M.C. Tierney, J. Zecevic, W.J. Bettger, R.H. Fisher. 2000. Fatty acid analysis of blood plasma of patients with Alzheimer's disease, other types of dementia, and cognitive impairment. *Lipids.* 35:1305–1312.

Corell J. et al. 1998. The risk of Parkinson's disease with exposure to pesticides, farming, well water and rural living. *Neurology.* 67:1210–1218.

Durga, J., B.M.P. Van, E.G. Schouten et al. 2007. The effect of 3-year folic acid supplementation on cognitive function in older adults in the FACIT trial: A randomized, double blind, controlled trial. *Lancet.* 369(1):208–216.

Duthie, S.J.et al. 2002. Homocysteine, B vitamin status, and cognitive function in the elderly. *Am. J. Clin. Nutr.* 75(5):908–913.

Eussen S. J. et al. 2005. Oral cyanocobalamin supplementation in older people with vitamin B12 deficiency: A dose-finding trial. *Arch. Intern. Med.* 165(10):1167–1172.

Feart, C., C. Samieri, P. Barberger-Gateau. 2010. Mediterranean diet and cognitive function in older adults. *Curr. Opin. Clin. Nutr. Metab. Care.* 13(1):14–18. doi:10.1097/MCO.0b013e 3283331fe4.

George, E. 2006. *Managing Stress: "Physiology of Stress".* Seaward, B.L. (Ed.). pp. 34–35. Jones & Bartlett Publishers, Sudbury, MA.

Grace, E. 2013. How to choose the best supplement. *Health Beacon.* http://healthbeacon.co.uk/articles/featured/health-beacon/2013/08/how-to-choose-the-best-supplement.aspx (accessed on August 6, 2014). Retrieved October 3, 2013.

Hartman, R.E., A. Shah, A.M. Fagan, K.E. Schwetye, M. Parsadanian, R.N. Schulman et al. 2006. Pomegranate juice decreases amyloid load and improves behavior in a mouse model of Alzheimer's disease. *Neurobiol. Dis.* 24:506–515.

Holden, K. 2005. *Parkinson's Disease: Nutrition Matters.* National Parkinson Foundation, Miami, FL. pp. 1–59. www.parkinson.org (accessed on July 17, 2014).

Institute of Medicine and National Research Council of the National Academies (IMNRC) 2004. *Dietary Supplements a Framework for Evaluating Safety.* Washington, DC: National Academies Press. pp. ES-1–ES-3. ISBN 0-309-09206-X.

Kalmijn, S., E.J. Feskens, L.J. Launer, D. Kromhout. 1997. Polyunsaturated fatty acids, antioxidants, and cognitive function in very old men. *Am. J. Epidemiol.* 145:33–41.

Keservani, R.K., A.K. Sharma. 2014. Flavonoids: Emerging trends and potential health benefits. *J Chin. Pharm. Sci.* 23 (12):815–822.

Keservani, R.K., R.K. Kesharwani, A.K. Sharma, N. Vyas, A. Chadoker. 2010a. Nutritional supplements: An overview. *Int. J. Curr. Pharm. Rev. Res.* 1:59–75.

Keservani, R. K., R.K. Kesharwani, N. Vyas, S. Jain, R. Raghuvanshi, A.K. Sharma. 2010b. Nutraceutical and functional food as future food: A review. *Der. Pharmacia. Lett.* 2:106–116.

Kish, S.J., C. Morito, O. Hornykiewicz. 1985. Glutathione peroxidase activity in Parkinson's disease brain. *Neurosci. Lett.* 58:343–346.

Li, J. et al. 2008. Huperzine A for Alzheimer's disease. *Cochrane Database Syst. Rev.* 16(2):CD005592.

Nagamatsu, M. et al. 1995. Lipoic acid improves nerve blood flow, reduces oxidative stress, and improves distal nerve conduction in experimental diabetic neuropathy. *Diabetes Care.* 18:1160–1167.

Oken, B.S., D.M. Storzbach, J.A. Kaye. 1998. The efficacy of *Ginkgo biloba* on cognitive function in Alzheimer disease. *Arch. Neurol.* 55:1409–1415.

Oulhaj, A., H. Refsum, H. Beaumont et al. 2010. Homocysteine as a predictor of cognitive decline in Alzheimer's disease. *Int. J. Geriatr. Psychiatry.* 25(1):82–90.

Oyama, Y., L. Chikahisa, T. Ueha, K. Kanemaru, K. Noda. 1996. *Ginkgo biloba* extract protects brain neurons against oxidative stress induced by hydrogen peroxide. *Brain Res.* 712:349–352.

Park, M. 2011. Half of Americans use supplements. *CNN.* http://edition.cnn.com/2011/HEALTH/04/13/supplements.dietary/ (accessed on July 24, 2014). Retrieved October 3, 2013.

Paus, S. et al. 2007. Bright light therapy in Parkinson's disease: A pilot study. *Mov. Disord.* 22:1495–1498.

Postuma, R.B. et al. 2006. Vitamins and entacapone in levodopa-induced hyperhomocysteinemia: A randomized controlled study. *Neurology.* 66(12):1941–1943.

Riederer, P., E. Sofic, W.D. Rausch, B. Schmidt, G.P. Reynolds, K. Jellinger et al. 1989. Transition metals, ferritin, glutathione, and ascorbic acid in Parkinsonian brains. *J. Neurochem.* 52:515–520.

Ritchie J. Combating Stress with a Balanced Nutritional Diet. Stress Management Society. http://www.stress.org.uk/files/combat-nutritional-stress.pdf (accessed on August 11, 2014).

Sachdev, P.S. et al. 2002. Relationship between plasma homocysteine levels and brain atrophy in healthy elderly individuals. *Neurology.* 58:1539–1541.

Seshadri, S. et al. 2002. Plasma homocysteine as a risk factor for dementia and AD. *N. Engl. J. Med.* 346(7):476–483.

da Silva T.M., Munhoz R.P., Alvarez C., Naliwaiko K., Kiss A., Andreatini R., Ferraz A. C. 2008. Depression in Parkinson's disease: A double-blind, randomized, placebo-controlled pilot study of omega-3 fatty-acid supplementation. *J. Affect Disord.* 111:351–359.

Smith, A.D. 2008. The worldwide challenge of the dementias: A role for B vitamins and homocysteine. *Food Nutr. Bull.* 29(2 Suppl): S143–S172.

Smith, A.D., H. Refsum. 2009. Vitamin B-12 and cognition in the elderly. *Am. J. Clin. Nutr.* 89(2):707S–711S.

Smith, A.D., S.M. Smith, C.A. de Jager et al. 2010. Homocysteine-lowering by B vitamins slows the rate of accelerated brain atrophy in mild cognitive impairment: A randomized controlled trial. *PLoS One.* 5(9):1–10.

Swanson, D., R. Block, S.A. Mousa. 2012. Omega-3 fatty acids EPA and DHA: Health benefits throughout life. *Adv. Nutr.* 3(1):1–7. doi: 10.3945/an.111.000893. Epub January 5, 2012.

Szatmari, S.Z., P.J. Whitehouse. 2003. Vinpocetine for cognitive impairment and dementia. *Cochrane Database Syst Rev.*1:CD003119.

Tangney, C. et al. 2009. Biochemical indicators of vitamin B12 and folate insufficiency and cognitive decline. *Neurology.* 72(4):361–367.

Tapias, V., J.R. Cannon, J.T. Greenamyre. 2013. Pomegranate juice exacerbates oxidative stress and nigrostriatal degeneration in Parkinson's disease. *Neurobiol. Aging.* 35:1162–1176.

Thiruchevlvam, M. et al. 2000. The Nigrostriatal Dopaminergic System as a preferential target of repeated exposures to combined paraquat and maneb: Implications for Parkinson's disease. *J. Neurosci.* 20(24):9207–9214.

Tripathi, K.D. 2009. *Essentials of Medical Pharmacology*. Jaypee Brothers Medical Publishers (P) Ltd, New Delhi, India.

Uttara, B., A.V. Singh, P. Zamboni, R.T. Mahajan. 2009. Oxidative stress and neurodegenerative diseases: A review of upstream and downstream antioxidant therapeutic options. *Curr. Neuropharmacol.* 7:65–74.

Van, D.F., W.A. Van Gool. 2009. Hyperhomocysteinemia and Alzheimer's disease: A systematic review. *Arch. Gerentol. Geratr.* 48:425–430.

15 Nutraceuticals and Functional Foods in the Prevention of Mental Disorders

Raj K. Keservani, Swati Singh, Virendra Singh, Rajesh K. Kesharwani, and Anil K. Sharma

CONTENTS

15.1 INTRODUCTION

The term "nutraceuticals," coined by Stephen L. DeFelice in 1989, is derived from the words "nutrition" and "pharmaceutical." Nutraceutical is a food or food product that provides health and medical benefits, including the prevention and treatment of disease (Biesalski 2001, Kalra 2003, Keservani et al. 2010a). Such products may range from isolated nutrients, dietary supplements and specific diets to genetically engineered foods, herbal products, and processed foods such as cereals, soups, and beverages. A nutraceutical is demonstrated to have a physiological benefit or provide protection against chronic disease. Their bioactive ingredients, the phytochemicals, sustain or promote health and occur at the intersection of food and pharmaceutical industries. Such substances may range from isolated nutrients, dietary supplements, and specific diets to genetically engineered designer foods, herbal products, processed foods, and beverages (Kalra 2003, Prakash et al. 2004). They play a crucial role in maintaining optimal immune response, such that deficient or excessive intakes can have negative impact on health. "Nutrigenomics" is the subsequent cutting edge in nutraceutical therapy progressing in the battle against aging, diseases, and sufferings by the availability of genomic information. The interface between the nutritional environment and cellular/genetic processes is being referred to as nutrigenomics (Kaput and Rodriguez 2004). It provides a molecular genetics understanding of phytochemicals/phytonutrients (Keservani and Sharma 2014) that affect health by altering the expression and/or structure of an individual's genetic makeup. This in turn may alter initiation, development, and/or progression of specific diseases. The recent notion of "customized" or "personalized" medicine and diet is being comprehensive to the field of nutrition that can be used to delay the onset of disease and to sustain optimum human health (Dijsselbloem et al. 2004, Kaput and Rodriguez 2004).

The nutraceuticals industry is now expending billions of dollars each year for the purchase of health-related foods and supplements. The respective health benefits are based on science and ethics, for health claims for functional foods, and presence of certain phytochemicals. They are constituents of plants and have certain pharmacological and/or physiological effects in the ethnomedical treatment of various disorders. Phytochemicals (Keservani and Sharma 2014) play an important role in human health as antioxidants, antibacterial, antifungal, anti-inflammatory, anti-allergic, antispasmodic, chemopreventive, hepatoprotective, hypolipidemic, neuroprotective, hypotensive, prevent aging, diabetes, osteoporosis, cancer and heart diseases, induce apoptosis, diuretic, CNS stimulant, analgesic, protects from UVB-induced carcinogenesis, immunomodulator, and carminative (Dillard and German 2000, Packer and Weber 2001, Nichenametla et al. 2006, Prakash and Kumar 2011). The diet of people with serious mental disorders is often inadequate, so there is obvious interest in exploring the possibility that metabolic brain diseases like schizophrenia and depression are aggravated by concurrent nutritional deficiencies (Hoffer 2012).

Mental illness is any disease or condition, which strangely affects the manner a person speculates, perceives, behaves, or associates with others and with his or her ambience. Though the signs of mental illness may spread over mild to severe and are diverse based on the kind of mental illness, a person with an unattended mental illness generally faces trouble while dealing with life's routines and requirements (Faraone 1995). Mental illnesses are of different types and degrees of severity. Some of the major types are depression, anxiety, schizophrenia, bipolar mood disorder, personality disorders, trauma, and eating disorders (Tripathi 2009). The most common mental illnesses are anxiety and depressive disorders (Tripathi 2009).

15.2 CAUSES OF MENTAL ILLNESS

The proper etiology of majority mental illnesses is unknown. It is, although, being apparent via research that several of these conditions are due to a combination of genetic, biological, psychological, and environmental determinants, not individual weakness or a character flaw, and recovery from a mental illness is not merely subject to willpower and austerity.

15.2.1 Heredity (Genetics)

Several mental illnesses may be in families, heralding they may be carried on from parents to their siblings via genes. Genes have a set of directions for the role of every cell in the body and are accountable for our look, act, speculate, etc. Nevertheless, simply because your mother or father may have or had a mental illness does not say you will have one of such illness. Hereditary only matters such that you are more prone toward the condition than if you did not have a diseased family member. Experts trust that most of the mental conditions are associated with problems in multiple genes not just single, as with many diseases; that is why a person has a legacy to have a mental disorder but does not always progress the condition (Jeffery 1999, Shiveley and Patrick 2000, Westermarck and Antila 2000, Katz 2001). The disorder itself takes place from the complex interaction of such genes and other variables such as psychological impact and environmental stress-causing factors, which can affect, or kick off, the illness in a person who has inherited a tendency to develop it.

15.2.2 Biology

A few mental illnesses have been related to a diverse activity of brain networks, which articulates various brain regions that regulate functions such as thinking, mood, and behavior. Nerve cells confined in those brain circuits carry information along from one cell to the next via brain chemicals called neurotransmitters. Scientists speculate that by changing the function of certain neurotransmitters (through medicines, psychotherapy, brain stimulation, or other measures), these abnormal brain circuits can work with more efficiency, thereby managing signs. Besides, defects in or injury to certain regions of the brain have also been associated with several mental conditions. Furthermore, recent studies exhibit that inflammation can have a role in the progression of mental illness (Jeffery 1999, Shiveley and Patrick 2000, Westermarck and Antila 2000, Katz 2001).

15.2.3 Psychological Trauma

Trauma, which means wound in Greek, is often the result of an overwhelming amount of stress that exceeds one's ability to cope or integrate the emotions involved with that experience. A few mental illnesses can be caused by psychological trauma suffered as a child or teenager, like severe emotional, physical, or sexual abuse, and an importantly early loss, such as the loss of a parent.

15.2.4 Mental Health

Some functional foods could potentially promote optimal mental state and mental performance and influence behavior. They may influence cognitive performance, mood and vitality, reaction to stress, short-term memory, vigilance and attention, changes in memory, and other mental processes. There has been a recent increase in research looking at mental health and diet, particularly in older people. A Mediterranean-type diet (rich in nuts, fish, and vegetables) has been shown to reduce the risk of developing Alzheimer's disease (Gu et al. 2010). A Mediterranean diet contains folate, which reduces homocysteine (an amino acid linked to Alzheimer's), vitamin E, which has an antioxidant effect, and is low in saturated fat, which can increase dementia risk by encouraging clot formation (Gu et al. 2010). It should be noted, however, that homocysteine has a stronger association with vascular disease as clinical studies have shown that even moderately increased homocysteine levels increase the risk of atherothrombotic vascular events (Hankey and Eikelboom 1999, McCulley 2007).

15.2.5 Aging

Glucose may have a beneficial influence on aspects of mental performance, including memory and decision time. Sucrose may reduce pain perception. Caffeine can lead to the improvement in cognitive performance with effects on reaction time, vigilance, memory, and psychomotor performance (Tripathi 2009). Cognitive performance and maintenance of mental health in older people may be improved with B vitamins. People often find that meals high in carbohydrate are associated with sleepiness and calmness. The amino acid tryptophan can reduce the time taken to fall asleep, while tyrosine and tryptophan may help recovery from jet lag. Several ingredients, such as n-3 fatty acids, *S*-adenosylmethione (SAMe), and folic acid (FA), have attracted attention as potential functional ingredients for improving depression.

15.3 ROLE OF NUTRACEUTICAL AND FUNCTIONAL FOODS IN MENTAL PERFORMANCE

The cognitive functions are mental activities that allow organisms, including humans, to perceive, understand, and act upon the environment, thereby optimizing adaptation and performance. The development of cognitive abilities through evolution has permitted certain species to master their environment. Today, foods are intended not only to provide necessary nutrients for humans but also to prevent nutrition-related diseases and improve the physical and mental well-being of consumers (Roberfroid 2002, Menrad 2003). Many dietary supplements derived from plants have benefits to the body or may supply the body with essential fatty acids (*glycerols, omega 6, and omega 3*), proteins (*globulins, methionine, cysteine, tryptophan, and lysine*), and other macronutrients and micronutrients (*zinc, calcium, cobalt, iron, sodium, etc.*). These foods with medicinal benefits are termed as nutraceuticals (Khan et al. 2011). Various nutraceutical and functional foods used in the prevention of mental disorder and its effects on mental performance are presented in Table 15.1 and naturally occurring functional foods are presented in Table 15.2 (Keservani et al. 2010a,b).

15.3.1 Carbohydrates and Mental Health

Carbohydrates (Figure 15.1): for instance, starches, naturally present and refined sugars, and dietary fiber. Foods high in starches and dietary fiber cover grain products such as breads, rice, etc. Carbohydrates significantly affect mood and behavior. Eating a meal high in carbohydrates triggers release of a hormone called insulin in the body. Insulin helps let blood sugar into cells where it can be used for energy, but insulin also has other effects in the body. As insulin levels rise, more tryptophan enters the brain (Lichtenstein 2006). Tryptophan is an amino acid, or a building block of protein, that affects the levels of neurotransmitters in the brain. As more tryptophan enters the

TABLE 15.1
Functional Food and Their Effects on Mental Performance

Functional Foods	Effect on Mental Performance
Glucose	Increases memory and decision time
Sucrose	Reduces pain perception
Caffeine	Improves cognitive performance with effect on reaction time, vigilance time, memory, and psychomotor performance
Carbohydrate	Sleepiness and calmness
Tryptophan	Reduces time taken to fall asleep
n-3 Fatty acid	Depression
S-Adenosylmethionine (SAMe)	Depression
FA	Depression

TABLE 15.2
Naturally Occurring Functional Foods Containing the Substances

Naturally Occurring Substances	Foods Containing the Substance
Dietary fibers	Fruits, grains, legumes, vegetables
Probiotics	Many naturally fermented foods
Prebiotics	Bananas, tomato
Polyunsaturated fats	Fatty fishes
Antioxidant vitamins	Citrus fruits, peppers, nuts, carrots
Polyphenols	Tea, dry legumes, berries

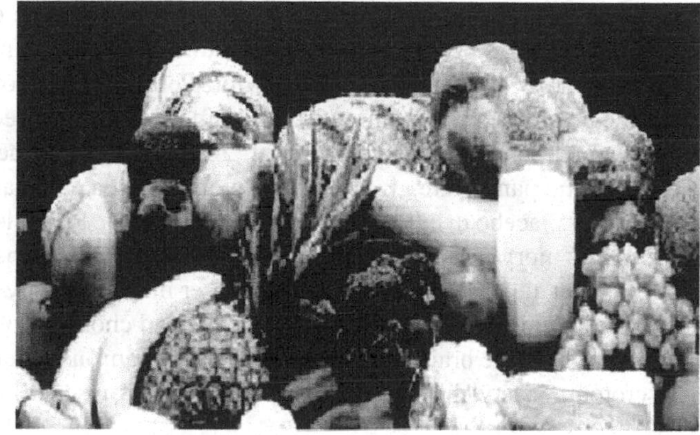

FIGURE 15.1 Food source of carbohydrate.

brain, more of the neurotransmitter serotonin is produced. Higher serotonin levels in the brain enhance mood and have a sedating effect, promoting sleepiness. This effect is partly responsible for the drowsiness some people experience after a large meal.

Glucose is the only metabolic fuel available to the brain. It is required for the synthesis of neurotransmitters such as serotonin (5-hydroxytryptamine [5-HT]), noradrenaline (NA), and acetylcholine (ACh). Other mechanisms influence cognition, for example 5-HT availability, which in turn may be influenced by CHO/protein intake, by altering the ratio of tryptophan: large neutral amino acids. Numerous reports suggest that memory is particularly affected by changes in glucose availability (Blundell et al. 2003). Glucose administration has reportedly been shown to benefit memory in young adults and the elderly (Hall et al. 1989).

15.3.2 Proteins and Mental Health

Proteins are made up of amino acids linked together in various sequences and amounts. Protein intake and intake of each unitary amino acids may influence brain functioning and mental health. Most of the neurotransmitters in the brain are derived from amino acids. The neurotransmitter dopamine is synthesized from the amino acid tyrosine. The neurotransmitter serotonin is synthesized from the amino acid tryptophan (Lichtenstein 2006). If the essential amino acid is not available, concentration of that particular neurotransmitter in the brain will go down, and brain functioning and mood will be affected. For instance, if there is a deficiency of tryptophan in the body, not enough serotonin will be generated, and low brain levels of serotonin are linked with low mood and even aggression in few individuals. Similarly, some diseases may cause a buildup of certain amino acids in the blood, causing brain damage and mental defects: for example a buildup of the amino acid phenylalanine in individuals with a disease called phenylketonuria (Lichtenstein 2006).

Protein is one of the most popular dietary supplements marketed to athletes and physically active individuals. Protein supplements have been recommended to athletes to enhance nitrogen retention and increase muscle mass, to prevent protein catabolism during prolonged exercise, to promote muscle glycogen resynthesis following exercise, and to prevent *sports anemia* by promoting an increased synthesis of hemoglobin, myoglobin, oxidative enzymes, and mitochondria during aerobic training (Williams 2005). Tryptophan (Segura and Ventura 1988) and glutamine (Williams 2005) promote glycogen synthesis and were used in mood supports. Sports nutrition scientists do note that even if athletes need more protein, the recommended amounts are compatible with the current Acceptable Macronutrient Dietary Recommendations (10%–35% of energy from protein) and may be easily obtained from natural foods in the diet (Lambert et al. 2004, Tipton et al. 2004). In general, protein supplements are not necessary (Phillips 2004, Williams 2005).

Studying meals is important, because it represents the way that people actually eat. Although studies examining the effects of single nutrients on mental performance may be easier to interpret and produce larger effects than studies using mixed meals, results of studies using single nutrients are difficult to frame in the context of normal eating behavior. People do not consume individual nutrients; rather, they eat meals or snacks containing varying amounts of the three energy-containing nutrients protein, fat, and carbohydrate (Mahoney et al. 2005). A study done by Kaplan et al. (2001) examined this issue. Participants were given a pure protein drink, a pure carbohydrate drink, a pure fat drink, or a nonenergy placebo drink on four separate mornings. Pure dietary protein, carbohydrate, and fat enhanced memory performance 15 min after ingestion, independently of elevations of blood glucose (Kaplan et al. 2001). However, 60 min after ingestion, only the glucose drink was associated with improved memory. Brain needs amino acids and choline from outside sources (dietary intake) in order to maintain the brain's necessary amount of neurons to release other necessary chemicals such as serotonin, acetylcholine, and norepinephrine (Rausch 2013).

15.3.3 Fats and Mental Health

Fatty acids are a primary portion of human nutritional requirements, subdivided into saturated, monounsaturated, polyunsaturated, and *trans*- varieties. In this terminology, the term *saturated* means a fat molecule with no double bonds between the carbon atoms (Parker et al. 2006), the distinction is important, because when they are packed together, molecules with double bonds resist compacting. The long chain, omega-3 and omega-6 polyunsaturated fatty acids, are called "essential" fatty acids, because they or their precursors cannot be made by human bodies and must be found in our diet (Enig 2000). These fatty acids are carbon chain compounds with several double bonds, subdivided into those whose first double bond occurs on the third carbon from the methyl end (omega-3 essential fatty acids) and those whose first double bond occurs on the sixth carbon from the methyl end (omega-6 essential fatty acids).

Dietary intake of fats can also play a role in controlling mood and brain activity. Dietary fats are present in animal as well as in plant foods. Meats, daily fat dairy products, butter, margarine, and plant oils are rich in fats; omega-3 fatty acids are present in fish oils and affect brain working. However, some studies recommend that omega-3 fatty acids are beneficial in bipolar affective disorder and stress; results are inconclusive (Lichtenstein 2006). Erikson also noted that certain fats are necessary, such as omega-3, in order to keep the brain well nourished and stave off feelings of depression and inflammation, and increase memory and mood with an increase in serotonin, which is also known for creating the feeling of pleasure. The brain comprises 60% fat, and brain cells help regulate aspects of the immune system (Erikson 2006).

15.3.4 Vitamins and Mental Health

Vitamins are dietary components other than carbohydrates, fats, minerals, and proteins that are necessary for life. B vitamins are required for proper functioning of the methylation cycle, monoamine production, DNA synthesis, and maintenance of phospholipids such as myelin. Fat-soluble vitamins A, D, and E play important roles in genetic transcription, antioxidant recycling, and inflammatory regulation in the brain. To help clinicians recognize and treat vitamin deficiencies among psychiatric patients, this chapter reviews the role of the six essential water-soluble vitamins (B1, B2, B6, B9, B12, and C) and three fat-soluble vitamins (A, D, and E) in brain metabolism and psychiatric pathology (Ramsey and Muskin 2013).

Subclinical vitamin C deficiency causes fatigue and psychological abnormalities (Evans-Olders et al. 2010). Folic acid (FA) deficiency precipitates depression and inhibits the response to antidepressant drugs (Das 2008, Farah 2009). In some cases, the first clinical manifestation of vitamin B12 deficiency is a psychiatric disorder (Hector and Burton 1988). Subclinical vitamin B12 deficiency is relatively common in old age and is associated with cognitive dysfunction (Smith and Refsum 2009, Tangney et al. 2009). Thiamine and niacin deficiency may first come to medical attention as stupor, confusion, psychosis, or neurocognitive dysfunction in the absence of the classic signs of beriberi and pellagra (Sydenstricker and Cleckley 1941, Botez et al. 1993). Epidemiologic and some clinical data suggest that biochemical vitamin D deficiency can precipitate or predispose to depression (Wilkins et al. 2006, Jorde et al. 2008). Subclinical zinc deficiency in children (Gardner et al. 2005) and iron deficiency, even in adults (Tu et al. 1994, Murray-Kolb and Beard 2007), can cause neurocognitive dysfunction. There is evidence that sufficient long-term consumption of FA and omega-3 fatty acids helps preserve cognitive function in old age and could prevent or delay the progression of early dementia (Das 2008, Cole et al. 2009, Vogel et al. 2009).

15.3.4.1 Vitamin A

Vitamin A is a fat-soluble vitamin present in meats, fish, and eggs. A type of vitamin A, beta-carotene, is present in orange as well as green leafy vegetables such as carrots, yellow squash, and spinach. Headache and rise in pressure of the head is related with both lack and extra vitamin A intake. Among other impacts, excess vitamin A intake may cause fatigue, irritability, and loss of appetite (Jeffery 1999, Shiveley and Patrick 2000, Westermarck and Antila 2000, Katz 2001).

15.3.4.2 Vitamin B1 (Thiamin)

Thiamin is a B vitamin occurring in fortified grain products, pork, legumes, nuts, seeds, and organ meats. Thiamin is involved in a complex manner with metabolizing glucose, or blood sugar, inside the body. Glucose is the brain's first energy source. Thiamin is also required to make variety of neurotransmitters. Alcoholism is generally linked with thiamin deficiency. Alcohol impairs thiamin metabolism in the body, and diets rich in alcohol are often lacking in vitamins and minerals. Persons with a thiamin deficiency may progress to Wernicke–Korsakoff syndrome, which is manifested by confusion, mental changes, abnormal eye movements, and unsteadiness that can lead to severe memory loss (Jeffery 1999, Shiveley and Patrick 2000, Westermarck and Antila 2000, Katz 2001).

15.3.4.3 Vitamin B2

Vitamin B2 (riboflavin) is essential for oxidative pathways, monoamine synthesis, and the methylation cycle. It is needed to create the essential flavoprotein coenzymes for the synthesis of L-methylfolate the active form of folate and for proper utilization of B6. Top dietary sources of B2 are dairy products, meat and fish, eggs, mushrooms, almonds, leafy greens, and legumes. Although generally B2 deficiency is rare, surveys in the United States have found that 10%–27% of older adults (age ≥ 65) are deficient (Powers 2003).

15.3.4.4 Vitamin B6

Vitamin B6, also known as pyridoxine, is found in many plant and animal foods, including chicken, fish, pork, whole wheat products, brown rice, and some fruits and vegetables. Vitamin B6 is required by the body to synthesize majority of the brain's neurotransmitters. It has also role in hormone production. Though rare, vitamin B6 deficiency is identified by mental changes such as fatigue, nervousness, irritability, depression, insomnia, dizziness, and nerve changes. Such mental changes are associated with the body's reduced ability to produce neurotransmitters with vitamin B6 deficiency (Jeffery 1999, Shiveley and Patrick 2000, Westermarck and Antila 2000, Katz 2001).

15.3.4.5 Vitamin B9 (Folate)

Folate is needed for proper one-carbon metabolism and thus requisite in synthesis of serotonin, norepinephrine, dopamine, and DNA and in phospholipid production. Low maternal folate status increases the risk of neural tube defects in newborns. Folate deficiency and insufficiency are common among patients with mood disorders and correlate with illness severity (Coppen and Bolander-Gouaille 2005). Dietary folate must be converted to L-methylfolate for use in the brain. Patients with a methylenetetrahydrofolate reductase (MTHFR) C677T polymorphism produce a less active form of the enzyme. The TT genotype is associated with major depression and bipolar disorder (Gilbody et al. 2007). Leafy greens and legumes such as lentils are top dietary sources of folate; supplemental FA has been linked to an increased risk of cancer and overall mortality (Ramsey and Muskin 2013).

15.3.4.6 Vitamin B12

Vitamin B12 is found only in foods of animal origin like milk, meat, or eggs. Vitamin B12 is required to keep the outermost layer, called the myelin sheath, intact on nerve cells. Improper myelin leads to nerve damage and hampered brain function. Vitamin B12 deficiency may go undiagnosed in individuals for years, but it finally causes low blood iron, irreversible nerve damage, dementia, and brain atrophy (Jeffery 1999, Shiveley and Patrick 2000, Westermarck and Antila 2000, Katz 2001).

15.3.4.7 Niacin

The B vitamin niacin is found in enriched grains, meat, fish, wheat bran, asparagus, and peanuts. Niacin is involved in releasing energy in the body from carbohydrates, proteins, and fats. A deficiency of niacin produces many mental symptoms such as irritability, headaches, loss of memory, inability to sleep, and emotional instability; deficiency can lower levels of serotonin in the brain (Jeffery 1999, Shiveley and Patrick 2000, Westermarck and Antila 2000, Katz 2001).

15.3.4.8 Vitamin C

Many fruits and vegetables are high in vitamin C. Citrus fruits (such as oranges, lemons, and limes), potatoes, strawberries, tomatoes, kiwi fruit, broccoli, spinach and other leafy greens, cabbage, green and red peppers, and cauliflower are excellent sources of vitamin C (Zee et al. 1991). Fortified beverages and cereals are also good sources. Dairy foods, meats, and nonfortified cereals and grains provide little or no vitamin C. By eating the recommended amounts of fruits and vegetables daily, we can easily meet the body's requirement for vitamin C. Vitamin C assists in the synthesis of DNA, bile, neurotransmitters such as serotonin (which helps regulate mood), and carnitine (Weber and Ernst 2006), which transports long-chain fatty acids from the cytosol into the mitochondria for energy production (Boothby and Doering 2005). Vitamin C also helps ensure that appropriate levels of thyroxine, a hormone produced by the thyroid gland, are produced to support basal metabolic rate and to maintain body temperature. Other hormones that are synthesized with assistance from vitamin C include epinephrine, norepinephrine, and steroid hormones (Yeomans et al. 2005). Vitamin C has been shown to protect the body from the damage caused by excess vanadium. A double-blind, placebo-controlled study that involved controlling elevated vanadium levels showed that a single 3 g dose of vitamin C decreases manic symptoms in comparison to placebo (Naylor and Smith 1981).

15.3.4.9 Vitamin E

Vitamin E is a fat-soluble vitamin that is plentiful in the diet, particularly in plant oils, green leafy vegetables, and fortified breakfast cereals. Vitamin E deficiency causes changes in red blood cells and nerve tissues. It progresses to dizziness, vision changes, muscle weakness, and sensory changes (Boothby and Doering 2005). If remains untreated, the nerve damage from vitamin E deficiency may be irreversible. Since it is an antioxidant, vitamin E has also been investigated for the treatment of neurological conditions viz—Parkinson's and Alzheimer's disease. Though findings are inconclusive, vitamin E exhibits some promise in retarding the development of Parkinson's disease (Jeffery 1999, Shiveley and Patrick 2000, Westermarck and Antila 2000, Katz 2001).

Studies have shown that tocotrienols exert more significant neuroprotective, anticancer, and cholesterol-lowering properties than do tocopherols (Qureshi et al. 2001, Sun et al. 2008).

One vitamin E deficiency symptom is *erythrocyte hemolysis.* This rupturing of red blood cells leads to *anemia,* a condition in which the red blood cells cannot carry and transport enough oxygen to the tissues, leading to fatigue, weakness, and a diminished ability to perform physical and mental work (IMFNB 2000).

15.3.4.10 Vitamin D

Vitamin D is produced from cholesterol in the epidermis through exposure to sunlight, namely, ultraviolet B radiation (Ramsey and Muskin 2013). Although vitamin D is known for its role in bone growth and mineralization, increasing evidence reveals vitamin D's role in brain function and development. Both glial and neuronal cells possess vitamin D receptors in the hippocampus, prefrontal cortex, hypothalamus, thalamus, and substantia nigra, all regions theorized to be linked to depression pathophysiology (Eyles et al. 2005). Limited but provocative biological, epidemiological, and clinical data suggest that vitamin D could play a role in preventing or treating depression (Wilkins et al. 2006, McCann and Ames 2008).

15.3.5 Folic Acid

FA is another B vitamin found in foods such as liver, yeast, asparagus, fried beans and peas, wheat, broccoli, and some nuts. FA plays a key role in protein metabolism within the body and in the metabolism of some amino acids, in particular the amino acid methionine. When FA concentration in the body is low, methionine cannot be metabolized adequately and the level of other chemical, homocysteine, rises in the blood. High blood homocysteine levels increase the danger of heart disease and stroke. Even mild FA deficiency in women leads to an increased risk of neural tube defects, such as spina bifida, in developing fetuses (Jeffery 1999, Shiveley and Patrick 2000, Westermarck and Antila 2000, Katz 2001).

In Spain where no mandatory fortification policy exists, we have shown that overages are a current practice in FA-fortified breakfast cereals and milk products, and total folate values were higher than those declared by manufacturers in most cases (Samaniego-Vaesken et al. 2009, Samaniego-Vaesken et al. 2010). The most well-known adverse effect of supplementation and for food fortification with FA is the masking of the diagnosis of B12 deficiency, because megaloblastic anemia caused by cobalamin deficiency can be reversed, but not the potential long-term neurological effects (Mills 2000). Morris et al. (2007) observed that low B12 status and high serum folate levels were associated with cognitive impairment and anemia in the elderly. By contrast, adequate B12 status and high serum folate levels were associated with protection against cognitive impairment. This has led to a controversy about the effects of supplementation and/or fortification with FA in subjects with vitamin B12 deficiency (Morris et al. 2007).

15.3.6 Caffeine and Mental Health

Caffeine is a bitter, white crystalline xanthine alkaloid that acts as a psychoactive stimulant drug and a mild diuretic (Maughan and Griffin 2003). In humans, caffeine is a central nervous system (CNS) stimulant (Nehlig et al 1992), having the effect of temporarily warding off drowsiness and restoring alertness. Caffeine (present in coffee, tea, cola- and guarana-based soft drinks, as well as in chocolate at a low dose) is the most widely consumed stimulant drug in the world (Benowitz 1990). Energy drinks are a group of beverages used by consumers to provide an extra boost in energy, promote wakefulness, maintain alertness, and provide cognitive and mood enhancement. These beverages have stimulant effects on the CNS, because it contains caffeine and their consumption is accompanied by an expectation of improving user's performance physically and mentally (Oteri et al. 2007, Seifert et al. 2011). Caffeine is one of the most commonly consumed alkaloids worldwide in the form of coffee, tea, or soft drinks, and in high doses may cause abnormal stimulation of the nervous system (Dworzariski et al. 2009).

15.3.7 Minerals and Mental Health

Minerals such as iron, magnesium, copper, and zinc, which are present in vegetables, meat and fish, etc., were taken by diet and were used in the prevention of mental disorder.

15.3.7.1 Iron

Iron is found in meat, poultry, and fish. Another form of iron that is not as well absorbed as the form in animal foods is found in whole or enriched grains, green leafy vegetables, dried beans and peas, and dried fruits. Iron deficiency eventually leads to severe anemia, decreased cognitive function (Grantham-McGregor and Ani 2001) with insufficient oxygen reaching the brain. The anemia can cause fatigue and impair mental functioning. Iron deficiency during the first 2 years of life can lead to permanent brain damage (Jeffery 1999, Shiveley and Patrick 2000, Westermarck and Antila 2000, Katz 2001). Iron is essential for ensuring brain oxygenation and producing energy for brain cells. Iron deficiency anemia can cause apathy, fatigue, etc., and persons land up in psychiatry with depression with somatic complaints (Kaur et al. 2014). Iron deficiency alters myelination, neurotransmitter metabolism, and function (Beard and Connor 2003), cellular and oxidative processes (Beard 1995), and thyroid hormone metabolism (Zimmermann and Kohrle 2002). Further studies have concluded that iron deficiency occurring with and without anemia can lead to defects in attention and cognitive functions, minimal brain dysfunction, and hyperactivity (Watts 1988).

15.3.7.2 Magnesium

The mineral magnesium occurs in green leafy vegetables, whole grains, nuts, seeds, and bananas. In regions with hard water, the water can avail a significant quantum of magnesium. Magnesium helps in the transmission of nerve impulses. Magnesium deficiency may lead to restlessness, nervousness, muscular twitching, and unsteadiness. Acute magnesium deficiency can develop to apathy, delirium, convulsions, coma, and death (Jeffery 1999, Shiveley and Patrick 2000, Westermarck and Antila 2000, Katz 2001). Magnesium deficiency disrupts the biochemical function in the human body, especially the nervous system. Studies indicate that magnesium, rather than pharmaceuticals, is the best treatment for patients suffering from major depression. This mineral helped participants to recover from traumatic brain injuries, headaches, suicidal thoughts, anxiety, and postpartum depression (Faryadi 2012).

15.3.7.3 Copper

The richest sources of the trace mineral copper in the diet are organ meats, seafood, nuts, seeds, whole grain breads and cereals, and chocolate. In addition to other functions, copper is involved in iron metabolism in the body and in brain function. Deficiency of copper causes anemia, with inadequate oxygen delivery to the brain and other organs. Copper deficiency also impairs brain functioning and immune system response, including changes in certain chemical receptors in the brain and lowered levels of neurotransmitters (Jeffery 1999, Shiveley and Patrick 2000, Westermarck and Antila 2000, Katz 2001). Copper is an essential trace element for living cells and plays an important role in redox reactions. Copper is mainly transported in the bloodstream by ceruloplasmin, in Cu-binding antioxidant protein. Ceruloplasmin is synthesized in several tissues, including the brain (Geir 2013).

15.3.7.4 Zinc

The trace mineral zinc is present in red meats, liver, eggs, dairy products, vegetables, and some sea foods. Among other functions, zinc is part of maintaining cell membranes and shielding cells from damage. Lack of zinc can cause neurological impairment, affecting appetite, taste, smell, and vision (Jeffery 1999, Shiveley and Patrick 2000, Westermarck and Antila 2000, Katz 2001). After iron, zinc has the second highest concentration of all transition metals in the brain (Huang 1997). Zinc is also needed for DNA synthesis and cell membrane stabilization. It is essential to the structure and function of regulatory, structural, and enzymatic proteins. Zinc deficiency causes immunosuppression (Maes et al. 1991).

15.4 OTHER PLANT- AND FRUIT-DERIVED NUTRACEUTICAL AND FUNCTIONAL FOODS USED IN THE PREVENTION OF MENTAL DISORDER

The fruit juice of *M. citrifolia* L. is in high demand in alternative medicine for mental depression (Wang et al. 2002, Kamiya et al. 2004). Therefore, one of the challenges in recent years has been to process fruit juice so as to make a more modern drug from a traditional product (Chunhieng 2003). Asian ginseng (*Panax ginseng*) has been a part of Chinese medicine for over 2000 years and was traditionally used to improve mental and physical vitality (Gleeson 2012).

Ginkgo biloba has been used for several thousand years by the Chinese for various maladies, including vertigo, short-term memory loss, and lack of attention or vigilance. Standardized extracts of ginkgo have been shown to possess antioxidant (Oyama et al. 1996) and neuroprotective properties, including slowing the progression of dementia (Le et al. 2000). Recent studies have shown ginkgo to possess antistress properties as well (Jezova et al. 2002). *Ocimum sanctum* (Holy basil or tulsi) is used in ayurvedic medicine and has been shown to have antistressor effects (Sembulingam and Sembulingam 1997).

15.5 CONCLUSIONS

Nutraceuticals have received considerable interest because of their presumed safety and potential nutritional and therapeutic effects. Various preparations either in the form of foods, capsules, and powder under the food supplement category making health claims are still being marketed in the country. The exploration and exploitation of the disease-fighting properties of a multitude of phytochemicals found in both food and nonfood plants have created a renaissance in human health and nutrition research. It is finally concluded that carbohydrates, caffeine, fats, proteins, vitamins, and minerals in food are essential parts of any diet that provide specific mental benefits for the human body. A lack of any of these nutritional components can lead to physical difficulties, increased mental health problems, and even changes in brain functioning.

REFERENCES

Beard, J. 1995. One person's view of iron deficiency, development, and cognitive function. *Am J Clin Nutr* 62:709–710.

Beard, J.L., J.R. Connor. 2003. Iron status and neural functioning. *Annu Rev Nutr* 23:41–58.

Benowitz, N. 1990. Clinical pharmacology of caffeine. *Ann Rev Med* 41:277–288.

Biesalski, H.K. 2001. Nutraceuticals: The link between nutrition and medicine. In: K. Kramer, P.P. Hoppe, L. Packer, eds. *Nutraceuticals in Health and Disease Prevention.* New York: Marcel Deckker Inc. pp. 1–26.

Blundell, J., D. Gumaste, R. Handley, L. Dye. 2003. Diet, behaviour and cognitive functions: A psychobiological view. *Scand J Nutr* 47(2):85–91.

Boothby, L.A., P.L. Doering. 2005. Vitamin C and vitamin E for Alzheimer's disase. *Ann Pharmacother* 39(2005):2073–2080.

Botez, M. I. et al. 1993. Thiamine and folate treatment of chronic epileptic patients: A controlled study with the Wechsler IQ scale. *Epilepsy Res* 16:157–163.

Chunhieng, M.T. (2003). Developpement de nouveaux aliments santé tropicale: application a la moix du Bresil Bertholettia excelsa et au fruit de Cambodge Morinda citrifolia. Ph.D thesis, INOL, France.

Cole, G.M., Q.L. Ma, S.A. Frautschy. 2009. Omega-3 fatty acids and dementia. *Prostaglandins Leukot Essent Fatty Acids* 81:213–221.

Coppen, A., C. Bolander-Gouaille. 2005. Treatment of depression: Time to consider folic acid and vitamin B12. *J Psychopharmacol* 19(1):59–65.

Das, U.N. 2008. Folic acid and polyunsaturated fatty acids improve cognitive function and prevent depression, dementia, and Alzheimer's disease but how and why? *Prostaglandins Leukot Essent Fatty Acids* 78:11–19.

Dijsselbloem, N., W.V. Berghe, A.D. Naeyer, G. Haegeman. 2004. Soy isoflavone phyto-pharmaceuticals in interleukin-6 affections: Multi-purpose nutraceuticals at the crossroad of hormone replacement, anti-cancer and anti-inflammatory therapy. *Biochem Pharmacol* 68:1171–1185.

Dillard, C.J., J.B. German. 2000. Review. Phytochemicals: Nutraceuticals and human health. *J Sci Food Agric* 80:1744–1756.

Dworzariski, W. et al. 2009. Side effects of caffeine. *Pol Merkurlekarski* 27(161):357–361.

Enig, M.G. 2000. *Know Your Fats*. Silver Spring, MD: Bethesda Press p. 64.

Erikson, J. 2006. Brain food: The real dish on nutrition and brain function. *WisKids J.* November/December. Retrieved from http://www.wccf.org/wkj/1106/story7.htm (accessed on May 12, 2014).

Evans-Olders, R., S. Eintracht, L.J. Hoffer. 2010. Metabolic origin of hypovitaminosis C in acutely hospitalized patients. *Nutrition* 26:1070–1074.

Eyles, D.W. et al. 2005. Distribution of the vitamin D receptor and 1 alpha-hydroxylase in human brain. *J Chem Neuroanat* 29(1):21–30.

Farah, A. 2009. The role of L-methylfolate in depressive disorders. *CNS Spectr* 14(1 Suppl 2):2–7.

Faraone, S.V. 1995. Genetic heterogeneity in attention-deficit hyperactivity disorder (ADHD): Gender, psychiatric comorbidity, and maternal ADHD. *J Abnorm Psychol* 104:334–345.

Faryadi, Q. 2012. The magnificent effect of magnesium to human health: A critical review. *Int J Appl Sci Technol* 2(3):118–126.

Gardner, J.M. et al. 2005. Zinc supplementation and psychosocial stimulation: Effects on the development of undernourished Jamaican children. *Am J Clin Nutr* 82:399–405.

Geir, B. 2013. The role of zinc and copper in autism spectrum disorders. *Acta Neurobiol Exp* 73:225–236.

Gilbody, S, S. Lewis, T. Lightfoot. 2007. Methylenetetrahydrofolate reductase (MTHFR) genetic polymorphisms and psychiatric disorders: A HuGE review. *Am J Epidemiol* 165(1):1–13.

Gleeson, M. 2012. Exercise, nutrition and immunity. In: P.C. Calder, P. Yaqoob, eds. *Diet, Immunity and Inflammation*. Cambridge, U.K.: Woodhead Publishing, pp. 652–685.

Grantham-Mcgregor, S., C. Ani. 2001. A review of studies on the effect of iron deficiency on cognitive development in children. *J Nutr* 131(2):649S–666S.

Gu, Y., J.W. Nieves, Y. Stern, J.A. Luchsinger, N. Scarmeas. 2010. Food combination and Alzheimer's disease risk. *Arch Neurol* 67(6):1–6.

Hall, J.L. et al. 1989. Glucose enhancement of performance on memory tests in young and aged humans. *Neuropsychologia* 27:1129–1138.

Hankey, G.J., J.W. Eikelboom. 1999. Homocysteine and vascular disease, *Lancet* 354:407–413.

Hector, M., J.R. Burton. 1988. What are the psychiatric manifestations of vitamin B12 deficiency? *J Am Geriatr Soc* 36:1105–1112.

Hoffer, L.J. 2012. Micronutrients and mental disorders. *J Orthomol Med* 27(4):157–161.

Huang, E.P. 1997. Metal ions and synaptic transmission: Think zinc. *Proc Natl Acad Sci USA* 94:13386–13387.

Institute of Medicine, Food and Nutrition Board (IMFNB). 2000. *Dietary Reference Intakes for Vitamin C, Vitamin E, Selenium, and Carotenoids*. Washington, DC: The National Academy of Sciences.

Jeffery, D.R. 1999. Nutrition and diseases of the nervous system. In: M.E. Shils, J.A. Olson, M. Shike, A.C. Ross, eds. *Modern Nutrition in Health and Disease*. 9th edn. Baltimore, MD: Williams & Wilkins, pp. 1552–1553.

Jezova, D., R. Duncko, M. Lassanova, M. Kriska, F. Moncek. 2002. Reduction of rise in blood pressure and cortisol release during stress by *Ginkgo biloba* extract (EGb761) in healthy volunteers. *J Phys Pharmacol* 53(3):337–348.

Jorde, R. et al. 2008. Effects of vitamin D supplementation on symptoms of depression in overweight and obese subjects: Randomized double blind trial. *J Intern Med* 264:599–609.

Kalra, E.K. 2003. Nutraceutical—Definition and introduction. *AAPS Pharm Sci* 5:1–2.

Kamiya, K., Y. Tanaka, H. Endang, M. Umar, T. Satake. 2004. Chemical constituents of *Morinda citrifolia* fruits inhibit copper-induced low-density lipoprotein oxidation, *J Agric Food Chem* 52:5843–5848.

Kaplan, R.J., C.E. Greenwood, G. Winocur, T.M.S. Wolever. 2001. Dietary protein, carbohydrate and fat enhance memory performance in the healthy elderly. *Am J Clin Nutr* 74:687–693.

Kaput, J., R.L. Rodriguez. 2004. Nutritional genomics: The next frontier in the postgenomic era. *Physiol Genomics* 16:166–177.

Katz, D.L. 2001. *Nutrition in Clinical Practice*. New York: Lippincott, Williams, & Wilkins.

Kaur, J., M.S. Bhatia, P. Gautam. 2014. Role of dietary factors in psychiatry. *Delhi Psychiatry J* 17(2):452–457.

Keservani, R.K., A.K. Sharma. 2014. Flavonoids: Emerging trends and potential health benefits. *J Chin Pharm Sci* 23(12):815–822.

Keservani, R.K., R.K. Kesharwani, A.K. Sharma, N. Vyas, A. Chadoker. 2010b. Nutritional supplements: An overview. *Int J Curr Pharm Rev Res* 1:59–75.

Keservani, R.K., R.K. Kesharwani, N. Vyas, S. Jain, R. Raghuvanshi, A.K. Sharma. 2010a. Nutraceutical and functional food as future food: A review. *Der Pharmacia Lett* 2:106–116.

Khan, T.M. et al. 2011. Nutraceuticals use among the inhabitants of Penang, Malaysia. *Int J Collab Res Int Med Public Health* 3(5):402–414.

Lambert, C. et al. 2004. Macronutrient considerations for the sport of bodybuilding. *Sports Med* 34:317–327.

Le, B.P.L., M. Keiser, K.Z. Itil. 2000. A 26-week analysis of a double-blind, placebo-controlled trial of the *Ginkgo biloba* extract EGb 761 in dementia. *Dement Geriatr Cogn Disord* 11(4):230–237.

Lichtenstein, A.H. 2006. Dietary fat, carbohydrate, and protein: Effects on plasma lipoprotein patterns. *J Lipid Res* 47:1661–1667.

Maes, M., E. Bosmans, E. Suy, C. Vandervorst, C. DeJonckheere, J. Raus. 1991. Depression-related disturbances in mitogen-induced lymphocyte responses and interleukin-1 beta and soluble interleukin-2 receptor production. *Acta Psychiatr Scand* 84:379–386.

Mahoney, C.R. et al. 2005. *The Acute Effects of Meals on Cognitive Performance*. Boca Raton, FL: Taylor & Francis Group, LLC.

Maughan, R.J., J. Griffin. 2003. Caffeine ingestion and fluid balance: A review. *J Hum Nutr Diet* 16: 411–420.

McCann, J.C., B.N. Ames. 2008. Is there convincing biological or behavioral evidence linking vitamin D deficiency to brain dysfunction? *FASEB J* 22:982–1001.

McCulley, K.S. 2007. Homocysteine, vitamins and vascular disease prevention. *Am J Clin Nutr* 86:S1563–S1568.

Menrad, K. 2003. Market and marketing of functional food in Europe. *J Food Eng* 56:181–188.

Mills, J.L. 2000. Fortification of foods with folic acid: How much is enough? *N Engl J Med* 342:1442–1445.

Morris, M.S., P.F. Jacques, I.H. Rosenberg, J. Selhub. 2007. Folate and vitamin B-12 status in relation to anemia, macrocytosis, and cognitive impairment in older Americans in the age of folic acid fortification. *Am J Clin Nutr* 85:193–200.

Murray-Kolb, L.E., J.L. Beard. 2007. Iron treatment normalizes cognitive functioning in young women. *Am J Clin Nutr* 85:778–787.

Naylor, G.J., A.H. Smith. 1981. Vanadium: A possible aetiological factor in manic depressive illness. *Psychol Med* 11:249–256.

Nehlig, A. et al. 1992. Caffeine and the central nervous system: Mechanisms of action, biochemical, metabolic, and psychostimulant effects. *Brain Res Rev* 17(2):139–170.

Nichenametla, S.N., T.G. Taruscio, D.L. Barney, J.H. Exon. 2006. A review of the effects and mechanism of polyphenolics in cancer. *Crit Rev Food Sci Nutr* 46:161–183.

Oteri, A. et al. 2007. Intake of energy drinks in association with alcoholic beverages in cohort of students of the School of Medicine of the University of Messina. *Alcohol Clin Exp Res* 31(10):1677–1809.

Oyama, Y., L. Chikahisa, T. Ueha, K. Kanemaru, K. Noda. 1996. *Ginkgo biloba* extract protects brain neurons against oxidative stress induced by hydrogen peroxide. *Brain Res.* 712(2):349–352.

Packer, L., S.U. Weber. 2001. *The Role of Vitamin E in the Emerging Field of Nutraceuticals*. New York: Marcel Dekker. pp. 27–43.

Parker, G. et al. 2006. Omega-3 fatty acids and mood disorders. *Am J Psychiatry* 163:969–978.

Phillips, S. 2004. Protein requirements and supplementation in strength sports. *Nutrition* 20:689–695.

Powers, H.J. 2003. Riboflavin (vitamin B-2) and health. *Am J Clin Nutr* 77(6):1352–1360.

Prakash, D., N. Kumar. 2011. Cost effective natural antioxidants. In: R.R. Watson, J.K. Gerald, V.R. Preedy, eds. *Nutrients, Dietary Supplements and Nutriceuticals*. New York: Humana Press, Springer. pp. 163–188.

Prakash, D., R. Dhakarey, A. Mishra. 2004. Carotenoids: The phytochemicals of nutraceutical importance. *Ind J Agric Biochem* 17:1–8.

Qureshi, A.A., W.A. Salser, R. Parmar, E.E. Emeson. 2001. Novel tocotrienols of rice bran inhibit atherosclerotic lesions in C57Bl/6 apoe-deficient mice. *J Nutr* 131:2606–2618.

Ramsey, D., P.R. Muskin. 2013. Vitamin deficiencies and mental health: How are they linked. *Curr Psychiatry* 12(1):37–44.

Rausch, R. 2013. Nutrition and academic performance in school-age children the relation to obesity and food insufficiency. *J Nutr Food Sci* 3(2):1–3.

Roberfroid, M. B. 2002. Global view on functional foods: European perspectives. *Br J Nutr.* 88:S133–S138.

Samaniego-Vaesken, M.L., E. Alonso-Aperte, G. Varela-Moreiras. 2009. Elaboraci6n de una base de datos del contenido en folatos de los alismentos: Fortificaci6n voluntaria con acido folico en España. *Nutr Hosp* 24:459–466.

Samaniego-Vaesken, M.L., E. Alonso-Aperte, G. Varela-Moreiras. 2010. Analysis and evaluation of voluntary folic acid fortification of breakfast cereals in the Spanish market. *J Food Compos Anal* 23:419–423.

Segura, R., J. Ventura, 1988. Effect of L-tryptophan supplementation on exercise performance. *Int J Sports Med* 9: 301–305.

Seifert, S. et al. 2011. Health effects of energy drinks on children, adolescents, and young adults. *Pediatrics* 127(3):511–528.

Sembulingam, K., P. Sembulingam, A. Nanasivayam. 1997. Effect of *Ocimum sanctum* Linn on noise induced changes in plasma corticosterone level. *Ind J Physiol Pharmacol* 41(2):139–143.

Shiveley, L.R., J.P. Connolly. 2000. Medical nutrition therapy for neurologic disorders. In: L.K. Mahan, S. Escott-Stump, eds. *Krause's Food, Nutrition, & Diet Therapy.* 10th edn. New York: W. B. Saunders Company, pp. 935–969.

Smith, A.D., H. Refsum. 2009. Vitamin B12 and cognition in the elderly. *Am J Clin Nutr* 89:707S–711S.

Sun, W., Q. Wang, B. Chen, J. Liu, H. Liu, W. Xu. 2008. γ-Tocotrienol-induced apoptosis in human gastric cancer SGC-7901 cells is associated with a suppression in mitogen-activated protein kinase signaling. *Br J Nutr* 99:1247–1254.

Sydenstricker, V.P., H.M. Cleckley. 1941. The effect of nicotinic acid in stupor, lethargy and various other psychiatric disorders. *Am J Psychiatry* 98:83–92.

Tangney, C.C. et al. 2009. Biochemical indicators of vitamin B12 and folate insuficiency and cognitive decline. *Neurology* 72:361–367.

Tipton, K. et al. 2004. Ingestion of casein and whey proteins result in muscle anabolism after resistance exercise. *Med Sci Sports Exerc* 36:2073–2081.

Tripathi, K.D. 2009. *Essentials of Medical Pharmacology.* New Delhi, India: Jaypee Brothers Medical Publishers (P) ltd.

Tu, J.B., H. Shafey, C. Van Dewetering. 1994. Iron deficiency in two adolescents with conduct, dysthymic and movement disorders. *Can J Psychiatry* 39:371–375.

Vogel, T. et al. 2009. Homocysteine, vitamin B12, folate and cognitive functions: A systematic and critical review of the literature. *Int J Clin Pract* 63:1061–1067.

Wang, M.Y. et al. 2002. *Morinda citrifolia* (Noni): A literature review and recent advances in Noni research. *Acta Pharmacol Sin* 23:1127–1141.

Watts, D.L. 1988. The nutritional relationships of iron. *J Orthomol Med* 3(3):110–116.

Weber, C.A., E.M. Ernst. 2006. Antioxidants, supplements, and Parkinson's disease. *Ann Pharmacother* 40:935–938.

Westermarck, T., E. Antila. 2000. Diet in relation to the nervous system. In: J.S. Garrow, W.P.T. James, A. Ralph, eds. *Human Nutrition and Dietetics.* 10th edn. New York: Churchill Livingstone, pp. 715–730.

Wilkins, C.H. et al. 2006. Vitamin D deficiency is associated with low mood and worse cognitive performance in older adults. *Am J Geriatr Psychiatry* 14:1032–1040.

Williams, M. 2005. Dietary supplements and sports performance: Amino acids. *J Int Soc Sports Nutr* 2(2):63–67.

Williams, M.H. 2005. *Nutrition for Health, Fitness & Sports.* Boston, MA: McGraw-Hill.

Yeomans, V.C., J. Linseisen, G. Wolfram. 2005. Interactive effects of polyphenols, tocopherol, and ascorbic acid on the Cu_2-mediated oxidative modification of human low density lipoproteins. *Eur J Nutr.* Epub April 15. DOI 10.1007/s00394-005-0546-y.

Zee, J. et al. 1991. Effect of storage conditions on the stability of vitamin C in various fruits and vegetables produced and consumed in Quebec. *J Food Compos Anal* 4:77.

Zimmermann, M.B., J. Kohrle. 2002. The impact of iron and selenium deficiencies on iodine and thyroid metabolism: Biochemistry and relevance to public health. *Thyroid* 12:867–878.

Section VI

Pulmonary Diseases

16 Prebiotics, Probiotics, and Synbiotics for the Management of Respiratory Disease

Seil Sagar, Gert Folkerts, and Johan Garssen

CONTENTS

16.1 INTRODUCTION

Respiratory diseases are among the leading causes of death worldwide. In 2008, chronic obstructive pulmonary disease (COPD), lung infections, and lung cancer together attributed to 9.5 million deaths worldwide (Gibson et al. 2013). In parallel, the increase in the prevalence of allergic diseases including asthma is becoming a major global health concern (Devereux 2006, Gibson et al. 2013). According to the classical "hygiene hypothesis," this increase in prevalence of allergic diseases can be attributed at least in part to reduced microbial exposure in early life (Devereux 2006). There is an unmet need for novel respiratory allergies and airway disease prevention strategies (Prescott and Nowak-Wegrzyn 2011). In this regard, understanding the relationships between the microbial populations and microbial diversity and the host in health and disease has gained a lot of attention in the last 10 years (Charlson et al. 2012a, Erb-Downward et al. 2011, Madan et al. 2012). In the last 3 years, a new frontier in pulmonary research noted as "airway microbiome" has emerged (Huang 2013, Huang and Lynch 2011, Marsland et al. 2013). There is increasing evidence that the composition of the airway microbiome varies under healthy and diseased conditions (Huang and Lynch 2011). Studies in this research field revealed that the bacterial diversity is affected by the severity of the chronic respiratory disease (Blainey et al. 2012, Erb-Downward et al. 2011, Gollwitzer and Marsland 2014, Marri et al. 2013). However, it should be realized that it is not clear yet whether a change in microbiome is the chicken or the egg in relation to symptoms of respiratory disease. Interestingly, the concept of the airway microbiome also holds promise for lung transplantation research as lower microbiota diversity was found in the respiratory tract of transplant recipient (Charlson et al. 2012b).

In this chapter, current knowledge on the airway microbiome is highlighted. The potential of beneficial bacteria-based therapies for respiratory diseases (i.e. allergic asthma, chronic obstructive pulmonary disease [COPD], and cystic fibrosis [CF]) is discussed. The clinical implications of the use of prebiotics, probiotics, and synbiotics in asthma will be assessed.

16.2 AIRWAY MICROBIOTA

Partly due to the fact that many bacterial species in the airways are nonculturable, the airways were thought to be sterile (Marsland et al. 2013). Recently, various studies using advanced sequencing technologies have confirmed the existence of a microbiome in the airways. In this regard, a study by Charlson et al. (2012a) emphasized the importance of avoiding the "carry over" of bacterial species from the upper to the lower respiratory tract during the collection of the specimen.

The respiratory tract of healthy subjects was shown to have a homogeneous microbiota with no consistent distinct microbiome (Charlson et al. 2011). In 2010, the composition of the airway microbiome was for the first time shown to be different between healthy subjects and those with asthma or COPD (Hilty et al. 2010). Asthmatic airways have disordered microbial communities compared with healthy subjects. Aligning with this work, other studies in humans have shown differences between the microbial composition of the intestine and airways of healthy people and subjects with chronic lung diseases (e.g. asthma, COPD, and CF). Interestingly, the microbial composition of expectorated sputum from asthmatic and nonasthmatic subjects was shown to be different as well. A higher bacterial diversity was found in sputum samples from asthmatics (Marri et al. 2013).

Patients with severe COPD have reduced bacterial diversity in the airways as compared with milder cases of COPD and healthy subjects (Erb-Downward et al. 2011). In this same study, the authors reported diversity in the composition of the microbiota in different regions of the airways. Consistent with these findings, a study by Sze et al. (2012) indicated that lung tissue samples from very severe COPD subjects have different airway microbiota compositions compared with those from nonsmokers and smokers without COPD. In regard to CF, microbial diversity was diminished in the airways of subjects with the severe type of the disease (Blainey et al. 2012). Compared with healthy controls, sputum from CF patients revealed a characteristic "signature" microbial profile. Additionally, a study in infants with CF indicated that microbial development in the respiratory tract of those patients may be influenced by gut colonization patterns and nutritional factors suggesting a potential for beneficial bacteria-based approaches in CF (Madan et al. 2012).

It is now well established that the diversity of the lung microbiome is reduced in the diseased state (Marsland et al. 2013). Changes in the composition of the intestinal microbiota, upon administration of beneficial bacteria, might modulate the composition of the airway microbiota. This can take place either indirectly via stimulation of the growth of probiotic bacteria in the lung by the released products or directly by microaspiration of the beneficial bacteria from the intestinal tract to the airways (Gollwitzer and Marsland 2014).

16.3 GUT–AIRWAY CROSS TALK

Under homeostasis, the gut microbiome fulfills an important metabolic role, prevents the colonization of the gut by pathogens, and exerts many immunologic effects (Quigley 2013). Additionally, the gut microbiome plays a crucial role in the development of mucosal tolerance to allergen exposure, including the airways and is therefore considered as a major regulator of the immune system (Noverr and Huffnagle 2004). Early-life exposure to environmental microbes is thought to influence the gut colonization pattern, which in turn can have a major impact on regulating immune responses associated with atopy and asthma (Kozyrskyj et al. 2011, Russell and Finlay 2012). One possible mechanism underlying the tolerogenic immunomodulatory property of the gut microbiota is possibly driven by the activation of specific dendritic cells (tolerogenic), which in turn stimulate the differentiation of regulatory T cells (Tregs) (McLoughlin and Mills 2011).

Interestingly, changes in the composition of the gut microbiome are suggested to be implicated in the pathogenesis of various inflammatory diseases including asthma (Kranich et al. 2011, Noverr and Huffnagle 2004). The gut microbiome diversity in atopic children is different from this in nonatopic children and in countries of high and low prevalence of allergy (Bjorksten et al. 1999, 2001, Kalliomaki et al. 2001, Ouwehand et al. 2001, Penders et al. 2007, Watanabe et al. 2003).

Although this hypothesis needs to be validated, the airways, lungs, and the gastrointestinal tract were suggested to be affected in the same pathophysiological manner under the condition of bronchial asthma (Vieira and Pretorius 2010). Literature overviewed in this section and Section 16.2 indicates that restoring the microbial balance and bacterial load in the airways and gut may be beneficial in the treatment of respiratory disorders.

16.4 PRE-, PRO-, AND SYNBIOTIC-BASED THERAPIES

Prebiotics are oligosaccharides that resist digestion but are fermentable by the intestinal microbiome and those nondigestible oligosaccharides may be metabolized by probiotics. Additionally, prebiotics are also suggested to stimulate the survival of probiotics (Gourbeyre et al. 2011). Probiotics are defined as "live microorganisms which, when consumed in adequate amounts, confer a health benefit on the host" (Gourbeyre et al. 2011, Guarner and Schaafsma 1998). Synbiotics is the combination of both (Gourbeyre et al. 2011).

In the past 10 years, there has been a growing interest in shaping the gut microbiome by potentially beneficial bacteria-based intervention strategies for a broad range of disorders (Forsythe et al. 2007, Kranich et al. 2011, Prescott and Nowak-Wegrzyn 2011, Vyas and Ranganathan 2012). Interestingly, evidence from studies in germ-free mice has highlighted a new hope for the potential of pre-, pro-, and synbiotics strategies in shaping the allergic airway response in the gut but also in the airways (Herbst et al. 2011, Noverr and Huffnagle 2004). Compared with mice having normal microbiota, mice lacking exposure of bacteria, viruses and fungi showed an exaggerated type 2 helper T cells (Th2)-dominated allergic airway immune response upon exposure to an allergen along with other characteristics of pulmonary inflammation. However, administration of innocuous bacteria via the airways protected mice with normal microbiome against the development of an allergic airway response. Accordingly, beneficial bacteria alone or in combination with nondigestible oligosaccharides modulated the intestinal microbiota and mucosal and systemic immune responses in human and rodents (Gourbeyre et al. 2011, Vyas and Ranganathan 2012).

To date, little has been reported regarding the therapeutic potential of prebiotics in pulmonary diseases.

In regard to allergic asthma, bacterial species of *Lactobacillus* were reported to prevent asthma in mice by inhibiting allergic airway hyperresponsiveness and modulation of the Th1/Th2 immunobalance (Ezendam et al. 2008, Forsythe et al. 2007, Li et al. 2010, Yu et al. 2010). Animal and clinical studies with probiotics in allergic asthmatic subjects revealed conflicting outcomes. The latter seem to be confounded by different factors including the bacterial species used, route of administration, duration of the treatment, and the used mixture of prebiotics and probiotics (Jeurink et al. 2012). Ovalbumin (OVA)-induced allergic airway inflammation was decreased in allergen-sensitized and challenged mice administered with probiotics orally (Kim et al. 2005). We recently demonstrated in a murine ovalbumin-induced chronic allergic asthma model that *Bifidobacterium breve* M-16V and *Lactobacillus rhamnosus* NutRes1 are as effective as corticosteroids (budesonide) in suppressing airway allergic response (Sagar et al. 2014a). Although different probiotic species and strains and mouse models were used in the literature, oral probiotic administration has similarly been effective in other animal studies (Feleszko et al. 2007, Jang et al. 2012, Karimi et al. 2009). In contrast to clinical studies reporting no impact on disease symptoms (Giovannini et al. 2007, Wheeler et al. 1997), Gutkowski et al. (2010) demonstrated beneficial effects of probiotics in allergic asthmatics.

One possible explanation for the superior effect of a combination therapy (synbiotics) on prebiotics or probiotics treatment alone may be the fact that prebiotics strengthen the immunomodulatory effect of probiotics by prolonging their survival in the intestinal tract (Gourbeyre et al. 2011). A combination therapy consisting of *B. breve* M-16V and a specific mixture of short-chain and long-chain nondigestible oligosaccharides was reported to reduce allergic responses in mice (Schouten 2009). The same mixture reduced the Th2 immune response and improved the lung function in allergic asthmatics (van de Pol et al. 2011). *B. breve* M-16V bacteria combined with a specific mixture of short-chain and long-chain nondigestible oligosaccharides and pectin-derived acidic oligosaccharides were shown to reduce several parameters of allergic asthma in mice and to prevent asthma-like symptoms in infants with atopic dermatitis (Vos et al. 2007). In a murine OVA-induced chronic asthma model, we demonstrated that a combination of *B. breve* M-16V with a specific mixture of short-chain and long-chain fructo-oligosaccharides, and pectin-derived acidic oligosaccharides was effective in suppressing airway inflammation in mice (Sagar et al. 2014b).

16.5 MECHANISM OF ACTION OF PRE-, PRO-, AND SYNBIOTICS

While the exact mechanism of action of beneficial bacteria remains to be elucidated, a number of possible mechanisms are proposed. Dietary oligosaccharides (prebiotics) are suggested to modify the intestinal microbiota or interact directly on immune cells (Jeurink 2013). Probiotic bacteria can act within the gut lumen, interact with the gut mucus and the epithelium, and/or have an effect on the systemic immune system beyond the gut (Rijkers 2010). Additionally, those Gram-positive bacteria can exert their immunomodulatory effects by shifting the immune balance from a Th2 to a Th1 as well as enhance a toll-like receptor (TLR)-driven immune response (Georgiou 2011). Regarding the possible cross talk between the gut and the lung microbiota, a gut–lung axis is proposed. Lactic acid bacteria are suggested to induce Tregs in the gut that can spread to the airways upon immune challenge and inflammation (Forsythe 2011). Another possible mechanism is through the induction of galectines. A combination of *B. breve* M-16V with a specific mixture of galacto- and fructo-oligosaccharides suppressed allergic symptoms in mice and human via the induction of gelectin-9 (de Kivit 2013).

16.6 CONCLUDING COMMENTS

Although the airway microbiome research has recently emerged and is still in its infancy, there is accumulating evidence that the composition and the bacterial load of the lung microbiome are altered in the diseased state. More in-depth studies are warranted to address the issue of whether the observed change in the composition of the microbiome is the cause of the disease or is a consequence of the inflammation in the airways. In regard to asthma, these studies may pose the critical challenge that asthma is a heterogeneous disorder with many different phenotypes underlined by different disease mechanisms.

Additionally, the function of the airway microbiome in health and disease remains to be elucidated. Further investigation is also needed to explore the mechanism underlying the possible communication/cross talk between the gut and the airway microbiome.

Gut and airway microbiome studies hold much promise that restoring the microbial balance in the gut and the airways might have therapeutic potential in respiratory diseases. This suggests that beneficial bacteria-based therapies can be a novel approach for the treatment of respiratory diseases. The exact mechanism of action of prebiotics, probiotics, and synbiotics still needs to be elucidated. More studies investigating the immunomodulatory effects of beneficial bacteria in a therapeutic setup are required.

REFERENCES

Bjorksten, B., P. Naaber, E. Sepp, and M. Mikelsaar. 1999. The intestinal microflora in allergic Estonian and Swedish 2-year-old children. *Clin Exp Allergy* 29 (3):342–346.

Bjorksten, B., E. Sepp, K. Julge, T. Voor, and M. Mikelsaar. 2001. Allergy development and the intestinal microflora during the first year of life. *J Allergy Clin Immunol* 108 (4):516–520. doi: 10.1067/mai.2001.118130.

Blainey, P. C., C. E. Milla, D. N. Cornfield, and S. R. Quake. 2012. Quantitative analysis of the human airway microbial ecology reveals a pervasive signature for cystic fibrosis. *Sci Transl Med* 4 (153):153ra130. doi: 10.1126/scitranslmed.3004458.

Charlson, E. S., K. Bittinger, J. Chen, J. M. Diamond, H. Li, R. G. Collman, and F. D. Bushman. 2012a. Assessing bacterial populations in the lung by replicate analysis of samples from the upper and lower respiratory tracts. *PLoS One* 7 (9):e42786. doi: 10.1371/journal.pone.0042786.

Charlson, E. S., K. Bittinger, A. R. Haas, A. S. Fitzgerald, I. Frank, A. Yadav, F. D. Bushman, and R. G. Collman. 2011. Topographical continuity of bacterial populations in the healthy human respiratory tract. *Am J Respir Crit Care Med* 184 (8):957–963. doi: 10.1164/rccm.201104-0655OC.

Charlson, E. S., J. M. Diamond, K. Bittinger, A. S. Fitzgerald, A. Yadav, A. R. Haas, F. D. Bushman, and R. G. Collman. 2012b. Lung-enriched organisms and aberrant bacterial and fungal respiratory microbiota after lung transplant. *Am J Respir Crit Care Med* 186 (6):536–545. doi: 10.1164/rccm.201204-0693OC.

de Kivit, S. 2013. Galectin-9 induced by dietary synbiotics is involved in suppression of allergic symptoms in mice and humans. *J Innate Immun* 5(6):625–638.

Devereux, G. 2006. The increase in the prevalence of asthma and allergy: Food for thought. *Nat Rev Immunol* 6 (11):869–874. doi: 10.1038/nri1958.

Erb-Downward, J. R., D. L. Thompson, M. K. Han, C. M. Freeman, L. McCloskey, L. A. Schmidt, V. B. Young et al. 2011. Analysis of the lung microbiome in the "healthy" smoker and in COPD. *PLoS One* 6 (2):e16384. doi: 10.1371/journal.pone.0016384.

Ezendam, J., A. de Klerk, E. R. Gremmer, and H. van Loveren. 2008. Effects of *Bifidobacterium animalis* administered during lactation on allergic and autoimmune responses in rodents. *Clin Exp Immunol* 154 (3):424–431. doi: 10.1111/j.1365-2249.2008.03788.x.

Feleszko, W., J. Jaworska, R. D. Rha, S. Steinhausen, A. Avagyan, A. Jaudszus, B. Ahrens, D. A. Groneberg, U. Wahn, and E. Hamelmann. 2007. Probiotic-induced suppression of allergic sensitization and airway inflammation is associated with an increase of T regulatory-dependent mechanisms in a murine model of asthma. *Clin Exp Allergy* 37 (4):498–505. doi: 10.1111/j.1365-2222.2006.02629.x.

Forsythe, P. 2011. Probiotics and lung diseases. *Chest* 139(4):901–908.

Forsythe, P., M. D. Inman, and J. Bienenstock. 2007. Oral treatment with live *Lactobacillus reuteri* inhibits the allergic airway response in mice. *Am J Respir Crit Care Med* 175 (6):561–569. doi: 10.1164/rccm.200606-821OC.

Georgiou, N. A. 2011. Pharma-nutrition interface: The gap is narrowing. *Eur J Pharmacol* 25:651(1–3):1–8.

Gibson, G. J., R. Loddenkemper, B. Lundback, and Y. Sibille. 2013. Respiratory health and disease in Europe: The new European Lung White Book. *Eur Respir J* 42 (3):559–563. doi: 10.1183/09031936.00105513.

Giovannini, M., C. Agostoni, E. Riva, F. Salvini, A. Ruscitto, G. V. Zuccotti, G. Radaelli, and Group Felicita Study. 2007. A randomized prospective double blind controlled trial on effects of long-term consumption of fermented milk containing *Lactobacillus casei* in pre-school children with allergic asthma and/or rhinitis. *Pediatr Res* 62 (2):215–220. doi: 10.1203/PDR.0b013e3180a76d94.

Gollwitzer, E. S. and B. J. Marsland. 2014. Microbiota abnormalities in inflammatory airway diseases—Potential for therapy. *Pharmacol Ther* 141 (1):32–39. doi: 10.1016/j.pharmthera.2013.08.002.

Gourbeyre, P., S. Denery, and M. Bodinier. 2011. Probiotics, prebiotics, and synbiotics: Impact on the gut immune system and allergic reactions. *J Leukoc Biol* 89 (5):685–695. doi: 10.1189/jlb.1109753.

Guarner, F. and G. J. Schaafsma. 1998. Probiotics. *Int J Food Microbiol* 39 (3):237–238.

Gutkowski, P., K. Madalinski, M. Grek, H. Dmenska, M. Syczewska, and J. Michalkiewicz. 2010. Effect of orally administered probiotic strains Lactobacillus and Bifidobacterium in children with atopic asthma. *Central Eur J Immunol* 35 (4):233–238.

Herbst, T., A. Sichelstiel, C. Schar, K. Yadava, K. Burki, J. Cahenzli, K. McCoy, B. J. Marsland, and N. L. Harris. 2011. Dysregulation of allergic airway inflammation in the absence of microbial colonization. *Am J Respir Crit Care Med* 184 (2):198–205. doi: 10.1164/rccm.201010-1574OC.

Hilty, M., C. Burke, H. Pedro, P. Cardenas, A. Bush, C. Bossley, J. Davies et al. 2010. Disordered microbial communities in asthmatic airways. *PLoS One* 5 (1):e8578. doi: 10.1371/journal.pone.0008578.

Huang, Y. J. 2013. Asthma microbiome studies and the potential for new therapeutic strategies. *Curr Allergy Asthma Rep* 13 (5):453–461. doi: 10.1007/s11882-013-0355-y.

Huang, Y. J. and S. V. Lynch. 2011. The emerging relationship between the airway microbiota and chronic respiratory disease: Clinical implications. *Expert Rev Respir Med* 5 (6):809–821. doi: 10.1586/ers.11.76.

Jang, S. O., H. J. Kim, Y. J. Kim, M. J. Kang, J. W. Kwon, J. H. Seo, H. Y. Kim, B. J. Kim, J. Yu, and S. J. Hong. 2012. Asthma prevention by *Lactobacillus rhamnosus* in a mouse model is associated with CD4(+) CD25(+)Foxp3(+) T cells. *Allergy Asthma Immunol Res* 4 (3):150–156. doi: 10.4168/aair.2012.4.3.150.

Jeurink, P. V. 2013. Mechanisms underlying immune effects of dietary oligosaccharides. *Am J Clin Nutr* 98(2):572S-577S.

Jeurink, P. V., A. Rijnierse, R. Martin, J. Garssen, and L. M. Knippels. 2012. Difficulties in describing allergic disease modulation by pre-, pro- and synbiotics. *Curr Pharm Des* 18 (16):2369–2374.

Kalliomaki, M., P. Kirjavainen, E. Eerola, P. Kero, S. Salminen, and E. Isolauri. 2001. Distinct patterns of neonatal gut microflora in infants in whom atopy was and was not developing. *J Allergy Clin Immunol* 107 (1):129–134. doi: 10.1067/mai.2001.111237.

Karimi, K., M. D. Inman, J. Bienenstock, and P. Forsythe. 2009. *Lactobacillus reuteri*-induced regulatory T cells protect against an allergic airway response in mice. *Am J Respir Crit Care Med* 179 (3):186–193. doi: 10.1164/rccm.200806-951OC.

Kim, H., K. Kwack, D. Y. Kim, and G. E. Ji. 2005. Oral probiotic bacterial administration suppressed allergic responses in an ovalbumin-induced allergy mouse model. *FEMS Immunol Med Microbiol* 45 (2):259–267. doi: 10.1016/j.femsim.2005.05.005.

Kozyrskyj, A. L., S. Bahreinian, and M. B. Azad. 2011. Early life exposures: Impact on asthma and allergic disease. *Curr Opin Allergy Clin Immunol* 11 (5):400–406. doi: 10.1097/ACI.0b013e328349b166.

Kranich, J., K. M. Maslowski, and C. R. Mackay. 2011. Commensal flora and the regulation of inflammatory and autoimmune responses. *Semin Immunol* 23 (2):139–145. doi: 10.1016/j.smim.2011.01.011.

Li, C. Y., H. C. Lin, K. C. Hsueh, S. F. Wu, and S. H. Fang. 2010. Oral administration of *Lactobacillus salivarius* inhibits the allergic airway response in mice. *Can J Microbiol* 56 (5):373–379. doi: 10.1139/w10-024.

Madan, J. C., D. C. Koestler, B. A. Stanton, L. Davidson, L. A. Moulton, M. L. Housman, J. H. Moore et al. 2012. Serial analysis of the gut and respiratory microbiome in cystic fibrosis in infancy: Interaction between intestinal and respiratory tracts and impact of nutritional exposures. *mBio* 3 (4), e00251–e00212. doi: 10.1128/mBio.00251-12.

Marri, P. R., D. A. Stern, A. L. Wright, D. Billheimer, and F. D. Martinez. 2013. Asthma-associated differences in microbial composition of induced sputum. *J Allergy Clin Immunol* 131 (2):346–352, e1–e3. doi: 10.1016/j.jaci.2012.11.013.

Marsland, B. J., K. Yadava, and L. P. Nicod. 2013. The airway microbiome and disease. *Chest* 144 (2):632–637. doi: 10.1378/chest.12-2854.

McLoughlin, R. M. and K. H. Mills. 2011. Influence of gastrointestinal commensal bacteria on the immune responses that mediate allergy and asthma. *J Allergy Clin Immunol* 127 (5):1097–1107; quiz 1108–1109. doi: 10.1016/j.jaci.2011.02.012.

Noverr, M. C. and G. B. Huffnagle. 2004. Does the microbiota regulate immune responses outside the gut? *Trends Microbiol* 12 (12):562–568. doi: 10.1016/j.tim.2004.10.008.

Ouwehand, A. C., E. Isolauri, F. He, H. Hashimoto, Y. Benno, and S. Salminen. 2001. Differences in *Bifidobacterium flora* composition in allergic and healthy infants. *J Allergy Clin Immunol* 108 (1): 144–145.

Penders, J., C. Thijs, P. A. van den Brandt, I. Kummeling, B. Snijders, F. Stelma, H. Adams, R. van Ree, and E. E. Stobberingh. 2007. Gut microbiota composition and development of atopic manifestations in infancy: The KOALA Birth Cohort Study. *Gut* 56 (5):661–667. doi: 10.1136/gut.2006.100164.

Prescott, S. and A. Nowak-Wegrzyn. 2011. Strategies to prevent or reduce allergic disease. *Ann Nutr Metab* 59 (Suppl 1):28–42. doi: 10.1159/000334150.

Quigley, E. M. 2013. Gut bacteria in health and disease. *Gastroenterol Hepatol (NY)* 9 (9):560–569.

Rijkers, G. T. 2010. Guidance for substantiating the evidence for beneficial effects of probiotics: current status and recommendations for future research. *J Nutr* 140(3):671S–676S.

Russell, S. L. and B. B. Finlay. 2012. The impact of gut microbes in allergic diseases. *Curr Opin Gastroenterol* 28 (6):563–569. doi: 10.1097/MOG.0b013e3283573017.

Sagar, S., M. E. Morgan, S. Chen, A. P. Vos, J. Garssen, J. van Bergenhenegouwen, L. Boon, N. A. Georgiou, A. D. Kraneveld, and G. Folkerts. 2014a. *Bifidobacterium breve* and *Lactobacillus rhamnosus* treatment is as effective as budesonide at reducing inflammation in a murine model for chronic asthma. *Respir Res* 15:46. doi: 10.1186/1465-9921-15-46.

Sagar, S., A. P. Vos, M. E. Morgan, J. Garssen, N. A. Georgiou, L. Boon, A. D. Kraneveld, and G. Folkerts. 2014b. The combination of *Bifidobacterium breve* with non-digestible oligosaccharides suppresses airway inflammation in a murine model for chronic asthma. *Biochim Biophys Acta* 1842 (4):573–583. doi: 10.1016/j.bbadis.2014.01.005.

Schouten, B. 2009. Cow milk allergy symptoms are reduced in mice fed dietary synbiotics during oral sensitization with whey. *J Nutr* 139(7):1398–1403.

Sze, M. A., P. A. Dimitriu, S. Hayashi, W. M. Elliott, J. E. McDonough, J. V. Gosselink, J. Cooper, D. D. Sin, W. W. Mohn, and J. C. Hogg. 2012. The lung tissue microbiome in chronic obstructive pulmonary disease. *Am J Respir Crit Care Med* 185 (10):1073–1080. doi: 10.1164/rccm.201111-2075OC.

van de Pol, M. A., R. Lutter, B. S. Smids, E. J. Weersink, and J. S. van der Zee. 2011. Synbiotics reduce allergen-induced T-helper 2 response and improve peak expiratory flow in allergic asthmatics. *Allergy* 66 (1):39–47. doi: 10.1111/j.1398-9995.2010.02454.x.

Vieira, W. A. and E. Pretorius. 2010. The impact of asthma on the gastrointestinal tract (GIT). *J Asthma Allergy* 3:123–130. doi: 10.2147/JAA.S10592.

Vos, A. P., B. C. van Esch, B. Stahl, L. M'Rabet, G. Folkerts, F. P. Nijkamp, and J. Garssen. 2007. Dietary supplementation with specific oligosaccharide mixtures decreases parameters of allergic asthma in mice. *Int Immunopharmacol* 7 (12):1582–1587. doi: 10.1016/j.intimp.2007.07.024.

Vyas, U. and N. Ranganathan. 2012. Probiotics, prebiotics, and synbiotics: Gut and beyond. *Gastroenterol Res Pract* 2012:872716. doi: 10.1155/2012/872716.

Watanabe, S., Y. Narisawa, S. Arase, H. Okamatsu, T. Ikenaga, Y. Tajiri, and M. Kumemura. 2003. Differences in fecal microflora between patients with atopic dermatitis and healthy control subjects. *J Allergy Clin Immunol* 111 (3):587–591.

Wheeler, J. G., S. J. Shema, M. L. Bogle, M. A. Shirrell, A. W. Burks, A. Pittler, and R. M. Helm. 1997. Immune and clinical impact of *Lactobacillus acidophilus* on asthma. *Ann Allergy Asthma Immunol* 79 (3):229–233. doi: 10.1016/S1081-1206(10)63007-4.

Yu, J., S. O. Jang, B. J. Kim, Y. H. Song, J. W. Kwon, M. J. Kang, W. A. Choi, H. D. Jung, and S. J. Hong. 2010. The effects of *Lactobacillus rhamnosus* on the prevention of asthma in a murine model. *Allergy Asthma Immunol Res* 2 (3):199–205. doi: 10.4168/aair.2010.2.3.199.

[illegible]

17 Pulmonary and Respiratory Health

Antioxidants and Nutraceuticals

Raj K. Keservani, Rajesh K. Kesharwani, and Anil K. Sharma

CONTENTS

17.1 INTRODUCTION

Asthma (MMWR 2007) and chronic obstructive pulmonary disease (COPD) (MMWR 2002) are significant public health burdens. Specific methods of detection, intervention, and treatment exist that may reduce this burden and promote health (Rabe et al. 2007, GOLD 2010). Asthma is a chronic inflammatory disorder of the airways characterized by episodes of reversible breathing problems due to airway narrowing and obstruction. These episodes can range in severity from mild to life threatening. Symptoms of asthma include wheezing, coughing, chest tightness, and shortness of breath. Daily preventive treatment can prevent symptoms and attacks and enable individuals who have asthma to lead active lives.

COPD is a preventable and treatable disease characterized by airflow limitation that is not fully reversible (Agusti 2001, MacNee 2001, Rennard 2002). The airflow limitation is usually progressive and associated with an abnormal inflammatory response of the lung to noxious particles or gases (typically from exposure to cigarette smoke) (GOLD 2010). Treatment can lessen symptoms and improve the quality of life for those with COPD. COPD is the fourth leading cause of death in the

United States. In 2006, approximately 120,000 individuals died from COPD, a number very close to that reported for lung cancer deaths (approximately 158,600) in the same year (CDC 2009). In nearly 8 out of 10 cases, COPD is caused by exposure to cigarette smoke. In addition, other environmental exposures (such as those in the workplace) may cause COPD. The prevalence of asthma has increased since 1980. However, deaths from asthma have decreased since the mid-1990s. The causes of asthma are an active area of research and involve both genetic and environmental factors. Risk factors for asthma currently being investigated include having a parent with asthma, sensitization to irritants and allergens, respiratory infections in childhood, and overweight. Asthma affects people of every race, sex, and age. However, significant disparities in asthma morbidity and mortality exist, particularly for low-income and minority populations. Populations with higher rates of asthma include children, women (among adults), and boys (among children), African Americans, Puerto Ricans, people living in the Northeast United States, people living below the federal poverty level, and employees with certain exposures in the workplace. While there is not a cure for asthma yet, there are diagnoses and treatment guidelines that are aimed at ensuring that all people with asthma live full and active lives (NHLBI 2007).

An antioxidant is a molecule that inhibits the oxidation of other molecules. Oxidation is a chemical reaction that transfers electrons or hydrogen from a substance to an oxidizing agent. Oxidation reactions can produce free radicals. Stable atoms have an even number of electrons orbiting in pairs at successive distances (called *shells* or *rings*) from the nucleus. When a stable atom loses an electron during oxidation, it is left with an odd number of electrons in its outermost shell. In other words, it now has an *unpaired electron*. In most exchange reactions, two atoms with unpaired electrons immediately pair up, making newly stabilized molecules, but in rare cases, atoms with unpaired electrons in their outermost shell remain unpaired. Such atoms are highly unstable and are called free radicals. Free radical is a highly unstable atom with an unpaired electron in its outermost shell (Yeomans et al. 2005). When an oxygen molecule becomes a free radical, it is specifically referred to as a reactive oxygen species (ROS). In turn, these radicals can start chain reactions. When the chain reaction occurs in a cell, it can cause damage or death to the cell. Antioxidants terminate these chain reactions by removing free radical intermediates and inhibit other oxidation reactions. They do this by being oxidized themselves, so antioxidants are often reducing agents such as thiols, ascorbic acid, or polyphenols (Helmut 1997). Although oxidation reactions are crucial for life, they can also be damaging; plants and animals maintain complex systems of multiple types of antioxidants, such as glutathione, vitamin C, vitamin A, and vitamin E, as well as enzymes such as catalase, superoxide dismutase, and various peroxidases. The use of antioxidants in pharmacology is intensively studied, particularly as treatments for stroke and neurodegenerative diseases. Antioxidants are widely used in dietary supplements and have been investigated for the prevention of diseases such as cancer, coronary heart disease, and even altitude sickness (Baillie et al. 2009). Antioxidants (Keservani et al. 2010b) also have many industrial uses, such as preservatives in food and cosmetics and can prevent the degradation of rubber and gasoline (Dabelstein et al. 2007).

Nutraceutical is hybrid of "nutrition" and "pharmaceutical," was coined in 1989 by Stephen L. DeFelice, founder and chairman of the Foundation of Innovation Medicine (Kalra 2003), and defined as "Food, or parts of food, that provide medical or health benefits, including the prevention and treatment of disease" (Keservani et al. 2010a). There are many functional foods and nutraceuticals that are becoming increasingly available in the marketplace, but there is a challenge for the functional food producers because such products should address the issue of sensory acceptability that is not necessary for the nutraceutical or pharmaceutical products (Shahidi 2012). Functional, health-enhancing foods, or nutraceuticals (Figure 17.1) are food-type products that influence specific physiological functions in the body. This function provides benefits to health, well-being, or performance beyond regular nutrition, and products of this nature are marketed and consumed for these value-added properties (Kasbia 2005).

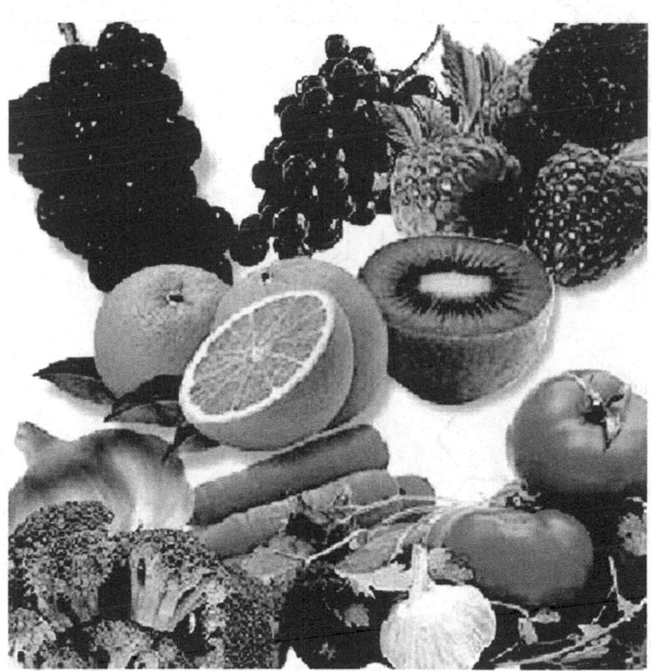

FIGURE 17.1 Nutraceuticals used in the prevention of pulmonary and respiratory disease.

17.2 ANTIOXIDANTS AND NUTRACEUTICALS IN PULMONARY AND RESPIRATORY HEALTH

The human body is provided with a variety of antioxidants that help to counterbalance the influence of oxidants. For all practical objectives, these may be divided into two classes, viz. enzymatic (Table 17.1) and nonenzymatic (Table 17.2). Nutraceuticals used in the prevention of pulmonary and respiratory diseases are briefly discussed in Tables 17.1 and 17.2.

TABLE 17.1
Antioxidant Defense for Enzymatic Scavenger

Name of Scavenger	Acronym	Catalyzed Reaction
Superoxide dismutase	SOD	$M^{(n+1)+}$-SOD+ O_2^- → M^{n+}-SOD + O_2
		M^{n+}-SOD+ O_2^- + $2H^+$ → $M^{(n+1)+}$-SOD + H_2O_2
Catalase	CAT	$2H_2O_2$ → O_2 + $2H_2O$
		H_2O_2 + Fe(III)-E → H_2O + O = Fe(IV)-E(·+)
		H_2O_2 + O = Fe(IV)-E(·+) → H_2O + Fe(III)-E + O_2
Glutathione peroxidase	GTPs	2GSH + H_2O_2 → GSSG + $2H_2O$
		2GSH + ROOH → GSSG + ROH + H_2O
Thioredoxin	TRX	Adenosine monophosphate + sulfite + thioredoxin disulfide = 5′-adenyly + sulfate + thioredoxin
		Adenosine 3′,5′-bisphosphate + sulfite + thioredoxin disulfide = 3′-phosphoadenylyl sulfate + thioredoxin
Peroxiredoxin	PRX	2R′-SH + ROOH = R′-S-S-R′ + H_2O + ROH
Glutathione transferase	GST	RX + GSH = HX + R-S-GSH

TABLE 17.2
Antioxidant Defense for Nonenzymatic Scavenger

Chemical Name of Scavenger	Name of Scavenger	Structure
All trans retinol 2	Vitamin A	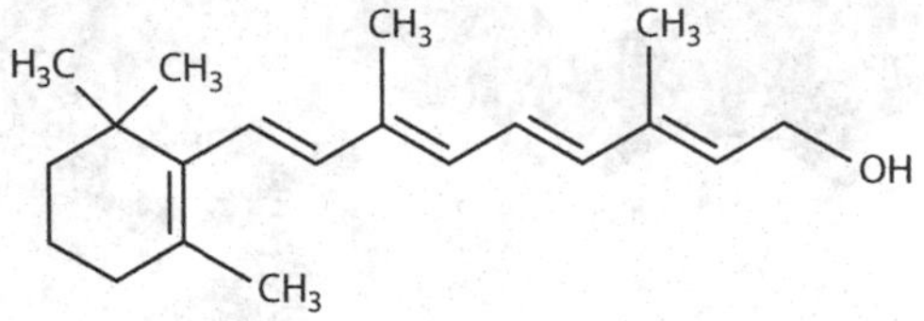
Ascorbic acid	Vitamin C	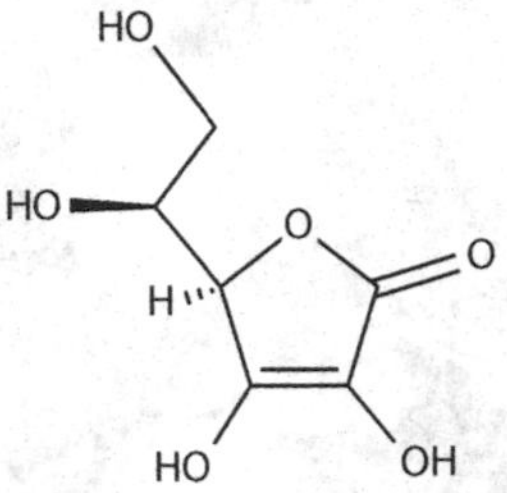
α-Tocopherol	Vitamin E	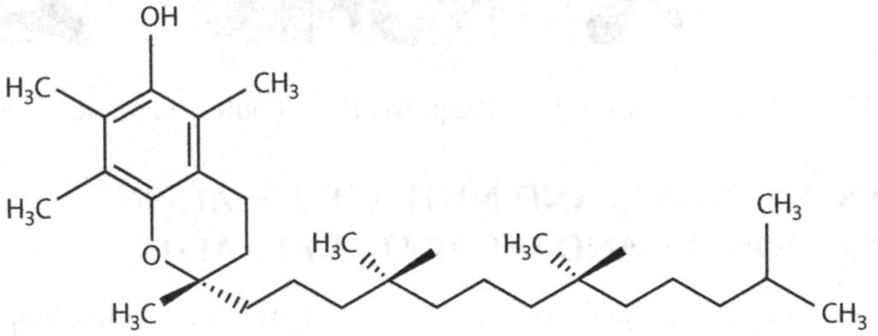
β-Carotene		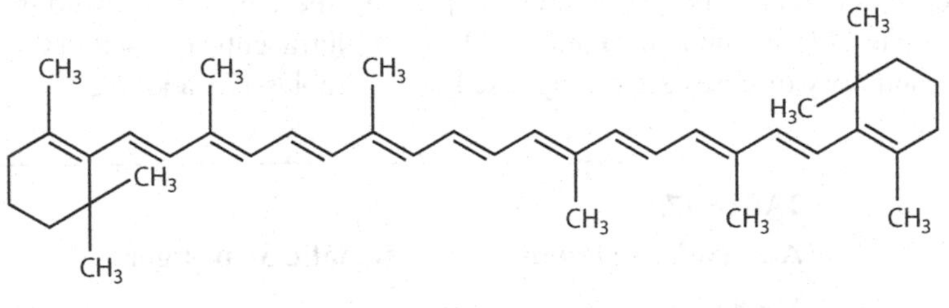
Glutathione		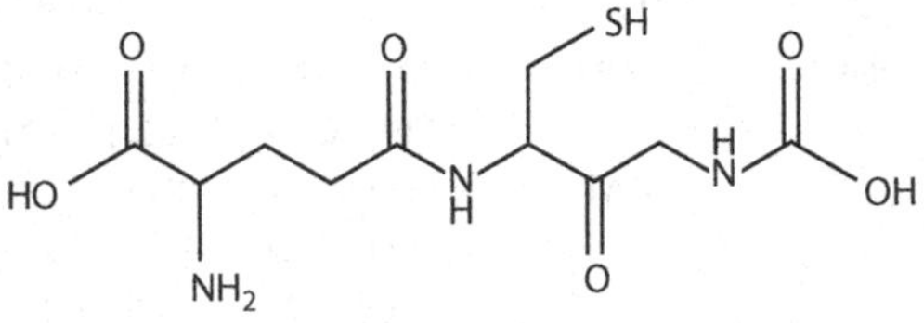

17.2.1 Enzymatic Antioxidants

The main enzymatic antioxidants of the pulmonary setup are superoxide dismutases (SODs) (EC 1.15.1.11), catalase (EC 1.11.1.6), and glutathione peroxidase (GSH-Px) (EC 1.11.1.9). Besides these major enzymes, other antioxidants, including heme oxygenase-1 (EC 1.14.99.3), and redox proteins, such as thioredoxins (TRXs, EC 1.8.4.10), peroxiredoxins (PRXs, EC 1.11.1.15), and glutaredoxins have also been observed significantly in the pulmonary antioxidant protection. Since superoxide is the prime ROS manufactured from different sources, its dismutation by SOD is of paramount importance for every cell. All three types of SOD, that is CuZn-SOD, Mn-SOD, and extracellular-SOD (EC-SOD), are broadly expressed in the human lung. Mn-SOD is localized within the mitochondrial matrix. EC-SOD is essentially localized in the extracellular matrix, particularly in zones containing high amounts of type I collagen fibers and surrounding pulmonary and systemic vessels. It has also been identified in the bronchial epithelium, alveolar epithelium, and alveolar macrophages (Kinnula 2005, Kinnula and Crapo 2003). The relatively high EC-SOD concentration in the lung with its specific binding to the extracellular matrix components may suggest a fundamental portion of lung matrix defense (Zelko et al. 2002).

H_2O_2 that is produced by the action of SODs or the action of oxidases, such as xanthine oxidase, is reduced to water by catalase and the GSH-Px. Catalase exists as a tetramer composed of four identical monomers, each of which contains a heme group at the active site. Degradation of H_2O_2 is accomplished via the conversion between two conformations of catalase–ferricatalase (iron coordinated to water) and compound I (iron complexed with an oxygen atom). Catalase also binds NADPH as a reducing equivalent to prevent oxidative inactivation of the enzyme (formation of compound II) by H_2O_2 as it is reduced to water (Kirkman et al. 1999). Enzymes in the redox cycle responsible for the reduction of H_2O_2 and lipid hydroperoxides (generated as a result of membrane lipid peroxidation) include the GSH-Pxs (Flohe 2000). The GSH-Pxs are a family of tetrameric enzymes that contain the unique amino acid selenocysteine within the active sites and use low-molecular-weight thiols, such as GSH, to reduce H_2O_2 and lipid peroxides to their corresponding alcohols. Four GSH-Pxs have been described, encoded by different genes: GSH-Px-1 (cellular GSH-Px) is ubiquitous and reduces H_2O_2 and fatty acid peroxides, but not esterified peroxyl lipids (Arthur 2000). Esterified lipids are reduced by membrane-bound GSH-Px-4 (phospholipid hydroperoxide GSH-Px), which may utilize many different low-molecular-weight thiols as reducing equivalents. GSH-Px-2 (gastrointestinal GSH-Px) is localized in gastrointestinal epithelial cells where it works to reduce dietary peroxides (Chu et al. 1993). GSH-Px-3 (extracellular GSH-Px) is the sole member of the GSH-Px family that dwells in the extracellular compartment and is trusted to be one of the most significant extracellular antioxidant enzymes in mammals. Of these, extracellular GSH-Px is most broadly studied in the human lung (Comhair et al. 2001).

Also, disposal of H_2O_2 is keenly linked with many thiol-containing enzymes, namely TRXs (TRX1 and TRX2), thioredoxin reductases (EC 1.8.1.9) (TRRs), PRXs (which are thioredoxin peroxidases), and glutaredoxins (Gromer et al. 2004). Two TRXs and TRRs have been authenticated in human cells, existing in cytosol as well as mitochondria. In the lung, TRX and TRR are expressed in bronchial and alveolar epithelium and macrophages. Six different PRXs have been seen in human cells, varying in their ultrastructural compartmentalization. Experimental investigations have revealed the significance of PRX VI in the shielding of alveolar epithelium. Human lung expresses all PRXs in bronchial epithelium, alveolar epithelium, and macrophages (Kinnula et al. 2002). PRX V has recently been observed to function as a peroxynitrite reductase (Dubuisson et al. 2004), which means that it may function as a potential defense yielding compound in the development of ROS-mediated lung injury (Holmgren 2000).

Common to these antioxidants is the need of NADPH as a reducing equivalent. NADPH keeps catalase in the active form and is utilized as a cofactor by TRX and GSH reductase (EC 1.6.4.2), which transforms GSSG to GSH, a co-substrate for the GSH-Pxs. Intracellular NADPH, in exchange, is produced by the reduction of NADP1 by glucose-6-phosphate dehydrogenase, the first and rate-limiting enzyme of the pentose phosphate pathway, during the conversion of glucose-6-phosphate to 6-phosphogluconolactone. By producing NADPH, glucose-6-phosphate dehydrogenase is a crucial determinant of cytosolic GSH buffering ability (GSH/GSSG) and, hence, can be considered an essential, regulatory antioxidant enzyme (Dickinson and Forman 1999, Sies 1999).

Glutathione-S-transferases (GSTs) (EC 2.5.1.18), other antioxidant enzyme class, inactivate secondary metabolites, viz. unsaturated aldehydes, epoxides, and hydroperoxides. Three main categories of GSTs have been explained: cytosolic GST, mitochondrial GST (Ladner et al. 2004, Robinson et al. 2004), and membrane-associated microsomal GST that plays a role in eicosanoid and GSH metabolism (Jakobsson et al. 1999). Seven families of cytosolic GST are located in mammalian, designated alpha, mu, pi, sigma, theta, omega, and zeta (Hayes and Pulford 1995, Hayes and McLellan 1999, Armstrong 1997, Sheehan et al. 2001). During stress-free circumstances, class Mu and Pi GSTs interact with kinases Ask1 and JNK, respectively, and inhibit these kinases (Adler et al. 1999, Cho et al. 2001, Dorion et al. 2002). It has been exhibited that GSTP1 dissociates from JNK in reply to oxidative stress (Adler et al. 1999). GSTP1 too physically interacts with PRX VI and causes the recovery of PRX enzyme activity via glutathionylation of the oxidized protein (Manevich et al. 2004).

17.2.2 Nonenzymatic Antioxidants

Nonenzymatic antioxidants cover low-molecular-weight substances, like vitamins (vitamins C and E), β-carotene, uric acid, and glutathione (GSH), a tripeptide (L-g-glutamyl-L-cysteinyl-glycine) that has a thiol (sulfhydryl) group. Dietary antioxidants supplementation is one of the simplest approaches to boost antioxidant defense systems. Supplementation of vitamin C, vitamin E, and β-carotene has been attempted in cigarette smokers and patients with COPD (Allard et al. 1994, Cross et al. 1994, Rautalahti et al. 1997, Steinberg and Chait 1998, Aghdassi et al. 1999, Habib et al. 1999, Lykkesfeldt et al. 2000).

17.2.2.1 Vitamin C (Ascorbic Acid)

Water-soluble vitamin C (ascorbic acid) provides intracellular and extracellular aqueous-phase antioxidant capacity primarily by scavenging oxygen free radicals. It converts vitamin E free radicals back to vitamin E. Its plasma levels have been shown to decrease with age (Bunker 1992, Mezzetti et al. 1996). All fruits and vegetables contain some amount of vitamin C. Fruits with the highest sources of vitamin C include cantaloupe, citrus fruits, and juices, such as orange and grapefruit, kiwi fruit, mango, papaya, pineapple, strawberries, raspberries, blueberries, cranberries, and watermelon. Vegetables with the highest sources of vitamin C include broccoli, Brussels sprouts, cauliflower, green and red peppers, spinach, cabbage, turnip greens, and other leafy greens, sweet and white potatoes, tomatoes and tomato juice, and winter squash. Some cereals and other foods and beverages are fortified with vitamin C. Fortified means a vitamin or mineral has been added to the food (Douglas et al. 2007, Sarubin and Thomson 2007, Escott-Stump 2008).

17.2.2.2 Vitamin E (α-Tocopherol)

Lipid-soluble vitamin E is concentrated in the hydrophobic interior site of cell membrane and is the major defense versus oxidant-induced membrane damage. Vitamin E donates electron to peroxyl radical, which is generated during lipid peroxidation. α-Tocopherol is the most active form of vitamin E and the main membrane-bound antioxidant in cell. Vitamin E kicks off apoptosis of cancer cells and prevents free radical productions (White et al. 1997). The best way to get the daily requirement of vitamin E is by eating food sources. Vitamin E is found in the following foods: vegetable oils (such as wheat germ, sunflower, safflower, corn, and soybean oils), nuts (such as almonds, peanuts, and hazelnuts/filberts), seeds (such as sunflower seeds), green leafy vegetables (such as spinach and broccoli), fortified breakfast cereals, fruit juices, margarine, and spreads. Fortified means that vitamins have been added to the food. Check the Nutrition Fact Panel on the food label. Products made from these foods, such as margarine, also contain vitamin E (Douglas et al. 2007, Sarubin and Thomson 2007).

17.2.2.3 Glutathione

GSH is profoundly present in all cell compartments and is the principal soluble antioxidant. GSH/GSSG ratio is a key determinant of oxidative stress. GSH exhibits its antioxidant effects in different manners (Masella et al. 2005). It detoxifies hydrogen peroxide and lipid peroxides via the activity of GSH-Px. GSH donates its electron to H_2O_2 to reduce it into H_2O and O_2. GSSG is again reduced into GSH by GSH reductase that utilizes NAD(P)H as the electron donor. GSH-Pxs are important for the defense of cell membrane from lipid peroxidation too. Reduced glutathione donates protons to membrane lipids and shields them from oxidant stress (Curello et al. 1985). GSH is a cofactor for a variety of detoxifying enzymes like GSH-Px and transferase. It has a part to play in converting vitamins C and E back to their active types. GSH defenses cells to combat apoptosis by interacting with proapoptotic and antiapoptotic signaling pathways (Masella et al. 2005). It also controls and activates various transcription factors, such as AP-1, NF-κB, and Sp-1.

17.2.2.4 Carotenoids (β-Carotene)

Fruits and vegetables that are red, orange, yellow, and deep green are generally high in β-carotene and other carotenoids such as lutein and lycopene. Tomatoes, carrots, cantaloupe, sweet potatoes, apricots, leafy greens such as kale and spinach, and pumpkin are good sources of β-carotene (Figure 17.2). Eating the recommended amounts of fruits and vegetables each day ensures an adequate intake of β-carotene and other carotenoids. Because of its color, β-carotene issued as a natural coloring agent for many foods, including margarine, yellow cheddar cheese, cereal, cake mixes, gelatins, and soft drinks (USDA 2004). Carotenoids are pigments occurring in plants. At first, β-carotene has been shown to react with peroxyl (ROO), hydroxyl (OH), and superoxide (O_2^-) radicals (El-Agamey et al. 2004). Carotenoids exhibit their antioxidant effects in lower oxygen partial pressure; however, they may have pro-oxidant effects at higher oxygen levels (Rice-Evans et al. 1997). Both carotenoids and retinoic acids are able of controlling transcription factors (Niles 2004). β-Carotene inhibits the oxidant-induced NF-κB activation and interleukin (IL)-6 and tumor necrosis factor-a production. Carotenoids influence the apoptosis of cells too. Antiproliferative effects of RA have been observed in many studies. This impact of RA is channeled principally by retinoic acid receptors and differs among cell types. In mammary carcinoma cells, retinoic acid receptor was found to kick off growth inhibition by inducing cell cycle arrest, apoptosis, or both (Donato and Noy 2005, Niizuma et al. 2006).

Concentrations of these nonenzymatic antioxidants vary in the lungs. Glutathione is more concentrated in epithelial lining fluid compared to plasma (Van der Vliet et al. 1999) and others, such as albumin, are found in high concentrations in serum, but at much lower concentrations in the epithelial lining fluid (Reynolds and Newball 1974).

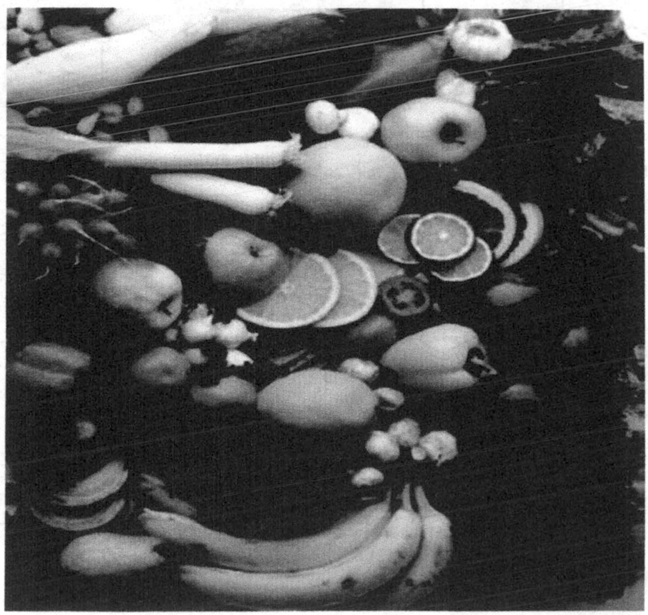

FIGURE 17.2 High food source of carotenoids.

17.2.2.5 Lycopene

Lycopene is a carotenoid (a natural pigment made by plants). Lycopene protects plants from stress and helps them use the energy of the sun to make nutrients. Lycopene is found in fruits and vegetables like tomatoes, apricots, guavas, and watermelons.

The main source of lycopene in the American diet is tomato-based products. Lycopene is more bioavailable (easier for the body to use) in processed tomato products like tomato paste and tomato puree than in raw tomatoes. Lycopene may be consumed in the diet or taken in dietary supplements. Lycopene (Figure 17.3) in the diet may affect antioxidant activity and communication between cells. Lycopene is available in the United States in food products and dietary supplements because dietary supplements are regulated as foods, not as drugs (Li et al. 1997, Rao and Agarwal 1999, PCNDS 2014).

17.2.2.6 Tannins

Tannins (commonly referred to as tannic acid) are water-soluble polyphenols that are present in many plant foods. They have been reported to be responsible for decreases in feed intake, growth rate, feed efficiency, net metabolizable energy, and protein digestibility in experimental animals. Therefore, foods rich in tannins are considered to be of low nutritional value. However, recent findings indicate that the major effect of tannins was not due to their inhibition on food consumption or digestion but rather the decreased efficiency in converting the absorbed nutrients to new body substances (Chung et al. 1998). The antioxidant property of tannins (Figure 17.4) is important in protecting cellular oxidative damage, including lipid peroxidation. The generation of superoxide radicals was reported to be inhibited by tannins and related compounds. Black tea contains chemicals called tannins (Leigh 2000).

17.2.2.7 Catechins

Catechin is a flavan-3-ol, a type of natural phenol and antioxidant. It is a plant secondary metabolite. It belongs to the group of flavan-3-ols (or simply flavanols), part of the chemical family of flavonoids. The name of the catechin chemical family derives from catechu, which is the tannic juice or boiled extract of *Mimosa catechu* (Acaciacatechu L.f) (Zheng et al. 2008).

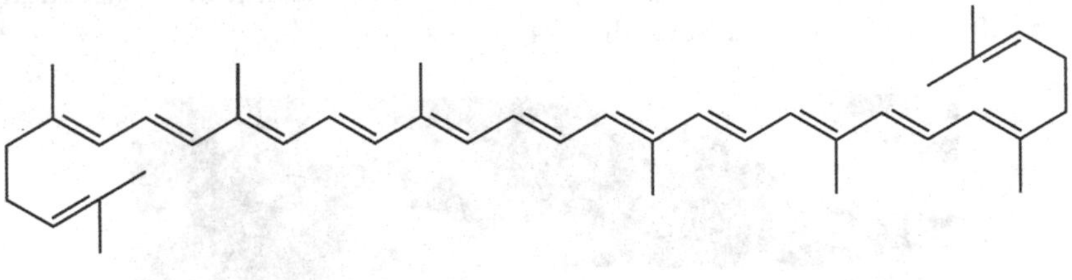

FIGURE 17.3 Structure of lycopene.

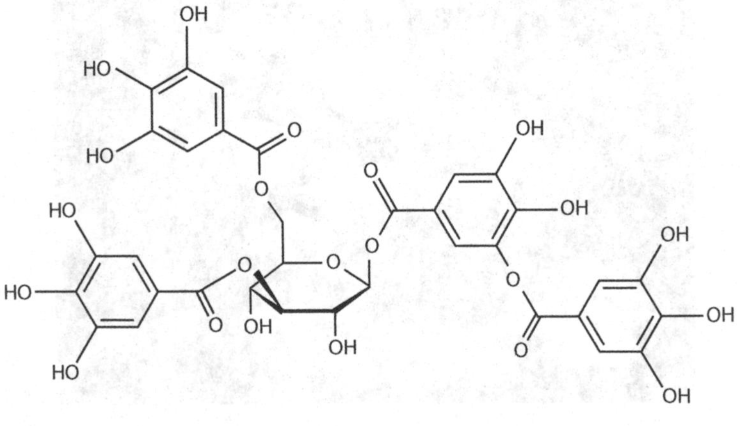

FIGURE 17.4 Structure of tannic acid.

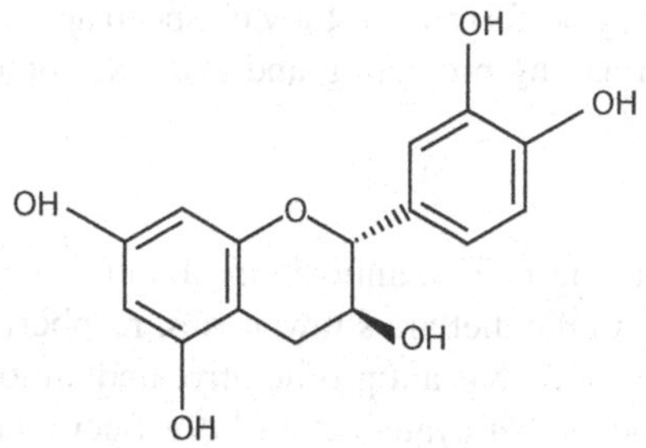

FIGURE 17.5 Structure of catechin.

Catechins and epicatechins are found in cocoa (Kwik-Uribe and Bektash 2008), which, according to one database, has the highest content (108 mg/100 g) of catechins among foods analyzed, followed by prune juice (25 mg/100 mL) and broad bean pod (16 mg/100 g). Açaí oil, obtained from the fruit of the açai palm (*Euterpe oleracea*), contains (+)-catechins (67 mg/kg) (Pacheco-Palencia et al. 2008). (–)-Epicatechin and (+)-catechin are among the main natural phenols in argan oil (Charrouf and Guillaume 2007). Catechins (Figure 17.5) are diverse among foods, from peaches (Cheng and Crisosto 1995) to green tea and vinegar (Galvez et al. 1994). Catechins are found in barley grain where they are the main phenolic compound responsible for dough discoloration (Zory and Byung-Kee 2006). Catechin inhibits the oxidation of low-density lipoprotein (Mangiapane et al. 1992). Catechin has been found to outperform vitamin C and β-carotene 10 times in scavenging the alkyl peroxyl radical. One study found green tea polyphenols to be more potent antioxidants than vitamin C, vitamin E, rosemary extract, and even curcumin in some systems (Green Tea, White Tea, 2014).

17.2.2.8 Luteolin

Luteolin is a flavone, a type of flavonoid. Like all flavonoids, it has a yellow crystalline appearance. Luteolin can be found in *Terminalia chebula*. It is most often found in leaves, but it is also seen in rinds, barks, clover blossom, and ragweed pollen. It has also been isolated from the aromatic flowering plant, *Salvia tomentosa* in mint family *Lamiaceae* (Ulubelen et al. 1979). Dietary sources include celery, broccoli, green pepper, parsley, thyme, dandelion, perilla, chamomile tea, carrots, olive oil, peppermint, rosemary, navel oranges, and oregano (Kayoko et al. 1998, Lopez-Lazaro 2009).) It can also be found in the seeds of the palm *Aiphanes aculeata* (Lee et al. 2001). Many luteolin-containing plants ((Figure 17.6) possess antioxidant properties. The antioxidant activity of luteolin and its glycosides has been associated with their capacity to scavange reactive oxygen and nitrogen species. The antioxidant activity of luteolin has been observed not only in vitro but also in vivo (Lopez-Lazaro 2009).

In the observation of luteolin, kaempferol, and apigenin and its binding to calf thymus (ct)-DNA found that in the cell culture medium. Luteolin, followed by apigenin and kaempferol, was shown to be the most effective in protecting DNA from oxidative damage induced by hydrogen peroxide,

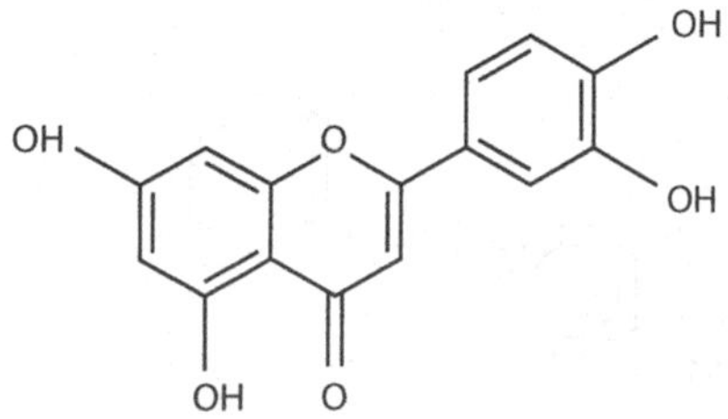

FIGURE 17.6 Structure of luteolin.

according to Rusak et al. (2010) by performing a study on spectrophotometric analysis of flavonoid–DNA interactions and DNA damaging/protecting and cytotoxic potential of flavonoids in human peripheral blood lymphocytes.

17.2.2.9 Ellagic Acid

Ellagic acid is a naturally occurring phenol antioxidant found in numerous fruits and vegetables. The best sources of ellagic acid in the diet are strawberries, raspberries, blackberries, and walnuts (ACS 2008). Ellagic acid (Figure 17.7) has antiproliferative and antioxidant properties in a number of in vitro and small animal models (Narayanan et al. 1999, Seerama et al. 2005). Like other polyphenol antioxidants, ellagic acid has also a chemoprotective effect in cellular models by reducing oxidative stress (Vattem and Shetty 2005).

17.2.2.10 Gingerol

Gingerol (Figure 17.8), or sometimes [6]-gingerol, is the active constituent of fresh ginger and variety of other plants. Chemically, gingerol is a relative of capsaicin and piperine, the compounds that give chilli peppers and black pepper their respective spiciness (McGee 2004). It is normally found as a pungent yellow oil, but also can form a low-melting crystalline solid.

In the investigation of the effectiveness of chemical constituents of *Zingiber officinale* Rosc. (Zingiberaceae) in treating oxidative stress found that compounds [6]-gingerol, [8]-gingerol, [10]-gingerol, and [6]-shogaol of the herb scavenges of 1,1-diphenyl-2-picyrlhydrazyl (DPPH), superoxide and hydroxyl radicals (Dugasani et al. 2010), inhibits of *N*-formyl-methionyl-leucyl-phenylalanine (f-MLP) induced reactive oxygen species (ROS) production in human polymorphonuclear neutrophils (PMN), lipopolysaccharide induced nitrite and prostaglandin E(2) production in RAW 264.7 cells, according to the study of "Comparative antioxidant and anti-inflammatory effects of [6]-gingerol, [8]-gingerol, [10]-gingerol and [6]-shogaol" by Dugasani et al. In the evaluation of [6]-shogaol, [6]-gingerol, [8]-gingerol, and [10]-gingerol of gingerol and its human bronchial smooth muscle cells (BSMC) effects found that they suppress phthalate ester-mediated airway remodeling by depleting both IL-8 and RANTES completely reversed the effect of DBP-BEAS-2B-CM and DBP-HBE-CM-mediated BSMC proliferation and migration, according to "Ginger suppresses phthalate ester-induced airway remodeling" by Kuo et al.

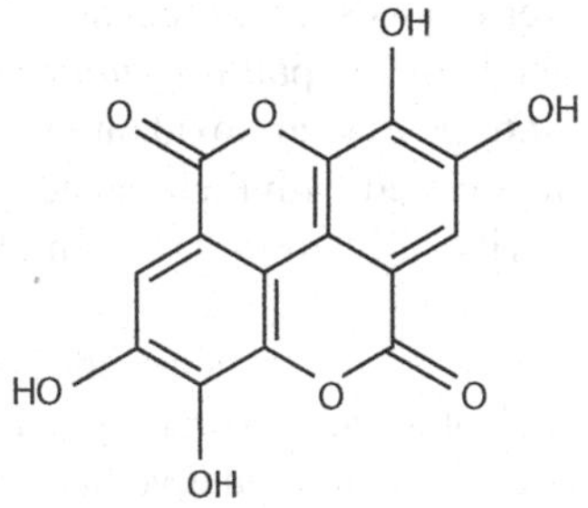

FIGURE 17.7 Structure of ellagic acid.

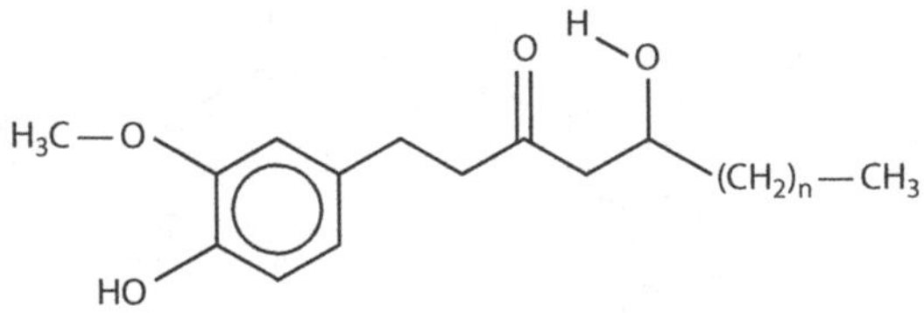

FIGURE 17.8 Structure of gingerol.

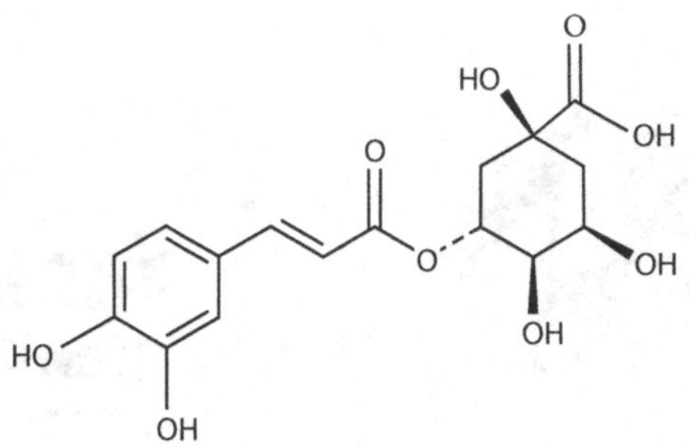

FIGURE 17.9 Structure of chlorogenic acid.

17.2.2.11 Chlorogenic Acid

Chlorogenic acid (CGA) is a natural chemical compound that is the ester of caffeic acid and (−)-quinic acid. It is an important biosynthetic intermediate (Boerjan et al. 2003). Chlorogenic acid is an important intermediate in lignin biosynthesis. This compound, known as an antioxidant, may also slow the release of glucose into the bloodstream after a meal (Johnston et al. 2003). Chlorogenic acid (Figure 17.9) is marketed under the trade name Svetol, a standardized green coffee extract, as a food additive used in coffee products, chewing gum, and mints, and also as a stand-alone product. Chlorogenic acid is reported to be a chemical sensitizer responsible for human respiratory allergy to certain types of plant materials (Freedman et al. 1964).

17.3 THERAPEUTIC INTERVENTION WITH ANTIOXIDANTS

Oxidative stress is implicitly involved with the pathogenesis of chronic airway diseases. A rational approach for the treatment of COPD would therefore consider antioxidant intervention not only to neutralize the increased oxidative stress and the subsequent inflammatory response, but also to identify the source of oxidants and overwhelm their generation. This can be achieved through two approaches, either by increasing the endogenous antioxidant enzyme defenses or by enhancing the nonenzymatic defenses through dietary or pharmacological means. Several small molecular weight compounds that target oxidant signaling or quench cigarette smoke-derived oxidants and reactive aldehydes are currently being tested clinically (Rahman and MacNee 2000a). Antioxidant agents, such as thiol donors and analogues (GSH and mucolytic drugs, such as *N*-acetyl-L-cysteine, nacystelyn, erdosteine, and carbocysteine lysine salt), dietary polyphenols and flavonoids (curcumin, green tea, resveratrol, quercetin [Figure 17.10]) (Keservani and Sharma 2014), all have been reported to scavenge/detoxify free radicals/oxidants, increase intracellular thiol levels, and control NF-κB activation and consequently inhibit inflammatory gene expression. Flavonoids are potent scavengers of free radicals in vitro (Keservani and Sharma 2014). Faruk et al. (2010) studied and reported the usefulness of antioxidants drugs in bronchial asthma.

Antioxidant vitamins (C, E, retinol, and carotenoids) not only improve the pulmonary function of COPD patients but also support the hypothesis that antioxidant vitamins may play an important role in respiratory health (Schunemann et al. 2001).

17.4 POLYPHENOLS AS ANTIOXIDANT

Several epidemiological studies have established a beneficial link between polyphenol intake and reduced risk of disease, which were attributed to both the antioxidant and anti-inflammatory properties of polyphenols (Arts and Hollman 2005). In one Finnish study with over 10,000 participants, a significant inverse correlation was observed between polyphenol intake and the incidence of

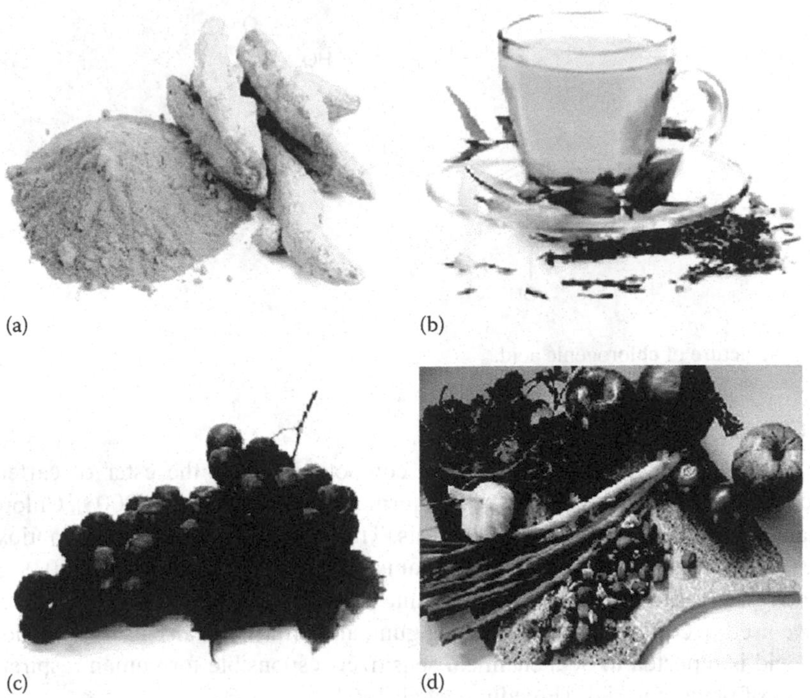

FIGURE 17.10 Flavonoid source with antioxidants potentials used in the prevention of pulmonary and respiratory disease: (a) curcumin, (b) green tea, (c) resveratrol, and (d) quercetin.

asthma (Knekt et al. 2002). Similar beneficial associations were also observed for COPD in a study encompassing over 13,000 adults. This study reported that increased polyphenols, such as catechin (e.g. green tea polyphenols, and epigallocatechin gallate), flavonol (e.g. quercetin and kaempferol), and flavone (such as apigenin and luteolin) intake correlated with improved symptoms, as assessed by cough, phlegm production, and breathlessness and improved lung function as measured by FEV1 (Tabak et al. 2001). Flavonol and flavone intake was independently associated with chronic cough only.

One study showed a beneficial protective effect against COPD symptoms after increased intake of fruits high in polyphenol and vitamin E content (Walda et al. 2002). Recently, researchers found that a standardized polyphenol extract administered orally was shown to be effective in reducing oxidant stress and increasing PaO_2 as well as improvements in FEV1 between enrolment and the end of the study (Santus et al. 2005).

Other studies have demonstrated a direct impact of specific polyphenolic compounds on inflammation in vitro and in vivo. For example the flavonoid resveratrol, a constituent of red wine, inhibits inflammatory cytokine release from macrophages isolated from COPD patients (Culpitt et al. 2003). Birrel et al. (2005) have confirmed this effect of resveratrol in rat lungs challenged with LPS. Furthermore, in both monocytic U937 cells and alveolar epithelial A549 cells, resveratrol inhibits NF-κB and AP-1 activation (Manna et al. 2000, Donnelly et al. 2004).

Another well-studied polyphenol is curcumin. It is the active constituent of *Curcuma longa*, commonly known as turmeric. Like resveratrol, it has also been reported to inhibit NF-κB activation, along with IL-8 release, cyclooxygenase-2 expression, and neutrophil recruitment in the lungs (Biswas et al. 2005). Leaf of *Kalanchoe integra* contains flavonoids (quercetin) and tannins that have been found to have beneficial effects in the management of bronchial asthma (Park et al. 2009, Joskova et al. 2011, Fortunato et al. 2012, Aseidu-Gyekye et al. 2013).

17.5 OTHER PLANT-DERIVED NUTRACEUTICALS USED IN THE PREVENTION OF PULMONARY AND RESPIRATORY DISEASE

Plant-derived medicines in recent time have immensely contributed to the management of disease conditions in humans (Pandey et al. 2011). *K. integra* (syn. *Kalanchoe spanthulata*, *Bryophyllum pinnata*) (Dymock et al. 1890, Dokosi 1998) is an emerging plant of interest of multipurpose use. Boiled leaf extracts are useful in the management of acute and chronic bronchitis, pneumonia, bronchial asthma, and palpitation (Cruz et al. 2008, Biswas et al. 2011, Ghasi et al. 2011).

17.6 CONCLUSIONS

There is now considerable evidence of increased oxidative stress in COPD, which is pivotal in the pathogenesis and progression of the disease. Several small molecule compounds under clinical trials have either targeted component(s) of oxidant signaling or quench oxidants derived from cigarette smoke. Antioxidant and/or anti-inflammatory agents such as thiol molecules/donors, spin traps, dietary polyphenols, and inhibitors of oxidative stress-induced signaling pathways present potential means by which to treat this element of COPD. Antioxidant defense biomarkers constitute the first step in search for a healthy body status. Antioxidants and antioxidant vitamins improve lung function and respiratory health lending overwhelming support for antioxidant supplementation in COPD. Finally, it is concluded that flavonoids, large numbers of antioxidants like vitamin C, glutathione, carotenoids, etc., and nutraceutical antioxidants such as lycopene, gingerol, chlorogenic acid, etc., play an important role in the prevention of pulmonary and respiratory disease and maintained health pulmonary and respiratory health.

REFERENCES

Adler, V. et al., 1999. Regulation of JNK signalling by GSTp. *EMBO J.* 18:1321–1334.

Aghdassi, E. et al., 1999. Oxidative stress in smokers supplemented with vitamin C. *Int J Vitam Nutr Res.* 69:45–51.

Agusti, A.G., 2001. Systemic effects of chronic obstructive pulmonary disease. *Novartis Found Symp.* 234:242–254.

Allard, J.P. et al., 1994. Critical assessment of body-composition measurements in malnourished subjects with Crohn's disease: The role of bioelectric impedance analysis. *Am J Clin Nutr.* 59:884–890.

Armstrong, R.N., 1997. Structure, catalytic mechanism, and evolution of the glutathione transferases. *Chem Res Toxicol.* 10:2–18.

Arthur, J.R., 2000. The glutathione peroxidases. *Cell Mol Life Sci.* 57:1825–1835.

Arts, I.C., P.C. Hollman., 2005. Polyphenols and disease risk in epidemiologic studies. *Am J Clin Nutr.* 81 (1 Suppl):317S–325S.

Asiedu-Gyekye, I.J. et al., 2013. Comparative study of two *kalanchoe* species: Total flavonoid, phenolic contents and antioxidant properties. *Afr J Pure Appl Chem.* 6:65–73.

Baillie, J.K., A.A.R. Thompson, J.B. Irving, M.G.D. Bates, A.I. Sutherland, W. MacNee, S.R.J. Maxwell, D.J. Webb, 2009. Oral antioxidant supplementation does not prevent acute mountain sickness: Double blind, randomized placebo-controlled trial. *QJM.* 102 (5):341–348.

Birrell, M.A. et al., 2005. Resveratrol, an extract of red wine, inhibits lipopolysaccharide induced airway neutrophilia and inflammatory mediators through an NF-kappaB-independent mechanism. *FASEB J.* 19 (7):840–841.

Biswas, S.K. et al., 2005. Curcumin induces glutathione biosynthesis and inhibits NF-kappaB activation and interleukin-8 release in alveolar epithelial cells: Mechanism of free radical scavenging activity. *Antioxid Redox Signal.* 7 (1–2):32–41.

Biswas, S.K., A. Chowdhury, J. Das, S.Z. Hosen, R. Uddin, M.S. Rahaman 2011. Literature review on pharmacological potentials of *Kalanchoe pinnata* (Crassulaceae). *Afr J Pharm Pharmacol.* 5:1258–1262.

Boerjan, W., J. Ralph, M. Baucher, 2003. Lignin biosynthesis. *Annu Rev Plant Biol.* 54:519–546.

Bunker, V.W., 1992. Free radicals, antioxidants and ageing. *Med Lab Sci.* 49:299–312.

Centers for Disease Control and Prevention, 2002. Chronic obstructive pulmonary disease surveillance—United States, 1970–2000: Surveillance summaries, August 2, 2002. *MMWR.* 51(SS-06).

Centers for Disease Control and Prevention, 2007. National surveillance for asthma—United States, 1980–2004: Surveillance summaries, October 19, 2007. *MMWR.* 5(SS-8).

Centers for Disease Control and Prevention (CDC), National Center for Health Statistics, 2009. Compressed mortality file 1999–2006. CDC WONDER on-line database, compiled from Compressed Mortality File 1999–2006 Series 20 No. 2L. CDC, Atlanta, GA (cited March 5, 2010). Available from: http://wonder.cdc.gov/cmf-icd10.html.

Charrouf, Z., D. Guillaume, 2007. Phenols and polyphenols from argania spinosa. *Am J Food Technol.* 2 (7):679.

Cheng, G.W., C.H. Crisosto, 1995. Browning potential, phenolic composition, and polyphenol oxidase activity of buffer extracts of peach and nectarine skin tissue. *J Am Soc Hort Sci.* 120 (5):835–838.

Chu, F.F., J.H. Doroshow, R.S. Esworthy, 1993. Expression, characterization, and tissue distribution of a new cellular selenium-dependent glutathione peroxidase, *GSHPx-GI. J Biol Chem.* 268:2571.

Chung, K.T., T.Y. Wong, C.I. Wei, Y.W. Huang, Y. Lin, 1998. Tannins and human health: A review. *Crit Rev Food Sci Nutr.* 38 (6):421–464.

Cho, S.G. et al., 2001. Glutathione S-transferase Mu modulates the stress activated signals by suppressing apoptosis signal-regulating kinase. *J Biol Chem.* 276:12749–12755.

Comhair, S.A., P.R. Bhathena, C. Farver, F.B. Thunnissen, S.C. Erzurum, 2001. Extracellular glutathione peroxidase induction in asthmatic lungs: Evidence for redox regulation of expression in human airway epithelial cells. *FASEB J.* 15:70–78.

Cross, C.E. et al., 1994. Oxidants, antioxidants, and respiratory tract lining fluids. *Environ Health Perspec.* 102:185–191.

Cruz, E., S. Da-silva, M. Muzitano, P. Silva, S. Costa, B. Rossi-Bergmann, 2008. Immunomodulatory pretreatment with *Kalanchoe pinnata* extract and its quercitrin flavonoid effectively protects mice against fatal anaphylactic shock. *Int Immunopharmacol.* 8:1616–1621.

Culpitt, S.V. et al., 2003. Inhibition by red wine extract, resveratrol, of cytokine release by alveolar macrophagesin COPD. *Thorax.* 58 (11):942–946.

Curello, S., C. Ceconi, C. Bigoli, R. Ferrari, A. Albertini, C. Guarnieri, 1985. Changes in the cardiac glutathione status after ischemia and reperfusion. *Experientia.* 41:42–43.

Dabelstein, W., A. Reglitzky, A. Schütze, K. Reders, 2007. Automotive Fuels. *Ullmann's Encyclopedia of Industrial Chemistry.* doi: 10.1002/14356007.a16_719. ISBN: 3527306730.

Dickinson, D.A., H.J. Forman, 1999. Glutathione in defense and signaling: Lessons from a small thiol. *Ann NY Acad Sci.* 973:488–504.

Dokosi, O.B. (ed.), 1998. *Herbs of Ghana.* Ghana University Press, Accra, Ghana, pp. 32–33.

Donato, L.J., N. Noy, 2005. Suppression of mammary carcinoma growth by retinoic acid: Proapoptotic genes are targets for retinoic acid receptor and cellular retinoic acid-binding protein II signaling. *Cancer Res.* 65:8193–8199.

Donnelly, L.E. et al., 2004. Anti-inflammatory effects of resveratrol in lung epithelial cells: Molecular mechanisms. *Am J Physiol Lung Cell Mol Physiol.* 287 (4):L774–L783.

Dorion, S., H. Lambert, J. Landry, 2002. Activation of the p38 signaling pathway by heat shock involves the dissociation of glutathione S-transferase Mu from Ask1. *J Biol Chem.* 277:30792–30797.

Douglas, R.M., H. Hemila, E. Chalker, B. Treacy, 2007. Vitamin C for preventing and treating the common cold. *Cochrane Database Syst Rev.* 18(3):CD000980.

Dubuisson, M. et al., 2004. Human peroxiredoxin 5 is a peroxynitrite reductase. *FEBS Lett.* 571:161–165.

Dugasani, S., M.R. Pichika, V.D. Nadarajah, M.K. Balijepalli, S. Tandra, J.N. Korlakunta, 2010. Comparative antioxidant and anti-inflammatory effects of [6]-gingerol, [8]-gingerol, [10]-gingerol and [6]-shogaol. *J Ethnopharmacol.* 127 (2):515–520.

Dymock, W., C.J.H. Warden, D. Hooper, 1890. *Pharmacographica Indica*, Vol. 1. Trubner & Co., London, U.K., Educational Society's Press, Calcutta, India, p. 590.

El-Agamey, A., G.M. Lowe, D.J. McGarvey, A. Mortensen, D.M. Phillip, T.G. Truscott, 2004. Carotenoid radical chemistry and antioxidant/pro-oxidant properties. *Arch Biochem Biophys.* 430:37–48.

American Cancer Society (ACS), 2008. Ellagic acid, November 2008. http://www.cancer.org/. Retrieved August 2014.

Escott-Stump, S., 2008. *Nutrition and Diagnosis-Related Care.* Lippincott Williams & Wilkins, Philadelphia, PA.

Faruk, H., A. Jawad, G. Hayder, A. Atabee, S.S. Ahmed, 2010. Usefulness of antioxidants drugs in bronchial asthma. *Pak J Physiol.* 6 (2):18–21.

Flohe, L., 2000. Glutathione peroxidase. *Basic Life Sci.* 1988;49:663–668.

Fortunato, L.R., C. de Freitas Alves, M.M. Teixeira, A.P. Rogerio, 2012. Quercetin: A flavonoid with the potential to treat asthma. *Braz J Pharmaceut Sci.* 48:4.

Freedman, S.O., R. Shulman, J. Krupey, A.H. Sehon, 1964. Antigenic properties of chlorogenic acid. *J Allergy.* 35 (2):97–107.

Galvez, M.C., C.G. Barroso, J.A. Perez-Bustamante, 1994. Analysis of polyphenolic compounds of different vinegar samples. *Z Lebensm Unters Forsch.* 199 (1):29–31.

Ghasi, S., C. Egwuib, P. Achukwu, J. Onyeanusi, 2011. Assessment of the medical benefit in the folkloric use of *Bryophyllum pinnatum* Leaf among the Igbos of Nigeria for the treatment of hypertension. *Afr J Pharm Pharmacol.* 5:83–92.

Global Initiative for Chronic Obstructive Lung Disease (GOLD), 2010. Strategy for the diagnosis, management, and prevention of chronic obstructive pulmonary lung disease: Executive summary [Internet] (cited March 12, 2010). Available from: http://www.goldcopd.com.

Green Tea, White Tea: Catechin Health Benefits. http://greentealovers.com/greenteahealthcatechin. htm. Accessed on July 25, 2014.

Gromer, S., S. Urig, K. Becker, 2004. The thioredoxin systemdfrom science to clinic. *Med Res Rev.* 24:40–89.

Habib, M.P. et al., 1999. Effect of vitamin E on exhaled ethane in cigarette smokers. *Chest.* 115:684–690.

Hayes, J.D., D.J. Pulford 1995. The glutathione S-transferase supergene family: Regulation of GST and the contribution of the isoenzymes to cancer chemoprotection and drug resistance. *Crit Rev Biochem Mol Biol.* 30:445–600.

Hayes, J.D., L.I. McLellan, 1999. Glutathione and glutathione-dependent enzymes represent a co-ordinately regulated defence against oxidative stress. *Free Radic Res.* 31:273–300.

Helmut, S., 1997. Oxidative stress: Oxidants and antioxidants. *Exp Physiol.* 82 (2):291–295.

Holmgren, A., 2000. Antioxidant function of thioredoxin and glutaredoxin systems. *Antioxid Redox Signal.* 2:811–820.

Jakobsson, P.J., R. Morgenstern, J. Mancini, H.A. Ford, B. Persson, 1999. Common structural features of MAPEGda widespread superfamily of membrane associated proteins with highly divergent functions in eicosanoid and glutathione metabolism. *Protein Sci.* 8:689–692.

Johnston, K.L., M.N. Clifford, L.M. Morgan, 2003. Coffee acutely modifies gastrointestinal hormone secretion and glucose tolerance in humans: Glycemic effects of chlorogenic acid and caffeine. *Am J Clin Nutr.* 78 (4):728–733.

Joskova, M., S. Franova, V. Sadlonova, 2011. Acute bronchodilator effect of quercetin in experimental allergic asthma. *Bratislavské Lekárske Listy.* 112:9–12.

Kalra, E.K., 2003. Nutraceutical-definition and introduction. *AAPS Pharm Sci.* 5 (3):27–28.

Kasbia, G.S., 2005. Functional foods and nutraceuticals in the management of obesity. *Nutr Food Sci.* 35:344–351.

Kayoko, S., O. Hisae, F. Michiyo, G. Toshinao, T. Sachiko, S. Masayuki, H. Yukihiko, Y. Hiroyo, K. Naohide 1998. Intestinal absorption of luteolin and luteolin 7-O-[beta]-glucoside in rats and humans. *FEBS Lett.* 438 (3):220–224.

Keservani, R.K., A.K. Sharma, 2014. Flavonoids: Emerging trends and potential health benefits. *J Chin Pharm Sci.* 23(12):815–822.

Keservani, R.K., R.K. Kesharwani, A.K. Sharma, N. Vyas, A. Chadoker, 2010b. Nutritional supplements: An overview. *Int J Curr Pharm Rev Res.* 1:59–75.

Keservani, R.K., R.K. Kesharwani, N. Vyas, S. Jain, R. Raghuvanshi, A.K. Sharma, 2010a. Nutraceutical and functional food as future food: A review. *Der Pharm Lett.* 2:106–116.

Kinnula, V.L., 2005. Production and degradation of oxygen metabolites during inflammatory states in the human lung. *Curr Drug Targets Inflamm Allergy.* 4:465–470.

Kinnula, V.L., J.D. Crapo, 2003. Superoxide dismutases in the lung and human lung diseases. *Am J Respir Crit Care Med.* 167:1600–1619.

Kinnula, V.L. et al., 2002. Cell specific expression of peroxiredoxins in human lung and pulmonary sarcoidosis. *Thorax.* 57:157–164.

Kirkman, H.N., M. Rolfo, A.M. Ferraris, G.F. Gaetani, 1999. Mechanisms of protection of catalase by NADPH. Kinetics and stoichiometry. *J Biol Chem.* 274:13908–13914.

Knekt, P. et al., 2002. Flavonoid intake and risk of chronic diseases. *Am J Clin Nutr.* 76 (3):560–568.

Kuo, P.L., Y.L. Hsu, M.S. Huang, M.J. Tsai, Y.C. Ko, 2011. *J Agric Food Chem.* 59(7):3429–3438.

Kwik-Uribe, C., R.M. Bektash, 2008. Cocoa flavanols-measurement, bioavailability and bioactivity. *Asia Pac J Clin Nutr.* 17 (Suppl 1):280–283.

Ladner, J.E., J.F. Parsons, C.L. Rife, G.L. Gilliland, R.N. Armstrong, 2004. Parallel evolutionary pathways for glutathione transferases: Structure and mechanism of the mitochondrial class kappa enzyme rGSTK1-1. *Biochemistry*. 43:52–61.

Lee, D., M. Cuendet, J.S. Vigo, J.G. Graham, F. Cabieses, H.H. Fong, J.M. Pezzuto, A.D. Kinghorn, 2001. A novel cyclooxygenase-inhibitory stilbenolignan from the seeds of aiphanes aculeata. *Org Lett*. 3 (14):2169–2171.

Leigh, E., 2000. Antioxidant activity of tea unaffected by milk. *Herbal Gram*. 50:25–26.

Li, Y. et al., 1997. Lycopene, smoking and lung cancer. *Proc Am Assoc Cancer Res*. 38:113.

Lopez-Lazaro, M., 2009. Distribution and biological activities of the flavonoid luteolin. *MRMC*. 9:31–59.

Lykkesfeldt, J. et al., 2000. Ascorbate is depleted by smoking and repleted by moderate supplementation: A study in male smokers and nonsmokers with matched dietary antioxidant intakes. *Am J Clin Nutr*. 71:530–536.

MacNee, W., 2001. Oxidative stress and lung inflammation in airways disease. *Eur J Pharmacol*. 429:195–207.

Manevich, Y., S.I. Feinstein, A.B. Fisher, 2004. Activation of the antioxidant enzyme 1-CYS peroxiredoxin requires glutathionylation mediated by heterodimerization with pGST. *Proc Natl Acad Sci USA*. 101:3780–3785.

Mangiapane, H., J. Thomson, A. Salter, S. Brown, G.D. Bell, D.A. White, 1992. The inhibition of the oxidation of low density lipoprotein by (+)-catechin, a naturally occurring flavonoid. *Biochem Pharmacol*. 43 (3):445–450.

Mann, J., 1992. *Secondary Metabolism*. Oxford University Press, Oxford, U.K., pp. 279–280.

Manna, S.K. et al., 2000. Resveratrol suppresses TNF-induced activation of nuclear transcription factors NFkappa B, activator protein-1, and apoptosis: Potential role of reactive oxygen intermediates and lipid peroxidation. *J Immunol*. 164 (12):6509–6519.

Masella, R., D.R. Benedetto, R. Vari, C. Filesi, C. Giovannini, 2005. Novel mechanisms of natural antioxidant compounds in biological systems: Involvement of glutathione and glutathione-related enzymes. *J Nutr Biochem*. 16:577–586.

McGee, H., 2004. A survey of tropical spices. *McGee on Food and Cooking*. Hodder and Stoughton, p. 426.

Mezzetti, A. et al., 1996. Systemic oxidative stress and its relationship with age and illness. *J Am Geriatr Soc*. 44:823–827.

Narayanan, B.A., O. Geoffroy., M.C. Willingham, G.G. Re, D.W. Nixon, 1999. p53/p21(WAF1/CIP1) expression and its possible role in G1 arrest and apoptosis in ellagic acid treated cancer cells. *Cancer Lett*. 136 (2):215–221.

National Institutes of Health, National Heart, Lung, and Blood Institute (NHLBI), 2007. National asthma education and prevention program expert panel report 3 (EPR3): Guidelines for the diagnosis and management of asthma. NHLBI, Bethesda, MD (cited March 29, 2010). Available from: http://www.nhlbi.nih.gov/guidelines/asthma/asthgdln.htm.

Niizuma, H. et al., 2006. Bcl-2 is a key regulator for the retinoic acid-induced apoptotic cell death in neuroblastoma. *Oncogene*. 25:5046–5055.

Niles, R.M., 2004. Signaling pathways in retinoid chemoprevention and treatment of cancer. *Mutat Res*. 555:81–96.

Pandey, M., M. Debnath, S. Gupta, S.K. Chikara, 2011. Phytomedicine: An ancient approach turning into future potential source of therapeutics. *J Pharmacol Phytother*. 3:27–37.

Pacheco-Palencia, L.A., S. Mertens-Talcott, S.T. Talcott, 2008. Chemical composition, antioxidant properties, and thermal stability of a phytochemical enriched oil from Acai (*Euterpe oleracea* Mart.). *J Agric Food Chem*. 56 (12):4631–4636.

Park, H.J. et al., 2009. Quercetin regulates Th1/Th2 balance in a murine model of asthma. *Int Immunopharmacol*. 9:261–267.

Prostate Cancer, Nutrition, and Dietary Supplements (PCNDS), 2014. Lycopene for prostate cancer. http://www.cancer.gov/cancertopics/pdq/cam/prostatesupplements/Patient/page4.

Rabe, K.F. et al., 2007. Global initiative for chronic obstructive lung disease. *Am J Respir Crit Care Med*. 176 (6):532–555.

Rahman, I., W. MacNee, 2000a. Regulation of redox glutathione levels and gene transcription in lung inflammation: Therapeutic approaches. *Free Radic Biol Med*. 28:1405–1420.

Rao, A.V., S. Agarwal, 1999. Role of lycopene as antioxidant carotenoid in the prevention of chronic diseases: A review. *Nutr Res*. 19:305–323.

Rautalahti, M. et al., 1997. The effect of alpha-tocopherol and beta-carotene supplementation on COPD symptoms. *Am J Respir Crit Care Med*. 156:1447–1452.

Rennard, S.I., 2002. Overview of causes of COPD. New understanding of pathogenesis and mechanisms can guide future therapy. *Postgrad Med.* 111:28–38.

Reynolds, H.Y., H.H. Newball, 1974. Analysis of proteins and respiratory cells obtained from human lungs by bronchial lavage. *J Lab Clin Med.* 84:559–573.

Rice-Evans, C.A., J. Sampson, P.M. Bramley, D.E. Holloway, 1997. Why do we expect carotenoids to be antioxidants in vivo? *Free Radic Res.* 26:381–398.

Robinson, A, G.A. Huttley, H.S. Booth, P.G. Board, 2004. Modelling and bioinformatics studies of the human kappa class glutathione transferase predict a novel third transferase family with homology to prokaryotic 2-hydroxychromene-2-carboxylate isomerases. *Biochem J.* 379:541–552.

Rusak, G., I. Piantanida, L. Masic, K. Kapuralin, K. Durgo, N. Kopjar, 2010. Spectrophotometric analysis of flavonoid-DNA interactions and DNA damaging/protecting and cytotoxic potential of flavonoids in human peripheral blood lymphocytes. *Chem Biol Interact.* 188 (1):181–189.

Santus, P. et al., 2005. Lipid peroxidation and 5-lipoxygenase activity in chronic obstructive pulmonary disease. *Am J Respir Crit Care Med.* 171 (8):838–843.

Sarubin, F.A., C. Thomson, 2007. *The Health Professional's Guide to Popular Dietary Supplements.* American Dietetic Association, Chicago, Illinois.

Schunemann, H.J., B.J.B. Grant, J. Freudenheim, 2001. The relation of serum levels of antioxidant vitamins C, E, retinol and carotinoids with pulmonary function in the general population. *Am J Respir Crit Care Med.* 163:1246–1255.

Seerama, N.P. et al., 2005. In vitro antiproliferative, apoptotic and antioxidant activities of punicalagin, ellagic acid and a total pomegranate tannin extract are enhanced in combination with other polyphenols as found in pomegranate juice. *J Nutr Biochem.* 16 (6):360–367.

Shahidi, F., 2012. Nutraceuticals, functional foods and dietary supplements in health and disease. *J Food Drug Anal.* 20 (1):226–230.

Sheehan, D., G. Meade, V.M. Foley, C.A. Dowd, 2001. Structure, function and evolution of glutathione transferases: Implications for classification of nonmammalian members of an ancient enzyme superfamily. *Biochem J.* 360:1–16.

Sies, H., 1999. Glutathione and its role in cellular functions. *Free Radic Biol Med.* 27:916–921.

Steinberg, F.M., A. Chait, 1998. Antioxidant vitamin supplementation and lipid peroxidation in smokers. *Am J Clin Nutr.* 68:319–327.

Tabak, C. et al., 2001. Chronic obstructive pulmonary disease and intake of catechins, flavonols, and flavones: The MORGEN study. *Am J Respir Crit Care Med.* 164:61–64.

Ulubelen, A., M. Miski, P. Neuman, T.J. Mabry, 1979. Flavonoids of *Salvia tomentosa* (Labiatae). *J Natural Prod.* 42 (4):261–263.

U.S. Department of Agriculture (USDA), Agricultural Research Service, 2004. USDA National Nutrient Database for Standard Reference, Release 17. Available at www.nal.usda.gov/fnic/foodcomp. Accessed on August 5, 2014.

Van der Vliet, A., C.A. O'Neill, C.E. Cross, J.M. Koostra, W.G. Volz, B. Halliwell, S. Louie, 1999. Determination of low molecular mass antioxidant concentrations in human respiratory tract lining fluids. *Am J Physiol.* 276:289–296.

Vattem, D.A., K. Shetty, 2005. Biological function of ellagic acid: A review. *J Food Biochem.* 29 (3):234–266.

Walda, I.C. et al., 2002. Diet and 20-year chronic obstructive pulmonary disease mortality in middle-aged men from three European countries. *Eur J Clin Nutr.* 56 (7):638–643.

White, E., J.S. Shannon, R.E. Patterson, 1997. Relationship between vitamin and calcium supplement use and colon cancer. *Cancer Epidemiol Biomark Prev.* 6:769–774.

Yeomans, V.C., J. Linseisen, G. Wolfram, 2005. Interactive effects of polyphenols, tocopherol, and ascorbic acid on the Cu_2-mediated oxidative modification of human low density lipoproteins. *Eur J Nutr.* 44 (7):422–428.

Zelko, I.N., T.J. Mariani, R.J. Folz, 2002. Superoxide dismutase multigene family: A comparison of the CuZn-SOD (SOD1), Mn-SOD (SOD2), and EC-SOD (SOD3) gene structures, evolution, and expression. *Free Radic Biol Med.* 33:337–349.

Zheng, L.T., G.M. Ryu, B.M. Kwon, W.H. Lee, K. Suk, 2008. Anti-inflammatory effects of catechols in lipopolysaccharide-stimulated microglia cells: Inhibition of microglial neurotoxicity. *Eur J Pharmacol.* 588 (1):106–113.

Zory, Q.A., B. Byung-Kee, 2006. Phenolic compounds of barley grain and their implication in food product discoloration. *J Agric Food Chem.* 54 (26):9978–9984.

Section VII

Hypertension

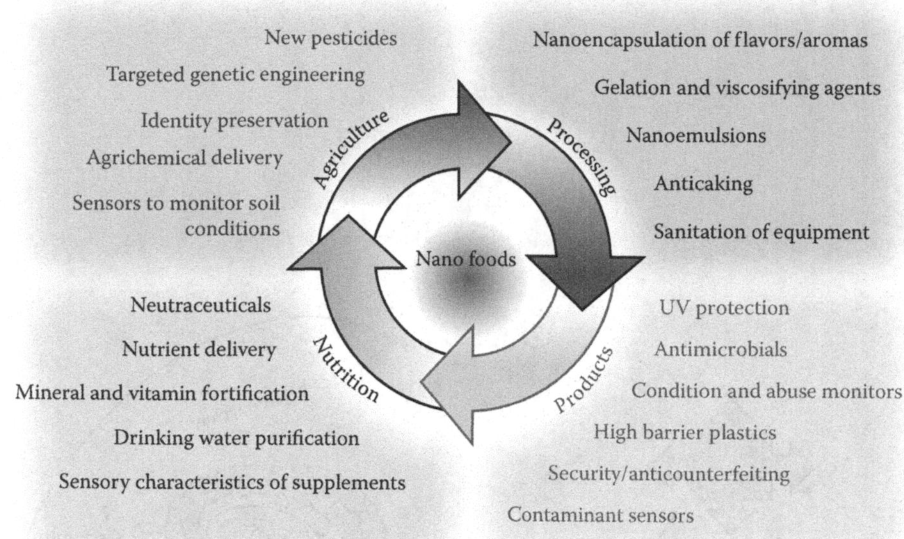

FIGURE 2.1 Food nanotechnology applications in the food production, processing, and delivery pipeline. (From Saba, N., et al., *Polymers*, 6(8), 2247, 2014.)

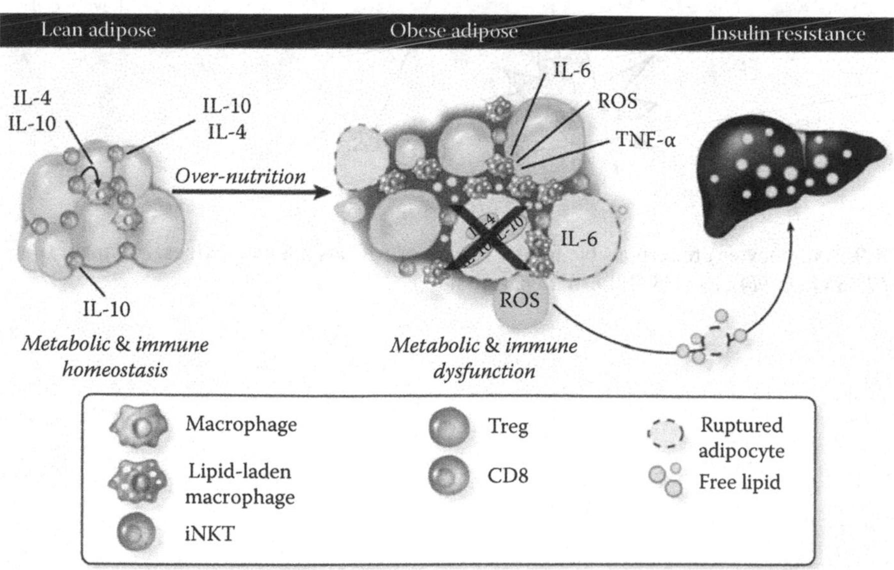

FIGURE 5.5 The role of iNKT cells in lipid handling and metabolic regulation. (Adapted from Lynch, L., *Immunology*, 142(3), 337, 2014. With permission.)

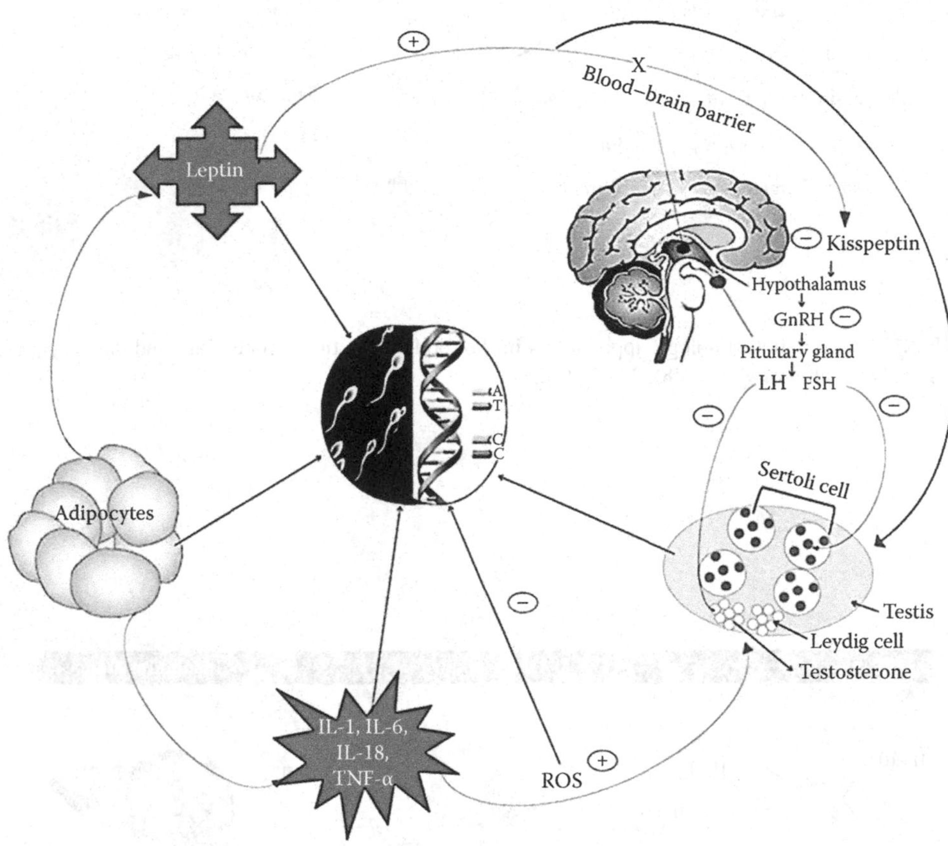

FIGURE 5.9 Adipocytes are responsible for the release of various adipocytokines. (Adapted from Shukla, A. et al., *PLoS ONE*, 9(4), e94433, 2014. With permission.)

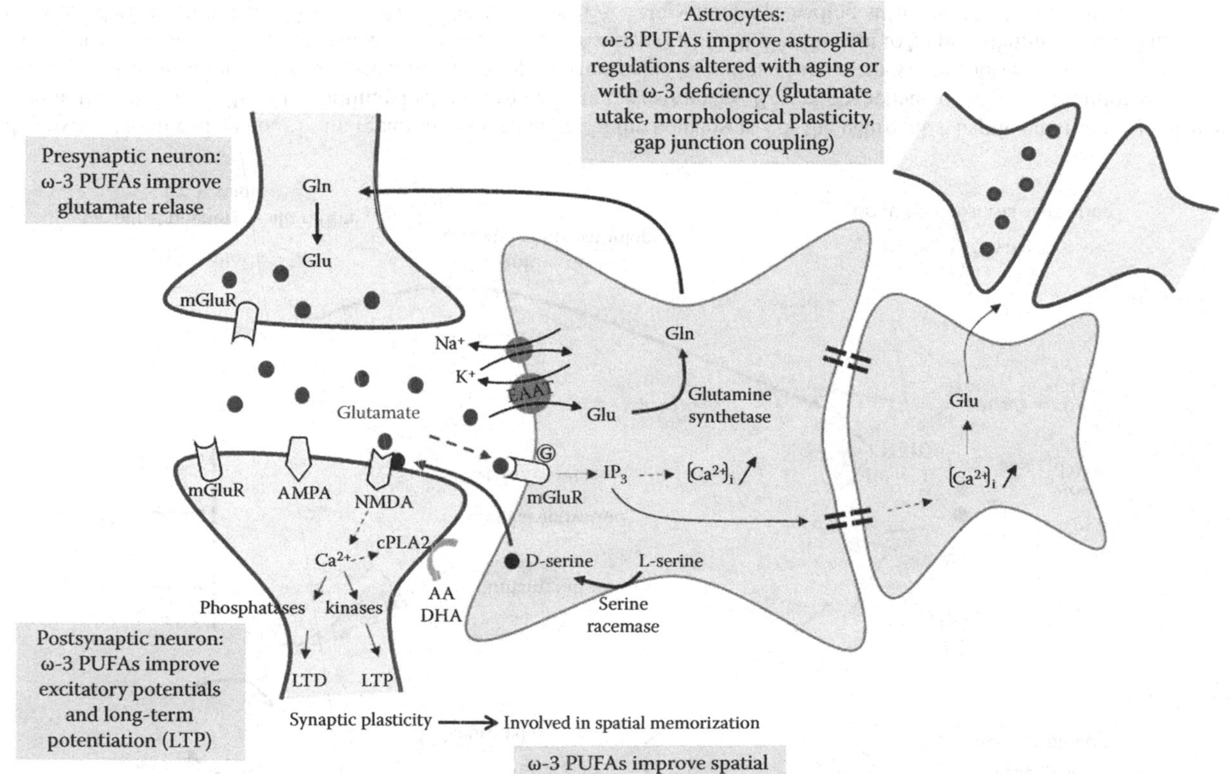

FIGURE 13.2 ω-3 PUFA implication in the synaptic activity and regulation: Glutamatergic neurotransmission relies on a finely regulated cross-talk between the presynaptic and postsynaptic neurons and the astrocytes. Notably, the presynaptic release of glutamate (Glu) is controlled by the feedback activation of metabotropic receptors (mGluR), its postsynaptic binding on ionotropic receptors (AMPA and NMDA) is modified by gliotransmitters (such as D-serine), its concentration in the synaptic cleft depends on the astroglial glutamate uptake activity, and its extrasynaptic leakage varies according to the extent of the astroglial sheath around the synapse. The changes in synaptic efficiency, called long-term potentiation (LTP) and long-term depression (LTD), are considered to sustain memory formation and are notably involved in spatial learning. Several of these mechanisms are affected directly by DHA or by the ω-3 PUFA status of brain cell membranes Gln (Glutamine).

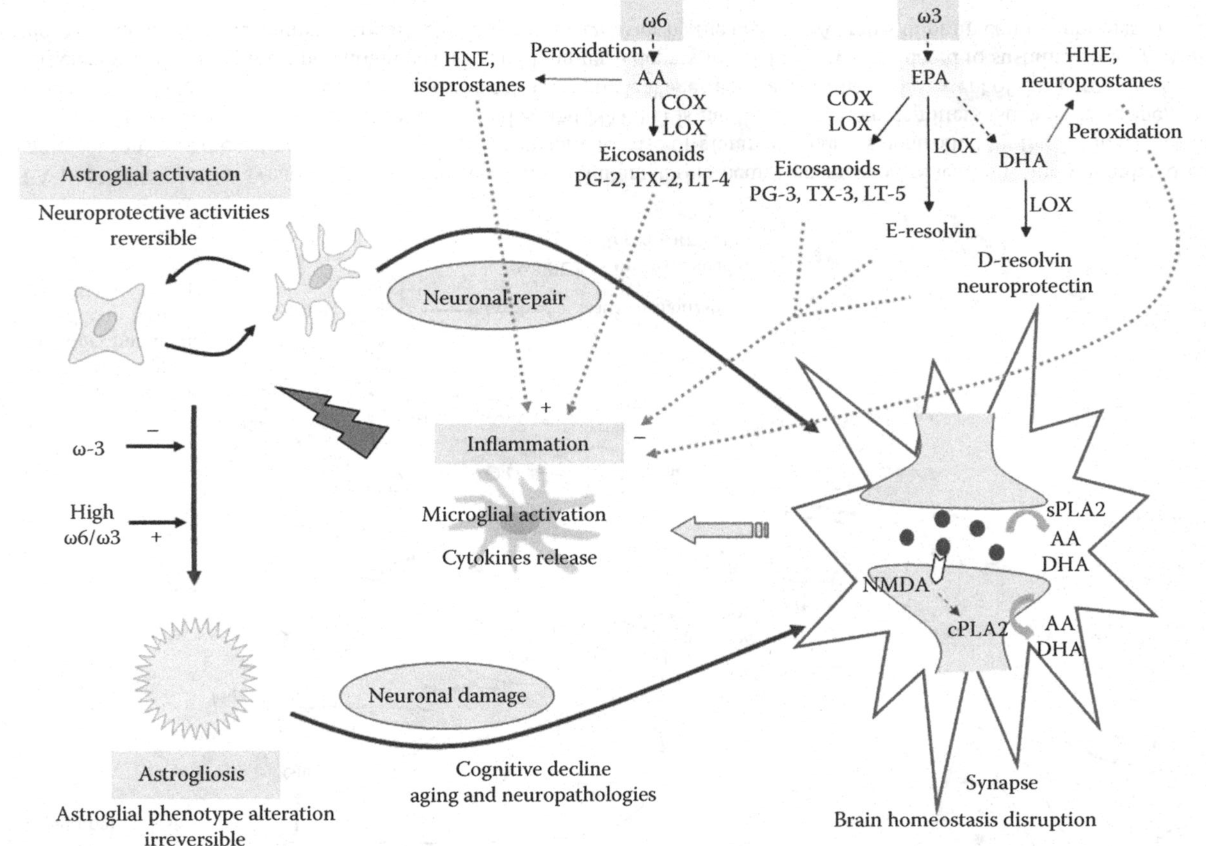

FIGURE 13.3 Glial activation—an endogenous brain repair system: Changes in the homeostasis of the neuronal/synaptic environment (such as increased glutamate release) activate microglia, the immune cells of the brain, which in turn activate the astrocytes. Reversibly activated astrocytes reinforce their neuroprotective activities to restore the homeostasis. During aging, astrocyte activation turns to an irreversible alteration of the astrocyte phenotype called astrogliosis, resulting in impaired synaptic regulations. The underlying signaling pathways involve oxygenated derivatives of LC-PUFA, thought to be proinflammatory when derived from the ω-6 series and anti-inflammatory when derived from the ω-3 series. An adequate ω-3 PUFA dietary intake providing sufficient DHA to the brain may, therefore, limit the glial activation and slow down the age-induced brain damages.

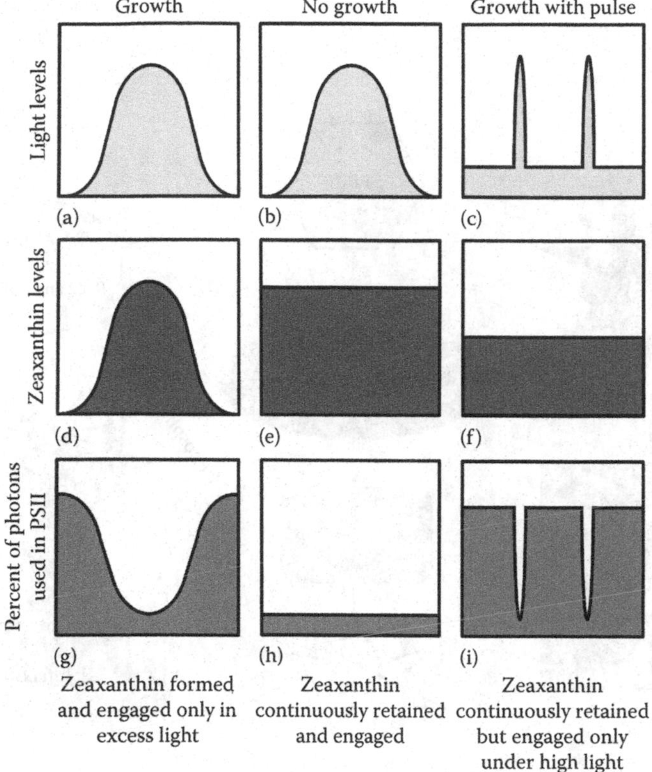

FIGURE 23.3 Changes in the intensity of light (yellow; a–c) striking a horizontal leaf surface, changes in leaf zeaxanthin concentration (blue; d–f), and changes in the percentage of photons absorbed in photosystem II (PSII) and used in PSII photochemistry (green; g–i). Different panels depict light absorption in a natural setting on a sunny day (a, b) or in a growth chamber providing low background light supplemented with two short pulses of high light (c) and depict zeaxanthin levels and utilization of absorbed photons for a growing plant (d, g), a plant impeded in its growth due to harsh environmental conditions (e, h), or a plant growing under growth chamber conditions conducive for growth (f, i).

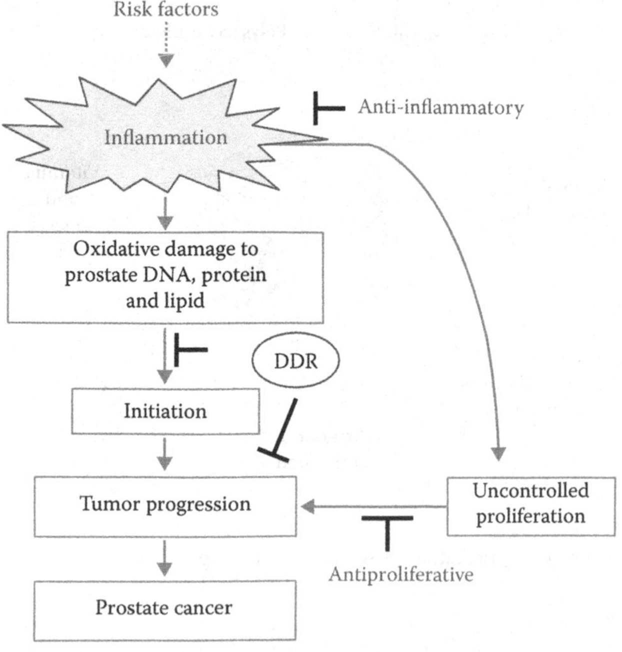

FIGURE 24.3 Chemopreventive actions of soy isoflavones and curcumin.

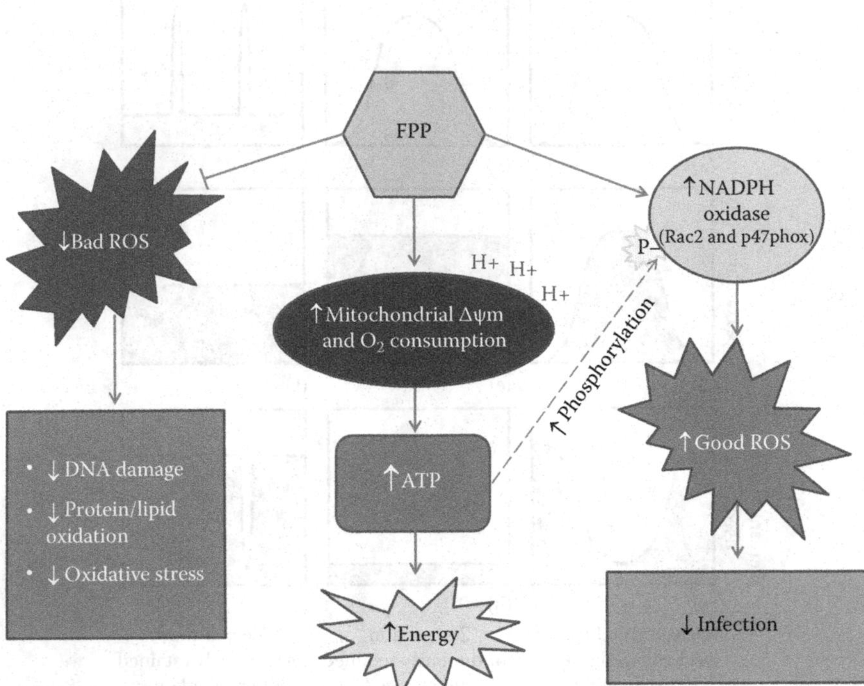

FIGURE 26.1 FPP corrects T2DM-mediated aberrant ROS in innate immune cells. FPP's antioxidant properties combat harmful "bad" ROS thereby reducing the negative effects of elevated oxidative stress (DNA damage, protein and lipid oxidation, etc.). FPP supplementation increases mitochondrial membrane potential leading to elevated ATP levels, which may be used in phosphorylation reactions to activate NADPH oxidase, rescuing compromised useful "good" ROS production via respiratory burst, reducing the infection.

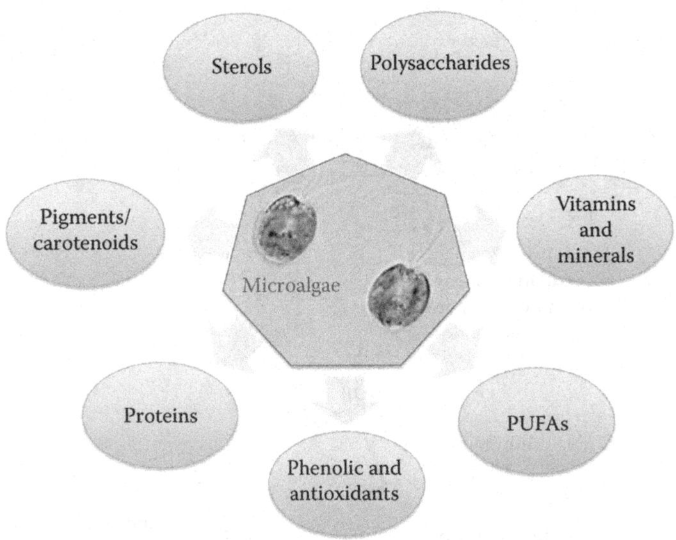

FIGURE 39.1 An overview of nutraceuticals used from microalgae.

18 Nutrition and Nutraceutical Supplements for the Treatment of Hypertension

Mark Houston

CONTENTS

18.1 INTRODUCTION

Vascular biology, endothelial and vascular smooth muscle, and cardiac dysfunction play a primary role in the initiation and perpetuation of hypertension, cardiovascular disease (CVD), and target-organ damage (TOD). Nutrient–gene interactions and epigenetics are predominant factors in promoting beneficial or detrimental effects in cardiovascular health and hypertension. Macronutrients and micronutrients may be able to prevent, control, or treat hypertension through numerous mechanisms related to vascular biology or other mechanisms. Oxidative stress, inflammation, and autoimmune dysfunction are some of the primary factors that initiate and propagate hypertension and CVD. The literature suggests that there may be a complementary role of single and component nutraceutical supplements, vitamins, antioxidants, and minerals in the treatment of hypertension when combined with optimal nutrition and other lifestyle modifications. However, many of these studies are small and do not have long-term follow-up for efficacy and safety. The role of these nutrition and nutraceutical supplements will require a careful review and additional studies to determine their exact role in the management of hypertension.

Vascular disease is a balance between vascular injury and repair [1]. The endothelium is strategically located between the blood and the vascular smooth muscle where it secretes various substances to maintain vascular homeostasis and health including mediators that control vasodilation or vasoconstriction, inflammation or anti-inflammation, oxidative stress or defense, thrombosis or antithrombosis, and growth or antigrowth [1]. Various insults that lead to endothelial dysfunction (ED) may cause hypertension and CVD. Hypertension may be a hemodynamic marker of injured endothelium and vascular smooth muscle related to at least three finite responses of inflammation, oxidative stress, and immune dysfunction of the arteries. Hypertension is in part a consequence of the interaction of genetics and environment. Macronutrients and micronutrients that may be crucial in the regulation of blood pressure (BP) are often deficient in hypertensive patients due to genetics, environment, and prescription drugs.

These deficiencies may have an impact on present and future cardiovascular health outcomes such as hypertension, myocardial infarction (MI), stroke, and renal disease. The diagnosis and treatment of these nutrient deficiencies may reduce BP and improve vascular health, ED, vascular biology, and cardiovascular events when coupled with proper nutrition, lifestyle, and antihypertensive therapy.

18.2 EPIDEMIOLOGY

Epidemiology underscores the etiological role of diet and associated nutrient intake in hypertension. The transition from the Paleolithic diet to our modern diet may have contributed to an epidemic of nutritionally related diseases such as hypertension and coronary heart disease (CHD) (Table 18.1) [1,2]. Table 18.1 contrasts intake of nutrients involved in BP regulation during the Paleolithic era and in modern time.

The human genetic makeup is 99.9% that of our Paleolithic ancestors, yet our nutritional, vitamin, and mineral intakes are vastly different [3]. The macronutrient and micronutrient variations may have a link to some of the proposed mechanisms that could possibly lead to vascular dysfunction, ED, and hypertension. Oxidative stress from radical oxygen species (ROS) and radical nitrogen species (RNS) inflammatory mediators and autoimmune vascular dysfunction contribute to hypertension. Cell adhesion molecules (CAMs) that promote leukocyte adhesion to the endothelium as well as numerous cytokines, chemokines, signaling molecules, and altered T-cell and B-cell functions have been suggested to contribute to hypertension and other CVD through complex nutrient–gene

TABLE 18.1
Dietary Intake of Nutrients Involved in Vascular Biology: Comparing and Contrasting the Diet of Paleolithic and Contemporary Humans

Nutrients and Dietary Characteristics	Paleolithic Intake	Modern Intake
Sodium	<50 mmol/day (1.2 g)	175 mmol/day (4 g)
Potassium	>10,000 meq/day (256 g)	150 meq/day (6 g)
Sodium/potassium ratio	<0.13/day	>0.67/day
Protein	37%	20%
Carbohydrate	41%	40%–50%
Fat	22%	30%–40%
Polyunsaturated/saturated fat ratio	1.4	0.4
Fiber	>100 g/day	9 g/day

interactions and epigenetics. Many cell surface receptors such as caveolae (lipid microdomains in the cell membrane) and pattern recognition receptors (PRR) interact with external environmental insults that promote intracellular signaling and vascular function. The nutrient–caveolae interactions and nutrient reactions with PRR (toll-like receptors [TLR] and Nod-like receptors [NLR]) in the endothelium [4–9] may promote ED and hypertension. Nitric oxide (NO) is the primary vasodilator, antihypertensive, and antiatherosclerotic mediator produced in the endothelium. Angiotensin II and endothelin are potent vasoconstrictors that promote hypertension and atherosclerosis. Reduction in NO bioavailability, increase in angiotensin II, and endothelin coupled with endothelial activation initiate the vascular and cardiac dysfunction and hypertension. In particular, the high Na^+/K^+ ratio of modern diets has contributed to hypertension [3,10] as have the relatively low intake of omega-3 PUFA, increase in omega-6 PUFA, saturated fat, and trans fatty acids [9].

18.3 PATHOPHYSIOLOGY

Vascular biology assumes a pivotal role in the initiation and perpetuation of hypertension and cardiovascular TOD [1]. Oxidative stress (ROS and RNS), inflammation (increased expression of redox-sensitive pro-inflammatory genes, CAMS, and recruitment migration and infiltration of circulating cells) and autoimmune vascular dysfunction (T cells and B cells) are the primary pathophysiological and functional mechanisms that induce vascular disease [1,11–13]. All three of these are closely interrelated and establish a deadly combination that leads to ED, vascular smooth muscle and cardiac dysfunction, hypertension, vascular disease, atherosclerosis, and CVD. Hypertension may be a correct but chronically dysregulated responses to infinite vascular insults and environmental–genetic expression patterns in which the vascular system becomes an innocent bystander. This response may become a maladaptive vascular response that was initially intended to provide vascular defense to the endothelial insults [1,12–14]. Hypertension is a vasculopathy characterized by ED, structural remodeling, vascular inflammation, increased arterial stiffness, reduced distensibility, and loss of elasticity [12]. These insults are biomechanical (BP, pulse pressure, blood flow, oscillatory flow, turbulence, augmentation, pulse wave velocity, and reflected waves) and biohumoral or biochemical, which includes all the nonmechanical causes such as metabolic, endocrine, nutritional, toxic, infectious, and other etiologies [1]. In addition to the very well-established connections for endocrine and nutritional causes of hypertension, toxins and infections also increase BP [15–19]. Various toxins such as polychlorinated biphenyls (PCBs), mercury, lead, cadmium, arsenic, and iron also increase BP and CVD [15,16]. Numerous microbial organisms have been implicated in hypertension and CHD [17–19]. All of these insults lead to impaired microvascular structure and function that manifests clinically as hypertension [11–13]. The level of BP may not give an accurate indication of the microvascular involvement and impairment in hypertension [11–13]. Hypertensive patients have abnormal microvasculature in the form of inward eutrophic remodeling of the small resistance arteries. This may lead to impaired vasodilatory capacity, increased vascular resistance, increased media to lumen ratio (MLR), decreased maximal organ perfusion, and reduced flow reserve, especially in the heart with decreased coronary flow reserve (CFR) [11–13]. Significant functional then structural microvascular impairment occurs even before the BP begins to rise in normotensive offspring of hypertensive parents. This is evidenced by ED, impaired vasodilation, forearm vascular resistance, diastolic dysfunction, increased left ventricular mass index, increased septal and posterior wall thickness, and left ventricular hypertrophy (LVH) [11,14]. Thus, the cellular processes underlying the vascular perturbations constitute a vascular phenotype of hypertension that may be determined by early life programming and imprinting, which is compounded by vascular aging [11–13].

18.3.1 Oxidative Stress

Oxidative stress, with an imbalance between ROS and RNS and antioxidant defense mechanisms, contributes to the etiology of hypertension in animals [20] and humans [21–26]. ROS and RNS are generated by multiple cellular sources, including nicotinamide adenine dinucleotide phosphate (NADPH) oxidase, mitochondria, xanthine oxidase, uncoupled endothelium-derived NO synthase (U-eNOS), cyclo-oxygenase, and lipo-oxygenase [27]. Superoxide anion is produced by the stimulation of the AT1R and NADPH oxidase by A-II. Superoxide anion is the predominant ROS species produced by these tissues, neutralizes NO, and leads to downstream production of other ROS such as hydrogen peroxide, hydroxyl radical, and peroxynitrite. Hypertensive patients have impaired endogenous and exogenous antioxidant defense mechanisms [23], an increased plasma oxidative stress, and an exaggerated oxidative stress response to various stimuli [23,24]. Hypertensive subjects also have lower plasma FRAP (ferric reducing ability of plasma), lower vitamin C levels, and increased plasma 8-isoprostanes, which correlate with both systolic and diastolic BP. Various single-nucleotide polymorphisms (SNPs) in genes that codify for antioxidant enzymes are directly related to hypertension [25], including NADPH oxidase, xanthine oxidase, SOD 3 (superoxide dismutase), catalase, GPx 1 (glutathione peroxidase), and thioredoxin. ROS directly damage endothelial cells and degrade NO [1,21–24]. Various neurohormonal systems including the RAAS and sympathetic nervous system (SNS) also contribute to oxidative stress, inflammation, and vascular immune dysfunction. The increased oxidative stress, inflammation, and autoimmune vascular dysfunction in human hypertension results from a combination of increased generation of ROS and RNS, an exacerbated response to ROS and RNS, and a decreased antioxidant reserve [23–26,28,29]. There are direct interactions of the central nervous system, inflammation, and BP. Increased oxidative stress in the rostral ventrolateral medulla (RVLM) enhances glutamatergic excitatory inputs and attenuates GABA-ergic inhibitory inputs to the RVLM, which contributes to increased SNS activity from the paraventricular nucleus [30]. Activation of the AT1R in the RVLM increases NADPH oxidase and increases oxidative stress and superoxide anion, increases SNS outflow causing an imbalance of SNS/PNS activity with elevation of BP, increased heart rate and alterations in heart rate variability and heart rate recovery time, which can be blocked by AT1R blockers [30,31].

18.3.2 Inflammation

The link between inflammation and hypertension has been suggested in both cross-sectional and longitudinal studies [32]. The inflammation can be from a myriad of causes. One of the best markers of vascular inflammation is high-sensitivity C-reactive protein (HS-CRP). Increases in HS-CRP as well as other inflammatory cytokines such as interleukin 1B (IL-1B), interleukin 6 (IL-6), tumor necrosis alpha (TNF-alpha), and chronic leukocytosis occur in hypertension and hypertensive-related TOD [33]. HS-CRP predicts future CV events [32,33] and is both a risk marker and a risk factor for hypertension and CVD [34,35]. Increases in HS-CRP of over

3 μg/mL may increase BP in just a few days that is directly proportional to the increase in HS-CRP [34,35]. NO and eNOS are inhibited by HS-CRP [34,35]. The AT2R, which normally counterbalances AT1R, is downregulated by HS-CRP [34,35]. Both of these effects result in reduction in NO bioavailability and increased BP. Angiotensin II (A-II) upregulates many of the cytokines, especially IL-6, CAMs, and chemokines by activating nuclear factor kappa B (NF-κB), leading to vasoconstriction and inflammation. These events, along with the increase in oxidative stress and endothelin-1, elevate BP [32].

18.3.3 Autoimmune Dysfunction

Innate and adaptive immune responses are linked to hypertension and hypertension-induced CVD through at least three mechanisms: cytokine production, central nervous system stimulation, and renal damage. An imbalance of T-cell and B-cell function, especially a loss of T regulatory cells that normally decrease autoimmune reactions, is involved in hypertension and vascular damage. This includes salt-sensitive hypertension with increased renal inflammation as a result of T-cell imbalance, dysregulation of CD4+ and CD8+ lymphocytes, and chronic leukocytosis with increased neutrophils and reduced lymphocytes [36–38]. Leukocytosis, especially increased neutrophils and decreased lymphocyte count, increase BP in Blacks by 6/2 mm Hg in the highest versus the lowest tertile [38]. Macrophages and various T-cell subtypes regulate BP, invade the arterial wall, activate TLRs, and induce autoimmune vascular damage [38,39]. Angiotensin II directly activates immune cells (T cells, macrophages, and dendritic cells) and promotes cell infiltration into target organs [39]. CD4+ T lymphocytes express AT1R and PPAR gamma receptors and release TNF-alpha, interferon, and interleukins within the vascular wall when activated [39]. IL-17 produced by T cells may play a pivotal role in the genesis of hypertension caused by angiotensin II [39]. Hypertensive patients have significantly higher TLR 4 mRNA in monocytes compared to normal subjects [40]. Intensive reduction in BP to systolic BP (SBP) less than 130 mm Hg versus SBP to only 140 mm Hg lowers the TLR 4 more [40]. Angiotensin II activates the TLR expression, leading to inflammation and activation of the innate immune system. When TLR 4 is activated, there is downstream macrophage activation, migration, increased metalloproteinase 9 (MMP 9), vascular remodeling, collagen accumulation in the artery, LVH, and cardiac fibrosis [40]. The autonomic nervous system is critical in increasing or decreasing immune dysfunction and inflammation [42]. Efferent cholinergic anti-inflammatory pathways via the vagal nerve innervate the spleen, nicotine acetylcholine receptor subunits, and cytokine producing immune cells to influence vasoconstriction and BP [42]. Local CNS inflammation or ischemia may mediate vascular inflammation and hypertension [39].

Aldosterone is associated with increased adaptive immunity and autoimmune responses with CD4+ T-cell activation and Th 17 polarization with increased IL-17, TGF-β and TNF-alpha, which modulate over 30 inflammatory genes [43,44]. Increased serum aldosterone is an independent risk factor for CVD and CHD through nonhemodynamic effects as well as through increased BP [43,44]. Blockade of mineralocorticoid receptors in the heart, brain, blood vessels, and immune cells reduces CV risk even with the persistence of hypertension [43,44].

18.4 TREATMENT

Many of the natural compounds in food, nutraceutical supplements, or minerals function in a similar fashion to a specific class of antihypertensive drugs. Although the potency of these natural compounds may be less than the antihypertensive drug, when used in combination with proper nutrition, lifestyle modifications, other macro- or micronutrients, nutraceutical supplements or with antihypertensive drugs, the antihypertensive effect is additive or synergistic. It should be noted that the role of supplements in hypertension does not yet have clinical outcome trials that conventional drugs have. At this time, there is a possible role for supplements in hypertension to improve cardiovascular outcomes, but this remains to be proven. Table 18.2 summarizes these natural compounds

TABLE 18.2
Natural Antihypertensive Compounds Categorized by Antihypertensive Class

Antihypertensive Therapeutic Class (Alphabetical Listing)	Foods and Ingredients Listed by Therapeutic Class	Nutrients and Other Supplements Listed by Therapeutic Class
Angiotensin-converting enzyme inhibitors	Egg yolk Fish (specific): Bonito Dried salted fish Fish sauce Sardine muscle/protein Tuna Garlic Gelatin Hawthorn berry Milk products (specific): Casein Sour milk Whey (hydrolyzed) Sake Sea vegetables (kelp) Sea weed (Wakame) Wheat germ (hydrolyzed) Zein (corn protein)	Melatonin Omega-3 fatty acids Pomegranate Pycnogenol Zinc
Angiotensin receptor blockers	Celery Fiber Garlic MUFA	Coenzyme Q10 Gamma linolenic acid NAC Oleic acid Resveratrol Potassium Taurine Vitamin C Vitamin B6 (pyridoxine)
Beta blockers	Hawthorn berry	
Calcium channel blockers	Celery Garlic Hawthorn berry MUFA	Alpha lipoic acid Calcium Magnesium *N*-Acetyl cysteine Oleic acid Omega-3 fatty acids: Eicosapentaenoic acid Docosahexaenoic acid Taurine Vitamin B6 Vitamin C Vitamin E
Central alpha agonists (reduce sympathetic nervous system activity)	Celery Fiber Garlic Protein	Coenzyme Q10 Gamma linolenic acid Potassium Restriction of sodium Taurine Vitamin C Vitamin B6 Zinc

(Continued)

TABLE 18.2 (*Continued*)
Natural Antihypertensive Compounds Categorized by Antihypertensive Class

Antihypertensive Therapeutic Class (Alphabetical Listing)	Foods and Ingredients Listed by Therapeutic Class	Nutrients and Other Supplements Listed by Therapeutic Class
Direct renin inhibitors		Vitamin D
Direct vasodilators	Celery	Alpha linolenic acid
	Cooking oils with monounsaturated fats	Arginine
	Fiber	Calcium
	Garlic	Flavonoids
	MUFA	Magnesium
	Soy	Omega-3 fatty acids
		Potassium
		Taurine
		Vitamin C
		Vitamin E
Diuretics	Celery	Calcium
	Hawthorn berry	Coenzyme Q10
	Protein	Fiber
		Gamma linolenic acid
		L-Carnitine
		Magnesium
		Potassium
		Taurine
		Vitamin B6
		Vitamin C
		Vitamin E: high gamma/delta tocopherols and tocotrienols

into the major antihypertensive drug classes such as diuretics, beta blockers, central alpha agonists, direct vasodilators, calcium channel blockers (CCBs), angiotensin-converting enzyme inhibitors (ACEIs), angiotensin receptor blockers (ARBs), and direct renin inhibitors (DRI).

18.4.1 DASH Diets

The DASH I and II diets conclusively demonstrated significant reductions in BP in borderline and stage I hypertensive patients [45,46]. At 2 weeks, the BP was decreased by 10.7/5.2 mm Hg in the hypertensive patients in DASH I and 11.5/6.8 mm Hg in the hypertensive patients in DASH II. The DASH diet increases plasma renin activity (PRA) and serum aldosterone levels in response to the BP reductions [47,48]. There was an associated response with the G46A polymorphism of β2-AR (beta 2 adrenergic receptor). The A allele of G46A had a greater BP reduction and blunted PRA and aldosterone. The AA genotype had the best response and the GG genotype had no response. Adding an ARB, ACEI, or DRI improved BP response to the DASH diet in the GG group due to blockade of the increase in PRA. A low sodium DASH diet decreases oxidative stress (urine F2-isoprostanes), improves vascular function (augmentation index), and lowers BP in salt-sensitive subjects [49]. In addition, plasma nitrite increased and pulse wave velocity decreased at week 2 on the DASH diet [50].

18.4.1.1 Sodium (Na^+) Reduction

The average sodium intake in the United States is 5,000 mg/day with some areas of the country consuming 15,000–20,000 mg/day [26]. Epidemiological, observational, and controlled clinical trials demonstrate that an increased sodium intake is associated with higher BP as well as increased risk for

CVD, cerebral vascular accident (CVA), LVH, CHD, MI, renal insufficiency, proteinuria, and increased SNS activity [26]. A reduction in sodium intake in hypertensive patients, especially the salt-sensitive patients, significantly lowers BP by 4–6/2–3 mm Hg that is proportional to the degree of sodium restriction and may prevent or delay hypertension in high-risk patients and reduce future CV events [28].

Salt sensitivity (≥10% increase in MAP with salt loading) occurs in about 51% of hypertensive patients [29]. Cardiovascular events are more common in the salt-sensitive patients than in salt-resistant ones, independent of BP [29]. An increased sodium intake has a direct positive correlation with BP and the risk of CVA and CHD [29]. The risk is independent of BP for CVA with a relative risk of 1.04–1.25 from the lowest to the highest quartile [26,29]. In addition, patients will convert to a nondipping BP pattern with increases in nocturnal BP as the sodium intake increases [26,29].

Increased sodium intake has a direct adverse effect on endothelial cells [30]. Sodium promotes cutaneous lymphangiogenesis; increases endothelial cell stiffness; reduces size, surface area, volume, cytoskeleton, deformability, and pliability; reduces eNOS and NO production; and increases ADMA, oxidative stress, and TGF-β. All of these abnormal vascular responses are increased in the presence of aldosterone [30,31]. These changes occur independent of BP and may be partially counteract by dietary potassium. The endothelial cells act as vascular salt sensors [30,31]. Endothelial cells are targets for aldosterone that activate epithelial sodium channels and have negative effects on the release of NO and on endothelial function. The mechanical stiffness of the cell plasma membrane and the submembranous actin network (endothelial glycocalyx) ("shell") serve as a "firewall" to protect the endothelial cells and are regulated by serum sodium, potassium, and aldosterone within the physiological range [30,31]. Changes in shear stress–dependent activity of the endothelial NO synthase located in the caveolae regulate the viscosity in this "shell" [30,31]. High plasma sodium gelates the shell of the endothelial cell, whereas the shell is fluidized by high potassium. Blockade of the epithelial sodium channel (ENaC) with spironolactone (100%) or amiloride (84%) minimizes or stops many of these vascular endothelial responses and increases NO [30,31]. NO release follows endothelial nanomechanics and not vice versa and membrane depolarization decreases vascular endothelial cell stiffness that improves flow-mediated nitric oxide–dependent vasodilation [32]. In the presence of vascular inflammation and increased HSCRP, the effects of aldosterone on the ENaC are enhanced further increasing vascular stiffness and BP [33]. High sodium intake also abolishes the AT2R-mediated vasodilation immediately with complete abolition of endothelial vasodilation (EDV) within 30 days [34]. Thus, it has become clear that increased dietary sodium has adverse effects on the vascular system, BP and CVD, by altering the endothelial glycocalyx, which is a negatively charged biopolymer that lines the blood vessels and serves as a protective barrier against sodium overload, increased sodium permeability, and sodium-induced TOD [46]. Certain SNPs of SIK1 (salt-inducible kinase I), which alter Na^+/K^+ ATPase, determine sodium-induced hypertension and LVH [35].

The sodium intake per day in hypertensive patients should be between 1500 and 2000 mg. Sodium restriction improves BP reduction in those on patients that are on pharmacological treatment and the decrease in BP is additive with restriction of refined carbohydrates [36]. Reducing dietary sodium intake may reduce damage to the brain, heart, kidney, and vasculature through mechanisms dependent on the small BP reduction as well as those independent of the decreased BP [36].

A balance of sodium with other nutrients, especially potassium, magnesium, and calcium, is important, not only in reducing and controlling BP, but also in decreasing cardiovascular and cerebrovascular events [36]. An increase in the sodium to potassium ratio is associated with significantly increased risk of CVD and all-cause mortality [36].

18.4.1.2 Potassium

The average U.S. dietary intake of potassium (K^+) is 45 mmol/day with a potassium to sodium (K^+/Na^+) ratio of less than 1:2 [10]. The recommended intake of K^+ is 4700 mg day (120 mmol) with a K^+/Na^+ ratio of about 4–5 to 1 [10]. Numerous epidemiological, observational, and clinical trials have demonstrated a significant reduction in BP with increased dietary K^+ intake in both normotensive and hypertensive patients [10]. The average BP reduction with a K^+ supplementation of 60–120 mmol/day is 4.4/2.5 mm Hg in hypertensive patients but may be as much as 8/4.1 mm Hg with 120 mmol/day (4700 mg) [10,37,38]. In hypertensive patients, the linear dose–response relationship is 1.0 mm Hg reduction in SBP and 0.52 mm Hg reduction in diastolic BP per 0.6 g/day increase in dietary potassium intake that is independent of baseline dietary potassium ingestion [38]. The response depends on race (black > white), sodium, magnesium, and calcium intake [10]. Alteration of the K^+/Na^+ ratio to a higher level is important for both antihypertensive as well as cardiovascular and cerebrovascular effects [37,38]. High potassium intake reduces the incidence of cardiovascular (CHD, MI) and cerebrovascular accidents independent of the BP reduction [37,38]. If the serum potassium is less than 4.0 meq/dL, there is an increased risk of CVD mortality, ventricular tachycardia, ventricular fibrillation, and CHF [10]. Red blood cell potassium is a better indication of total body stores and CVD risk than is serum potassium [10].

Potassium increases natriuresis, modulates baroreflex sensitivity, vasodilates, decreases the sensitivity to catecholamines and angiotensin II, increases sodium potassium ATPase and DNA synthesis in the vascular smooth muscle cells, and decreases SNS activity in cells with improved vascular function [38]. In addition, potassium increases bradykinin and urinary kallikrein, decreases NADPH oxidase, which lowers oxidative stress and inflammation, improves insulin sensitivity, decreases ADMA, reduces intracellular sodium, and lowers the production of TGF-β [38].

Each 1000 mg increase in potassium intake per day reduces all-cause mortality by approximately 20%. Potassium intake of 4.7 g/day is estimated to decrease CVA by 8%–15% and MI by 6%–11% [38]. Numerous SNPs such as nuclear receptor subfamily 3 group C (NR3C2), angiotensin II type receptor (AGTR1), and hydroxysteroid 11 beta dehydrogenase (HSD11β1 and β2) determine an individual's response to dietary potassium intake [39]. Each 1000 mg decrease in sodium intake per day will decrease all-cause mortality by 20% [38]. A recent analysis suggested a dose-related response to CVA with urinary potassium excretion [40]. There was a RRR of CVA of 23% at 1.5–1.99 g, 27% at 2.0–2.49 g, 29% at 2.5–3 g, and 32% over 3 g/day of potassium urinary excretion [40]. The recommended daily dietary intake for patients with hypertension is 4.7–5.0 g of potassium and less than 1500 mg of sodium [10,38]. Potassium in food or from supplementation should be reduced or used with caution in those patients with renal impairment or those on medications that increase renal potassium retention such as ACEI, ARB, DRI, and SARA (serum aldosterone receptor antagonists) [41].

18.4.1.3 Magnesium (Mg^{2+})

A high dietary intake of magnesium of at least 500–1000 mg/day reduces BP, but the results are less consistent than those seen with Na^+ and K^+ [42]. In most epidemiological studies, there is an inverse relationship between dietary magnesium intake and BP [42,43]. The maximum reduction in clinical trials has been 5.6/2.8 mm Hg but some studies have shown no change in BP [43]. The combination of high potassium and low sodium intake with increased magnesium intake had additive antihypertensive effects [43]. Magnesium also increases the effectiveness of all antihypertensive drug classes [43].

Magnesium competes with Na^+ for binding sites on vascular smooth muscle and acts as a direct vasodilator, like a CCB. Magnesium increases PGE (prostaglandin E), regulates intracellular calcium, sodium, potassium, and pH, increases NO, improves endothelial function, reduces HS CRP, A-II, and norepinephrine. Magnesium binds in a necessary-cooperative manner with potassium, inducing EDV and BP reduction, inhibits nuclear factor Kb, and reduces oxidative stress [43–45].

A meta-analysis of 241,378 patients with 6,477 strokes showed an inverse relationship of dietary magnesium to the incidence of ischemic stroke [46]. For each 100 mg of dietary magnesium intake, ischemic stroke was decreased by 8%. A meta-analysis showed reductions in BP of 3–4/2–3 mm Hg in 22 trials of 1173 patients [46]. Magnesium may be supplemented in doses of 500–1000 mg/day chelated to an amino acid to improve absorption and decrease the incidence of diarrhea [43]. Adding taurine at 1000–2000 mg/day will enhance the antihypertensive effects of magnesium [43].

Magnesium supplements should be avoided or used with caution in patients with known renal insufficiency or in those taking medications that induce magnesium retention [43].

18.4.1.4 Zinc (Zn^{2+})

Low serum zinc levels in observational studies correlate with hypertension as well as CHD [47]. Zinc is transported into cardiac and vascular muscle and other tissues by metallothionein [47]. Genetic deficiencies of metallothionein with intramuscular zinc deficiencies may lead to hypertension [47]. There is an inverse correlation of BP and serum Zn^{2+} and Zn^{2+}-dependent enzyme-lysyl oxidase activity. Zn^{2+} inhibits gene expression and transcription through NF-κB and activated protein-1 (AP-1) and is an important cofactor for superoxide dismutase [47]. These effects as well as those on the RAAS and SNS effects may account for Zn^{2+} antihypertensive effects [47]. Zinc intake should be 50 mg/day.

18.4.2 Protein

Observational and epidemiologic studies demonstrate a consistent association between a high protein intake and a reduction in BP, incident BP, and stroke [48,49]. Animal protein is less effective than nonanimal or plant protein [48,49]. In the Inter-Salt Study of over 10,000 subjects, those with a dietary protein intake 30% above the mean had a lower BP by 3.0/2.5 mm Hg compared to those that were 30% below the mean (81 g versus 44 g/day) [48]. However, lean or wild animal protein with less saturated fat and more essential omega-3 fatty acids may reduce BP, lipids, and CHD risk [72,75]. Soy protein and milk protein also reduce BP [48,49]. Office BP was decreased by 4.9/2.7 mm Hg in those given a combination of 25% protein intake versus the control group given 15% protein in an isocaloric manner [50]. The daily recommended intake of protein from all sources is 1.0–1.5 g/kg body weight, varying with exercise level, age, renal function, and other factors [36].

Fermented milk supplemented with whey protein concentrate significantly reduces BP in human studies [51,52]. Administration of 20–30 g/day of hydrolyzed whey protein supplement rich in bioactive peptides significantly reduced BP over 6–8 weeks by 8–11/6–7 mm Hg [51–53]. Milk peptides that contain both caseins and whey proteins are a rich source of ACEI peptides. Val–Pro–Pro and Ile–Pro–Pro given at 5–60 mg/day have variable reductions in BP with an average decrease in pooled studies of about 1.28–4.8/0.59–2.2 mm Hg [51–53]. Milk peptides are beneficial in treating metabolic syndrome [53]. The clinical response is attributed to fermented milk's active peptides that inhibit ACE. Bovine casein–derived peptides and whey protein–derived peptides exhibit ACEI activity [51–53]. These components include B-caseins, B-lg fractions, B2-microglobulin, and serum albumin. The enzymatic hydrolysis of whey protein isolates releases ACEI peptides.

Marine collagen peptides (MCPs) from deep sea fish have antihypertensive activity [53,54]. Bonito protein (*Sarda orientalis*), from the tuna and mackerel family, has natural ACEI inhibitory peptides and reduces BP 10.2/7 mm Hg at 1.5 g/day [53,54].

Sardine muscle protein, which contains Valyl-Tyrosine (Val-Tyr), significantly lowers BP in hypertensive subjects [55]. Kawasaki et al. treated 29 hypertensive subjects with 3 mg of Valyl-Tyrosine sardine muscle concentrated extract for 4 weeks and lowered BP 9.7/5.3 mm Hg ($p < 0.05$) [55]. Valyl-Tyrosine is a natural ACEI. A similar study with a vegetable drink with sardine protein hydrolysates significantly lowered BP by 8/5 mm Hg in 13 weeks [56].

Soy protein lowers BP in hypertensive patients in most studies [57–59]. Soy protein intake was significantly and inversely associated with both SBP and DBP in 45,694 Chinese women consuming 25 g/day or more of soy protein over 3 years and the association increased with age [57]. The SBP reduction was 1.9–4.9 mm lower and the DBP 0.9–2.2 mm Hg lower [57]. However, randomized clinical trials and meta-analysis have shown mixed results on BP with no change in BP to reductions of 7%–10% for SBP and DBP [57–59]. The recent meta-analysis of 27 trials found a significant reduction in BP of 2.21/1.44 mm Hg [58]. Fermented soy at about 25 g/day is recommended. The optimal protein intake, depending on the level of activity, renal function, stress and other factors, is about 1.0–1.5 g/kg/day.

18.4.3 Amino Acids and Related Compounds

18.4.3.1 L-Arginine

L-Arginine and endogenous methylarginines are the primary precursors for the production of NO, which has numerous beneficial cardiovascular effects, mediated through the conversion of L-arginine to NO by eNOS. Patients with hypertension have increased levels of HSCRP and inflammation, increased microalbumin, low levels of apelin (stimulates NO in the endothelium), increased levels of arginase (breaks down arginine), and elevated serum levels of ADMA, which inactivates NO [108–112].

Human studies in hypertensive and normotensive subjects of parenteral and oral administrations of L-arginine demonstrate an antihypertensive effect given alone or with NAC [60,61]. The BP decreases by 6.2/6.8 mm Hg on 10 g/day of L-arginine when provided as a supplement or though natural foods to a group of hypertensive subjects [60,61]. Arginine produces a statistically and biologically significant decrease in BP and improved metabolic effect in normotensive and hypertensive humans that is similar in magnitude to that seen in the DASH-I diet [60,61]. A meta-analysis of 11 trials with 383 subjects administered arginine 4–24 g/day found average reduction in BP of 5.39/2.66 mm Hg ($p < 0.001$) in 4 weeks [62]. Although these doses of L-arginine appear to be safe, no long-term studies in humans have been published at this time and there are concerns of a pro-oxidative effect or even an increase in mortality in patients who may have severely dysfunctional endothelium, advanced atherosclerosis, CHD, ACS, or MI [63]. In addition to the arginine-NO path, there exists a nitrate/nitrite pathway that is related to dietary nitrates from vegetables, beetroot juice, and the DASH diet that are converted to nitrites by symbiotic, salivary, GI, and oral bacteria [64]. Administration of beetroot juice or extract at 500 mg/day will increase nitrites and lower BP, improve endothelial function, and increase cerebral, coronary, and peripheral blood flow [64].

18.4.3.2 L-Carnitine and Acetyl-L-Carnitine

L-Carnitine is a nitrogenous constituent of muscle primarily involved in the oxidation of fatty acids in mammals that improves endothelial function, NO, and oxidative defense, while oxidative stress and BP are reduced [65,66].

Human studies on the effects of L-carnitine and acetyl-L-carnitine are limited, with minimal to no change in BP [67–69]. In patients with metabolic syndrome, acetyl-L-carnitine at 1 g bid over 8 weeks reduced SBP by 7–9 mm Hg, but diastolic BP was significantly decreased only in those with higher glucose [69]. Low carnitine levels are associated with a nondipping BP pattern in type 2 DM [70]. Doses of 2–3 g twice/day are recommended.

18.4.3.3 Taurine

Taurine is a sulfonic beta-amino acid that is considered a conditionally essential amino acid, with its highest concentration in the brain, retina, and myocardium [71]. In cardiomyocytes, it represents about 50% of the free amino acids and has a role of an osmoregulator, inotropic factor, and antihypertensive agent [72].

Human studies have noted that essential hypertensive subjects have reduced urinary taurine as well as other sulfur amino acids [71,72]. Taurine lowers BP, SVR HR, and SNS activity, increases urinary sodium and water excretion, increases NO, improves endothelial function, decreases A-II, PRA, aldosterone, intracellular calcium and sodium, and has antioxidant, antiatherosclerotic and anti-inflammatory activities [71]. Fujita et al. [72] demonstrated a reduction in BP of 9/4.1 mm Hg ($p < 0.05$) in 19 hypertension subjects given 6 g of taurine for 7 days. The BP reductions range from 9–14.8/4.1 to 6.6 mm Hg [71,72]. The recommended dose of taurine is 2–3 g/day at which no adverse effects are noted, but higher doses up to 6 g/day may be needed to reduce BP significantly [71,72].

18.4.4 Omega-3 Fats

The omega-3 fatty acids found in cold water fish, fish oils, flax, flax seed, flax oil, and nuts lower BP in observational, epidemiological, and in prospective clinical trials [73–80].

DHA at 2 g/day reduced BP 8/5 mm Hg and heart rate by 6 beats/min in 6 weeks [73]. Fish oil at 4–9 g/day or combination of DHA and EPA at 3–5 g/day reduces BP [73–80]. Eating cold water fish 3 times/week may be as effective as high-dose fish oil in reducing BP in hypertensive patients, and the protein in the fish may also have antihypertensive effects [73].

The omega-3 FA increase eNOS and NO, improve ED, reduce calcium influx, reduce plasma norepinephrine, increase parasympathetic nervous system tone, and suppress ACE activity [73–80]. The recommended daily dose is 3000–5000 mg/day of combined DHA and EPA in a ratio of three parts EPA to two parts DHA and about 50% of this dose as GLA combined with gamma/delta tocopherol at 100 mg/g of DHA and EPA to get the omega-3 index to 8% to reduce BP and provide optimal cardioprotection [78]. DHA is more effective than EPA for reducing BP and should be given at 2 g/day if administered alone [73,74].

18.4.4.1 Omega-9 Fats

Olive oil is rich in the omega-9 monounsaturated fat (MUFA) oleic acid, which has been associated with BP reduction in Mediterranean and other diets [81–86]. Olive oil and monounsaturated fats have shown consistent reductions in BP in most clinical studies in humans [81–86]. The SBP is reduced 8 mm Hg ($p \leq 0.05$) and the DBP is decreased by 6 mm Hg ($p \leq 0.01$) in both clinic and 24 h ambulatory BP monitoring in the MUFA-treated subjects compared to the PUFA-treated subjects [81–86]. In stage I hypertensive patients, oleuropein-olive leaf (*Olea eurpoaea*) extract 500 mg bid for 8 weeks reduced BP 11.5/4.8 mm Hg, which was similar to captopril 25 mg bid [85]. Olive oil intake in the EPIC study of 20,343 subjects was inversely associated with both systolic and diastolic BP [82]. Olive oil inhibits the AT1R receptor, exerts L-type calcium channel antagonist effects, and improves wave reflections and augmentation index [86].

Extra virgin olive oil (EVOO) also contains lipid-soluble phytonutrients such as polyphenols. Approximately 5 mg of phenols are found in 10 g of EVOO. About 4 tablespoons of extra virgin olive oil are equal to 40 g of EVOO, which is the amount required to get significant reductions in BP.

18.4.4.2 Fiber

The clinical trials with various types of fiber to reduce BP have been inconsistent [87,88]. Soluble fiber, guar gum, guava, psyllium, and oat bran may reduce BP and reduce the need for antihypertensive medications in hypertensive subjects, diabetic subjects, and hypertensive-diabetic subjects [87,88]. The average reduction in BP is about 7.5/5.5 mm Hg on 40–50 g/day of a mixed fiber. There is improvement in insulin sensitivity, endothelial function, reduction in SNS activity, and increase in renal sodium loss [87,88].

18.4.4.3 Vitamin C

Vitamin C is a potent water-soluble electron donor. At physiological doses, vitamin C recycles vitamin E, improves ED, and produces a diuresis [89–95]. Dietary intake of vitamin C and plasma ascorbate concentration in humans is inversely correlated to SBP, DBP, and heart rate [89–95].

An evaluation of published clinical trials indicates that vitamin C dosing at 250 mg twice daily will significantly lower BP 5–7/2–4 mm Hg over 8 weeks [89–95]. Vitamin C will induce a sodium water diuresis, improve arterial compliance, improve endothelial function, increase NO and PGI2, decrease adrenal steroid production, improve sympathovagal balance, increase RBC Na/K ATPase, increase superoxide dismutase, improve aortic elasticity and compliance, improve flow-mediated vasodilation, decrease pulse wave velocity and augmentation index, increase cyclic GMP, activate potassium channels, reduce cytosolic calcium, and reduce serum aldehydes [89–95].

Vitamin C enhances the efficacy of amlodipine, decreases the binding affinity of the AT1 receptor for angiotensin II by disrupting the ATR1 disulfide bridges, and enhances the antihypertensive effects of medications in the elderly with refractory hypertension [92–94]. In elderly patients with refractory hypertension already on maximum pharmacologic therapy, 600 mg of vitamin C daily lowered the BP by 20/16 mm Hg [94]. The lower the initial ascorbate serum level, the better is the BP response. A serum level of 100 μmol/L is recommended [89–95]. The SBP and 24 ABM show the most significant reductions with chronic oral administration of vitamin C [89–95]. In a meta-analysis of 13 clinical trials with 284 patients, vitamin C at 500 mg/day over 6 weeks reduced BP 3.9/2.1 mm Hg [95].

18.4.4.4 Vitamin E

Most studies have not shown reductions in BP with most forms of tocopherols or tocotrienols [36]. Patients with type 2 diabetes mellitus and controlled hypertension (130/76 mm Hg) on prescription medications with an average BP of 136/76 mm Hg were administered mixed tocopherols containing 60% gamma, 25% delta, and 15% alpha tocopherols [96]. The BP actually increased by 6.8/3.6 mm Hg in the study patients ($p < 0.0001$) but was less compared to those that received alpha tocopherol (7/5.3 mm Hg, $p < 0.0001$). This may be a reflection of drug interactions with tocopherols via cytochrome P 450 (3A4 and 4F2) and reduction in the serum levels of the pharmacological treatments that were simultaneously being given [96]. Gamma tocopherol may have natriuretic effects by the inhibition of the 70pS potassium channel in the thick ascending limb of the loop of Henle and lower BP [97]. Both alpha and gamma tocopherol improve insulin sensitivity and enhance adiponectin expression via PPAR gamma-dependent processes, which have the potential to lower BP and serum glucose [98]. If vitamin E has an antihypertensive effect, it is probably small.

18.4.4.5 Vitamin D

Vitamin D3 may have an independent and direct role in the regulation of BP [99–104]. If the vitamin D level is below 30 ng/mL, the circulating PRA levels and angiotensin II are higher [99–185]. The lower the level of vitamin D, the greater the risk of hypertension, with the lowest quartile of serum vitamin D having a 52% incidence of hypertension and the highest quartile having a 20% incidence [99–104]. Vitamin D3 markedly suppresses renin transcription by a VDR-mediated mechanism via the JGA apparatus. Vitamin D lowers asymmetric dimethyl arginine (ADMA), suppresses pro-inflammatory cytokines such as TNF alpha, increases NO, improves endothelial function and arterial elasticity, decreases vascular smooth muscle hypertrophy, regulates electrolytes and blood volume, and lowers HS-CRP [99–104].

Although vitamin D deficiency is associated with hypertension in observational studies, randomized clinical trials and their meta-analysis have yielded inconclusive results [103]. In addition, vitamin D receptor gene polymorphisms may affect the risk of hypertension in men [104]. A 25 hydroxyvitamin D level of 60 ng/mL is recommended.

18.4.4.6 Vitamin B6 (Pyridoxine)

Low serum vitamin B6 (pyridoxine) levels are associated with hypertension in humans [105]. One human study by Aybak et al. [106] proved that high-dose vitamin B6 at 5 mg/kg/day for 4 weeks significantly lowered BP by 14/10 mm Hg. Pyridoxine (vitamin B6) is a cofactor in neurotransmitter and hormone synthesis in the central nervous system (norepinephrine, epinephrine, serotonin, GABA, and kynurenine), increases cysteine synthesis to neutralize aldehydes, enhances the production of glutathione, blocks calcium channels, decreases central sympathetic tone, and reduces end organ responsiveness to glucocorticoids and mineralocorticoids [107,108]. Vitamin B6 is reduced with chronic diuretic therapy and heme pyrollactams (HPU). Vitamin B6 thus has similar action to central alpha agonists, diuretics, and CCB. The recommended dose is 200 mg/day orally.

18.4.4.7 Flavonoids

Over 4000 naturally occurring flavonoids have been identified in such diverse substances as fruits, vegetables, red wine, tea, soy, and licorice [109]. Flavonoids (flavonols, flavones, and isoflavones) are potent free radical scavengers that inhibit lipid peroxidation, prevent atherosclerosis, promote vascular relaxation, and have antihypertensive properties [109,110].

Resveratrol is a potent antioxidant and antihypertensive found in the skin of red grapes and in red wine. Resveratrol administration to humans reduces augmentation index, improves arterial compliance, and lowers central arterial pressure when administered as 250 mL of either regular or dealcoholized red wine [111]. The central arterial pressure was significantly reduced by dealcoholized red wine at 7.4 and 5.4 mm Hg by regular red wine. Resveratrol increases flow-mediated vasodilation in a dose-related manner, improves ED, prevents uncoupling of eNOS, increases adiponectin, lowers HS-CRP, and blocks the effects of angiotensin II [112,113]. The recommended dose is 250 mg/day of *trans* resveratrol [112].

18.4.4.8 Lycopene

Lycopene is a fat-soluble carotenoid found in tomatoes, guava, pink grapefruit, watermelon, apricots, and papaya in high concentrations that show a significant reduction in BP and oxidative stress markers in most studies [114–117]. Paran and Engelhard [117] administered 10 mg of lycopene to subjects with Grade I hypertension over 8 weeks with a reduction in BP of 9/7 mm Hg ($p < 0.01$). A tomato extract given to 31 hypertensive subjects reduced BP reduction 10/4 mm Hg [114]. Patients on various antihypertensive agents including ACEI, CCB, and diuretics had additional BP reduction of 5.4/3 mm Hg in 6 weeks when administered a standardized tomato extract [115]. Lycopene and tomato extract improve ED and reduce plasma total oxidative stress [114–117]. The recommended daily intake of lycopene is 10–20 mg in food or supplement form.

18.4.4.9 Pycnogenol

Pycnogenol, a bark extract from the French maritime pine, at doses of 200 mg/day reduced BP 7.2/1.8 mm Hg ($p < 0.05$) [118–120]. Pycnogenol acts as a natural ACEI, protects cell membranes from oxidative stress, increases NO and improves endothelial function, and decreases HS-CRP [118–120]. Other studies have shown reductions in BP and a decreased need for ACEI and CCB and decreased endothelin-1 and myeloperoxidase [118–120].

18.4.4.10 Garlic

Clinical trials have shown consistent reductions in BP with garlic in hypertensive patients with an average reduction in BP of 8.4/7.3 mm Hg [121–123]. Cultivated garlic (*Allium sativum*), wild uncultivated garlic or bear garlic (*Allium urisinum*), and aged garlic are the most effective [121–123]. Garlic is also effective in reducing BP in patients with uncontrolled hypertension already on antihypertensive medication [121–123]. A garlic homogenate-based supplement was administered to 34 prehypertensive and stage I hypertensive patients at 300 mg/day over 12 weeks with a reduction in BP of 6.6–7.5/4.6–5.2 mm Hg [122]. Aged garlic at doses of 240–960 mg/day given to 79 hypertensive subjects over 12 weeks significantly lowered SBP 11.8 ± 5.4 mm Hg in the high-dose garlic group [123]. The overall net reduction in BP of 10–12/6–9 mm Hg in all clinical trials with garlic [121–123]. Garlic has ACEI activity, CCB activity, reduces catecholamine sensitivity, improves arterial compliance, and increases bradykinin and NO [121–123].

18.4.4.11 Seaweed

Wakame seaweed (*Undaria pinnatifida*) the most popular, edible seaweed in Japan [124–126] at doses of 3.3 g/day significantly reduced BP 14/5 mm Hg ($p < 0.01$) [125]. A potassium-loaded, ion-exchange, sodium-adsorbing, potassium-releasing seaweed preparation reduced the MAP 11.2 mm Hg ($p < 0.001$) in the sodium-sensitive subjects and 5.7 mm Hg ($p < 0.05$) in the sodium-insensitive subjects [126].

Seaweed and sea vegetables contain most all of the seawater's 77I minerals and rare earth elements, fiber, and alginate in a colloidal form [124–126]. The primary effect of Wakame appears to be through its ACEI activity [127]. Its long-term use in Japan has demonstrated its safety.

18.4.4.12 Sesame

Sesame has been shown to reduce BP [128–135] when given alone [169–173] or in combination with nifedipine [132] diuretics and beta blockers [129]. A dose of 60 mg of sesamin for 4 weeks lowered BP 3.5/1.9 mm Hg ($p < 0.045$) [130]. Black sesame meal at 2.52 g/day reduced SBP by 8.3 mm Hg ($p < 0.05$) but there was a nonsignificant reduction in DBP of 4.2 mm Hg [131]. Sesame oil at 35 g/day significantly lowered central BP within 1 h and also maintained BP reduction chronically in 30 hypertensive subjects with reduced heart rate, arterial stiffness, augmentation index, pulse wave velocity, HSCRP and ET-1 with increased NO and antioxidant capacity [135]. The active ingredients are natural ACEIs such as sesamin, sesamolin, sesaminol glucosides, and furoufuran lignans that are also suppressors of NF-κB [134].

18.4.4.13 Beverages: Tea, Coffee, and Cocoa

Green tea, black tea, and extracts of active components in both have demonstrated reduction in BP in humans [136–140]. In a double-blind placebo-controlled trial of 379 hypertensive subjects given green tea extract 370 mg/day for 3 months, BP was reduced significantly at 4/4 mm Hg with simultaneous decrease in HS CRP [139].

Dark chocolate (100 g) and *cocoa* with a high content of polyphenols (30 mg or more) have been shown to significantly reduce BP in humans [141–147]. A meta-analysis of 173 hypertensive subjects given cocoa for a mean duration of 2 weeks had a significant reduction in BP 4.7/2.8 mm Hg ($p = 0.002$) [141]. Cocoa at 30 mg of polyphenols reduced BP in prehypertensive and stage I hypertensive patients by 2.9/1.9 mm Hg at 18 weeks ($p < 0.001$) [142]. Two more recent meta-analysis of 13 trials and 10 trials with 297 patients found a significant reduction in BP of 3.2/2.0 and 4.5/3.2 mm Hg, respectively [143,145]. The BP reduction is the greatest in those with the highest baseline BP and those with at least 50%–70% cocoa at doses of 6–100 g/day [143,145,146]. Cocoa may also improve insulin resistance and endothelial function [147].

Polyphenols, chlorogenic acids (CGAs), the ferulic acid metabolite of CGAs, and dihydrocaffeic acids decrease BP in a dose-dependent manner, increase eNOS, and improve endothelial function in humans [148–150]. CGAs in green coffee been extract at doses of 140 mg/day significantly reduced BP in 28 subjects in a placebo-controlled randomized clinical trial [148]. A study of 122 male subjects demonstrated a dose response in BP with doses of CGA from 46 to 185 mg/day [149]. The group that received the 185 mg dose had a significant reduction in BP of 5.6/3.9 mm Hg ($p < 0.01$). Hydroxyhydroquinone is another component of coffee beans, which reduces the efficacy of CGAs in a dose-dependent manner that partially explains the conflicting results of coffee ingestion on BP [150]. Furthermore, there is genetic variation in the enzyme responsible for the metabolism of caffeine modifies the association between coffee intake, amount of coffee ingested and the risk of hypertension, heart rate, MI, arterial stiffness, arterial wave reflections, and urinary catecholamine levels [151]. Fifty-nine percent of the population has the IF/IA allele of the CYP1A2 genotype that confers slow metabolism of caffeine. Heavy coffee drinkers who are slow metabolizers had a 3.00 hazard ratio (HR) for developing hypertension. In contrast, fast metabolizers with the IA/IA allele have a 0.36 HR for incident hypertension [151].

18.4.4.14 Additional Compounds

Melatonin demonstrates significant antihypertensive effects in humans in a numerous double-blind randomized placebo-controlled clinical trials at 3–5 mg/day [152–155]. The average reduction in BP is 6/3 mm Hg. Melatonin stimulates GABA receptors in the CNS and vascular melatonin receptors, inhibits plasma A II levels, improves endothelial function, increases NO, vasodilates, improves nocturnal dipping, lowers cortisol, and is additive with ARBs. Beta blockers reduce melatonin secretion [155].

Hesperidin significantly lowered DBP 3–4 mm Hg ($p < 0.02$) and improved microvascular endothelial reactivity in 24 obese hypertensive male subjects in a randomized, controlled crossover study over 4 weeks for each of three treatment groups consuming 500 mL of orange juice, hesperidin, or placebo [156].

Pomegranate juice is rich in tannins and has numerous other properties that improve vascular health and reduce the SBP by 5%–12% [157,158]. A study of 51 healthy subjects given 330 mg/day of pomegranate juice had reduction in BP of 3.14/2.33 mm Hg ($p < 0.001$) [158]. Pomegranate juice also suppresses the postprandial increase in SBP following a high-fat meal [158]. Pomegranate juice reduces serum ACE activity by 36% and has antiatherogenic, antioxidant, and anti-inflammatory effects [157–159]. Pomegranate juice at 50 mL/day reduced carotid IMT by 30% over 1 year, increased PON 83%, decreased oxLDL by 59%–90%, decreased antibodies to oxLDL by 19%, increased total antioxidant status by 130%, reduced TGF-β, increased catalase, SOD, and GPx, increased eNOS and NO, and improved endothelial function [157–159]. Pomegranate juice works like an ACEI.

Grape seed extract (GSE) was administered to subjects in nine randomized trials, meta-analysis of 390 subjects, and demonstrated a significant reduction in SBP of 1.54 mm Hg ($p < 0.02$) [160–162]. Significant reduction in BP of 11/8 mm Hg ($p < 0.05$) was seen in another dose–response study with 150–300 mg/day of GSE over 4 weeks [161]. GSE has high phenolic content that activates the PI3K/Akt signaling pathway that phosphorylates eNOS and increases NO [161,162].

18.4.4.15 Coenzyme Q10 (Ubiquinone)

Coenzyme Q10 has consistent and significant antihypertensive effects in patients with essential hypertension [163–168]. Compared to normotensive patients, essential hypertensive patients have a higher incidence (sixfold) of coenzyme Q10 deficiency documented by serum levels [163–168]. Doses of 120–225 mg/day of coenzyme Q10 are necessary to achieve a therapeutic level of 3 μg/mL [163–168]. This dose is usually 3–5 mg/kg/day of coenzyme Q10. Patients with the lowest coenzyme Q10 serum levels may have the best antihypertensive response to supplementation [163–168]. The average reduction in BP is about 15/10 mm Hg and heart rate falls 5 beats/min based on reported studies and meta-analysis [163–168]. The antihypertensive effect takes time to reach its peak level at 4 weeks. Then the BP remains stable during long-term treatment. The antihypertensive effect is gone within 2 weeks after discontinuation of coenzyme Q10. The reductions in BP and SVR are correlated with the pretreatment and posttreatment serum levels of CoQ10. About 50% of patients respond to oral CoQ10 supplementation for BP [164].

Approximately 50% of patients on antihypertensive drugs may be able to stop between one and three agents. Both total dose and frequency of administration may be reduced.

Patients administered CoQ10 with enalapril improved the 24 h ABM better than with enalapril monotherapy and also normalized endothelial function [169]. CoQ10 is a lipid-phase antioxidant and free radical scavenger, increases eNOS and NO, reduces inflammation and NF-κB, and improves endothelial function and vascular elasticity [165,166].

18.4.4.16 Alpha Lipoic Acid

Alpha lipoic acid (ALA) is a sulfur-containing compound with antioxidant activity that is effective in hypertension, especially as part of the metabolic syndrome [170–173]. In a double-blind crossover study of 36 patients over 8 weeks with CHD and hypertension, 200 mg of lipoic acid with 500 mg of acetyl-L-carnitine significantly reduced BP 7/3 mm Hg and increased brachial artery diameter [170]. The QUALITY study of 40 patients with DM and stage I hypertension showed significant improvements in BP, urinary albumin excretion and with a combination of quinapril (40 mg/day) and lipoic acid (600 mg/day) that was greater than either alone [172]. Lipoic acid increases levels of glutathione, cysteine, vitamin C and vitamin E, inhibits NF-κB, reduces endothelin-1, tissue factor and VCAM-1, increases cAMP, downregulates CD4 immune expression on mononuclear cells, reduces oxidative stress, inflammation, reduces atherosclerosis in animal models, decreases serum aldehydes, and closes calcium channels that improve vasodilation, increases NO and nitrosothiols, improves endothelial function, and lowers BP [170–173]. Lipoic acid normalizes membrane calcium channels by providing sulfhydryl groups, decreasing cytosolic free calcium, and lowering SVR. Morcos et al. [173] showed the stabilization of urinary albumin excretion in DM subjects given 600 mg of ALA compared to placebo for 18 months ($p < 0.05$). The recommended dose is 100–200 mg/day of R-lipoic acid with biotin 2–4 mg/day to prevent biotin depletion with long-term use of lipoic acid.

18.4.5 *N*-Acetyl Cysteine

N-Acetyl cysteine (NAC) and L-arginine (ARG) in combination significantly reduce endothelial activation and BP in hypertensive patients with type 2 DM [174]. In addition, HSCRP, ICAM, and VCAM were decreased while NO and endothelial postischemic vasodilation increased [174]. NAC increases NO via IL-1B and increases iNOS mRNA, increases glutathione by increasing cysteine levels, reduces the affinity for the AT1 receptor by disrupting disulfide groups, and blocks the L-type calcium channel [174–176]. The recommended dose is 500–1000 mg bid.

18.4.6 Hawthorn

Hawthorn extract has been used for centuries for the treatment of hypertension, CHF, and other CVDs [177–179]. A recent 4-period crossover design, dose–response study in 21 subjects with pre-hypertension or mild hypertension over 3½ days did not show changes in FMD or BP on standardized extract with 50 mg of oligomeric procyanidin/250 mg extract with 1000, 1500 or 2500 mg of the extract [177]. Patients with hypertension and type 2 DM on medications for BP and DM were randomized to 1200 mg of hawthorn extract for 16 weeks showing significant reductions in DBP of 2.6 mm Hg ($p = 0.035$) [178]. Thirty-six mildly hypertensive patients were administered 500 mg of hawthorn extract for 10 weeks and showed a nonsignificant trend in DBP reduction ($p = 0.081$) compared to placebo [179]. Hawthorn acts like an ACEI, BB, CCB, and diuretic. More studies are needed to determine the efficacy, long-term effects, and dose of Hawthorn for the treatment of hypertension.

18.4.7 Quercetin

Quercetin is an antioxidant flavonol found in apples, berries, and onions, which reduces BP in hypertensive individuals [180–182], but the hypotensive effects do not appear to be mediated by changes in HSCRP, TNF-alpha, ACE activity, ET-1, NO, vascular reactivity, or FMD [180]. Quercetin was administered to 12 hypertensive men at an oral dose of 1095 mg with reduction BP by 7/3 mm Hg [180]. Forty-one pre-hypertensive and stage I hypertensive subjects were enrolled in a randomized, double-blind, placebo-controlled, crossover study with 730 mg of quercetin per day versus placebo [181]. In the stage I hypertensive patients, the BP was reduced by 7/5 mm Hg ($p < 0.05$). Quercetin administered to 93 overweight or obese subjects at 150 mg/day over 6 weeks lowered SBP 2.9 mm Hg in the hypertensive group and up to 3.7 mm Hg in SBP in the patients 25–50 years of age [182]. The recommended dose of quercetin is 500 mg bid.

18.5 CLINICAL CONSIDERATIONS

18.5.1 Combining Food and Nutrients with Medications

Several of the strategic combinations of nutraceutical supplements together or with antihypertensive drugs have been shown to lower BP more than the medication alone:

- Sesame with beta blockers, diuretics, and nifedipine
- Pycnogenol with ACEI and CCB
- Lycopene with ACEI, CCB, and diuretics
- Alpha lipoic acid with ACEI or acetyl-L-carnitine
- Vitamin C with CCB
- *N*-Acetyl cysteine with arginine
- Garlic with ACEI, diuretics, and beta blockers
- Coenzyme Q10 with ACEI and CCB
- Taurine with magnesium
- Potassium with all antihypertensive agents
- Magnesium with all antihypertensive agents

Many antihypertensive drugs may cause nutrient depletions that can actually interfere with their antihypertensive action or cause other metabolic adverse effects manifest through the lab or with clinical symptoms [183–185]. Diuretics decrease potassium, magnesium, phosphorous, sodium, chloride, folate, vitamin B6, zinc, iodine, and coenzyme Q10; increase homocysteine, calcium and creatinine; and elevate serum glucose by inducing insulin resistance. Beta blockers reduce coenzyme Q10. ACEI and ARBs reduce zinc.

18.6 SUMMARY

- Vascular biology such as endothelial and vascular smooth muscle dysfunction plays a primary role in the initiation and perpetuation of hypertension, CVD, and TOD.
- Nutrient–gene interactions and epigenetics are a predominant factor in promoting beneficial or detrimental effects in cardiovascular health and hypertension.
- Food and nutrients can prevent, control, and treat hypertension through numerous vascular biology mechanisms.
- Oxidative stress, inflammation, and autoimmune dysfunction initiate and propagate hypertension and CVD.
- There is a role for the selected use of single and component nutraceutical supplements vitamins, antioxidants, and minerals in the treatment of hypertension based on scientifically controlled studies as a complement to optimal nutritional, dietary intake from food, and other lifestyle modifications.
- A clinical approach that incorporates diet, foods, nutrients, exercise, weight reduction, smoking cessation, alcohol and caffeine restriction, and other lifestyle strategies can be systematically and successfully incorporated into clinical practice (Table 18.3).

TABLE 18.3
An Integrative Approach to the Treatment of Hypertension

Intervention Category	Therapeutic Intervention	Daily Intake
Diet characteristics	DASH I, DASH II-Na+, or PREMIER diet	Diet type
	Sodium restriction	1500 mg
	Potassium	5000 mg
	Potassium/sodium ratio	>3:1
	Magnesium	1000 mg
	Zinc	50 mg
Macronutrients	*Protein*: Total intake from nonanimal sources, organic lean or wild animal protein, or coldwater fish	30% of total calories, which 1.5–1.8 g/kg body weight
	Whey protein	30 g
	Soy protein (fermented sources are preferred)	30 g
	Sardine muscle concentrate extract	3 g
	Milk peptides (VPP and IPP)	30–60 mg
	Fat	30% of total calories
	Omega-3 fatty acids	2–3 g
	Omega-6 fatty acids	1 g
	Omega-9 fatty acids	2–4 tablespoons of olive or nut oil or 10–20 olives
	Saturated fatty acids from wild game, bison, or other lean meat	<10% total calories
	Polyunsaturated to saturated fat ratio	>2.0
	Omega 3 to omega 6 ratio	1.1–1.2
	Synthetic *trans* fatty acids	None (completely remove from diet)
	Nuts in variety	*Ad libitum*
	Carbohydrates as primarily complex carbohydrates and fiber	40% of total calories
	Oatmeal or	60 g
	Oatbran or	40 g
	Beta-glucan or	3 g
	Psyllium	7 g
Specific foods	Garlic as fresh cloves or aged Kyolic garlic	4 fresh cloves (4 g) or 600 mg aged garlic taken twice daily
	Sea vegetables, specifically dried wakame	3.0–3.5 g
	Lycopene as tomato products, guava, watermelon, apricots, pink grapefruit, papaya or supplements	10–20 mg
	Dark chocolate	100 g
	Pomegranate juice or seeds	8 ounces or one cup
	Sesame	60 mg sesamin or 2.5 g sesame meal
Exercise	Aerobic	20 min daily at 4200 kJ/week
	Resistance	40 min/day
Weight reduction	Body mass index < 25 Waist circumference: <35 in. for women <40 in. for men Total body fat: <22% for women <16% for men	Lose 1–2 lb/week and increasing the proportion of lean muscle

(Continued)

TABLE 18.3 (*Continued*)
An Integrative Approach to the Treatment of Hypertension

Intervention Category	Therapeutic Intervention	Daily Intake
Other lifestyle recommendations	Alcohol restriction:	<20 g/day
	Among the choice of alcohol red wine is preferred due to its vasoactive phytonutrients	Wine < 10 ounces
		Beer < 24 ounces
		Liquor < 2 ounces
	Caffeine restriction or elimination depending on CYP 450 type	<100 mg/day
	Tobacco and smoking	Stop
Medical considerations	Medications that may increase blood pressure.	Minimize use when possible, such as by using disease-specific nutritional interventions
Supplemental foods and nutrients	Alpha lipoic acid with biotin	100–200 mg twice daily
	Amino acids:	
	Arginine	5 g twice daily
	Carnitine	1–2 g twice daily
	Taurine	1–3 g twice daily
	Chlorogenic acids	150–200 mg
	Coenzyme Q10	100 mg once to twice daily
	Grape seed extract	300 mg
	Hawthorn extract	500 mg twice a day
	Melatonin	2.5 mg
	N-acetyl cysteine (NAC)	500 mg twice a day
	Olive leaf extract (oleuropein)	500 mg twice a day
	Pycnogenol	200 mg
	Quercetin	500 mg twice a day
	Resveratrol (*trans*)	250 mg
	Vitamin B6	100 mg once to twice daily
	Vitamin C	250–500 mg twice daily
	Vitamin D3	Dose to raise 25-hydroxyvitamin D serum level to 60 ng/mL
	Vitamin E as mixed tocopherols	400 IU

REFERENCES

1. Houston MC. Treatment of hypertension with nutraceuticals. Vitamins, antioxidants and minerals. *Exp Rev Cardiovasc Ther* 2007;5(4):681–691.
2. Eaton SB, Eaton SB III, Konner MJ. Paleolithic nutrition revisited: A twelve-year retrospective on its nature and implications. *Eur J Clin Nutr* 1997;51:207–216.
3. Houston MC, Harper KJ. Potassium, magnesium, and calcium: Their role in both the cause and treatment of hypertension. *J Clin Hypertens* 2008;10(7 Suppl 2):3–11.
4. Layne J, Majkova Z, Smart EJ, Toborek M, Hennig B. Caveolae: A regulatory platform for nutritional modulation of inflammatory diseases. *J Nutr Biochem* 2011;22:807–811.
5. Dandona P, Ghanim H, Chaudhuri A, Dhindsa S, Kim SS. Macronutrient intake induces oxidative and inflammatory stress: Potential relevance to atherosclerosis and insulin resistance. *Exp Mol Med* 2010;42(4):245–253.
6. Berdanier CD. Nutrient-gene interactions. In: Ziegler EE, Filer LJ Jr, eds. *Present Knowledge in Nutrition*, 7th edn. ILSI Press, Washington, DC, 1996, pp. 574–580.

7. Talmud PJ, Waterworth DM. In-vivo and in-vitro nutrient-gene interactions. *Curr Opin Lipidol* 2000;11:31–36.
8. Lundberg AM, Yan ZQ. Innate immune recognition receptors and damage-associated molecular patterns in plaque inflammation. *Curr Opin Lipidol* 2011;22(5):343–349.
9. Zhao L, Lee JY, Hwang DH. Inhibition of pattern recognition receptor-mediated inflammation by bioactive phytochemicals. *Nutr Rev* 2011;69(6):310–320.
10. Houston MC. The importance of potassium in managing hypertension. *Curr Hypertens Rep* 2011;13(4):309–317.
11. Eftekhari A, Mathiassen ON, Buus NH, Gotzsche O, Mulvany MJ, Christensen KL. Disproportionally impaired microvascular structure in essential hypertension. *J Hypertens* 2011;29(5):896–905.
12. Touyz RM. New insights into mechanisms of hypertension. *Curr Opin Nephrol Hypertens* 2012;21(2):119–121.
13. Xing T, Wang F, Li J, Wang N. Hypertension: An immunologic disease? *J Hypertens* 2012;30(12):2440–2441.
14. Giannattasio C, Cattaneo BM, Mangoni AA, Carugo S, Stella ML, Failla M, Trazzi S, Sega R, Grassi G, Mancia G. Cardiac and vascular structural changes in normotensive subjects with parental hypertension. *J Hypertens* 1995;13(2):259–264.
15. Goncharov A, Bloom M, Pavuk M, Birman I. Carpenter blood pressure and hypertension in relation to levels of serum polychlorinated biphenyls in residents of Anniston, Alabama. *DO Hypertens* 2010;28(10):2053–2060.
16. Houston MC. Role of mercury toxicity in hypertension, cardiovascular disease, and stroke. *J Clin Hypertens (Greenwich)* 2011;13(8):621–627.
17. Al-Ghamdi A. Role of herpes simplex virus-1, cytomegalovirus and Epstein-Barr virus in atherosclerosis. *Pak J Pharm Sci* January 2012;25(1):89–97.
18. Kotronias D, Kapranos N. Herpes simplex virus as a determinant risk factor for coronary artery atherosclerosis and myocardial infarction. *In Vivo* 2005;19(2):351–357.
19. Grahame-Clarke C, Chan NN, Andrew D, Ridgway GL, Betteridge DJ, Emery V, Colhoun HM, Vallance P. Human cytomegalovirus seropositivity is associated with impaired vascular function. *Circulation* August 12, 2003;108(6):678–683 [Epub August 4, 2003].
20. Nayak DU, Karmen C, Frishman WH, Vakili BA. Antioxidant vitamins and enzymatic and synthetic oxygen-derived free radical scavengers in the prevention and treatment of cardiovascular disease. *Heart Disease* 2001;3:28–45.
21. Kizhakekuttu TJ, Widlansky ME. Natural antioxidants and hypertension: Promise and challenges. *Cardiovasc Ther* 2010;28(4):e20–e32.
22. Kitiyakara C, Wilcox C. Antioxidants for hypertension. *Curr Opin Nephrol Hypertens* 1998;7:531–538.
23. Russo C, Olivieri O, Girelli D, Faccini G, Zenari ML, Lombardi S, Corrocher R. Antioxidant status and lipid peroxidation in patients with essential hypertension. *J Hypertens* 1998;16:1267–1271.
24. Tse WY, Maxwell SR, Thomason H, Blann A, Thorpe GH, Waite M, Holder R. Antioxidant status in controlled and uncontrolled hypertension and its relationship to endothelial damage. *J Hum Hypertens* 1994;8:843–849.
25. Mansego ML , Solar Gde M, Alonso MP, Martinez F, Saez GT, Escudero JC, Redon J, Chaves FJ. Polymorphisms of antioxidant enzymes, blood pressure and risk of hypertension. *J Hypertens* 2011;29(3):492–500.
26. Galley HF, Thornton J, Howdle PD, Walker BE, Webster NR. Combination oral antioxidant supplementation reduces blood pressure. *Clin Sci* 1997;92:361–365.
27. Broadhurst CL. Balanced intakes of natural triglycerides for optimum nutrition: An evolutionary and phytochemical perspective. *Med Hypotheses* 1997;49:247–261.
28. Dhalla NS, Temsah RM, Netticadam T. The role of oxidative stress in cardiovascular diseases. *J Hypertens* 2000;18:655–673.
29. Saez G, Tormos MC, Giner V, Lorano JV, Chaves FJ. Oxidative stress and enzymatic antioxidant mechanisms in essential hypertension. *Am J Hypertens* 2001;14:248A (Abstract P-653).
30. Nishihara M, Hirooka Y, Matsukawa R, Kishi T, Sunagawa K. Oxidative stress in the rostral ventrolateral medulla modulates excitatory and inhibitory inputs in spontaneously hypertensive rats. *J Hypertens* 2012;30(1):97–106.
31. Konno S, Hirooka Y, Kishi T, Sunagawa K. Sympathoinhibitory effects of telmisartan through the reduction of oxidative stress in the rostral ventrolateral medulla of obesity-induced hypertensive rats. *J Hypertens* 2012;30(10):1992–1999.

32. Ghanem FA, Movahed A. Inflammation in high blood pressure: A clinician perspective. *J Am Soc Hypertens* 2007;1(2):113–119.
33. Amer MS, Elawam AE, Khater MS, Omar OH, Mabrouk RA, Taha HM. Association of high-sensitivity C reactive protein with carotid artery intima-media thickness in hypertensive older adults. *J Am Soc Hypertens* April 23, 2011;5:395–400.
34. Vongpatanasin W, Thomas GD, Schwartz R, Cassis LA, Osborne-Lawrence S, Hahner L, Gibson LL, Black S, Samois D, Shaul PW. C-reactive protein causes downregulation of vascular angiotensin subtype 2 receptors and systolic hypertension in mice. *Circulation* 2007;115(8):1020–1028.
35. Razzouk , Munter P, Bansilal S, Kini AS, Aneja A, Mozes J, Ivan O, Jakkula M, Sharma S, Farkouh ME. C reactive protein predicts long-term mortality independently of low-density lipoprotein cholesterol in patients undergoing percutaneous coronary intervention. *Am Heart J* 2009;158(2):277–283.
36. Kvakan H, Luft FC, Muller DN. Role of the immune system in hypertensive target organ damage. *Trends Cardiovasc Med* 2009;19(7):242–246.
37. Rodriquez-Iturbe B, Franco M, Tapia E, Quiroz Y, Johnson RJ. Renal inflammation, autoimmunity and salt-sensitive hypertension. *Clin Exp Pharmacol Physiol* 2012;39(1):96–103.
38. Tian N, Penman AD, Mawson AR, Manning RD Jr, Flessner MF. Association between circulating specific leukocyte types and blood pressure The Atherosclerosis risk in communities (ARIC) study. *J Am Soc Hypertens* 2010;4(6):272–283.
39. Muller DN, Kvakan H, Luft FC. Immune-related effects in hypertension on and target-organ damage. *Curr Opin Nephrol Hypertens* 2011;20(2):113–117.
40. Marketou ME, Kontaraki JE, Zacharis EA, Kochiadakis GE, Giaouzaki A, Chlouverakis G, Vardas PE. TLR2 and TLR4 gene expression in peripheral monocytes in nondiabetic hypertensive patients: The effect of intensive blood pressure-lowering. *J Clin Hypertens* (*Greenwich*) 2012;14(5):330–335.
41. Lordan S, Ross P, Stanton C. Marine bioactives as functional food ingredients: Potential to reduce the incidence of chronic disease. *Drugs* 2011;9(6):1056–1100.
42. Luft FC. Neural regulation of the immune system modulates hypertension-induced target-organ damage. *J Am Soc Hypertens* 2012;6(1):23–26.
43. Herrada AA, Campino C, Amador CA, Michea LF, Fardella CE, Kalergis AM. Aldosterone as a modulator of immunity: Implications in the organ damage. *J Hypertens* 2011;29(9):1684–1692.
44. Colussi G, Catena C, Sechi LA. Spironolactone, eplerenone and the new aldosterone blockers in endocrine and primary hypertension. *J Hypertens* January 2013;31(1):3–15.
45. Appel LJ, Moore TJ, Obarzanek E et al., DASH Collaborative Research Group. A clinical trial of the effects of dietary patterns on blood pressure. *N Engl J Med* April 17, 1997;336(16):1117–1124.
46. Sacks FM, Svetkey LP, Vollmer WM et al., DASH-Sodium Collaborative Research Group. Effects on blood pressure of reduced dietary sodium and the Dietary Approaches to Stop Hypertension (DASH) diet. *N Engl J Med* January 4, 2001;344(1):3–10.
47. Sun B, Williams JS, Svetkey LP, Kolatkar NS, Conlin PR. Beta2-adrenergic receptor genotype affects the renin-angiotensin-aldosterone system response to the Dietary Approaches to Stop Hypertension (DASH) dietary pattern. *Am J Clin Nutr* 2010;92(2):444–449.
48. Chen Q, Turban S, Miller ER, Appel LJ. The effects of dietary patterns on plasma renin activity: Results from the Dietary Approaches to Stop Hypertension trial. *J Hum Hypertens* 2012;26(11):664–669.
49. Al-Solaiman Y, Jesri A, Zhao Y, Morrow JD, Egan BM. Low-sodium DASH reduces oxidative stress and improves vascular function in salt-sensitive humans. *J Hum Hypertens* 2009;23(12):826–835.
50. Lin PH, Allen JD, Li YJ, Yu M, Lien LF, Svetkey LP. Blood pressure-lowering mechanisms of the DASH dietary pattern. *J Nutr Metab* 2012;2012:472396.
51. Gemino FW, Neutel J, Nonaka M, Hendler SS. The impact of lactotripeptides on blood pressure response in stage 1 and stage 2 hypertensives. *J Clin Hypertens* 2010;12(3):153–159.
52. Cicero AF, Aubin F, Azais-Braesco V, Borghi C. Do the lactotripeptides isoleucine-proline-proline and valine-proline-proline reduce systolic blood pressure in European subjects? A meta-analysis of randomized controlled trials. *Am J Hypertens* 2013;26(3):442–449.
53. Pal S, Radavelli-Bagatini S. The effects of whey protein on cardiometabolic risk factors. *Obes Rev* 2013;14(4):324–343.
54. Zhu CF, Li GZ, Peng HB, Zhang F, Chen Y, Li Y. Therapeutic effects of marine collagen peptides on Chinese patients with type 2 diabetes mellitus and primary hypertension. *Am J Med Sci* 2010;340(5):360–366.
55. Kawasaki T, Seki E, Osajima K, Yoshida M, Asada K, Matsui T, Osajima Y. Antihypertensive effect of valyl-tyrosine, a short chain peptide derived from sardine muscle hydrolyzate, on mild hypertensive subjects. *J Hum Hypertens* 2000;14:519–523.

56. Kawasaki T, Jun CJ, Fukushima Y, Seki E. Antihypertensive effect and safety evaluation of vegetable drink with peptides derived from sardine protein hydrolysates on mild hypertensive, high-normal and normal blood pressure subjects. *Fukuoka Igaku Zasshi* 2002;93(10):208–218.
57. Yang G, Shu XO, Jin F, Zhang X, Li HL, Li Q, Gao YT, Zheng W. Longitudinal study of soy food intake and blood pressure among middle-aged and elderly Chinese women. *Am J Clin Nutr* 2005;81(5):1012–1017.
58. Teunissen-Beekman KF, Dopheide J, Geleijnse JM, Bakker SJ, Brink EJ, de Leeuw PW, van Baak MA. Protein supplementation lowers blood pressure in overweight adults: Effect of dietary proteins on blood pressure (PROPRES), a randomized trial. *Am J Clin Nutr* 2012;95(4):966–971.
59. Dong JY, Tong X, Wu ZW, Xun PC, He K, Qin LQ. Effect of soya protein on blood pressure: A meta-analysis of randomised controlled trials. *Br J Nutr* 2011;106(3):317–326.
60. Rajapakse NW, Mattson DL. Role of L-arginine in nitric oxide production in health and hypertension. *Clin Exp Pharmacol Physiol* 2009;36(3):249–255.
61. Ast J, Jablecka A, Bogdanski I, Krauss H, Chmara E. Evaluation of the antihypertensive effect of L-arginine supplementation in patients with mild hypertension assessed with ambulatory blood pressure monitoring. *Med Sci Monit* 2010;16(5):CR266–CR271.
62. Dong JY, Qin LQ, Zhang Z, Zhao Y, Wang J, Arigoni F, Zhang W. Effect of oral L-arginine supplementation on blood pressure: A meta-analysis of randomized, double-blind, placebo-controlled trials. *Am Heart J* 2011;162(6):959–965.
63. Schulman SP, Becker LC, Kass DA et al. L arginine therapy in acute myocardial infraction: The vascular interaction with age in myocardial infarction (VINTAGE MI) randomized clinical trial. *JAMA* 2006;295(1):58–64.
64. Miller GD, Marsh AP, Dove RW, Beavers D, Presley T, Helms C, Bechtold E, King SB, Kim-Shapiro D. Plasma nitrate and nitrite are increased by a high-nitrate supplement but not by high-nitrate foods in older adults. *Nutr Res* 2012;32(3):160–168.
65. Vilskersts R, Kuka J, Svalbe B, Cirule H, Liepinsh E, Grinberga S, Kalvinsh I, Dambrova M. Administration of L-carnitine and mildronate improves endothelial function and decreases mortality in hypertensive Dahl rats. *Pharmacol Rep* 2011;63(3):752–762.
66. Mate A, Miguel-Carrasco JL, Monserrat MT, Vázquez CM. Systemic antioxidant properties of L-carnitine in two different models of arterial hypertension. *J Physiol Biochem* June 2010;66(2):127–136.
67. Digiesi V, Cantini F, Bisi G, Guarino G, Brodbeck B. L-Carnitine adjuvant therapy in essential hypertension. *Clin Ter* 1994;144:391–395.
68. Digiesi V, Palchetti R, Cantini F. The benefits of L-carnitine therapy in essential arterial hypertension with diabetes mellitus type II. *Minerva Med* 1989;80(3):227–231.
69 Ruggenenti P, Cattaneo D, Loriga G, Ledda F, Motterlini N, Gherardi G, Orisio S, Remuzzi G. Ameliorating hypertension and insulin resistance in subjects at increased cardiovascular risk: Effects of acetyl-L-carnitine therapy. *Hypertension* 2009;54(3):567–574.
70. Korkmaz S, Yıldız G, Kılıçlı F, Yılmaz A, Aydın H, Içağasıoğlu S, Candan F. [Low L-carnitine levels: Can it be a cause of nocturnal blood pressure changes in patients with type 2 diabetes mellitus?]. *Anadolu Kardiyol Derg* 2011;11(1):57–63.
71. Huxtable RJ. Physiologic actions of taurine. *Physiol Rev* 1992;72:101–163.
72. Fujita T, Ando K, Noda H, Ito Y, Sato Y. Effects of increased adrenomedullary activity and taurine in young patients with borderline hypertension. *Circulation* 1987;75:525–532.
73. Mori TA, Bao DQ, Burke V, Puddey IB, Beilin LJ. Docosahexaenoic acid but not eicosapentaenoic acid lowers ambulatory blood pressure and heart rate in humans. *Hypertension* 1999;34:253–260.
74. Bønaa KH, Bjerve KS, Straume B, Gram IT, Thelle D. Effect of eicosapentaenoic and docosahexanoic acids on blood pressure in hypertension: A population-based intervention trial from the Tromso study. *N Engl J Med* 1990;322:795–801.
75. Ueshima H, Stamler J, Elliot B, Brown CQ. Food Omega 3 fatty acid intake of individuals (total, linolenic acid, long chain) and their blood pressure: INTERMAP study. *Hypertension* 2007;50(20):313–319.
76. Mon TA. Omega 3 fatty acids and hypertension in humans. *Clin Exp Pharmacol Physiol* 2006; 33(9):842–846.
77. Cabo J, Alonso R, Mata P. Omega-3 fatty acids and blood pressure. *Br J Nutr* June 2012;107(Suppl 2):S195–S200.
78. Sagara M, Njelekela M, Teramoto T, Taguchi T, Mori M, Armitage L, Birt N, Birt C, Yamori Y. Effects of docosahexaenoic acid supplementation on blood pressure, heart rate, and serum lipids in Scottish men with hypertension and hypercholesterolemia. *Int J Hypertens* 2011;2011:809198.
79. Liu JC, Conklin SM, Manuck SB, Yao JK, Muldoon MF. Long-chain omega-3 fatty acids and blood pressure. *Am J Hypertens* 2011;24(10):1121–1126.

80. Saravanan P, Davidson NC, Schmidt EB, Calder PC. Cardiovascular effects of marine omega-3 fatty acids. *Lancet* 2010;376(9740):540–550.
81. Alonso A, Ruiz-Gutierrez V, Martínez-González MA. Monounsaturated fatty acids, olive oil and blood pressure: Epidemiological, clinical and experimental evidence. *Public Health Nutr* 2006;9(2): 251–257.
82. Psaltopoulou T, Naska A, Orfanos P, Trichopoulos D, Mountokalakis T, Trichopoulou A. Olive oil, the Mediterranean diet, and arterial blood pressure: The Greek European Prospective Investigation into Cancer and Nutrition (EPIC) study. *Am J Clin Nutr* 2004;80(4):1012–1018.
83. Perrinjaquet-Moccetti T, Busjahn A, Schmidlin C, Schmidt A, Bradl B, Aydogan C. Food supplementation with an olive (*Olea europaea* L.) leaf extract reduces blood pressure in borderline hypertensive monozygotic twins. *Phytother Res* 2008;22(9):1239–1242.
84. Moreno-Luna R, Muñoz-Hernandez R, Miranda ML, Costa AF, Jimenez-Jimenez L, Vallejo-Vaz AJ, Muriana FJ, Villar J, Stiefel P. Olive oil polyphenols decrease blood pressure and improve endothelial function in young women with mild hypertension. *Am J Hypertens* 2012;25(12):1299–1304.
85. Susalit E, Agus N, Effendi I, Tjandrawinata RR, Nofiarny D, Perrinjaquet-Moccetti T, Verbruggen M. Olive (*Olea europaea*) leaf extract effective in patients with stage-1 hypertension: Comparison with Captopril. *Phytomedicine* 2011;18(4):251–258.
86. Papamichael CM, Karatzi KN, Papaioannou TG, Karatzis EN, Katsichti P, Sideris V, Zakopoulos N, Zampelas A, Lekakis JP. Acute combined effects of olive oil and wine on pressure wave reflections: Another beneficial influence of the Mediterranean diet antioxidants? *J Hypertens* 2008;26(2): 223–229.
87. He J, Whelton PK. Effect of dietary fiber and protein intake on blood pressure: A review of epidemiologic evidence. *Clin Exp Hypertens* 1999;21:785–796.
88. Pruijm M, Wuerzer G, Forni V, Bochud M, Pechere-Bertschi A, Burnier M. Nutrition and hypertension: More than table salt. *Rev Med Suisse* 2010;6(282):1715–1720.
89. Sherman DL, Keaney JF, Biegelsen ES et al. Pharmacological concentrations of ascorbic acid are required for the beneficial effect on endothelial vasomotor function in hypertension. *Hypertension* 2000;35:936–941.
90. Ness AR, Khaw K-T, Bingham S, Day NE. Vitamin C status and blood pressure. *J Hypertens* 1996;14:503–508.
91. Duffy SJ, Bokce N, Holbrook M. Treatment of hypertension with ascorbic acid. *Lancet* 1999; 354:2048–2049.
92. Mahajan AS, Babbar R, Kansai N, Agarwai SK, Ray PC. Antihypertensive and antioxidant action of amlodipine and vitamin C in patients of essential hypertension. *J Clin Biochem Nutr* 2007; 402:141–147.
93. Ledlerc PC, Proulx, CD, Arquin G, Belanger S. Ascorbic Acid decreases the binding affinity of the AT! Receptor for angiotensin II. *Am J Hypertens* 2008;21(1):67–71.
94. Sato K, Dohi Y, Kojima M, Miyagawa K. Effects of ascorbic acid on ambulatory blood pressure in elderly patients with refractory hypertension. *Arzneimittelforschung* 2006;56(7):535–540.
95. McRae MP. Is Vitamin C an effective antihypertensive supplement? A review and analysis of the literature. *J Chiropr Med* 2006;5(2):60–64.
96. Ward NC, Wu JH, Clarke MW, Buddy IB. Vitamin E effects on the treatment of hypertension in type 2 diabetics. *J Hypertens* 2007;227:227–234.
97. Murray ED, Wechter WJ, Kantoci D, Wang WH, Pham T, Quiggle DD, Gibson KM, Leipold D, Anner BM. Endogenous natriuretic factors 7: Biospecificity of a natriuetic gamma-tocopherol metabolite LLU alpha. *J Pharmacol Exp Ther* 1997;282(2):657–662.
98. Gray B, Swick J, Ronnenberg AG. Vitamin E and adiponectin: Proposed mechanism for vitamin E-induced improvement in insulin sensitivity. *Nutr Rev* 2011;69(3):155–161.
99. Rosen CJ. Clinical practice. Vitamin D insufficiency. *N Engl J Med* 2011;364(3):248–254.
100. Pittas AG, Chung M, Trikalinos T, Mitri J, Brendel M, Patel K, Lichtenstein HA, Lau J, Balk EM. Systematic review: Vitamin D and cardiometabolic outcomes. *Ann Intern Med* 2010;152(5):307–314.
101. Motiwala SR, Want TJ. Vitamin D and cardiovascular disease. *Curr Opin Nephrol Hypertens* 2011;20(4):345–353.
102. Kienreich K, Tomaschitz A, Verheyen N, Pieber TR, Pilz S. Vitamin D and arterial hypertension: Treat the deficiency! *Am J Hypertens* 2013;26(2):158.
103. Tamez H, Kalim S, Thadhani RI. Does vitamin D modulate blood pressure? *Curr Opin Nephrol Hypertens* 2013;22(2):204–209.

104. Wang L, Ma J, Manson JE, Buring JE, Gaziano JM, Sesso HD. A prospective study of plasma vitamin D metabolites, vitamin D receptor gene polymorphisms, and risk of hypertension in men. *Eur J Nutr* 2013;52(7):1771–1779.
105. Keniston R, Enriquez JI Sr. Relationship between blood pressure and plasma vitamin B6 levels in healthy middle-aged adults. *Ann N Y Acad Sci* 1990;585:499–501.
106. Aybak M, Sermet A, Ayyildiz MO, Karakilcik AZ. Effect of oral pyridoxine hydrochloride supplementation on arterial blood pressure in patients with essential hypertension. *Arzneimittelforschung* 1995;45:1271–1273.
107. Paulose CS, Dakshinamurti K, Packer S, Stephens NL. Sympathetic stimulation and hypertension in the pyridoxine-deficient adult rat. *Hypertension* 1988;11(4):387–391.
108. Dakshinamurti K, Lal KJ, Ganguly PK. Hypertension, calcium channel and pyridoxine (vitamin B6). *Mol Cell Biochem* 1998;188(1–2):137–148.
109. Moline J, Bukharovich IF, Wolff MS, Phillips R. Dietary flavonoids and hypertension: is there a link? *Med Hypotheses* 2000;55:306–309.
110. Knekt P, Reunanen A, Järvinen R, Seppänen R, Heliövaara M, Aromaa A. Antioxidant vitamin intake and coronary mortality in a longitudinal population study. *Am J Epidemiol* 1994;139:1180–1189.
111. Karatzi KN, Papamichael CM Karatizis EN, Papaioannou TG, Aznaouridis KA, Katsichti PP, Stamatelopuolous KS. Red Wine acutely induces favorable effects on wave reflections and central pressures in coronary artery disease patients. *Am J Hypertens* 2005;18(9):1161–1167.
112. Wong RH, Howe PR, Buckley JD, Coates AM, Kunz L, Berry NM. Acute resveratrol supplementation improves flow-mediated dilatation in overweight obese individuals with mildly elevated blood pressure. *Nutr Metab Cardiovasc Dis* November 2011;21(11):851–856.
113. Rivera L, Moron R, Zarzuelo A, Galisteo M. Long-term resveratrol administration reduces metabolic disturbances and lowers blood pressure in obese Zucker rats. *Biochem Pharmacol* 2009; 77(6):1053–1063.
114. Engelhard YN, Gazer B, Paran E. Natural antioxidants from tomato extract reduce blood pressure in patients with grade-1 hypertension: A double blind placebo controlled pilot study. *Am Heart J* 2006;151(1):100.
115. Paran E, Novac C, Engelhard YN, Hazan-Halevy I. The effects of natural antioxidants form tomato extract in treated but uncontrolled hypertensive patients. *Cardiovasc Drugs Ther* 2009;23(2):145–151.
116. Reid K, Frank OR, Stocks NP. Dark chocolate or tomato extract for prehypertension: A randomized controlled trial. *BMC Complement Altern Med* 2009;9:22.
117. Paran E, Engelhard Y. Effect of tomato's lycopene on blood pressure, serum lipoproteins, plasma homocysteine and oxidative stress markers in grade I hypertensive patients. *Am J Hypertens* 2001;14:141A (Abstract P-333).
118. Hosseini S, Lee J, Sepulveda RT et al. A randomized, double-blind, placebo-controlled, prospective 16 week crossover study to determine the role of pycnogenol in modifying blood pressure in mildly hypertensive patients. *Nutr Res* 2001;21:1251–1260.
119. Zibadi S, Rohdewald PJ, Park D, Watson RR. Reduction of cardiovascular risk factors in subjects with type 2 diabetes by pycnogenol supplementation. *Nutr Res* 2008;28(5):315–320.
120. Liu X, Wei J, Tan F, Zhou S, Wurthwein G, Rohdewald P. Pycnogenol French maritime pine bark extract improves endothelial function of hypertensive patients. *Life Sci* 2004;74(7):855–862.
121. Simons S, Wollersheim H, Thien T. A systematic review on the influence of trial quality on the effects of garlic on blood pressure. *Neth J Med* 2009;67(6):212–219.
122. Reinhard KM, Coleman CI, Teevan C, Vacchani P. Effects of garlic on blood pressure in patients with and without systolic hypertension: A meta-analysis. *Ann Pharmacother* 2008;42(12):1766–1771.
123. Reid K, Frank OR, Stocks NP. Aged garlic extract lowers blood pressure in patients with treated but uncontrolled hypertension: A randomized controlled trial. *Maturitas* 2010;67(2):144–150.
124. Suetsuna K, Nakano T. Identification of an antihypertensive peptide from peptic digest of wakame (*Undaria pinnatifida*). *J Nutr Biochem* 2000;11:450–454.
125. Nakano T, Hidaka H, Uchida J, Nakajima K, Hata Y. Hypotensive effects of wakame. *J Jpn Soc Clin Nutr* 1998;20:92.
126. Krotkiewski M, Aurell M, Holm G, Grimby G, Szckepanik J. Effects of a sodium-potassium ion-exchanging seaweed preparation in mild hypertension. *Am J Hypertens* 1991;4:483–488.
127. Sato M, Oba T, Yamaguchi T, Nakano T, Kahara T, Funayama K, Kobayashi A, Nakano T. Antihypertensive effects of hydrolysates of wakame (*Undaria pinnatifida*) and their angiotensin-1-converting inhibitory activity. *Ann Nutr Metab* 2002;46(6):259–267.

128. Sankar D, Sambandam G, Ramskrishna Rao M, Pugalendi KV. Modulation of blood pressure, lipid profiles and redox status in hypertensive patients taking different edible oils. *Clin Chim Acta* 2005;355(1–2):97–104.
129. Sankar D, Rao MR, Sambandam G, Pugalendi KV. Effect of sesame oil on diuretics or beta-blockers in the modulation of blood pressure, athropometry, lipid profile and redox status. *Yale J Biol Med* 2006;79(1):19–26.
130. Miyawaki T, Aono H, Toyoda-Ono Y, Maeda H, Kiso Y, Moriyama K. Anti-hypertensive effects of sesamin in humans. *J Nutr Sci Vitaminol (Toyko)* 2009;55(1):87–91.
131. Wichitsranoi J, Weerapreeyakui N, Boonsiri P, Settasatian N, Komanasin N, Sirjaichingkul S, Teerajetgul Y, Rangkadilok N, Leelayuwat N. Antihypertensive and antioxidant effects of dietary black sesame meal in pre-hypertensive humans. *Nutr J* 2011;10(1):82–88.
132. Sudhakar B, Kalaiarasi P, Al-Numair KS, Chandramohan G, Rao RK, Pugalendi KV. Effect of combination of edible oils on blood pressure, lipid profile, lipid peroxidative markers, antioxidant status, and electrolytes in patients with hypertension on nifedipine treatment. *Saudi Med J* 2011; 32(4):379–385.
133. Sankar D, Rao MR, Sambandam G, Pugalendi KV. A pilot study of open label sesame oil in hypertensive diabetics. *J Med Food* 2006;9(3):408–412.
134. Nakano D, Ogura K, Miyakoshi M et al. Antihyptensive effect of angiotensin-I-converting enzyme inhibitory peptides from a sesame protein hydrolysate in spontaneously hypertensive rats. *Biosci Biotechnol Biochem* 206;70(5):1118–1126.
135. Karatzi K, Stamatelopoulos K, Lykka M, Mantzouratou P, Skalidi S, Manios E, Georgiopoulos G, Zakopoulos N, Papamichael C, Sidossis LS. Acute and long-term hemodynamic effects of sesame oil consumption in hypertensive men. *J Clin Hypertens (Greenwich)* 2012;14(9):630–636.
136. Hodgson JM, Puddey IB, Burke V, Beilin LJ, Jordan N. Effects on blood pressure of drinking green and black tea. *J Hypertens* 1999;17:457–463.
137. Kurita I, Maeda-Yamamoto M, Tachibana H, Kamei M. Anti-hypertensive effect of Benifuuki tea containing O-methylated EGCG. *J Agric Food Chem* 2010;58(3):1903–1908.
138. McKay DL, Chen CY, Saltzman E, Blumberg JB. *Hibiscus sabdariffa* L. tea (tisane) lowers blood pressure in pre-hypertensive and mildly hypertensive adults. *J Nutr* 2010;140(2):298–303.
139. Bogdanski P, Suliburska J, Szulinska M, Stepien M, Pupek-Musialik D, Jablecka A. Green tea extract reduces blood pressure, inflammatory biomarkers, and oxidative stress and improves parameters associated with insulin resistance in obese, hypertensive patients. *Nutr Res* June 2012;32(6):421–427.
140. Hodgson JM, Woodman RJ, Puddey IB, Mulder T, Fuchs D, Croft KD. Short-term effects of polyphenol-rich black tea on blood pressure in men and women. *Food Funct* January 19, 2013;4(1):111–115.
141. Taubert D, Roesen R, Schomig E. Effect of cocoa and tea intake on blood pressure: A meta-analysis. *Arch Intern Med* 2007;167(7):626–634.
142. Taubert D, Roesen R, Lehmann C, Jung N, Schomig E. Effects of low habitual cocoa intake on blood pressure and bioactive nitric oxide: A randomized controlled trial. *JAMA* 2007;298(1):49–60.
143. Reid I, Sullivan T, Fakler P, Frank OR, Stocks NP. Does chocolate reduce blood pressure? A meta-analysis. *BMC Med* 2010;8:39–46.
144. Desch S, Kobler D, Schmidt J, Sonnabend M, Adams V, Sareben M, Eitel I, Bluher M, Shuler G, Thiele H. Low vs higher-dose dark chocolate and blood pressure in cardiovascular high-risk patients. *Am J Hypertens* 2010;23(6):694–700.
145. Desch S, Schmidt J, Sonnabend M, Eitel I, Sareban M, Rahimi K, Schuler G, Thiele H. Effect of cocoa products on blood pressure: Systematic review and meta-analysis. *Am J Hypertens* 2010;23(1): 97–103.
146. Ellinger S, Reusch A, Stehle P, Helfrich HP. Epicatechin ingested via cocoa products reduces blood pressure in humans: A nonlinear regression model with a Bayesian approach. *Am J Clin Nutr* 2012;95(6):1365–1377.
147. Hooper L, Kay C, Abdelhamid A, Kroon PA, Cohn JS, Rimm EB, Cassidy A. Effects of chocolate, cocoa, and flavan-3-ols on cardiovascular health: A systematic review and meta-analysis of randomized trials. *Am J Clin Nutr* March 2012;95(3):740–751.
148. Yamaquchi T, Chikama A, Mori K, Watanabe T, Shiova Y, Katsuraqi Y, Tokimitsu I. Hydroxyhydroquinone-free coffee: A double-blind, randomized controlled dose-response study of blood pressure. *Nutr Metab Cardiovasc Dis* 2008;18(6):408–414.
149. Chen ZY, Peng C, Jiao R, Wong YM, Yang N, Huang Y. Anti-hypertensive nutraceuticals and functional foods. *J Agric Food Chem* 2009;57(11):4485–4499.

150. Ochiai R, Chikama A, Kataoka K, Tokimitsu I, Maekawa Y Ohsihi M, Rakugi H, MIkmai H. Effects of hydroxyhydroquinone-reduce coffee on vasoreactivity and blood pressure. *Hypertens Res* 2009;32(11):969–974.
151. Palatini P, Ceolotto G, Ragazzo F, Donigatti F, Saladini, F, Papparella I, Mos L, Zanata G, Santonastaso M. CYP 1A2 genotype modifies the association between coffee intake and the risk of hypertension. *J Hypertens* 2008;27(8):1594–1601.
152. Scheer FA, Van Montfrans GA, van Someren EJ, Mairuhu G, Buijs RM. Daily nighttime melatonin reduces blood pressure in male patients with essential hypertension. *Hypertension* 2004;43(2): 192–197.
153. Grossman E, Laudon M, Yalcin R, Zengil H, Peleg E, Sharabi Y, Kamari Y, Shen-Orr Z, Zisapel N. Melatonin reduces night blood pressure in patients with nocturnal hypertension. *Am J Med* 2006;119(10):898–902.
154. Kozirog M, Poliwczak AR, Duchnowicz P, Koter-Michalak M, Sikora J, Broncel M. Melatonin treatment improves blood pressure, lipid profile and parameters of oxidative stress in patients with metabolic syndrome. *J Pineal Res* 2011;50(3):261–266.
155. De-Leersnyder H, de Biois MC, Vekemans M, Sidi D, Villain E, Kindermans C, Munnich A. Beta (1) adrenergic antagonists improve sleep and behavioural disturbances in a circadian disorder, Smith-Magenis syndrome. *J Med Genet* 2110;38(9):586–590.
156. Morand C, Dubray C, Milenkovic D, Lioger D, Martin JF, Scalber A, Mazur A. Hesperidin contributes to the vascular protective effects of orange juice: A randomized crossover study in healthy volunteers. *Am J Clin Nutr* 2011;93(1):73–80.
157. Basu A, Penugonda K. Pomegranate juice: A heart-healthy fruit juice. *Nutr Rev* 2009;67(1):49–56.
158. Aviram M, Rosenblat M, Gaitine D, Nitecki S, Hoffman A, Dorndeld L, Volkova N, Presser D, Attias J, Liker H, Hayek T. Pomegranate juice consumption for 3 years by patients with carotid artery stenosis reduces common carotid intima-media thickness, blood pressure and LDL oxidation. *Clin Nutr* 2004;23(3):423–433.
159. Aviram M, Dornfeld L. Pomegranate juice inhibits serum angiotensin converting enzyme activity and reduces systolic blood pressure. *Atherosclerosis* 2001;18(1):195–198.
160. Feringa HH, Laskey DA, Dickson JE, Coleman CI. The effect of grape seed extract on cardiovascular risk markers: A meta-analysis of randomized controlled tirals. *J Am Diet Assoc* 2011;111(8):1173–1181.
161. Sivaprakasapillai B, Edirsinghe K, Randolph J, Steinberg F, Kappagoda T. Effect of grape seed extract on blood pressure in subjects with the metabolic syndrome. *Metabolism* 2009;58(12):1743–176.
162. Edirisinghe I, Burton-Freeman B, Tissa Kappagoda C. Mechanism of the endothelium-dependent relaxation evoked by grape seed extract. *Clin Sci (Lond)* 2008;114(4):331–337.
163. Rosenfeldt FL, Haas SJ, Krum H, Hadu A. Coenzyme Q10 in the treatment of hypertension: A meta-analysis of the clinical trials. *J Hum Hypertens* 2007;21(4):297–306.
164. Burke BE, Neuenschwander R, Olson RD. Randomized, double-blind, placebo-controlled trial of coenzyme Q10 in isolated systolic hypertension. *South Med J* 2001;94(11):1112–1117.
165. Tsai KL, Huang YH, Kao CL et al. A novel mechanism of coenzyme Q10 protects against human endothelial cells from oxidative stress-induced injury by modulating NO-related pathways. *J Nutr Biochem* 2012;23(5):458–468.
166. Sohet FM, Delzenne NM. Is there a place for coenzyme Q in the management of metabolic disorders associated with obesity? *Nutr Rev* 2012;70(11):631–641.
167. Trimarco V, Cimmino CS, Santoro M, Pagnano G, Manzi MV, Piglia A, Giudice CA, De Luca N, Izzo R. Nutraceuticals for blood pressure control in patients with high-normal or grade 1 hypertension. *High Blood Press Cardiovasc Prev* 2012;19(3):117–122.
168. Young JM, Florkowski CM, Molyneux SL, McEwan RG, Frampton CM, Nicholls MG, Scott RS, George PM. A randomized, double-blind, placebo-controlled crossover study of coenzyme Q10 therapy in hypertensive patients with the metabolic syndrome. *Am J Hypertens* 2012;(2):261–270.
169. Mikhin VP, Kharchenko AV, Rosliakova EA, Cherniatina MA. [Application of coenzyme Q(10) in combination therapy of arterial hypertension]. *Kardiologiia* 2011;51(6):26–31.
170. McMackin CJ, Widlansky ME, Hambury NM, Haung AL. Effect of combined treatment with alpha lipoic acid and acetyl carnitine on vascular function and blood pressure in patients with coronary artery disease. *J Clin Hypertens* 2007;9:249–255.
171. Salinthone S, Schillace RV, Tsang C, Regan JW, Burdette DN, Carr DW. Lipoic acid stimulates cAMP production via G protein-coupled receptor-dependent and -independent mechanisms. *J Nutr Biochem* 2011;22(7):681–690.

172. Rahman ST, Merchant N, Haque T, Wahi J, Bhaheetharan S, Ferdinand KC, Khan BV. The impact of lipoic acid on endothelial function and proteinuria in quinapril-treated diabetic patients with stage I hypertension: Results from the QUALITY study. *J Cardiovasc Pharmacol Ther* June 2012;17(2):139–145.
173. Morcos M, Borcea V, Isermann B et al. Effect of alpha-lipoic acid on the progression of endothelial cell damage and albuminuria in patients with diabetes mellitus: An exploratory study. *Diab Res Clin Prac* 2001;52(3):175–183.
174. Martina V, Masha A, Gigliardi VR, Brocato L, Manzato E, Berchio A, Massarenti P, Settanni F, Della Casa L, Bergamini S, Iannone A. Long-term *N*-acetylcysteine and L-arginine administration reduces endothelial activation and systolic blood pressure in hypertensive patients with type 2 diabetes. *Diab Care* 2008;31(5):940–944.
175. Jiang B, Haverty M, Brecher P. *N*-acetyl-L-cysteine enhances interleukin-1beta-induced nitric oxide synthase expression. *Hypertension* 1999;34(4 Pt 1):574–579.
176. Vasdev S, Singal P, Gill V. The antihypertensive effect of cysteine. *Int J Angiol* 2009;18(1):7–21.
177. Asher GN, Viera AJ, Weaver MA, Dominik R, Caughey M, Hinderliter AL. Effect of hawthorn standardized extract on flow mediated dilation in prehypertensive and mildly hypertensive adults: A randomized, controlled cross-over trial. *BMC Complement Altern Med* 2012;12:26.
178. Walker AF, Marakis G, Simpson E, Hope JL, Robinson PA, Hassanein M, Simpson HC. Hypotensive effects of hawthorn for patients with diabetes taking prescription drugs: A randomised controlled trial. *Br J Gen Pract* 2006;56(527):437–443.
179. Walker AF, Marakis G, Morris AP, Robinson PA. Promising hypotensive effect of hawthorn extract: A randomized double-blind pilot study of mild, essential hypertension. *Phytother Res* 2002;16(1):48–54.
180. Larson A, Witman MA, Guo Y, Ives S, Richardson RS, Bruno RS, Jalili T, Symons JD. Acute, quercetin-induced reductions in blood pressure in hypertensive individuals are not secondary to lower plasma angiotensin-converting enzyme activity or endothelin-1: Nitric oxide. *Nutr Res* 2012; 32(8):557–564.
181. Edwards RL, Lyon T, Litwin SE, Rabovsky A, Symons JD, Jalili T. Quercetin reduces blood pressure in hypertensive subjects. *J Nutr* 2007;137(11):2405–2411.
182. Egert S, Bosy-Westphal A, Seiberl J et al. Quercetin reduces systolic blood pressure and plasma oxidised low-density lipoprotein concentrations in overweight subjects with a high-cardiovascular disease risk phenotype: A double-blinded, placebo-controlled cross-over study. *Br J Nutr* October 2009;102(7):1065–1074.
183. Trovato A, Nuhlicek DN, Midtling JE. Drug-nutrient interactions. *Am Fam Phys* 1991;44(5):1651–1658.
184. McCabe BJ, Frankel EH, Wolfe JJ, eds. *Handbook of Food-Drug Interactions*. CRC Press, Boca Raton, FL, 2003.
185. Houston MC. The role of cellular micronutrient analysis and minerals in the prevention and treatment of hypertension and cardiovascular disease. *Therap Adv Cardiovasc Dis* 2010;4:165–183.

19 Effects of Different Dietary Fibers on Sugar-Induced Blood Pressure Elevations in Hypertensive Rats

Focus on Viscosity

Harry G. Preuss, Debasis Bagchi, Dallas Clouatre, Anand Swaroop, and Nicholas V. Perricone

CONTENTS

ABBREVIATIONS

BW	Body weight
Cel	Cellulose
CHO	Carbohydrates
CMC	Carboxymethylcellulose
HG	Hydrolyzed guar
MM	Mustard mucilage
Pec	Pectin
Psy	Psyllium
SBP	Systolic blood pressure
SHR	Spontaneously hypertensive rats

19.1 INTRODUCTION

Recently, more and more attention has been given to the likelihood that consumption of dietary sugars and other refined carbohydrates (CHO) in amounts characteristic of modern times causes or at least contributes in some way to many regulatory dysfunctions associated with age-related, deleterious changes in the human health status [1–9]. Hypertension and obesity can be included among these. Despite such revelations, the intake of refined CHO like sugars remains high and continues on the rise [10–12].

Much of this increased interest in sugar consumption is encouraged by laboratory investigations performed in animals where, unlike clinical studies, compliance to a regimen does not become a compromising factor. To give a well-studied example, ingestion of common sugars like sucrose and fructose in certain rat strains provided in a concentration calculated to be in the range consumed by the average human has been linked to significant SBP elevations [13,14], insulin resistance [15], and many other perturbations such as distinct entities in the so-called metabolic syndrome [16–20]. Because the use of drugs to prevent or treat such disorders has been too frequently associated with many harmful adverse reactions [21], safe, easy-to-implement, and effective dietary means to prevent, lessen, or even overcome these metabolic disturbances warrant serious investigation.

While animal models have consistently shown that excess oral intake of certain sugars significantly increases systolic blood pressure (SBP), concomitant intake of some soluble fibers has been reported to overcome this phenomenon [22–26]. Similar associations are now becoming more apparent at a clinical level [27,28]. Accordingly, the primary purpose of the present investigation was to examine and compare the abilities of a variety of fibers to prevent and/or ameliorate "sugar-induced" blood pressure elevations. Additional objectives were to observe the influence of the various fibers on weight changes and to begin to discern potential mechanisms behind the encountered developments.

19.2 MATERIALS AND METHODS

19.2.1 Protocol

The Animal Welfare Board at Georgetown University Medical Center approved the protocol for this investigation. Sixty-four mature male spontaneously hypertensive rats (SHR) obtained from Taconic Farms, Germantown, NY, were used. At initiation of study, SHR weighed an average of 294 ± 5.0 g (SEM) with a range between 280 and 378 g. Rats were housed two in a cage in a constant temperature room with a light-dark phase of 12 h each. The SHR were divided into eight groups, each containing eight rats that consumed a diet differing mainly in the fiber content. The eight groups were selected so that among them the average starting body weight and SBP of all groups were reasonably close.

The eight diets obtained from Food-Tek Inc., Morris Plains, NJ, are listed in Table 19.1. Diets among the eight groups differed only in carbohydrate (CHO) content—sugar, starch, and fiber. Concerning consumable CHO, diet 1 contained only cornstarch (St 57%, w/w), while diets 2–8 consisted of a mixture of cornstarch (St 37%, w/w) and sucrose (Su 20%, w/w). Also, diet 1 contained the insoluble fiber cellulose as did diet 2. Diets 3–8 contained the following soluble fibers, respectively: mustard mucilage (MM), hydrolyzed guar (HG), psyllium (Psy), carboxymethylcellulose (CMC), pectin (Pec), and guar (Guar). The SHR were followed for 71 days while consuming their particular diets. Body weights (BWs) and SBP were regularly measured.

19.2.2 Body Weight

BW was estimated by routine measurements on the same scale throughout the study. Two reading taken minutes apart on the given day had to be within 2 g of each other or the procedure was repeated until the weights were consistently within the 2 g range.

TABLE 19.1
Diets

Ingredient	Group 1 Percentage[a]	Groups 2–8 Percentage[a]
Vegetable oil	16.44	16.44
Protein	13.00	13.00
Mineral mix, AIN 76A	4.00	4.00
Vitamin mix, AIN 76A	1.20	1.20
Cholesterol	1.10	1.10
Salt	0.50	0.50
Choline bitartrate	0.50	0.50
DL-Methionine	0.20	0.20
Sodium cholate	0.02	0.02
Ethoxyquin	0.04	0.04
Fiber	6.00	6.00
Cornstarch	57.00	37.00
Sucrose		20.00
	Fiber Content (6%, w/w)	**Designations**
Diets 1	Cellulose	St Cel
Diet 2	Cellulose	Su Cel
Diet 3	Mustard mucilage	Su MM
Diet 4	Hydrolyzed guar	Su HG
Diet 5	Psyllium	Su Psy
Diet 6	Carboxymethylcellulose	Su CMC
Diet 7	Pectin	Su Pec
Diet 8	Guar	Su Guar

[a] Based on g/100 g.

19.2.3 Food Intake

Food intakes were estimated on day 64 of the study by subtracting the weight of the remaining food from the amounts premeasured 24 h earlier. SHR were housed two in a cage, so the results for average daily intake per rat were obtained for each cage dividing by two.

19.2.4 Systolic Blood Pressure

SBP was measured by tail plethysmography [29] using an instrument obtained from Narco Biosciences (Houston, TX) [13,30]. This allowed for rapid measurement of SBP with a beeper sound system. Rats were allowed free access to their diet and water until SBP readings were obtained after a slight warming between 13.00 and 17.00 h. Multiple readings on individual rats at each reading were taken. To be accepted, SBP measurements on a given rat had to be virtually stable. Over the 71 days of study, multiple SBP and BW readings were recorded.

19.2.5 Viscosity Measurements

Pure fibers and diets added to water were measured for viscosity using a Cannon Ubbelohde Viscometer (Cannon Instrument Co., P.O. Box 16, State College, PA 16804). Fibers added to water were examined at a concentration of 0.5% (w/v), and feeds were added to the water at a weight that brought the content of the contained fiber of interest to 0.5% (w/v).

19.2.6 Xylose Test

Gavaged rats received 4.0 mL water containing 240 mg of a given fiber and 200 mg xylose orally. Urine was collected over 6 h in a metabolism cage. Volume and xylose concentration were measured [31,32].

19.2.7 Statistical Analyses

Results are presented as average ± SEM using KaleidaGraph graphing and data analysis Version 3.6. BW was examined by repeated measures and two-way analyses of variance (one factor being group and the second factor being time of examination). Where a significant effect of regimen was detected by analysis of variance (ANOVA) ($p < 0.05$), Dunnett's *t*-test was used to establish which differences between averages reached statistical significance [33]. In the case of SBP, some groups (those receiving the fiber with intermediate viscosity) showed two outcomes. Over the initial time period, the SBP resembled those from the SHR receiving Guar (high viscosity); however, later, their SBP resembled SHR receiving Cel, MM, and HG (low viscosity). Accordingly, one-way ANOVA was performed at two time points representing periods where the different responses were noted (days 34 and 71).

19.3 RESULTS

The primary purpose of the study was to determine and compare the effects of a variety of fibers on sugar-induced SBP elevations. In so doing, three distinct effective patterns on SBP and BW from the six soluble fibers were discerned.

19.3.1 Systolic Blood Pressure (Figure 19.1a through c)

In the two Cel groups, SHR receiving sucrose (Su Cel—group 2) compared to cornstarch (St Cel—group 1) consistently displayed after the initial 2 weeks significantly higher SBPs over the course of study. Because the two cellulose groups (groups 1 and 2) are used as low and high baselines for comparing the effects of various soluble fibers on sugar-induced SBP, these data will be depicted in bold type in all three figures comprising Figure 19.1. In the case of the MM and the HG groups (Figure 19.1a), SBP from the beginning resembled the Su Cel group.

Psy, CMC, and Pec provided an interesting SBP pattern (Figure 19.1b). For approximately the initial 40 days, SBP readings coincided with the St Cel group. However, somewhere near that time point, SBP values rose rapidly so that by the second month SBP values of all three fiber groups (Su Psy, Su CMC, and Su Pec) resembled the values of the Su Cel group, that is sugar-induction took place. Interestingly, the SBP elevation above the pure starch control resembled those brought on by the sucrose alone—no more, but also no less.

In the case of highly viscous Guar, SBP readings simulated those of the St Cel group throughout the 71 days of study (Figure 19.1c).

Because of the different early and late SBP responses to the intermediate viscous soluble fibers that took place around 40 days (Figure 19.1b), Figure 19.2a and b depicts SBP results at 34 (early) and 71 (late) days for further clarity. At both time points, SHR in the Cel group consuming sucrose (Su Cel) displayed significantly higher SBPs compared to SHR ingesting cornstarch (St Cel). At day 34, compared to the SBP of Su Cel, the SBPs of groups consuming Suc Pec, Su CMC, and Su Guar were significantly lower (Figure 19.2a). The Su Psy group showed a trend toward a lower pressure, whereas the Su MM and Su HG groups showed little difference from the Su Cel group. By day 71, only the Su Guar group still maintained a lower pressure compared to the Su Cel group (Figure 19.2b).

19.3.2 Food Consumption (Table 19.2)

Food consumption by weight estimated in the second month of study was similar among the groups. There were no statistically significant differences in the 24 h food consumption.

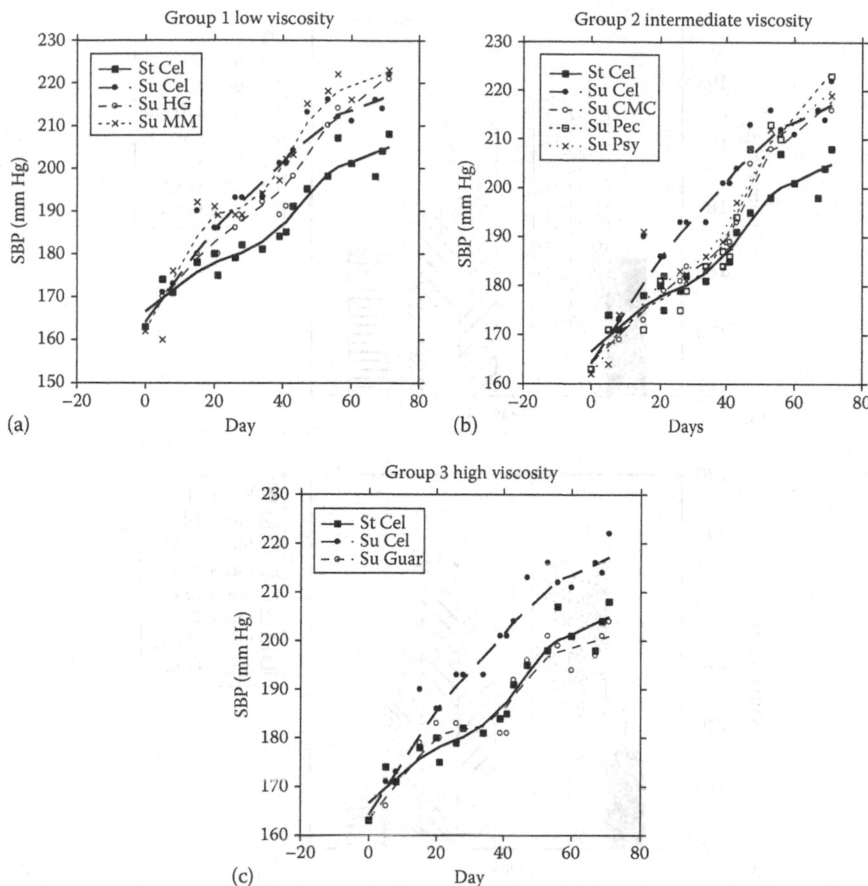

FIGURE 19.1 (a through c) Compared to SHR ingesting all CHO as cornstarch (52% total calories—group 1), those ingesting 1/3 of their CHO calories as sucrose (18% Su/34% cornstarch—group 2) showed a significantly increased SBP approximately 2–3 weeks after starting their respective diets. These two groups depicted in heavier lines are used for comparison with those groups consuming different soluble fibers. (a) From 3 weeks on, SBP of SHR ingesting HG and MM was closer to the sucrose eaters (group 2) than to the starch eaters (group 1). (b) The addition of CMC, Pec, and Psy delayed the onset of the sucrose-induced elevation of SBP until about 6 weeks after initiation of the diets. Then, a sharp rise in SBP occurred so that the SBP values mimicked those of group 2. (c) The SHR ingesting Guar did not show the sucrose-induced rise in SBP over the 2 months of study. Accordingly, the sucrose ingesting Guar group resembled group 1—SHR receiving no sucrose.

19.3.3 Body Weight (Figure 19.3a through c)

The two groups of SHR consuming the insoluble fiber Cel (groups 1 and 2) had a reasonably similar weight gain over 2 months whether they consumed sucrose or cornstarch (Figure 19.3). These two groups depicted with thick lines are used as baseline for comparison with the other six soluble fibers depicted with thin lines in Figure 19.3a through c. The body weights were compared along the lines of the SBP findings in Figure 19.1a through c, that is in three groupings. The first group consisted of MM and HG (Figure 19.3a), the second of Psy, CMC, and Pec (Figure 19.3b), and the final of Guar alone (Figure 19.3c). In general, the group consuming Guar showed the lowest average weight gain over the course of study ($p < 0.0001$ compared with the Cel groups) (Figure 19.3c). In contrast, HG and MM showed essentially no change in weight gain relative to the Cel groups (Figure 19.3a). HG tended to have lower body weights initially; however, by the end of the experiment, there were no statistically significant differences compared to Cel groups in

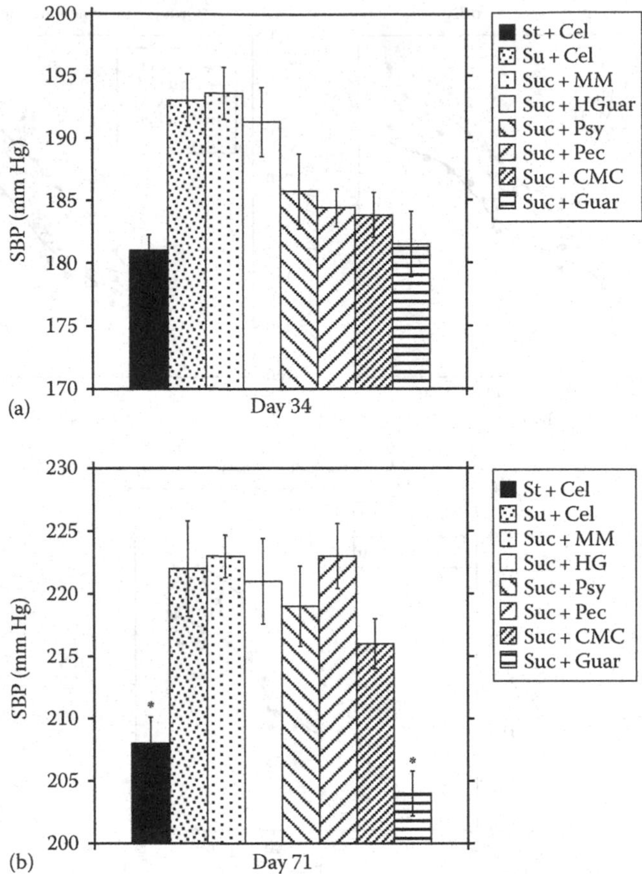

FIGURE 19.2 (a and b) The St Cel group has a significantly lower SBP compared to the Su Cel group by day 34. The Su MM and Su HG groups showed virtually the same SBP as Su Cel. The SBP of the groups consuming Pec, CMC, and Guar was significantly lower than that of Su Cel. SHR ingesting Psy showed a lower trend. At day 71, the Su Guar group continued to show a significantly lower SBP compared to the Suc Cel group. With the exception of St Cel, no other group showed a significantly lower SBP compared to Su Cel.

TABLE 19.2
Estimated Average Individual Food Intake of Eight SHR per Group (Day 64)

Fiber (6%, w/w)	Average (g/24 h)
St Cel	20
Su Cel	20
Su MM	18
Su HG	19
Su Psy	20
Su Pec	19
Su CMC	21
Su Guar	19

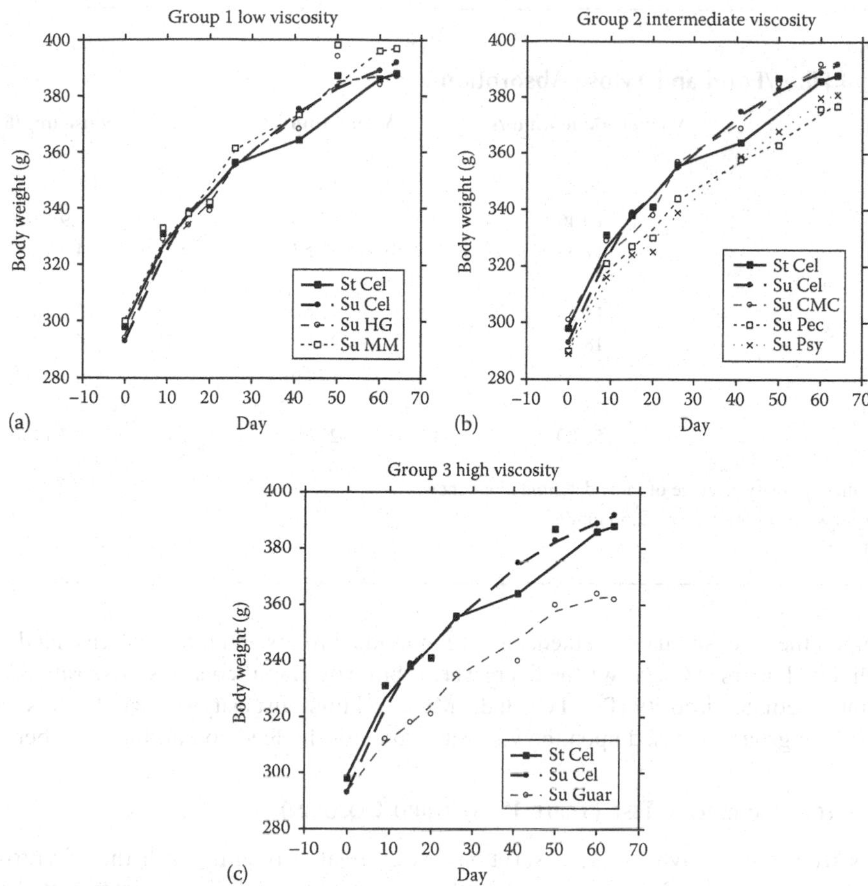

FIGURE 19.3 (a through c) In general, comparing groups 1 and 2, both receiving the insoluble fiber cellulose, where the only dissimilarity between the two groups was the presence of sucrose in the diet of the second, little difference in average body weights occurred over the 2 months of study. The data of these two initial groups distinguished by heavier lines are used for comparison in all subsets of the figure. The other groups ate different soluble fibers with varying viscosities (groups 3–8). (a) Effects of low-viscosity fibers HG and MM. Similar body weight patterns comparable to the Cel groups were found. (b) Results gathered from the intermediate viscous fibers. Although CMC displayed a weight pattern similar to the first two groups receiving Cel, the presence of Pec and Psy was associated with a significantly lower weight gain. Examining the effects of highly viscous Guar in (c), a definitely lower rate of weight gain is apparent.

body weight. Among the remaining fibers, those ingesting Pec and Psy showed statistically lower average weight gains over the course of study compared to the Cel groups ($p < 0.0001$), while CMC did not (Figure 19.3b).

19.3.4 Viscosity Measurements of Fiber and Fiber-Containing Feed (Table 19.3)

When viscosities of the fibers were measured in vitro (see column 1), addition of Cel to water did not significantly alter viscosity (9.58 vs. 9.56 $mm^2 s^2$). The soluble fibers MM, HG, and Psy added to water changed viscosity only slightly (Table 19.3). CMC and Pec showed intermediate viscosity when compared to the other fibers, while Guar proved markedly viscous. When powdered diets containing the respective fibers were checked (see column 2), viscosity generally increased with the exception of CMC. Psy proved to be much more viscous in the diet than alone.

TABLE 19.3
Viscosity of Fiber/Food and Xylose Absorption

Group	V Fiber Alone (mm^2/s^2)	V Diet (mm^2/s^2)	Xylose (mg/6 h)[a]
Low viscosity			
2. Su Cel	9.58	10.53	5.5 ± 1.0
3. Su MM	10.46	14.00	4.9 ± 0.8
4. Su HG	11.63	12.54	4.0 ± 0.6
Intermediate viscosity			
5. Su Psy	11.58	17.60	3.8 ± 0.5
6. Su Pec	18.33	24.10	4.2 ± 0.8
7. Su CMC	24.33	23.56	4.4 ± 0.8
High viscosity			
8. Su Guar	55.00	127.00	3.7 ± 0.6

For fiber and diet viscosity, average of three determinations shown.
Viscosity for Su water without fiber = 9.56 mm^2/s^2.
[a] Ave ± SEM.

Based upon the viscosity measurements for the individual fibers and the respective feed containing the individual fibers at 6% (w/w), the fibers were arbitrarily classified as low viscosity (Cel, MM, and HG), intermediate viscosity (Psy, Pec, and CMC), and high viscosity (Guar). Psy was placed in the intermediate grouping based upon the viscosity value for the feed containing this fiber.

19.3.5 Xylose Excretory Test (Table 19.3, Third Column)

The results from the in vivo xylose absorption test correlated roughly with the in vitro studies using the viscometer. After 2 months ingesting the respective special diets, the greatest absorption of xylose over 6 h based upon urinary excretion was found in the presence of Cel and MM, while the least absorption was seen with Guar. The presence of Psy, Pec, and CMC was associated with intermediate values of absorption. A slight deviation from the expected occurred in the hydrolyzed guar group that resembled the intermediate group more than low-viscosity group.

19.4 DISCUSSION

The concept that excess sugar consumption contributes significantly to a multitude of prevalent metabolic perturbations largely arose from epidemiological observations made during the two world wars. The incidences of diabetes mellitus and serious heart disorders were dramatically decreased in countries where food was scarce all through World War I. Paton attributed these unexpected benefits to a reduced supply of dietary sugar [1]. Differently, Aschoff and Himsworth favored low-fat intake as an alternative explanation behind the favorable wartime responses [34,35]. Additional data from World War II failed to settle the debate since both low-sugar and low-fat intakes once more preceded the decreased incidences of type 2 diabetes and cardiovascular disorders [36].

An obvious question is—while both sugars and fats could contribute to the perturbations, was one a more significant factor than the other? After World War II, the major dietary focus was directed toward fats especially saturated fats due mainly to the work of Keys [37–39]. Although a plethora of early evidence existed for sugar being the primary culprit, it is only relatively recently that the major emphasis began to switch from saturated fats to dietary sugars [9,40–42].

Aside from the recent epidemiological associations given earlier, knowledge relating to the ability of dietary sugars like sucrose, fructose, and HFCS to harm the regulation of many metabolic events has been available for a number of years [1–9]. In the 1960s, 1970s, and 1980s, reports arising from both animal studies and clinical observations mainly by John Yudkin's group contributed notably to a hypothesis that the augmented rate of sugar consumption worldwide was a major factor in the more frequent occurrence of several severe metabolic disorders—particularly, glucose-insulin perturbations and cardiovascular risk factors [2,3,6]. Included in the latter perturbations was hypertension. In 1964, attempting to explain the increased incidence of hypertension in the Western world, Ahrens reported, "the most striking recent dietary change has been the marked increase in consumption of sucrose." [36]

Numerous early findings concerning the role of sugars in influencing blood pressure were more suggestive than conclusive [36]. However, in the late 1970s, a study using three different strains of rats (SHR, WKy, and regular Wistars) examined sugar-induced SBP elevations [13]. SHR displayed a marked increase in SBP following sucrose challenge, Wky, a normotensive control for SHR, had an intermediate but significant rise, and a regular Wistar strain showed essentially no elevation when drinking a sucrose solution. The increase did not relate to the amount of fluid consumed, and later studies where sucrose was placed in food rather than water strengthened the conclusion that augmented fluid intake was not behind "sugar-induced" SBP elevations. Interestingly, time and again, sugar-induced hypertension in rats occurred despite virtually no body weight gain. This further suggested that factors other than or in addition to weight gain played a significant role in the pathogenesis.

In this study, eight rodent diets were assessed that differed in two important respects: (1) the presence of cornstarch alone or the presence of sucrose in addition to cornstarch and (2) the presence of different fibers with a wide range of viscosities. The first dietary variations with cellulose (St Cel, Su Cel) not only tested the effects of sucrose compared to cornstarch consumption on SBP of SHR to corroborate previous published findings [22–26] but established reasonable baseline values to compare the effects of soluble fibers with varying viscosities on sugar-induced SBP elevations.

Concerning the major CHO content, the baseline control diet (diet 1) contained only cornstarch—no sucrose, whereas the other seven contained sucrose replacing some of the starch—added at a concentration reasonably close to that contained in the average adult American diet [10–12]. Comparing the SBP of group 1 to that of group 2, where the only major difference was the presence of sucrose in the diet in the latter (Table 19.1), corroborates the "sucrose effect" by showing a statistically significant increased SBP of group 2 vs. group 1 (Figure 19.1a through c). Establishing baseline values for SBP in virtually a nonviscous environment provided by cellulose addition allowed us to compare the effects of a number of soluble fibers with different viscosities on sugar-induced SBP elevations [22–26].

Common reasoning dictates that rats do not always respond similarly as humans do; yet, in the case of sugar-induced blood pressure elevations, many early findings in rats heralded today's experiences in human clinical trials. In rodent models, the ability of sucrose to increase SBP was ameliorated by the simultaneous intake of soluble fibers such as beta glucan (oat bran), Psy, and guar [24–26]. Despite knowledge that animal studies produce results under strictly controlled situations not compromised by compliance issues, the general tendency among clinicians was and still is to overlook them. However, poor compliance is a major problem in the interpretation of data obtained in clinical trials and often not considered in interpretation of findings [43]. Nevertheless, previous clinical trials have also reported that soluble fibers can lower blood pressure [27,28]. The earlier reports attributed much of the favorable effects derived from soluble fiber to their ability to slow sugar absorption in a viscous environment. Reasoning would conclude that the more viscous the environment the slower the sugar absorption and the greater the beneficial effects would be such as ameliorating hyperglycemia, hyperinsulinemia, and insulin resistance [44,45].

This study suggests that viscosity of fiber has a significant influence on sugar-enhanced SBP. Of the six soluble fibers tested, guar showed by far the greatest viscosity both in water and in the rodent feed (Table 19.3); this soluble fiber also showed the greatest inhibition of both sucrose-induced SBP and body weight (Figures 19.1c, 19.2, and 19.3c). Furthermore, the effect of guar in overcoming of sucrose-induced SBP elevations lasted for the entire 2 months of the study, unlike the other fibers. The xylose test examining guar also revealed the lowest excretory rate compared to the other fibers.

In correlating viscosity with the xylose test in this study, the only exception between the tests occurred with hydrolyzed guar. We have no explanation for the workings of hydrolyzed guar here, as the latter did show relatively low viscosity when tested in water and feed (Table 19.3). The other soluble fiber placed in the low-viscosity category (MM) did show a relatively high excretory rate of xylose. Both soluble fibers placed in the low-viscosity category had little effect on sugar-induced SBP elevation and virtually no effect on body weight.

The results with the intermediate viscous grouping of fibers were most interesting. Psy, Pec, and CMC were placed in the intermediate viscosity grouping based on the data shown in Table 19.3. Psy presented a slight dilemma in its categorization because it displayed low viscosity in water. However, it fell into an intermediate viscosity range in feed. We have no ready explanation for this difference. Nevertheless, Psy was placed in the intermediate grouping because we judged the results in feed to be more important in determining outcome.

Psy and Pec lessened the rate of weight gain, whereas CMC did not show this at any time (Figure 19.3b). Effects of these intermediate viscous fibers on sugar-induced SBP elevations were indeed worthy of note. For approximately 40 days, no sugar-induced SBP elevations were observed in their presence. Then the suppressive effects were lost. Between 40 and 60 days, SBP reached levels seen in the sucrose cellulose group despite continuance of the fiber in the diet and despite no marked deviations in weight gain (Figure 19.3b). Therefore in this grouping, the fiber effects on sugar-enhanced SBP differed markedly depending on whether these measurements were checked early or late in the course of intake (Figure 19.2a and b). In the case of guar, its presence prevented sugar-enhanced SBP elevations for the length of study. However, it is uncertain what would have happened had the study with the guar group been carried out much beyond 2 months.

The explanation for this time-related effect of intermediate viscous fibers on SBP (Figure 19.1b) may relate to the known characteristic pattern of sugar-induced elevations of SBP in rats. Although the species and age of rat as well as the type of CHO challenge often determines the extent of response, dose also plays a significant role [13,30,47–48]. In the rodent model, rats have a sudden takeoff of SBP elevation in response to sugar that is dependent on the dose—at high levels this response may occur within days [13]. In contrast, low-level challenge of sucrose may take weeks or even months to augment SBP [49]. In this study, although the young SHR had a steady rise in SBP based on genetics, examining Figure 19.1 closely shows the "sugar effect" at the 20% (w/w) level occurred around day 7 and reached a peak around day 14. Accordingly, we offer the following possibility to explain Figure 19.1b. Soluble fiber affects sugar dosing—the more viscous the fiber, the lower the sugar challenge. Thus, soluble fibers "lower" the sugar challenge and cause the sugar influence on SBP to take longer [49].

Several mechanisms seem to be involved to some degree in the sugar-induced SBP elevation of rats [50]. These include augmented catecholamine levels [17], disturbed vasodilatory function via perturbations in NO signaling in blood vessels [18], alterations in fluid and electrolyte balance [19], and disturbances in the renin–angiotensin system (RAS) manifested by elevated circulating levels of angiotensin-2 [20,50]. These mechanisms useful in the animal model may help explain the pathogenesis behind sugar-induced SBP elevations at the clinical level. If this turns out to be true, these mechanisms also should suggest preventive and treatment regimens.

To prevent or treat sugar-induced SBP elevations, diet is the obvious first approach. Rodent studies, similar to findings depicted in Figures 19.1 and 19.2, suggest that carbohydrates more slowly absorbed compared to sucrose are associated with lower SBP [30]. Many recent clinical studies incriminate rapidly absorbed CHO as nutritional elements that can augment blood pressure [51]. The majority of reported relevant clinical studies indicate that avoidance can be beneficial [52–59]. Unfortunately, it seems reasonable to state that a majority of individuals would have extreme difficulty adhering to such a diet. To make matters worse, sugars may even be addictive according to some investigators [60].

If a reasonable portion of sugars is to remain in the diet of many for the sake of palatability and reducing fat intake, the addition of soluble, viscous fibers could still provide some therapeutic relief because the effect of soluble fibers slowing sugar absorption is healthful [45]. Nutritionists long have implored the public to eat more dietary fiber, especially soluble fiber [61,62]. In carefully controlled animal studies, the ability of soluble fiber to delay sugar absorption is associated with the lowering of elevated blood pressures, a major cardiovascular risk factor [24,25].

Unfortunately, the general public has significantly resisted increasing dietary fiber intake, probably for taste reasons and because of perturbations created in the gastrointestinal tract—gas, cramps, and frequent bowel movements. An alternative to viscous soluble fiber would be "carb-blockers" like white bean extract and l arabinose that can also slow sugar absorption in the gastrointestinal tract [63].

REFERENCES

1. Paton JHP: Relation of excessive carbohydrate ingestion to catarrhs and other diseases. *Brit Med J* 1:738, 1933.
2. Yudkin J: Patterns and trends in carbohydrate consumption and their relation to disease. *Proc Nutr Soc* 23:149–162, 1964.
3. Yudkin J: Sucrose and cardiovascular disease. *Proc Nutr Soc* 31:331–337, 1972.
4. Preuss HG, Fournier RD: Effects of sucrose ingestion on blood pressure. *Life Sci* 30:879–886, 1982.
5. Israel KD, Michelis OE IV, Reiser S, Keeney M: Serum uric acid, inorganic phosphorus, and glutamic-oxalacetic transaminase and blood pressure in carbohydrates-sensitive adults consuming three different levels of sucrose. *Ann Nutr Metab* 27:425–435, 1983.
6. Yudkin J: Sucrose, coronary heart disease, diabetes and obesity. Do hormones provide a link? *Am Heart J* 115:493–498, 1988.
7. Preuss HG: Effects of glucose/insulin perturbations on aging and chronic disorders of aging: The evidence. *J Am Coll Nutr* 16:397–403, 1997.
8. Ferrannini E, Natali A, Bell P et al.: Insulin resistance and hypersecretion in obesity. *J Clin Invest* 100:1166–1173, 1997.
9. Vartanian LR, Schwartz MB, Brownell KD: Effects of soft drink consumption on nutrition and health. A systematic review and meta-analysis. *Am J Public Health* 97:667–675, 2007.
10. Bowman SA: Diets of individuals based on energy intakes from added sugars. *Family Econ Nutr Rev* 12:31–38, 1999.
11. Ervin RB, Ogden CL: *Consumption of Added Sugars Among US Adults, 2005–2010.* NCHS data brief, no 122. Hyattsville, MD: National Center for Health Statistics. May 2013.
12. Marriott BP, Olsho L, Hadden L, Conner P: Intake of added sugars and selected nutrients in the United States, National Health and Nutrition Examination Survey (NHANES) 2003–2006. *Crit Rev Food Sci Nutr* 50:228–258, 2010.
13. Preuss MB, Preuss HG: Effects of sucrose on the blood pressure of various strains of Wistar rats. *Lab Invest* 43:101–107, 1980.
14. Preuss HG, Fournier RD, Chieuh CC et al.: Refined carbohydrates affect blood pressure and retinal vasculature in SHR and WKY. *J Hypertens* 4:S459–S462, 1986.
15. Tobey TA, Nondon CE, Zavaroni I, Reaven GM: Mechanism of insulin resistance in fructose-fed rats. *Metabolism* 31:608–612, 1982.
16. Reaven GM, Ho H, Hoffman BB: Effects of a fructose-enriched diet on plasma insulin and triglyceride concentration in SHR and WKY rats. *Horm Metab Res* 22:363–365, 1990.
17. Fournier RD, Chiueh CC, Kopin IJ et al.: The interrelationship between excess CHO ingestion, blood pressure and catecholamine excretion in SHR and WKY. *Am J Physiol* 250:E381–E385, 1986.
18. Kopilas MA, Dang LNT, Anderson HDI: Effect of dietary chromium on resistance artery function and nitric oxide signaling in the sucrose-fed spontaneously hypertensive rat. *Vasc Res* 44:110–118, 2007.
19. Preuss HG, Memon S, Dadgar A, Jiang G: Effects of diets high in sugar on renal fluid, electrolyte, and mineral handling in SHR: Relationship to blood pressure. *J Am Coll Nutr* 13:73–82, 1994.
20. Shi S-J, Preuss HG, Abernathy DR et al.: Elevated blood pressure in spontaneously hypertensive rats consuming a high sucrose diet is associated with elevated angiotensin II and is reversed by vanadium. *J Hypertens* 15:857–862, 1997.
21. Krentz AJ, Bailey CJ: Oral antidiabetic agents: Current role in type 2 diabetes mellitus. *Drugs* 65:385–411, 2005.

22. Vachon C, Jones JD, Wood PJ, Savoie L: Concentration effect of soluble dietary fibers on postprandial glucose and insulin in the rat. *Can J Physiol Pharmacol* 66:801–806, 1987.
23. Tinker LF, Schneeman BO: The effects of guar gum or wheat bran on the disappearance of 14C-labeled starch from the rat. *J Nutr* 119:403–408, 1989.
24. El Zein M, Areas J, Knapka J et al.: Influence of oat bran on sucrose-induced blood pressure elevations in SHR. *Life Sci* 47:1121–1128, 1990.
25. Preuss HG, Gondal JA, Bustos E et al.: Effects of chromium and guar on sugar-induce hypertension in rats. *Clin Nephrol* 44:170–177, 1995.
26. Gondal JA, MacArthy P, Myers AK, Preuss HG: Effects of dietary sucrose and fibers on blood pressure in hypertensive rats. *Clin Nephrol* 45:163–168, 1996.
27. Papathanasopoulos A, Camilleri M: Dietary fiber supplements: Effects in obesity and metabolic syndrome and relationship to gastrointestinal function. *Gastroenterology* 138:65–72, 2010.
28. Cicero AF, Derosa G, Manca M et al.: Different effect of psyllium and guar dietary supplementation on blood pressure control in hypertensive overweight patients: A six-month, randomized clinical trial. *Clin Exp Hypertens* 29:383–394, 2007.
29. Bunag RD: Validation in awake rats of a tail-cuff method measuring systolic pressure. *J Appl Physiol* 34:279–282, 1973.
30. Preuss HG, Fournier RD, Preuss J et al.: Effects of different refined carbohydrates on the blood pressure of SH and WKY Rats. *J Clin Biochem Nutr* 5:9–20, 1988.
31. Harris AL: Determination of D-xylose in urine for the D-xylose absorption test. *Clin Chem* 15:65–71, 1969.
32. Benson Jr. JA, Culver PJ, Ragland S et al.: The D-xylose absorption test in malabsorption syndrome. *NEJM* 256:335–339, 1957.
33. Dunnett C: A multiple comparison procedure for comparing several treatments with control. *J Am Stat Assoc* 50:1096–1121, 1955.
34. Aschoff L: Observations concerning the relationship between cholesterol metabolism and vascular disease. *Br Med J* 2:1131–1134, 1932.
35. Himsworth HP: Diet and the incidence of diabetes mellitus. *Clin Sci* 2:117–148, 1935.
36. Ahrens RA: Sucrose, hypertension, and heart disease: An historical perspective. *Am J Clin Nutr* 27:403–422, 1974.
37. Keys A, Aravanis C, Blackburn HW et al.: Epidemiologic studies related to coronary heart disease: Characteristics of men aged 40–59 in seven countries. *Acta Med Scand* (Suppl to vol. 460) 1–392, 1967.
38. Keys A, Aravanis C, Blackburn, H et al.: *Seven Countries. Multivariate Analysis of Death and Coronary Heart Disease*. Harvard University Press, Cambridge, MA, pp. 1–381, 1980.
39. Keys A: Coronary heart disease in seven countries 1970. *Nutrition* 13:250–252, 1997.
40. Bray GA, Popkin BM: Calorie-sweetened beverages and fructose: What have we learned 10 years later? *Pediatr Obes* 15:182–189, 2013.
41. Fagherazzi G, Vilier A, Sartorelli DS et al.: Consumption of artificially and sugar-sweetened beverages and incident type 2 diabetes in the Etude Epidemiologique aupres des femmes del la Mutuelle Generale de L'Education Nationale-European Prospective investigation into cancer and nutrition cohort. *Am J Clin Nutr* 97:517–523, 2013.
42. Taubes G, Kearns-Couzens K: Big sugar's sweet little lies. *Mother Jones*, November/December, 2012, pp. 1–3, www.motherjones.com/environment/2012/10/sugar-industry-lies-campaign, accessed May 24, 2015.
43. Kaats GR, Preuss HG: Challenges to the conduct and interpretation of weight loss research. In: Bagchi D, Preuss HG (eds.). *Obesity: Epidemiology, Pathophysiology, Prevention*, 2nd edn. Taylor & Francis Group, Boca Raton, FL, pp. 833–852, 2012.
44. Blackburn NA, Johnson IT: The effect of guar gum on the viscosity of the gastrointestinal contents and on glucose uptake from the perfused jejunum in the rat. *Br J Nutr* 46:239–246, 1981.
45. Jenkins DJA, Wolever TMS, Leeds AR et al.: Dietary fibres, fibre analogues, and glucose tolerance: Importance of viscosity. *Br Med J* 1:1392–1394, 1978.
46. Zein M, Areas JL, Knapka J et al.: Excess sucrose and glucose ingestion acutely elevate blood pressure in spontaneously hypertensive rats. *Am J Hypertens* 3:380–386, 1990.
47. Preuss HG, Zein M, Knapka J et al.: Blood pressure responses to sucrose ingestion in four strains of rats. *Am J Hypertens* 5:244–250, 1992.
48. Preuss HG, Knapka JJ: Sugar-induced hypertension in Fischer 344 and F1-hybrid rats (F244/BN) at different ages. *Geriatric Nephrol Urol* 4:15–21, 1994.

49. Preuss HG, Echard B, Clouatre D et al: Niacin-bound chromium (NBC) increases life span in Zucker rats. *J Inorg Chem* 105:1344–1349, 2011.
50. Perricone NV, Echard B, Preuss HG: Blood pressure lowering effects of niacin-bound chromium in sucrose-fed rats: Renin-angiotensin system. *J Inorg Biochem* 102:1541–1548, 2008.
51. Jenkins DJA, Srichaikul K, Mirrahimi A et al.: Glycemic index. In: Bagchi D, Preuss HG (eds.). *Obesity. Epidemiology, Pathophysiology, and Prevention*, 2nd edn. CRC Press, Boca Raton, FL, pp. 212–238, 2012.
52. Nordmann AJ, Nordmann A, Briel M et al.: Effects of low-carbohydrate vs. low-fat diets on weight loss and cardiovascular risk factors: A meta-analysis of randomized controlled trials. *Arch Intern Med* 166:285–293, 2006.
53. Thomas DE, Elliott EJ, Baur L: Low glycaemic index or low glycaemic load diets for overweight and obesity. *Cochrane Database Syst Rev* (3):CD005105, July 18, 2007.
54. Samaha FF, Iqbal N, Seshadri P et al.: A low-carbohydrate as compared with a low-fat diet in severe obesity. *N Engl J Med* 348:2074–2081, 2003.
55. Stern L, Iqbal N, Seshadri P et al.: The effects of low-carbohydrate versus conventional weight loss diets in severely obese adults: One-year follow-up of a randomized trial. *Ann Int Med* 18:778–785, 2004.
56. McAuley KA, Hopkins CM, Smith KJ et al.: Comparison of high-fat and high-protein diets with a high-carbohydrate diet in insulin-resistant obese women. *Diabetologia* 48:8–16, 2005.
57. Hession M, Rolland C, Kulkarni U et al.: Systematic review of randomized controlled trials of low-carbohydrate vs. low-fat/low-calorie diets in the management of obesity and its comorbidities. *Obes Rev* 10:36–50, 2009.
58. Sacks FM, Bray GA, Carey VJ et al.: Comparison of weight-loss diets with different compositions of fat, protein, and carbohydrates. *N Engl J Med* 360:859–873, 2009.
59. Krebs JD, Bell D, Hall R et al.: Improvements in glucose metabolism and insulin sensitivity with a low-carbohydrate diet in obese patients with type 2 diabetes. *J Am Coll Nutr* 32:11–17, 2013.
60. Ifland JR, Sheppard K, Preuss HG et al.: Refined food addiction: A classic substance use disorder. *Med Hypotheses* 72:518–526, 2009.
61. Fukagawa NK, Anderson JW, Hageman G et al.: High-carbohydrate, high-fiber diets increase peripheral insulin sensitivity in healthy young and old adults. *Am J Clin Nutr* 52:524–528, 1990.
62. Jenkins DJ, Kendall CW, Marchie A et al.: Type 2 diabetes and the vegetarian diet. *Am J Clin Nutr* 78(3 Suppl.):610S–616S, 2003.
63. Preuss HG: Bean amylase inhibitor and other carbohydrate absorption blockers: Effects on diabesity and general health. *J Am Coll Nutr* 28:266–276, 2009.

Section VIII

Immune Health

20 Dietary Supplements, Nutraceutical, and Functional Foods in Immune Response (Immunomodulators)

Raj K. Keservani, Rajesh K. Kesharwani, Anil K. Sharma, and Urmila Jarouliya

CONTENTS

20.1 INTRODUCTION

Dietary supplements are also called food supplements, defined as any product (other than tobacco) that is intended to supplement the diet. It mainly contains one or more of the following: a vitamin, mineral, herb, or other botanical; an amino acid or metabolite; an extract; or any combination of the previously mentioned items. According to U.S. Food and Drug Administration (FDA) regulations, a dietary supplement may be marketed in food form if it is not *represented* as a conventional food and is clearly labeled as a dietary supplement (IFIC 1999, IMNRC 2004). Nutraceutical, which is a hybrid of *nutrition* and *pharmaceutical*, was coined in 1989 by Stephen L. DeFelice, founder and chairman of the Foundation of Innovation Medicine (Kalra 2003), and defined as "Food, or parts of food, that provide medical or health benefits, including the prevention and treatment of disease" (Keservani et al. 2010a). Functional foods, according to their generally accepted definition, are "any food or food ingredient that may provide a health benefit beyond the traditional nutrients it contains" (IFIC 1999). There are indications for some beneficial effects of nutraceuticals such as antioxidant, mushrooms, vitamins, essential amino acids, phytochemicals, and polyunsaturated fatty acids in infant foods on the developing immune response (Keservani et al. 2010a, Chintale et al. 2013).

Immunomodulators may be defined as a substance, biological or synthetic, which can stimulate, suppress, or modulate any of the components of the immune system including both innate and adaptive arms of the immune response (Agarwal and Singh 1999, Simopoulos 2002). The active agents of immunotherapy are collectively called immunomodulators (Masihi 2001). Immunological reactions are divided into two parts by the specificity and the speed of the reaction, innate and adaptive responses, although in practice there is extensive interaction between them and it is often hard to describe where the innate immunity ends and the adaptive immunity starts (Parkin and Cohen 2001). The innate immunity provides the immediate but nonspecific host defense, and it includes physical, chemical, and microbiological barriers as well as many elements of the immune system (neutrophils, monocytes, macrophages, complement, cytokines, and acute-phase proteins). The adaptive immunity consists of antigen-specific reactions through T lymphocytes and B lymphocytes. The adaptive immune response is highly specific, and it develops an immunological memory, but its development requires several days or weeks.

20.2 DIETARY SUPPLEMENTS, NUTRACEUTICAL, AND FUNCTIONAL FOODS IN IMMUNE RESPONSE

The health benefits are primarily in various areas, such as atherosclerosis, cardiovascular disease, aging, respiratory, diabetes, mental health, and immune response–enhancing effects. Dietary supplements, nutraceutical, and functional food products mentioned later are used to enhance the body immune response to fight against environmental pathogens and possess immunomodulator effects on humans (Keservani et al. 2010a).

20.2.1 Dietary Fibers in Immune Response

Dietary fibers include cellulose, hemicellulose, polyfructoses, galacto-oligosaccharides, gums, mucilages, pectins, lignin, and resistant starches and are classically divided into soluble or insoluble. More recently, some are proposing the use of the terms "viscous" and "fermentability" in place of soluble and insoluble to describe the functions and health benefits of dietary fiber. Functional fiber is something that manufacturers deliberately add to food products to provide similar health benefits to those of dietary fiber, without adding significant calories. Some examples of functional fibers are cellulose, maltodextran, polydextrose, and inulin, and these are isolated from foods where they occur naturally. The consumption of dietary and functional fibers has many potential health benefits in constipation (Castillejo et al. 2006), irritable bowel syndrome (Malhotra et al. 2004), lowering of cholesterol, diminishing the incidence of coronary and cardiovascular heart diseases (Romero et al. 2002, Van Rosendaal et al. 2004, Otles and Ozgoz 2014), preventing obesity (Murakami et al. 2007) and diabetes (Hannan et al. 2007), avoiding colon cancer (Wakai et al. 2007), and increasing survival in breast cancer (McEligot et al. 2006).

Inulin and other oligofructoses have been the most extensively studied dietary fibers. They act to stimulate the growth of bifidobacteria in the colon. Bifidobacteria and lactobacilli are health-promoting bacteria that generate short-chain fatty acids and stimulate the immune system (Otles and Ozgoz 2014). The proposed health benefits of bifidobacteria include the following:

1. Protection from intestinal infection
2. Lowering of intestinal pH for formation of acids after assimilation of carbohydrates
3. Reduction of the number of potentially harmful bacteria and production of vitamins and antioxidants
4. Activation of intestinal function and assistance in digestion and absorption, especially of calcium
5. Bulking activity to prevent and treat constipation
6. Stimulation of the immune response
7. Potential reduction in the risk for colorectal cancer

Limited studies in humans have indicated that inulin supplementation increases the fecal bacterial contents of bifidobacteria and has favorable effects on the types and amounts of circulating lymphocytes.

20.2.2 Probiotics in Immune Responses

Probiotics are organisms such as bacteria or yeast that are believed to improve health when consumed. They are available in supplements and foods (Rijkers et al. 2011). The rationale for probiotics is that many gastrointestinal dysfunctions are based on disturbances or imbalances of intestinal microflora (Salminen et al. 1999, Floch and Hong-Curtiss 2001, Lin 2003). Laparra and Sanz note that microbial imbalances are associated with metabolic and immune-mediated disorders and that diet is considered a major driver for changes in the diversity of the microbiota (Laparra and Sanz 2007). Some probiotic strains such as bifidobacteria are used to correct unbalanced intestinal microbiota (Floch and Hong-Curtiss 2001, Isolauri et al. 2004). In order for these probiotic strains to have a beneficial effect on microbial balance, a number of actions are suggested as necessary including increased digestive capacity, enhanced mucosal barrier, reduced inflammation, and lowered allergic sensitivity (German et al. 1999, Lesvos-Pantoflickova et al. 2007). Sanders (2008), however, notes that while probiotic strains have been shown to alter populations or activities of colonizing microbes, it is difficult to say with accuracy that this improves the balance as there is no agreement on what is a healthy microbiota composition (Sanders 2008).

Commensal bacteria can modulate the immune system at both a systemic and a local level. Signals mediated by commensal bacteria or their ligands are essential to develop optimal mucosal and immune system and to maintain and repair the gut. In the intestine, immunosensory cells, such as enterocytes, M cells, and dendritic cells (DCs), are continually sampling and responding to intestinal bacteria. These immunocytes express pattern recognition receptors including toll-like receptors that engage bacterial signals, such as lipopolysaccharide, lipoteichoic acid, bacterial DNA, and flagellin. This contributes to the activation of transcription factors and proinflammatory cascades in immunosensory cells.

Some strains of probiotic bacteria, such as *Lactobacillus casei* or *Lactobacillus reuteri*, but not *Lactobacillus plantarum*, can promote tolerance-inducing DCs by priming DCs to drive the development of regulatory T cells (O'Hara and Shanahan 2007). Ribeiro et al. (2007) studied the effects of prebiotics and probiotics on the colonization and immune response of broiler chickens challenged with *Salmonella enteritidis*. Ashgan and Samah (2011) also studied the impact of symbiotic on the immune response of broiler chickens against Newcastle disease virus (NDV) and infectious bronchitis virus (IBV) vaccines and reported that high concentration of symbiotic improves the antibody response to NDV and IBV vaccines. Aghaee et al. (2014) studied the effect of probiotic supplement on immune response in male athletes, a randomized clinical trial, and concluded that probiotics play a role in the development of immune system.

Nutrition is known to influence immunity and host resistance to illness. Widespread interest exists in the use of probiotics to enhance host resistance to illness. Probiotics can enhance epithelial barrier function in vitro and animal models (Madsen et al. 2001). Probiotics protect human epithelial cell cultures (HT29) and T84 cells against damage resulting from exposure to *Escherichia coli* (Resta-Lenert and Barrett 2006, Zyrek et al. 2007). Probiotics also enhance immunity beyond the gastrointestinal (GI) tract through interactions with the common mucosal immune system.

To function as effective prophylactic agents against common illnesses, probiotics must enhance innate and acquired elements of the mucosal immune system (Rosenthal 2006). Experimental evidence suggests that probiotics can modulate GI permeability. The GI barrier comprises mainly of individual epithelial cell membranes that are impermeable to hydrophilic solutes except at sites of specific transporters (Turner 2006).

A number of studies have addressed the effects of supplementation with various probiotic strains in healthy volunteers. Increases in natural killer (NK) activity have been observed after supplementation with *L. casei* Shirota, *L. casei* DN114001, *Lactobacillus rhamnosus* HN001, or *Bifidobacterium lactis* HN019 (Borchers et al. 2009). Probiotic organisms are used in a variety of foods, the main category being dairy products, but they are also present as food supplements in capsule or tablet form. Since viability is an essential property of a probiotic, the final product must contain an adequate amount of living probiotic(s) until the end of its shelf life (Binns 2013).

20.2.3 Antioxidants in Immune Response

Antioxidants are effective via various mechanisms including (1) preventive antioxidants, (2) free radical scavengers, (3) sequestration of elements by chelation, and (4) quenching active oxygen species (Dunnet 2003). Oxidative stress occurs when production of free radicals exceeds the capacity of the antioxidant system of body cells (McDowell et al. 2007). Antioxidants have been defined as substances or a compound that prevents damage of cell against excess free radicals and are critical for maintaining optimal health in both animals and humans. The cell of living systems requires optimum levels of substances in order to protect or nullify the harmful effect of an excessively produced reactive oxygen species (ROS) and maintain the homeostasis (Puertollano et al. 2011). Certain nutrients such as lipid, iron, selinium, zinc, vitamin A, vitamin C, vitamin D, and vitamin E with oxidants and antioxidant action, their food sources, and effects in the immune system are mentioned in Table 20.1 (Weiss 2005, McDowell et al. 2007, Vazquez et al. 2014).

Several metalloenzymes, which include glutathione peroxidase (Se), catalase (Fe), and superoxide dismutase (Cu, Zn, and Mn), are also critical in protecting the internal cellular constituents from oxidative damage. Only when these metals are delivered in the diet in sufficient amounts can the animal body synthesize these antioxidant enzymes. In contrast, deficiency of those elements causes oxidative stress and damage to biological molecules and membranes. Zinc deficiency in the elderly is also associated with impaired immune responses, which can be restored by zinc supplementation. Dietary selenium occurs in protein-rich foods such as meat, fish, nuts, and seeds (Gredel 2011).

TABLE 20.1
Nutrients with Their Food Source, Function, and Role in Immune Response

Nutrients	Food Source	Function	Role in Immune System
Lipid	Vegetable oils, olive oil, almonds, walnuts, peanuts, coconut, and avocado	Assists in the transport and absorption of liposoluble vitamins and cell membrane component	Production of cytokine IL-1 and IL-6. Production of TNF- and inflammatory response.
Iron	Liver, seafood, and lean meat	Component of hemoglobin and myoglobin and important in oxygen transfer	Involvement of Fenton reaction with the production of free radicals with antimicrobial action.
Selenium	Giblets, fish, seafood, wheat germ, and brazil nut	Involved in the metabolism of fat and vitamin E	Component of glutathione peroxides.
Zinc	Meat, fish, poultry, and dairy	Acts on growth and cell replication	Structural and catalytic components of the superoxide dismutase.
Vitamin A	Liver, egg, milk, and carrots	Protective action on the skin and mucus and essential role in retinal function	Inhibition of the lipid peroxidation and the generation of hydroperoxides.
Vitamin C	Citrus fruits, tomatoes, peppers, and leafy vegetables	Increases the absorption of nonheme iron	Enzymatic cofactor with redox properties.
Vitamin D	Fish (oil liver), egg yolk, butter, cheeses, and meats	Maintaining homeostasis of calcium and phosphorus	Expression of antimicrobial peptides.
Vitamin E	Vegetable oils, olive oil, almonds, and avocados	Protection of cell membrane–unsaturated phospholipids	Decreased lipid peroxidation.

Selenium is essential for an optimal immune response and influences both the innate and acquired immune systems. Iron is an example of a nutrient, which is required not only for an adequate immune response but also for an optimal growth of pathogens. As long as iron deficiency does not impair immune function, iron supplementation may benefit only pathogenic bacteria (Gredel 2011). Zinc and vitamin E with Se could improve the immunity of animals and protect them from the appearance of clinical signs of disease although pathogenic bacterium was detected. Combination of vitamin E and selenium improve cell-mediated and humoral immune response and increased resistance to *E. coli* infection (Hala et al. 2013).

Vitamin E is an important lipid-soluble antioxidant that protects against free radical–initiated lipid peroxidation. Fresh green forage is an excellent source of vitamin E. However, concentrates and stored forages (hays, haylages, and silages) are generally low in vitamin E (Spears and Weiss 2008). It is the most common naturally occurring antioxidant. It has a phytyl chain that is attached to its chromanol nucleus. The principal vitamin E form with antioxidant and immune functions is α-tocopherol. However, although studies are limited, non-α-tocopherol and tocotrienols have important functions. γ-Tocopherol has been shown to be a more effective inhibitor of peroxy nitrite–induced lipid peroxidation (McCormick and Parker 2004).

Vitamin C (Figure 20.1) is a water-soluble electron donor vitamin. It donates two electrons from C-2 and C-3 double bond carbons to act as an antioxidant that results in the formation of an intermediate free radical, semi-dehydroascorbic acid E. The resulting ascorbate free radicals reduce to a neutral ascorbate molecule (Spears and Weiss 2008). Vitamin C is the most important antioxidant in extracellular fluids and can protect biomembranes against lipid peroxidation damage by eliminating peroxyl radicals in the aqueous phase before the latter can initiate peroxidation. Vitamin C is located in the aqueous phase of cells, where it contributes to radical scavenging (McDowell et al. 2007).

Carotenoids are among the most widespread and important ones, especially due to their varied functions. These are fat-soluble pigments found mostly in plants, fruits, flowers, algae, and photosynthetic bacteria, and they also occur in some nonphotosynthetic bacteria, yeasts, and molds. Carotenoids have extensive applications as antioxidants in dietary supplements and as colors in foods and beverages as well as pigments in poultry and fish. The carotenoids used as food ingredients include astaxanthin, beta-apo-carotenal, canthaxanthin, beta-carotene, lutein, zeaxanthin, and lycopene. Protective effects of carotenoids against serious disorders such as cancer (Donaldson 2004, Kantoff 2006), heart disease (Lonn and Yusuf 1999, Sesso et al. 2003), and degenerative eye disease (Mozaffarieh et al. 2003) have been recognized and have stimulated intensive research into the role of carotenoids as antioxidants and as regulators of the immune response system.

Carotenoids are a large group of compounds with the basic skeleton of a polyisoprenoid carbon chain with a number of conjugated double bonds (Chakraborty et al. 2009). The traditional concept

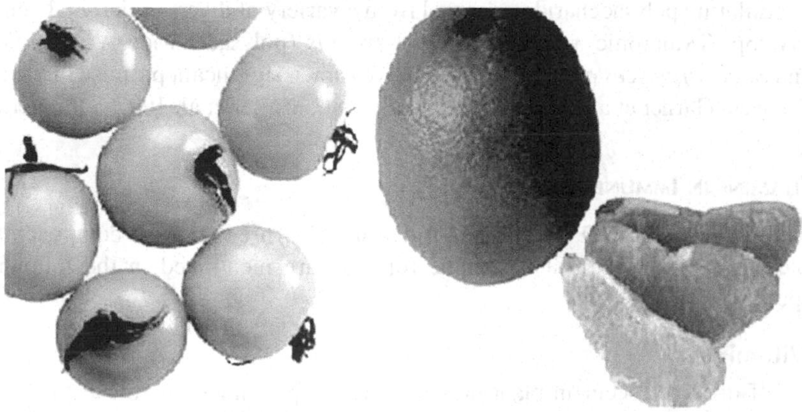

FIGURE 20.1 Food sources containing vitamin C with antioxidant potentials.

of ROS function is that they indiscriminately destroy cell components. However, exciting research has more recently elucidated the role of these reactive species in signal transduction, gene regulation, and disease etiology. This has infused new excitement and challenges into research on the possible role of carotenoids as antioxidants in disease prevention.

Spirulina is blue-green algae due to the presence of both chlorophyll (green) and phycocyanin (blue) pigments in its cellular structure. We review here the beneficial effects of spirulina as a nutritional and dietary supplement covering all major areas of health benefits, with special focus on its immunomodulatory and antioxidant effects. The aqueous extract of spirulina was found to have a major impact on the immune system by increasing the phagocytic activity of macrophages, stimulating the NK cells. It also played a role in the activation and mobilization of T and B cells due to its stimulatory effects in the production of cytokines and antibodies (Maddaly et al. 2010).

20.2.4 Mushrooms in Immune Response

Mushrooms have been valued by humankind as an edible and medical resource. A number of bioactive molecules, including antitumor substances, have been identified in many mushroom species. Polysaccharides are the best known and most potent mushroom-derived substances with antitumor and immunomodulating properties (Wasser 2002). Qualitative and quantitative analyses of these mushrooms showed that they contained some biologically active compounds and nutrients such as sugars and amino acids. These bioactive compounds belong to the group of polysaccharides and antioxidants; the presence of polysaccharides in mushrooms (which are polymers of sugar molecules) suggests that they can be useful as natural health promoters against parasites, bacteria, and viruses (Oei 2003).

Mushrooms such as *Ganoderma lucidum* (Reishi), *Lentinus edodes* (Shiitake), *Inonotus obliquus* (Chaga), and many others have been collected and used for hundreds of years in Korea, China, Japan, and eastern Russia. Those practices still form the basis of modern scientific studies of fungal medical activities, especially in the field of stomach, prostate, and lung cancers. Mushrooms cataloged worldwide, barely a hundred can be cultivated, and little research has been conducted in developing countries like Nigeria on strictly local species. Tanzania is reported as one of the countries in Africa that is actively exploring *Ganoderma* species of mushroom, which are highly prized as supplementary dietary feed (Anon 2008). Yu et al. (2009) carried out research on the effects of whole mushrooms during inflammation and concludes that edible mushrooms regulate immunity in vitro. Yang et al. (2014) studied the effect of mushroom beta glucan (MBG) on immune and hemocyte response in pacific white shrimp (*Litopenaeus vannamei*) and reported that MBG administration through dietary administration is also a convenient and useful practical technique in the future.

Immunomodulating polysaccharides, derived from a variety of diverse microbial genera, include *Streptococcus* spp. (hyaluronic acid), *Bacteroides fragilis* (polysaccharide A), *Candida albicans* (Mannan), and *Saccharomyces cerevisiae*, which have shown significant promise in the treatment of infectious diseases (Garner et al. 1990, Shapiro et al. 1986, Muller et al. 1997, Schrager et al. 1998).

20.2.5 Vitamins in Immune Response

Vitamin E, vitamin C, vitamin D, and vitamin A (carotenoids) are important components of animal, and their roles in animal health and immune function are mentioned in the following in each vitamin, respectively.

20.2.5.1 Vitamin A

Vitamin A itself does not occur in plant products, but its precursors, carotenes, do occur in several forms. These compounds (carotenoids) are commonly referred to as provitamin A because the body can transform them into active vitamin A. The combined potency in a feed, represented by its vitamin A and carotene content, is referred to as its vitamin A value. Vitamin A occurs in three forms: retinol, retinal, and retinoic acid. Retinol is the alcohol form of vitamin A (Olson 1984). Carotenoids enhance the immune system and boost the body's ability to fight illness and disease (Burri 1997).

Adequate dietary vitamin A is necessary to help maintain normal resistance to stress and disease. An animal's ability to resist infectious disease depends on a responsive immune system, with a vitamin A deficiency causing a reduced immune response. In many experiments with laboratory and domestic animals, the effects of both clinical and subclinical deficiencies of vitamin A on the production of antibodies and on the resistance of different tissues against microbial infection or parasitic infestation have frequently been demonstrated (Kelley and Easter 1987, Lessard et al. 1997). Supplemental vitamin A improved the health of animals infected with roundworms, of hens infected with the genus *Capillaria*, and of rats with hookworms (Herrick 1972). Vitamin A is a valuable nutritional aid in the management of ringworm (*Trichophyton verrucosum*) infection in cattle. Vitamin A deficiency affects immune function, particularly the antibody response to T cell–dependent antigens (Ross 1992). The RAR-alpha mRNA expression and antigen-specific proliferative responses to T lymphocytes are influenced by vitamin A status in vivo and directly modulated by retinoic acid (Halevy et al. 1994). Vitamin A deficiency affects a number of cells of the immune system, and repletion with retinoic acid effectively reestablishes the number of circulating lymphocytes (Zhao and Ross 1995). A diminished primary antibody response could also increase the severity and/or duration of an episode of infection, whereas a diminished secondary response could increase the risk of developing a second episode of infection. Vitamin A deficiency causes decreased phagocytic activity in macrophages and neutrophils. The secretory immunoglobulin A (IgA) system is an important first line of defense against infections of mucosal surfaces (McGhee et al. 1992). Several studies in animal models have shown that the intestinal IgA response is impaired by vitamin A deficiency (Wiedermann et al. 1993, Stephensen et al. 1996). Recent animal studies indicate that certain carotenoids without vitamin A activity have antioxidant capacities and can enhance many aspects of immune functions, act directly as antimutagens and anticarcinogens, protect against radiation damage, and block the damaging effects of photosensitizers (Chew 1995, Koutsos et al. 2006, Lindshield and Erdman 2006).

20.2.5.2 Vitamin C

Vitamin C is a water-soluble vitamin. We must therefore consume it on a regular basis, as any excess is excreted (primarily in the urine) rather than stored. There are two active forms of vitamin C: ascorbic acid and dehydroascorbic acid. Most animals can make their own vitamin C from glucose. Humans and guinea pigs are two groups that cannot synthesize their own vitamin C and must consume it in the diet (IMFNB 2000). Many fruits and vegetables are high in vitamin C. Citrus fruits (such as oranges, lemons, and limes), potatoes, strawberries, tomatoes, kiwi fruit, broccoli, spinach and other leafy greens, cabbage, green and red peppers, and cauliflower are excellent sources of vitamin C (Zee et al. 1991). Fortified beverages and cereals are also good sources. Dairy foods, meats, and nonfortified cereals and grains provide little or no vitamin C. Consuming a healthful diet that includes excellent sources of vitamin C will assist with maintaining a strong immune system (Gredel 2011).

Vitamin C also acts as an antioxidant. In addition to collagen, vitamin C assists in the synthesis of DNA, bile, neurotransmitters such as serotonin (which helps regulate mood), and carnitine, which transports long-chain fatty acids from the cytosol into the mitochondria for energy production. It also enhances immune function by protecting the white blood cells from the oxidative damage that occurs in response to fighting illness and infection (IMFNB 2000). Biochemical and physiological functions of vitamin C have been reviewed (Moser and Bendich 1991, Padh 1991, Gershoff 1993, Johnston 2006, Johnston et al. 2007).

20.2.5.3 Vitamin D

Vitamin D is found in two forms: ergocalciferol (vitamin D_2) and cholecalciferol (vitamin D_3), and on the basis of function, they are closely related compounds that possess antirachitic activity. Both vitamin

D_2 and D_3 may be supplied through the diet or, specifically, D_3 is formed by irradiation of the skin of the body. Vitamin D, in the pure form, occurs as colorless crystals that are insoluble in water but readily soluble in alcohol and other organic solvents (Braun 1986). Sources of vitamin D are feedstuff, irradiation, sebaceous material licked from skin or hair or directly absorbed products, or irradiation formed on or in the skin. For dogs and cats (and presumably other carnivores), vitamin D must be obtained from dietary sources due to the inability of these species to synthesize and utilize vitamin D from precursors in the skin (How et al. 1995). Vitamin D supplementation may be needed for an optimum immune response. Vitamin D deficiency results in a marked depression in the cellular immune responses of young broiler chicks with negligible apparent impact on humoral immunity (Aslam et al. 1998).

Vitamin D has many important functions other than calcium and bone homeostasis, which include modulation of the adaptive and innate immunity. The most prevalent disease related to vitamin D deficiency is autoimmune disease. Cells of the immune system are capable of synthesizing and responding to vitamin D. Immune cells in autoimmune diseases are responsive to the ameliorative effects of vitamin D suggesting that the beneficial effects of supplementing vitamin D–deficient individuals with autoimmune disease may extend beyond the effects on bone and calcium homeostasis (Aranow 2011). Besides the effects in calcium and bone metabolism, vitamin D and especially its biologically active metabolite 1,25-dihydroxycholecalciferol (1,25(OH)2D3) act as powerful immunoregulators (Maggini et al. 2007).

20.2.5.4 Vitamin E

Vitamin E is widespread in foods. Much of the vitamin E that we consume comes from vegetable oils, safflower oil, sunflower oil, canola oil, and soybean oil, which are good sources (McDowell 2000, Traber 2006). Mayonnaise and salad dressings made from these oils also contain vitamin E. Nuts, seeds, and some vegetables also contribute vitamin E to our diet. Although no single fruit or vegetable contains very high amounts of vitamin E, eating the recommended amounts of fruits and vegetables each day will help ensure adequate intake of this nutrient. Cereals (Traber 2006) are often fortified with vitamin E, and other grain products contribute modest amounts to our diet. Wheat germ and soybeans are also good sources of vitamin E. Vitamin E is one of the fat-soluble vitamins; thus, dietary fats carry it from the intestines through the lymph system and eventually transport it to the cells. Vitamin E is absorbed with dietary fat and incorporated into the chylomicrons. As the chylomicrons are broken down, most of the vitamin E remains in the remnants of the chylomicrons and is transported to the liver. There, vitamin E is incorporated into very-low-density lipoproteins (VLDLs) and released into the blood. After VLDLs release their triglyceride load, they become LDLs. Vitamin E is a part of both VLDLs and LDLs and is transported to the tissues and cells by both these lipoproteins. The liver serves as a storage site for vitamins A and D, and about 90% of the vitamin E in the body is stored in our adipose tissue. The remaining vitamin E is found in cell membranes (Winklhofer-Roob et al. 2004, Yeomans et al. 2005).

Vitamin E is actually two separate families of compounds, tocotrienols and tocopherols. None of the four different tocotrienol compounds, alpha, beta, gamma, and delta, appear to play an active role in the body. The tocopherol compounds are the biologically active forms of vitamin E in the body (Upadhyay et al. 2009b). Four different tocopherol compounds have been discovered: as with tocotrienol, these have been designated alpha, beta, gamma, and delta. Of these, the most active, or potent, vitamin E compound found in food and supplements is α-tocopherol.

The primary function of vitamin E is as an antioxidant (Upadhyay et al. 2009a Keservani et al. 2010b). As described earlier in this chapter, this means that vitamin E donates an electron to free radicals, stabilizing them and preventing them from destabilizing other molecules. Vitamin E serves many other roles essential to human health. Vitamin E is critical for normal fetal and early childhood development of nerves and muscles as well as for maintenance of their functions. It enhances immune function by protecting white blood cells and other components of the immune system, thereby helping the body to defend against illness and disease (Winklhofer-Roob et al. 2004, Yeomans et al. 2005).

20.2.6 Folic Acid in Immune Response

Folic acid is widely distributed in nature; only limited amounts of free folic acid occur in natural products, and most feed sources contain predominantly polyglutamyl folic acid. Soybeans, other beans, nuts, some animals, products, and citrus fruits are good sources. Folic acid is abundant in green leafy materials and organ meats. The abundance of folic acid in green forages is shown by the higher concentrations of folic acid in milk from grazing herds than from herds fed dry hay (Dong and Oace 1975). Folacin is the generic descriptor not only for the original vitamin, folic acid, but also for related compounds that qualitatively show folic acid activity, the pure substance being designated pteroylmonoglutamic acid. Its chemical structure contains three distinct parts, consisting of glutamic acid, a *para*-aminobenzoic acid residue, and a pteridine nucleus (Wagner 1984).

Folic acid, in the form 5,6,7,8-tetrahydrofolic acid, is indispensable in the transfer of single-carbon units in various reactions, a role analogous to that of pantothenic acid in the transfer of two-carbon units (Bailey and Gregory 2006). Folic acid requirements are related to the type and the level of production. Growth rate, age, and pregnancy influence folic acid requirements. The requirement decreases with age because diminished growth rate reduces the need for DNA synthesis. Increased catabolism of folic acid is a feature of pregnancy. Studies with humans (McPartlin et al. 1993) demonstrated enhanced folic acid catabolism; this was a feature of pregnancy per se and not simply due to increased weight.

The role of folic acid in biochemical reactions, such as metabolism of amino acids and synthesis of DNA, renders it a critical nutrient in embryogenesis (Almeida and Cardoso 2011). Folic acid supplementation was primarily indicated for the prevention and treatment of megaloblastic and maternal anemia (Almeida and Cardoso 2011). Supplementation is also indicated in individuals with a genetic defect requiring greater amounts of folate than that can be derived from the diet (Ashfield-Watt et al. 2002). Recent findings on folic acid supply and effects during pregnancy, lactation, and infancy were presented (Hermoso et al. 2011). Liu et al. (2011) studied and reported that supplementation of micronutrients might increase immune function and reduce the incidence of common infections in type 2 diabetic outpatients. Folic acid fortification of wheat has become widespread in the Americans, a strategy adopted by Canada and the United States and about 20 Latin American countries (Lindsay et al. 2006). Susumu et al. (2012) studied folate deficiency among aged patients and its amelioration through the consumption of folic acid–fortified rice and concluded the nutritional benefits of folic acid in geriatric patients.

20.2.7 Polysaccharides in Immune Response

Polysaccharides isolated from many medicinal plants represent a large class of biopolymers with a structure variability, which is the basis for their biological activities. This enormous potential of proprieties can play a role in the various applications of the polysaccharides in the broad field of pharmacy and medicine by Franz (1989). Polysaccharides possess immunological properties ranging from nonspecific stimulation of host immune system, resulting in antitumor, antiviral, and anti-infection effects to antioxidant, antimutagenic, or hematopoietic activity. These properties were found in the blue-green filamentous alga *Spirulina* extract, which can inhibit viral replications and cancer development and enhance antibody production. The antiviral polysaccharides should have very low cytotoxicity toward mammalian cells if they are to be used for medicinal purpose. Polysaccharides have shown good immunomodulatory properties associated with antitumor effects (Katarzyna et al. 2012).

Dalila et al. (2010) studied immunologically active polysaccharides isolated from *Anacyclus pyrethrum* and reported that three polysaccharides extracted from *A. pyrethrum* have immunostimulating activity that could be used clinically for the modulation of immune systems. Polysaccharide content of *Echinacea purpurea* L. (EP) is a plant originally used by native Americans to treat respiratory infections and have long been used to aid in wound healing and to enhance the immune system reported by Lee et al. (2010) and Kumar and Ramaiah (2011). Nair et al. (2004) studied immune-stimulating properties of a novel polysaccharide from the medicinal plant *Tinospora cordifolia*. Koffi et al. (2013) studied and reported immunomodulatory activity of polysaccharides isolated from *Clerodendrum splendens* and its beneficial effects in experimental autoimmune encephalomyelitis. Ghildyal et al. (2010) studied and reported chemical composition and immunological activities of polysaccharides isolated from the malian medicinal plant *Syzygium guineense*.

Research shows that astragalus root stimulates the immune system in many ways. It has been identified as glucans, and polysaccharide D as a heteropolysaccharide increases the number of stem cells in bone marrow and lymph tissue and encourages their development into active immune cells (Das et al. 2014). Polysaccharide components of ginseng have received much attention recently because of the emergence of different biological activities, such as immunomodulatory, antibacterial, antimutagenic, radioprotective, antioxidative, antiulcer, antidepressant, antisepticemic, and anti-inflammatory activities (Sun 2011).

20.2.8 Phytochemicals in Immune Response

Phytochemicals are nonnutritive naturally occurring plant chemicals that have either defensive or disease-protective properties. Dietary intake of phytochemicals may promote health benefits, protecting against chronic degenerative disorders, such as cancer, immune response, cardiovascular, and neurodegenerative diseases. Phytochemicals (Figure 20.2) are found in abundance in fruits, vegetables, whole grains, legumes, seeds, soy products, garlic, onion, and green, and black teas (Greenwald et al. 2001, Keservani and Sharma 2014).

Food sources of various phytochemicals are presented in Table 20.2. These phytochemicals, either alone and/or in combination, have tremendous therapeutic potential in curing various ailments. Phytochemicals with nutraceutical properties present in food are of enormous significance due to their beneficial effects on human health since they offer protection against numerous diseases or disorders such as cancers, coronary heart disease, diabetes, high blood pressure, inflammation, microbial, viral and parasitic infections, psychotic diseases, spasmodic conditions, ulcers, osteoporosis, and associated disorders (Prakash et al. 2012).

Carotenoids and flavonoids have been investigated for their immunomodulatory potential (Gredel 2011). Carotenoids (such as beta-carotene, lycopene, lutein, and zeaxanthin) may inhibit cancer cell growth, work as antioxidants, and improve immune response. Flavonoids (such as anthocyanins and quercetin) may inhibit inflammation and tumor growth and may aid immunity and boost the production of detoxifying enzymes in the body (www.preventcancer.aicr.org/site/PageServer?pagename=elements_phytochemicals). The flavonoid kaempferol has been shown to be suppressive toward $CD8^+$ cell activities including interferon-gamma production and may be

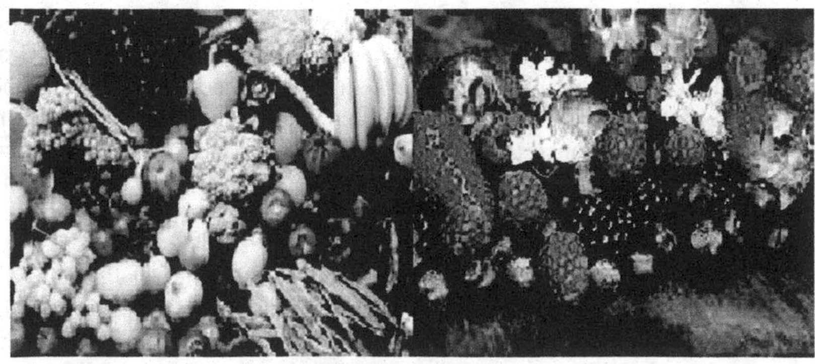

FIGURE 20.2 Food sources of phytochemicals.

TABLE 20.2
Food Sources of Various Phytochemicals

Phytochemicals	Examples	Food Sources
Carotenoids	Alpha-carotene, beta-carotene, lycopene, lutein	Yellow-red, red, orange, and dark green vegetables and fruits such as carrots, cantaloupe, sweet potatoes, apricots, kale, spinach, pumpkin, and tomatoes
Glucosinolates, isothiocyanates, indoles	Glucobrassicin, indole-3-carbinol	Cruciferous vegetables such as broccoli, cabbage, cauliflower, and Brussels sprouts
Organosulfur compounds	Diallyl sulfide, allyl methyl trisulfide, dithiolthiones	Allium vegetables, including onion and garlic, and cruciferous vegetables such as broccoli, cabbage, cauliflower, and Brussels sprouts
Polyphenols	Flavonoids and phenolic acids	Apple skins, berries, broccoli, citrus fruit, red wine, and black and green teas
Phytoestrogens	Isoflavones, lignans	Soybeans and soy-based foods, vegetables, rye

counterproductive in cell-mediated cancer immunotherapy (Okamoto et al. 2002). This polyphenol does attenuate adhesion molecule expression in vascular cells (Ferrero et al. 1998, Aggarwal and Shishodia 2006) and may thus be more effective in preventing metastatic spread of cancers. Asgand showed a significant modulation of immune reactivity in animal models (Uddin et al. 2012).

Camellia sinensis, commonly used for the preparation of the product green tea, belongs to Theaceae family, which is grown throughout Asia, Middle East, and Africa (Zahra 2011). Green tea reduced autoimmune symptoms in the rat adjuvant arthritis, a model of human rheumatoid arthritis. Epigallocatechin-3-gallate is a component of green tea with anti-inflammatory and immunomodulatory activities (Kawaguchi et al. 2011). This compound has shown effective immunosuppressive effects on T-cell-mediated immune responses (Yoneyama et al. 2008). Flavonoid content of *E. purpurea* L. (EP) is a plant originally used by native Americans to treat respiratory infections and have long been used to aid in wound healing and to enhance the immune system reported by Lee et al. (2010).

20.3 CONCLUSIONS

Inadequate intake and status of vitamins and trace elements may lead to suppressed immunity, which predisposes to infections and aggravates undernutrition. An increased understanding of the unique effects of strain-specific probiotics on the immune system will help health-care professionals to be more specific with their therapeutic intent and select certain probiotic supplements based on the diagnosed condition and the desired direction needed to positively influence the immune system. Nutraceutical companies also can formulate safe, effective probiotic supplements with unique effects on the immune system that can be more effectively used to reduce pathogenesis and maintain intestinal homeostasis. This valuable knowledge of the effect of specific strains of probiotics to boost the immunity has widespread medical implications. Antioxidants are emerging as prophylactic and therapeutic agents and due to their immunomodulation action used as immunomodulator in humans. Several antioxidants have been found to be pharmacologically active as prophylactic and therapeutic agents for several diseases finally concluded that dietary fiber, probiotics, vitamins, antioxidants, folic acid, etc., were used as immunomodulators in humans.

REFERENCES

Agarwal, S.S., V.K. Singh. 1999. Immunomodulators: A review of studies on Indian medicinal plants and synthetic peptides. *PINSA*. B65(3 and 4):179–204.

Aggarwal, B.B., S. Shishodia. 2006. Molecular targets of dietary agents for prevention and therapy of cancer. *Biochem. Pharmacol.* 71:1397–1421.

Aghaee, M., N. Khosravi, P. Hanachi, M.R. Kordi, R. Aghaee. 2014. *Qom Univ. Med. Sci. J.* 7(6):5.

Almeida, L.C., M.A. Cardoso. 2011. Recommendations for folate intake in women: Implications for public health strategies. *Cad. Public Health, Rio de Janeiro* 26(11):2011–2026.

Anon. 2008. Mushrooms, a delicacy worth cultivating. Spore 134 CTA. 11. As Anti-infectives. *Can. J. Infect. Dis. Med. Microbiol.* 17:307–314.

Ashfield-Watt, P.A. et al. 2002. Methylenetetrahydrofolate reductase 677C-->T genotype modulates homocysteine responses to a folate-rich diet or a low-dose folic acid supplement: A randomized controlled trial. *Am. J. Clin. Nutr.* 76:180–186.

Ashgan F.E., H.M. Samah. 2011. Impact of symbiotic on the immune response of broiler chickens against NDV and IBV vaccines. *Global J. Biotechnol. Biochem.* 6(4):186–191.

Aslam, S.M., J.D. Garlich, M.A. Quershi. 1998. Vitamin D deficiency alters the immune responses of broiler chicks. *Poult. Sci.* 77:842–849.

Bailey, L.B., J.F. Gregory III. 2006. Folate. In: B.A. Bowman, R.M. Russel, eds. *Present Knowledge in Nutrition*, 9th edn. International Life Science Institute, Washington, DC, pp. 278–301.

Binns, N. 2013. *Probiotics, Prebiotics and the Gut Microbiota*. International Life Sciences Institute, Brussels, Belgium, pp. 1–31.

Borchers A.T., C. Selmi, F.J. Meyers, C. Keen, M.E. Gershwin. 2009. Probiotics and immunity. *J. Gastroenterol.* 44:26–46.

Braun, F. 1986. The effect of bile on intestinal absorption of calcium and vitamin D. *Wiener Klinische Wochenschrift*. 98(166):23.

Burri B.J. 1997. Beta-carotene and human health: A review of current research. *Nutr. Res.* 17:547–580.

Castillejo, G., M. Bullo, A. Anguera, J. Escribano, J. Salas-Salvado. 2006. A controlled, randomized, double-blind trial to evaluate the effect of a supplement of cocoa husk that is rich in dietary fiber on colonic transit in constipated pediatric patients. *Pediatrics* 118(3):e641–e648.

Chakraborty, P., S. Kumar, D. Dutta, V. Gupta. 2009. Role of antioxidants in common health diseases. *Res. J. Pharm. Technol.* 2(2):238–244.

Chew, B.P. 1995. Antioxidant vitamins affect food animal immunity and health. *J. Nutr.* 125:1804S.

Chintale, A.G., V.S. Kadam, R.S. Sakhare, G.O. Birajdar, D.N. Nalwad. 2013. Role of nutraceuticals in various diseases: A comprehensive review. *IJRPC* 3(2):290–299.

Dalila, B., L. Korrichi, S. Dalila. 2010. Immunologically active polysaccharides isolated from *Anacyclus pyrethrum. Libyan Agric. Res. Center J. Int.* 1(3):128–133.

Das, S. et al. 2014. A review on immune modulatory effect of some traditional medicinal herbs. *J. Pharm. Chem. Biol. Sci.* 2(1):33–42.

Donaldson, M.S. 2004. Nutrition and cancer: A review of the evidence for an anti-cancer diet. *Nutr. J.* 3:19.

Dong, F.M., S.M. Oace. 1975. Folate concentration and pattern in ovine milk. *J. Agric. Food Chem.* 23:534.

Dunnett, C.E. 2003. Antioxidants in physiology and nutrition of exercising horses. In: T.P. Lyons, K.P. Jacques, eds. *Nutritional Biotechnology in the Feed and Food Industries*. Nottingham University Press, Nottingham, U.K., pp. 439–448.

Ferrero, M.E., A.A. Bertelli, F. Pelegatta. 1998. Phytoalexin resveratrol (3,4,5-trihydroxystilbene) modulates granulocyte and monocyte endothelial cell adhesion. *Transplant Proc.* 30:4191-4193.

Floch, M.H., J.A. Hong-Curtiss. 2001. Probiotics and functional foods in gastrointestinal disorders. *Curr. Gastroenterol. Rep.* 3:343–350.

Franz, G. 1989. Polysaccharides in pharmacy: Current application and future concepts. *Planta Med.* 55:493–497.

Garner R.E., A.M. Childress, L.G. Human, J.E. Domer. 1990. Characterization of *Candida albicans* mannan-induced, mannan-specific delayed-hypersensitivity suppressor cells. *Infect. Immun.* 58:2613–2620.

German, B. et al. 1999. The development of functional foods: Lesson from the gut. *Tibtech.* 17:492–499.

Gershoff, S.N. 1993. Vitamin C (ascorbic acid): New roles, new requirements? *Nutr. Rev.* 51:313.

Ghildyal, P. et al. 2010. Chemical composition and immunological activities of polysaccharides isolated from the malian medicinal plant *Syzygium guineense. J. Pharmacog. Phytother.* 2(6):6–85.

Gredel, S. 2011. *Nutrition and Immunity in Man*, 2nd edn. ILSI Europe, pp. 1–40.

Greenwald, P., C.K. Clifford, J.A. Milner. 2001. Diet and cancer prevention. *Eur. J. Cancer* 37:948–965.

Hala, A.A. et al. 2013. Effects of dietary antioxidants supplementation on cellular immune response and evaluation of their antimicrobial activity against some enteric pathogens in goats. *Global Vet.* 11(2):145–154.

Hannan, J.M. et al. 2007. Soluble dietary fibre fraction of *Trigonella foenum-graecum* (fenugreek) seed improves glucose homeostasis in animal models of type 1 and type 2 diabetes by delaying carbohydrate digestion and absorption, and enhancing insulin action. *Br. J. Nutr.* 97(3):514–521.

Hermoso, M., C. Vollhardt, K. Bergmann, B. Koletzko. 2011. Critical micronutrients in pregnancy, lactation, and infancy: Considerations on vitamin D, folic acid, and iron, and priorities for future research. *Ann. Nutr. Metab.* 59:5–9.

Herrick, J.B. 1972. The influence of vitamin A on disease states. *Vet. Med.* 67:906.

How, K.L., H.A.W. Hazewinkel, J.A. Mol. 1995. Photosynthesis of vitamin D in the skin of dogs, cats, and rats. In: H.P. Meyer, H.A.W. Hazewinkel, eds. *Proceedings of the Voorjaarsdagen Congress*, Amsterdam, the Netherlands, p. 1.

Institute of Medicine and National Research Council of the National Academies (IMNRC). 2004. *Dietary Supplements a Framework for Evaluating Safety.* National Academies Press, Washington, DC, pp. ES-1–ES-3. ISBN: 0-309-09206-X.

Institute of Medicine, Food and Nutrition Board (IMFNB). 2000. *Dietary Reference Intakes for Vitamin C, Vitamin E, Selenium, and Carotenoids.* The National Academy of Sciences, Washington, DC.

International Food Information Council (IFIC). 1999. *Functional Foods Now.* Washington, DC.

Isolauri, E. et al. 2004. Probiotics. *Best Pract. Res. Clin. Gastroenterol.* 18(2):299–313.

Johnston, C.S. 2006. Vitamin C. In: B.A. Bowman, R.M. Russell, eds. *Present Knowledge in Nutrition*, 9th edn. International Life Sciences Institute, Washington, DC, pp. 233–241.

Johnston, C.S., F.M. Steinberg, R.B. Rucker. 2007. Ascorbic acid. In: J. Zempleni, R.B. Rucker, D.B. McCormick, J.W. Suttle, eds. *Handbook of Vitamins*, 4th edn. CRC Press, Boca Raton, FL, pp. 489–520.

Kantoff, P. 2006. Prevention, complementary therapies, and new scientific developments in the field of prostate cancer. *Rev. Urol.* 8(2):S9–S14.

Katarzyna, C. et al. 2012. Biologically active compounds in seaweed extracts—The prospects for the application. *Open Conf. Proc. J.* 3(1):20–28.

Kawaguchi, K., T. Matsumoto, Y. Kumazawa. 2011. Effects of antioxidant polyphenols on TNF-alpha-related diseases. *Curr Top Med Chem.* 11:1767–1779.

Kelley, K., R. Easter. 1987. Nutritional factors can influence immune response of swine. *Feedstuffs* 59(22):14.

Keservani, R.K., R.K. Kesharwani, A.K. Sharma N. Vyas, A. Chadoker. 2010b. Nutritional supplements: An overview. *Int. J. Curr. Pharm. Rev. Res.* 1:59–75.

Keservani, R.K., R.K. Kesharwani, N. Vyas, S. Jain, R. Raghuvanshi, A.K. Sharma. 2010a. Nutraccutical and functional food as future food: A review. *Der Pharm. Lett.* 2:106–116.

Keservani, R.K., A.K. Sharma. 2014. Flavonoids: Emerging trends and potential health benefits. *J Chin. Pharm. Sci.*, in press. http://dx.doi.org/10.5246/jcps.2014.12.103.

Koffi, K. et al. 2013. Immunomodulatory activity of polysaccharides isolated from *Clerodendrum splendens*: Beneficial effects in experimental autoimmune encephalomyelitis. *BMC Complem. Altern. Med.* 13:1–19.

Koutsos, E.A., J.C. García López, K.C. Klasing. 2006. Carotenoids from in ovo or dietary sources blunt systemic indicies of the inflammatory response in growing chicks (*Gellur gallus domesticus*). *J. Nutr.* 136:1027–1031.

Kumar, K.M., S. Ramaiah. 2011. Pharmacological importance of *Echinacea purpurea. Int. J. Pharma Biosci.* 2(4):304–314.

Laparra, J.M., Y. Sanz. 2007. Comparison of in vitro models to study bacterial adhesion to the intestinal epithelium. *Lett. Appl. Microbiol.* 49(6):695–701.

Lee, T.T. et al. 2010. Flavonoid, phenol and polysaccharide contents of *Echinacea Purpurea* L. and its immunostimulant capacity *in vitro. Int. J. Environ. Sci. Dev.* 1(1):1–9.

Lessard, M., D. Hutchings, N.A. Cave. 1997. Cell-mediated and humoral immune responses in broiler chickens maintained on diets containing different levels of vitamin A. *Poult. Sci.* 76:1368.

Lesvos-Pantoflikova, D. et al. 2007. *Helicobacter pylori* and probiotics. *J. Nutr.* 137:812S–818S.

Lin, D.C. 2003. Probiotics as functional foods. *Nutr. Clin. Pract.* 18:497–506.

Lindsay, A. et al. 2006. *Guidelines on Food Fortification with Micronutrients.* WHO Library Catalouging-in-Publication.

Lindshield, B.L., J.W. Erdman. 2006. Carotenoids. In: B.A. Bowman, R.M. Russell, eds. *Present Knowledge in Nutrition*, 9th edn. International Life Sciences Institute, Washington, DC, pp. 184–197.

Liu, Y. et al. 2011. Micronutrients decrease incidence of common infections in type 2 diabetes outpatients. *Asia Pac. J. Clin. Nutr.* 20(3):375–382.

Lonn, E.M., S. Yusuf. 1999 Clinical evidence: Emerging approaches in preventing cardiovascular disease. *West. J. Med.* 171(4):247–252.

Maddaly, R., S.L. De, A. Syed, F.D.P. Solomon. 2010. The beneficial effects of spirulina focusing on its immunomodulatory and antioxidant properties. *Nutr. Diet. Suppl.* 2:73–83.

Madsen, K., A. Cornish, P. Soper, C. McKaigney, H. Jijon, C. Yachimec, J. Doyle, L. Jewell, S.C. De. 2001. Probiotic bacteria enhance murine and human intestinal epithelial barrier function. *Gastroenterology.* 121:580–591.

Maggini, S. et al. 2007. Selected vitamins and trace elements support immune function by strengthening epithelial barriers and cellular and humoral immune responses. *Br. J. Nutr.* 98(1):S29–S35.

Malhotra, S., S.V. Rana, S.K. Sinha, S. Khurana. 2004. Dietary fiber assessment of patients with irritable bowel syndrome from Northern India. *Indian J. Gastroenterol.* 23(6):217–218.

Masihi, K.N. 2001. Fighting infection using immunomodulatory agents. *Exp. Opin. Biol. Ther.* 1(4):641–653.

McCormick, C.C., R.S. Parker. 2004. The cytotoxicity of vitamin E is both vitamer and cell specific and involves a selectable trait. *J. Nutr.* 134:3335.

McDowell, L.R., N. Wilkinson, R. Madison, T. Felix. 2007. Vitamins and minerals functioning as antioxidants with supplementation considerations. *Florida Ruminant Nutrition Symposium*, Best Western Gateway Grand, Gainesville, FL, pp. 1–17.

McEligot, A.J., J. Largent, A. Ziogas, D. Peel, H. Anton-Culver. 2006. Dietary fat, fiber, vegetable, and micronutrients are associated with overall survival in postmenopausal women diagnosed with breast cancer. *Nutr. Cancer.* 55(2):132–140.

McGhee, J.R., J. Mestecky, M.T. Dertzbaugh, J.H. Eldridge, M. Hirasawa, H. Kiyono. 1992. The mucosal immune system: From fundamental concepts to vaccinal development. *Vaccine* 10:75.

McPartlin, J., J.M. Scott, A. Halligan, M. Darling, D.G. Weir. 1993. Accelerated folate breakdown in pregnancy. *Lancet.* 341:148.

Moser, U., A. Bendich. 1991. Vitamin C. In: L.J. Machlin, ed. *Handbook of Vitamins*, 2nd edn. Marcel Dekker, New York, p. 195.

Mozaffarieh, M., S. Sacu, A. Wedrich. 2003. The role of the carotenoids, lutein and zeaxanthin, in protecting against age-related macular degeneration: A review based on controversial evidence. *Nutr. J.* 2:20.

Muller, A., H. Ensely, H. Pretus, R. McNameee, El Jones, E. McLaughlin, W. Chandley, W. Browder, D. Lowman, D. Williams. 1997. The application of various protic acids in the extraction of (1–3)-beta-D-glucan from *Saccharomyces cerevisiae*. *Carbohyd. Res.* 299:203–208.

Murakami, K., S. Sasaki, H. Okubo, Y. Takahashi, Y. Hosoi, M. Itabashi. 2007. Dietary fiber intake, dietary glycemic index and load, and body mass index: A cross-sectional study of 3931 Japanese women aged 18–20 years. *Eur. J. Clin. Nutr.* 61:986–995.

Nair, P.K.R. et al. 2004. Studied immune stimulating properties of a novel polysaccharide from the medicinal plant *Tinospora cordifolia*. *Int. Immunopharm.* 4:1645–1659.

O'Hara, A.M., F. Shanahan. 2007. Mechanisms of action of probiotics in intestinal diseases. *Scient. World J.* 7:31–46.

Oei, P. 2003. Mushroom cultivation. In: CTA, ed. *Appropriate Technology for the Mushroom Growers*. Backhuys Publishers, Leiden, the Netherlands, pp. 1–7.

Okamoto, I. et al. 2002. The flavonoid Kaempferol suppresses the graft-versus-host reaction by inhibiting type 1 cytokine production and CD8+ T-cell engraftment. *Clin. Immunol.* 103:132– 44.

Olson, J.A. 1984. Vitamin A. In: L.J. Machlin, ed. *Handbook of Vitamins*. Marcel Dekker, Inc., New York.

Otles, S., S. Ozgoz. 2014. Health effects of dietary fiber. *Acta Sci. Pol. Technol. Aliment.* 13(2):191–202.

Padh, H. 1991. Vitamin C: Newer insights into its biochemical functions. *Nutr. Rev.* 49:65.

Parkin, J., B. Cohen. 2001. An overview of the immune system. *Lancet* 357:1777–1789.

Prakash, D. et al. 2012. Importance of phytochemicals in nutraceuticals. *J. Chin. Med. Res. Develop.* 1(3):70–78.

Puertollano, M.A., E. Puertollano, G.A. De Cienfuegos, M.A. De Pablo. 2011. Dietary antioxidants: Immunity and host defense. *Curr. Top. Med. Chem.* 11:1752–1766.

Resta-Lenert, S., K. Barrett. 2006. Probiotics and commensals reverse TNF-alpha- and IFN-gamma-induced dysfunction in human intestinal epithelial cells. *Gastroenterology*. 130:731–746.

Ribeiro, A.M.L., L.K. Vogt, C.W. Canal, M.R.I. Cardoso, R.V. Labres, A.F. Streck, M.C. Bessa. 2007. Effects of prebiotics and probiotics on the colonization and immune response of broiler chickens challenged with *Salmonella* enteritidis. *Braz. J. Poult. Sci.* 9(3):193–200.

Rijkers, G.T., W.M. de Vos, R.J. Brummer, L. Morelli, G.P. Corthier Marteau. 2011. Health benefits and health claims of probiotics: Bridging science and marketing. *Br. J. Nutr.* 106(9):1291–1296.

Romero, A.L., K.L. West, T. Zern, M.L. Fernandez. 2002. The seeds from *Plantago ovata* lower plasma lipids by altering hepatic and bile acid metabolism in guinea pigs. *J. Nutr.* 132:1194–1198.

Rosenthal, K.L. 2006. Tweaking innate immunity: The promise of innate immunologicals to clinical application. *Am. J. Pathol.* 169:1901–1909.

Ross, A.C. 1992. Vitamin A status: Relationship to immunity and the antibody response. *Proc. Soc. Exp. Biol. Med.* 200:303.

Salminen, S. et al. 1999. Probiotics: How should they be defined. *Trends Food Sci. Technol.* 10:107–110.

Sanders, M.E. 2008. Probiotics: Definition, sources, selections and uses. *Clin. Infect. Disease*. 46(2): S58–S61.

Schrager H.J., S. Alberti, C. Cywes, B.J. Dougherty, M.R. Wessels. 1998. Hyaluronic acid capsule modulates M protein-mediated adherence and acts as a ligand for attachment of group A *Streptococcus* to CD44 on human keratinocytes. *J. Clin. Invest.* 101:1708–1716.

Sesso, H.D., S. Liu, J.M. Gaziano, J.E. Buring. 2003. Dietary lycopene, tomato-based food products and cardiovascular disease in women. *J. Nutr.* 133:2336–2341.

Shapiro, M.E., D.L. Kasper, D.F. Zaleznik, S. Spriggs, A.B. Onderdonk, R.W. Finberg. 1986. Cellular control of abscess formation: Role of T cells in the regulation of abscesses formed in response to *Bacterioides fragilis*. *J. Immunol.* 137:341–346.

Simopoulos, A.P. 2002. Omega-3 fatty acids in inflammation and autoimmune diseases: Review. *J. Am. Coll. Nutr.* 21:495–505.

Spears, J.W., Weiss, W.P. 2008. Role of antioxidants and trace elements in health and immunity of transition dairy cows. *Vet. J.* 176:70–76.

Stephensen, C.B., Z. Moldoveanu, N.N. Gangopadhyay. 1996. Vitamin deficiency diminishes the salivary immunoglobulin A response and enhances the serum immunoglobulin G response to influenza A virus infection in BALB/C mice. *J. Nutr.* 126:94.

Sun, Y. 2011. Structure and biological activities of the polysaccharides from the leaves, roots and fruits of *Panax ginseng* C.A. Meyer: An overview. *Carbohyd. Polym.* 85:490–499.

Susumu, A. et al. 2012. *Folate Deficiency among Aged Patients and Its Amelioration through Consumption of Folic Acid-Fortified Rice*, Vol. 13. House Foods Group Inc., pp. 123–137.

Traber, M.G. 2006. Vitamin E. In: B.A. Bowman, R.M. Russell, eds. *Present Knowledge in Nutrition*, 9th edn. ILSI, Washington, DC, pp. 211–219.

Turner, J.R. 2006. Molecular basis of epithelial barrier regulation: From basic mechanisms.

Uddin Q., L. Samiulla, V.K. Singh, S.S. Jamil. 2012. Phytochemical and pharmacological profile of *Withania somnifera* Dunal: A review. *J. Appl. Pharm. Sci.* 2(1):170–175.

Upadhyay, J. et al. 2009a. Comparative study of antioxidants as cancer preventives through inhibition of HIF-1 alpha activity. *Bioinformation*. 4(6):233–236.

Upadhyay, J. et al. 2009b. Metabolism, pharmacokinetics and bioavailability of ascorbic acid; synergistic effect with tocopherols and curcumin. *J. Comput. Intell. Bioinform.* 2(1):77–84.

Van Rosendaal, G.M.A, E.A. Shaffer, A.L. Edwards, R. Brant. 2004. Effect of time of administration on cholesterol-lowering by psyllium: A randomized cross-over study in normocholesterolemic or slightly hypercholesterolemic subjects. *Nutr. J.* 3:17.

Vazquez, C.M.P. et al. 2014. Micronutrients influencing the immune response in leprosy. *Nutr. Hosp.* 29(1):26–36.

Wagner, C. 1984. Folic acid. In: R.E. Olson, H.P. Broquist, C.O. Chichester, W.J. Drby, A.C. Kolbye, Jr., R.M. Stalvey, eds. *Nutrition Reviews: Present Knowledge in Nutrition*, 5th edn. The Nutrition Foundation Inc., Washington, DC, p. 332.

Wakai, K. et al. 2007. Dietary fiber and risk of colorectal cancer in the Japan Collaborative Cohort Study. *Cancer Epidemiol. Biomark. Prev.* 16(4):668–675.

Wasser, S.P. 2002. Medicinal mushrooms as a source of antitumor and immunomodulating polysaccharides. *Appl. Microbiol. Biotechnol.* 60:258–274.

Weiss, W.P. 2005. Antioxidants nutrients, cow health and milk quality. *Dairy Cattle Nutrition Workshop*, Department of Dairy and Animal Sciences, Pennsylvania State University, Grantville, PA, pp. 11–18.

Wiedermann, U., L.A. Hanson, J. Holmgren, H. Kahu, U.I. Dahlgren. 1993. Impaired mucosal antibody response to cholera toxin in vitamin A-deficient rats immunized with oral cholera vaccine. *Infect. Immun.* 61:3952.

Winklhofer-Roob, B.M., A. Meinitzer, M. Maritschnegg, J.M. Roob, G. Khoschsorur, J. Fibalta, I. Sundl, S. Wuga, W. Wonisch, B. Tiran, E. Rock. 2004. Effects of vitamin E depletion/repletion on biomarkers of oxidative stress in healthy aging. *Ann. N.Y. Acad. Sci.* 1031:361–364.

www.preventcancer.aicr.org/site/PageServer?pagename=elements_phytochemicals.

Yang, C.C. et al. 2014. Effect of mushroom beta glucan (MBG) on immune and haemocyte response in pacific white shrimp (*Litopenaeus vannamei*). *J. Aquac. Res. Develop.* 5:1–5.

Yeomans, V.C., J. Linseisen, G. Wolfram. 2005. Interactive effects of polyphenols, tocopherol, and ascorbic acid on the Cu_2-mediated oxidative modification of human low density lipoproteins. *Eur. J. Nutr.* doi: 10.1007/s00394-005-0546-y [Epub April 15].

Yoneyama, S. et al. 2008. Epigallocatechin gallate affects human dendritic cell differentiation and maturation. *J. Allergy Clin. Immunol.* 121(1):209–214.

Yu, S. et al. 2009. The effects of whole mushrooms during inflammation. *BMC Immunol.* 10:12.

Zahra, A. 2011. Herbal medicines for immunosuppression. *Iran J. Allergy Asthma Immunol.*, in press.

Zee, J. et al. 1991. Effect of storage conditions on the stability of vitamin C in various fruits and vegetables produced and consumed in Quebec. *J. Food Compos. Anal.* 4:77.

Zhao, Z., C. Ross. 1995. Retinoic acid repletion restores the number of leukocytes and their subsets and stimulates natural cytotoxicity in vitamin A-deficient rats. *J. Nutr.* 125:2064.

Zyrek, A.A., C. Cichon, S. Helms, C. Enders, U. Sonnenborn, M.A. Schmidt. 2007. Molecular mechanisms underlying the probiotic effects of *Escherichia coli* Nissle 1917 involve ZO-2 and PKCzeta redistribution resulting in tight junction and epithelial barrier repair. *Cell Microbiol.* 9:804–816.

Section IX

Cancer

21 Natural Products in the Prevention of Cancer
A Review

Kelly C. Heim and Michael J. Spinella

CONTENTS

21.1 INTRODUCTION

Cancer is the second leading cause of death in the United States, accounting for nearly one of every four deaths. An estimated 1,665,540 new cancer diagnoses and about 585,720 cancer-related mortalities were expected in 2014. According to the National Institutes of Health (NIH), total cancer costs were approximately $216.6 billion in 2009 (ACS Cancer Facts & Figures 2014). Longer life expectancies were accountable, in part, for the increasing prevalence of cancer and its financial burden. While considerable progress has been made in antineoplastic drug development, mitigation of existing cancers is limited by the toxicity of these agents. Despite a rapidly evolving repertoire of molecular therapeutics in clinical oncology, the majority of malignancies remain incurable.

Cancer develops in a ternary sequence of initiation, promotion, and progression that involves aberrant signal transduction and genetic and epigenetic changes. The multifactorial nature of this course, which typically requires 20–30 years or longer to culminate in malignancy, presents many opportunities at which preventive strategies might delay or prevent the disease (Figure 21.1). Chemoprevention, a term coined in 1976 by M.B. Sporn, refers to any natural or synthetic preventive modality that slows, stops, reverses, or prevents cancer development (Sporn et al. 1976). Prevention can be primary, which is aimed at the general, healthy population with emphasis on

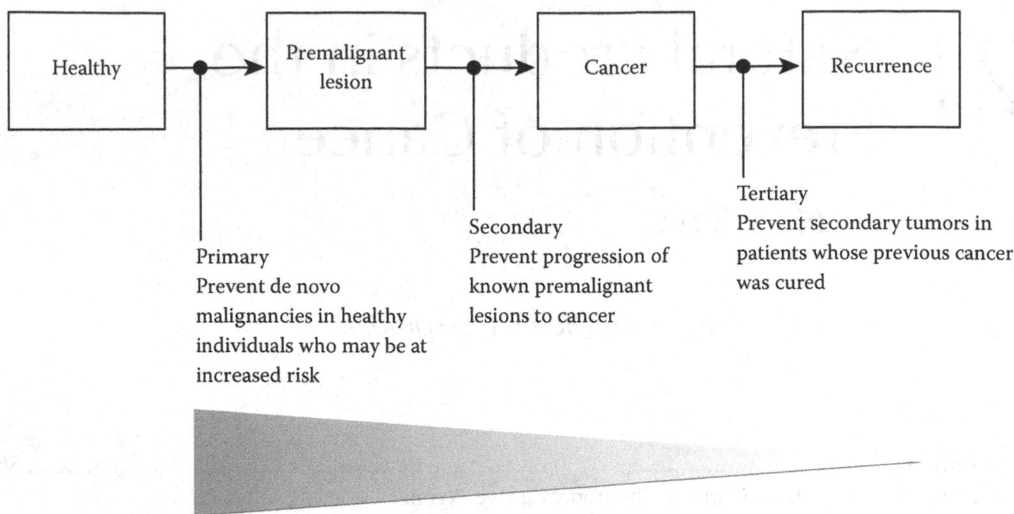

FIGURE 21.1 Cancer prevention at three stages with natural products.

individuals at increased risk. Secondary chemoprevention refers to an effort to preclude or attenuate progression to malignant disease in individuals carrying premalignant lesions. Tertiary prevention refers to strategies intended to block recurrence or to attenuate progression of cancer (Alberts and Hess 2008). Over the last three decades, more than 1000 agents have been investigated for chemopreventive activity by the National Cancer Institute. Of these, merely 40 compounds have proceeded to clinical trials. There remains a critical need to identify compounds that favorably moderate the elaborate, multifactorial, and variable molecular etiologies of cancer with safety profiles allowing lengthy durations of use in healthy individuals.

Epidemiologic investigations have inversely associated cancer incidence with fruit and vegetable consumption, and estimates suggest that one-third of all cancer mortalities could be prevented through dietary and lifestyle adjustments (Danaei et al. 2005). The salutary effects of fruits and vegetables were initially ascribed to familiar essential micronutrients such as vitamin E, selenium, folate, and beta-carotene. However, as isolates, all of these compounds have failed to demonstrate chemopreventive competence in the majority of controlled human trials (Lippman et al. 2009).

Plants are elaborate libraries of secondary metabolites—compounds that are dispensable for life-sustaining functions. In both plants and the herbivores that consume them, secondary metabolites serve no purpose in basic metabolism and are not required for viability. These phytochemicals, the majority belonging to the phenolic, terpenoid, alkaloid, indole, and organosulfur classes, exceed vitamins and minerals in fruits and vegetables in both quantity and diversity. In plants, they serve as defenses against highly erratic and even unprecedented environmental, pathogenic, mechanical, and predatory threats. In animal and human cells, they modulate variegated processes that are etiologically germane to the most prevalent and lethal Western diseases, including cancer. Phenolics and organosulfur compounds occurring in tea and broccoli, for example, inhibit all three stages of carcinogenesis in highly validated models (Landis-Piwowar and Iyer 2014). Importantly, as food has been consumed since the dawn of humankind, the self-evident safety of moderately dosed agents originating from common foods supports their potential value as chemopreventive measures suitable for long-term use in healthy individuals. The aim of this chapter is to summarize the current knowledge of the most extensively characterized natural chemopreventive products from plants, with special attention given to their molecular targets.

21.2 MOLECULAR TARGETS OF NATURAL CHEMOPREVENTIVE AGENTS

21.2.1 Oxidant and Xenobiotic Defense

Carcinogens, their electrophilic metabolites, and common oxidative insults originating from the environment or endogenous metabolism are capable of mutating DNA in the initiation stage of carcinogenesis. Accordingly, dual augmentation of antioxidant defenses and facilitation of carcinogen detoxification are powerful strategies to block or attenuate early initiating events. Nuclear transcription factor erythroid 2p45 (NF-E2)-related factor 2 (Nrf2) is a transcriptional inducer of endogenous antioxidant and phase II detoxification enzymes. When activated, Nrf2 binds to antioxidant response elements (AREs), *cis*-enhancer sequences flanking the promoters of genes encoding antioxidant and detoxification enzymes such as hemeoxygenase 1 (HO-1), NADPH:quinone oxidoreductase (NQO1), and glutathione sulfotransferases (GSTs) (Kobayashi et al. 2004).

Under homeostatic conditions, the Nrf2 transcription factor is restrained in the cytosol by Kelch-like ECH-associating protein 1 (Keapl). In the presence of oxidative, chemical, or electrophilic stress, Nrf2 translocates to the nucleus and heterodimerizes with Maf proteins to bind electrophile/AREs in the promoters of genes encoding antioxidant proteins, phase II enzymes, xenobiotic transporters, and other adaptive cellular defense proteins. The collective actions of this program protect many cell types against DNA damage and other electrophilic adversities that commonly permit cancer initiation. Phytochemicals activate Nrf2 by a variety of mechanisms, including redox modification of Keapl, and potentially through epigenetic mechanisms (Wu et al. 2013). Points where curcumin, a constituent of the spice turmeric, and sulforaphane, a compound in broccoli, inhibit the Nrf2 pathway are shown in Figure 21.2.

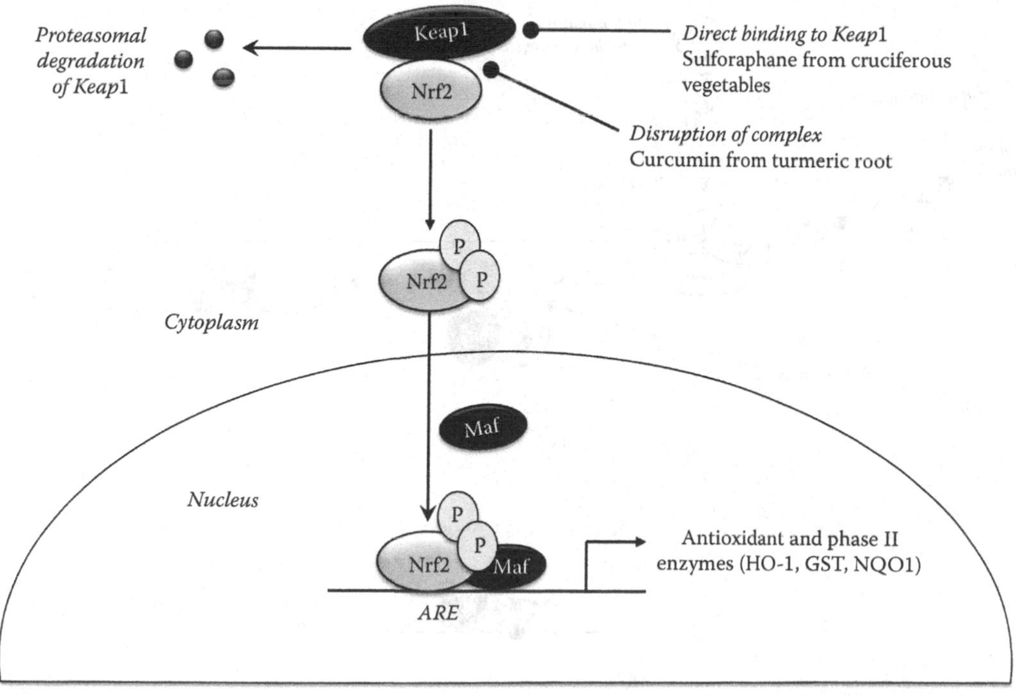

FIGURE 21.2 The Nrf2/Keapl pathway and activation by sulforaphane and curcumin. Arrows indicate activation, while bulbed lines indicate inhibition.

21.2.2 Inflammatory Signaling

Over the last two decades, inflammation has received considerable recognition as a contributor to the initiation and progression of cancer. Much of this attention has come from the evidence supporting cyclooxygenase-2 (COX-2) inhibitors as efficacious in the secondary chemoprevention of colorectal cancer, although attempts to demonstrate primary prevention have been disappointing (Giardiello et al. 1993; Steinbach et al. 2000; Baron et al. 2003). The metazoan transcription factor nuclear factor kappa-light-chain-enhancer of activated B cells (NFκB) is not only a focal conduit of inflammation but a positive regulator of tumor cell survival. COX-2 is among many key target genes of NFκB, which include oncogenic cytokines, chemokines, apoptotic regulators, trophic factors, transcription factors, and stress response regulators (Van Antwerp et al. 1996; Huang et al. 2001). Collectively, this gene expression program coordinates and sustains tumor cell survival, growth potential, and resistance to endogenous inhibitory factors and cytotoxic chemotherapeutics. Thus, it is an attractive and viable target for chemoprevention and reversal of antineoplastic drug resistance.

Under basal circumstances, NFκB is sequestered in the cytosol by IκB family proteins. Inductive stimuli, which include lipopolysaccharide (LPS) and pro-inflammatory cytokines (e.g. TNFα), activate IκB kinase complexes (IKK), which phosphorylate IκB. This permits ubiquitin tagging, proteasomal degradation, and exposure of the nuclear localization signal on NFκB. Upon translocation to the nucleus, NFκB binds to response elements in the promoters of target genes, enabling transcription (Figure 21.3). Examples of target genes include COX-2, inducible nitric oxide synthase (iNOS), cyclin D1, matrix metalloproteinases (MMPs), and cytokines such as interleukins and tumor necrosis factor alpha (TNFα) (Thanos and Maniatis 1995). Many genes induced by NFκB are involved in tumor promotion and progression.

The *raison d'être* of NFκB is to orchestrate an acute and robust response to unanticipated and potentially destabilizing immunologic, mitogenic, and oxidative challenges. This critical cellular

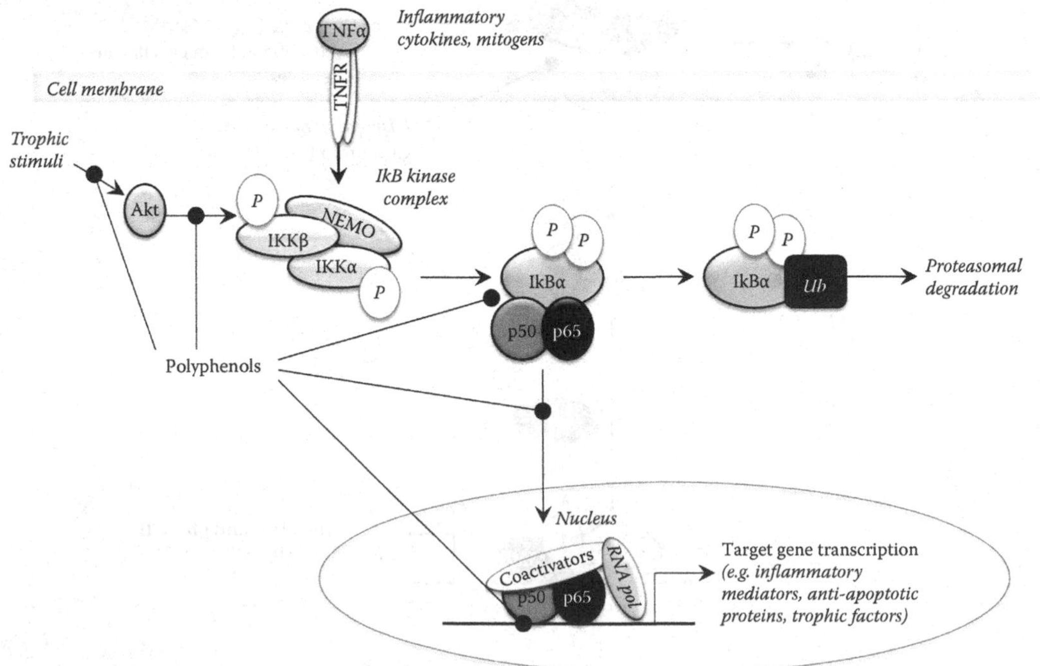

FIGURE 21.3 The canonical NFκB pathway and its multimodal inhibition by polyphenols, an abundant class of secondary plant metabolites present in fruits, vegetables, and spices. Arrows indicate activation, while bulbed lines indicate inhibition.

role of NFκB may explain why it can be modulated by structurally and functionally heterogeneous inhibitors. Many established natural product inhibitors belong to the highly variegated phenolic and isoprenoid classes of secondary plant metabolites. It is interesting to note that these *dispensable* plant compounds operate *in planta* on a similar conceptual premise as NFκB in metazoans, coordinating adjustments to unanticipated pathogenic, oxidative, and mechanical adversities. To the plant and its herbivore, these compounds are nutritionally dispensable, yet potentially physiologically important. These unexpected xenobiotics target the NFκB pathway at multiple steps, albeit with low affinity, and exhibit minimal toxicity in humans. Some single polyphenols have even been shown to inhibit three or more signaling proteins in the NFκB pathway in addition to NFκB target genes. Whether this multifarious behavior is operative in vivo has yet to be elucidated, but offers a potential advantage of phytochemicals over singularly targeted pharmaceuticals.

21.2.3 Growth Factor Signaling

Growth factors support multiple hallmarks of cancer via augmenting cell proliferation and inhibiting apoptosis. Familiar examples include insulin-like growth factor (IGF) and epidermal growth factor (EGF). Augmentation of circulating levels of these proteins and constitutive activation of their cognate transmembrane receptor kinases are common aberrations in human malignancies. Moreover, the downstream trophic and antiapoptotic signaling events from the activated receptor are often deregulated at multiple points.

The phosphatidylinositol-3-kinase (PI3K)/Akt pathway is an integral mediator of cellular responses to growth factors. Binding of ligand or constitutive activation of growth factor receptors induces the recruitment of PI3K to the membrane where it catalyzes the phosphorylation of phosphatidylinositol-4,5-bisphosphate (PIP2) to the oncogenic second messenger, phosphatidylinositol-3,4,5-triphosphate (PIP3). Akt (protein kinase B), a serine/threonine protein kinase, is activated upon PIP3-mediated membrane recruitment and phosphorylation at two sites. Active Akt phosphorylates proteins involved in trophic and anabolic cellular processes. The tumor suppressor phosphate and tensin homolog deleted on chromosome 10 (PTEN), which negatively regulates PI3K signaling, is one of the most frequently mutated tumor suppressor genes (Fruman and Rommel 2014).

Among the primary effectors of Akt is mammalian target of rapamycin (mTOR), a conserved serine/threonine protein kinase. mTOR occurs as two complexes—mTORC1, which is rapamycin sensitive and binds to Raptor, and mTORC2, which is rapamycin insensitive and interacts with Rictor. In a growth-stimulating climate, mTORC1 is activated and phosphorylates several proteins. Two of its main roles are to inhibit the repressor of mRNA translation, 4E-BP1, and to activate p70S6K, promoting translation and cell growth (Tan et al. 2014). In essence, mTOR supports protein synthesis and shifts metabolism toward an anabolic, anticatabolic state. The collective actions of Akt and mTOR positively regulate cell proliferation, survival, angiogenesis, and negatively regulate apoptosis (Houghton 2010; Tan et al. 2014) (Figure 21.4).

mTOR signaling is among the most frequently altered pathways in human malignancies (Tan et al. 2014). Many points in the PI3K/Akt/mTOR network, their upstream activators (e.g., RTKs), and cross talk with other pathways (e.g. NFκB) are deregulated in human malignancies, including breast, prostate, and colorectal cancer (Tan et al. 2014). Direct and indirect inhibition has been documented for various dietary polyphenols. Caloric restriction, which has been suggested to be a cardioprotective, neuroprotective, and potentially chemopreventive dietary modification, also downregulates the Akt and mTOR axes.

21.2.4 Apoptosis

By necessity, multicellular organisms are equipped to eliminate nonviable, damaged, and mutated cells in a decisive manner. A principal means of selective termination is programmed cell death, or apoptosis. Apoptosis is the culmination of coordinated signal transduction events involving

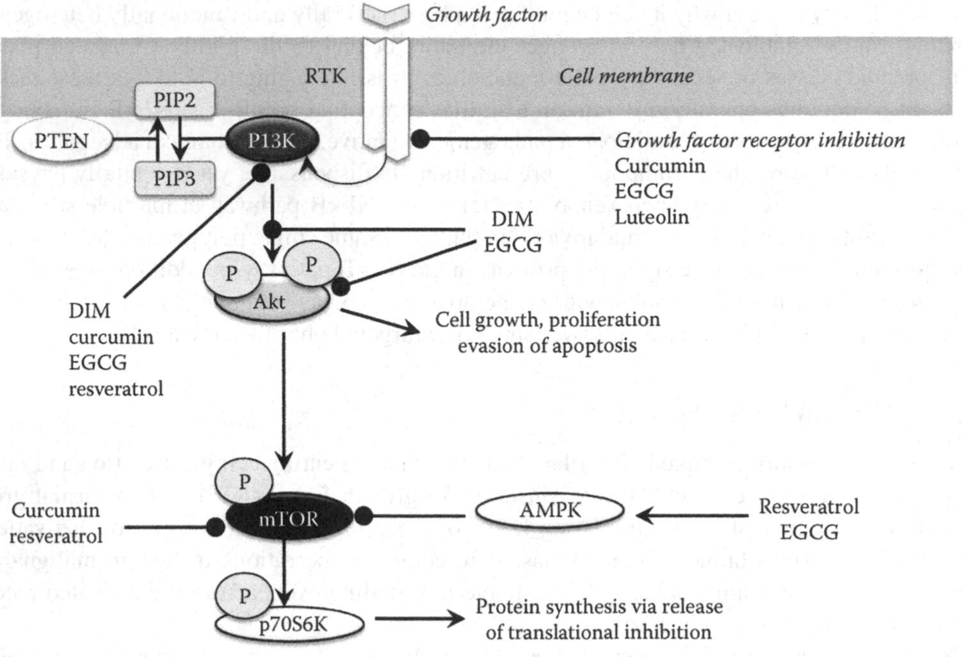

FIGURE 21.4 Growth factor signaling and inhibition by curcumin from turmeric, epigallocatechin gallate (EGCG) from green tea, 3,3′-diindolylmethane (DIM), a metabolite of sulforaphane, luteolin, a flavonoid from fruits, and resveratrol, a phenolic from grape skin. Arrows indicate activation, while bulbed lines indicate inhibition.

more than a hundred proteins, and aberrant downregulation of apoptosis is a hallmark of cancer. Deregulated apoptotic responses allow uncontrolled growth, death evasion in the presence of endogenous stimuli, and resistance to exogenous factors (e.g. cytotoxic chemotherapeutics). Since evasion of death sustains viability of newly damaged, preinitiated, or transformed cells, selective proapoptotic responses are desirable in chemopreventive agents.

Apoptosis is almost always driven by one of two canonical pathways—the intrinsic pathway, which involves the mitochondria, or the extrinsic pathway, which emanates from external signals via cell membrane receptors. The intrinsic pathway, which is engaged by cellular stress (e.g. oxidative injury, damage to DNA, or withdrawal of trophic signals), is controlled by the Bcl-2 family of proteins. The balance of inhibitory Bcl-2 members (e.g. Bcl-2, Bcl-xL) and pro-apoptotic members (Bax, Bad, Bak, Bid, Bim) determines whether apoptosis will ensue. A balance favoring the latter will cause mitochondrial membrane pores to open, altering membrane potential. This results in discharge of pro-apoptotic factors, such as cytochrome c and second mitochondrial activator of caspases (Smac/Diablo), from the mitochondrial intermembrane space into the cytosol. Smac/Diablo activates caspases through functional abrogation of the inhibitory action of inhibitor of apoptosis proteins (IAPs). Cell termination is finalized by cytochrome c-mediated sequential activation of the cysteine proteases, caspase-9 and caspase-3, and other enzymes that cleave indispensable structural and functional cellular components (Iannolo et al. 2008). The extrinsic pathway is incited by the cross-linking of extracellular death ligands, such as tumor necrosis factor (TNF), to transmembrane death receptors, followed by receptor clustering and recruitment of procaspase-8 by the Fas-associated death domain protein (FADD). Proteolytic activation of procaspase-8 initiates a cascade involving caspases 3 and 7, which orchestrate lethal degradative events.

In tumor cell lines, dietary phytochemicals are highly prone to supporting one or both pathways through pro-oxidant behavior and/or modulating multiple pro- and anti-apoptotic proteins (Figure 21.5). Polyphenols can upregulate Bax, Bim, and Bak with simultaneous downregulation of Bcl-2

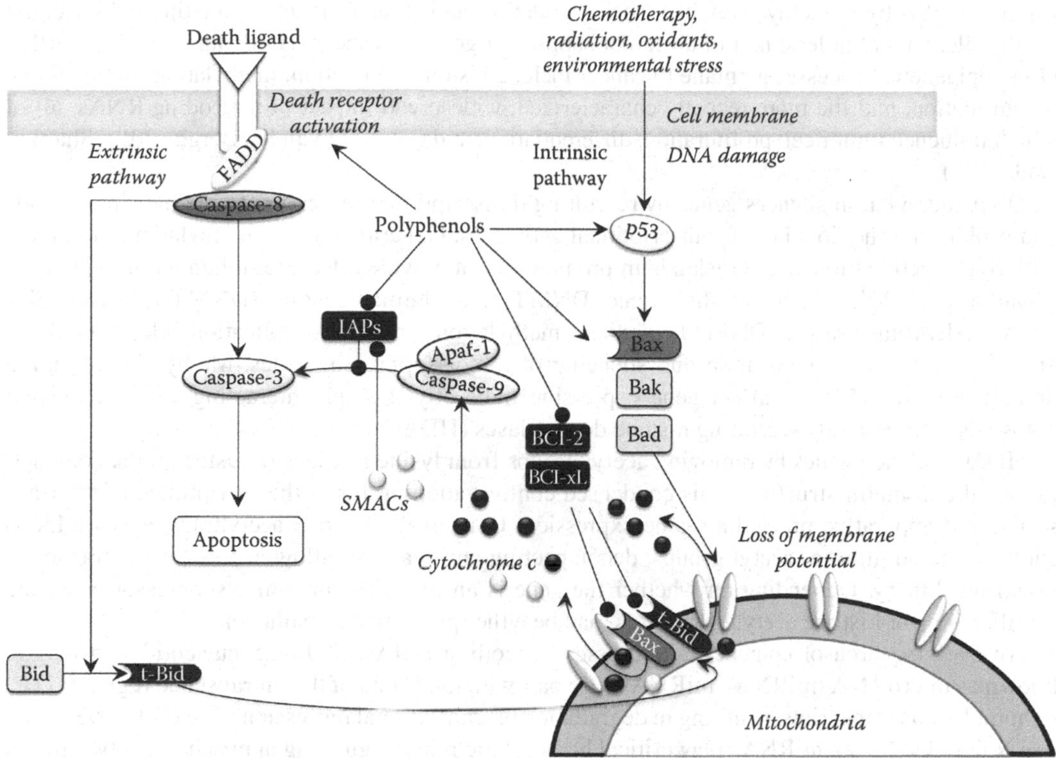

FIGURE 21.5 The extrinsic and intrinsic pathways of apoptosis. In the extrinsic pathway, extrinsic signals such as TNF (tumor necrosis factor) or Fas bind transmembrane death receptors, leading to caspase 8 activation via TNF receptor–associated death domain (TRADD) and Fas-associated death domain protein (FADD), respectively. In either event, this results in sequential activation of caspases 8 and 3. Bid, a pro-apoptotic member of the Bcl-2 family, is activated by caspase 8 and participates in mitochondrial membrane destabilization. In the intrinsic pathway, DNA-damaging stimuli activate p53 and pro-apoptotic Bcl-2 family members, which include Bax, Bak, Bid, and Bad. Channels form, increasing mitochondrial membrane permeability and release of cytochrome c and SMACs (small mitochondria-derived activator of caspases), which inactivate the inhibitor of apoptosis proteins (IAPs) that normally suppress caspases. Cytochrome c binds to apoptotic protease–activating factor 1 (Apaf-1) and pro-caspase-9, which is proteolytically activated to caspase 9, which activates caspase 3. Bax and/or Bak forms pores in the mitochondrial membrane. Activated t-Bid facilitates Bax insertion. The anti-apoptotic members Bcl-2 and Bcl-xL inhibit pore formation. Dietary polyphenols have been shown to inhibit multiple steps in this signaling network. Arrows indicate activation, while bulbed lines indicate inhibition.

and Bcl-xL (Shankar and Srivastava 2007). Some degree of selectivity for transformed cells versus normal cells has been documented. Polyphenols in green tea, for example, can induce apoptosis by increasing pro-apoptotic Bcl-2 family members in malignant cells without harming normal cells (Khan and Mukhtar 2008). Natural products can also sensitize death receptors to cytotoxic drugs in cancer therapy, enhancing efficacy and potentially mitigating or delaying the onset of drug resistance (Park et al. 2013). Sustainable pro-apoptotic efficacy is most probable with multitargeting agents, given the many death signals amenable to deregulation in cancer and the temporal changes in their prominence with disease progression.

21.2.5 Epigenome

Although 90% of cancers develop due to somatic mutations, epigenetic alterations, which affect gene expression without changing DNA sequence, are increasingly recognized as major contributing factors.

Promoter DNA hypermethylation, histone deacetylation, and other aberrant chromatin marks account for the silencing of at least half of all tumor suppressor genes in cancer (Hardy and Tollefsbol 2011). Other epigenetic processes germane to cancer include histone acetylation, methylation, sumoylation, ubiquitination, and the more recently characterized, widespread impact of noncoding RNAs, all of which influence tumor cell proliferation, differentiation, and survival (Vanden Berghe 2012; Shankar et al. 2013).

DNA methylation silences genes by recruiting transcriptional repressors to methyl CpG islands and prohibiting the docking of transcriptional activators. Generalized hypomethylation, in tandem with hypermethylation at CpG islands in promoters, is a prevalent feature in human malignancies (Shankar et al. 2013). There are three major DNMTs in the human genome (DNMT 1, 3A, and 3B). DNA methyltransferase 1 (DNMT1) mediates methylation after DNA replication, while DNMT3a and 3b catalyze the methylation and silencing of tumor suppressor genes. Methyl CpG-binding domain proteins (MBDs) affect gene expression indirectly through interacting with methylated cytosines, subsequently recruiting histone deacetylases (HDACs).

HDACs silence genes by removing acetyl groups from lysine residues of histone tails, compacting local chromatin structure. This condensed configuration prohibits the recruitment of the transcriptional apparatus, precluding gene expression. Conversely, histone acetyltransferases (HATs) catalyze the addition of acetyl groups, decompacting chromatin to allow access for the transcriptional machinery. Depending on whether the gene is an oncogene or tumor suppressor gene, the ramifications of histone acetylation status may be either protective or pathogenic.

An evolving area of epigenetics addresses noncoding RNAs, of 18–25 nucleotides in length, known as microRNA (miRNA). miRNAs base pair with the 3′ end of the untranslated region (UTR) of homologous transcripts, resulting in degradation or translational repression (Lee et al. 1993; Chen and Rajewsky 2007). miRNAs play critical homeostatic roles, regulating approximately two-thirds of human protein-coding genes (Friedman et al. 2009). Initially discovered in *Caenorhabditis elegans* in 1993, miRNAs went largely unrecognized in cancer research until a 2002 study in which 68% of cases of chronic lymphocytic leukemia featured deletion or downregulation of two specific miRNAs (Lee et al. 1993; Calin et al. 2002).

Over the last decade, a progressively expanding body of evidence has underscored the prevalence of deregulation of miRNAs in premalignant and malignant cells. miRNAs can act as oncogenes or tumor suppressors and are pertinent to the hallmarks of cancer—cell proliferation, growth, apoptosis, immortality, genomic instability, invasion, and metastasis. Noteworthy examples include miR-15a/16-1 and miR-34, which exert tumor suppressor functions, and the oncogenic miR-17-92 and miR-155 (Ling et al. 2011). By silencing DNMTs, HDACs, and other enzymes, miRNAs can indirectly impact the epigenome (Parasramka et al. 2012; Vanden Berghe 2012).

miRNAs have been the subject of intensive investigation across major topics in oncology, including molecular diagnostics, chemoprevention, therapy, and biomarker development (Cortez et al. 2011; Ling et al. 2013; Pichler et al. 2014). miRNAs are increasingly appreciated not only as viable molecular targets, but as prospective therapeutic and chemosensitizing agents, deliverable as antisense or mimetic oligonucleotides through vehicles such as nanoparticles. By virtue of their stability in plasma and tissue, miRNAs are also undergoing intense investigation as noninvasive biomarkers (Cortez et al. 2011; Ling et al. 2013, Pichler et al. 2014). Folate, vitamin D, retinoids, indoles, and phenolics are examples of dietary constituents that modulate miRNAs in human cancer cell lines (Ross and Davis 2011). An analysis of in vitro and animal studies found that polyphenols modulated over 100 different miRNAs involved in inflammation, apoptosis, and other processes highly relevant to cancer prevention and therapy (Milenkovic et al. 2013).

Epigenetic effects may account, in part, for the favorable effects of phytochemicals in preventing DNA damage, inhibiting inflammation, suppressing growth, and inducing apoptosis. As with the signal transduction pathways, epigenetic effects of phytochemicals often involve more than one mode of action. Polyphenols from tea, for example, can inhibit DNMT1, 3a, and 3b expression and catalytic activity in skin cancer cells, reactivating previously silenced tumor suppressor genes

(Nandakumar et al. 2011). The same compounds also inhibit HATs and alter miRNA expression profiles (Choi et al. 2009). Whether these interactions have any functional significance in vivo, however, remains elusive.

21.3 EFFICACY AND MECHANISMS OF CHEMOPREVENTIVE PHYTOCHEMICALS

21.3.1 Retinoids

Vitamin A is an essential nutrient with essential roles in regulating embryonic development, germ cell homeostasis, and maintenance of healthy tissue and epithelia (Clagett-Dame and Knutson 2011). In both preventive and therapeutic contexts, retinoids have undergone more extensive preclinical, epidemiological, and clinical interrogation and validation than any other chemopreventive phytochemical and comprise one of the first proofs of principles for chemoprevention (Sporn et al. 1976). Robust evidence for primary, secondary, and tertiary chemoprevention has been forthcoming over many years of clinical research (Bhutani and Koo 2011). In normal, premalignant, and malignant settings, the successes and lessons learned from the last 30 years of retinoid research are universally instructive to the characterization and successful clinical integration of chemopreventive agents (Yim et al. 2014). The use of retinoids in clinical cancer prevention and therapy is summarized in Table 21.1.

The inhibitory effects of retinoids on premalignant and malignant cells have been well established for many years. Like the more recently identified anticancer phytochemicals, the impetus to investigate retinoids as chemopreventive agents stemmed, in part, from epidemiologic evidence of cancer risk reduction with higher intakes of fruits and vegetables. These foods are rich sources of beta-carotene, the dietary precursor of vitamin A (Figure 21.6). It has since become apparent that beta-carotene cannot recapitulate the growth suppression and differentiation induction that typifies clinically validated retinoids.

Induction of differentiation and growth suppression are the canonical mechanisms of action of retinoids that are executed via a well-defined pharmacologic profile. Unlike other phytochemicals described in the most current evidence-based discourses of chemoprevention, retinoids exert their pleiotropic effects by well-defined, selective, high-affinity binding to nuclear retinoid receptors. Binding of ligand to these well-characterized transcription factors enlists complex programs of positive and negative gene regulation, which orchestrate the preventive and therapeutic actions of these compounds (Freemantle et al. 2003; Niles 2004; Tang and Gudas 2011; Duong and Rochette-Egly 2011). These genomic effects are linked with epigenetic alterations of histones, DNA, and miRNA (Stallings et al. 2011; Gudas 2013). Nongenomic inhibition of kinase

TABLE 21.1
Preventive and Therapeutic Uses of Retinoids in the Cancer Clinic

Cancer Type	Clinical Use	Retinoid	FDA Approved
Promyelocytic leukemia	Therapy	Ail-*trans* retinoic acid (tretinoin)	Yes
Neuroblastoma	Therapy	13-*cis* retinoic acid (isotretinoin)	Yes
Cutaneous T-cell lymphoma	Therapy	Bexarotene (targretin)	Yes
Kaposi's sarcoma	Therapy	9-*cis* retinoic acid (alitretinoin)	Yes
Breast cancer	Prevention	Fenretinide (4-HPR)	No
Xeroderma pigmentosum	Prevention	13-*cis* retinoic acid (isotretinoin)	No
Non-melanoma skin cancer	Prevention	Acitretin (soriatane)	No
Bladder cancer	Prevention	Etretinate (tigason)	No
Hepatocellular carcinoma	Prevention	Acyclic retinoid (polyprenoic acid)	No

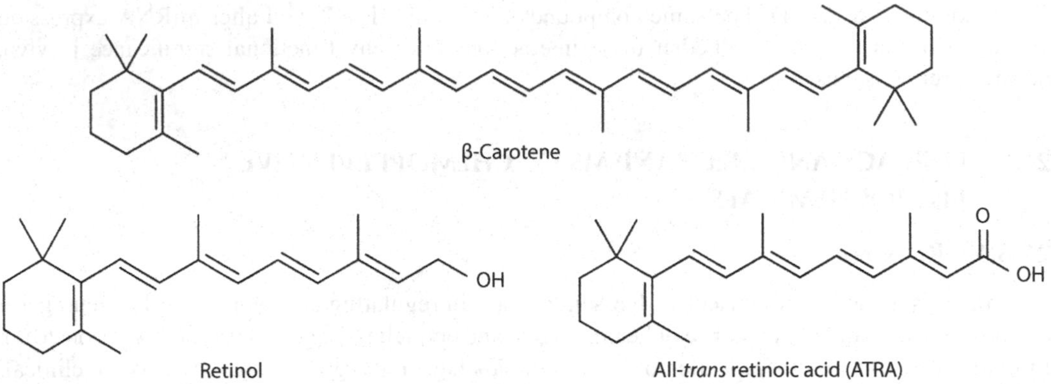

FIGURE 21.6 Beta-carotene is a dietary phytochemical precursor of vitamin A (retinol). Pleiotropic cellular effects are mediated by all-*trans* retinoic acid (ATRA), the active ligand of retinoid receptors.

cascades such as PI3K and NFκB comprises more recently identified noncanonical mechanisms (Al Tanoury et al. 2013). As forerunners of molecularly targeted cancer prevention, retinoids constitute a valuable paradigm for translation of dietary phytochemicals to the cancer clinic (Yim et al. 2014).

21.3.2 Phenolic Compounds

More than 8,000 phenolic compounds have been identified in leaves, fruits, flowers, seeds, and barks of plants, with molecular weights ranging from 100 Da for simple phenolics to 30,000 Da for complex polymers (Strack 1997; Crozier et al. 2009; Heim 2010). Examples include phenolic acids, flavonoids, stilbenes, curcuminoids, and tannins. *In planta*, the phenol functional group is uniquely amenable to diverse substitutions that facilitate adaptive, defensive, and reproductive processes, including pigmentation, photoprotection, deterrence of herbivores, and resistance to microbial invasion (Iwashina 2003; Buer et al. 2010). Owing to the facile donation of electrons by phenolic hydroxyl groups, the stability of the resulting phenolic radical, and indirect antioxidant effects such as divalent metal chelation and antioxidant gene induction, these compounds have been acclaimed for decades for their potent antioxidant activity (Heim et al. 2002). It has become clear, however, that phenolics exhibit other mechanisms of action that are operative throughout the course of transformation of a healthy cell to a malignant cell. Examples include induction of carcinogen detoxification, inhibition of trophic and survival signals, anti-inflammatory effects, and induction of programmed cell death.

The plant kingdom harbors thousands of simple phenolics, comprising one hydroxylated aromatic ring, and a much larger and relatively underexplored array of polyphenols, defined by two or more phenolic rings. Polyphenol diversity is considerable, owing to a wide variety of aromatic ring substitutions and polymerization to high-molecular-weight compounds with variable interphenolic linkage architectures (Crozier et al. 2009; Heim 2010).

21.3.2.1 Flavonoids

Characterized by the flavan (2-phenyl-1,4-benzopyrone) nucleus, flavonoids comprise the most prevalent, widely consumed and researched class of polyphenols, with more than 5000 identified to date (Andersen and Markham 2006). It is estimated that flavonoids account for 60% of dietary polyphenol intake. In plants, common substitutions in the flavan nucleus are hydroxyl, methoxy, galloyl, and glycosidic moieties (Heim et al. 2002). Flavonoid classification is summarized in Table 21.2. Condensation can generate oligomers and polymers, known as condensed tannins, or proanthocyanidins. Most of the compounds in Table 21.2 have been investigated for potential anticancer

TABLE 21.2
Classification of Dietary Flavonoids

Flavonoid Class	Structure	Examples	Substitution Pattern	Dietary Sources
Flavan-3-ol		(+)-Catechin (−)-Epicatechin EGCG	3,5,7,3′,4′-OH 3,5,7,3′,4′-OH 3,5,7,3′,4′,5′-OH, 3-gallate	Green tea, cocoa Green tea, cocoa Green tea
Flavone		Rutin Luteolin Apigenin Chrysin	5,7,3′,4′-OH, 3-rutinose 5,7,3′,4′-OH 5,7,4′-OH 5,7-OH	Citrus, red wine, Red pepper Parsley, celery Fruit skins
Flavonol		Quercetin Myricetin	3,5,7,3′,4′-OH 3,5,7,3′,4′,5′-OH	Citrus, berries, onion Berries, grapes, wine
Flavanone		Naringenin Taxifolin Hesperidin	5,7,4′-OH 3,5,7,3′,4′-OH 3,5,3′-OH, 4′-OMe, 7-rutinose	Citrus Citrus Citrus
Isoflavone		Genistein Daidzein	5,7,4′-OH 7,4′-OH	Soy Soy
Anthocyanidin		Cyanidin Apigenidin	3,5,7,4′-OH,3,5-OMe 5,7,4′-OH	Berries, red wine Berries, red wine

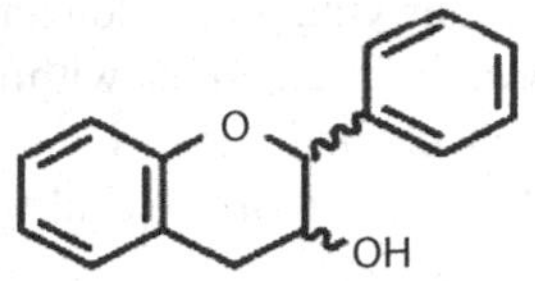

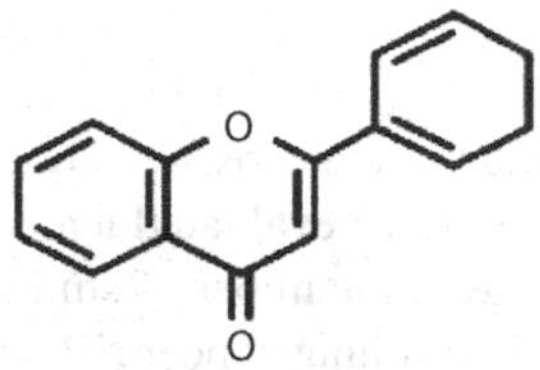

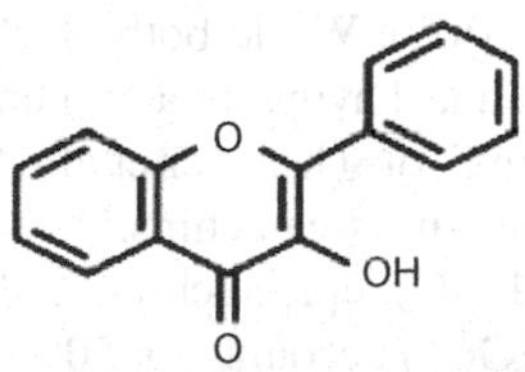

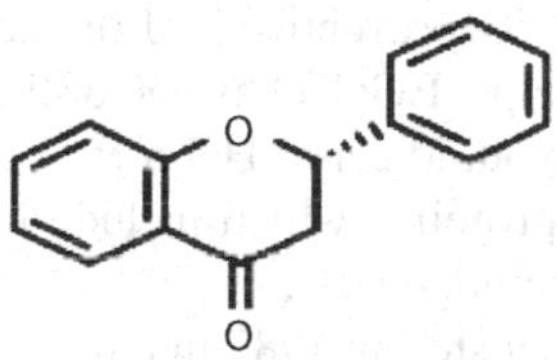

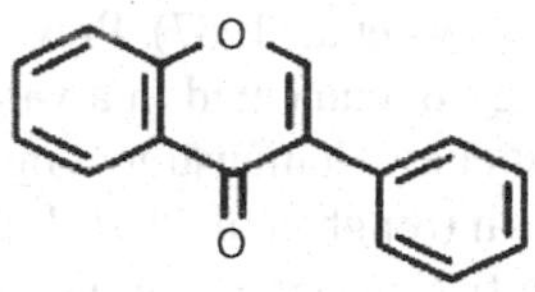

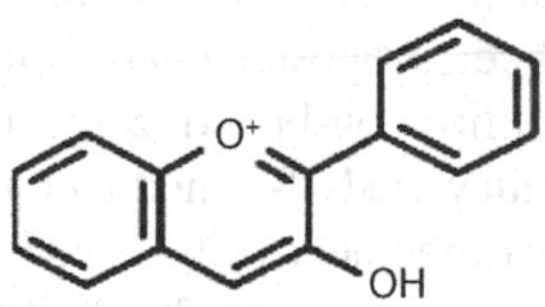

actions, with nearly universal success in tumor cell culture experiments. Those with the strongest evidence supporting chemopreventive utility are catechins, quercetin, and isoflavones from green tea, fruits, and soy, respectively.

Although the cumulative epidemiological record is inconsistent (Hertog et al. 1993; De Stefani et al. 1999; Bosetti et al. 2005), considerable evidence supports the preventive effects of flavonoid-rich diets against lung, breast, prostate, pancreatic, and colorectal cancers (Lin et al. 2006; Theodoratou et al. 2007; Cui et al. 2008; Romagnolo and Selmin 2012). Interpretation of epidemiological studies is challenged by many factors, particularly the enormous variability in total intake, especially across continents, limited quantitative data on food content, extreme variability of flavonoid composition in foods owing to agrarian, processing and preparation differences, and the intractable and probable pharmacodynamic and pharmacokinetic interactions between flavonoids and other constituents.

The antioxidant actions of flavonoids are mediated not only by direct scavenging of reactive oxygen and nitrogen species, but by chelation of redox-active metals, direct inhibition of radical-generating enzymes, and induction of cytoprotective genes (Bors and Michel 2002; Heim et al. 2002; Heim 2010). In these capacities, flavonoids are adept "blocking agents," intercepting ROS from many angles to protect DNA from electrophilic insults and blocking genetic alterations that might initiate carcinogenesis. Suppression of signaling pathways underlying promotion and progression by flavonoids is underpinned by redox-mediated and direct protein interactions within multiple signal transduction networks that regulate gene expression (e.g. NFκB and Nrf2). However, direct binding to proteins such as receptors and enzymes in vitro and in cell culture typically occurs with low affinity and limited selectivity.

21.3.2.1.1 Catechins

Tea, made from the leaves of *Camellia sinensis*, is the oldest and most widely consumed beverage in the world. Since 2006, over 50 epidemiologic studies have evaluated tea consumption with respect to cancer risk. Although results have been inconsistent, a number of studies have inversely associated green tea intake with breast, prostate, colorectal, and lung cancer risk (Yang et al. 2007; Kurahashi et al. 2008; Shrubsole et al. 2009; Tang et al. 2009). While both black and green teas have demonstrated anticancer potential, the latter is regarded as having greater therapeutic promise, owing to its high concentration of unique monomeric flavan-3-ols (Kanwar et al. 2012).

Contrary to black tea, green tea contains flavanols known as catechins. The four major species in green tea are epicatechin (EC), epigallocatechin (EGC), epicatechin-3-gallate (ECG), and epigallocatechin-3-gallate (EGCG) (Kanwar et al. 2012). EGCG accounts for 50%–75% of catechin content of green tea and is thought to mediate many of its preventive and therapeutic properties (Du et al. 2012). By virtue of eight aromatic hydroxyl groups, EGCG has one of the greatest hydrogen bonding and radical quenching capabilities of the flavonoid class (Heim et al. 2002). Hydrogen bonding mediates direct inhibition of an assortment of proteins, which include receptors, growth factors, and enzymes implicated in all three stages of carcinogenesis.

The chemopreventive potential of EGCG was first suggested in 1987 in a report of inhibition of teleocidin-induced tumor promotion in mouse skin (Yoshizawa et al. 1987). Prevention or attenuation of initiation, promotion, and progression has since been documented in a variety of cell lines and animal models, and observational and clinical trial data have demonstrated inhibition of tumor incidence and multiplicity in the breast, colon liver, and skin (Singh et al. 2011; Lambert 2013).

EGCG downregulates signaling pathways involved in initiation and postinitiation stages of carcinogenesis (Khan et al. 2006). Mechanisms of action have been proposed, but the molecular pharmacology of EGCG remains vague (Beltz et al. 2006). As an initiation-blocking agent, EGCG induces carcinogen detoxification and protection from oxidative injury via Nrf-2-mediated induction of antioxidant and phase II enzymes. By virtue of its unique arrangement of hydroxyl groups, together with the gallate moiety, it is a potent free radical scavenger (Heim et al. 2002). As a postinitiation suppressor, EGCG inhibits proliferation in many human tumor cell lines, including cervical, melanoma, and lung cancer cells (Nihal et al. 2009; Philips et al. 2009; Qiao et al. 2009; Yamauchi et al. 2009). Growth suppressive effects involve direct interactions with receptors, such as IGF-1R (Li et al. 2007), in tandem with inhibition of Akt/PI3K/mTOR signaling (Van Aller et al. 2011). EGCG has recently been identified as a dual competitive inhibitor of PI3K and mTOR with *Ki* values of 380 and 320 nM, respectively (Van Aller et al. 2011). In animal models of prostate cancer, growth suppression is attributable to inhibition of the EGF/EGFR and IGF-1/IGF-1R axes and attenuation of the PI3K/Akt/mTOR pathways. In lung cancer cells, EGCG suppresses EGFR expression, activation, and downstream trophic signaling events (Ma et al. 2014). In SW480 colon cancer cells, EGCG suppresses growth via EGFR internalization, degradation, and p38 MAPK-mediated phosphorylation (Adachi et al. 2009). EGCG can also suppress constitutive activity of growth factor receptors, as observed with Her-2/neu, a member of the EGFR family that is overexpressed in approximately 30% of breast cancers and correlates with high mortality (Pianetti et al. 2002).

EGCG can induce apoptosis through the intrinsic or extrinsic pathway (Nihal et al. 2009; Philips et al. 2009; Qiao et al. 2009; Yamauchi et al. 2009). Activation of pro-apoptotic Bcl-2 proteins may be selective for malignant cells (Khan and Mukhtar 2008). In lung cancer xenografts, EGCG induced apoptosis of A549 cells, inhibited markers of proliferation and apoptosis, repressed Bcl-xL, and induced Bax expression and protein accumulation. EGCG also repressed Ku70, a negative regulator of Bax (Li et al. 2013).

At physiologically attainable concentrations, EGCG is a natural ligand of the 67 kDa laminin receptor (67LR), which plays important roles in cell growth, death, metastasis, and chemoresistance (Tachibana et al. 2004). As a mediator of cell adhesion to the basement membrane, 67LR is instrumental in tumor cell metastasis (Castronovo 1993). 67LR is also regarded as a death receptor, although the cGMP-mediated PKCδ/acid sphingomyelinase (PKCδ/ASM) pathway accountable for its activation is aberrantly regulated in several cancers (Kumazoe et al. 2013). Its overexpression is common in human colorectal, cervical, and breast carcinomas, and downregulation of 67LR is an attractive target in secondary and tertiary chemoprevention (Tachibana 2009; Fujimura et al. 2012). In myeloma cells, RNAi-mediated silencing of 67LR abrogates EGCG-induced apoptosis (Shammas et al. 2006). Selectivity is another potential advantage of targeting 67LR, as it appears to have differential roles in normal versus malignant cells. Selective 67LR-mediated apoptosis by EGCG has been demonstrated in acute myeloid leukemia cells (AML) (Kumazoe et al. 2013).

Despite these advances in the pharmacology of EGCG, its anticancer mechanisms remain unclear. Target resolution and mechanistic validation in vivo will be essential for the development of chemoprevention strategies featuring EGCG. Current knowledge is complicated by the historical and widespread preference to use EGCC in vitro at high concentrations (50–200 μM) that are not easily attainable with consumption of green tea as a beverage. Plasma EGCG levels in humans consuming green tea extract as a supplement reach the low micromolar range (Chow et al. 2001). Polyphenon E, a well-defined, commonly used formulation in cancer research, can yield peak plasma EGCG levels of 17.4 and 32.7 μM following a single oral dose of 400 and 800 mg in humans (Chow et al. 2001). However, intersubject variability is considerable, most likely owing to the poorly understood metabolic fates of EGCG. Since a considerable fraction of the oral dose is removed by phase II conjugation alone, slight changes in other determinants of bioavailability can dramatically impact exposure (Chow et al. 2001).

21.3.2.1.2 Quercetin

Being the subject of over 10,000 published studies and scholarly reviews, quercetin is the most extensively researched flavonoid. Its clinical applications are diverse, with cardiovascular, neurocognitive, and immune health at the forefront of an expanding therapeutic profile. Initially acclaimed for its antioxidant activity, the past decade of research has underscored cellular signal transduction, enzyme activity, and gene expression as major targets of its health benefits. Quercetin is ubiquitous in edible plants and is the most abundant monomeric flavonoid in fruits and vegetables, with apples and onions providing the majority of dietary intake in the United States. The anticarcinogenic utility of quercetin in primary chemoprevention is supported by considerable in vitro and in vivo data (Gibellini et al. 2011; Li et al. 2012). In rodents, quercetin inhibits chemically induced colon, mammary, and prostate tumor formation (Deschner et al. 1991; Volate et al. 2005; Devipriya et al. 2006; Kamaraj et al. 2007). In humans, high intake has been inversely associated with gastric adenocarcinoma, one of the leading causes of cancer deaths worldwide (Ekström et al. 2011). In two prospective cohort studies and two case–control studies, quercetin significantly reduced lung cancer risk (Stefani et al. 1999; Hirvonen et al. 2001; Knekt et al. 2002; Cui et al. 2008).

Quercetin exceeds most flavonoids in the number of aromatic hydroxyl groups. As with EGCG, these attributes enable potent radical scavenging in addition to the ability to interact with proteins via hydrogen bonding (Heim et al. 2002). The presence of a 2,3-double bond and 4-oxo group also account for the potent antioxidant properties of quercetin. However, it is these features that also underlie pro-oxidant tendencies, which may contribute to pro-apoptotic effects and induction of redox-sensitive signaling pathways such as Nrf2. Like other chemopreventive phenolics, mechanisms of action are multifaceted and include direct protein binding and indirect redox regulation of anti-inflammatory and cytoprotective pathways (e.g. NFκB inhibition and Nrf2 activation, respectively). Inhibition of tumor growth in murine melanoma is mediated in part by the inhibition of STAT3 signaling, which is often constitutively active in melanoma and other human malignancies (Cao et al. 2014). Quercetin also inhibits PI3K/Akt signal transduction with multiple putative protein targets (Bruning 2013; Firdous et al. 2014; Ko et al. 2014).

Induction of apoptosis is perhaps the most thoroughly researched molecular mechanism of quercetin in tumor cell lines. In androgen-independent PC-3 prostate cancer cells, quercetin elevated cytochrome c concentrations and apoptosis, mediated by both the intrinsic and extrinsic pathways (Senthilkumar et al. 2010). In HT-29 cells, quercetin-induced apoptosis via the intrinsic pathway was accompanied by the activation of the tumor suppressors p53 and p21 (Kim et al. 2010). In HepG2 cells, an immortalized cancer cell line, apoptosis was mediated by caspase-3 and -9 activation, downregulation of anti-apoptotic Bcl-2 members, translocation of Bax to the mitochondrial membrane, and inhibition of Akt and ERK signals (Granado-Serrano et al. 2006). Activation of AMP-activated protein kinase (AMPK) and inhibition of PI3K and NFκB signaling have been reported to mediate quercetin-induced apoptosis in HT-29 colon cancer and salivary adenoid cystic carcinoma cells, respectively (Kim et al. 2010; Sun et al. 2010). Apoptotic induction in human CLL is mediated by the downregulation of the anti-apoptotic protein, Mcl-1 (Spagnuolo et al. 2012; Russo et al. 2014). Direct binding of quercetin to Bcl-2 family proteins has been demonstrated (Primikyri et al. 2014).

The radiosensitizing and chemosensitizing effects of quercetin suggest that it may be a valuable adjuvant to cytotoxic drugs (Spagnuolo et al. 2012). Low doses, however, may be cytoprotective and support chemoresistance (Li et al. 2014). The dose- and context-dependent antioxidant and pro-oxidant behavior of quercetin necessitate future dose–response investigations in each specific tumor type. Whether quercetin will behave as a cytoprotective antioxidant or pro-apoptotic pro-oxidant is likely contingent upon dose and cell context. Monitoring of oxidative stress biomarkers such as F_2-isoprostanes should be considered in human clinical trials of quercetin and other phenolics with known pro-oxidant tendencies.

Typical dietary intake of quercetin affords plasma concentrations in the nanomolar range, which falls far below the 1–100 μM doses validated by preclinical cancer research. Orally administering quercetin as an unformulated isolate at doses commonly provided by dietary supplements allows plasma levels to exceed 10 μM, which is consistent with mechanistic and animal experiments (Russo et al. 2012). Whether the aggressive attempts to increase bioavailability are beneficial is unclear, as pro-oxidant effects are observed with cellular levels as low as 40 μM (Heim et al. 2002; Vargas and Burd 2010). Nonetheless, efforts have been undertaken to overcome the limited 20%–30% absorption that is ascribed to poor solubility, instability, and limited membrane permeability. In the foregoing capacities, liposomes, inclusion complexes, and nanoparticles have been successful (Cai et al. 2013).

It is important to note that in contrast to most dietary supplements and study preparations, quercetin occurs in food predominantly as water-soluble 3′ or 4′-*O*-glucosides, which are more bioavailable than the aglycone. The glycosidic moiety of naturally occurring flavonoids accelerates absorption via the intestinal sodium-dependent glucose transporter 1 (SGLT1), circumventing the physicochemical limitations of passive diffusion. Brush border lactase phlorizin hydrolase (LPH), which recruits flavonoid glycosides to the mucosal membrane, also enhances cellular uptake by cleaving the sugar and allowing the aglycone, now in close proximity to the membrane, to permeate and access the portal blood more effectively. In humans, absorption from onions is 52%, compared to 24% from a standard quercetin aglycone supplement (Hollman et al. 1997). Animal studies have documented superior bioavailability of the glucosides relative to the aglycone (Manach et al. 1997). Collectively, the evidence suggests that the glucoside is twofold–sixfold more bioavailable than its aglycone. Also known as isoquercetin, the 3′-*O*-glucoside has recently become available as a dietary supplement, although clinical knowledge remains limited to preliminary pharmacokinetics.

EGCG and other tea catechins are vulnerable to extensive methylation in vivo, which restricts systemic exposure. Quercetin is a direct inhibitor of catechol-*O*-methyltransferase (COMT), which methylates catechins in vivo and compromises their efficacy in tumor cell lines. Wang et al. (2012) reported significant reductions in COMT protein levels and activity with quercetin cotreatment in 786-O and A549 cells, resulting in a twofold and fourfold increase in cellular uptake of EGCG, respectively. In a SCID mouse model, supplementation of brewed green tea combined with 0.4% quercetin produced twofold–threefold elevation in total and unmethylated EGCG in lung and kidney relative to green tea alone (Wang et al. 2012). From this evidence, it is rational to speculate that combinations of phytochemicals at moderate doses may optimize pharmacokinetic parameters. Coformulations may allow lower, safer doses. Given the redundancy of putative chemopreventive molecular targets of quercetin and EGCG, pharmacodynamic synergy is another potential advantage. Further investigation of EGCG and quercetin should consider the high prevalence of the Val-Met COMT polymorphism, which decreases catalytic activity by twofold–fourfold. Individuals with the variant allele would be expected to retain higher EGCG levels, obviating the need for a COMT-inhibiting adjuvant.

21.3.2.2 Stilbenes

Stilbenes are diarylethene phytoalexins produced by over 70 plant species in response to pathogenic stress. The grape (*Vitis vinifera*) is best characterized with respect to stilbene biosynthesis. When cultivated in damp climates, microbial burden induces the accumulation of the dietary prototype, 3,5,4′-trihydroxy-*trans*-stilbene (resveratrol) in the fruit skin. Stilbenes are of restricted botanical occurrence, and relative to other phenolics are poorly represented in the human diet. Peanuts, grapes, and berries are among the main sources. Red grape skins and red wine are the most widely consumed sources of dietary resveratrol (Burns et al. 2002) (Figure 21.7).

Resveratrol first received widespread recognition with reports of life span prolongation in *C. elegans* and other model organisms (Wood et al. 2004). It has since been heralded as an activator of sirtuin (SIRT)-1, a histone deacetylase (HDAC) with far-reaching metabolic and homeostatic roles that are theoretically pertinent to many Western diseases. SIRT-1 functionally intersects many of the molecular aberrations underlying carcinogenesis, including DNA repair, cell cycle regulation, inflammation, cell survival, and apoptosis (Haigis and Sinclair 2010). Recognition of resveratrol as a potential chemopreventive modality began in 1997 with efficacy documented in experiments reflecting all three stages of carcinogenesis (Jang et al. 1997).

Numerous studies in tumor cell lines, animals, and humans have since supported multimodal chemopreventive effects of resveratrol. Resveratrol decreases the number of preneoplastic lesions, tumor incidence, and multiplicity in animal models of melanoma, prostate, mammary, and colon carcinomas (Juan et al. 2012; Singh et al. 2013). Like ECGC and quercetin, growth suppressive, anti-inflammatory, and pro-apoptotic effects have been demonstrated in preclinical studies. Growing evidence indicates considerable mechanistic redundancy of resveratrol with EGCG and quercetin, including targeting NFκB, Nrf2, growth factor receptors, PI3K/Akt/mTOR signaling, and Bcl-2 family members. The potency of resveratrol relative to other polyphenols at these targets is yet to be elucidated. The more pressing challenge is to overcome the poor bioavailability of resveratrol so that it can reach its target tissues in vivo.

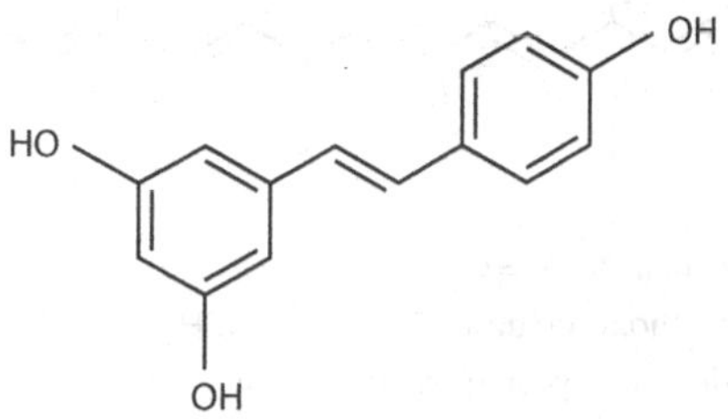

OH
HO
OH

FIGURE 21.7 *Trans*-resveratrol, the most prevalent dietary stilbene.

The oral bioavailability of resveratrol is perhaps the poorest of the chemopreventive polyphenols, with the unconjugated parent compound often being undetectable in human plasma following a single oral dose. Most of the mechanistic studies in tumor cell lines are with resveratrol at concentrations of 1–10 mM (Scott et al. 2012). Even at oral doses of 1 g, these levels are unattainable in human plasma (Scott et al. 2012). At 2.5 g/day, unconjugated resveratrol accumulated to micromolar concentrations in plasma (Brown et al. 2010). Gastrointestinal cancers are more likely to respond because of high luminal concentrations, and the fact that exposure to tumor cells precedes the hepatic phase II conjugation that is largely responsible for poor systemic bioavailability. Doses of 500–1000 mg have been effective in reducing cell proliferation in colorectal cancer tissue (Patel et al. 2010).

Efforts to improve upon the pharmacokinetics of resveratrol encompass an array of synthetic and natural analogs, along with adjuvants, cyclodextrin conjugates, colloidal systems, and nanoparticles. There is concern, however, regarding the safety of prolonged exposure to high concentrations in healthy individuals, as resveratrol is a hormetic agent with paradoxical, dose-dependent salutary, and toxic effects (Borriello et al. 2013). Thus, it is not prudent to assume that higher plasma levels will yield superior clinical outcomes. Moreover, free resveratrol should not be regarded as the only analyte of interest. New evidence indicates that its relatively abundant circulating glucuronides and sulfates can access tissues and liberate the free compound locally. Ideally, metabolites or biomarkers should be developed to determine exposure and efficacy in future clinical trials.

21.3.2.3 Curcuminoids

The rhizomes of turmeric (*Curcuma longa*) contain three polyphenolic diarylheptanoids—curcumin demethoxycurcumin, and bisdemethoxycurcumin. Curcumin (*bis*-α,β-unsaturated β-diketone) (Figure 21.8) is the most abundant, potent, widely accessible, and studied constituent (Amin et al. 2009). Curcumin has received extensive recognition over the last two decades for its multifaceted and salutary effects in diverse cancer cell lines and animal models. Preclinical investigations support efficacy at initiation and postinitiation phases of carcinogenesis, in which curcumin exerts multitargeted effects in carcinogen blockade, attenuation of oxidative stress, inhibition of cell proliferation, and induction of apoptosis. Molecular targets include growth factors, receptors, signal transduction pathways, transcription factors, and epigenetic-modifying enzymes (Amin et al. 2009; Park et al. 2013).

Curcumin mitigates survival signals, induces apoptosis, alters redox state, moderates immune factors, and alters cell metabolism (Park et al. 2013). Initiation of blockade is mediated, at least in part, by direct antioxidant effects and induction of the Nrf2 pathway, inducing detoxifying and cytoprotective genes. Curcumin is a well-established anti-inflammatory, inhibiting IKK, augmenting IκB degradation, suppressing nuclear translocation of NFκB, and inhibiting its binding to DNA (Surh et al. 2001). Curcumin can engage apoptosis by upregulating Bax, Bim, and Bak while downregulating the anti-apoptotic Bcl-2 and Bcl-xL proteins (Shankar and Srivastava 2007). Pro-apoptotic effects have also been ascribed to induction of miRNAs that downregulate

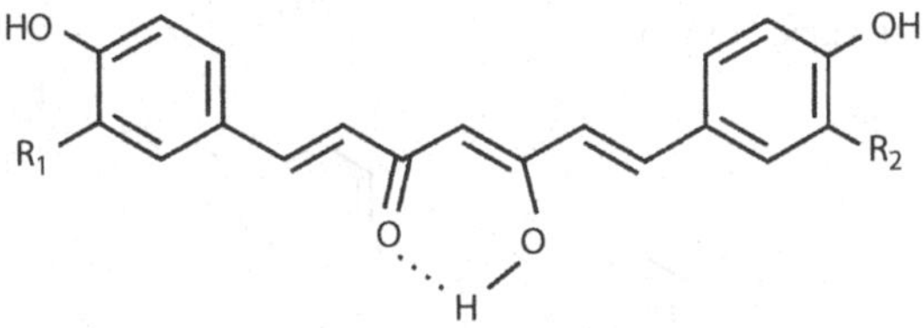

Curcumin: $R_1, R_2 = OCH_3$
Demethoxycurcumin: $R_1 = H, R_2 = OCH_3$
Bisdemethoxycurcumin: $R_1, R_2 = H$

FIGURE 21.8 The major curcuminoids in turmeric (*C. longa*) rhizomes.

Bcl-2 (Yang et al. 2010b). Suppression of transcriptional regulation of miR-21 also plays a role in inhibition of tumor growth, invasion, and metastasis in vivo by curcumin (Mudduluru et al. 2011). miR-21 is one of the most studied miRNAs and has been associated with poor cancer outcomes (Nair et al. 2012).

Antiproliferative actions of curcumin include cell cycle arrest via upregulation of p53 and p21 and suppression of growth factor receptors and trophic effectors (Korutla et al. 1995; Cho et al. 2007; Watson et al. 2010; Sun et al. 2012; Jiang et al. 2014). The EGF/EGFR and IGF-1/IGF-1R axes are both implicated in curcumin-induced growth suppression and apoptosis with multiple points of inhibition in cell culture studies. In MCF-7 breast cancer cells, growth suppression and apoptosis involve (1) reduction of IGF-1 secretion, (2) increased IGFBP-3, (3) IGF-1R tyrosine kinase inhibition, and (4) transcriptional repression of the IGF1R gene (Xia et al. 2007). Curcumin represses EGFR expression and kinase function, blocking both ligand-induced and constitutive activation of EGFR, inhibiting its intrinsic kinase activity by up to 90% (Korutla et al. 1995; Sun et al. 2012). Recently, Jiang et al. (2014) reported induction of ubiquitin-activating enzyme E1 (UBE1L), which is often lost in human lung carcinomas, as a novel mechanism of curcumin-induced EGFR transcriptional repression. Downstream Akt and NFκB signaling was mitigated concomitantly (Jiang et al. 2014).

In animal studies, curcumin is inhibitory at initiation and postinitiation phases. In a rat model of DMBA-induced mammary adenocarcinoma, initiation was suppressed by prior intraperitoneal administration of curcumin (Singletary et al. 1996). In a mouse model of familial adenomatous polyposis (FAP), daily oral administration of curcumin prevented intestinal adenoma formation (Perkins et al. 2002). In a xenograft model of squamous cell carcinoma of the head and neck (SCCHN), curcumin attenuated nuclear and cytosolic IκB-beta kinase (IKKβ) in the tumors, with marked growth attenuation (Duarte et al. 2010).

Curcumin is available as a dietary supplement of high purity (>95%) as standardized turmeric extract or as a synthetic isolate. In phase I human clinical trials, curcumin was well tolerated and nontoxic up to 12 g/day (Cheng et al. 2001; Sharma et al. 2001). As with resveratrol, the oral bioavailability of curcumin in humans is 1% or less, owing to poor solubility, limited absorption, and extensive phase II glucuronidation and sulfation in the enterocytes and liver. An early phase I study reported peak concentrations of 0.51, 0.63, and 1.77 μM with daily doses of 4, 6, and 8 g (Cheng et al. 2001). The majority of subsequent trials using doses up to 8 g have failed to detect free curcumin in blood. Since curcumin suffers many of the same pharmacokinetic limitations as resveratrol, many of the same bioavailability technologies (e.g. liposomes, phospholipids, and nanoparticles) are being applied and tested. Natural approaches include adjuvants and phytosomes. Piperine, an alkaloid from black pepper, augments metabolic stability by inhibiting UDP-glucuronosyltransferase (UGT), enhancing plasma accumulation of free curcumin. In a phase I trial of 10 patients, piperine (20 mg/kg) coadministered with curcumin (2 g/day) resulted in a 20-fold increase in bioavailability (Shoba et al. 1998). Encapsulation in nanoparticles can increase peak plasma concentrations of curcumin bioavailability by over 50-fold (Duan et al. 2010; Khalil et al. 2013). Improvements in water solubility and/or reductions in particle size with polymeric micelles, hydrogels, and liposomes produce robust enhancements in pharmacokinetic performance (Belkacemi et al. 2011; Gupta and Dixit 2011).

The colon is exposed to high concentrations of ingested curcumin. It has also been suggested that malignant mucosa accumulates curcumin more readily than normal tissue (Sharma et al. 2001). Sharma et al. (2001) reported radiologically stable disease in 5 of 15 colorectal cancer patients after 2–4 months of low-dose curcumin treatment, despite undetectable levels of curcumin or its metabolites in plasma or urine. In a more recent study, colorectal cancer patients given 4 g curcumin for 30 days exhibited a 40% reduction in the number of aberrant crypt foci (Carroll et al. 2011). In a phase II trial of 5 FAP patients, 480 mg curcumin and 20 mg quercetin given orally t.i.d. for 180 days decreased the number of polyps in 60.4% and reduced the mass of polyps in 50.9% of subjects (Cruz-Correa et al. 2006). This suggests that combinations of polyphenols with overlapping modes of action may have enhanced efficacy through pharmacokinetic and/or pharmacodynamic synergy.

21.3.3 Glucosinolates

Cruciferous vegetables, which include broccoli, cauliflower, Brussels sprouts, watercress, and bok choy, contain high levels of glucosinolates, a family of over 130 water-soluble, sulfur-containing secondary metabolites that impart the distinct pungency and bitter character to these vegetables. Upon mechanical perturbation of the plant structure by chewing, chopping, or processing, glucosinolates are ephemeral molecules. Hydrolysis ensues upon contact with the plant enzyme myrosinase, which is released from adjacent cell walls upon breaching of the cell structure. If myrosinase is thermally inactivated by cooking, hydrolysis can occur in the gut by microbial enzymes. Glucosinolate hydrolysis yields an assortment of biologically active isothiocyanates and indoles. Cleavage of glucoraphanin and glucobrassicin, two major dietary glucosinolates, yields the isothiocyanate sulforaphane (SFN) and indole-3-carbinol (I3C), respectively (Figure 21.9). I3C spontaneously undergoes acid condensation and polymerization, giving rise to numerous acid condensation products in the stomach, the most abundant and well characterized of which is the dimer 3,3′-diindoylmethane (DIM) (Watson et al. 2013).

Evidence from cohort and case–control studies in the United States and Europe supports an inverse association between cruciferous vegetable consumption and the risk of prostate, breast, renal, lung, and colorectal carcinomas (Steinbrecher et al. 2009; Liu and Lv 2013; Watson et al. 2013; Wu et al. 2013; Tse and Eslick 2014). In a prospective evaluation of 11,405 male participants of the EPIC-Heidelberg cohort study, dietary glucosinolate intake significantly reduced prostate cancer risk (Steinbrecher et al. 2009). Although several cohort studies have failed to document reduced prostate or colon cancer risk with higher daily cruciferous vegetable intakes, several case–control studies support significant risk reduction (Jain et al. 1999; Kolonel et al. 2000). In the Netherlands Cohort Study on Diet and Cancer, women with higher crucifer intake showed significant colon cancer risk reduction (Voorrips et al. 2000). In two case–control studies, women with higher crucifer intakes exhibited reduced risk of breast cancer (Zhang et al. 1999; Terry et al. 2001). However, pooled analysis of cohort studies failed to support breast cancer risk reduction (Smith-Warner et al. 2001).

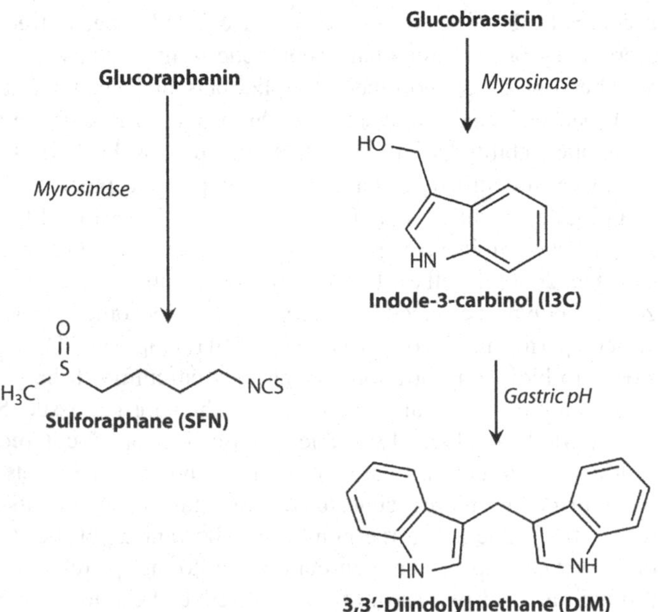

FIGURE 21.9 Formation of indole-3-carbinol and sulforaphane from glucosinolates. SFN, I3C, and DIM have individually been investigated as chemopreventive agents.

The inconsistent data have been ascribed to multiple factors. Foremost, considerable vagaries persist regarding the relationship between glucosinolate content in food with the corresponding levels of its bioactive derivatives in plasma and tissues. Other poorly tractable variables include (1) high natural variation in glucosinolate content of foods, (2) impact of both mechanical preparation methodology and temperature range on myrosinase activity, and (3) interindividual heterogeneity at multiple steps in the metabolism to bioactive compounds. Genetic variations can affect both exposure and responses to crucifers. For example common polymorphisms in glutathione S-transferases (GSTs), which detoxify both isothiocyanates and carcinogenic xenobiotics, dually impact isothiocyanate bioavailability and cancer risk reduction (Yang et al. 2010a).

Sulforaphane (SFN) is the most extensively studied dietary isothiocyanate. Its anticarcinogenic efficacy has been documented in carcinogen-induced genetic and xenograft animal models (Lenzi et al. 2014). SFN is inhibitory at pre- and postinitiation stages. Its carcinogen-blocking capability is ascribed primarily to the activation of the Nrf2 pathway. Its postinitiation actions involve attenuation of Akt and NFκB signaling and induction of apoptosis (Watson et al. 2013). Following ingestion, peak plasma SFN levels are typically achieved within 2 h with complete elimination occurring within 24 h. SFN accumulates in tissues such as the stomach and genitourinary tract, where it may potentially exert protective effects with minimal detection in plasma (Veeranki et al. 2013; Watson et al. 2013).

Relative to SFN, the pharmacology of the more durable metabolite, I3C, is better understood, as most cell culture and animal models of breast, prostate, pancreatic, hepatic, and colon cancer have evaluated I3C, and more recently, DIM (Maruthanila et al. 2014). In cellular and animal experiments recapitulating various aspects of initiation, promotion, and progression, I3C exerts inhibitory activity mediated by similar pathways as with polyphenols. Induction of carcinogen detoxification, cell cycle arrest, inhibition of Akt and NFκB pathways, attenuation of tumor invasion, and antiangiogenic actions are among the most salient chemopreventive actions of I3C and DIM in preclinical studies (Higdon et al. 2007).

The role of epigenetic modifications in the chemopreventive actions of SFN, I3C, and DIM comprises an area of intensive investigation in tumor cell lines, animal models, and human subjects. The Nrf2 pathway is influenced by epigenetic effects of SFN (Gerhauser 2013). Inhibition of HDACs and HATs and bidirectional effects on miRNAs have been demonstrated in vivo. For example a dose of 68 g of broccoli sprouts inhibited HDAC activity in peripheral blood mononucleocytes up to 6 h following consumption (Myzak et al. 2007). EGCG combined with SFN resulted in re-expression of the estrogen receptor (ER) in ER-negative breast carcinoma cells (Meeran et al. 2012). In ER-positive MCF-7 breast cancer cells, DIM increases miR-21 expression with concomitant repression of the cell cycle–promoting phosphatase, Cdc25A, suppressing growth (Jin 2011). In pancreatic cancer cells, DIM augments miR-146a, resulting in downregulation of EGFR, metastasis-associated protein 2 (MTA-2), interleukin-1 receptor–associated kinase 1 (IRAK-1), and NFκB, with concomitant inhibition of cell invasion (Li et al. 2010). miRNA modulation by natural products including SFN, I3C, and DIM has been reviewed at length by Phuah and Nagoor (2014).

The recent shift in focus on DIM as a chemopreventive compound resulted from observations that oral doses as high as 1200 mg I3C failed to produce detectable levels of parent compound in plasma (Reed et al. 2006; Maruthanila et al. 2014). Conversely, recovery of DIM, which is more stable in vivo, has been clearly documented (Reed et al. 2006; Maruthanila et al. 2014). The pharmacokinetics of SFN and I3C suggests that DIM, and possibly other acid condensation derivatives of I3C, is instrumental in the protective effects of crucifer-derived organosulfur compounds. DIM, when administered as the study compound in TRAMP mice, inhibited prostate tumor growth and proliferation markers and elevated markers of apoptosis (Cho et al. 2011). Other examples of the potential of DIM to recapitulate known molecular pharmacologic actions of I3C are Nrf2 activation, NFκB inhibition, and blockade of Akt signaling (Chen et al. 2013). DIM concentrations evaluated in many in vitro investigations exceed the peak plasma levels (<2 μM) reported in men after a single oral 300 mg dose (Heath et al. 2010; Watson et al. 2013). It is critical to acknowledge that the vast majority of studies of SFN and I3C have not assessed DIM nor considered the potential biological activities of other condensation products. If DIM is the sole biologically active condensation product, further optimization of DIM (e.g. enhancing bioavailability) may be justified. Given the structural similarities between DIM and other acid condensation products, however, this is unlikely to be the case, and characterization of the bioactivity of these compounds will be imperative.

21.4 OVERCOMING CHALLENGES IN THE DEVELOPMENT OF CHEMOPREVENTIVE MODALITIES

21.4.1 Bioavailability

Secondary plant metabolites are recognized and handled as toxins by the body and therefore have poor solubility, limited absorption, and rapid efflux and clearance. Accordingly, bioavailability optimization of chemopreventive natural products is a large area of research focus. According to Lipinski's rule of 5, many polyphenols display flagrant hindrances to permeation and absorption (Lipinski et al., 2001). Quercetin and EGCG have hydrogen bond donors and limited membrane-partitioning capacity. Resveratrol and curcumin are particularly subject to extensive presystemic glucuronide and sulfate conjugation in the intestinal mucosa and liver. Many phytochemicals are prone to efflux via multidrug resistance protein (MRP) and p-glycoprotein. Thus, discrepancies between experimental concentrations and levels detected in the human circulation after an oral dose are often quite large.

Many attempts to enhance the solubility, reduce particle size, and/or improve metabolic stability of these compounds have been successful in elevating peak plasma levels, durability, elimination half-life, and area under the curve. Why take the trouble of investigating chemopreventive efficacy if the only alteration was encapsulation of the same compound in an enhanced delivery system? Both safety and pharmacologic profiles are dependent on the level of exposure. For hormetic agents such as resveratrol, "too much of a good thing" may produce paradoxical outcomes. Moving forward, chemopreventive phytochemicals with bioavailability enhancements should proceed methodically with attention given to their potentially unique effects against well-defined clinical safety and efficacy biomarkers and other endpoints.

A historically significant oversight that is creating much confusion in the current literature is the fact that many phytochemicals are putative prodrugs. This has been evident in observations that, despite modest or absent plasma concentrations of resveratrol, cardiovascular and neurological efficacy has been clearly demonstrated in human clinical trials. The sequential genesis of I3C and DIM from SFN is relatively well defined, but is highly erratic and poorly tractable. The complex biotransformation of phenolics by colonic microbiota to an extensive litany of phenylpropionic, phenylvaleric, and phenolic acids remains an understudied area (Crozier et al. 2009; Heim 2010). Which metabolites, in what concentrations, in what tissues, and in which genotypes, mediate the anticancer legacies of their ephemeral parent compounds? Far from trivial, research investigating the possible chemopreventive effects of phytochemical metabolites is underway. Until those efforts reach fruition, mechanistic and pharmacokinetic studies may continue evaluating the wrong compound at an irrelevant dose.

21.4.2 Individualization

The underpinnings of what has been previously dismissed as "biochemical individuality" are now being delineated by an expanding catalog of genetic polymorphisms affecting cancer risk, the pharmacodynamics and pharmacokinetics of therapeutics, and the molecular characteristics of individual tumors. Ideally, the continued development of clinical genotyping methods will evaluate and adjust dose and schedule of phytochemicals to maximize the efficacy on an individual basis. It is a future goal that large sets of data pertaining to the influence of genotypes on dietary requirements, cancer risk, and the efficacy and safety of specific chemopreventive strategies in subpopulations will become accessible to clinicians.

Ideally, a chemopreventive agent should be developed by (1) identifying candidates through screening in cellular assays, (2) applying modern methods such as OMICs technologies to identify molecular target candidates for individual compounds, (3) identifying individuals most likely to respond to the agent, and (4) designing clinical trials with consideration of the pathways altered in a participants' tumor type (Gonzáles-Vallinas et al. 2013). The current repertoire of promising natural products has not followed this course. While there is a wealth of cell culture studies with phenolics and organosulfur compounds, attempts to confirm *real* mechanisms of action have been met with limited success. More ominously, the individuals most likely to respond to one agent versus another remains uncharacterized. To date, the vast majority of clinical trials have not been designed to consider molecular target expression and pathological relevance in study population. Instead, we have an assortment of phytochemicals that are mechanistically vague, poorly bioavailable, and uncategorized based on tumor type and other parameters of patient individuality.

Future attempts to gather data on phytochemical intake in relation to cancer incidence should consider *profiles* and *patterns* of phytochemical intakes and their corresponding metabolomes in humans. The 5000 different species of flavonoids likely impart structure- and metabolite-dependent protection; moreover, phytochemicals are invariably consumed in complex combinations. From both pharmacodynamics and pharmacokinetics perspective, the interactive pharmacologic profiles of phytochemicals, for example synergy and antagonism, comprise an incipient, vital, and extraordinarily complicated area of study that demands a systems biology approach. Since polyphenols are subject to a variety of agrarian and food production variables that dramatically impact total content and composition in rich dietary sources such as tea, cocoa, and fruits, refinement of qualitative and quantitative methods toward accurate composition profiling will be essential. Since phytochemicals in vivo are prone to modifying the pharmacokinetics and functions of one another, metabolomics analyses may provide insight as to what profiles correlate with efficacy. Biomarkers that reflect collective actions correlated to chemoprevention outcomes may make obsolete the need to characterize each individual metabolite.

Biomarkers should first be identified thorough preclinical investigation, followed by animal studies to identify markers predictive of response. Subsequent validation of markers can be accomplished in the phase 0 window of opportunity trials (Dragnev et al. 2005, 2011). It should be confirmed that the compound or relevant metabolites (1) access the preneoplastic lesion or tumor and (2) display the predicted effects on molecular targets. Retrospective pharmacogenomics studies can correlate single nucleotide polymorphisms with outcomes to allow determination of loci to use for selecting patients for specific chemopreventive approaches. Patients should be prospectively stratified to receive a phytochemical based on the individual tumor's molecular characteristics.

21.5 PERSPECTIVE

How will the practitioner of evidence-based medicine rationally select the most efficacious chemopreventive agents, at the proper dosage, according to a personalized risk assessment utilizing reliable, thoroughly validated measurements? Poor and variable bioavailability, unknowns regarding metabolites and mechanistic complexity, and limited, realistic clinical risk assessment tools (e.g. biomarkers) are among the major challenges in the translation of current knowledge into clinical practice. The global burden of cancer embodies an extraordinary array of different tumor types, and in the realm of personalized medicine, identification of assessment methods to characterize an individual's risk is critical, but difficult.

Understanding which molecular targets are operative in vivo is essential, but difficult. This course of investigation should be preceded by the identification of bioactive metabolites. The potential value of combining phytochemicals alone or in tandem with pharmaceuticals, supported by an evolving body of clinical evidence, should enhance efficacy and minimize toxicity. The overwhelming nature of the complexities of phytochemical diversity, metabolism, variability, and mechanistic pleiotropy can be combated with OMICs technologies and biomarkers.

Existing data from epidemiological and observational studies have largely been from healthy populations. Whether the benefit extends to high-risk groups, in which the initiation stage has passed, is uncertain. Although difficult, it will be ideal to evaluate chemopreventive agents in groups with uniform risk factors or stage of carcinogenesis. Surrogate markers will be indispensable, and expensive trials with large groups and lengthy durations will be required. Long study durations are necessary to clearly define long-term safety. Natural products are more likely to work in the early stages of the disease, yet this is when toxicity may be least tolerated.

This chapter has illustrated a cohesive theme in the molecular pharmacology of dietary phytochemicals—redundancy of actions across structurally disparate classes. In contrast to conventional pharmaceutical agents, the compounds reviewed in the foregoing sections operate on multiple molecular targets, often with low affinity. This striking mechanistic pluralism may be advantageous to inhibit the elaborate biochemical changes associated with each stage of carcinogenesis. The most straightforward advantage of a multitargeted agent is better efficacy. Initiation, promotion, and progression of cancer stems from the aberration of multiple pathways, and on an individual basis, those most pertinent to a given patient's tumor are almost always uncertain. The contribution of these pathways to cancer pathology may change over the course of the disease. The broad action of a single agent, or mechanistic expansion through combining broad-acting agents, improves the likelihood of success against the hurdles of genetic individuality, etiologic and pathologic heterogeneity of tumors, pharmacokinetic variability among patients, and the threat of compensatory biochemical alterations with prolonged exposure to drugs (e.g. drug resistance). The current paucity of reliable biomarkers for fine-tuned, individualized clinical assessment is also a hurdle for multi-targeted agents. The functional redundancy and promiscuity of natural products that frustrate many medicinal chemists and pharmacologists call for a reappraisal of the pejorative tone of "dirty drug," an apt descriptor of food and its phytochemical constituents—even in their most purified forms.

REFERENCES

Adachi, S., M. Shimizu, Y. Shirakami et al. 2009. (–)-Epigallocatechin gallate downregulates EGF receptor via phosphorylation at Ser1046/1047 by p38 MAPK in colon cancer cells. *Carcinogenesis* 30:1544–1552.

Al Tanoury, Z., A. Piskunov, and C. Rochette-Egly. 2013. Vitamin A and retinoid signaling: Genomic and nongenomic effects. *J Lipid Res* 54:1761–1775.

Alberts, D.S. and L.M. Hess. 2008. *Fundamentals of Cancer Prevention*. New York: Springer Verlag.

American Cancer Society. 2014. Cancer Facts & Figures 2014. http://www.cancer.org/acs/groups/content/@research/documents/webcontent/acspc-042151.pdf. Accessed on 1 October 2014.

Amin, A.R., O. Kucuk, F.R. Khuri, and D.M. Shin. 2009. Perspectives for cancer prevention with natural compounds. *J Clin Oncol* 27:2712–2725.

Andersen, O.M. and K.R. Markham. 2006. *Flavonoids: Chemistry, Biochemistry and Applications*. Boca Raton, FL: Taylor & Francis.

Baron, J.A., B.F. Cole, R.S. Sandler et al. 2003. A randomized trial of aspirin to prevent colorectal adenomas. *N Engl J Med* 348:891–899.

Belkacemi, A., S. Doggui, L. Dao, and C. Ramassamy. 2011. Challenges associated with curcumin therapy in Alzheimer disease. *Expert Rev Mol Med* 13:e34.

Beltz, L.A., D.K. Bayer, A.L. Moss, and I.M. Simet. 2006. Mechanisms of cancer prevention by green and black tea polyphenols. *Anticancer Agents Med Chem* 6:389–406.

Bhutani, T. and J. Koo. 2011. A review of the chemopreventative effects of oral retinoids for internal neoplasms. *J Drugs Dermatol* 10:1292–1298.

Borriello, A., D. Bencivenga, I. Caldarelli et al. 2013. Resveratrol and cancer treatment: Is hormesis a yet unsolved matter? *Curr Pharm Des* 19:5384–5393.

Bors, W. and C. Michel. 2002. Chemistry of the antioxidant effect of polyphenols. *Ann N Y Acad Sci* 957:57–69.

Bosetti, C., L. Spertini, M. Parpinel et al. 2005. Flavonoids and breast cancer risk in Italy. *Cancer Epidemiol Biomarkers Prev* 14:805–808.

Brown, V.A., K.R. Patel, M. Viskaduraki et al. 2010. Repeat dose study of the cancer chemopreventive agent resveratrol in healthy volunteers: Safety, pharmacokinetics, and effect on the insulin-like growth factor axis. *Cancer Res* 70:9003–9011.

Bruning, A. 2013. Inhibition of mTOR signaling by quercetin in cancer treatment and prevention. *Anticancer Agents Med Chem* 13:1025–1031.

Buer, C.S., N. Imin, and M.A. Djordjevic. 2010. Flavonoids: New roles for old molecules. *J Integr Plant Biol* 52: 98–111.

Burns J., T. Yokota, H. Ashihara, M.E. Lean, and A. Crozier. 2002. Plant foods and herbal sources of resveratrol. *J Agric Food Chem* 50:3337–3340.

Cai, X., Z. Fang, J. Dou, A. Yu, and G. Zhai. 2013. Bioavailability of quercetin: Problems and promises. *Curr Med Chem* 20:2572–2582.

Calin, G.A., C.D. Dumitru, M. Shimizu et al. 2002. Frequent deletions and down-regulation of micro-RNA genes miR15 and miR16 at 13q14 in chronic lymphocytic leukemia. *Proc Natl Acad Sci USA* 99:15524–15529.

Cao, H.H., A.K. Tse, H.Y. Kwan et al. 2014. Quercetin exerts anti-melanoma activities and inhibits STAT3 signaling. *Biochem Pharmacol* 87:424–434.

Carroll, R.E., R.V. Benya, D.K. Turgeon et al. 2011. Phase IIa clinical trial of curcumin for the prevention of colorectal neoplasia. *Cancer Prev Res (Phila)* 4:354–364.

Castronovo, V. 1993. Laminin receptors and laminin binding proteins during tumor invasion and metastasis. *Invasion Metastasis* 13:1–30.

Chen, C., S.M. Chen, B. Xu et al. 2013. In vivo and in vitro study on the role of 3,3′-diindolylmethane in treatment and prevention of nasopharyngeal carcinoma. *Carcinogenesis* 34:1815–1821.

Chen, K. and N. Rajewsky. 2007. The evolution of gene regulation by transcription factors and microRNAs. *Nat Rev Genet* 8:93–103.

Cheng, A.L., C.H. Hsu, J.K. Lin et al. 2001. Phase I clinical trial of curcumin, a chemopreventive agent, in patients with high-risk or pre-malignant lesions. *Anticancer Res* 21:2895–2900.

Cho, H.J., S.Y. Park, E.J. Kim, J.K. Kim, and J.H. Park. 2011. 3,3′-Diindolylmethane inhibits prostate cancer development in the transgenic adenocarcinoma mouse prostate model. *Mol Carcinog* 50:100–112.

Cho, J.W., K.S. Lee, and C.W. Kim. 2007. Curcumin attenuates the expression of IL-1beta, IL-6, and TNF-alpha as well as cyclin E in TNF-alpha-treated HaCaT cells; NF-kappaB and MAPKs as potential upstream targets. *Int J Mol Med* 19:469–474.

Choi, K.C., M.G. Jung, Y.H. Lee et al. 2009. Epigallocatechin-3-gallate, a histone acetyltransferase inhibitor, inhibits EBV-induced B lymphocyte transformation via suppression of RelA acetylation. *Cancer Res* 69:583–592.

Chow, H.H., Y. Cai, D.S. Alberts et al. 2001. Phase I pharmacokinetic study of tea polyphenols following single-dose administration of epigallocatechin gallate and polyphenon E. *Cancer Epidemiol Biomarkers Prev* 10:53–58.

Clagett-Dame, M. and D. Knutson. 2011. Vitamin A in reproduction and development. *Nutrients* 3:385–428.

Cortez, M.A., C. Bueso-Ramos, J. Ferdin, G. Lopez-Berestein, A.K. Sood, and G.A. Calin. 2011. MicroRNAs in body fluids—The mix of hormones and biomarkers. *Nat Rev Clin Oncol* 8:467–477.

Crozier, A., I.B. Jaganath, and M.N. Clifford. 2009. Dietary phenolics: Chemistry, bioavailability and effects on health. *Nat Prod Rep* 26:1001–1043.

Cruz-Correa, M., D.A. Shoskes, P. Sanchez et al. 2006. Combination treatment with curcumin and quercetin of adenomas in familial adenomatous polyposis. *Clin Gastroenterol Hepatol* 4:1035–1038.

Cui, Y., H. Morgenstern, S. Greenland et al. 2008. Dietary flavonoid intake and lung cancer—A population-based case–control study. *Cancer* 112:2241–2248.

Danaei G., S. Vander Hoorn, A.D. Lopez, C.J. Murray, and M. Ezzati. 2005. Comparative risk assessment collaborating group (Cancers). Causes of cancer in the world: Comparative risk assessment of nine behavioural and environmental risk factors. *Lancet* 366:1784–1793.

De Stefani, E., P. Boffetta, H. Deneo-Pellegrini et al. 1999. Dietary antioxidants and lung cancer risk: A case–control study in Uruguay. *Nutr Cancer* 34:100–110.

Deschner, E.E., J. Ruperto, G. Wong, and H.H. Newmark. 1991. Quercetin and rutin as inhibitors of azoxymethanol-induced colonic neoplasia. *Carcinogenesis* 12:1193–1196.

Devipriya, S., V. Ganapathy, and C.S. Shyamaladevi. 2006. Suppression of tumor growth and invasion in 9,10 dimethyl benz(a) anthracene induced mammary carcinoma by the plant bioflavonoid quercetin. *Chem Biol Interact* 162:106–113.

Dragnev, K.H., T. Ma, J. Cyrus et al. 2011. Bexarotene plus erlotinib suppress lung carcinogenesis independent of KRAS mutations in two clinical trials and transgenic models. *Cancer Prev Res* 4:818–828.

Dragnev, K.H., W.J. Petty, S. Shah et al. 2005. Bexarotene and erlotinib for aerodigestive tract cancer. *J Clin Oncol* 23:8757–8764.

Du, G.J., Z. Zhang, X.D. Wen et al. 2012. Epigallocatechin Gallate (EGCG) is the most effective cancer chemopreventive polyphenol in green tea. *Nutrients* 4:1679–1691.

Duan, J., Y. Zhang, S. Han et al. 2010. Synthesis and in vitro/in vivo anti-cancer evaluation of curcumin-loaded chitosan/poly(butyl cyanoacrylate) nanoparticles. *Int J Pharm* 400:211–220.

Duarte, V.M., E. Han, M.S. Veena et al. 2010. Curcumin enhances the effect of cisplatin in suppression of head and neck squamous cell carcinoma via inhibition of IKKbeta protein of the NFkappaB pathway. *Mol Cancer Ther* 9:2665–2675.

Duong, V. and C. Rochette-Egly. 2011. The molecular physiology of nuclear retinoic acid receptors: From health to disease. *Biochim Biophys Acta* 1812:1023–1031.

Ekström, A.M., M. Serafini, O. Nyrén, A. Wolk, C. Bosetti, and R. Bellocco. 2011. Dietary quercetin intake and risk of gastric cancer: Results from a population-based study in Sweden. *Ann Oncol* 22:438–443.

Firdous, A.B., G. Sharmila, S. Balakrishnan et al. 2014. Quercetin, a natural dietary flavonoid, acts as a chemopreventive agent against prostate cancer in an in vivo model by inhibiting the EGFR signaling pathway. *Food Funct* 5:2632–2645.

Freemantle, S.J., M.J. Spinella, and E. Dmitrovsky. 2003. Retinoids in cancer therapy and chemoprevention: Promise meets resistance. *Oncogene* 22:7305–7315.

Friedman, R.C., K.K. Farh, C.B. Burge, and D.P. Bartel. 2009. Most mammalian mRNAs are conserved targets of microRNAs. *Genome Res* 19:92–105.

Fruman, D.A. and C. Rommel. 2014. PI3K and cancer: Lessons, challenges and opportunities. *Nat Rev Drug Discov* 13:140–156.

Fujimura, Y., M. Sumida, K. Sugihara, S. Tsukamoto, K. Yamada, and H. Tachibana. 2012. Green tea polyphenol EGCG sensing motif on the 67-kDa laminin receptor. *PLoS ONE* 7(5):e37942. http://www.plosone.org/article/info%3Adoi%2F10.1371%2Fjournal.pone.0037942.

Gerhauser, C. 2013. Epigenetic impact of dietary isothiocyanates in cancer chemoprevention. *Curr Opin Clin Nutr Metab Care* 16:405–410.

Giardiello, F.M., S.R. Hamilton, A.J. Krush et al. 1993. Treatment of colonic and rectal adenomas with sulindac in familial adenomatous polyposis. *N Engl J Med* 328:1313–1316.

Gibellini, L., M. Pinti, M. Nasi et al. 2011. Quercetin and cancer chemoprevention. *Evid Based Complement Alternat Med* 2011:1–15. http://dx.doi.org/10.1093/ecam/neq053.

González-Vallinas, M., M. González-Castejón, A. Rodríguez-Casado, and A. Ramírez de Molina. 2013. Dietary phytochemicals in cancer prevention and therapy: A complementary approach with promising perspectives. *Nutr Rev* 71:585–599.

Granado-Serrano, A.B., M.A. Martín, L. Bravo, L. Goya, and S. Ramos. 2006. Quercetin induces apoptosis via caspase activation, regulation of Bcl-2, and inhibition of PI-3-kinase/Akt and ERK pathways in a human hepatoma cell line (HepG2). *J Nutr* 136:2715–2721.

Gudas, L.J. 2013. Retinoids induce stem cell differentiation via epigenetic changes. *Semin Cell Dev Biol* 24:701–705.

Gupta, N.K. and V.K. Dixit. 2011. Bioavailability enhancement of curcumin by complexation with phosphatidyl choline. *J Pharm Sci* 100:1987–1995.

Haigis, M.C. and D.A. Sinclair. 2010. Mammalian sirtuins: Biological insights and disease relevance. *Ann Rev Pathol* 5:253–295.

Hardy, T.M. and T.O. Tollefsbol. 2011. Epigenetic diet: Impact on the epigenome and cancer. *Epigenomics* 3:503–518.

Heath, E.I., L.K. Heilbrun, J. Li et al. 2010. A phase I dose-escalation study of oral BR-DIM (BioResponse 3,3′-Diindolylmethane) in castrate-resistant, non-metastatic prostate cancer. *Am J Transl Res* 2:402–411.

Heim, K. 2010. Natural polyphenol and flavonoid polymers. In *Antioxidant Polymers: Synthesis, Properties and Applications*, G. Cirillo and F. Iemma (eds.), pp. 23–53. Salem, MA: Scrivener Publishing LLC.

Heim, K., A.R. Tagliaferro, and D.J. Bobilya. 2002. Flavonoid antioxidants: Chemistry, metabolism and structure–activity relationships. *J Nutr Biochem* 13:572–584.

Hertog, M.G., P.C. Hollman, M.B. Katan, and D. Kromhout. 1993. Intake of potentially anticarcinogenic flavonoids and their determinants in adults in the Netherlands. *Nutr Cancer* 20:21–29.

Higdon, J.V., B. Delage, D.E. Williams, and R.H. Dashwood. 2007. Cruciferous vegetables and human cancer risk: Epidemiologic evidence and mechanistic basis. *Pharmacol Res* 55:224–236.

Hirvonen, T., J. Virtamo, P. Korhonen, D. Albanes, and P. Pietinen. 2001. Flavonol and flavone intake and the risk of cancer in male smokers (Finland). *Cancer Causes Control* 12:789–796.

Hollman, P.C., J.M. van Trijp, M.N. Buysman et al. 1997. Relative bioavailability of the antioxidant flavonoid quercetin from various foods in man. *FEBS Lett* 418:152–156.

Houghton, P.J. 2010. mTOR and cancer therapy: General principles. In *mTOR Pathway and mTOR Inhibitors in Cancer Therapy*, V.A. Polunovsky and P.J. Houghton (eds.), pp. 113–31. New York, Humana Press, Springer.

Huang, S., C.A. Pettaway, H. Uehara, C.D. Bucana, and I.J. Fidler. 2001. Blockade of NF-kappaB activity in human prostate cancer cells is associated with suppression of angiogenesis, invasion, and metastasis. *Oncogene* 20:4188–4197.

Iannolo, G., C. Conticello, L. Memeo, and R. De Maria. 2008. Apoptosis in normal and cancer stem cells. *Crit Rev Oncol Hematol* 66:42–51.

Iwashina, T. 2003. Flavonoid function and activity to plants and other organisms. *Biol Sci Space* 17:24–44.

Jain, M.G., G.T. Hislop, G.R. Howe, and P. Ghadirian. 1999. Plant foods, antioxidants, and prostate cancer risk: Findings from case–control studies in Canada. *Nutr Cancer* 34:173–184.

Jang, M., L. Cai, G.O. Udeani et al. 1997. Cancer chemopreventive activity of resveratrol, a natural product derived from grapes. *Science* 275:218–220.

Jiang, A.P., D.H. Zhou, X.L. Meng et al. 2014. Down-regulation of epidermal growth factor receptor by curcumin-induced UBE1L in human bronchial epithelial cells. *J Nutr Biochem* 25:241–249.

Jin, Y. 2011. 3,39-Diindolylmethane inhibits breast cancer cell growth via miR-21-mediated Cdc25A degradation. *Mol Cell Biochem* 358:345–354.

Juan, M.E., I. Alfaras, and J.M. Planas. 2012. Colorectal cancer chemoprevention by trans-resveratrol. *Pharmacol Res* 65:584–591.

Kamaraj, S., R. Vinodhkumar, P. Anandakumar, S. Jagan, G. Ramakrishnan, and T. Devaki. 2007. The effects of quercetin on antioxidant status and tumor markers in the lung and serum of mice treated with benzo(a)pyrene. *Biol Pharm Bull* 30:2268–2273.

Kanwar, J., M. Taskeen, I. Mohammad, C. Huo, T.H. Chan, and Q.P. Dou. 2012. Recent advances on tea polyphenols. *Front Biosci (Elite Ed)*. 4:111–131.

Khalil, N.M., T.C. do Nascimento, D.M. Casa et al. 2013. Pharmacokinetics of curcumin-loaded PLGA and PLGA–PEG blend nanoparticles after oral administration in rats. *Colloids Surf B Biointerfaces* 101:353–360.

Khan, N., F. Afaq, M. Saleem, N. Ahmad, and H. Mukhtar. 2006. Targeting multiple signaling pathways by green tea polyphenol (–)-epigallocatechin-3-gallate. *Cancer Res* 66:2500–2505.

Khan, N. and H. Mukhtar. 2008. Multitargeted therapy of cancer by green tea polyphenols. *Cancer Lett* 269:269–280.

Kim, H.J., S.K. Kim, B.S. Kim et al. 2010. Apoptotic effect of quercetin on HT-29 colon cancer cells via the AMPK signaling pathway. *J Agric Food Chem* 58:8643–8650.

Knekt, P., J. Kumpulainen, R. Järvinen et al. 2002. Flavonoid intake and risk of chronic diseases. *Am J Clin Nutr* 76:560–568.

Ko, C.C., Y.J. Chen, C.T. Chen et al. 2014. Chemical proteomics identifies heterogeneous nuclear ribonucleoprotein (hnRNP) A1 as the molecular target of quercetin in its anti-cancer effects in PC-3 cells. *J Biol Chem* 289:22078–22089.

Kobayashi, A., T. Ohta, and M. Yamamoto. 2004. Unique function of the Nrf2-Keapl pathway in the inducible expression of antioxidant and detoxifying enzymes. *Methods Enzymol* 378:273–286.

Kolonel, L.N., J.H. Hankin, A.S. Whittemore et al. 2000. Vegetables, fruits, legumes and prostate cancer: A multiethnic case–control study. *Cancer Epidemiol Biomarkers Prev* 9:795–804.

Korutla, L., J.Y. Cheung, J. Mendelsohn, and R. Kumar. 1995. Inhibition of ligand-induced activation of epidermal growth factor receptor tyrosine phosphorylation by curcumin. *Carcinogenesis* 16:1741–1745.

Kumazoe, M., K. Sugihara, S. Tsukamoto et al. 2013. 67-kDa laminin receptor increases cGMP to induce cancer-selective apoptosis. *J Clin Invest* 123:787–799.

Kurahashi, N., S. Sasazuki, M. Iwasaki, M. Inoue, and S. Tsugane. 2008. Green tea consumption and prostate cancer risk in Japanese men: A prospective study. *Am J Epidemiol* 167:71–77.

Lambert, J.D. 2013. Does tea prevent cancer? Evidence from laboratory and human intervention studies. *Am J Clin Nutr* 98:1667S–1675S.

Landis-Piwowar, K.R. and N.R. Iyer. 2014. Cancer chemoprevention: Current state of the art. *Cancer Growth Metastasis* 7:19–25.

Lee, R.C., R.L. Feinbaum, and V. Ambros. 1993. The *C. elegans* heterochronic gene lin-4 encodes small RNAs with antisense complementarity to lin-14. *Cell* 75:843–854.

Lenzi, M., C. Fimognari, and P. Hrelia. 2014. Sulforaphane as a promising molecule for fighting cancer. *Cancer Treat Res* 159:207–223.

Li, J., M. Mottamal, H. Li et al. 2012. Quercetin-3-methyl ether suppresses proliferation of mouse epidermal JB6 P+ cells by targeting ERKs. *Carcinogenesis* 33:459–465.

Li, J.J., Q.H. Gu, M. Li, H.P. Yang, L.M. Cao, and C.P. Hu. 2013. Role of Ku70 and Bax in epigallocatechin-3-gallate-induced apoptosis of A549 cells in vivo. *Oncol Lett.* 5:101–106.

Li, M., Z. He, S. Ermakova et al. 2007. Direct inhibition of insulin-like growth factor-I receptor kinase activity by (–)-epigallocatechin-3-gallate regulates cell transformation. *Cancer Epidemiol Biomarkers Prev* 16:598–605.

Li, N., C. Sun, B. Zhou et al. 2014. Low concentration of quercetin antagonizes the cytotoxic effects of anti-neoplastic drugs in ovarian cancer. *PLoS One* 9(7):e100314 (July). http://www.plosone.org/article/info%3Adoi%2F10.1371%2Fjournal.pone.0100314.

Li, Y., T.G. Vandenboom II, Z. Wang et al. 2010. miR-146a suppresses invasion of pancreatic cancer cells. *Cancer Res* 70:1486–1495.

Lin, J., S.M. Zhang, K. Wu, W.C. Willett, C.S. Fuchs, and E. Giovannucci. 2006. Flavonoid intake and colorectal cancer risk in men and women. *Am J Epidemiol* 164:644–651.

Ling, H., M. Fabbri, and G.A. Calin. 2013. MicroRNAs and other non-coding RNAs as targets for anticancer drug development. *Nat Rev Drug Discov* 12:847–865.

Ling, H., W. Zhang, and G.A. Calin. 2011. Principles of microRNA involvement in human cancers. *Chin J Cancer* 30:739–748.

Lipinski, C.A., F. Lombardo, B.W. Dominy, and P.J. Feeney. 2001. Experimental and computational approaches to estimate solubility and permeability in drug discovery and development settings. *Adv Drug Deliv Rev* 46:3–26.

Lippman, S.M., E.A. Klein, P.J. Goodman et al. 2009. Effect of selenium and vitamin E on risk of prostate cancer and other cancers: The Selenium and Vitamin E Cancer Prevention Trial (SELECT). *JAMA* 301:39–51.

Liu, X. and K. Lv. 2013. Cruciferous vegetables intake is inversely associated with risk of breast cancer: A meta-analysis. *Breast* 22:309–313.

Ma, Y.C., C. Li, F. Gao et al. 2014. Epigallocatechin gallate inhibits the growth of human lung cancer by directly targeting the EGFR signaling pathway. *Oncol Rep* 31:1343–1349.

Manach, C., C. Morand, C. Demigné, O. Texier, F. Régérat, and C. Rémésy. 1997. Bioavailability of rutin and quercetin in rats. *FEBS Lett* 409:12–16.

Maruthanila, V.L., J. Poornima, and S. Mirunalini. 2014. Attenuation of carcinogenesis and the mechanism underlying by the influence of indole-3-carbinol and its metabolite 3,3′-diindolylmethane: A therapeutic marvel. *Adv Pharmacol Sci* 2104:1–5. Advance online publication. doi: 10.1155/2014/832161.

Meeran, S.M., S.N. Patel, Y. Li, S. Shukla, and T.O. Tollefsbol. 2012. Bioactive dietary supplements reactivate ER expression in ER-negative breast cancer cells by active chromatin modifications. *PLoS ONE* 7(5), http://www.plosone.org/article/info%3Adoi%2F10.1371%2Fjournal.pone.0037748.

Milenkovic, D., B. Jude, and C. Morand. 2013. miRNA as molecular target of polyphenols underlying their biological effects. *Free Radic Biol Med* 64:40–51.

Mudduluru, G., J.N. George-William, S. Muppala et al. 2011. Curcumin regulates miR-1 expression and inhibits invasion and metastasis in colorectal cancer. *Biosci Rep* 31:185–197.

Myzak, M.C., P. Tong, W.M. Dashwood, R.H. Dashwood, and E. Ho. 2007. Sulforaphane retards the growth of human PC-3 xenografts and inhibits HDAC activity in human subjects. *Exp Biol Med* (*Maywood*) 232:227–234.

Nair, V.S., L.S. Maeda, and J.P. Ioannidis. 2012. Clinical outcome prediction by microRNAs in human cancer: A systematic review. *J Natl Cancer Inst* 104:528–540.

Nandakumar, V., M. Vaid, and S.K. Katiyar. 2011. (–)-Epigallocatechin-3-gallate reactivates silenced tumor suppressor genes, Cipl/p21 and p16INK4a, by reducing DNA methylation and increasing histones acetylation in human skin cancer cells. *Carcinogenesis* 32:537–544.

Nihal, M., H. Ahsan, I.A. Siddiqui, H. Mukhtar, N. Ahmad, and G.S. Wood. 2009. (–)-Epigallocatechin-3-gallate (EGCG) sensitizes melanoma cells to interferon induced growth inhibition in a mouse model of human melanoma. *Cell Cycle* 8:2057–2063.

Niles, R.M. 2004. Signaling pathways in retinoid chemoprevention and treatment of cancer. *Mutat Res* 555:81–96.

Parasramka, M.A., E. Ho, D.E. Williams, and R.H. Dashwood. 2012. MicroRNAs, diet, and cancer: New mechanistic insights on the epigenetic actions of phytochemicals. *Mol Carcinog* 51:213–230.

Park, S., D.H. Cho, L. Andera, N. Suh, and I. Kim. 2013. Curcumin enhances TRAIL-induced apoptosis of breast cancer cells by regulating apoptosis-related proteins. *Mol Cell Biochem* 383:39–48.

Patel, K.R., V.A. Brown, D.J. Jones et al. 2010. Clinical pharmacology of resveratrol and its metabolites in colorectal cancer patients. *Cancer Res* 70:7392–7399.

Perkins, S., R.D. Verschoyle, K. Hill et al. 2002. Chemopreventive efficacy and pharmacokinetics of curcumin in the min/+ mouse, a model of familial adenomatous polyposis. *Cancer Epidemiol Biomarkers Prev* 11:535–540.

Philips, B.J., C.H. Coyle, S.N. Morrisroe, M.B. Chancellor, and N. Yoshimura. 2009. Induction of apoptosis in human bladder cancer cells by green tea catechins. *Biomed Res* 30:207–215.

Phuah, N.H. and N.H. Nagoor. 2014. Regulation of microRNAs by natural agents: New strategies in cancer therapies. *Biomed Res Int* 2014:1–17. Advance online publication. doi: 10.1155/2014/804510.

Pianetti, S., S. Guo, K.T. Kavanagh, and G.E. Sonenshein. 2002. Green tea polyphenol epigallocatechin-3 gallate inhibits Her-2/neu signaling, proliferation, and transformed phenotype of breast cancer cells. *Cancer Res* 62:652–655.

Pichler, M., A.L. Ress, E. Winter et al. 2014. MiR-200a regulates epithelial to mesenchymal transition-related gene expression and determines prognosis in colorectal cancer patients. *Br J Cancer* 110:1614–1621.

Primikyri, A., M.V. Chatziathanasiadou, E. Karali et al. 2014. Direct binding of Bcl-2 family proteins by quercetin triggers its pro-apoptotic activity. *ACS Chem Biol* 9:2737–2741. Advance online publication. doi: 10.1021/cb500259e.

Qiao, Y., J. Cao, L. Xie, and X. Shi. 2009. Cell growth inhibition and gene expression regulation by (–) epigallocatechin-3-gallate in human cervical cancer cells. *Arch Pharm Res* 32:1309–1315.

Reed, G.A., D.W. Arneson, W.C. Putnam et al. 2006. Single-dose and multiple-dose administration of indole-3-carbinol to women: Pharmacokinetics based on 3,3′-diindolylmethane. *Cancer Epidemiol Biomarkers Prev* 15:2477–2481.

Romagnolo, D.F. and O.I. Selmin. 2012. Flavonoids and cancer prevention: A review of the evidence. *J Nutr Gerontol Geriatr* 31:206–238.

Ross, S.A. and C.D. Davis. 2011. MicroRNA, nutrition, and cancer prevention. *Adv Nutr* 2:472–485.

Russo, G.L., M. Russo, and C. Spagnuolo. 2014. The pleiotropic flavonoid quercetin: From its metabolism to the inhibition of protein kinases in chronic lymphocytic leukemia. *Food Funct* 5:2393–2401.

Russo, M., C. Spagnuolo, I. Tedesco, S. Bilotto, and G.L. Russo. 2012. The flavonoid quercetin in disease prevention and therapy: Facts and fancies. *Biochem Pharmacol* 83:6–15.

Scott, E., W.P. Steward, A.J. Gescher, and K. Brown. 2012. Resveratrol in human cancer chemoprevention—Choosing the 'right' dose. *Mol Nutr Food Res* 56:7–13.

Senthilkumar, K., P. Elumalai, R. Arunkumar et al. 2010. Quercetin regulates insulin like growth factor signaling and induces intrinsic and extrinsic pathway mediated apoptosis in androgen independent prostate cancer cells (PC-3). *Mol Cell Biochem* 344:173–184.

Shammas, M.A., P. Neri, H. Koley et al. 2006. Specific killing of multiple myeloma cells by (–)-epigallocatechin-3-gallate extracted from green tea: Biologic activity and therapeutic implications. *Blood* 108:2804–2810.

Shankar, S., D. Kumar, and R.K. Srivastava. 2013. Epigenetic modifications by dietary phytochemicals: Implications for personalized nutrition. *Pharmacol Ther* 138:1–17.

Shankar, S. and Srivastava, R.K. 2007. Involvement of Bcl-2 family members, phosphatidylinositol 30-kinase/AKT and mitochondrial p53 in curcumin (diferuloylmethane)-induced apoptosis in prostate cancer. *Int J Oncol* 30:905–918.

Sharma, R.A., H.R. McLelland, K.A. Hill et al. 2001. Pharmacodynamic and pharmacokinetic study of oral Curcuma extract in patients with colorectal cancer. *Clin Cancer Res* 7:1894–1900.

Shoba, G., D. Joy, T. Joseph, M. Majeed, R. Rajendran, and P.S. Srinivas. 1998. Influence of piperine on the pharmacokinetics of curcumin in animals and human volunteers. *Planta Med* 64:353–356.

Shrubsole, M.J., W. Lu, Z. Chen et al. 2009. Drinking green tea modestly reduces breast cancer risk. *J Nutr* 139:310–316.

Singh, B.N., S. Shankar, and R.K. Srivastava. 2011. Green tea catechin, epigallocatechin-3-gallate (EGCG): Mechanisms, perspectives and clinical applications. *Biochem Pharmacol* 82:1807–1821.

Singh, C.K., J. George, and N. Ahmad. 2013. Resveratrol-based combinatorial strategies for cancer management. *Ann N Y Acad Sci* 1290:113–121.

Singletary, K., C. MacDonald, M. Wallig, and C. Fisher. 1996. Inhibition of 7,12-dimethylbenz[a]anthracene (DMBA)-induced mammary tumorigenesis and DMBA-DNA adduct formation by curcumin. *Cancer Lett* 103:137–141.

Smith-Warner, S.A., D. Spiegelman, S.S. Yaun et al. 2001. Intake of fruits and vegetables and risk of breast cancer: A pooled analysis of cohort studies. *JAMA* 285:769–776.

Spagnuolo, C., M. Russo, S. Bilotto, I. Tedesco, B. Laratta, and G.L. Russo. 2012. Dietary polyphenols in cancer prevention: The example of the flavonoid quercetin in leukemia. *Ann N Y Acad Sci* 1259:95–103.

Sporn, M.B., N.M. Dunlop, D.L. Newton, and J.M. Smith. 1976. Prevention of chemical carcinogenesis by vitamin A and its synthetic analogs (retinoids). *Fed Proc* 35:1332–1338.

Stallings, R.L., N.H. Foley, I.M. Bray, S. Das, and P.G. Buckley. 2011. MicroRNA and DNA methylation alterations mediating retinoic acid induced neuroblastoma cell differentiation. *Semin Cancer Biol* 21:283–290.

Stefani, E.D., P. Boffetta, H. Deneo-Pellegrini et al. 1999. Dietary antioxidants and lung cancer risk: A case–control study in Uruguay. *Nutr Cancer* 34:100–110.

Steinbach, G., P.M. Lynch, R.K. Phillips et al. 2000. The effect of celecoxib, a cyclooxygenase-2 inhibitor, in familial adenomatous polyposis. *N Engl J Med* 342:1946–1952.

Steinbrecher, A., K. Nimptsch, A. Hüsing, S. Rohrmann, and J. Linseisen. 2009. Dietary glucosinolate intake and risk of prostate cancer in the EPIC-Heidelberg cohort study. *Int J Cancer* 125:2179–2186.

Sun, X.D., X.E. Liu, and D.S. Huang. 2012. Curcumin induces apoptosis of triple-negative breast cancer cells by inhibition of EGFR expression. *Mol Med Rep* 6:1267–1270.

Sun, Z.J., G. Chen, X. Hu et al. 2010. Activation of PI3K/Akt/IKK-alpha/NF-kappaB signaling pathway is required for the apoptosis-evasion in human salivary adenoid cystic carcinoma: Its inhibition by quercetin. *Apoptosis* 15:850–863.

Surh, Y.J., K.S. Chun, H.H. Cha et al. 2001. Molecular mechanisms underlying chemopreventive activities of anti-inflammatory phytochemicals: Down-regulation of COX-2 and iNOS through suppression of NF-kB activation. *Mutat Res* 243–268.

Strack, D. 1997. Phenolic metabolism. In: *Plant Biochemistry*, P.M. Dey and J.B. Harborne (eds.), pp.397–416. London, U.K.: Academic Press.

Tachibana, H. 2009. Molecular basis for cancer chemoprevention by green tea polyphenol EGCG. *Forum Nutr* 61:156–169.

Tachibana, H., K. Koga, Y. Fujimura, and K. Yamada. 2004. A receptor for green tea polyphenol EGCG. *Nat Struct Mol Biol* 11:380–381.

Tan, H.K., A.I. Moad, and M.L. Tan. 2014. The mTOR signaling pathway in cancer and the potential mTOR inhibitory activities of natural phytochemicals. *Asian Pac J Cancer Prev* 15:6463–6475.

Tang, N., Y. Wu, B. Zhou, B. Wang, and R. Yu. 2009. Green tea, black tea consumption and risk of lung cancer: A meta-analysis. *Lung Cancer* 65:274–283.

Tang, X.H. and L.J. Gudas. 2011. Retinoids, retinoic acid receptors, and cancer. *Annu Rev Pathol* 6:345–364.

Terry, P., A. Wolk, I. Persson, and C. Magnusson. 2001. Brassica vegetables and breast cancer risk. *JAMA* 285:2975–2977.

Thanos, D. and T. Maniatis. 1995. NF-kappa B: A lesson in family values. *Cell* 80:529–532.

Theodoratou, E., J. Kyle, R. Cetnarskyj et al. 2007. Dietary flavonoids and the risk of colorectal cancer. *Cancer Epidem Biomarkers Prev* 16:684–693.

Tse, G. and G.D. Eslick. 2014. Cruciferous vegetables and risk of colorectal neoplasms: A systematic review and meta-analysis. *Nutr Cancer* 66:128–139.

Van Aller, G.S., J.D. Carson, W. Tang et al. 2011. Epigallocatechin gallate (EGCG), a major component of green tea, is a dual phosphoinositide-3-kinase/mTOR inhibitor. *Biochem Biophys Res Commun* 406:194–199.

Van Antwerp, D.J., S.J. Martin, T. Kafri, D.R. Green, and I.M. Verma. 1996. Suppression of TNF[alpha]-induced apoptosis by NF-[kappa]B. *Science* 274:787–789.

Vanden Berghe, W. 2012. Epigenetic impact of dietary polyphenols in cancer chemoprevention: Lifelong remodeling of our epigenomes. *Pharmacol Res* 65:565–576.

Vargas, A.J. and R. Burd. July 2010. Hormesis and synergy: Pathways and mechanisms of quercetin in cancer prevention and management. *Nutr Rev* 68(7):418–428.

Veeranki, O.L., A. Bhattacharya, J.R. Marshall, and Y. Zhang. 2013. Organ-specific exposure and response to sulforaphane, a key chemopreventive ingredient in broccoli: Implications for cancer prevention. *Br J Nutr* 109:25–32.

Volate, S.R., D.M. Davenport, S.J. Muga, and M.J. Wargovich. 2005. Modulation of aberrant crypt foci and apoptosis by dietary herbal supplements (quercetin, curcumin, silymarin, ginseng and rutin). *Carcinogenesis* 26:1450–1456.

Voorrips, L.E., R.A. Goldbohm, G. van Poppel, F. Sturmans, R.J. Hermus, and P.A. van den Brandt. 2000. Vegetable and fruit consumption and risks of colon and rectal cancer in a prospective cohort study: The Netherlands Cohort Study on Diet and Cancer. *Am J Epidemiol* 152:1081–1092.

Wang, P., D. Heber, and S.M. Henning. 2012. Quercetin increased bioavailability and decreased methylation of green tea polyphenols in vitro and in vivo. *Food Funct* 3:635–642.

Watson, G.W., L.M. Beaver, D.E. Williams, R.H. Dashwood, and E. Ho. 2013. Phytochemicals from Cruciferous Vegetables, Epigenetics, and Prostate Cancer Prevention. *AAPS J* 15:951–961.

Watson, J.L., A. Greenshields, R. Hill et al. 2010. Curcumin-induced apoptosis in ovarian carcinoma cells is p53-independent and involves p38 mitogen-activated protein kinase activation and downregulation of Bcl-2 and survivin expression and Akt signaling. *Mol Carcinog* 49:13–24.

Wood, J.G., B. Rogina, S. Lavu et al. 2004. Sirtuin activators mimic caloric restriction and delay ageing in metazoans. *Nature* 430:686–689.

Wu, Q.J., L. Xie, W. Zheng et al. 2013. Cruciferous vegetables consumption and the risk of female lung cancer: A prospective study and a meta-analysis. *Ann Oncol* 24:1918–1924.

Xia, Y., L. Jin, B. Zhang, H. Xue, Q. Li, and Y. Xu. 2007. The potentiation of curcumin on insulin-like growth factor-1 action in MCF-7 human breast carcinoma cells. *Life Sci* 80:2161–2169.

Yamauchi, R., K. Sasaki, and K. Yoshida. 2009. Identification of epigallocatechin-3-gallate in green tea polyphenols as a potent inducer of p53-dependent apoptosis in the human lung cancer cell line A549. *Toxicol In Vitro* 23:834–839.

Yang, G., X.O. Shu, H. Li et al. 2007. Prospective cohort study of green tea consumption and colorectal cancer risk in women. *Cancer Epidemiol Biomarkers Prev* 16:1219–1223.

Yang, G., Y.T. Gao, X.O. Shu et al. 2010a. Isothiocyanate exposure, glutathione S-transferase polymorphisms, and colorectal cancer risk. *Am J Clin Nutr* 91:704–711.

Yang, J., Y. Cao, J. Sun, and Y. Zhang. 2010b. Curcumin reduces the expression of Bcl-2 by upregulating miR-15a and miR-16 in MCF-7 cells. *Med Oncol* 27:1114–1118.

Yim, C.Y., P. Mao, and M.J. Spinella. 2014. Headway and hurdles in the clinical development of dietary phytochemicals for cancer therapy and prevention: Lessons learned from vitamin A derivatives. *AAPS J* 16:281–288.

Yoshizawa, H.T., H. Fujiki, T. Yoshida, T. Okuda, and T. Sugimura. 1987. Antitumor promoting activity of (−)-epigallocatechin gallate, the main constituent of "Tannin" in green tea. *Phytother Res* 1:44–47.

Zhang, S., D.J. Hunter, M.R. Forman et al. 1999. Dietary carotenoids and vitamins A, C, and E and risk of breast cancer. *J Natl Cancer Inst* 91:547–556.

22 *Helicobacter pylori* Infection and Phytochemicals

Archana Chatterjee

CONTENTS

22.1 INTRODUCTION

Helicobacter pylori is a microaerophilic, flagellated, spiral, gram-negative bacterium, which colonizes the surface of the gastric mucosa and can cause gastric inflammation, chronic active gastritis as well as peptic ulcer disease (PUD), and increased risk of gastric cancer [1]. About half of the world's population is infected with *H. pylori* [2]. Most *H. pylori* infections are contracted in early childhood, and colonization may last for a lifetime [3,4]. Chronic colonization with *H. pylori* has been implicated in increased risk for gastric cancer including adenocarcinoma and a form of lymphoma involving the mucosa-associated lymphoid tissue [5]. The International Agency for Research on Cancer has classified *H. pylori* infection as a Group 1 human carcinogen in 1994 and reconfirmed this classification in 2009 [6]. Successful treatment and eradication of *H. pylori* has the potential to decrease the subsequent risk of gastric cancer by 30%–40% [6]. The goal of management of *H. pylori* infections is to induce eradication with the first-line therapy prescribed, preventing the need for further treatments or procedures for the patient, the development of antibiotic resistance, and the spread of resistant *H. pylori* within the community. There has been increasing resistance reported to many of the antibiotics such as clarithromycin and metronidazole that are recommended for the first-line treatment of *H. pylori* infection [7,8]. In light of this emerging resistance, there is a need for new remedies effective against *H. pylori*. The traditional use and anecdotal evidence of plants as medicine provide the basis for suggesting that plant extracts may be useful for specific medical conditions [9]. In recent years, phytochemicals derived from various fruits and vegetables have been shown to have *in vitro* and *in vivo* antibacterial, anti-inflammatory, and antioxidant activities. This chapter provides a review of selected published literature on the impact of these phytochemicals on *H. pylori* infection.

22.2 PATHOGENICITY OF *H. pylori*

Infection with *H. pylori* leads to chronic inflammation because of the failure of the host to eradicate the infection. Chronic inflammation leads to oxidative stress, arising both from immune cells attracted to the site of infection and from within gastric epithelial cells. This in turn results in DNA damage, apoptosis, and neoplastic transformation. Both pathogen and host factors contribute to oxidative stress, including *H. pylori* virulence factors, as well as pathways involving DNA damage and repair, polyamine synthesis and metabolism, and oxidative stress response [10].

Several virulence factors have been described, which mediate pathogenicity and disease outcomes of *H. pylori* infection [11]. These include the flagella (important for mobility), urease (necessary for acid tolerance), and adhesins, which not only mediate *H. pylori* colonization and persistence, but also direct progression of the infection and incidence of the disease. Other virulence factors include the cytotoxin-associated gene pathogenicity island (cagPAI), vacuolating cytotoxin (VacA), and γ-glutamyl transferase (GGT). Each of these important mediators of *H. pylori* pathogenicity will now be briefly discussed.

Urease and neutrophil-activating protein A (NapA) are two *H. pylori* virulence factors that contribute to neutrophil infiltration and reactive oxygen species (ROS) production [10]. In experimental models, the infiltrating neutrophils demonstrated increased resistance to apoptosis and an enhanced life span, potential contributing factors to the chronic inflammation associated with *H. pylori* infection, leading to cellular stress and oxidative DNA damage [12].

The adherence of *H. pylori* to the gastric mucosa is important for protection from mechanisms such as acidic pH, mucus, and exfoliation [13]. Recognition of and adhesion to epithelial cells by *H. pylori* as well as its persistence in the stomach are primarily mediated by several outer membrane proteins from the *Helicobacter* outer membrane protein (Hop) group [14]. Members of the Hop group implicated in *H. pylori* pathogenesis include the blood group antigen-binding adhesin (BabA, also known as HopS) and the sialic acid–binding adhesin (SabA, also known as HopP) [14]. Fucosylated and sialylated blood group antigens favor the colonization of the gastric mucosa by *H. pylori*. The adherence-associated lipoproteins (AlpA and AlpB, also known as HopB and HopC), outer inflammatory protein (OipA, also known as HopH), and HopZ are also associated with bacterial adhesion [15–17]. Extracellular matrix proteins such as laminin, fibronectin, and type IV collagen have been described to function as receptors for *H. pylori* in the gastric region [18–20]. These highly complex interactions and the importance of *H. pylori* adherence for the development of its pathogenicity highlight the potential benefits of antiadhesive compounds that could provide a preventive, cytoprotective strategy to control *H. pylori* colonization, especially to prevent its recurrence after antibiotic eradication therapy.

Bacterial virulence factors contribute to the inflammatory response toward *H. pylori* either by altering host-signaling pathways important to maintain tissue homeostasis in epithelial cells or by differentially stimulating innate immune cells [15]. CagA and VacA are the best characterized of these virulence factors. However, other bacterial determinants such as γ-glutamyltranspeptidase (gGT) have been also shown to be important inducers of gastric inflammation [10]. A recent report indicates that cagA+ strains of *H. pylori* induce greater levels of hydrogen peroxide (H_2O_2) production and oxidative DNA damage [21]. Moreover, cagA positivity is significantly associated with increased expression of tumor necrosis factor α (TNFα) and interleukin (IL)-8, both of which are markers of inflammation and oxidative stress [22–24]. VacA enhances colonization by *H. pylori* and correlates with increased inflammation and risk for gastric carcinogenesis [25]. It has been demonstrated that VacA induces Ca^{2+} influx and ROS generation, subsequently leading to nuclear factor kappa-light-chain enhancer of B-cell activation (NF-κB) activation and upregulation of chemokine expression, enhancing the influx of pro-inflammatory immunocytes to the site of *H. pylori* infection and contributing to the pro-tumorigenic environment [26–28]. Purified GGT elicits H_2O_2 production in gastric epithelial cells resulting in oxidative DNA damage, as well as a corresponding increase in NF-κB activation and IL-8 production [29,30]. IL-8 is a pro-inflammatory cytokine that signifies the establishment of inflammation at the site of infection and also has pro-tumorigenic properties [31]. The immune response of the host is a key determinant in the development of gastric cancer [32]. *H. pylori* upregulates several inflammatory molecules including IL-1β, IL-32, IL-10, and TNFα, and this plays a key role in *H. pylori*–induced disease progression [33]. Natural antioxidants and phytochemicals with antibacterial and anti-inflammatory properties may therefore serve as novel therapeutic tools in alleviating *H. pylori*–induced ROS and pro-inflammatory cytokine production, leading to the diminution of DNA damage and tumor development.

22.3 EPIDEMIOLOGICAL STUDIES SUPPORTING THE ROLE OF PHYTOCHEMICALS

Due to the elucidation of the mechanisms of *H. pylori*–induced gastric inflammation and damage outlined earlier, and its emerging resistance to many first-line antibiotics, in the past two decades, there has been increasing interest in alternative/adjunct compounds with antioxidant, free radical scavenging, antibacterial, antimutagen, and anticarcinogen properties that could potentially mitigate its effects. The standard treatment for *H. pylori*–related disease is a combination of antimicrobial agents and anti-acid agents [3]. However, adverse effects of these regimens are common, and a major concern is the development of antimicrobial resistance resulting in treatment failures [34]. In fact, no therapeutic regimen is able to cure the infection in all treated patients, and in many, the infection persists despite the administration of several consecutive standard therapies, resulting in significant costs. As a result, several naturally occurring substances have been investigated as potential alternatives/adjuncts for the treatment of *H. pylori* infection, and emerging epidemiological evidence is increasingly pointing to the beneficial effects of fruits and vegetables in managing many chronic and infectious diseases [35,36] including *H. pylori*.

Studies of the association between dietary factors and *H. pylori* infection/disease have produced conflicting results. For example in a study of 383 Sherpa residents of the Upper Khumbu region of Nepal, where *H. pylori* is highly prevalent, it was not significantly associated with any of the lifestyle and health measures collected, including dyspeptic symptoms, medication, smoking, alcohol intake, and dietary factors such as salt, smoked food, fruit/vegetable, and pickle consumption [37]. However, in a study of 1358 Japanese adults, among *H. pylori*–positive nonelderly subjects, anti-*H. pylori* IgG antibody titers were significantly lower in the group with high intake of Japanese apricots that are rich in polyphenols and have significant antioxidant activity ($p = 0.041$) [38]. Endoscopic tissue biopsy from 68 volunteers in the study showed less *H. pylori* bacterial load and mononuclear infiltration overall, with antral neutrophil infiltration significantly less pronounced and corporal atrophy less extensive in the high-intake group [38]. The authors concluded that there was a strong preventive effect of Japanese apricot intake on chronic active gastritis due to its inhibition of *H. pylori* infection and reduction in active mucosal inflammation. A case–control study of dietary habits in a Portuguese urban population revealed a lower risk of gastric cancer in the group with high consumption of fruits and dairy products, but no effect modification of *H. pylori* infection was observed [39]. A large cohort study of 521,457 men and women participating in the European Prospective Investigation into Cancer and Nutrition (EPIC-EURGAST) cohort in 10 European countries followed participants for an average of 6.5 years and found no association with total vegetable intake or specific groups of vegetables and gastric cancer risk, except for the intestinal type, where a negative association was noted with total vegetable as well as onion and garlic intake [40]. Interestingly, no evidence of association between fresh fruit intake and gastric cancer risk was observed in this study, except for citrus fruit intake and cancer of the gastric cardia [40]. The authors of this study concluded that intake of fresh fruits and vegetables did not modify *H. pylori* infection, but supported a possible protective role of vegetable intake in the intestinal type of gastric cancer and adenocarcinoma of the esophagus [40]. They also noted that citrus fruit consumption may have a role in the protection against cardia gastric cancer and adenocarcinoma of the esophagus [40].

In a systematic review of gastric cancer risk and protective factors, beta-carotene below 20 mg/day, fruits, vegetables, non-fermented soy foods, whole-grain, and dairy products were found to decrease the risk of gastric cancer, based upon which the authors recommend increasing the consumption of food containing protective components [41]. Another review of the literature also supports the argument that high intake of salted, pickled, or smoked foods, as well as dried fish and meat and refined carbohydrates significantly increased the risk of developing gastric cancer while fibers, fresh vegetables, and fruit were found to be inversely associated with gastric cancer risk [42]. These authors also recommend improving dietary habits from childhood onward by increasing vegetable and fruit intake. A review of several ecological, case–control, and cohort studies strongly suggests that the risk of gastric cancer may be increased with a high intake of various traditional salt-preserved foods and salt per se and decreased with a high intake of fruit and vegetables, particularly fruit [43]. The authors conclude that dietary modification by reducing salt and salted food intake, as well as by increasing intake of fruits, is a practical strategy to prevent gastric cancer.

22.4 *IN VITRO* STUDIES

The beneficial effects of plant food sources are suggested to be due to the constituent phenolic phytochemicals such as anthocyanins, proanthocyanidins, phenolic acids, flavonoids, and ellagic acid that have antioxidant activity [36]. One of the most intensely studied organisms in this field is *H. pylori*, and among the various fruit and vegetable sources of phytochemicals, perhaps the most promising have been berries and their extracts, particularly cranberries. A summary of the *in vitro* data supports a beneficial effect of cranberry or its proanthocyanin constituents by blocking adhesion to and biofilm formation on target tissues of pathogens such as *H. pylori* [44]. In one study, polyphenol-rich fractions from cranberry juice concentrate suppressed bacterial proliferation of *H. pylori* in a dose-dependent manner [45]. When compared with other juices, polyphenol-rich fruits (cranberries, blueberries, and red grapes) showed similar growth inhibitory activity, whereas polyphenol-poor fruits (oranges, pineapples, apples, and white grapes) did not show such activity [45]. More bacteria in a coccoid form were observed after culture with cranberry, indicating bacteriostatic growth inhibition [45].

In studies examining the beneficial effects of extracts of wild blueberry, bilberry, cranberry, elderberry, raspberry seeds, strawberry, and a novel combination of all six berry extracts known as OptiBerry®, it was found that the latter exhibited superior antioxidant efficacy due to its high oxygen radical absorbance capacity values and showed potential cytotoxicity toward *H. pylori*, as compared to the individual berry extracts [46]. OptiBerry also significantly inhibited basal MCP-1 and inducible NF-κB transcriptions as well as the inflammatory biomarker IL-8 [46]. In a study evaluating the effects of various berry extracts, with and without clarithromycin on *H. pylori*, all berry extracts significantly inhibited *H. pylori* compared with controls and also increased the susceptibility of *H. pylori* to clarithromycin, with OptiBerry demonstrating maximal effects [47]. This study also showed the synergistic effects of berry extracts with antibiotics against *H. pylori*.

The antimicrobial activity and mechanisms of action of phenolic extracts of 12 Nordic berries were evaluated against selected human pathogenic microbes [48]. Among the most sensitive bacteria for berry phenolics was *H. pylori* [48]. The antimicrobial activity and antimicrobial-linked urease inhibition of phenolic extract mixtures from oregano and cranberry alone and in combination were studied and indicated that the antimicrobial activity was greater in extract mixtures than in individual extracts of each species [49]. The authors concluded that the likely mode of action may be through urease inhibition and disruption of energy production by inhibition of proline dehydrogenase at the plasma membrane [49]. Several studies of antibiotic-resistant and nonresistant *H. pylori* isolates from antibiotic-treated and untreated patients have shown that adhesion to gastric cells was inhibited by a high-molecular-mass, nondialysable constituent of cranberry juice [50–52], suggesting that a combination of antibiotics and a cranberry preparation may improve *H. pylori* eradication.

A novel study examined the anti-*H. pylori* activity of silver nanoparticles using a methanolic extract from *Solanum xanthocarpum* against 34 clinical isolates and two reference strains of *H. pylori* [53]. This first-of-its-kind study showed that the extract effectively inhibited the growth of *H. pylori* by inhibiting urease production and had a stronger anti-*H. pylori* activity than that of metronidazole, while being almost equally potent to tetracycline [53]. The antibacterial activity of the extract against amoxicillin-resistant, clarithromycin-resistant, tetracycline-resistant, and metronidazole-resistant clinical isolates was nearly comparable to those against susceptible isolates [53]. Most importantly, it was also found to be equally effective against the strains showing double and triple drug resistance [53], opening up the possibility of using the extract to treat *H. pylori* in patients with multiply resistant strains.

For centuries, herbals have been used in traditional medicine to treat a wide range of ailments, including gastrointestinal (GI) disorders such as dyspepsia, gastritis, and PUD [54,55]. A study evaluating the *in vitro* susceptibility of 15 *H. pylori* strains to botanical extracts from multiple plant sources showed that *Myristica fragrans* (seed) had a minimum inhibitory concentration (MIC) of 12.5 μg/mL; *Zingiber officinale* (ginger rhizome/root) and *Rosmarinus officinalis* (rosemary leaf) had an MIC of 25 μg/mL; extracts with an MIC of 50 μg/mL included *Achillea millefolium, Foeniculum vulgare* (seed), *Passiflora incarnata* (herb), *Origanum majorana* (herb), and a (1:1) combination of *Curcuma longa* (root) and *ginger rhizome*; extracts with an MIC of 100 μg/mL included *Carum carvi* (seed), *Elettaria cardamomum* (seed), *Gentiana lutea* (roots), *Juniperus communis* (berry), *Lavandula angustifolia* (flowers), *Melissa officinalis* (leaves), *Mentha piperita* (leaves), and *Pimpinella anisum* (seed); extracts of *Matricaria recutita* (flowers) and *Ginkgo biloba* (leaves) had an MIC > 100 μg/mL [54].

Garcinol, a polyisoprenylated benzophenone derivative, and resveratrol, a phytoalexin, are phytochemicals with free radical–scavenging, antibacterial, and chemopreventative properties [56–58]. In a study evaluating the antimicrobial activity of five solvent extracts of *Garcinia kola* seeds against 30 clinical strains of *H. pylori* and a standard control strain, with metronidazole and amoxicillin as positive control antibiotics, the ethanol extract demonstrated considerable anti-*H. pylori* activity with a percentage susceptibility of 53.3%, similar to that of metronidazole [59]. The killing rate increased with increasing concentrations of the extract to 100% at 5 mg/mL [59]. Both garcinol and resveratrol with and without clarithromycin have been shown to have potent *in vitro* activity against a laboratory strain of *H. pylori* [60,61]. In addition, multiple studies have demonstrated the antibacterial effects of resveratrol and on *H. pylori*–induced interleukin-8 secretion, ROS generation, and morphological changes in human gastric epithelial cells [58,62–65].

A number of studies have shown the anti-*H. pylori* activities of extracts from various fruits—chief among these being from the citrus family [66–68]. 4′-Geranyloxyferulic (GOFA) and boropinic acid derived from Citrus and Fortunella fruits are phytochemicals having valuable pharmacological effects as cancer chemopreventive, anti-inflammatory, and anti-*H. pylori* agents [66]. Methanol extracts of the peels of *Citrus sudachi* have yielded two compounds sudachitin and 3′-demethoxysudachitin, which showed significant anti-*H. pylori* activity [68]. Ethanol and ethyl acetate extracts of noni fruit (*Morinda citrifolia*), which is known to possess antibacterial, anti-inflammatory, and antioxidant activities were studied for their inhibitory effects on CagA and *H. pylori*–induced IL-8, inducible nitric oxide (iNOS), cyclooxygenase 2 (COX-2), and neutrophil chemotaxis [69]. Both extracts of noni fruit showed weak inhibition of *H. pylori* and provided antiadhesion of *H. pylori* to gastric adenocarcinoma cells, as well as downregulation of the CagA, IL-8, COX-2, and iNOS expressions, along with decreased neutrophil chemotaxis [69]. Noni fruit extracts thus downregulated inflammatory responses during *H. pylori* infection, and its phenolic compounds played a key role in antiadhesion [69]. The active compound of *Feijoa sellowiana* fruit flavone showed high antibacterial activity against nine standard bacterial strains and matched clinically isolated strains of *H. pylori* and was significantly more active against *H. pylori* than metronidazole [70]. The *in vitro* effect of a standardized extract of apple peel APPE (60% of total polyphenols; 58% of flavonoids; 30% of flavan-3-ols and procyanidins) was evaluated with regard to the viability of *H. pylori* [71]. APPE showed an early cytotoxic effect, which was both concentration- and time-dependent on the multiplication of two *H. pylori* strains (ATCC 43504 and TX136) with an MIC value of 112.5 μg gallic acid equivalent (GAE)/mL [71]. In addition, APPE inhibited the respiratory burst of neutrophils induced by *H. pylori* in a concentration-dependent manner [71]. The authors conclude that apple peel polyphenols have an attenuating effect on the damage to gastric mucosa caused by neutrophil-generated ROS secondary to *H. pylori* infection [71]. Carotenoid fractions extracted from red paprika, Valencia orange peel, and the peel of Golden delicious apples were studied for their anti-*H. pylori* and free radical–scavenging activity [72]. The apple peel extract demonstrated potent anti-*H. pylori* activity (MIC50 = 36 μg/mL), comparable to metronidazole (MIC50 = 45 μg/mL), while both red paprika and apple peel extracts scavenged oxygen free radicals efficiently [72].

Other parts of plants besides fruits also yield a number of phytochemicals shown to be active *in vitro* against *H. pylori*–induced infection and its effects. Apigenin (4′,5,7-trihydroxyflavone) is widely distributed in fruits and vegetables, and is a well-known anti-inflammatory supplement with low cytotoxicity [73]. In *H. pylori*–infected MKN45 cells, apigenin treatments effectively inhibited NF-κB activation and the related inflammatory factor expression of COX-2, intercellular adhesion molecule-1 (ICAM-1), ROS, IL-8, IL-6, IL-1β, as well as increased mucin-2 (MUC-2) expression, showing great potential as a candidate agent for the inhibition of *H. pylori*–induced extensive gastric epithelial cell inflammation [73]. Antiadhesive peptides against *H. pylori* obtained by enzymatic hydrolysis of seed proteins from *Pisum sativum* L. were evaluated using a quantitative *in vitro* assay on human gastric adenocarcinoma cells along with a semiquantitative in situ adhesion assay using FITC-labeled *H. pylori* on human stomach tissue sections [74]. Two anti-adhesive peptides that bound *H. pylori* adhesins were identified [74]. The authors concluded that bioactive peptides from pea protein could be applied as functional ingredients for protecting patients against *H. pylori* [74]. A crude alcoholic extract of celery seeds (*Apium graveolens*) had potent bactericidal effects against *H. pylori*—the MIC and minimum bactericidal concentration (MBC) were 3.15 and 6.25–12.5 μg/mL, respectively [75]. The anti-*H. pylori* activity of *Impatiens balsamina* L. was investigated through MIC, MBC, and time-kill assays with strains resistant to clarithromycin, metronidazole, and levofloxacin [76]. Extracts of all parts (root/stem/leaf, seed, and pod) of *I. balsamina* L. exhibited bactericidal *H. pylori* activity. Specifically, the pod extract had significantly lower MICs and MBCs (1.25–2.5 and 1.25–5.0 μg/mL, respectively) [76]. This activity exceeded that of metronidazole and approximated to that of amoxicillin [76]. Capsidiol, a terpenoid compound isolated from the fresh sweet pepper fruits of *Capsicum annuum* L., showed bacteriostatic properties *in vitro* against *H. pylori* with an MIC of 200 μg/mL when compared with metronidazole (MIC, 250 μg/mL) [77]. A 70% ethanol extract of *Mallotus philippinensis* was found to have strong bactericidal activity at the concentration of 15.6–31.2 mg/L against eight *H. pylori* strains [78]. A further purified compound from the extract named rottlerin exhibited the most potent bactericidal activity with an MBC value of 3.12–6.25 mg/L against several clinical *H. pylori* isolates including Japanese and Pakistani strains, with nine being clarithromycin resistant and seven metronidazole resistant [78]. The additive and synergistic effects of *Eucalyptus torelliana* leaf extracts, in combination with clarithromycin, were investigated using two types of *H. pylori* strains (ATCC 43629, ATCC 43579) and four clinical isolates of *H. pylori* [79]. *E. torelliana* extract inhibited the growth of all *H. pylori* strains, and the addition of one of its isolated active compounds, a substituted pyrenyl ester, enhanced the activity of clarithromycin [79]. The MIC values of clarithromycin and the botanical compound were reduced twofold (from 0.125 to 0.0625 μg/mL and > 100 to 50 μg/mL, respectively). A 100% reduction in CFU/mL of *H. pylori* ATCC 43579 was observed with the combination of 0.25 μg/mL clarithromycin and 100 and 200 μg/mL of the compound after 3 h of exposure [79]. This investigation showed that the combination of botanical compounds and antibiotics may be beneficial in the treatment of *H. pylori* infections [79]. Traditional Asian and African medicine use immature okra fruits (*Abelmoschus esculentus*) as a mucilaginous food to combat gastritis [80]. Its effectiveness is due to polysaccharides that inhibit the adhesion of *H. pylori* to stomach tissue [80]. A standardized aqueous fresh extract (Okra FE) from immature okra fruits was used for a quantitative *in vitro* adhesion assay with FITC-labeled *H. pylori* J99, two clinical isolates and gastric adenocarcinoma cells [80]. Okra FE dose dependently (0.2–2 mg/mL) inhibited *H. pylori* binding to gastric adenocarcinoma cells [80]. FE inhibited the adhesive binding of membrane proteins BabA, SabA, and HpA to its specific ligands [80]. Okra FE did not lead to subsequent feedback regulation or increased expression of adhesins or virulence factors [80]. The authors concluded that nonspecific interactions between high molecular compounds from okra fruits and the *H. pylori* surface lead to strong antiadhesive effects [80]. Polyphenols from almond skins were studied *in vitro* against *H. pylori*, with natural almond skin being the most effective compound (MIC range, 64–128 μg/mL) and the pure flavonoid compound protocatechuic acid showing the MIC range 128–512 μg/mL [81].

The studies cited earlier indicate the growing repertoire of phytochemicals from various plant sources that may have activity against *H. pylori*–induced infection and disease. The next section will highlight some *in vivo* studies of these botanical compounds.

22.5 *IN VIVO* STUDIES

In vivo data from human clinical trials and animal models support the beneficial effects of phytochemicals against *H. pylori* as well. For example consumption of various cranberry products in conjunction with antibiotic treatment resulted in eradicating *H. pylori* infections in women [44]. A multicenter, randomized, controlled, double-blind trial with cranberry juice treatment carried out in 295 asymptomatic children (6–16 years of age) who tested positive for *H. pylori* showed that eradication rates were significantly higher in the groups that received cranberry juice: 1.5% in the control group compared with 16.9% and 22.9% in the groups that were treated with cranberry juice, respectively ($p < 0.01$) [82]. In a placebo-controlled trial of cranberry juice in 177 patients with *H. pylori* infection treated with standard triple antibiotic therapy, for female subjects, the eradication rate was higher in the cranberry–antibiotic arm ($n = 42$, 95.2%) than in the placebo–antibiotic arm ($n = 53$, 86.8%) [83]. The addition of cranberry juice to triple therapy improved the rate of *H. pylori* eradication in females [83]. Another prospective, randomized, double-blind, placebo-controlled trial in 189 Chinese adults showed that cranberry juice consumption significantly reduced *H. pylori* infection [84], while in a case–control study among Chinese men, of 226 cases and 451 controls nested within a prospective cohort with over 90% prevalence of CagA-positive *H. pylori* infection, increasing intake of fruit decreased gastric cancer risk [85]. The oral administration of β-myrcene (a minor constituent of essential oil from *Citrus aurantium*) at a dose of 7.5 mg/kg showed important antiulcer activity with significantly decreased gastric and duodenal lesions as well as increased gastric mucus production [86]. Treatment with β-myrcene caused a significant increase in mucosal malondialdehyde level, an important index of oxidative tissue damage accompanied by decreased activity of superoxide dismutase (SOD) and increased levels of glutathione peroxidase (GPx), glutathione reductase (GR), and total glutathione in gastric tissue [86]. This study established the importance of β-myrcene as an inhibitor of gastric and duodenal ulcers and demonstrated that an increase in the levels of gastric mucosa defense factors is involved in the antiulcer activity of β-myrcene [86]. In a case–control study of 257 Chinese men and women with histologically diagnosed primary noncardia gastric cancer and 514 sex- and age-matched control subjects, high consumption of vegetables (OR: 0.3; 95% CI: 0.1–0.89), fruits (OR: 0.2; 95% CI: 0.09–0.81), and soy products (OR: 0.04; 95% CI: 0.01–0.3) appeared to decrease the risk [87]. A statistically significant lower frequency of vegetables ($p = 0.02$) and fruit ($p = 0.008$) consumption was noted among patients in Poland with *H. pylori* reinfection ($n = 111$) as compared to those who had not been reinfected ($n = 175$) [88]. In a case–control study conducted at the University Teaching Hospital in Zambia, gastric cancer cases were compared with age- and sex-matched controls [89]. Fifty cases with gastric cancer (mean age: 61 years; $n = 31$ males) and 90 controls (mean age: 54 years; $n = 41$ males) were enrolled [89]. On univariate analysis, habitual fruit intake was lower in cases than in controls during the dry season ($p = 0.02$), while on multivariate analysis, higher fruit intake was protective (OR: 0.44; IQR: 0.20–0.95) [89].

Bioactive compounds with anti-*H. pylori* activity have also been studied in various animal models. Momordicae Semen extract derived from *Momordica cochinchinensis* Springer (Cucurbitaceae) has demonstrated anti-gastritis effects in various rodent models including ethanol- and diclofenac-induced acute gastritis models and an *H. pylori*–induced chronic gastritis model [90]. Citrus lemon fruit bark essential oil and limonene derived from it both showed gastroprotection through increased mucus secretion in a rat model with induced gastric ulcers due to ethanol or indomethacin [67]. An extract of the seed from celery (*Apium graveolens*) (CSE), and fractions thereof, has been found to possess anti-inflammatory, gastroprotective, and anti-*H. pylori* activity [91]. A 28-day toxicity study performed in rats dosed orally with CSE resulted in no visible or behavioral signs of toxicity being observed during the study, indicating its safety profile [91]. The efficacy of a fruit juice concentrate of Japanese apricot (CJA) in the glandular stomach of *H. pylori*–infected Mongolian gerbils was evaluated by giving infected gerbils CJA in their drinking water at concentrations of 1% and 3% for 10 weeks [92]. The microscopic scores for gastritis and mucosal hyperplasia in the CJA groups were significantly lower than that in the *H. pylori*–inoculated control group, with dose dependence [92]. Real-time PCR was performed to quantitate *H. pylori* by demonstrating the urease A gene amount [92]. Average urease A gene dosage in the glandular stomach in the 1% and 3% CJA and *H. pylori*–inoculated control groups was 26.6% ± 11.6% (average ± SE), 30.3% ± 10.5%, 100% ± 40.9%, respectively, the fruit juice concentrate causing significant lowering ($p < 0.01$ and $p < 0.05$, respectively, with 1% and 3%) [92]. In summary, animal models confirm the anti-*H. pylori* activity of many botanicals and their extracts.

22.6 COMBINED *IN VITRO* AND *IN VIVO* STUDIES

A few reports provide information regarding the anti–*H. pylori* activity of phytochemicals through both *in vitro* and in vivo studies [44,93,94]. To evaluate the effects of ellagitannins from Rubus berries on gastric inflammation, ellagitannin-enriched extracts (ETs) were prepared from *Rubus fruticosus* L. (blackberry) and *Rubus idaeus* L. (raspberry) [93]. The anti-inflammatory activity was tested on a gastric adenocarcinoma cell line stimulated by TNFα and IL-1β for evaluating the effect on NF-κB driven transcription, nuclear translocation, and IL-8 secretion [93]. *In vivo*, the protective effect of ellagitannins was evaluated in a rat model of ethanol-induced gastric lesions [93]. Rats were treated orally for 10 days with 20 mg/kg/day of ETs, and ethanol was given 1 h before they were sacrificed [93]. Gastric mucosa was isolated and used for the determination of IL-8 release, NF-κB nuclear translocation, Trolox equivalents, and SOD and catalase activities [93]. *In vitro*, ETs inhibited TNFα-induced NF-κB-driven transcription (IC50: 0.67–1.73 mg/mL) and reduced TNFα-induced NF-κB nuclear translocation (57%–67% at 2 mg/mL) [93]. ETs inhibited IL-8 secretion induced by TNFα and IL-1β at low concentrations (IC50 range of 0.7–4 mg/mL) [93]. Sanguiin H-6 and lambertianin C, the major ETs present in the extracts, were found to be responsible, at least in part, for the effect of the mixtures [93]. ETs of blackberry and raspberry decreased Ulcer Index by 88% and 75%, respectively, and protected from the ethanol-induced oxidative stress in rats [93]. CINC-1 (the rat homologue of IL-8) secretion in the gastric mucosa was reduced in the animals receiving blackberry and raspberry ETs [93]. The effect of ETs on CINC-1 was associated with a decrease in NF-κB nuclear translocation in ET-treated animals [93]. The authors concluded that the results of their study demonstrated the preventive effect of ETs in gastric inflammation and support for their use in dietary regimens against peptic ulcer [93]. The susceptibility to resveratrol of 26 *H. pylori* strains representing nine CagA+ strains from patients with gastric carcinoma and eight CagA– and nine CagA+ strains from patients with chronic gastritis only was evaluated [94]. The mean MBC of resveratrol for CagA-positive gastric carcinoma strains was significantly lower than those for both CagA-positive and CagA-negative chronic gastritis strains [94].

22.7 CONCLUSION/FUTURE DIRECTION

The earlier review of selected published literature on *H. pylori* and phytochemicals indicates that while much more research is needed to further elucidate the mechanisms of *H. pylori*–related gastric injury and the role that these compounds may have in its mitigation, the balance of evidence clearly favors the recommendation that a diet rich in plant foods/extracts not only reduces the risks of *H. pylori*–induced GI diseases, but may be helpful in the treatment of these diseases as well. Exciting new data are emerging on the role of *H. pylori* in other diseases such as pancreatic cancer, colorectal cancer, diabetes, obesity, and asthma [95–103]. It will be interesting to see the impact on these conditions of "phytoceuticals" as well [104].

REFERENCES

1. Marshall BJ, Armstrong JA, McGechie DB, Glancy RJ. 1985. Attempt to fulfill Koch's postulates for pyloric *Campylobacter. Med J Aust* 142(8):436–439.
2. Santacroce L. 2014. *Helicobacter pylori* infection. *Medscape,* http://emedicine.medscape.com/article/176938-overview, Accessed December 17, 2014.
3. *Helicobacter pylori* infections. 2012. In *Red Book: 2012 Report of the Committee on Infectious Diseases.* Pickering LK (ed.), 29th edn. Elk Grove Village, IL: American Academy of Pediatrics, pp. 354–356.
4. Ertem D. 2013. Clinical practice: *Helicobacter pylori* infection in childhood. *Eur J Pediatr* 172(11):1427–1434.
5. Pereira MI, Medeiros JA. 2014. Role of *Helicobacter pylori* in gastric mucosa-associated lymphoid tissue lymphomas. *World J Gastroenterol* 20(3):684–698.
6. World Health Organization International Agency for Research on Cancer, IARC Working Group Reports, Vol. 8. 2013. *Helicobacter pylori* eradication as a strategy for preventing gastric cancer. http://www.iarc.fr/en/publications/pdfs-online/wrk/wrk8/Helicobacter_pylori_Eradication.pdf, Accessed December 17, 2014.
7. Picoli SU, Mazzoleni LE, Fernández H, De Bona LR, Neuhauss E, Longo L, Prolla JC. 2014. Resistance to amoxicillin, clarithromycin and ciprofloxacin of *Helicobacter pylori* isolated from Southern Brazil patients. *Rev Inst Med Trop Sao Paulo* 56(3):197–200.
8. Peretz A, Paritsky M, Nasser O, Brodsky D, Glyatman T, Segal S, On A. 2014. Resistance of *Helicobacter pylori* to tetracycline, amoxicillin, clarithromycin and metronidazole in Israeli children and adults. *J Antibiot (Tokyo)* 67(8):555–557.
9. Salem EM, Yar T, Bamosa AO, Al-Quorain A, Yasawy MI, Alsulaiman RM, Randhawa MA. 2010. Comparative study of *Nigella sativa* and triple therapy in eradication of *Helicobacter pylori* in patients with non-ulcer dyspepsia. *Saudi J Gastroenterol* 16(3):207–214.
10. Hardbower DM, de Sablet T, Chaturvedi R, Wilson KT. 2013. Chronic inflammation and oxidative stress. The smoking gun for *Helicobacter pylori*-induced gastric cancer? *Gut Microbes* 4(6):475–481.
11. Shiota S, Suzuki R, Yamaoka Y. 2013. The significance of virulence factors in *Helicobacter pylori. J Dig Dis* 14(7):341–349.
12. Uberti AF, Olivera-Severo D, Wassermann GE, Scopel-Guerra A, Moraes JA, Barcellos-de-Souza P et al. 2013. Pro-inflammatory properties and neutrophil activation by *Helicobacter pylori* urease. *Toxicon* 69:240–249.
13. Smolka AJ, Backert S. 2012. How *Helicobacter pylori* infection controls gastric acid secretion. *J Gastroenterol* 47(6):609–618.
14. Messing J, Niehues M, Shevtsova A, Borén T, Hensel A. 2014. Antiadhesive properties of arabinogalactan protein from *Ribes nigrum* seeds against bacterial adhesion of *Helicobacter pylori. Molecules* 19:3696–3717.
15. Kalali B, Mejías-Luque R, Javaheri A, Gerhard M. 2014. *H. pylori* virulence factors: Influence on immune system and pathology. *Mediators Inflamm* 2014:426309.
16. Oleastro M, Ménard A. 2013. The role of *Helicobacter pylori* outer membrane proteins in adherence and pathogenesis. *Biology* 2(3):1110–1134.
17. Yamaoka Y, Alm RA. 2008. *Helicobacter pylori* outer membrane proteins. In *Helicobacter pylori: Molecular Genetics and Cellular Biology.* Yamaoka Y (ed.), 1st edn. Norfolk, U.K.: Caister Academic Press, pp. 37–60.
18. Senkovich OA, Yin J, Ekshyyan V, Conant C, Traylor J, Adegboyega P, McGee DJ, Rhoads RE, Slepenkov S, Testerman TL. 2011. *Helicobacter pylori* AlpA and AlpB bind host laminin and influence gastric inflammation in gerbils. *Infect Immun* 79(8):3106–3116.
19. Hennig EE, Godlewski MM, Butruk E, Ostrowski J. 2005. *Helicobacter pylori* VacA cytotoxin interacts with fibronectin and alters HeLa cell adhesion and cytoskeletal organization *in vitro. FEMS Immunol Med Microbiol* 44(2):143–150.
20. Trust TJ, Doig P, Emödy L, Kienle Z, Wadström T, O'Toole P. 1991. High-affinity binding of the basement membrane proteins collagen type IV and laminin to the gastric pathogen *Helicobacter pylori. Infect Immun* 59(12):4398–4404.
21. Chaturvedi R, Asim M, Romero-Gallo J, Barry DP, Hoge S, de Sablet T et al. 2011. Spermine oxidase mediates the gastric cancer risk associated with *Helicobacter pylori* CagA. *Gastroenterology* 141:1696, e1–e2.
22. Augusto AC, Miguel F, Mendonça S, Pedrazzoli J Jr, Gurgueira SA. 2007. Oxidative stress expression status associated to *Helicobacter pylori* virulence in gastric diseases. *Clin Biochem* 40:615–622.

23. Lamb A, Chen LF. 2013. Role of the *Helicobacter pylori*-induced inflammatory response in the development of gastric cancer. *J Cell Biochem* 114(3):491–497.
24. Lee KE, Khoi PN, Xia Y, Park JS, Joo YE, Kim KK, Choi SY, Jung YD. 2013. *Helicobacter pylori* and interleukin-8 in gastric cancer. *World J Gastroenterol* 19(45):8192–8202.
25. Raju D, Hussey S, Ang M, Terebiznik MR, Sibony M, Galindo-Mata E et al. 2012. Vacuolating cytotoxin and variants in Atg16L1 that disrupt autophagy promote *Helicobacter pylori* infection in humans. *Gastroenterology* 142:1160–1171.
26. Eruslanov E, Kusmartsev S. 2010. Identification of ROS using oxidized DCFDA and flow-cytometry. *Methods Mol Biol* 594:57–72.
27. Kim JM, Kim JS, Lee JY, Kim YJ, Youn HJ, Kim IY et al. 2007. Vacuolating cytotoxin in *Helicobacter pylori* watersoluble proteins upregulates chemokine expression in human eosinophils via Ca^{2+} influx, mitochondrial reactive oxygen intermediates, and NF-kappaB activation. *Infect Immun* 75:3373–3381.
28. Tsugawa H, Suzuki H, Saya H, Hatakeyama M, Hirayama T, Hirata K et al. 2012. Reactive oxygen species induced autophagic degradation of *Helicobacter pylori* CagA is specifically suppressed in cancer stem-like cells. *Cell Host Microbe* 12:764–777.
29. Gong M, Ling SSM, Lui SY, Yeoh KG, Ho B. 2010. *Helicobacter pylori* γ-glutamyl transpeptidase is a pathogenic factor in the development of peptic ulcer disease. *Gastroenterology* 139:564–573.
30. Berg K, Chatterjee A, Yasmin T, Shara M, Bagchi D. 2007. Cytokine expression due to *Helicobacter pylori* in a tissue culture model. *Mol Cell Biochem* 300(1–2):171–175.
31. Eftang LL, Esbensen Y, Tannæs TM, Bukholm IR, Bukholm G. 2012. Interleukin-8 is the single most up-regulated gene in whole genome profiling of *H. pylori* exposed gastric epithelial cells. *BMC Microbiol* 12:9.
32. Wroblewski LE, Peek RM Jr. 2013. *Helicobacter pylori* in gastric carcinogenesis: Mechanisms. *Gastroenterol Clin North Am* 42(2):285–298.
33. Wroblewski LE, Peek RM Jr, Wilson KT. 2010. *Helicobacter pylori* and gastric cancer: Factors that modulate disease risk. *Clin Microbiol Rev* 23(4):713–739.
34. Ierardi E, Giorgio F, Losurdo G, Di Leo A, Principi M. 2013. How antibiotic resistances could change *Helicobacter pylori* treatment: A matter of geography? *World J Gastroenterol* 19(45):8168–8180.
35. Vattem DA, Ghaedian R, Shetty K. 2005. Enhancing health benefits of berries through phenolic antioxidant enrichment: Focus on cranberry. *Asia Pac J Clin Nutr* 14(2):120–130.
36. Côté J, Caillet S, Doyon G, Sylvain JF, Lacroix M. 2010. Bioactive compounds in cranberries and their biological properties. *Crit Rev Food Sci Nutr* 50(7):666–679.
37. Sherpa TW, Sherpa KT, Nixon G, Heydon J, Heydon E, Dovey S. 2012. The prevalence of *Helicobacter pylori* infection in Sherpa residents of the Upper Khumbu, an isolated community in Eastern Nepal. *N Z Med J* 125(1365):30–37.
38. Enomoto S, Yanaoka K, Utsunomiya H, Niwa T, Inada K, Deguchi H et al. 2010. Inhibitory effects of Japanese apricot (Prunus mume Siebold et Zucc.; Ume) on *Helicobacter pylori*-related chronic gastritis. *Eur J Clin Nutr* 64(7):714–719.
39. Bastos J, Lunet N, Peleteiro B, Lopes C, Barros H. 2010. Dietary patterns and gastric cancer in a Portuguese urban population. *Int J Cancer* 127(2):433–441.
40. González CA, Pera G, Agudo A, Bueno-de-Mesquita HB, Ceroti M, Boeing H et al. 2006. Fruit and vegetable intake and the risk of stomach and oesophagus adenocarcinoma in the European Prospective Investigation into Cancer and Nutrition (EPIC-EURGAST). *Int J Cancer* 118(10):2559–2566.
41. Li L, Ying XJ, Sun TT, Yi K, Tian HL, Sun R, Tian JH, Yang KH. 2012. Overview of methodological quality of systematic reviews about gastric cancer risk and protective factors. *Asian Pac J Cancer Prev* 13(5):2069–2079.
42. Compare D, Rocco A, Nardone G. 2010. Risk factors in gastric cancer. *Eur Rev Med Pharmacol Sci* 14(4):302–308.
43. Tsugane S, Sasazuki S. 2007. Diet and the risk of gastric cancer: Review of epidemiological evidence. *Gastric Cancer* 10(2):75–83.
44. Shmuely H, Ofek I, Weiss EI, Rones Z, Houri-Haddad Y. 2012. Cranberry components for the therapy of infectious disease. *Curr Opin Biotechnol* 23(2):148–152.
45. Matsushima M, Suzuki T, Masui A, Kasai K, Kouchi T, Takagi A, Shirai T, Mine T. 2008. Growth inhibitory action of cranberry on *Helicobacter pylori*. *J Gastroenterol Hepatol* 23 (Suppl. 2):S175–S180.
46. Zafra-Stone S, Yasmin T, Bagchi M, Chatterjee A, Vinson JA, Bagchi D. 2007. Berry anthocyanins as novel antioxidants in human health and disease prevention. *Mol Nutr Food Res* 51(6):675–683.
47. Chatterjee A, Yasmin T, Bagchi D, Stohs SJ. 2004. Inhibition of *Helicobacter pylori in vitro* by various berry extracts, with enhanced susceptibility to clarithromycin. *Mol Cell Biochem* 265(1–2):19–26.

48. Nohynek LJ, Alakomi HL, Kähkönen MP, Heinonen M, Helander IM, Oksman-Caldentey KM, Puupponen-Pimiä RH. 2006. Berry phenolics: Antimicrobial properties and mechanisms of action against severe human pathogens. *Nutr Cancer* 54(1):18–32.
49. Lin YT, Kwon YI, Labbe RG, Shetty K. 2005. Inhibition of *Helicobacter pylori* and associated urease by oregano and cranberry phytochemical synergies. *Appl Environ Microbiol* 71(12):8558–8564.
50. Shmuely H, Burger O, Neeman I, Yahav J, Samra Z, Niv Y, Sharon N, Weiss E, Athamna A, Tabak M, Ofek I. 2004. Susceptibility of *Helicobacter pylori* isolates to the antiadhesion activity of a high-molecular-weight constituent of cranberry. *Diagn Microbiol Infect Dis* 50(4):231–235.
51. Burger O, Weiss E, Sharon N, Tabak M, Neeman I, Ofek I. 2002. Inhibition of *Helicobacter pylori* adhesion to human gastric mucus by a high-molecular-weight constituent of cranberry juice. *Crit Rev Food Sci Nutr* 42(3 Suppl.):279–284.
52. Burger O, Ofek I, Tabak M, Weiss EI, Sharon N, Neeman I. 2000. A high molecular mass constituent of cranberry juice inhibits *Helicobacter pylori* adhesion to human gastric mucus. *FEMS Immunol Med Microbiol* 29(4):295–301.
53. Amin M, Anwar F, Janjua MR, Iqbal MA, Rashid U. 2012. Green synthesis of silver nanoparticles through reduction with *Solanum xanthocarpum* L. berry extract: Characterization, antimicrobial and urease inhibitory activities against *Helicobacter pylori*. *Int J Mol Sci* 13(8):9923–9941.
54. Mahady GB, Pendland SL, Stoia A, Hamill FA, Fabricant D, Dietz BM, Chadwick LR. 2005. *In vitro* susceptibility of *Helicobacter pylori* to botanical extracts used traditionally for the treatment of gastrointestinal disorders. *Phytother Res* 19(11):988–991.
55. Mahady GB, Pendland S. 2000. Garlic and *Helicobacter pylori*. *Am J Gastroenterol* 95(1):309.
56. Yamaguchi F, Ariga T, Yoshimura Y, Nakazawa H. 2000. Antioxidative and anti-glycation activity of garcinol from *Garcinia indica* fruit rind. *J Agric Food Chem* 48(2):180–185.
57. Yamaguchi F, Saito M, Ariga T, Yoshimura Y, Nakazawa H. 2000. Free radical scavenging activity and antiulcer activity of garcinol from *Garcinia indica* fruit rind. *J Agric Food Chem* 48(6):2320–2325.
58. Mahady GB, Pendland SL. 2000. Resveratrol inhibits the growth of *Helicobacter pylori in vitro*. *Am J Gastroenterol* 95(7):1849.
59. Njume C, Afolayan AJ, Clarke AM, Ndip RN. 2011. Crude ethanolic extracts of *Garcinia kola* seeds Heckel (Guttiferae) prolong the lag phase of *Helicobacter pylori*: Inhibitory and bactericidal potential. *J Med Food* 14(7–8):822–827.
60. Chatterjee A, Bagchi D, Yasmin T, Stohs SJ. 2005. Antimicrobial effects of antioxidants with and without clarithromycin on *Helicobacter pylori*. *Mol Cell Biochem* 270(1–2):125–130.
61. Chatterjee A, Yasmin T, Bagchi D, Stohs SJ. 2003. The bactericidal effects of Lactobacillus acidophilus, garcinol and Protykin compared to clarithromycin, on *Helicobacter pylori*. *Mol Cell Biochem* 243(1–2):29–35.
62. Brown JC, Jiang X. 2013. Activities of muscadine grape skin and polyphenolic constituents against *Helicobacter pylori*. *J Appl Microbiol* 114(4):982–991.
63. Martini S, D'Addario C, Braconi D, Bernardini G, Salvini L, Bonechi C, Figura N, Santucci A, Rossi C. 2009. Antibacterial activity of grape extracts on cagA-positive and -negative *Helicobacter pylori* clinical isolates. *J Chemother* 21(5):507–513.
64. Zaidi SF, Ahmed K, Yamamoto T, Kondo T, Usmanghani K, Kadowaki M, Sugiyama T. 2009. Effect of resveratrol on *Helicobacter pylori*-induced interleukin-8 secretion, reactive oxygen species generation and morphological changes in human gastric epithelial cells. *Biol Pharm Bull* 32(11):1931–1935.
65. Mahady GB, Pendland SL, Chadwick LR. 2003. Resveratrol and red wine extracts inhibit the growth of CagA+ strains of *Helicobacter pylori in vitro*. *Am J Gastroenterol* 98(6):1440–1441.
66. Genovese S, Fiorito S, Locatelli M, Carlucci G, Epifano F. 2014. Analysis of biologically active oxyprenylated ferulic acid derivatives in Citrus fruits. *Plant Foods Hum Nutr* 69(3):255–260.
67. Rozza AL, Moraes Tde M, Kushima H, Tanimoto A, Marques MO, Bauab TM, Hiruma-Lima CA, Pellizzon CH. 2011. Gastroprotective mechanisms of *Citrus lemon* (Rutaceae) essential oil and its majority compounds limonene and β-pinene: Involvement of heat-shock protein-70, vasoactive intestinal peptide, glutathione, sulfhydryl compounds, nitric oxide and prostaglandin E_2. *Chem Biol Interact* 189(1–2):82–89.
68. Nakagawa H, Takaishi Y, Tanaka N, Tsuchiya K, Shibata H, Higuti T. 2006. Chemical constituents from the peels of *Citrus sudachi*. *J Nat Prod* 69(8):1177–1179.
69. Huang HL, Ko CH, Yan YY, Wang CK. 2014. Antiadhesion and anti-inflammation effects of noni (*Morinda citrifolia*) fruit extracts on AGS cells during *Helicobacter pylori* infection. *J Agric Food Chem* 62(11):2374–2383.

70. Basile A, Conte B, Rigano D, Senatore F, Sorbo S. 2010. Antibacterial and antifungal properties of acetonic extract of *Feijoa sellowiana* fruits and its effect on *Helicobacter pylori* growth. *J Med Food* 13(1):189–195.
71. Pastene E, Speisky H, Troncoso M, Alarcón J, Figueroa G. 2009. *In vitro* inhibitory effect of apple peel extract on the growth of *Helicobacter pylori* and respiratory burst induced on human neutrophils. *J Agric Food Chem* 57(17):7743–7749.
72. Molnár P, Kawase M, Satoh K, Sohara Y, Tanaka T, Tani S, Sakagami H, Nakashima H, Motohashi N, Gyémánt N, Molnár J. 2005. Biological activity of carotenoids in red paprika, Valencia orange and Golden delicious apple. *Phytother Res* 19(8):700–707.
73. Wang YC, Huang KM. 2013. *In vitro* anti-inflammatory effect of apigenin in the *Helicobacter pylori*-infected gastric adenocarcinoma cells. *Food Chem Toxicol* 53:376–383.
74. Niehues M, Euler M, Georgi G, Mank M, Stahl B, Hensel A. 2010. Peptides from *Pisum sativum* L. enzymatic protein digest with anti-adhesive activity against *Helicobacter pylori*: Structure-activity and inhibitory activity against BabA, SabA, HpaA and a fibronectin-binding adhesin. *Mol Nutr Food Res* 54(12):1851–1861.
75. Zhou Y, Taylor B, Smith TJ, Liu ZP, Clench M, Davies NW, Rainsford KD. 2009. A novel compound from celery seed with a bactericidal effect against *Helicobacter pylori. J Pharm Pharmacol* 61(8):1067–1077.
76. Wang YC, Wu DC, Liao JJ, Wu CH, Li WY, Weng BC. 2009. *In vitro* activity of *Impatiens balsamina* L. against multiple antibiotic-resistant *Helicobacter pylori. Am J Chin Med* 37(4):713–722.
77. De Marino S, Borbone N, Gala F, Zollo F, Fico G, Pagiotti R, Iorizzi M. 2006. New constituents of sweet *Capsicum annuum* L. fruits and evaluation of their biological activity. *J Agric Food Chem* 54(20):7508–7516.
78. Zaidi SF, Yoshida I, Butt F, Yusuf MA, Usmanghani K, Kadowaki M, Sugiyama T. 2009. Potent bactericidal constituents from *Mallotus philippinensis* against clarithromycin and metronidazole resistant strains of Japanese and Pakistani *Helicobacter pylori. Biol Pharm Bull* 32(4):631–636.
79. Lawal TO, Adeniyi BA, Moody JO, Mahady GB. 2012. Combination studies of *Eucalyptus torelliana* F. Muell. leaf extracts and clarithromycin on *Helicobacter pylori. Phytother Res* 26(9):1393–1398.
80. Messing J, Thöle C, Niehues M, Shevtsova A, Glocker E, Borén T, Hensel A. 2014. Antiadhesive properties of *Abelmoschus esculentus* (Okra) immature fruit extract against *Helicobacter pylori* adhesion. *PLoS ONE* 9(1):e84836.
81. Bisignano C, Filocamo A, La Camera E, Zummo S, Fera MT, Mandalari G. 2013. Antibacterial activities of almond skins on cagA-positive and-negative clinical isolates of *Helicobacter pylori. BMC Microbiol* 13:103.
82. Gotteland M, Andrews M, Toledo M, Muñoz L, Caceres P, Anziani A, Wittig E, Speisky H, Salazar G. 2008. Modulation of *Helicobacter pylori* colonization with cranberry juice and *Lactobacillus johnsonii* La1 in children. *Nutrition* 24(5):421–426.
83. Shmuely H, Yahav J, Samra Z, Chodick G, Koren R, Niv Y, Ofek I. 2007. Effect of cranberry juice on eradication of *Helicobacter pylori* in patients treated with antibiotics and a proton pump inhibitor. *Mol Nutr Food Res* 51(6):746–751.
84. Zhang L, Ma J, Pan K, Go VL, Chen J, You WC. 2005. Efficacy of cranberry juice on *Helicobacter pylori* infection: A double-blind, randomized placebo-controlled trial. *Helicobacter* 10(2):139–145.
85. Epplein M, Zheng W, Li H, Peek RM Jr, Correa P, Gao J, Michel A, Pawlita M, Cai Q, Xiang YB, Shu XO. 2014. Diet, *Helicobacter pylori* strain-specific infection, and gastric cancer risk among Chinese men. *Nutr Cancer* 66(4):550–557.
86. Bonamin F, Moraes TM, Dos Santos RC, Kushima H, Faria FM, Silva MA et al. 2014. The effect of a minor constituent of essential oil from *Citrus aurantium*: The role of β-myrcene in preventing peptic ulcer disease. *Chem Biol Interact* 212:11–19.
87. Wang XQ, Yan H, Terry PD, Wang JS, Cheng L, Wu WA, Hu SK. 2012. Interaction between dietary factors and *Helicobacter pylori* infection in noncardia gastric cancer: A population-based case-control study in China. *J Am Coll Nutr* 31(5):375–384.
88. Jarosz M, Rychli E, Siuba M, Respondek W, Ryzko-Skiba M, Sajór I, Gugała S, Błazejczyk T, Ciok J. 2009. Dietary and socio-economic factors in relation to *Helicobacter pylori* re-infection. *World J Gastroenterol* 15(9):1119–1125.
89. Asombang AW, Kayamba V, Mwanza-Lisulo M, Colditz G, Mudenda V, Yarasheski K et al. 2013. Gastric cancer in Zambian adults: A prospective case-control study that assessed dietary intake and antioxidant status by using urinary isoprostane excretion. *Am J Clin Nutr* 97(5):1029–1035.

90. Jung K, Chin YW, Chung YH, Park YH, Yoo H, Min DS, Lee B, Kim J. 2013. Anti-gastritis and wound healing effects of Momordicae Semen extract and its active component. *Immunopharmacol Immunotoxicol* 35(1):126–132.
91. Powanda MC, Rainsford KD. 2011. A toxicological investigation of a celery seed extract having anti-inflammatory activity. *Inflammopharmacology* 19(4):227–233.
92. Otsuka T, Tsukamoto T, Tanaka H, Inada K, Utsunomiya H, Mizoshita T, Kumagai T, Katsuyama T, Miki K, Tatematsu M. 2005. Suppressive effects of fruit-juice concentrate of *Prunus mume* Sieb. et Zucc. (Japanese apricot, Ume) on *Helicobacter pylori*-induced glandular stomach lesions in Mongolian gerbils. *Asian Pac J Cancer Prev* 6(3):337–341.
93. Sangiovanni E, Vrhovsek U, Rossoni G, Colombo E, Brunelli C, Brembati L, Trivulzio S, Gasperotti M, Mattivi F, Bosisio E, Dell'Agli M. 2013. Ellagitannins from Rubus berries for the control of gastric inflammation: *In vitro* and *in vivo studies. PLoS ONE* 8(8):e71762.
94. Martini S, Bonechi C, Rossi C, Figura N. 2011. Increased susceptibility to resveratrol of *Helicobacter pylori* strains isolated from patients with gastric carcinoma. *J Nat Prod* 74(10):2257–2260.
95. Testerman TL, Morris J. 2014. Beyond the stomach: An updated view of *Helicobacter pylori* pathogenesis, diagnosis, and treatment. *World J Gastroenterol* 20(36):12781–12808.
96. Rokkas T, Sechopoulos P, Pistiolas D, Kothonas F, Margantinis G, Koukoulis G. 2013. The relationship of *Helicobacter pylori* infection and colon neoplasia, on the basis of meta-analysis. *Eur J Gastroenterol Hepatol* 25:1286–1294.
97. Sonnenberg A, Genta RM. 2013. *Helicobacter pylori* is a risk factor for colonic neoplasms. *Am J Gastroenterol* 108:208–215.
98. Shmuely H, Melzer E, Braverman M, Domniz N, Yahav J. 2014. *Helicobacter pylori* infection is associated with advanced colorectal neoplasia. *Scand J Gastroenterol* 49:35–42.
99. Zhou X, Zhang C, Wu J, Zhang G. 2013. Association between *Helicobacter pylori* infection and diabetes mellitus: A meta-analysis of observational studies. *Diabetes Res Clin Pract* 99:200–208.
100. Gunji T, Matsuhashi N, Sato H, Fujibayashi K, Okumura M, Sasabe N, Urabe A. 2008. *Helicobacter pylori* infection is significantly associated with metabolic syndrome in the Japanese population. *Am J Gastroenterol* 103:3005–3010.
101. Agrawal RP, Sharma R, Garg D, Pokharna R, Kochar DK, Kothari RP. 2010. Role of *Helicobacter pylori* in causation of diabetic gastropathies and non-gastrointestinal complications in type 2 diabetes. *J Indian Med Assoc* 108:140–143.
102. Wang F, Fu Y, Lv Z. 2014. Association of *Helicobacter pylori* infection with diabetic complications: A meta-analysis. *Endocr Res* 39:7–12.
103. Maisonneuve P, Lowenfels AB. 2015. Risk factors for pancreatic cancer: A summary review of meta-analytical studies. *Int J Epidemiol* 44(1):186–198.
104. Lee SY, Shin YW, Hahm KB. 2008. Phytoceuticals: Mighty but ignored weapons against *Helicobacter pylori* infection. *J Dig Dis* 9(3):129–139.

Section X

Ocular Health and Vision

23 Integrative View of the Nutrition of the Eye

S.K. Polutchko, J.J. Stewart, and B. Demmig-Adams

CONTENTS

23.1 HANDLING SUNLIGHT: PARALLELS BETWEEN THE HUMAN EYE AND PHOTOSYNTHESIS

23.1.1 Introduction

Several similarities exist between human vision and photosynthesis. Both systems must be able to (1) maximize light absorption under low-light conditions and (2) cope with exposure to intense light that has the potential to cause damage. This requires the ability to not only absorb enough photons to discern the visual nature of objects at extremely low levels of visible light, for example at night, on part of the eye and to energize the photochemistry of photosynthesis during early morning or afternoon/evening hours on part of the leaves, respectively, but also minimize photodamage from the intense light of a cloudless day via photoprotective mechanisms employed by both eyes and leaves. Despite the fact that information is derived from the photons gathered for vision whereas a source of chemical energy (for sugar production) is derived from the photons gathered by leaves' chloroplasts, the solutions to the challenge of flexibly switching from efficient light harvesting under low light to powerful photoprotection in high light are remarkably similar in eyes and photosynthesis.

Moreover, one particular class of molecules plays a key role in these solutions. Colorful carotenoid pigments are involved in light processing as well as in photoprotection in the processes of *both* vision and photosynthesis (Demmig-Adams and Adams 2010, 2013; Demmig-Adams et al. 2012b). Some carotenoids or their derivatives collect light as a source of information in vision and as a source of chemical energy in photosynthesis, while other carotenoids play a crucial role in safely removing potentially damaging excitation energy. Light energy absorbed by the light-absorbing photoreceptors and not consumed in the production of sugars in photosynthesis, or used for the production of visual signals in the eye, has the potential to be transferred to oxygen resulting in the formation of highly reactive and potentially damaging reactive oxygen species (ROS; Demmig-Adams and Adams 2002, 2013).

ROS play a dual role in both plants and animals, while massive ROS formation leads to damage, small quantities of ROS are vital to the regulation of genes (Demmig-Adams et al. 2013, 2014). In both plants and animals, carotenoids play an important role as gene regulators by controlling ROS formation and preventing massive ROS formation. Since neither carotenoids nor the antioxidant vitamins complementing carotenoid function can be synthesized in the human body, eye function is dependent on the consumption of these nutrients with the diet. Carotenoids are thus a vital part of the human diet; they are thought to lower the risk of vision loss via cataracts and age-related macular degeneration (AMD; Richer et al. 2011; SanGiovanni and Neuringer 2012) as well as additional diseases caused by oxidative stress and inflammation such as heart disease and diabetes (Mares-Perlman et al. 2002).

Two important carotenoids for human eye health, zeaxanthin and lutein, are pigments synthesized by plants as well as some other photosynthetic organisms, and they participate in those organisms' own control of ROS formation (Demmig-Adams and Adams 2002). The class of carotenoids includes the subcategories of (oxygen-free) carotenes and (oxygen-containing) xanthophylls. Zeaxanthin and lutein belong to the latter group. The present review will summarize the current understanding of the role of various carotenoids, with a focus on zeaxanthin and lutein, in helping organisms deal with sunlight over a wide range of light intensities—from collecting sufficient light to safely dealing with intense light. Insight from both humans and photosynthetic organisms is synthesized to provide (1) a more complete mechanistic picture, (2) directions for the production of zeaxanthin-enhanced leafy greens for human consumption, and (3) recommendations for health management and for future research. Mechanistically, the roles of carotenoids in humans and photosynthetic organisms have many striking parallels; however, research on the human eye and on photosynthetic organisms has thus far focused on different, but complementary aspects of the mechanisms involved.

While the present review will focus on carotenoids with similar physiological functions in both human vision and photosynthesis, it should be noted that both eyes and leaves also employ similar macromolecular physical approaches to avoid intense light. Just as eyes can be shut, leaves of certain plants turn away from intense light; just as pupils can contract, leaves' chloroplasts can assume light-absorption-minimizing positions in the cells.

23.1.2 Structures of Carotenoids with Important Biological Function

Photosynthetic organisms are referred to as producers—able to produce not only sugars (that serve as both an energy source and building blocks for many cell components) but also vital chemicals such as carotenoids and other antioxidants (e.g. the antioxidant vitamins E and C that are essential to humans). In contrast, humans are consumers that rely on the consumption of other organisms for food, building blocks, and essential nutrients, including carotenoids and vitamins. The earlier-mentioned carotenoids zeaxanthin and lutein, with a critical role in eye protection, have to be consumed by humans with their diet.

Many carotenoids are named after the plant species from which they were first isolated and characterized. For instance, high concentrations of zeaxanthin (Figure 23.1) are present in the kernels of corn (*Zea mays*). Concerning the human diet, copious amounts of the yellow carotenoids zeaxanthin and lutein (Figure 23.1) are found in egg yolks, yellow peppers, and yellow corn; the intensity of these food's yellow coloration is an indication of the concentration of zeaxanthin + lutein (Demmig-Adams and Adams 2010). Carotenoids are pigments possessing a color (the color of light they reflect rather than absorb) because they absorb some, but not other, portions of the solar spectrum. As pigments, carotenoids lend their color to the plant tissue in which they are found and can thereby serve as a source of information to other organisms that typically benefit the plant. Examples include the attraction of a pollinator to a flower or a fruit consumer to a ripe seeded fruit, thereby enhancing the plant's reproductive success (Demmig-Adams et al. 2012b). One may ask: why do the kernels of

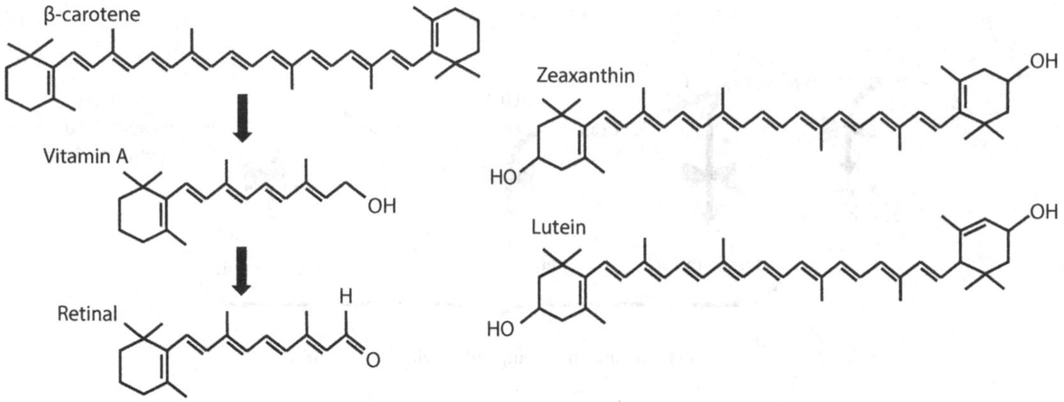

FIGURE 23.1 Structures of the carotenoid β-carotene, of its derivatives vitamin A and retinal, as well as of the xanthophylls zeaxanthin and lutein.

corn possess high levels of carotenoids with a role in photoprotection when the husks already shelter the ear from the sun? Zeaxanthin and lutein presumably serve as antioxidants that enhance seed viability. In conclusion, phytochemicals (plant chemicals) like the latter carotenoids serve in multiple vital functions (Demmig-Adams and Adams 2002, 2010, 2013; Demmig-Adams et al. 2012b).

23.1.3 Carotenoids and Light Harvesting

There are several factors and carotenoids that must be present to allow optimal function of the human eye. After consumption by humans, the carotenoid β-carotene (Figure 23.1), also referred to as provitamin A, can be cleaved into two molecules of vitamin A (Figure 23.1). Vitamin A is converted to retinal, light-absorbing component of the visual purple rhodopsin, the photoreceptor in human vision (Figure 23.1). Three other carotenoids (fucoxanthin, siphonoxanthin, and peridinin) serve as accessory light-harvesting pigments (in addition to the ubiquitous photosynthetic photoreceptor chlorophyll) in photosynthetic algae (Demmig-Adams et al. 2012b). Furthermore, even the two carotenoids zeaxanthin and lutein (Figure 23.1) that serve as photoprotectants against eye damage by intense light (see later) have an additional role in light collection in the human eye—they improve visual acuity via an unknown mechanism (Richer et al. 2011).

23.1.4 Carotenoids and Photoprotection

Photoprotection (against damage by intense light) of the light-harvesting systems in the human eye and in photosynthetic organisms involves multiple, synergistically acting factors: the xanthophylls zeaxanthin and lutein, the antioxidant vitamins E and C, and polyunsaturated fatty acids (Demmig-Adams and Adams 2013). Two principal mechanisms involved in photoprotection are (1) limitation of oxidation events in the membranes housing light receptors and (2) regulation of redox-controlled genes (regulated by the balance of oxidants and antioxidants in the cell) controlling light-receptor survival and light-receptor death. While much recent research in photosynthetic organisms has focused on the limitation of oxidation events, research on the human eye has elucidated signal-transduction events in the prevention of photoreceptor death (Demmig-Adams and Adams 2013).

23.2 OVERVIEW OF CAROTENOID FUNCTION IN PLANTS

Figure 23.2 depicts the cascade of photoprotective responses of plants—from (1) the adjustments in light absorption by modulation of photoreceptor levels over days to weeks to several fast-acting protective mechanisms involving xanthophylls (zeaxanthin and lutein) and/or vitamins E and C, that

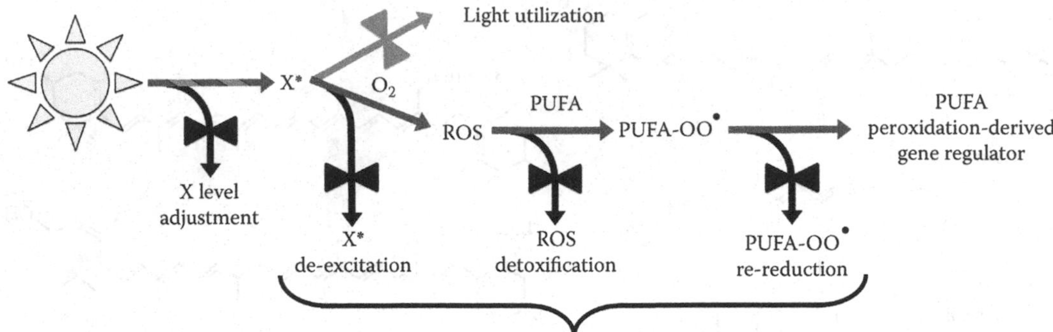

FIGURE 23.2 Schematic depiction of the fate of excitation energy resulting from the absorption of sunlight (yellow sun symbol), leading to the production of an excited-state photoreceptor (X*). Excitation energy is either utilized for (light-gray arrows) photosynthesis or (medium-gray arrows) transferred to oxygen, which can result in the formation of reactive oxygen species (ROS) that can oxidize polyunsaturated fatty acids (PUFA) to PUFA peroxyl radicals (PUFA-OO•) that can, in turn, be converted to PUFA peroxidation-based gene regulators. Photoprotective processes (dark-gray arrows) can prevent damage by excess light via modulating photoreceptor levels (adjusting the levels of the photoreceptor X) and by several additional processes catalyzed by the xanthophylls zeaxanthin and lutein and/or vitamins E and C, with the latter processes including dissipation of excitation energy from excess excited-state photoreceptors (X* de-excitation), detoxification of ROS, and/or recycling (re-reduction) of PUFA peroxyl radicals (PUFA-OO• re-reduction).

range from (2) photoreceptor de-excitation via thermal dissipation of excess absorbed light (X* de-excitation via xanthophylls) that proactively prevents ROS formation to (3) detoxification of ROS once formed (via xanthophylls and/or vitamins E and C), and finally, (4) recycling of the peroxyl radicals of polyunsaturated fatty acids by re-reduction (PUFA-OO• re-reduction; also via xanthophyll and/or vitamins E and C). These various steps of the photoprotective cascade in plants will be further detailed in Sections 23.2.1 and 23.2.2, and similarities between these photoprotective processes in plants and those in the human eye will be emphasized in Section 23.3 and throughout.

23.2.1 Photoprotection by Prevention of ROS Formation

Carotenoids in leaves play a key role in a highly regulated process that safely removes absorbed light energy *only* during times when more light is absorbed than can be utilized (Figures 23.2 and 23.3). Most of the harmless dissipation of excess absorbed light occurs during exposure of leaves to full sunlight at midday and is a preemptive step to limit the formation of reactive oxygen.

Zeaxanthin, and to a lesser extent lutein, catalyzes the safe removal of excess light absorbed by chlorophyll as harmless heat energy (Figures 23.2 and 23.3; Demmig-Adams and Adams 2006; Li et al. 2009). Since it is advantageous to remove only excess light, a highly sophisticated, two-step system has evolved to control energy dissipation without limiting the ability of the plant to exploit light for photosynthesis. This two-step system involves (1) biochemical regulation of zeaxanthin concentration in leaves (Figure 23.3d–f) and (2) biophysical regulation of zeaxanthin engagement in the actual dissipation of those photons that cannot be used for photochemistry (Figure 23.3g–i). Together, these two control steps give plants a remarkable degree of control (Demmig-Adams et al. 2012a) over the extent of energy dissipation and the speed with which dissipation rates increase under intense light and decrease again when light becomes limiting to the plant's performance. The control of zeaxanthin formation, furthermore, provides plants with a *biochemical memory* (García-Plazaola et al. 2012) of how much excess light was experienced during the previous day. Under ideal conditions that promote plant growth, zeaxanthin is formed from a biochemical precursor (violaxanthin, a carotenoid not active in energy dissipation and not playing any known role in eye

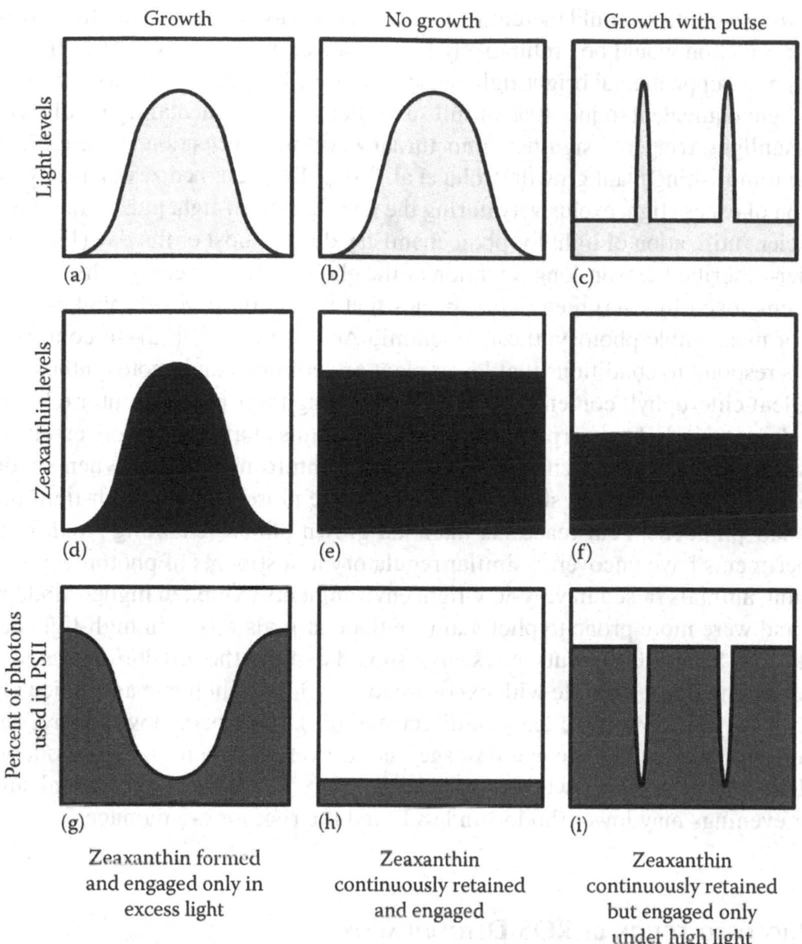

FIGURE 23.3 **(See color insert.)** Changes in the intensity of light (yellow; a–c) striking a horizontal leaf surface, changes in leaf zeaxanthin concentration (blue; d–f), and changes in the percentage of photons absorbed in photosystem II (PSII) and used in PSII photochemistry (green; g–i). Different panels depict light absorption in a natural setting on a sunny day (a, b) or in a growth chamber providing low background light supplemented with two short pulses of high light (c) and depict zeaxanthin levels and utilization of absorbed photons for a growing plant (d, g), a plant impeded in its growth due to harsh environmental conditions (e, h), or a plant growing under growth chamber conditions conducive for growth (f, i).

health) under excess light and quickly reconverted to this precursor when light is no longer in excess (Figure 23.3d); the engagement of thermal dissipation (safely dissipating those photons that cannot be utilized in photochemistry; Figure 23.3g) follows the same pattern under conditions favorable for plant growth (Demmig-Adams and Adams 1996). Leaves removed from a plant and kept in low light therefore typically contain no, or only negligible amounts of, zeaxanthin. Leafy green vegetables thus typically do not contain zeaxanthin by the time they reach the human consumer.

Under harsh environmental conditions that arrest plant growth (e.g. drought or freezing temperatures), even low levels of absorbed light cannot be fully used by the plant for growth. Under harsh, growth-precluding conditions, many plants continuously retain high levels of zeaxanthin (Figure 23.3e), do not use any of light they absorb for photochemistry (Figure 23.3h), and instead remove (dissipate) all absorbed light. Such constantly high zeaxanthin levels are observed in overwintering conifers that retain green needles and dissipate all light absorbed by their needles whenever the trees are not growing (Demmig-Adams et al. 2012a). Cultivating certain crop plants under growth-retarding conditions could therefore produce leaves with higher zeaxanthin levels—but overall biomass production would be prohibitively low. However, we recently demonstrated that exposing plants to a few supplemental bright-light pulses (Figure 23.3c) per day (in a growth chamber with background light equivalent to just 10% of full sunlight and supplemental light pulses equivalent to 40% of full sunlight) triggered significant nocturnal zeaxanthin retention (Figure 23.3f) in a leafy plant without diminishing plant growth (Cohu et al. 2014). This retained zeaxanthin was engaged in the dissipation of excess light exclusively during the few short high-light pulses and did not interfere with the efficient utilization of light for photochemistry during most of the day (Figure 23.3i).

The earlier-described season-long retention of the photoprotective energy dissipater zeaxanthin in nature is employed by evergreen plant species that maintain leaves throughout seasons without growth or measurable photosynthesis (Demmig-Adams et al. 2012a). In contrast, short-lived annual plants respond to conditions that lower plant growth rates and photosynthesis rates mainly by lowering leaf chlorophyll content, that is by downsizing their photoreceptor (chlorophyll) pool and thereby decreasing light absorption (Figure 23.2; Adams et al. 2013). Conversely, plants growing in the shade produce larger chlorophyll pools to capture more light; when suddenly moved to high light environments, these shade-grown plants are more prone to high-light-induced inactivation of their photochemical reactions than sun-grown plants (Demmig-Adams et al. 2012a). Animal experiments have uncovered similar regulatory adjustments of photoreceptor (rhodopsin) levels in vision; animals raised in very-low-light environments exhibited higher rhodopsin levels in their retina and were more prone to photodamage than animals raised in high-light environments (Rozanowska and Sarna 2005). Future research should explore the possibility that acclimation of human vision to an indoor lifestyle with exposure to very-low-light home and office environments (office lighting is typically a mere 0.5% of direct sunlight), interspersed with infrequent exposure to bright sunlight, may encourage eye damage due to overexcitation of high rhodopsin levels in the retina. It should be explored whether regular exposure to low levels of natural sunlight in the mornings or evenings may lower rhodopsin levels and the risk for eye damage.

23.2.2 Photoprotection by ROS Detoxification

As will be discussed later, cellular redox balance (the balance between oxidants and antioxidants) controls vital processes in plants, animals, and microbes (Lavrovsky et al. 2000; Demmig-Adams and Adams 2002). In plants, the light-harvesting chloroplast provides important input into the cellular redox network (Demmig-Adams et al. 2014). The chloroplast of green leaves strikes a balance between allowing some oxidants to inform the cellular redox state (cf. Figure 23.2), while preventing the formation of massive oxidant (ROS) levels that could cause damage to cellular structures. Photoprotective energy dissipation in the chloroplast of green leaves typically dissipates most, but not all, of the excess light and thus allows the formation of low levels of ROS (Figure 23.2).

ROS oxidize the most oxidation-sensitive fatty acids in the photosynthetic membrane as well as in the human retina. Polyunsaturated (omega-6 and omega-3) fatty acids are highly susceptible to oxidation (Figure 23.2) and are found in high concentrations in both the leaf's chloroplasts and in the human eye (as sites of light collection). Why would the highly susceptible fatty acids be placed into these sites where they are vulnerable to oxidative attack? In fact, their presence in these sensitive sites presumably serves as an early warning system that evolved to signal the organism that dangerously high amounts of light are absorbed. In fact, low levels of ROS formed in photosynthetic membranes during the process of photosynthesis are used by ROS-activated (lipoxygenase) enzymes to actively oxidize the abundant polyunsaturated fatty acids of photosynthetic membranes, which convert these fatty acids to hormone-like messengers (Figure 23.2) that inform signaling networks controlling the production of antioxidants and photoreceptors and also regulating plant development, reproduction, and a host of defense responses (Demmig-Adams et al. 2013).

23.2.3 Trade-Offs

Reactive oxygen-derived signals induce the formation of antioxidant biosynthesis for plant defenses against many environmental stresses such as drought and extreme temperatures (Demmig-Adams et al. 2014). In addition, reactive oxygen-derived signals orchestrate plant defenses against herbivores (e.g. insects) and pathogenic viruses, fungi, and bacteria (Demmig-Adams et al. 2013, 2014). Care thus needs to be taken in efforts to produce (e.g. by genetic engineering) plants with increased antioxidant levels that could inadvertently diminish the plant's ability to upregulate its defenses against certain biological agents. A parallel scenario exists in human physiology, whereby excess dietary consumption of antioxidants (via high-dose supplements) has adverse effects through, for example, the prevention of ROS-triggered increases in the concentration of antioxidant enzymes synthesized in the human body and of ROS-triggered stimulation of muscle formation and repair after exercise (Adams et al. 2014).

23.3 OVERVIEW OF PHOTOPROTECTIVE CAROTENOID FUNCTIONS IN THE HUMAN EYE

23.3.1 Roles of Zeaxanthin versus Lutein in the Human Eye

While both zeaxanthin and lutein are important for the function of the eye, they each have specific distinct functions. Zeaxanthin (and not lutein) is apparently the primary photoprotectant in those regions of the eye that receive the most intense light. The argument supporting the latter conclusion is that zeaxanthin is preferentially accumulated compared to lutein: the ratio of zeaxanthin to lutein is lowest in the food, becomes greater as the two xanthophylls are extracted in the digestive tract and moved to the blood plasma, and the highest zeaxanthin/lutein ratio is found in the retina's fovea where light is focused and brightest (for a recent review, see Demmig-Adams and Adams 2013). Lutein, on the other hand, is preferentially accumulated in the peripheral regions of the retina and has been found to be important for low-light vision (low-contrast acuity) and is associated with reducing glare (Richer et al. 2011).

Zeaxanthin and lutein thus improve overall visional acuity (with zeaxanthin improving high-contrast acuity) and apparently lower the risk of cataracts and AMD (e.g. Mares-Perlman et al. 2002; Richer et al. 2011; SanGiovanni and Neuringer 2012). At the same time, the levels of zeaxanthin and lutein are predictive of a lower risk for many other chronic diseases such as various cancers (Demmig-Adams and Adams 2002; Mares-Perlman et al. 2002; Sajilata et al. 2008).

23.3.2 Role of Carotenoids in Redox-Modulated Gene Regulation

Since the human eye is a highly oxygenated environment, thus making the eye extremely susceptible to reactive oxygen formation, it is not surprising that the eye is a site where zeaxanthin and lutein, the antioxidant vitamins E and C, and omega-3 polyunsaturated fatty acids accumulate and act synergistically in both photoprotection and reactive oxygen signaling (cf. Figure 23.2; Demmig-Adams and Adams 2013). Carotenoids and antioxidants, in turn, interact with specific polyunsaturated fatty acids in the protection of eye health; while messengers derived from oxidized omega-6 fatty acids tend to stimulate programmed cell death, messengers derived from oxidized omega-3 fatty acids tend to prevent programmed cell death (Roncone et al. 2010; Bazan et al. 2011).

Furthermore, carotenoids and other antioxidants, polyunsaturated fatty acids, and ROS apparently play an important role throughout the entire body via the same processes of (1) modulating oxidation events and (2) regulating genes responsible for responses like programmed light-receptor death (see Maccarrone et al. 1996, 1999, 2001). Carotenoids thus serve as regulators of vital genes controlling the rate of cell division, the rate of programmed cell death, and the activity of the immune system (Demmig-Adams and Adams 2002, 2013). Much of this gene regulation by carotenoids is assumed to occur via carotenoids' antioxidant role (and via synergistic interaction with other antioxidants); other more direct functions of carotenoids as gene regulators have, however, also been discussed (e.g. Stahl et al. 2002).

Since carotenoids regulate genes at very low but critical concentrations—as hormones do—it is not difficult to see that balanced concentrations are important and that both deficiency and excess can have negative effects on human health as well as on plant growth and development. In fact, carotenoids control growth and development in both humans and plants by controlling the rates of cell division via modulation of the concentrations of reactive oxygen. The presence of oxygen, specifically reactive oxygen, stimulates cell division in most organisms—presumably because the presence of oxygen is a sign of ample energy availability for growth. This link plays a role in cancer, which is excessive cell division, and other pro-oxidative, pro-inflammatory diseases (diabetes, heart disease, Alzheimer's, depression, etc.) in humans (Demmig-Adams and Adams 2013).

Furthermore, the human immune system employs the production of reactive oxygen to destroy invading pathogens and as a signal for the organisms to destroy—by programmed cell death—its own cells that are invaded by pathogens. Effective modulation of the latter responses by carotenoids and other antioxidants thus requires the regulators in proper concentrations, with both deficiency and excess having negative effects on humans (and, as stated earlier, on plant growth development, and defense). A fundamental difference between photosynthetic organisms and animals/humans is that the latter depend on an appropriate, balanced dietary intake of these important regulators, while plants and other photosynthetic organisms synthesize carotenoids and other antioxidants as needed. A lack of antioxidants in the modern human diet (along with other dietary imbalances) causes a chronic overstimulation of the immune system, which has been found to be involved in chronic pro-inflammatory diseases and disorders that include eye disease, diabetes, heart disease, Alzheimer's, depression, and others (Lavrovsky et al. 2000).

23.4 MANAGEMENT OF EYE HEALTH

23.4.1 Diet for Eye Health

While carotenoid supplementation has the potential to alleviate blindness in developing countries, a balanced, whole-food based diet, rather than supplements taken alongside the modern Western diet, may be the best strategy for the prevention of eye disease in more developed countries (Demmig-Adams and Adams 2013). Diet, in combination with other wellness-promoting lifestyle factors, is likely to be more effective in the prevention than in the treatment of the latter chronic diseases.

A deficiency of vitamin A (and resulting photoreceptor deficiency) leads to blindness and death from vitamin A-deficiency-associated immunodeficiency, in children in developing countries (Solomon and Bulux 1997; Demmig-Adams et al. 2012b). Supplementation with provitamin A (β-carotene) or vitamin A (retinol) alleviates this deficiency. Conversely, possible adverse effects of an excess intake of vitamin A have been discussed, while emphasizing the importance of a balanced vitamin A intake (Amadieh and Arabi 2011). While high-dose supplements may provide an excess level of vitamins, a whole-food-based diet is unlikely to have such an effect. The role of carotene-rich food in the prevention of vitamin malnutrition in low-income nations is discussed further in Solomon and Bulux (1997).

Chronic eye diseases, such as cataracts and AMD, involve programmed photoreceptor death associated with imbalances in ROS production and in the intake of antioxidants (carotenoids, like zeaxanthin and lutein, and other antioxidants) and of polyunsaturated fatty acids (Demmig-Adams and Adams 2013). Since omega-3 and omega-6 fatty acids cannot be produced in the human body, a balanced intake of these essential fatty acids via the diet is critical (Simopoulos 2004). The term "vitamin" (as in the antioxidant vitamins E and C) is used for essential dietary nutrients that humans are unable to synthesize. The carotenoids zeaxanthin and lutein, as well as the essential polyunsaturated fatty acids, should also be specifically acknowledged as vitamin-like nutrients. However, the optimal doses for the consumption of these latter essential nutrients are currently unknown.

Specific foods that are high in zeaxanthin include yellow corn, yellow peppers, and egg yolks (Demmig-Adams and Adams 2013). Concerning the zeaxanthin/lutein content of egg yolks, it is important that the chickens laying these eggs receive feed (corn or alfalfa) high in zeaxanthin. Leafy greens are rich in lutein, but do not typically retain high zeaxanthin levels postharvest (see earlier). Freezing of greens freshly harvested in sunny locations should help retain zeaxanthin. Moreover, protocols to enhance leaf zeaxanthin content can be developed, such as the specific growth conditions outlined earlier, where brief daily pulses of supplemental light during plant growth increase leaf zeaxanthin concentrations without diminishing plant biomass production (Cohu et al. 2014). Genetic engineering may also serve to increase the zeaxanthin content of leaves, fruits, or vegetables (Demmig-Adams and Adams 2010).

For the treatment of AMD, recommendations have been made for specific zeaxanthin and lutein supplements (e.g. 8 mg zeaxanthin and 9 mg of lutein daily; Richer et al. 2011), but more work is needed. Some current supplements recommended for the treatment of AMD contain mixes (Bartlett and Eperjesi 2004) of zeaxanthin, lutein, antioxidant vitamins like C and E, and antioxidant minerals like zinc and selenium as well as the omega-3 fatty acid docosahexaenoic acid, or DHA (Roncone et al. 2010; Bazan et al. 2011). In a whole-food-based diet, omega-6 and omega-3 fatty acids should be consumed in a ratio below 10:1 (the Western diet provides excessively high ratios that increase the risk of chronic inflammation and programmed cell death; Demmig-Adams and Adams 2002, 2010; Simopoulos 2003, 2004, 2008). The most effective way for the body to take up nutrients is with whole food. When considering supplementing a whole-food diet, it is important to consider the uptake specifications of various supplements in the gut. Oil-soluble xanthophylls/vitamin E/fatty acids need to be consumed with a meal containing oils/fats, while water-soluble vitamin C (and other water-soluble antioxidants) should be consumed with water. A whole-food diet encourages uptake of dietary nutrients in the gut, while avoiding the nutrient excess provided by high-dose supplements (Adams et al. 2014).

23.4.2 Holistic Eye-Health Management through Nutrition and Lifestyle

Whole-food-based diets, such as the traditional Mediterranean diet, that feature balanced levels of omega-3 to omega-6 fatty acids, ample antioxidants from fruit, vegetables, herbs, and spices, along with a low glycemic load (low levels of free sugars and quick-burning starches) and a low consumption of saturated fat, have been shown to lower the risk of pro-inflammatory diseases like heart disease and diabetes (Herder and Demmig-Adams 2004; see Figure 23.4). Such diets should also aid in the prevention of chronic eye disease, especially when coupled with other wellness-promoting lifestyle factors (Figure 23.4).

There are a number of lifestyle-related factors that increase intracellular ROS levels and should thus be avoided; these include smoking, excessive alcohol consumption, excessive UV radiation/direct exposure to bright sunlight, exposure to silica dust/asbestos, excessive exercise, and psychological stress/lack of sleep (Figure 23.4; see e.g. Kushner and Sorensen 2013; Smilin Bell Aseervatham et al. 2013). Conversely, ROS levels can be decreased by regular moderate exercise and stress reduction (Figure 23.4). In conclusion, the key nutrients required for eye health (see Figure 23.2 and text earlier) thus act in synergy with a host of other lifestyle factors. In turn, the lifestyle factors that preserve eye health simultaneously lower the risk for a host of other chronic diseases and disorders.

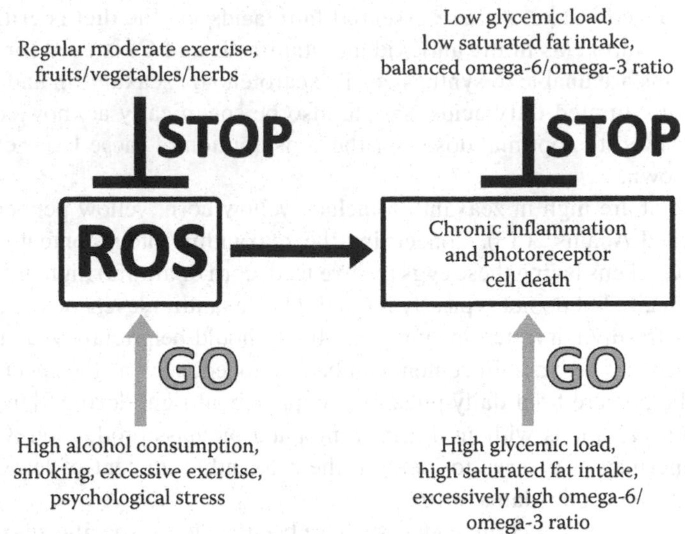

FIGURE 23.4 Schematic depiction of the effect of dietary and other lifestyle factors in modulating the levels of reactive oxygen species (ROS) and ROS effects in triggering chronic inflammation (as a cause of pro-inflammatory disease and disorders) as well as photoreceptor cell death. Light-light arrows (GO) depict triggering, while dark-gray lines (STOP) depict lessening of inflammation and cell death. Glycemic load is defined as the rapidity of the breakdown of carbohydrates into glucose multiplied by the amount in which the latter carbohydrates are consumed; omega-6/omega-3 ratio is the dietary ratio of omega-6 polyunsaturated fatty acids (typically converted to highly pro-inflammatory messengers) to omega-3-polyunsaturated fatty acids (typically converted to anti-inflammatory or only weakly pro-inflammatory messengers); cell death is programmed cell death induced by ROS and pro-inflammatory regulators.

REFERENCES

Adams, R.B., Egbo, K.N., and Demmig-Adams, B. 2014. High-dose vitamin C supplements diminish the benefits of exercise in athletic training and disease prevention. *Nutr Food Sci* 44:95–101. doi: 10.1108/NFS-03-2013-0038.

Adams, W.W. III, Muller, O., Cohu, C.M., and Demmig-Adams, B. 2013. May photoinhibition in plants be a consequence, rather than a cause, of limited productivity? *Photosynth Res* 117:31–44. doi: 10.1007/s11120-013-9849-7.

Amadieh, H. and Arabi, A. 2011. Vitamins and bone health: Beyond calcium and vitamin D. *Nutr Rev* 69:584–598.

Bartlett, H. and Eperjesi, F. 2004. An ideal ocular nutritional supplement? *Ophthalmic Physiol Opt* 24:339–349.

Bazan, N.G., Molina, M.F., and Gordon, W.C. 2011. Docosahexaenoic acid signalolipidomics in nutrition: Significance in aging, neuroinflammation, macular degeneration, Alzheimer's, and other neurodegenerative diseases. *Annu Rev Nutr* 31:321–351.

Cohu, C.M., Lombardi, E., Adams, W.W. III, and Demmig-Adams, B. 2014. Increased nutritional quality of plants for long-duration space missions through choice of plant variety and manipulation of growth conditions. *Acta Astronaut* 94:799–806.

Demmig-Adams, B. and Adams, R.B. 2013. Eye nutrition in context: Mechanisms, implementation, and future directions. *Nutrients* 5:2483–2501. doi: 10.3390/nu5072483.

Demmig-Adams, B. and Adams, W.W. III. 1996. The role of xanthophyll cycle carotenoids in the protection of photosynthesis. *Trends Plant Sci* 1:21–26. doi: 10.1016/S1360-1385(96)80019-7.

Demmig-Adams, B. and Adams, W.W. III. 2002. Antioxidants in photosynthesis and human nutrition. *Science* 298:2149–2153. doi: 10.1126/science.1078002.

Demmig-Adams, B. and Adams, W.W. III. 2006. Photoprotection in an ecological context: The remarkable complexity of thermal dissipation. *New Phytol* 172:11–21. doi: 10.1111/j.1469-8137.2006.01835.x.

Demmig-Adams, B. and Adams, W.W. III. 2010. Overview of diet-gene interaction and the example of xanthophylls. In *Bio-Farms for Nutraceuticals: Functional Food and Safety Control by Biosensors*, M.T. Giardi, G. Rea, B. Berra (eds.), Advances in Experimental Medicine and Biology, Vol. 698. Landes BioScience, Austin, TX, pp. 17–26. doi: 10.1007/978-1-4419-7347-4_2.

Demmig-Adams, B., Cohu, C.M., Amiard, V. et al. 2013. Emerging trade-offs—Impact of photoprotectants (PsbS, xanthophylls, and vitamin E) on oxylipins as regulators of development and defense. *New Phytol* 197:720–729. doi: 10.1111/nph.12100.

Demmig-Adams, B., Cohu, C.M., Muller, O., and Adams, W.W. III. 2012a. Modulation of photosynthetic energy conversion efficiency in nature: From seconds to seasons. *Photosynth Res* 113:75–88. doi: 10.1007/s11120-012-9761-6.

Demmig-Adams, B., Rixham, C.S., and Adams, W.W. III. 2012b. Carotenoids. In *McGraw-Hill Encyclopedia of Science & Technology*, 11th edn., Vol. 3. McGraw-Hill, New York, pp. 549–555. Available at http://www.accessscience.com/content/carotenoids/110600.

Demmig-Adams, B., Stewart, J.J., and Adams, W.W. III. 2014. Multiple feedbacks between chloroplast and whole plant in the context of plant adaptation and acclimation to the environment. *Philos Trans R Soc B Biol Sci* 369:20130244. Available at http://dx.doi.org/10.1098/rstb.2013.0244.

García-Plazaola, J.I., Esteban, R., Fernandez-Marin, B., Kranner, I., and Porcar-Castell, A. 2012. Thermal energy dissipation and xanthophyll cycles beyond the *Arabidopsis* model. *Photosynth Res* 113:89–103.

Herder, R. and Demmig-Adams, B. 2004. The power of a balanced diet and lifestyle in preventing cardiovascular disease. *Nutr Clin Care* 7:46–55. Available at http://web.ebscohost.com/ehost/detail?vid = 5&sid = fd413742-04f3-4dae-be00-5875e3e47fd1%40sessionmgr114&hid = 124&bdata = JnNpdGU9ZWhvc3QtbGl2ZQ%3d%3d#db = aph&AN = 22450621.

Kushner, R.F. and Sorensen, K.W. 2013. Lifestyle medicine: The future of chronic disease management. *Curr Opin Endocrinol Diabetes Obes* 20:389–395. doi:10.1097/01.med.0000433056.76699.5d.

Lavrovsky, Y., Chatterjee, B., Clark, R.A., and Roy, A.K. 2000. Role of redox-regulated transcription factors in inflammation, aging and age-related diseases. *Exp Gerontol* 35:521–532.

Li, Z.R., Ahn, T.K., Avenson, T.J. et al. 2009. Lutein accumulation in the absence of zeaxanthin restores non-photochemical quenching in the *Arabidopsis thaliana npq1* mutant. *Plant Cell* 21:1798–1812.

Maccarrone, M., Corasantini, M.T., Guerrieri, P., Nistico, G., and Finazzi-Agrò, A. 1996. Nitric oxide-donor compounds inhibit lipoxygenase activity. *Biochem Biophys Res Commun* 219:128–133.

Maccarrone, M., Lorenzon, T., Guerrieri, P., and Finazzi-Agrò, A. 1999. Resveratrol prevents apoptosis in K562 cells by inhibiting lipoxygenase and cyclooxygenase activity. *Eur J Biochem* 265:27–34.

Maccarrone, M., Melino, G., and Finazzi-Agrò, A. 2001. Lipoxygenases and their involvement in programmed cell death. *Cell Death Differ* 8:776–784.

Mares-Perlman, J.A., Millen, A.E., Ficek, T.L., Hankinson, S.E. 2002. The body of evidence to support a protective role for lutein and zeaxanthin in delaying chronic disease. Overview. *J Nutr* 132:518S–524S.

Richer, S.B., Stiles, W., Graham-Hoffman, K. et al. 2011. Randomized, double-blind, placebo-controlled study of zeaxanthin and visual function in patients with atrophic age-related macular degeneration. The zeaxanthin and visual function study (ZVF) FDA IND #78, 973. *Optometry* 82:667–680.

Roncone, M., Bartlett, H., and Eperjesi, F. 2010. Essential fatty acids for dry eye: A review. *Cont Lens Anterior Eye* 33:49–54.

Rozanowska, M. and Sarna, T. 2005. Light-induced damage to the retina: Role of the rhodopsin chromophore revisited. *Photochem Photobiol* 81:1305–1330.

Sajilata, M.G., Singhal, R.S., and Kamat, M.Y. 2008. The carotenoid pigment zeaxanthin—A review. *Compr Rev Food Sci Food Saf* 7:29–49.

SanGiovanni, J.P. and Neuringer, M. 2012. The putative role of lutein and zeaxanthin as protective agents against age-related macular degeneration: Promise of molecular genetics for guiding mechanistic and translational research in the field. *Am J Clin Nutr* 96:1223S–1233S.

Simopoulos, A.P. 2003. Omega-3 fatty acids and cancer. *Indoor Built Environ* 12:405–412.

Simopoulos, A.P. 2004. Omega-6/omega-3 essential fatty acid ratio and chronic disease. *Food Rev Int* 20:77–90.

Simopoulos, A.P. 2008. The omega-6/omega-3 fatty acid ratio, genetic variation and cardiovascular disease. *Asia Pac J Clin Nutr* 17:131–134.

Smilin Bell Aseervatham, G., Sivasudha, T., Jeyadevi R., and Arul Ananth, D. 2013. Environmental factors and unhealthy lifestyle influence oxidative stress in humans—An overview. *Environ Sci Pollut Res Int* 20:4356–4369.

Solomon, N.W. and Bulux, J. 1997. Identification and production of local carotene-rich foods to combat vitamin A malnutrition. *Eur J Clin Nutr* 51:S39–S45.

Stahl, W., Ale-Agha, N., and Polidori, M.C. 2002. Non-antioxidant properties of carotenoids. *Biol Chem* 383:553–558.

Section XI

Prostate Health

24 Nutraceuticals for Prostate Cancer

Shigeo Horie

CONTENTS

24.1 INTRODUCTION

Prostate cancer is a highly prevalent disease in Western cultures, in particular, North America, Europe, and Scandinavia. Even in Asian cultures, where the prevalence of this cancer was once low, cancer of the prostate now is a growing threat to men's health [1]. Age, race, and family history are long established risk factors of prostate cancer [2]. The evidence for diet and lifestyle is gaining, but less clear.

Although the incidence of prostate cancer is far greater in the West (120 per 100,000 in Northern America) compared with the East (less than 10 per 100,000 in Asia) [3], when Asians migrate to Western countries, their rate of prostate cancer incidence increases. This finding supports the notion that lifestyle and diet may promote the development of prostate cancer [4,5]. Indeed, there is a body of evidence, including epidemiologic surveys and laboratory, interventional and case-control studies, that diet and lifestyle play a crucial role in prostate tumorigenesis.

This observation has prompted investigators to identify whether certain dietary components, such as soy, a staple of the Asian diet, may have antitumorigenic properties. People in Asian countries, who consume a large amount of Omega-3 (v-3) polyunsaturated fatty acids (PUFA) from soy and phytochemicals from green tea, may experience a lower incidence of prostate cancer compared with people from Western countries who consume a Western-style diet [6]. The increasing burden of prostate cancer screening and the high cost of treatment have made primary prevention an attractive strategy for decreasing the incidence and slowing the progression of this disease [7].

Chemoprevention is a prophylactic method that uses nontoxic natural or synthetic compounds to reverse, inhibit, or prevent the development of cancer by impeding specific molecular steps in the carcinogenic pathway. Although race and family history are immutable factors, dietary components are amenable to alteration, and therefore, provide potential opportunities for prostate cancer chemoprevention. Diet can be modified either by controlling the intake of food or by adding natural foods or supplements with anticancer properties. The term "nutraceutical," derived from the words "nutrition" and "pharmaceutical," first coined in 1979, is commonly used to describe natural foods or supplements that have therapeutic effects, including the ability to prevent, delay, or treat disease [8].

It has become increasingly evident that diet plays a major role in the pathogenesis of prostate cancer and that general dietary modifications may benefit patients. Indeed, many prostate cancer patients attempt to modify diet on their own by taking nutraceuticals in the form of dietary supplements and vitamins [9,10]. The prevalence of nutraceutical use in this population ranges from 26% [11] to 73% [12]. However, at present, no single dietary factor has been shown conclusively to reduce risk or delay the progression of cancer. It is important to note that current evidence relating to the effects of specific nutraceuticals in prostate cancer is limited largely because of the heterogeneous nature of the studies, which vary greatly in design and quality. In addition, much of the current nutritional literature assumes a traditional linear cause–effect relationship, where a single dietary component is investigated for a particular effect. It may turn out that combined nutraceutical consumption is necessary to establish a measurable and beneficial effect. This chapter reviews the accumulated evidence for nutraceuticals, with emphasis on the molecular pathways and proteins implicated in prostate cancer, the DNA damage response (DDR), and the beneficial, synergistic effect of combined nutraceutical consumption.

24.1.1 Androgen Receptor and Prostate Cancer

Normal development and maintenance of the prostate is dependent on androgen hormone, which acts through the androgen receptor (AR) in cells. The AR protein is a key molecule in the development and progression of prostate cancer, and AR signaling is maintained throughout the course of the disease. Prostate cancer progression also has been associated with increased growth factor production, to which prostate cancer cells exhibit an altered response. The kinase signal transduction cascades, including mTOR, NF-KB, and PI3K, modulate the transcriptional activity of the *AR* gene. Inhibiting *AR* transcriptional activity, through mechanisms, such as androgen ablation and modulation of signal transduction pathways, may delay the progression of disease [13].

24.1.2 Inflammation and Prostate Cancer

Inflammation of the prostate gland (prostatitis) and proliferative inflammatory atrophy (PIA) are hypothesized to be precursors of high-grade prostatic intraepithelial neoplasia (HGPIN), which in turn is the precursor to prostate cancer [14,15]. Most cases of PIA and HGPIN represent chronic disease states and are associated with a lengthy period of development and progression [16]. The latency between the detection of localized lesions and the development of invasive cancer is similarly long [17].

Inflammation may signal early steps in carcinogenesis before the appearance of overt tumor. Inflammation is a common morphologic feature of prostate biopsies performed for increased PSA and/or abnormal digital rectal examination [18], and it is also commonly found in radical prostatectomy specimens [19]. Inflamed prostate tissue in the elderly often accompanies atrophy of the epithelium and, at times, stromal alterations [20]. These foci of inflammation contain cells with an increased proliferative index and are usually associated with inflammatory infiltrates, which explains the term, PIA [21]. Response to infection, cell trauma due to oxidant damage, autoimmunity, and hypoxia-related changes all are potential causes of PIA. PIA is also associated with enhanced expression of glutathione *S*-transferase (GST)-P1, the so-called antioxidative gene [21]. This finding suggests that PIA may be subject to increased oxidative stress. The presence of GST-P1 expression, as observed in PIA, is frequently absent in prostate adenocarcinoma [22] and HGPIN [23]. Loss of these defenses against reactive species generated during inflammation may enhance the likelihood of transition from PIA to HGPIN to prostate carcinoma. These features of the progression of prostate cancer have all the attributes of an ideal target disease for chemoprevention, including a long latency, high incidence, ample tumor marker availability, and identifiable pre-neoplastic lesions.

24.2 ANTITUMORIGENIC PROPERTIES OF NUTRACEUTICALS

Several nutraceuticals, including isoflavone, isothiocyanates, lycopene, (−)-epigallocatechin-3-gallete (EGCG), and curcumin, broadly classified as polyphenols, are known to modulate intracellular signaling pathways, including pathways for cellular proliferation, apoptosis, inflammation, and AR signaling, all of which have been implicated in cancer development and progression. Specifically, they are known to decrease signal transduction in AR, Akt, NF-κB, as well as other signal transduction pathways that are vital to the development and progression of prostate cancer in all of its forms, from androgen-sensitive to castrate-resistant disease [24–27].

These features make polyphenols promising chemopreventive agents for prostate cancer (Figure 24.1) [28,29]. The principal mechanisms for these preventive agents include hormone modulation, limiting the accumulation of genetic damage through anti-inflammatory and/or antioxidant properties, and modifying the epigenetic mechanism. Maintaining the integrity of the genome is fundamental to warding off cancer. Central to this process is the ability of cells to accurately recognize and correctly repair DNA damage in a timely manner to ensure the regulated and orderly progression of cells through the cell cycle. DNA damage caused by oxidative stress, chemical agents, or UV light triggers the DDR. Recent evidence has emerged that DDR is one of the earliest events capable of thwarting the multistep progression of human epithelial carcinomas to invasive malignancy [30,31]. Agents that can activate DDR are now appreciated to have potent cancer-preventive properties [32]. The evidence for individual nutraceutricals with demonstrated chemopreventive effects against prostate cancer is summarized in the following:

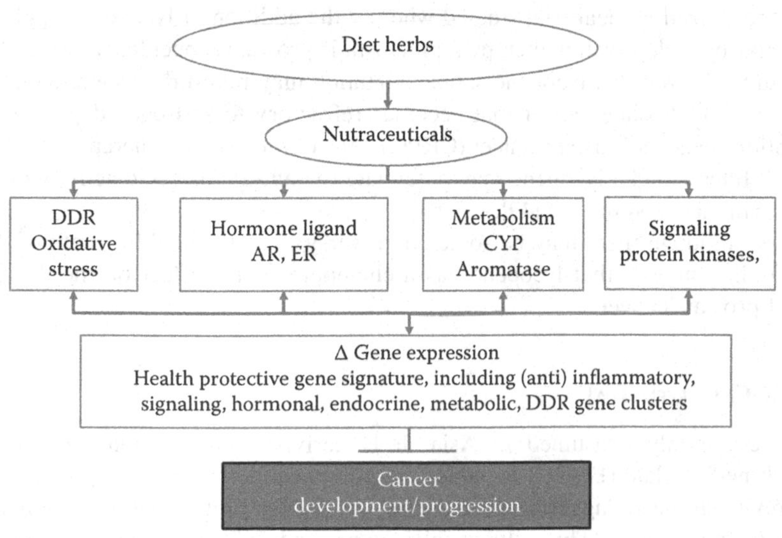

FIGURE 24.1 Action of neutraceuticals on the prevention of cancer.

24.2.1 Lycopene (Tomatoes)

Lycopene is a carotenoid antioxidant mainly found in tomatoes, which is thought to protect against free radicals that can damage DNA and initiate neoplasms. The molecular targets of lycopene are the HMG-CoA reductase, RAS oncogene, and NF-κB signaling pathways [33]. Of all the carotenoids, lycopene is the most efficient scavenger of oxygen radicals [34]. Experimental studies have revealed that lycopene may decrease the expression of RAS, NF-κB, cyclin D, p-Akt, and Bcl-2, whereas it may increase the expression of p21, p27, p53, and Bax in prostate cancer cells [33]. Lycopene also inhibits IGF-I signal transduction in normal prostate epithelial cells by downregulating DHT-stimulated IGF-I production [35]. Lycopene has been shown to exert antiproliferative effects by inhibiting the cell cycle at the G0/G1 phase [36]. Two prospective studies that correlate lycopene with the risk of prostate cancer have been reported. In a study of men from the Health Professionals' Follow Up Study, Giovannucci et al. found lycopene intake to be significantly associated with a decreased risk of prostate cancer (Relative risk [RR] 0.84; 95% CI, 0.73–0.96; p(trend) = 0.003) [37]. Similarly, Kirsh et al. found that increased intake of lycopene was associated with a decreased risk of prostate cancer, but only in men with a family history of disease [38].

Five case-control studies have been conducted on the effect of lycopene on prostate cancer. Of these, one reported a beneficial effect [39] and four reported no effect [40–43]. In the case-control study by McCann et al., high intake of lycopene was associated with a decreased risk of prostate cancer (OR 0.62; 95% CI, 0.42–0.92) [39]. A meta-analysis of 21 observational studies evaluating the role of lycopene in prostate cancer prevention reported that compared with infrequent consumers of tomato products, individuals who ate large amounts of raw tomato and cooked tomato products had a relative risk of developing prostate cancer of 0.89 (95% CI 0.80–1.00) and 0.81 (95% CI 0.71–0.92), respectively, suggesting that a high intake of tomato products had a modest role in preventing prostate cancer [44]. Conversely, the U.S. Food and Drug Administration (FDA) conducted a meta-analysis of 13 observational studies in 2007 and concluded that the evidence to support a role for tomato and lycopene consumption in reduction of prostate cancer is limited [45]. A clearer role for lycopene may lie in the *progression* of prostate cancer, where it has been observed to inhibit this process. A randomized, double-blind, placebo-controlled study, in which lycopene was administered for 1-year at a dose of 4 mg twice daily, was conducted in 40 patients with evidence of HGPIN at transurethral resection of the prostate. The rate of prostate cancer reduction after 1 year of treatment was 66%. Hence, lycopene was considered to be an effective chemopreventive agent for the treatment of HGPIN, with no toxicity and good tolerability [46].

Another randomized clinical trial studied whether the addition of lycopene supplementation to conventional androgen deprivation therapy for metastatic prostate cancer had any beneficial clinical effect. This study showed that lycopene supplementation may retard the progression of metastatic prostate cancer [47]. Prostate cancer that becomes refractory to androgen deprivation therapy is termed castration-resistant prostate cancer (CRPC). One of the primary therapies used for CRPC is docetaxel [48]. Interestingly, lycopene may potentiate the antitumorigenic activity of docetaxel in prostate cancer in vitro and in vivo [49].

In summary, although there may be some controversy as to the health benefit of lycopene, the majority of studies suggest that lycopene has a chemopreventive effect on the development and progression of prostate cancer.

24.2.2 EGCG (Green Tea)

Green tea is commonly consumed in Asia. It is derived from the plant *Camellia sinensis*. Epigallocatechine-3-gallate (EGCG) is one of the polyphenolic compounds produced from green tea. It has previously been suggested to decrease the risk and retard the progression of prostate cancer in vitro and in vivo. The polyphenolic compounds of green tea are termed catechins, which are comprised of four principal compounds: epicatechin (EC), epigallocatechin (EGC), epicatechin-3-gallate (ECG), and epigallocatechin-3-gallate (EGCG) [50,51]. The most abundant and the best studied polyphenolic compound is EGCG, an antioxidant with 25–100 times greater potency than vitamins C and E [52].

Suggested mechanisms of the antitumorigenic effects of catechin compounds include apoptosis and cell cycle arrest, which occur via alterations in the MAP kinase, phosphatidylinositol-3-kinase (PI3K)/Akt, and protein kinase C pathways; inhibition of the inflammatory pathways (NFκB and cyclooxygenase-2 [COX-2]); and modulation of the insulin-like growth factor (IGF) and AR axes [53,54]. Furthermore, EGCG and ECG have been shown to selectively inhibit type 1 5α-reductase, which converts testosterone into the more potent androgen, dihydrotestosterone [55].

The risk of prostate cancer was observed to decrease with increasing frequency, duration, and quantity of green tea consumption in a study reported by Jian et al. [56]. Moreover, a case-control study has been conducted using a combination of tea and lycopene. The results from the latter study showed that the protective effect of green tea or lycopene was significant and that the protective effect from consuming both green tea and lycopene was synergistic [57].

In a prospective study commencing in 1990 and ending in 2005, 49,920 Japanese men aged 40–69 years were examined for the effect of green tea consumption. This study found that green tea consumption was not correlated with localized prostate cancer; however, it was correlated with a dose-dependent reduction in the risk of advanced prostate cancer [58]. Bettuzzi et al. found that after 1 year of supplementation with green tea catechins, prostate cancer was significantly less prevalent compared to controls (3.3% vs. 30%, $p < 0.01$) [59]. In a follow-up to this study, men in the treatment group were found to have a significantly lower incidence of prostate cancer compared to those in the control group [60]. A meta-analysis supported these findings by showing that green tea but not black tea could exert protective effects against prostate cancer, especially in Asian populations [61].

A clinical trial was conducted to study the metabolism and bioactivity of green tea polyphenols in human prostate tissue. Men with clinically localized prostate cancer consumed six cups of green tea ($n = 8$) daily or water ($n = 9$) for 3–6 weeks before undergoing radical prostatectomy [62]. Using high-performance liquid chromatography, 4″-*O*-methyl EGCG (4″-MeEGCG) and EGCG were identified in comparable amounts, and EGCG was identified in lower amounts in prostatectomy tissue from men consuming green tea. Green tea polyphenols were not detected in prostate tissue or urine from men consuming water preoperatively. In the urine of men consuming green tea, 50%–60% of both EGC and EC were present in methylated form, with 4′-*O*-MeEGC being the major methylated form of (–)-epigallocatechin. When incubated with EGCG, LNCaP cells (cells from an androgen-sensitive human prostate adenocarcinoma cell line) were able to methylate EGCG to 4″-MeEGCG. The capacity of 4″-MeEGCG to inhibit proliferation and NF-κB activation and induce apoptosis in LNCaP cells was decreased significantly compared with EGCG. This study shows that methylated and nonmethylated forms of EGCG are detectable in prostate tissue following a short-term green tea intervention and that the methylation status of EGCG may potentially modulate its preventive effect on prostate cancer, possibly based on genetic polymorphisms of catechol *O*-methyltransferase [62].

In summary, green tea may have some benefit in the prevention of prostate cancer at normal daily doses (5–10 cups/day), and purified EGCG can be used as an alternative to brewed tea. However, a large randomized placebo-controlled trial is certainly needed before any clear recommendations can be made.

24.2.3 Isothiocyanates (Cruciferous Vegetables)

Cruciferous vegetables, which are named for their cross-shaped flowers, contain isothiocyanates, chemical compounds that impart a distinctive bitter taste. Some examples of the cruciferous vegetable group are cabbage, broccoli, brussel sprouts, cauliflower, and wasabi. Epidemiological studies suggest that the consumption of cruciferous vegetables, such as broccoli and cauliflower, is inversely related to prostate cancer risk [63–66].

The isothiocyanates have a marked effect on signal transduction. They induce cell cycle arrest, inhibit tumor invasion and angiogenesis, mediate extracellular signal-regulated kinases both in vitro and in vivo, and exhibit anti-inflammatory effects [67–69]. Recently, Bosetti et al. looked at seven cohort and six population-based case-control studies. They found that the overall risk for prostate cancer was significantly decreased in the cruciferous vegetable intake group (RR = 0.90; 95% confidence interval 0.85–0.96), but not in the subgroup of cohort studies [70].

Cruciferous vegetables also exert inhibitory effects on the progression of prostate cancer. The association between prostate cancer risk and intake of fruits and vegetables was evaluated in 1338 patients with prostate cancer among 29,361 men (average follow-up = 4.2 years) in the screening arm of the Prostate, Lung, Colorectal, and Ovarian Cancer Screening Trial. While vegetable and fruit consumption were not related to prostate cancer risk overall, the risk of extraprostatic prostate cancer (stage III or IV tumors) decreased with increasing vegetable intake (RR = 0.41, 95% CI = 0.22–0.74, for high vs. low intake; p(trend) = 0.01). This association was mainly accounted for by the intake of cruciferous vegetables (RR = 0.60, 95% CI = 0.36–0.98, for high vs. low intake; P(trend) = 0.02), in particular, broccoli (RR = 0.55, 95% CI = 0.34–0.89, for >1 serving per week vs. <1 serving per month; p(trend) = 0.02) and cauliflower (RR = 0.48, 95% CI = 0.25–0.89 for >1 serving per week vs. <1 serving per month; p(trend) = 0.03) [71].

Therefore, high intake of cruciferous vegetables, including broccoli and cauliflower, may be associated with reduced risk of aggressive prostate cancer, particularly extraprostatic disease. Another study prospectively examined whether intake of total vegetables, and specifically cruciferous vegetables, after diagnosis reduced the risk of prostate cancer progression among 1560 men diagnosed with nonmetastatic prostate cancer participating in the Cancer of the Prostate Strategic Urologic Research Endeavor, a United States prostate cancer registry. The participants were diagnosed primarily at community-based clinics and followed for 5 years. In this prospective analysis, 134 events of progression (i.e. 53 biochemical [only PSA] recurrences, 71 secondary treatments likely due to recurrence, six bone metastases, and four prostate cancer deaths) were shown during 3171 person-years. Men in the fourth (highest) quartile of post-diagnostic cruciferous vegetable intake had a statistically significant 59% decreased risk of prostate cancer progression compared with men in the lowest quartile (hazard ratio [HR]: 0.41; 95% confidence interval [CI]: 0.22, 0.76; p(trend): 0.003). No other vegetable or fruit group was statistically significantly associated with risk of prostate cancer progression. This study showed that post-diagnostic cruciferous vegetable intake significantly decreased the risk of prostate cancer progression [72]. This reduction in risk by cruciferous vegetable intake may be modulated by glutathione *S*-transferase mu 1 (GSTM1) genotype. One study showed that individuals who possessed at least one GSTM1 allele (i.e. approximately 50% of the population) gained more benefit than those who had a homozygous deletion of GSTM1 [73]. To see whether the genotype of GSTM1 indeed affects the preventive effects of cruciferous vegetables, a study investigating the changes of global gene expression patterns in the human prostate gland before, during, and after a 12-month broccoli-rich diet was conducted. Volunteers diagnosed with HGPIN were randomly assigned to either a broccoli-rich or a pea-rich diet. After 6 months, there were no differences in gene expression between glutathione *S*-transferase mu 1 (GSTM1) positive and null individuals on the pea-rich diet but significant differences between GSTM1 genotypes and null individuals on the broccoli-rich diet, associated with transforming growth factor beta 1 (TGF-β1) and epidermal growth factor (EGF) signaling pathways. Men on the broccoli diet had additional changes in mRNA processing, as well as TGF-β1, EGF, and insulin signaling. These findings suggest that broccoli consumption in subjects with GSTM1 genotype results in complex changes in signaling pathways associated with inflammation and carcinogenesis in the prostate. This unique study demonstrates that the effect of nutraceutical therapy differs based on the genotype of the specific gene [74].

24.2.4 Tocopherols (Vitamin E)

Vitamin E denotes a family of four tocopherols (alpha tocopherol is most active in humans) and four tocotrienols with antiproliferative properties. The tocopherols are most abundant in nuts and vegetable oils, whereas tocotrienols are found in palm oil, oat, rye, wheat, and rice bran. Their strong antioxidant and inhibitory properties have been postulated to play a chemopreventive role in the development of many cancers. The most abundant form of vitamin E in the Western diet is gamma tocopherol (found in soy oil); yet, alpha tocopherol (found in olive and sunflower oil) has been most studied as it is the biologically predominant form in humans and the most common form used in supplements. Multiple preclinical studies suggest that vitamin E slows tumor growth, partly by inhibiting DNA synthesis and inducing apoptotic pathways [75].

Data regarding the impact of alpha tocopherol supplementation on the prevention of prostate cancer come from the Alpha-Tocopherol, Beta-Carotene Cancer Prevention Study (ATBC) [76]. This study found that alpha tocopherol supplementation decreased both the risk and mortality of prostate cancer. After a median follow-up of 6 years, there was a 34% reduction in the incidence of prostate cancer and a 41% reduction in prostate cancer mortality among Finnish male smokers randomized to vitamin E (alpha tocopherol) supplementation. No significant difference was seen in nonsmokers given vitamin E and no beneficial effects were seen with vitamin A. However, this effect was later found to be attenuated [77]. Two observational studies (the Cancer Prevention Study II Nutrition Cohort and the NIH-AARP Diet and Health Study) both showed no association between vitamin E supplementation and prostate cancer risk [78,79].

A prospective randomized trial, the Selenium and Vitamin E Cancer Prevention Trial (SELECT), accrued 35,000 men and randomized them into four groups (selenium, vitamin E, selenium plus vitamin E, and placebo). Among the inclusion criteria were PSA level ≤4 ng/mL and negative digital rectal examination. After a follow-up period of 5.5 years, a total of 1758 men were diagnosed with prostate cancer, with no significant differences between groups. By contrast, an insignificant trend toward increased risk of prostate cancer was seen in the vitamin E group ($P = 0.06$) [80].

The Physicians' Health Study II randomized 14,641 male physicians in the United States to receive either vitamin E plus vitamin C, vitamin E (plus placebo), vitamin C (plus placebo), or placebo only. In contrast to SELECT, patients were not screened for prostate cancer before enrolment and 1307 men with a history of cancer were included [81]. After a mean follow-up of 8.0 years, 1008 new prostate cancers were diagnosed and no significant differences in incidence of prostate cancer (or other cancers) were noted between groups. Based on these studies, it should be fair to say that supplementation with alpha tocopherol has no preventive effects against the development of prostate cancer.

The NIH-AARP Diet and Health Study prospectively examined the relationships between supplemental vitamin E intake and dietary intake of alpha, beta, gamma, and delta tocopherols to prostate cancer risk among 295,344 men, ages 50–71 years. During 5 years of follow-up, 10,241 incident prostate cancers were identified. Supplemental vitamin E intake was not found to be related to prostate cancer risk. However, dietary gamma tocopherol, the most commonly consumed form of vitamin E in Western countries, was significantly inversely related to the risk of advanced prostate cancer (for highest vs. lowest quintile: RR, 0.68; 95% CI, 0.56–0.84; P(trend) = 0.001). This result indicated that increased consumption of gamma-tocopherol from foods is associated with a reduced risk of clinically relevant disease [82].

However, another study demonstrated that circulating gamma tocopherol levels may also be associated with an increased risk of high-grade disease at diagnosis [83]. This study measured circulating alpha and gamma tocopherol and genotyped 30 single nucleotide polymorphism (SNP) in SOD1, SOD2, SOD3, TTPA, and SEC14L2 among 573 men with organ-confined prostate cancer who underwent radical prostatectomy. Associations between circulating vitamin E, genotypes, and risk of high-grade prostate cancer (Gleason grade ≥8 or 7 with primary score ≥4; n = 117), and risk of recurrence (56 events; 3.7 years median follow-up) were evaluated. In this study, circulating gamma tocopherol was associated with an increased risk of high-grade prostate cancer (Q4 v. Q1 odds ratio [OR] = 1.87; 95% confidence intervals [CI]: 0.97–3.58; P(trend) = 0.02). The less common allele in SOD3 rs699473 was associated with an increased risk of high-grade disease (T > C: OR = 1.40, 95% CI: 1.04–1.89). Two independent SNPs in SOD1 were inversely associated with prostate cancer recurrence in additive models (rs17884057 hazard ratio [HR] = 0.49, 95% CI: 0.25–0.96;

rs9967983 HR = 0.62, 95% CI: 0.40–0.95). They found that germ line genetic variation in genes of enzymes associated with detoxification of free radicals may be associated with the risk of high-grade disease at diagnosis and disease recurrence, which might suggest consideration of such genotypes in the interpretation of vitamin E supplementation trials such as SELECT.

24.2.5 Isoflavones (Soy)

Soy products contain isoflavones. Soy isoflavones are classified as phytoestrogens. They have been suggested to modulate endogenous hormone homeostasis because their phenolic ring structures resemble estradiol and can bind to estrogen receptors, acting as either an estrogen agonist or antagonist [11]. Soy isoflavones alter the activities of enzymes involved in hormone metabolism [12]. The primary isoflavones in soybeans are genistein, daidzein, and glycitein. Genistein, the predominant isoflavone in the human diet, is derived mainly from soybeans but is also found in other legumes, including peas, lentils, or other bean varieties [84].

Several mechanisms have been proposed to explain the anticarcinogenic activity of genistein: inhibition of protein-tyrosine kinase (PTK), with the result of alleviating the growth of cancer cells by inhibiting PTK-mediated signaling mechanisms; inhibition of topoisomerase I and II and protein histidine kinase, which have antiproliferative or proapoptotic effects; antioxidant effects through inhibition of the expression of stress-response related genes; inhibition of NF-κB and Akt signaling pathways, both of which are important for cell survival; inhibition of angiogenesis; downregulation of TGF-β; and the inhibition of EGF [85–88].

Epidemiological studies have shown that Asian countries have low rates of prostate cancer incidence and high rates of soy consumption [1]. Daily isoflavone intake in Japan has been estimated to be 25–50 mg/day of aglycone equivalents [89], compared with <1 mg in Europe [90], and 3 mg/day in the UK [91].

In 2005, Yan and Spitznagel published a meta-analysis of papers on the relationship between soy and prostate cancer [92]. Collectively, the results show a relative risk/odds ratio for prostate cancer of 0.74 (95% CI 0.63–0.89; P = 0.01) with consumption of all types of soy products. Specifically, studies using nonfermented soy revealed a significant reduction in prostate cancer risk, whereas studies using fermented soy (miso soup or nattō) or isoflavone supplementation did not find significant results. In fact, the combined relative risk/odds ratio of fermented soy studies was 1.10 (95% CI 0.76–1.57) [93]. Additionally, soy consumption was correlated with a significantly lower mortality rate from prostate cancer.

The protective properties of soy against prostate cancer are not only apparent in low-intake populations, but also among high soy consumers. Even among Japanese men with a relatively high soy intake compared with Caucasians, higher soy consumption is associated with a decrease in localized prostate cancer [94]. In a population-based prospective study in 43,509 Japanese men, consumption of soy products and isoflavone supplements was found to be associated with a reduced risk of localized prostate cancer [94]. On further analysis of the isoflavone studies, significant risk reductions were found in Asian men, while studies in Western populations yielded no affect on prostate cancer risk [95].

The clinical effectiveness of soy protein may depend on the individual's ability to biotransform soy isoflavones to equol. Equol is converted from daidzein by human intestinal flora and is biologically more active than any other isoflavone aglycone, but only 35% of humans are equol-producers [96]. The capacity to produce equol has been found be to lower among American men compared with Japanese and Korean men [97]. Studies in Asian men have reported that lower concentrations of equol, a metabolite of daidzein in the gut, or a lower prevalence of equol-producers among men, are risk factors for prostate cancer [97–100]. Thus, the ability to produce equol or equol, itself, may be closely related to the low incidence of prostate cancer in Asia [97,98]. A significant association was found between decreased risk of prostate cancer and presence of isoflavones and/or equol-producers among Japanese men. The authors suggested that it may be possible to increase the proportion of equol-producers by altering the intestinal flora as a possible strategy for reducing the risk of prostate cancer [101]. Unfortunately, however, the proportion of equol producers is decreasing in younger generations of Korea and Japan, representing a potential new risk factor for prostate cancer [102].

The results of a meta-analysis of two case-controlled studies showed that higher doses of the isoflavone, genistein, were associated with a statistically significant lower risk of prostate cancer in one study and marginal significance in the other [1]. A recent systematic review included eight randomized controlled trials. Meta-analyses of the two studies that only included men with identified risk of prostate cancer found a significant reduction in prostate cancer diagnosis following administration of soy/soy isoflavones. The other six studies included patients already diagnosed with prostate cancer and no significant benefit was identified [103].

24.2.5.1 Mode of Action of Soy Isoflavones on Prostate Cancer

24.2.5.1.1 Androgen Receptor

Uncontrolled AR gene amplification, AR mutations, and increase of AR expression is a selective driving force for the progression of prostate cancer to the hormone refractory state. Soy isoflavones, or genistein, downregulate the AR and inhibit several steroid-metabolizing enzymes, such as 5-α-reductase or aromatase, thereby creating a more favorable hormonal milieu and a protective effect against prostate cancer. Soy isoflavones also block cell cycle progression at G1 and inhibit PSA expression [87,104]. Soy isoflavones inhibit PSA secretion in androgen-sensitive human prostate adenocarcinoma (LNCaP) cells [105].

Reduction of testosterone levels and downregulation of AR gene expression in the prostate have been observed [105] in animal models. Isoflavone could significantly inhibit the activation of AR, Akt, and NF-κB in prostate cancer cells and interrupt the cross talk between these three signaling pathways in vitro [106–113]. Isoflavone could also inhibit growth of the epithelial-to-mesenchymal transition (EMT) type of prostate cancer cells through inhibition of Wnt signaling [114].

24.2.5.1.2 Cell Proliferation and Apoptosis

The mechanisms of action of soy isoflavones include in vitro modulation of cell proliferation, cell cycle regulation, apoptosis, angiogenesis, tumor cell invasion, and tumor metastasis by genistein [115]. Soy isoflavones and curcumin inhibit the growth of LNCaP cells and DU 145 cells [116–118].

24.2.5.1.3 Cell Cycle

Soy isoflavones have an impact on the cell cycle of prostate cancer cells. In one study, genistein caused dose- and time-dependent G2/M phase cell cycle arrest with increased WAF1/p21 and decreased cyclin B1 expression [119]. In another study, genistein reduced MDM2 protein and mRNA levels in prostate cancer cells by inducing ubiquitination of MDM2, which leads to apoptosis, G2 arrest, and inhibition of cell proliferation [120]. Genistein also has been shown to upregulate p21 in prostate cancer cells [121]

24.2.5.1.4 Protein Kinases

Soy isoflavone functions as a tyrosine kinase inhibitor. It produces anticancer effects including apoptosis and inhibition of cell growth in prostate cancer cell lines and animal studies [122]. Genistein inhibits activation of p38 MAPK and FAK (promotility proteins) in vivo, and has been shown to block cell motility and prevent metastasis in an in vivo model [123]. The phosphatidylinositol 3-kinase (PI3 K)/Akt (protein kinase B)/mammalian target of rapamycin (mTOR) signaling pathway plays a central role in tumorigenesis and is often dysregulated in metastatic prostate cancers through the mutation of the phosphatase and tensin homolog (PTEN), which leads to the constitutive activation of Akt [124].

24.2.5.1.5 *Epigenetics*

Abnormalities in DNA methylation, histone modification, and microRNAs have been implicated in the carcinogenesis and progression of prostate cancer [125,126]. Genistein has been identified to target epigenetic regulation by modulating the expression of specific oncogenic microRNAs [127].

24.2.5.1.6 *Inflammation*

Inflammation is implicated as a major risk factor for prostate cancer. Cells that mediate inflammatory responses are major contributors to the in vivo production of reactive oxygen species (ROS), such as superoxide, nitric oxide, hydrogen peroxide, and hypochloric acid. High concentrations and the persistent presence of these ROS are mutagenic and can lead to tissue damage. Population studies have found an increased relative risk of prostate cancer in men with prior histories of prostatitis (inflammation of the prostate) [128]. Inflammatory pathways including the cyclooxygenase-2 (COX-2) and nuclear factor kappa B (NF-κB) are overexpressed in human prostate adenocarcinomas compared with normal prostate tissues [129,130]. The modulation of cellular signaling involved in the inflammatory response, especially targeting the NF-κB pathway, seems to be an important strategy for chemoprevention, since constitutive activation of NF-κB has been implicated in prostate cancer progression [131]. Genistein inhibits constitutive NF-κB/Ap-1 activities in prostate cancer PC3 cells [132]. These inhibitory effects are cancer cell specific because nontumorigenic prostate epithelial cells are not affected by genistein [132,133].

24.2.5.1.7 *Antioxidant Activity*

Oxygen radicals may cause damage to DNA and chromosomes, induce epigenetic alterations, interact with oncogenes or tumor suppressor genes, and impart changes in immunological mechanisms that promote carcinogenesis. Genistein confers an antioxidant effect on prostate cancer cells by inducing glutathione peroxidase [134].

24.2.5.1.8 *Animal Models*

Experiments with animal models of prostate carcinogenesis suggest that soy isoflavones reduce the risk of progression of prostate cancer [135–139].

24.2.5.2 Clinical Applications of Soy Isoflavones

Daily consumption of soy food has been shown to decrease prostate-specific antigen (PSA) levels in prostate cancer patients [140]. Short-term administration of soy isoflavones stimulated the production of serum equol and decreased serum DHT levels in healthy Japanese volunteers [141]. In a phase II, randomized, double-blind, placebo-controlled trial, isoflavone (60 mg/day) or placebo was administered for 12 months to Japanese men between 50 and 75 years of age who had serum PSA levels between 2.5 and 10.0 ng/mL, and a single negative prostate biopsy within 12 months prior to enrollment. In this study, the incidence of cancer in the isoflavone group was significantly lower than in the placebo group for patients aged 65 years or more [142].

The effect of soy supplementation on biologically significant prostate cancer in a randomized trial in men who were at high risk of recurrence after radical prostatectomy was investigated. The objective was to determine whether daily consumption of a soy protein-based supplement for 2 years reduced the rate of recurrence or delayed recurrence after radical prostatectomy using PSA failure as the intermediate end point. Participants were randomized to receive a daily serving of a beverage powder containing 20 g of protein in the form of either soy protein isolate ($n = 87$) or, as placebo, calcium caseinate ($n = 90$). The main outcomes were biochemical recurrence rate of prostate cancer (defined as development of PSA level $\geq$0.07 ng/mL) over the first 2 years following randomization and time to recurrence. However, the trial was stopped prematurely for lack of treatment effect at a planned interim analysis, with 81 evaluable participants in the intervention group and 78 in the placebo group. Overall, 28.3% of participants developed biochemical recurrence within 2 years of entering the trial (close to the a priori predicted recurrence rate of 30%). Among these, 22 (27.2%)

occurred in the intervention group and 23 (29.5%) in the placebo group. Daily consumption of a beverage powder supplement containing soy protein isolate for 2 years following radical prostatectomy did not reduce the biochemical recurrence of prostate cancer in men at high risk of PSA failure [143].

Prostate cancer chemoprevention treatments are likely to be initiated in middle-aged men, although as many as 50% already have small prostate cancers by this time [144,145]. Thus, it is plausible that soy is protective against prostate cancer when consumption begins early in life but not later or when prostate cancer is already present [143,145].

A pilot study to investigate the effects of soy isoflavone supplementation on acute and subacute toxicity (≤6 months) of external beam radiation therapy (EBRT) in patients with localized prostate cancer was conducted. Men with early stage prostate cancer undergoing EBRT received treatment to the entire prostate and the caudal portion of the seminal vesicles. The hypothesis was that since tissue toxicities of radiation are due to oxidation-induced vascular changes and inflammation, the antioxidant and anti-inflammatory effects of soy isoflavones would prevent radiation injury to normal tissues. In this study, patients with prostate cancer were randomly assigned to receive 200 mg soy isoflavone or placebo daily for 6 months beginning with the first day of radiation therapy. EBRT was administered in 1.8–2.5 Gy fractions for a total of 73.8–77.5 Gy. Patients receiving soy isoflavones during and after EBRT showed better PSA level reduction and decreased incidence of urinary, gastrointestinal, and erectile dysfunction compared to those patients receiving placebo [146]. The results suggested that soy isoflavones taken in conjunction with radiation therapy could mitigate radiation injury to adjacent normal tissues. This is a novel approach using safe dietary agents to enhance the efficacy of radiotherapy.

24.2.6 Curcumin (Diferuloylmethane)

Curcumin (diferuloylmethane) is a major chemical component of turmeric (*Curcuma longa* Linn.). Used as a spice in the Indian subcontinent, it adds flavor and yellow color to food. It has been used for centuries throughout Asia, not only as a food additive, but also in cosmetics and as a traditional herbal medicine, especially in the Ayurvedic, Chinese, and Hindu cultures, where it is used to treat a variety of inflammatory conditions and chronic diseases. Numerous studies have substantiated the anticarcinogenic properties and potential prophylactic or therapeutic value of curcumin [147]. Indeed, curcumin possesses antioxidant [148–150], anti-inflammatory [151], antiproliferative [152], and antiangiogenic [153] effects. Curcumin, therefore, may also be an effective chemopreventive agent when used as a nontoxic dietary supplement [154]. In prostate cancer cells, curcumin inhibits both constitutive and inducible activation of NF-κB, enhanced TNFα-induced apoptosis associated with decreased expression of Bcl-2 and Bcl-xL, and increased expression of procaspase-3 and -8 [155].

24.2.6.1 Mode of Action of Curcumin on Prostate Cancer

24.2.6.1.1 Androgen Receptor

Curcumin downregulates AR expression and AR-binding activity to the androgen response element of the PSA protein gene. It also downregulates PSA expression in LNCaP cells [104,156–158]. Curcumin interrupts the interaction between AR and Wnt/β-catenin signaling pathways in prostate cancer cells. The transcriptional activity of the AR is modulated by interaction with coregulators, one of which is β-catenin. Curcumin inhibits the Wnt/β-catenin signaling pathway and attenuates the phosphorylation of Akt and glycogen synthase kinase-3β [159].

Downregulation of AR expression and blockage of its DNA-binding activity by curcumin lead to the inhibition of the homeobox gene NKX3.1 [160]. This gene plays a pivotal role in normal prostate organogenesis and carcinogenesis [161].

24.2.6.1.2 Cell Proliferation and Apoptosis

Curcumin induces apoptosis in prostate cancer cells in response to cellular signals including stress or DNA damage. Curcumin is able to downregulate apoptosis suppressor proteins, such as Bcl-2 and

Bcl-xL, upregulate pro-apoptotic proteins from the Bcl-2 family (Bim, Bax, Bak, Puma, and Noxa), and activate caspases to induce apoptosis [155,156]. Curcumin also downregulates murine double minute 2 (MDM2) protein and mRNA, an important negative regulator of the p53 tumor suppressor that permits prostate cancer cells to undergo apoptosis [162]. The combination of isoflavones and curcumin has a more potent inhibitory effect on cell proliferation than isoflavones alone [118].

24.2.6.1.3 Protein Kinases

Curcumin inhibits the phosphorylation of mTOR in prostate cancer cells [162,163] and phosphatidyl-inositol-3 kinase (PI3K) [164]. Curcumin inhibits angiogenesis in vitro and in vivo [165,166]. The epithelial growth factor receptor (EGFR) family, including HER2, is an important mediator of cell proliferation and is highly expressed in prostate cancer cells where it is associated with poor prognosis [167]. Curcumin is a potent inhibitor of EGFR signaling as it downregulates EGFR expression and inhibits EGFR tyrosine kinase activity, as well as the ligand-induced activation of EGFR on LNCaP and PC-3 cells [164,168–170].

24.2.6.1.4 Cell Cycle

Cyclin D1 is a proto-oncogene that plays an important role in cell proliferation through the activation of cyclin-dependant kinases and is required for the progression of cells from the G1 to the S phase. Curcumin has been shown to downregulate cyclin D1 expression through activation of both transcriptional and post-transcriptional mechanisms in LNCaP prostate cancer cells [171]. A similar effect on cell cycle arrest in G1/S phase was also observed in DU145 and PC-3 cells. This effect was observed not only through the upregulation of the expression of cyclin-dependent kinase (CDK) inhibitors p16, p21, and p27 and the inhibition of the expression of cyclin E and cyclin D1, but also through the hyperphosphorylation of retinoblastoma (Rb) protein [172]. Curcumin inhibits prostate cell proliferation of LNCaP cell tumors implanted in nude mice, accompanying the induction of p21 and p27 and the inhibition of cyclin D1 [166,173]. Curcumin induces arrest in G2/M phase in PC-3 and LNCaP cells [174].

24.2.6.1.5 Antioxidant Activity and Inflammation

Curcumin confers its antioxidant properties through the induction of phase II enzymes (glutathione *S*-transferase, heme oxygenase), especially by the regulation of the transcription factor Nrf2 (nuclear factor-erythroid 2-related factor 2 erythroid) [148,175]. Curcumin inhibits NF-kB activation in prostate cancer cell lines [155,176].

24.2.6.2 Clinical Applications of Curcumin

Few clinical data about curcumin have been performed in humans, despite the large number of in vitro and animals studies. In a pilot study of a standardized oral *Curcuma* extract, doses of up to 180 mg of curcumin per day were administered to patients with advanced colorectal cancer for up to 4 months without overt toxicity or detectable systemic bioavailability [177]. A subsequent study has suggested that doses up to 8 g could be administered daily to patients with premalignant lesions for 3 months without overt toxicity [178]. The clinical advancement of this promising natural compound is hampered by its poor water solubility and short biological half-life, resulting in low bioavailability in both plasma and tissues [179]. In fact, after oral administration of free curcumin (up to 12 g/day), only nanomolar concentrations of curcumin or corresponding metabolites were found in patient serum [178,180]. On the other hand, low concentrations of curcumin were able to achieve a similar biological impact on NF-kB, COX-2, and phosphoSTAT-3 in peripheral blood mononuclear cells derived from treated patients compared with the ones observed in vitro with 5–50 μM of curcumin [181,182].

Curcumin has been shown to augment the antitumor efficacy of chemotherapeutics in prostate cancer cells. In combination with taxane, curcumin treatment decreased the resistance of prostate cancer cells to taxane and increased the inhibitory efficacy of taxane in hormone-refractory prostate cancer cells, suggesting that combination treatment with curcumin and taxane could have beneficial effects for the treatment of hormone-refractory prostate cancer [183]. Moreover, curcumin may also sensitize prostate cancer cells to radiotherapy. In prostate cancer cells, radiation could upregulate the expression of TNF-α and, in turn, induce NF-κB activity, leading to the induction of Bcl-2 protein and resistance to radiation. Importantly, curcumin in combination with radiation therapy caused significant inhibition of TNF-α-induced NF-κB activity with downregulation of Bcl-2, resulting in significant induction of apoptosis [184]. The limitation of curcumin for clinical use is its poor bioavailability. Therefore, it would be important to synthesize curcumin analogues or nanoparticles with high bioavailability and efficacy. Recent development of nanoparticle curcumin with increased water solubility (named THERACURMIN) shows promise for future clinical trials in the prevention or treatment of prostate cancer [185].

24.3 COMBINED TREATMENT WITH SOY ISOFLAVONES AND CURCUMIN

In a double-blind, placebo-controlled study, subjects with high PSA levels but negative pathologic findings on prostate biopsy received either isoflavones (40 mg) and curcumin (100 mg) or placebo for 6 months. Isoflavones contained 66% daidzen, 24% glycitin, and 10% genistein. PSA levels were significantly decreased in the supplement-treated subgroup compared with the placebo group but only in those subjects whose baseline PSA levels were over 10 ng/mL [104].

24.3.1 Effects of Soy Isoflavones and Curcumin on DNA Damage Response (DDR)

Recent evidence has emerged that the DDR is one of the earliest events to impede the multistep progression of human epithelial carcinomas to invasive malignancy. DNA damage can be due to a variety of factors, such as telomere dysfunction or oncogene-induced replication stress [30,31]. The signaling pathways activated during DDR have three critical goals: (1) halting cell cycle progression and division to prevent transfer of DNA damage to progeny cells; (2) increasing the accessibility of damage sites to, and engagement of, the DNA damage repair machinery, and (3) triggering apoptosis to exterminate cells with DNA damage that is beyond repair [186]. Early precursor lesions commonly express markers of an activated DDR [30,31]. These markers include phosphorylated kinases (i.e. ataxia-telangiectasia-mutated kinase [ATM] and checkpoint kinase2 [Chk2]), phosphorylated histone H2AX, and phosphorylated p53. Such activation of the DDR network leads to senescence or death of oncogene-transformed cells, which delays or prevents cancer progression. Epithelial cells within premalignant lesions that have markers of senescence maintain an intact response to cellular stress and are less likely to develop subsequent tumors. Conversely, the DDR is not only invoked, but also dysfunctional at an early stage in the development of neoplasia. Markers of double strand breaks (DSBs), such as nuclear γH2AX foci (a histone phosphorylation event that occurs on chromatin surrounding a DSB), are markedly elevated in some precancerous lesions [187,188]. One hypothesis proposes that the original cause of these effects is oncogene activation [188]. The activation of oncogenes such as MYC and RAS stimulates the firing of multiple replication forks as part of a proliferative program. For precancerous lesions to progress to mature tumors, it is thought that critical DSB signal transduction and cell-cycle checkpoint proteins, such as ataxia telangiectasia mutation (ATM), ataxia telangiectasis Rad3-related (ATR), and the master "gatekeeper" protein, p53, must become inactivated. With these DDR components rendered dysfunctional, collapsed forks are not effectively repaired and cells proceed through the cell cycle with DNA lesions intact, increasing the chance of mutagenesis [187,188]. The 370 kDa Serine (Ser)/Threonine (Thr) kinase ATM has begun to emerge as a central DNA damage checkpoint against cancer predisposition [189]. ATM is a member of the phosphoinositide 3-kinase-related protein kinase (PIKK) family to which the master regulator of cell growth and metabolism, the mammalian target of Rapamycin (mTOR) pathway, also belongs. ATM is a well-known primary regulator of the cellular response to DNA DSBs. Simultaneously, a number of studies have recently established that oxidative stress also

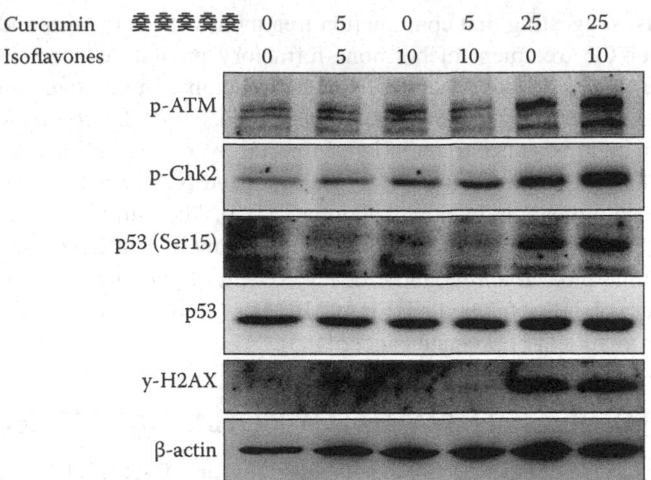

FIGURE 24.2 Isoflavones and curcumin synergistically induce phosphorylation of ataxia-telangiectasia-mutated kinase (ATM), checkpoint kinase2 (Chk2), p53 (Ser15) and H2AX in the LNCaP cells. (From Ide, H., et al., *Prostate*, 70, 1127, 2010.)

activates ATM, even in the absence of DSBs. In response to oxidative stress, ATM is phosphorylated at Ser-1981, which results in phosphorylation of its substrates, including p53, the master controller of DNA metabolic stresses, and AMP-activated protein kinase-α (AMPKα), the key sensor of fuel and energy status [190].

Type 2 diabetes has been associated with an elevated level of DNA damage and with the decreased efficacy of DNA repair [190]. This can contribute to genomic instability in type 2 diabetics and, consequently, to cancer promotion and progression. Indeed cancer risk in type 2 diabetic patients is high. However, recent studies show that metformin significantly diminishes the risk of developing cancer in type 2 diabetic patients [191]. One causal linkage between metformin's mechanism

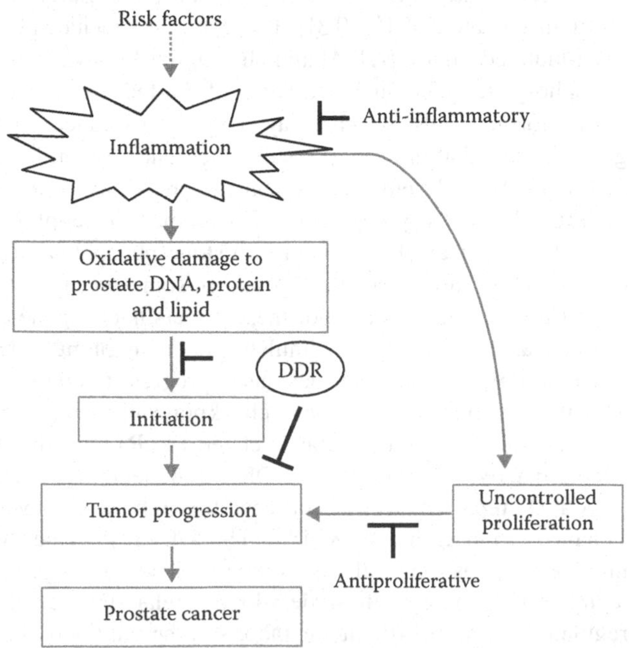

FIGURE 24.3 **(See color insert.)** Chemopreventive actions of soy isoflavones and curcumin.

of action and metformin's cancer-preventive effects might be the activation of DDR. Metformin promotes activation of ATM and ATM targets such as the protein kinase Chk2 [32].

We recently reported that soy isoflavones and curcumin activate the DDR in LNCaP cells by inducing phosphorylation of ATM, histone H2AX, Chk2, and p53, which leads to apoptosis. Combined treatment with isoflavones and curcumin conveys an additive effect. Interestingly, testosterone augments activation of the DDR as well as PARP cleavage induced by curcumin that is dependent on the AR. Thus, testosterone given in combination with this polyphenol may have suppressive effects on the progression of prostate cancer [118]. Similarly, resveratrol, a polyphenol found in berries, nuts, and red wine, has been shown to activate the DDR pathways in ovarian carcinoma cells [192] (Figure 24.2).

Because DDR is the major innate tumor suppressor barrier in early human tumorigenesis, selective activation of DDR surveillance mechanisms by polyphenols may therefore directly contribute to their cancer-preventive effects (Figure 24.3) [193]. This provides a rationale for the clinical application of curcumin and isoflavones for the chemoprevention of prostate cancer.

24.4 CONCLUSIONS

Identifying the key proteins involved in carcinogenesis is an essential prerequisite to establishing an effective chemoprevention strategy. Nutraceuticals have been shown to inhibit the growth of cell proliferation in prostate cancer by modulating specific targets. Epidemiological studies have shown the preventive effects of nutraceuticals on the development of prostate cancer in case-control, prospective, and interventional studies. However, the results of clinical studies are often inconsistent. The modalities and detection criteria of prostate cancer differ from time to time and from country to country. Furthermore, genetic or environmental variations also modulate the metabolism of nutraceuticals. Soy isoflavones and curcumin exert DDR effects in prostate cancer cells. Determining whether or not nutraceuticals are capable of inducing DDR in precancerous regions would provide a rationale for the clinical application of specific nutraceuticals for the chemoprevention of prostate cancer. To translate the demonstrated efficacy of dietary agents measured in vitro to clinical practice, attention should be given to defining physiologically relevant concentrations and chronic exposure times under in vivo conditions. To date, however, no single nutraceutical has been confirmed to have preventive effects for the development of prostate cancer in vivo. Indeed, it may be impractical to predict the chemopreventive effect of a single functional food factor, whereas increased focus on the synergistic effect of combining functional food factors or multiple nutrients may yield a more plausible approach.

REFERENCES

1. Namiki M, Akaza H, Lee SE et al. Prostate cancer working group report. *Jpn J Clin Oncol* 2010; 40:70–75.
2. Shavers VL, Underwood W, Moser RP. Race/ethnicity and the perception of the risk of developing prostate cancer. *Am J Prev Med* 2009; 37(1):64–67.
3. Parkin DM, Bray F, Ferlay J, Pisani P. Global cancer statistics, 2002. *CA Cancer J Clin* 2005; 55:74–108.
4. Gronberg H. Prostate cancer epidemiology. *Lancet* 2003; 361:859–864.
5. Whittemore AS, Kolonel LN, Wu AH et al. Prostate cancer in relation to diet, physical activity, and body size in blacks, whites, and Asians in the United States and Canada. *J Natl Cancer Inst* 1995; 87:652–661.
6. Baade PD, Youlden DR, Krnjacki LJ. International epidemiology of prostate cancer: Geographical distribution and secular trends. *Mol Nutr Food Res* 2009; 53:171–184.
7. Lieberman R, Bermejo C, Akaza H et al. Progress in prostate cancer chemoprevention: Modulators of promotion and progression. *Urology* 2001; 58:835–842.
8. Kalra EK. Nutraceutical definition and introduction. *AAPS Pharm Sci* 2003; 5, E25.
9. Grainger EM, Kim HS, Monk JP et al. Consumption of dietary supplements and over-the-counter and prescription medications in men participating in the prostate cancer prevention trial at an academic center. *Urol Oncol* 2008; 26(2):125–132.

10. Boon H, Brown JB, Gavin A, Westlake K. The use of complementary/alternative health care by men with prostate cancer. *Focus Alternat Complement Ther* 2002; 7(1):85–86.
11. Velicer CM, Ulrich CM. Vitamin and mineral supplement use among US adults after cancer diagnosis: A systematic review. *J Clin Oncol* 2008; 26(4):665–673.
12. Wiygul JB, Evans BR, Peterson BL et al. Supplement use among men with prostate cancer. *Urology* 2005; 66(1):161–166.
13. Heinlein CA, Chang C. Androgen receptor in prostate cancer. *Endocr Rev* Apr 2004; 25(2):276–308.
14. Nelson WG, De Marzo AM, Isaacs WB. Prostate cancer. *N Engl J Med* 2003; 349:366–381.
15. De Marzo AM, Platz EA, Sutcliffe S et al. Inflammation in prostate carcinogenesis. *Nat Rev Cancer* 2007; 7:256–269.
16. Sciarra A, Di Silverio F, Salciccia S et al. Inflammation and chronic prostatic diseases: Evidence for a link. *Eur Urol* 2007; 52:964–972.
17. Parnes HL, House MG, Tangrea JA. Prostate cancer prevention: Strategies for agent development. *Curr Opin Oncol* 2013; 25:242–251.
18. Schatteman PH, Hoekx L, Wyndaele JJ, Jeuris W, Van Marck E. Inflammation in prostate biopsies of men without prostatic malignancy or clinical prostatitis. *Eur Urol* 2000; 37:404.
19. Gerstenbluth RE, Seftel AD, MacLennan GT et al. Distribution of chronic prostatitis in radical prostatectomy specimens with up-regulation of bcl-2 in areas of inflammation. *J Urol* 2002; 167:2267.
20. Franks LM. Atrophy and hyperplasia in the prostate proper. *J Pathol Bacteriol* 1954; 68:617.
21. De Marzo VL, Marchi JI, Epstein WG. Nelson Proliferative inflammatory atrophy of the prostate: Implications for prostatic carcinogenesis. *Am J Pathol* 1999; 155:1985.
22. Lee WH, Morton RA, Epstein JI et al. Cytidine methylation of regulatory sequences near the π-class glutathione *S*-transferase gene accompanies human prostatic carcinogenesis. *Proc Natl Acad Sci USA* 1994; 91:11733.
23. Brooks JD, Weinstein M, Lin X et al. CG island methylation changes near the GSTP1 gene in prostatic intraepithelial neoplasia cancer. *Epidemiol Biomarkers Prev* 1998; 7:531.
24. Donovan MJ, Osman I, Khan FM et al. Androgen receptor expression is associated with prostate cancer-specific survival in castrate patients with metastatic disease. *BJU Int* 2010; 105:462–467.
25. Sircar K, Yoshimoto M, Monzon FA et al. PTEN genomic deletion is associated with p-Akt and AR signaling in poorer outcome, hormone refractory prostate cancer. *J Pathol* 2009; 218:505–513.
26. Attar RM, Takimoto CH, Gottardis MM. Castration-resistant prostate cancer: Locking up the molecular escape routes. *Clin Cancer Res* 2009; 15:3251–3255.
27. Debes JD, Tindall DJ. Mechanisms of androgenrefractory prostate cancer. *N Engl J Med* 2004; 351:1488–1490.
28. Singh RP, Agarwal R. Mechanisms of action of novel agents for prostate cancer chemoprevention. *Endocr Relat Cancer* 2006; 13:751–778.
29. Surh YJ. Cancer chemoprevention with dietary phytochemicals. *Nat Rev Cancer* 2003; 3:768–780.
30. Bartkova J, Horejsí Z, Koed K et al. DNA damage response as a candidate anti-cancer barrier in early human tumorigenesis. *Nature* 2005; 434:864–870.
31. Gorgoulis VG, Vassiliou LV, Karakaidos P et al. Activation of the DNA damage checkpoint and genomic instability in human precancerous lesions. *Nature* 2005; 434:907–913.
32. Vazquez-Martin A, Oliveras-Ferraros C, Cufí S, Martin-Castillo B, Menendez JA. Metformin activates an ataxia telangiectasia mutated (ATM)/Chk2-regulated DNA damage-like response. *Cell Cycle* 2011; 10:1499–1501.
33. Palozza P, Colangelo M, Simone R et al. Lycopene induces cell growth inhibition by altering mevalonate pathway and Ras signaling in cancer cell lines. *Carcinogenesis* 2010; 31:1813–1821.
34. Di Mascio P, Kaiser S, Sies H. Lycopene as the most efficient biological carotenoid singlet oxygen quencher. *Arch Biochem Biophys*1989; 274:532–538.
35. Liu X, Allen JD, Arnold JT et al. Lycopene inhibits IGF-I signal transduction and growth in normal prostate epithelial cells by decreasing DHT-modulated IGF-I production in co-cultured reactive stromal cells. *Carcinogenesis* 2008; 29:816–823.
36. Amir H, Karas M, Giat J et al. Lycopene and 1,25-dihydroxyvitamin D3 cooperate in the inhibition of cell cycle progression and induction of differentiation in HL-60 leukemic cells. *Nutr Cancer* 1999; 33:105–112.
37. Giovannucci E, Rimm EB, Liu Y, Stampfer MJ, Willett WC. A prospective study of tomato products, lycopene, and prostate cancer risk. *J Natl Cancer Inst* 2002; 94(5):391–398.
38. Kirsh VA, Mayne ST, Peters U et al. A prospective study of lycopene and tomato product intake and risk of prostate cancer. *Cancer Epidemiol Biomarkers Prev* 2006; 15(1):92–98.

39. McCann SE, Ambrosone CB, Moysich KB et al. Intakes of selected nutrients, foods, and phytochemicals and prostate cancer risk in western New York. *Nutr Cancer* 2005; 53(1):33–41.
40. Schuurman AG, Goldbohm RA, Brants HA, van den Brandt PA. A prospective cohort study on intake of retinol, vitamins C and E, and carotenoids and prostate cancer risk (Netherlands). *Cancer Causes Control* 2002; 13(6):573–582.
41. Deneo-Pellegrini H, De Stefani E, Ronco A, Mendilaharsu M. Foods, nutrients and prostate cancer: A case-control study in Uruguay. *Br J Cancer* 1999; 80(3–4):591–597.
42. Bidoli E, Talamini R, Zucchetto A et al. Dietary vitamins E and C and prostate cancer risk. *Acta Oncol* 2009; 48(6):890–894.
43. Hodge AM, English DR, McCredie MR et al. Foods, nutrients and prostate cancer. *Cancer Causes Control* 2004; 15(1):11–20
44. Etminan M, Takkouche B, Caamano-Isorna F. The role of tomato products and lycopene in the prevention of prostate cancer: A meta-analysis of observational studies. *Cancer Epidemiol Biomarkers Prev* 2004; 13:340–345.
45. Kavanaugh CJ, Trumbo PR, Ellwood KC: The U.S. Food and Drug Administration's evidence-based review for qualified health claims: Tomatoes, lycopene, and cancer. *J Natl Cancer Inst* 2007; 99:1074–1085.
46. Mohanty NK, Saxena S, Singh UP, Goyal NK, Arora RP: Lycopene as a chemopreventive agent in the treatment of high-grade prostate intraepithelial neoplasia. *Urol Oncol* 2005; 23:383–385.
47. Ansari MS, Gupta NP. A comparison of lycopene and orchidectomy vs orchidectomy alone in the management of advanced prostate cancer. *BJU Int* 2003; 92:375–378.
48. Tannock F, de Wit R, Berry WR et al. Docetaxel plus prednisone or mitoxantrone plus prednisone for advanced prostate cancer. *N Engl J Med* 2004; 351:1502–1512.
49. Tang Y, Parmakhtiar B, Simoneau AR et al. Lycopene enhances docetaxel's effect in castration-resistant prostate cancer associated with insulin-like growth factor I receptor levels. *Neoplasia* 2011; 13:108–119.
50. Adhami VM, Mukhtar H. Anti-oxidants from green tea and pomegranate for chemoprevention of prostate cancer. *Mol Biotechnol* 2007; 37:52–57.
51. Khan N, Adhami VM, Mukhtar H. Review: Green tea polyphenols in chemoprevention of prostate cancer: Preclinical and clinical studies. *Nutr Cancer* 2009; 61:836–841.
52. Cao Y, Cao R, Brakenhielm E. Antiangiogenic mechanisms of dietderived polyphenols. *J Nutr Biochem* 2002; 13:380–390.
53. Johnson JJ, Bailey HH, Mukhtar H. Green tea polyphenols for prostate cancer chemoprevention: A translational perspective. *Phytomedicine* 2010; 17:3–13.
54. Yang CS, Wang X, Lu G et al. Cancer prevention by tea: Animal studies, molecular mechanisms and human relevance. *Nat Rev Cancer* 2009; 9:429–439.
55. Liao S, Hiipakka RA. Selective inhibition of steroid 5 alpha-reductase isozymes by tea epicatechin-3-gallate and epigallocatechin-3-gallate. *Biochem Biophys Res Commun* 1995; 214:833–838.
56. Jian L, Xie LP, Lee AH et al. Protective effect of green tea against prostate cancer: A case–control study in southeast China. *Int J Cancer* 2004; 108:130–135.
57. Jian L, Lee AH, Binns CW. Tea and lycopene protect against prostate cancer. *Asia Pac J Clin Nutr* 2007; 16(Suppl 1):453–457.
58. Kurahashi N, Sasazuki S, Iwasaki M et al. Green tea consumption and prostate cancer risk in Japanese men: A prospective study. *Am J Epidemiol* 2008; 167:71–77.
59. Bettuzzi S, Brausi M, Rizzi F et al. Chemoprevention of human prostate cancer by oral administration of green tea catechins in volunteers with high-grade prostate intraepithelial neoplasia: A preliminary report from a one-year proof-of-principle study. *Cancer Res* 2006; 66(2):1234–1240.
60. Brausi M, Rizzi F, Bettuzzi S. Chemoprevention of human prostate cancer by green tea catechins: Two years later. A follow-up update. *Eur Urol* 2008; 54(2):472–473.
61. Zheng J, Yang B, Huang T et al. Green tea and black tea consumption and prostate cancer risk: An exploratory meta-analysis of observational studies. *Nutr Cancer* 2011; 63:663–672.
62. Wang P, Aronson WJ, Huang M et al. Green tea polyphenols and metabolites in prostatectomy tissue: Implications for cancer prevention. *Cancer Prev Res (Phila)* 2010; 3:985–993.
63. Kolonel LN, Hankin JH, Whittemore AS et al. Vegetables, fruits, legumes and prostate cancer: A multiethnic case-control study. *Cancer Epidemiol Biomarkers Prev* 2000; 9:795–804.
64. Cohen JH, Kristal AR, Stanford JL. Fruit and vegetable intakes and prostate cancer risk. *J Natl Cancer Inst* 2000; 92:61–68.
65. Liu B, Mao Q, Cao M et al. Cruciferous vegetables intake and risk of prostate cancer: A meta-analysis. *Int J Urol* 2012; 19:134–141.

66. Liu RH. Potential synergy of phytochemicals in cancer prevention: mechanism of action. *J Nutr* 2004; 134:3479S–3485S.
67. Singh SV, Srivastava SK, Choi S et al. Herman-Antosiewicz A: Sulforaphane-induced cell death in human prostate cancercells is initiated by reactive oxygen species. *J Biol Chem* 2005; 280:19911–19924.
68. Melchini A, Traka MH, Catania S, Miceli N, Taviano MF, Maimone P, Francisco M, Mithen RF, Costa C: Antiproliferative activity of the dietary isothiocyanate erucin, a bioactive compound from cruciferous vegetables, on human prostate cancer cells. *Nutr Cancer* 2013; 65:132–138.
69. Watson WG, Beaver ML, Williams ED, Dashwood HR, Ho E. Phytochemicals from cruciferous vegetables, epigenetics, and prostate cancer prevention. *AAPS J* 2013; 15:951–961.
70. Bosetti C, Filomeno M, Riso P, Polesel J, Levi F, Talamini R, Montella M, Negri E, Franceschi S, La Vecchia C. Cruciferous vegetables and cancer risk in a network of case–control studies. *Ann Oncol* 2012; 23:2198–2203.
71. Kirsh VA, Peters U, Mayne ST et al. Prospective study of fruit and vegetable intake and risk of prostate cancer. *J Natl Cancer Inst* 2007; 99:1200–1209.
72. Richman EL, Carroll PR, Chan JM. Vegetable and fruit intake after diagnosis and risk of prostate cancer progression. *Int J Cancer* 2012; 131:201–210.
73. Joseph MA, Moysich KB, Freudenheim JL et al. Cruciferous vegetables, genetic polymorphisms in glutathione Stransferases M1 and T1, and prostate cancer risk. *Nutr Cancer* 2004; 50:206–213.
74. Traka M, Gasper AV, Melchini A et al. Broccoli consumption interacts with gstm1 to perturb oncogenic signaling pathways in the prostate. *PLoS One* 2008; 3:e2568.
75. Basu A, Imrhan V. Vitamin E and prostate cancer: Is vitamin E succinate a superior chemopreventive agent? *Nutr Rev* 2005; 63:247–251.
76. Heinonen OP, Albanes D, Virtamo J et al. Prostate cancer and supplementation with alpha-tocopherol and beta-carotene: Incidence and mortality in a controlled trial. *J Natl Cancer Inst* 1998; 90(6):440–446.
77. Virtamo J, Pietinen P, Huttunen JK et al. Incidence of cancer and mortality following alpha-tocopherol and beta-carotene supplementation: A postintervention follow-up. *JAMA* 2003; 290(4):476–485.
78. Lawson KA, Wright ME, Subar A et al. Multivitamin use and risk of prostate cancer in the National Institutes of Health-AARP Diet and Health Study. *J Natl Cancer Inst* 2007; 99:754–764.
79. Calle EE, Rodriguez C, Jacobs EJ et al. The American Cancer Society Cancer Prevention Study II Nutrition Cohort: Rationale, study design, and baseline characteristics. *Cancer* 2002; 94:2490–2501.
80. Klein EA, Thompson Jr IM, Tangen CM et al. Vitamin E and the risk of prostate cancer: The Selenium and Vitamin E Cancer Prevention Trial (SELECT). *JAMA* 2011; 306:1549–1556.
81. Gaziano J, Glynn RJ, Christen WG et al. Vitamins E and C in the prevention of prostate and total cancer in men: The Physicians' Health Study II randomized controlled trial. *JAMA* 2009; 301:52–62.
82. Wright ME, Weinstein SJ, Lawson KA et al. Supplemental and dietary vitamin E intakes and risk of prostate cancer in a large prospective study. *Cancer Epidemiol Biomarkers Prev* 2007; 16(6):1128–1135.
83. Bauer SR, Richman EL, Sosa E, Weinberg V, Song X, Witte JS, Carroll PR, Chan JM. Antioxidant and vitamin E transport genes and risk of high-grade prostate cancer and prostate cancer recurrence. *Prostate* 2013; 73:1786–1795.
84. Jung W, Yu O, Lau SM, et al. Identification and expression of isoflavone synthase, the key enzyme for biosynthesis of isoflavones in legumes. *Nat Biotechnol* 2000; 18:208– 212.
85. Andres S, Abraham K, Appel KE, Lampen A. Risks and benefits of dietary isoflavones for cancer. *Crit Rev Toxicol* 2011; 41:463–506.
86. Makela S, Poutanen M, Kostian ML et al. Inhibition of 17beta-hydroxysteroid oxidoreductase by flavonoids in breast and prostate cancer cells. *Proc Soc Exp Biol Med* 1998; 217:310–316.
87. Perabo FGE, Von Löw EC, Ellinger J et al. Soy isoflavone genistein in prevention and treatment of prostate cancer. *Prostate Cancer Prostatic Dis* 2008; 11:6–12.
88. Banerjee S, Li Y, Wang Z, Sarkar FH. Multi-targeted therapy of cancer by genistein. *Cancer Lett* 2008; 269:226–242.
89. Messina M, Nagata C, Wu AH. Estimated Asian adult soy protein and isoflavone intakes. *Nutr Cancer* 2006; 55:1–12.
90. Zamora-Ros R, Knaze V, Lujan-Barroso L et al. Dietary intakes and food sources of phytoestrogens in the European Prospective Investigation into Cancer and Nutrition (EPIC) 24-hour dietary recall cohort. *Eur J Clin Nutr* 2012; 66:932–941.
91. Mulligan AA, Welch AA, McTaggart AA, Bhaniani A, Bingham SA. Intakes and sources of soya foods and isoflavones in a UK population cohort study (EPIC-Norfolk). *Eur J Clin Nutr* 2007; 61:248–254.

92. Yan L, Spitznagel EL. Meta-analysis of soy food and risk of prostate cancer in men. *Int J Cancer* 2005; 117:667–669.
93. Yan L, Spitznagel EL. Soy consumption and prostate cancer risk in men: A revisit of a meta-analysis. *Am J Clin Nutr* 2009; 89:1155–1163.
94. Kurahashi N, Iwasaki M, Sasazuki S et al. Soy product and isoflavone consumption in relation to prostate cancer in Japanese men. *Cancer Epidemiol Biomarkers Prev* 2007; 16:538–545.
95. Jacobsen BK, Knutsen SF, Fraser GE. Does high soy milk intake reduce prostate cancer incidence? The Adventist Health Study (United States). *Cancer Causes Control* 1998; 9:553–557.
96. Lampe JW, Karr SC, Hutchins AM, Slavin JL. Urinary equol excretion with a soy challenge: Influence of habitual diet. *Proc Soc Exp Biol Med* 1998; 217:335–339.
97. Akaza H, Miyanaga N, Takashima N et al. Comparisons of percent equol producers between prostate cancer patients and controls: Case-controlled studies of isoflavones in Japanese, Korean and American residents. *Jpn J Clin Oncol* 2004; 34:86–89.
98. Akaza H, Miyanaga N, Takashima N et al. Is daidzein non-metabolizer a high risk for prostate cancer? A case-controlled study of serum soybean isoflavone concentration. *Jpn J Clin Oncol* 2002; 32:296–300.
99. Ozasa K, Nakao M, Watanabe Y et al. Serum phytoestrogens and prostate cancer risk in a nested case-control study among Japanese men. *Cancer Sci* 2004; 95:65–71.
100. Kurahashi N, Iwasaki M, Inoue M, Sasazuki S, Tsugane S. Plasma isoflavones and subsequent risk of prostate cancer in a nested case-control study: The Japan Public Health Center. *J Clin Oncol* 2008; 26:5923–5929.
101. Sugiyama Y, Masumori N, Fukuta F et al. Influence of isoflavone intake and equol-producing intestinal flora on prostate cancer risk. *Asian Pac J Cancer Prev* 2013; 14:1–4.
102. Fujimoto K, Tanaka M, Hirao Y et al. Age-stratified serum levels of isoflavones and proportion of equol producers in Japanese and Korean healthy men. *Prostate Cancer Prostatic Dis* 2008; 11:252–257.
103. Van Die MD, Bone KM, Williams SG, Pirotta MV. Soy and soy isoflavones in prostate cancer: A systematic review and meta-analysis of randomized controlled trials. *BJU Int* 2014; 113:E119–E130.
104. Ide H, Tokiwa S, Sakamaki K et al. Combined inhibitory effects of soy isoflavones and curcumin on the production of prostate-specific antigen. *Prostate* 2010; 70:1127–1133.
105. Wuttke W, Jarry H, Seidlova-Wuttke D. Plant-derived alternative treatments for the aging male: Facts and myths. *Aging Male* 2010; 13:75–81.
106. Oh HY, Leem J, Yoon SJ et al. Lipid raft cholesterol and genistein inhibit the cell viability of prostate cancer cells via the partial contribution of EGFR-Akt/p70S6k pathway and downregulation of androgen receptor. *Biochem Biophys Res Commun* 2010; 393:319–324.
107. Basak S, Pookot D, Noonan EJ et al. Genistein downregulates androgen receptor by modulating HDAC6-Hsp90 chaperone function. *Mol Cancer Ther* 2008; 7:3195–3202.
108. Li Y, Wang Z, Kong D et al. Regulation of Akt/FOXO3a/GSK-3beta/AR signaling network by isoflavone in prostate cancer cells. *J Biol Chem* 2008; 283:27707–27716.
109. Jagadeesh S, Kyo S, Banerjee PP. Genistein represses telomerase activity via both transcriptional and posttranslational mechanisms in human prostate cancer cells. *Cancer Res* 2006; 66:2107–2115.
110. Li Y, Ahmed F, Ali S et al. Inactivation of nuclear factor kappaB by soy isoflavone genistein contributes to increased apoptosis induced by chemotherapeutic agents in human cancer cells. *Cancer Res* 2005; 65:6934–6942.
111. Wang Y, Wang H, Zhang W et al. Genistein sensitizes bladder cancer cells to HCPT treatment in vitro and in vivo via ATM/NF-kappaB/IKK pathway-induced apoptosis. *PLoS One* 2013; 8:e50175.
112. Legg RL, Tolman JR, Lovinger CT et al. Diets high in selenium and isoflavones decrease androgen-regulated gene expression in healthy rat dorsolateral prostate. *Reprod Biol Endocrinol* 2008; 6:57.
113. Fritz WA, Wang J, Eltoum IE et al. Dietary genistein downregulates androgen and estrogen receptor expression in the rat prostate. *Mol Cell Endocrinol* 2002; 186:89–99.
114. Phillip CJ, Giardina CK, Bilir B et al. Genistein cooperates with the histone deacetylase inhibitor vorinostat to induce cell death in prostate cancer cells. *BMC Cancer* 2012; 12:145.
115. Wuttke W, Jarry H, Seidlova-Wuttke D. Isoflavones–safe food additives or dangerous drugs? *Ageing Res Rev* 2007; 6:150–188.
116. Onozawa M, Fukuda K, Ohtani M et al. Effects of soybean isoflavones on cell growth and apoptosis of the human prostatic cancer cell line LNCaP. *Jpn J Clin Oncol* 1998; 28:360–363.
117. Yuan-Jing F, Nan-Shan H, Lian X. Genistein synergizes with RNA interference inhibiting survivin for inducing DU-145 of prostate cancer cells to apoptosis. *Cancer Lett* 2009; 284:189–197.
118. Ide H, Yu J, Lu Y et al. Testosterone augments polyphenol-induced DNA damage response in prostate cancer cell line, LNCaP. *Cancer Sci* 2011; 102:468–471.

119. Raffoul JJ, Wang Y, Kucuk O et al. Genistein inhibits radiation-induced activation of NF-kappaB in prostate cancer cells promoting apoptosis and G2/M cell cycle arrest. *BMC Cancer* 2006; 6:107.
120. Li M, Zhang Z, Hill DL et al. Genistein, a dietary isoflavone, down-regulates the MDM2 oncogene at both transcriptional and posttranslational levels. *Cancer Res* 2005; 65:8200–8208.
121. Choi YH, Lee WH, Park KY, Zhang L. p53-independent induction of p21 (WAF1/CIP1), reduction of cyclin B1 and G2/M arrest by the isoflavone genistein in human prostate carcinoma cells. *Jpn J Cancer Res* 2000; 91:164–173.
122. Jian L. Soy, isoflavones, and prostate cancer. *Mol Nutr Food Res* 2009; 53:217–226.
123. Lakshman M, Xu L, Ananthanarayanan V et al. Dietary genistein inhibits metastasis of human prostate cancer in mice. *Cancer Res* 2008; 68:2024–2032.
124. Steelman LS, Stadelman KM, Chappell WH et al. Akt as a therapeutic target in cancer. *Expert Opin Ther Targets* 2008; 12:1139–1165.
125. Parasramka MA, Ho E, Williams DE et al. Micrornas, diet, and cancer: New mechanistic insights on the epigenetic actions of phytochemicals. *Mol Carcinog* 2012; 51:213–230.
126. Abbas A, Gupta S. The role of histone deacetylases in prostate cancer. *Epigenetics* 2008; 3:300–309.
127. Chiyomaru T, Yamamura S, Zaman MS et al. Genistein suppresses prostate cancer growth through inhibition of oncogenic microRNA-151. *PLoS One* 2012; 7(8):e43812.
128. Palapattu GS, Sutcliffe S, Bastian PJ et al. Prostate carcinogenesis and inflammation: Emerging insights. *Carcinogenesis* 2005; 26:1170–1181.
129. Yoshimura R, Sano H, Masuda C et al. Expression of cyclooxygenase-2 in prostate carcinoma. *Cancer* 2000; 89:589–596.
130. Fujita H, Koshida K, Keller ET et al. Cyclooxygenase-2 promotes prostate cancer progression. *Prostate* 2002; 53:232–240.
131. Zerbini LF, Wang Y, Cho JY, Libermann TA. Constitutive activation of nuclear factor kappaB p50/p65 and Fra-1 and JunD is essential for deregulated interleukin 6 expression in prostate cancer. *Cancer Res* 2003; 63:2206–2215.
132. Davis JN, Kucuk O, Sarkar FH. Genistein inhibits NF-kappa B activation in prostate cancer cells. *Nutr Cancer* 1999; 35:167–174.
133. Li Y, Sarkar FH. Inhibition of nuclear factor kappaB activation in PC3 cells by genistein is mediated via Akt signaling pathway. *Clin Cancer Res* 2002; 8:2369–2377.
134. Suzuki K, Koike H, Matsui H et al. Genistein, a soy isoflavone, induces glutathione peroxidase in the human prostate cancer cell lines LNCaP and PC-3. *Int J Cancer* 2002; 99:846–852.
135. Ozten-Kandaş N, Bosland MC. Chemoprevention of prostate cancer: Natural compounds, antiandrogens, and antioxidants—In vivo evidence. *J Carcinog* 2011; 10:27.
136. McCormick DL, Johnson WD, Bosland MC, Lubet RA, Steele VE. Chemoprevention of rat prostate carcinogenesis by soy isoflavones and by Bowman-Birk inhibitor. *Nutr Cancer* 2007; 57(2):184–193.
137. Pollard M, Wolter W, Sun L. Prevention of induced prostate-related cancer by soy protein isolate/isoflavone-supplemented diet in Lobund-Wistar rats. *In Vivo* 2000; 14(3):389–392.
138. Wang J, Eltoum IE, Lamartiniere CA. Genistein chemoprevention of prostate cancer in TRAMP mice. *J Carcinog* 2007; 6:3.
139. Arper CE, Cook LM, Patel BB et al. Genistein and resveratrol, alone and in combination, suppress prostate cancer in SV-40 tag rats. *Prostate* 2009; 69(15):1668–1682.
140. Dalais FS, Meliala A, Wattanapenpaiboon N et al. Effects of a diet rich in phytoestrogens on prostate-specific antigen and sex hormones in men diagnosed with prostate cancer. *Urology* 2004; 64:510–515.
141. Tanaka M, Fujimoto K, Chihara Y et al. Isoflavone supplements stimulated the production of serum equol and decreased the serum dihydrotestosterone levels in healthy male volunteers. *Prostate Cancer Prostatic Dis* 2009; 12:247–252.
142. Miyanaga N, Akaza H, Hinotsu S et al. Prostate cancer chemoprevention study: An investigative randomized control study using purified isoflavones in men with rising prostate-specific antigen. *Cancer Sci* 2012; 103:125–130.
143. Bosland MC, Kato I, Zeleniuch-Jacquotte A et al. Effect of soy protein isolate supplementation on biochemical recurrence of prostate cancer after radical prostatectomy: A randomized trial. *JAMA* Jul 10, 2013; 310(2):170–178.
144. loussard G, Epstein JI, Montironi R et al. The contemporary concept of significant vs insignificant prostate cancer. *Eur Urol* 2011; 60(2):291–303.
145. Sakr WA, Haas GP, Cassin BF, Pontes JE, Crissman JD. The frequency of carcinoma and intraepithelial neoplasia of the prostate in young male patients. *J Urol* 1993; 150(2 pt 1):379–385.

146. Ahmad IU, Forman JD, Sarkar FH, Hillman GG, Heath E, Vaishampayan U, Cher ML, Andic F, Rossi PJ, Kucuk O. Soy isoflavones in conjunction with radiation therapy in patients with prostate cancer. *Nutr Cancer* 2010; 62:996–1000.
147. Khan N, Adhami VM, Mukhtar H. Apoptosis by dietary agents for prevention and treatment of prostate cancer. *Endocr Relat Cancer* 2010; 17:R39–R52.
148. Balogun E, Hoque M, Gong P et al. Curcumin activates the haem oxygenase-1 gene via regulation of Nrf2 and the antioxidant-responsive element. *Biochem J* 2003; 71:887–895.
149. Iqbal M, Okazaki Y, Okada S. Curcumin attenuates oxidative damage in animals treated with a renal carcinogen, ferric nitrilotriacetate (Fe-NTA): Implications for cancer prevention. *Mol Cell Biochem* 2009; 324:157–164.
150. Sandur SK, Pandey MK, Sung B et al. Curcumin, demethoxycurcumin, bisdemethoxycurcumin, tetrahydrocurcumin and turmerones differentially regulate anti-inflammatory and anti-proliferative responses through a ROS-independent mechanism. *Carcinogenesis* 2007; 28:1765–1773.
151. Menon VP, Sudheer AR. Antioxidant and anti-inflammatory properties of curcumin. *Adv Exp Med Biol* 2007; 595:105–125.
152. Duvoix A, Blasius R, Delhalle S et al. Chemopreventive and therapeutic effects of curcumin. *Cancer Lett* 2005; 223:181–190.
153. Bhandarkar SS, Arbiser JL. Curcumin as an inhibitor of angiogenesis. *Adv Exp Med Biol* 2007; 595:185–195.
154. Hong JH, Ahn KS, Bae E, Jeon SS, Choi HY. The effects of curcumin on the invasiveness of prostate cancer in vitro and in vivo. *Prostate Cancer Prostatic Dis* 2006; 9:147–152.
155. Mukhopadhyay A, Bueso-Ramos C, Chatterjee D et al. Curcumin downregulates cell survival mechanisms in human prostate cancer cell lines. *Oncogene* 2001; 20:7597–7609.
156. Dorai T, Gehani N, Katz A. Therapeutic potential of curcumin in human prostate cancer-I. curcumin induces apoptosis in both androgen-dependent and androgen-independent prostate cancer cells. *Prostate Cancer Prostatic Dis* 2000; 3:84–93.
157. Nakamura K, Yasunaga Y, Segawa T et al. Curcumin down-regulates AR gene expression and activation in prostate cancer cell lines. *Int J Oncol* 2002; 21:825–830.
158. Tsui KH, Feng TH, Lin CM, Chang PL, Juang HH. Curcumin blocks the activation of androgen and interlukin-6 on prostate-specific antigen expression in human prostatic carcinoma cells. *J Androl* 2008; 29:661–668.
159. Choi HY, Lim JE, Hong JH. Curcumin interrupts the interaction between the androgen receptor and Wnt/beta-catenin signaling pathway in LNCaP prostate cancer cells. *Prostate Cancer Prostatic Dis* 2010; 13:343–349.
160. Zhang HN, Yu CX, Zhang PJ et al. Curcumin downregulates homeobox gene NKX3.1 in prostate cancer cell LNCaP. *Acta Pharmacol Sin* 2007; 28:423–430.
161. Bieberich CJ, Fujita K, He WW, Jay G. Prostate-specific and androgen-dependent expression of a novel homeobox gene. *J Biol Chem* 1996; 271:31779–31782.
162. Li M, Zhang Z, Hill DL, Wang H, Zhang R. Curcumin, a dietary component, has anticancer, chemosensitization, and radiosensitization effects by down-regulating the MDM2 oncogene through the PI3K/mTOR/ETS2 pathway. *Cancer Res* 2007; 67:1988–1996.
163. Beevers CS, Li F, Liu L, Huang S. Curcumin inhibits the mammalian target of rapamycin-mediated signaling pathways in cancer cells. *Int J Cancer* 2006; 119:757–764.
164. Thangapazham RL, Shaheduzzaman S, Kim KH et al. Androgen responsive and refractory prostate cancer cells exhibit distinct curcumin regulated transcriptome. *Cancer Biol Ther* 2008; 7:1427–1435.
165. Deng G, Yu JH, Ye ZQ, Hu ZQ. Curcumin inhibits the expression of vascular endothelial growth factor and androgen-independent prostate cancer cell line PC-3 in vitro. *Zhonghua Nan Ke Xue* 2008; 14:116–121.
166. Dorai T, Cao YC, Dorai B, Buttyan R, Katz AE. Therapeutic potential of curcumin in human prostate cancer. III. Curcumin inhibits proliferation, induces apoptosis, and inhibits angiogenesis of LNCaP prostate cancer cells in vivo. *Prostate* 2001; 47:293–303.
167. Edwards J, Mukherjee R, Munro AF et al. HER2 and COX2 expression in human prostate cancer. *Eur J Cancer* 2004; 40:50–55.
168. Dorai T, Gehani N, Katz A. Therapeutic potential of curcumin in human prostate cancer. II. Curcumin inhibits tyrosine kinase activity of epidermal growth factor receptor and depletes the protein. *Mol Urol* 2000; 4:1–6.
169. Kim JH, Xu C, Keum YS et al. Inhibition of EGFR signaling in human prostate cancer PC-3 cells by combination treatment with beta-phenylethyl isothiocyanate and curcumin. *Carcinogenesis* 2006; 27:475–482.

170. Dorai T, Dutcher JP, Dempster DW, Wiernik PH. Therapeutic potential of curcumin in prostate cancer—V: Interference with the osteomimetic properties of hormone refractory C4–2B prostate cancer cells. *Prostate* 2004; 60:1–17.
171. Mukhopadhyay A, Banerjee S, Stafford LJ et al. Curcumin-induced suppression of cell proliferation correlates with down-regulation of cyclin D1 expression and CDK4-mediated retinoblastoma protein phosphorylation. *Oncogene* 2002; 21:8852–8861.
172. Srivastava RK, Chen Q, Siddiqui I, Sarva K, Shankar S. Linkage of curcumin-induced cell cycle arrest and apoptosis by cyclin-dependent kinase inhibitor p21(/WAF1/CIP1). *Cell Cycle* 2007; 6:2953–2961.
173. Shankar S, Ganapathy S, Chen Q, Srivastava RK. Curcumin sensitizes TRAIL-resistant xenografts: Molecular mechanisms of apoptosis, metastasis and angiogenesis. *Mol Cancer* 2008; 7:16.
174. Shenouda NS, Zhou C, Browning JD et al. Phytoestrogens in common herbs regulate prostate cancer cell growth in vitro. *Nutr Cancer* 2004; 49:200–208.
175. Surh YJ, Na HK. NF-kappaB and Nrf2 as prime molecular targets for chemoprevention and cytoprotection with anti-inflammatory and antioxidant phytochemicals. *Genes Nutr* 2008; 2:313–317.
176. Hour TC, Chen J, Huang CY et al. Curcumin enhances cytotoxicity of chemotherapeutic agents in prostate cancer cells by inducing p21(WAF1/CIP1) and C/EBPbeta expressions and suppressing NF-kappaB activation. *Prostate* 2002; 51:211–218.
177. Sharma RA, McLelland HR, Hill KA et al. Pharmacodynamic and pharmacokinetic study of oral Curcuma extract in patients with colorectal cancer. *Clin Cancer Res* 2001; 7:1894–1900.
178. Cheng AL, Hsu CH, Lin JK et al. Phase I clinical trial of curcumin, a chemopreventive agent, in patients with high-risk or pre-malignant lesions. *Anticancer Res* 2001; 21:2895–2900.
179. Anand P, Kunnumakkara AB, Newman RA, Aggarwal BB. Bioavailability of curcumin: problems and promises. *Mol Pharm* 2007; 4:807–818.
180. Garcea G, Jones DJ, Singh R et al. Detection of curcumin and its metabolites in hepatic tissue and portal blood of patients following oral administration. *Br J Cancer* 2004; 90:1011–1015.
181. Dhillon N, Aggarwal BB, Newman RA et al. Phase II trial of curcumin in patients with advanced pancreatic cancer. *Clin Cancer Res* 2008; 14:4491–4499.
182. Li L, Aggarwal BB, Shishodia S, Abbruzzese J, Kurzrock R. Nuclear factor-kappaB and IkappaB kinase are constitutively active in human pancreatic cells, and their down-regulation by curcumin (diferuloylmethane) is associated with the suppression of proliferation and the induction of apoptosis. *Cancer* 2004; 101:2351–2362.
183. Cabrespine-Faugeras A, Bayet-Robert M, Bay JO et al. Possible benefits of curcumin regimen in combination with taxane chemotherapy for hormone-refractory prostate cancer treatment. *Nutr Cancer* 2010; 62:148–153.
184. Chendil D, Ranga RS, Meigooni D et al. Curcumin confers radiosensitizing effect in prostate cancer cell line PC-3. *Oncogene* 2004; 23:1599–1607.
185. Kanai M, Imaizumi A, Otsuka Y, Sasaki H, Hashiguchi M, Tsujiko K, Matsumoto S, Ishiguro H, Chiba T. Dose-escalation and pharmacokinetic study of nanoparticle curcumin, a potential anticancer agent with improved bioavailability, in healthy human volunteers. *Cancer Chemother Pharmacol* Jan 2012; 69(1):65–70.
186. Jackson SP, Bartek J. The DNA-damage response in human biology and disease. *Nature* 2009; 461:1071–1078.
187. Bartkova J, Horejsí Z, Koed K et al. Oncogene-induced senescence is part of the tumorigenesis barrier imposed by DNA damage checkpoints. *Nature* 2006; 444:633–637.
188. Halazonetis TD, Gorgoulis VG, Bartek J. An oncogene-induced DNA damage model for cancer development. *Science* 2008; 319:1352–1355.
189. Cosentino C, Grieco D, Costanzo V. ATM activates the pentose phosphate pathway promoting antioxidant defense and DNA repair. *EMBO* 2011; 30:546–555.
190. Blasiak J, Arabski M, Krupa R et al. DNA damage and repair in type 2 diabetes mellitus. *Mutat Res* 2004; 554:297–304.
191. Birnbaum MJ, Shaw RJ. Genomics: Drugs, diabetes and cancer. *Nature* 2011; 470:338–339.
192. Tyagi A, Singh RP, Agarwal C, Siriwardana S, Sclafani RA. Resveratrol causes Cdc2-tyr15 phosphorylation via ATM/ATR-Chk1/2-Cdc25C pathway as a central mechanism for S phase arrest in human ovarian carcinoma Ovcar-3 cells. *Carcinogenesis* 2005; 26:1978–1987.
193. Baur JA, Sinclair DA. Therapeutic potential of resveratrol: The in vivo evidence. *Nat Rev Drug Discov* 2006; 5:493–506.

Section XII

Sleeping Disorders

25 Nutrition and Sleep
An Overview

Glenda Lindseth, Ashley Murray, and Brian Helland

CONTENTS

25.1 INTRODUCTION

A good night's sleep is crucial to human health, productivity, and longevity. Sleep deprivation is increasingly seen as a major unmet public health problem (Altevogt and Colten 2006) with serious consequences on daily performance and functionality. However, the National Sleep Foundation (2009) reports that more than two-thirds of adults sleep less than the recommended 8 h each night; of those, approximately 20% sleep less than 6 h each night. Some research suggests that the details of a person's intake of macronutrients may affect sleep quality and quantity (Montgomery et al. 2014; Papandreou 2013; Scorza et al. 2013). Therefore, this chapter describes a review of existing literature focusing on the effects of macronutrient consumption on sleep.

25.1.1 Sleep Measures

Several measures of sleep and activity are used to measure sleep quantity and sleep quality. For clinical studies and in research, sleep is commonly measured using actigraphs, polysomnographs, and paper/pencil, psychometrically designed sleep-assessment questionnaires.

Polysomnography is the gold standard for measuring sleep. It involves the use of surface electrodes to gather physiologic and electroencephalographic (EEG) measurements, for example of eye movements and cardiac and respiratory activities (Marino et al. 2013). Typically, the patient is immobilized under supervision in a controlled setting as sleep data are collected over time; these data are subsequently analyzed.

Actigraphy measures sleep when a small, portable, wristwatch-type device is worn to digitally record integrated measures of gross-motor activity. The device estimates sleep time by recording immobility to mark the beginning of the sleep period. The sensitivity of actigraphs for correctly detecting sleep is higher than 90% for each participant. Actigraphs record variables such as sleep and wake patterns, bed and rise times, sleep efficiency, sleep and wake bouts, sleep latency, and wake episodes. A computer interface is used to analyze the sleep data (Marino et al. 2013).

Questionnaires are typically self-reporting tools for assessing sleep quality and acquiring sleep inventories. The most reliable and valid sleep questionnaires are psychometrically tested for accuracy. Additional data may be collected through sleep diaries, thus enabling researchers to visualize sleep patterns over time (Werner et al. 2008).

25.1.2 Sleep Terminology

The commonly accepted definition of sleep is "unconsciousness from which the person can be aroused by sensory or other stimuli" (Guyton and Hall 1996). Sleep is likely caused by an active inhibitory center of the brain that is located below the mid-pontile level of the brain stem. This area inhibits higher brain functions to induce sleep.

The two major types of sleep are slow-wave sleep and rapid eye movement (REM) sleep. Slow-wave sleep is considered to be the more restful of the two main types of sleep, with decreases in blood pressure, respiration, and basal metabolism. In this type of sleep, the brain is relatively inactive, but is still actively regulating a movable body (Carskadon and Dement 2000). Conversely, REM sleep consists of EEG activation, muscle atonia, and episodic bursts of REMs (Carskadon and Dement 2000). This type of sleep involves more dreaming and eye movement and is not as restful.

Natural sleep is induced via the raphe nuclei located in the medulla and the lower half of the pons in the brain. The endings of fibers from raphe neurons secrete serotonin, leading to the common assumption that serotonin encourages sleep. This assumption highlights the importance of serotonin and its precursors in assisting with the regulation of the sleep–wake cycle (Guyton and Hall 1996).

The following terms are frequently used in the sleep literature as defined by Carskadon and Dement (2000):

- *Restorative sleep* is generally defined as deep, slow-wave sleep considered to be the more restful type of sleep.
- *Nonrestorative sleep* is defined as a person feeling that they have experienced unrestful sleep or feeling unrefreshed upon awakening.

The following terms are frequently used in the sleep literature as defined by Keenan and Hirshkowitz (2011):

- *Sleep efficiency* is the amount of time asleep divided by the amount of time spent in bed.
- *Sleep latency* is the time taken by a person to fall asleep after lying down in bed for the night.
- *Wake episodes* are the number of awakenings between falling asleep and rising.

25.1.3 Macronutrients Associated with Sleep

Macronutrients are essential nutritional components, with protein, fats, and carbohydrates being the micronutrients consumed in larger quantities to obtain energy. Proteins consist of 20 amino acids. The primary categories of dietary fat are saturated fat, unsaturated fat, monounsaturated fatty acids (MUFAs), polyunsaturated fatty acids (PUFAs), trans fat, and cholesterol. Carbohydrates and water are also essential for health and survival. While alcohol is not considered to be a macronutrient, it will be discussed due to its effect on sleep. Vitamins and minerals are also essential micronutrients required for health and survival. Each of these major categories is addressed in the following:

25.2 DIETARY FAT AND SLEEP

25.2.1 Fatty Acids and Sleep

Various relationships among dietary fats and sleep have been uncovered through research (Crispim et al. 2011; Grandner et al. 2010; Shi et al. 2008). The effects of fat and sleep are usually tested by manipulating the types of fatty acids that are commonly consumed and measuring the resulting changes in sleep. Studies focusing on the consumption of higher levels of fat and their effects on sleep are described in this section.

Shorter sleep duration can lead to small changes in eating patterns and in nutritional content of foods consumed in the diet. These small changes can work cumulatively to alter the energy balance in adolescents, which may increase obesity risk. For example using sleep actigraphs and 24 h food recalls, 240 adolescents who consumed fewer carbohydrate kilocalories and more fat kilocalories slept less than 8 h/day on average compared to adolescents who slept 8 or more hours on average during weekdays (Weiss et al. 2010). Also, it was found that average daily increases in fat kilocalories and decreases in carbohydrate kilocalories led to shorter sleep duration.

In a Chinese study of 2828 adult participants who responded to a national health and nutrition survey, consumption of significantly higher percentages of fat intake was associated with participants sleeping less than 7 h/day in comparison to those who slept more than 7 h/day (Shi et al. 2008). In a cross-sectional study of 30 healthy Greek women using a Sleep Habits Questionnaire, a 7-day sleep diary, and two 24 h dietary recalls, a weak positive association between consuming saturated fat and shorter sleep duration was determined (Rontoyanni et al. 2007).

Using sleep actigraph measurements from 423 postmenopausal women who participated in the 2007–2008 National Health and Nutrition Examination Survey (NHANES), an increase in dietary fat consumption was correlated with a decrease in sleep duration (Grandner et al. 2010). Nocturnal polysomnography and 3-day food diaries were used in a study of 52 healthy young- to middle-aged men and women (Crispim et al. 2011). This study identified a significant relationship between increased sleep latency and high nighttime fat intakes in the women. There was also a significant, negative relationship between the women's nighttime fat intake and their sleep efficiency. However, the results for the male participants were not significant, and the type of fat consumed was not identified.

25.2.2 Saturated Fatty Acids and Sleep

Using data from the 2007–2008 NHANES, the relationship between sleeping habits and nutritional intake was examined in 5587 adults (Grandner et al. 2013). Duration of sleep was significantly associated with consumption of two saturated fatty acids: dodecanoic acid (found in coconut oil) and butanoic acid (found in cow's milk). Sleep was measured using sleep surveys. Other results mined from the NHANES of 4552 participants older than 18 years indicated that hexadecanoic acid, found in meat, dairy products, and coconut oil, was associated with increased difficulty in falling asleep and hexanoic acid (found in coconut oil) was associated with increased difficulty in maintaining sleep (Grandner et al. 2014,b). Sleep was measured with a sleep questionnaire that contained questions about the participants' sleep symptoms. A negative correlation was also noted between sleep duration and serum (hexadecanoic) saturated fatty acid levels in 118 depressed inpatients (Irmisch et al. 2007). This relationship was likely due to the role of these saturated fatty acids as precursors of palmitoleic acid, which significantly increased throughout inpatient depression treatment and correlated with sleep disturbances (Irmisch et al. 2007).

25.2.3 Monounsaturated Fatty Acids and Sleep

In a sample of 58 elderly obese men and women, lower levels of monounsaturated fatty acids in the diet resulted in more hours of sleep in a 24 h period in both men and women; however, monounsaturated fatty acids had a significant relationship with more hours of sleep in men (Santana et al. 2012). Sleep time was evaluated with a nocturnal sleep-duration questionnaire and food intake was determined by self-reported recall of food consumption (Santana et al. 2012).

Several fatty acids were previously related to sleep improvement in 118 depressed inpatients (Irmisch et al. 2007). Diets with monounsaturated fatty acids and omega-6 PUFAs had the most beneficial effects on sleep. Total lipids were extracted from blood serum from the study participants; palmitoleic and eicosadienoic acids displayed the strongest statistical relationships with sleep disturbance. While the mechanism underpinning these results is unclear (Irmisch et al. 2007), the relationship between omega-3 and omega-6 fatty acids and sleep is thought to be due to their role in the synthesis of prostaglandin D^2, a chemical that helps regulate sleep (Urade and Hayaishi 2011).

25.2.4 Polyunsaturated Fatty Acids and Sleep

Diets high in unsaturated fatty acids, particularly PUFAs, have been found to improve sleep quality in gender- and age-specific groups. Deficiencies in the consumption of PUFAs have also been linked to a variety of neuropsychiatric disorders, such as attention deficit hyperactivity disorder (ADHD) (Huss et al. 2010; Yehuda et al. 2011), depression (Irmisch et al. 2007), and Alzheimer's disease (Yehuda et al. 1996). Each of these disorders is often accompanied by sleep disturbances (Huss et al. 2010; Irmisch et al. 2007; Yehuda et al. 1996, 2011). In a sample of 78 boys (aged 9–12 years) with sleep deficits secondary to ADHD, PUFA supplementation significantly improved reported sleep quality (Yehuda et al. 2011). Similarly, in a longitudinal study of more than 800 children aged 5–12 years with ADHD, sleep disturbances reported by participants declined by 40% after supplementation with omega-3 and omega-6 fatty acids for 12 weeks (Huss et al. 2010). Because supplementation also included zinc and magnesium, the investigators questioned whether the observed improvements in sleep were solely due to PUFAs.

In a 4-week, double-blind study of 100 Alzheimer's disease patients (79 males and 21 females; 50–73 years of age) who complained of sleep disturbances, 60 patients received supplementation with a 1:4 ratio of omega-3/omega-6 fatty acid and 40 patients received a placebo (Yehuda et al. 1996). A Likert-scale questionnaire measured sleep disturbances. Of participants who received the omega-3/omega-6 treatments, 74% noted improvements in their sleep in comparison to receiving a placebo.

Consuming PUFAs during pregnancy has also been linked with benefits. For example at 20 weeks of gestation, 48 healthy pregnant women (aged 18–35 years) received a cereal-based bar enriched with 300 mg of docosahexaenoic acid (DHA) or a placebo bar for 5 days/week until delivery (Judge et al. 2012). In the early postpartum period, the infant's sleep was measured with a pressure-sensitive pad placed under the crib bedding to record respirations and body movement. Women who received prenatal DHA acid supplementation had babies with fewer sleep arousals.

Similarly, in a study subset of 43 healthy British school children, children who received omega-3 fatty-acid supplements showed improved sleep quality (Montgomery et al. 2014). When sleep was measured with actigraphs, children averaged seven fewer wake episodes (a total of 58 more min of sleep per night) when they consumed omega-3 (docosahexaenoic) fatty acid supplements.

In a study sample of 78 boys (9–12 years of age) with sleep deficits secondary to ADHD, Yehuda et al. (2011) found PUFA supplementation for 10 weeks at a ratio of 1:4 linolenic–linoleic acids. This mixture significantly improved reported sleep quality in the treatment group. Forty children received supplementation, 38 children received a placebo, and 22 non-ADHD children acted as a controlled diet group. Sleep questionnaires were completed twice: before and after the serum assay.

25.2.5 Cholesterol and Sleep

Excessive cholesterol consumption was shown to be detrimental to sleep quality and duration by both Gangwisch et al. (2010) and Santana et al. (2012). Gangwisch et al. (2010) noted that less sleep during adolescence increased the risk of hypercholesterolemia in early adulthood. Although data for both genders displayed a similar relationship, the results were only significant in female participants (Gangwisch et al. 2010). Conversely, when 58 elderly obese male and female participants consumed increased amounts of cholesterol, shorter sleep duration was noted in both genders (Santana et al. 2012), although in this investigation the results were only significant in men. Both studies relied on self-reporting methods alone (Gangwisch et al. 2010; Santana et al. 2012) instead of controlled, measured food intakes. A related study of 24 Swedish participants (30 years of age on average) used polysomnography to determine that serum lipids and total cholesterol were the investigated factors most significantly related to the number of sleep arousals per hour (Ekstedt et al. 2004).

In contrast, Aneja and Tierney (2008) found that cholesterol supplementation was associated with improved behavior and sleep in patients with social and behavioral problems, anxiety and mood disorders, and sleep disturbances. For example people with certain autism spectrum disorders benefited from dietary cholesterol supplementation, either in natural form (single egg yolk, cream, liver) or given as treatment doses of purified cholesterol (Aneja and Tierney 2008). Grandner et al. (2010), however, detected a decrease in sleep duration when 423 postmenopausal women reported increased cholesterol intakes on their food-frequency questionnaires. Actigraphs and sleep diaries were used to measure their sleep. Grandner et al. felt that increases in dietary cholesterol led to decreases in lipid and cholesterol synthesis within the body, thus decreasing the stimulus to sleep. However, in a 2014 study by the same investigators, cholesterol exhibited a positive relationship with nonrestorative sleep. The relationship between cholesterol intake and sleep suggests that both over- and underconsumptions may be detrimental to physiologic functioning (Grandner et al. 2014,b).

To summarize, studies of the relationships among dietary fats and sleep behaviors have produced conflicting results with PUFAs showing the most positive results related to enhancing sleep. Summaries of investigations of dietary fat and its impact on sleep are shown in Table 25.1.

25.3 PROTEIN AND SLEEP

High-protein diets (including tryptophan-manipulated diets) were found to significantly improve sleep quality in some studies (Markus et al. 2005), while other studies showed no significant relationship between protein-enhanced diets and sleep onset (Landström et al. 2000). For example 35 healthy subjects with some sleep difficulties participated in a repeated-measure, crossover designed study to determine whether consuming cereals with two different amounts of enriched tryptophan or a controlled cereal diet improved their sleep (Bravo et al. 2013). Sleep was measured using wrist actimeter devices over 3 weeks with diets changed each week. Consuming the cereals enhanced with the highest doses (60 mg) of tryptophan increased sleep efficiency and sleep time and improved sleep latency.

The essential amino acid, tryptophan, has a direct role in neurotransmission functions of the brain (Fernstrom 2013). Tryptophan is also considered to be a sleep-enhancing amino acid, as it is a precursor to serotonin and melatonin. The amount of tryptophan that is available to the brain is determined by the ratio of plasma tryptophan to the total amount of large neutral amino acids (LNNA); any changes to this ratio change the availability of tryptophan to the brain.

The synthesis of serotonin from tryptophan requires a two-step process. During the first step, hydroxylation, 5-hydroxytryptophan is decarboxylated to serotonin. Serotonin is then released from the nerve terminals after depolarization and reacts with the serotonin receptors. Melatonin is a derivative of serotonin. Both melatonin and serotonin are hormones that have an effect on body

TABLE 25.1
High-Fat Diet

Authors	Study Design/Instrumentation	Sample Size	Results Related to Sleep
Aneja and Tierney (2008)	Review article.	N/A	• Individuals with certain autism spectrum disorders who were treated with cholesterol showed improvements in sleep and social interactions.
Crispim et al. (2011)	*Nutrition Measures*: • Three-day food diary. *Sleep Measures*: • Polysomnography.	52 participants (25 men and 27 women) (19–45 years of age)	• Food intake during or close to the nocturnal period was negatively correlated with sleep efficiency in healthy individuals, especially women. • Intakes of high-fat and high-carbohydrate foods preceeding the sleeping period led to higher sleep latency.
Gangwisch et al. (2010)	(Multivariate longitudinal analysis) *Nutrition Measures*: • Interview question on cholesterol intake. *Sleep Measures*: • Sleep duration questions. *Other*: • National Longitudinal Study of Adolescent Health data.	14,257 adolescent volunteers • Grades 7–12 at baseline (1994–1995) • (18–26 years of age at follow-up; 2001–2002)	• Each additional hour of sleep during adolescence resulted in decreased odds of developing high cholesterol in early adulthood.
Grandner et al. (2010)	(Large, multisite, longitudinal study) Ancillary study of the Women's Health Initiative. *Nutrition Measures*: • Food frequency questionnaires. *Sleep Measures*: • Actigraphs. • Daily sleep diaries.	423 postmenopausal women (50–81 years of age)	• Sleep time was negatively related to fat intakes. • Subjective sleepiness was associated with fat and meat intakes. • Decreased sleep duration was related to increased cholesterol intake.
Grandner et al. (2013)	*Nutrition Measures*: • 2007–2008 National Health and Nutrition Examination Survey (NHANES) data. *Sleep Measures*: • Sleep duration survey questions.	5587 adults (18+ years of age)	• Diets enriched with saturated fatty acids had a significant association with a sleep duration of 7–8 h.
Grandner et al. (2014,b)	(Large-scale survey data) *Nutrition Measures*: • 2007–2008 National Health and Nutrition Examination Survey (NHANES). *Sleep Measures*: • Sleep surveys.	4548 participants in the 2007–2008 NHANES (29–62 years of age)	• Subjective sleep data were not significantly correlated with the fat variables. • Difficulty in falling asleep was associated with greater saturated fatty acid intakes and lower intakes of MUFAs (dodecanoic acid).

(*Continued*)

TABLE 25.1(*Continued*)
High-Fat Diet

Authors	Study Design/Instrumentation	Sample Size	Results Related to Sleep
Huss et al. (2010)	*Nutrition Measures*: • Omega-3 and omega-6 fatty acid capsules with zinc and magnesium. *Sleep Measures*: • Interview questions on sleep initiation, maintenance, and sleep quality.	810 children (5–12 years of age)	• A combination of omega-3 and omega-6 fatty acid supplements with magnesium and zinc had a significant effect on reducing sleep-related problems by more than 40%.
Irmisch et al. (2007)	*Nutrition Measures*: • Serum fatty acid levels measured during the first 3 days and during the last 3 days of hospital admission. *Sleep Measures*: • *Beck Depression Index*, sleep disturbance questions.	118 depressive inpatients (51 males; 67 females) (33–57 years of age)	• Increased consumption of palmitoleic and oleic fatty acids decreased sleep disturbances in neuropsychiatric disorders (e.g. ADHD, depression). • PUFA omega-6 fatty acids enhanced sleep performance. • Cholesterol was associated with nonrestorative sleep.
Judge et al. (2012)	*Nutrition Measures*: • Cereal-based food bar with 300 mg DHA or placebo for 5 days/week during pregnancy. *Sleep Measures*: • Infant sleep/wake states measured with a pressure-sensitive mattress recording respirations and body movements.	48 pregnant women with no complications (18–35 years of age)	• Increased prenatal dietary docosahexaenoic acid (DHA) can play a beneficial role in early neonatal sleep patterns. • Women consuming DHA supplemented food bars had babies with fewer sleep arousals in the early neonatal period.
Montgomery et al. (2014)	(Randomized controlled trial) *Nutrition Measures*: • 16 weeks of docosahexaenoic acid (omega-3) supplements. *Sleep Measures*: • Actigraphs. • Child Sleep Habits Questionnaire.	Subset of 43 healthy UK children (7–9 years of age)	• No significance observed with the subjective sleep measures. • Actigraphs showed seven fewer wake episodes and 58 min more sleep per night with omega-3 fatty acid supplements.
Rontoyanni et al. (2007)	*Nutrition Measures*: • Two 24 h dietary recall interviews. *Sleep Measures*: • Sleep Habits Questionnaire. • 7-day sleep diary.	30 healthy Greek women (30–60 years of age)	• A weak positive association between sleep duration and saturated fat was observed.

(*Continued*)

TABLE 25.1 (*Continued*)
High-Fat Diet

Authors	Study Design/Instrumentation	Sample Size	Results Related to Sleep
Santana et al. (2012)	*Nutrition Measures*: • High-fat foods were served. *Sleep Measures*: • Nocturnal sleep questionnaire.	58 men and women with obesity (60–80 years of age)	• Significant associations with less sleep and higher MUFA intakes and less sleep and higher cholesterol intakes.
Shi et al. (2008)	(Large cross-sectional study) National Survey of Nutrition and Health. *Nutrition Measures*: • Weighed food intakes. • 3-day food records. *Sleep Measures*: • Interview questions querying hours slept per day.	2828 adults from China (30–69 years of age)	• Significant associations were found between shorter sleep duration and increases in fat. • Higher fat intakes resulted in significantly higher energy levels after sleeping less than 7 h/day.
Urade and Hayaishi (2011)	Review article.	N/A	• This chapter describes the physiology and synthesis of prostaglandin D^2, a chemical that helps regulate sleep, and explains its role as a sleep hormone.
Weiss et al. (2010)	(Cross-sectional study design) *Nutrition Measures*: • 24 h food-recall questionnaires. *Sleep Measures*: • Actigraphs.	240 adolescents (17–18 years of age)	• Shorter sleep duration was associated with increases in fat intake and decreases in carbohydrate intakes (even after including potential confounders).
Yehuda et al. (1996)	(Short-term, double-blinded study) *Nutrition Measures*: • Compound of 1:4 linolenic and linoleic acid (omega-3 and omega-6 fatty acid; 1:4 ratio) mixture for 60 participants; placebo for 40 participants. *Sleep Measures*: • Neurology exam with *sleep problem* questions.	100 patients (79 males, 21 females) (50–73 years of age)	• Short-term treatments with linolenic and linoleic acid fatty acid mixture induced behavioral changes in the quality of life (including sleep) of Alzheimer's disease patients. • The effects of the1:4 linolenic and linoleic fatty acid treatments were significantly greater than the effects of the placebo.
Yehuda et al. (2011)	*Nutrition Measures*: • 10 weeks of treatment with a polyunsaturated acid mixture. *Sleep Measures*: • Fatigue and sleep quality measured on a *five-point scale*.	78 ADHD children (9–12 years of age)	• Increased consumption of polyunsaturated fatty acid mixture resulted in significant improvement in sleep quality.

functions such as sleep. Thus, fluctuating levels of serotonin in the body can be a precursor to disturbances in sleep (Fernstrom 2012). Because the body is unable to synthesize tryptophan, it is necessary to obtain this essential amino acid through the diet (Soh and Walter 2011). The role of diet in influencing the central nervous system through serotonin (5-HT) and melatonin production is described in Figure 25.1 (Grimmett and Sillence 2005).

Changing the level of tryptophan concentrations in the brain is one method of influencing the rate of serotonin synthesis (Fernstrom 2013). The same system of transport that carries several LNAAs across the blood–brain barrier also transports tryptophan across that barrier. This makes the tryptophan/LNAA ratio a critical factor in transporting tryptophan from the blood to the brain. Tryptophan is the least abundant of the amino acids. As a result, other LNAAs are preferred for transport into the brain. Therefore, ingestion of forms of protein other than α-lactalbumin act to decrease the amount of tryptophan that reaches the brain. Consuming either pure tryptophan or a tryptophan-rich protein can be used to increase the ratio between tryptophan and LNNA (Markus 2005). A whey-derived protein called α-lactalbumin has the highest level of tryptophan content and thus the most favorable tryptophan/LNAA ratio (Markus 2005). Therefore, when analyzing the effects of tryptophan on sleep, the type of tryptophan supplementation should also be considered. Tryptophan levels in the brain can also be increased by carbohydrates. The insulin stimulation of LNAAs in turn increases the amount of free tryptophan (Fernstrom 2013). Because the synthesis of niacin, a B vitamin, is also dependent upon tryptophan, the intake of niacin in the diet is also important for sleep.

The levels of tryptophan in blood plasma affect sleep, as revealed through dietary manipulation. For example in 18 females who received a placebo or 1.3 g tablets of tryptophan before bedtime, tryptophan reduced sleep latency and increased non-REM sleep during the night (Brown et al. 1979). However, in another study, when 12 male and female adults (35–65 years of age) consumed 1 g tryptophan pills or a placebo at bedtime, tryptophan did not shorten sleep latency (Adam and Oswald 1979). Also, in another study, eight middle-aged insomniacs were given a placebo or 2 g tryptophan

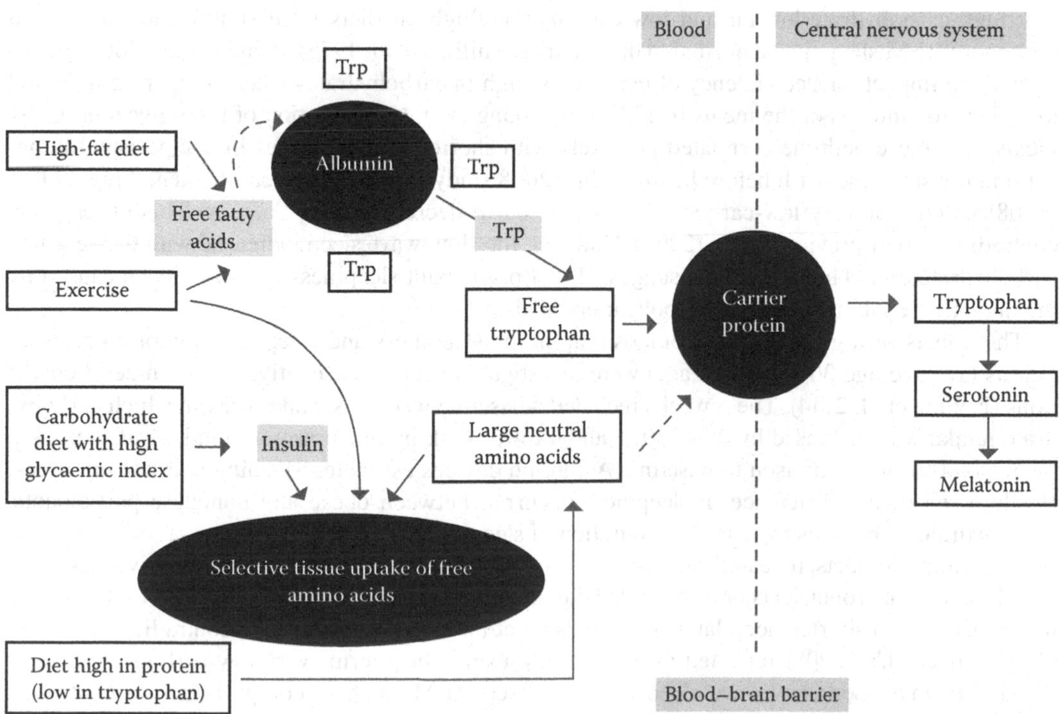

FIGURE 25.1 Effects of diet on tryptophan. (From Grimmett, A., and Sillence, M.N., *Vet. J.* 170, 26, 2005.)

pills 30 min before bedtime for 4 nights, resulting in increased sleep latency and non-REM sleep in the experimental group (Schneider-Helmert 1980). Hartmann and Spinweber (1979) found that sleep latencies could be significantly reduced in insomniacs using typical dietary intakes as low as one-fourth of a gram of dietary tryptophan per day. Furthermore, the daily nutritional requirement for tryptophan is 5 mg/kg of body weight. These results on the effects of lower tryptophan doses have significant implications since large tryptophan doses have typically been used without appropriate testing of the side effects. Also, published studies have been statistically underpowered.

Consumption of a high-protein diet produced significantly fewer wake episodes than a controlled diet in a study of healthy, young adults (Lindseth et al. 2013). These findings were similar to studies that showed sleep improvements with high-protein diets, especially diets rich in tryptophan (Markus et al. 2005). However, related work indicated that low-protein diets resulted in tryptophan depletion with subsequent reductions in brain serotonin levels (Voderholzer et al. 1998). Depleted tryptophan levels correlated with more wake periods and greater wake percentages than controlled conditions. In contrast, over an 8-week period, nine narcolepsy patients experienced modest improvements in daytime sleepiness on a low-carbohydrate, ketogenic diet (Atkin's diet) (Husain et al. 2004).

In summary, investigations into the impact of protein-rich diets on sleep quality have returned mixed results. Some research indicates that more protein in the diet significantly impacts sleep quality (Brown et al. 1979; Markus et al. 2005). However, other studies reached very different conclusions (Adam and Oswald 1979; Landström et al. 2000). Summaries of investigations of protein-rich diets and their impact on sleep are shown in Table 25.2.

25.4 CARBOHYDRATES AND SLEEP

"High-glycemic-index carbohydrate meals shorten sleep onset" (Afaghi et al. 2007). For example in a repeated-measure, within-subjects study of eight young healthy males, EEG measures indicated that high-carbohydrate/low-fat and low-carbohydrate/high-fat diets were significantly correlated with more REM sleep than a normal, balanced diet (Phillips et al. 1975). Afaghi et al. (2007) investigated the impact on sleep latency of meals very high in carbohydrates when comparing high and low glycemic indices of the meals in 12 healthy young men. Consumption of high-glycemic-index meals 4 h before bedtime correlated positively with shorter sleep latencies in comparison to consuming the same meal 1 h before bedtime. In a 2008 study involving 14 healthy men, Afaghi et al. (2008) noted that very low-carbohydrate meals led to decreased sleep latency. This observation contradicted their previous study (2007). However, the slow-wave sleep increased with the very low carbohydrate diet. The researchers suggested that participant sleepiness may have been caused by the higher fat content of the low-carbohydrate meals.

The effects of nighttime meal composition on the sleepiness and sleep duration of 24 security guards (average age 30.8 years of age) were investigated over 3 consecutive weeks under 3 conditions (Nehme et al. 2014). The 3 weeks included a baseline week, a second week in which carbohydrate intake was increased by 20%–30%, and a third week in which protein intake was increased by 30%–40% in comparison to baseline. Actigraph devices estimated sleeping and waking times. While a significant difference in sleepiness occurred between obese and nonobese participants, carbohydrate-rich meals increased the duration of sleep in obese workers.

In a within-subjects, repeated-measure study of 40 young adults randomized to receive diets with high levels of macronutrients or a controlled diet for 4 days each, consumption of high-carbohydrate meals resulted in shorter sleep latencies (Lindseth et al. 2013). These results contradict the results of Afaghi et al.'s (2008) repeated-measure study using short-term, very-low-carbohydrate diets that led to increased slow-wave sleep and decreased REM sleep in comparison to a controlled diet. Participants were fed isocaloric evening test meals 4 h before their normal bedtimes. Sleep was measured using a computerized sleep system. However, Afaghi et al. (2007) noted that very-low-carbohydrate meals led to decreased sleep latency. Further, Malone (2001) studied 19 healthy

TABLE 25.2
High-Protein Diet

Reference	Study Design and Instrumentation	Sample Size	Results Related to Sleep Implications
Adam and Oswald (1979)	*Nutrition Measures*: • For two nights, 1 g of tryptophan pills given. • For two nights, inert pills given. • Low-carbohydrate diets for two nights. • High-carbohydrate diets for two nights. *Sleep Measure*: • EEG sleep spindles.	12 participants: • 5 men • 7 women (38–65 years of age)	• There were no differences in the effects of placebo or tryptophan supplements and high-carbohydrate or low-carbohydrate foods on sleep latency.
Bravo et al. (2013)	(Experimental design) *Nutrition Measurements*: • Diet of 22.5 mg tryptophan in cereal. • Diet of 60 mg tryptophan in cereal. • Controlled diet cereal. *Sleep Measurements*: • Actigraphs.	35 middle-age volunteers with sleep difficulties.	• Cereals with higher amounts of tryptophan led to increases in sleep efficiency, sleep time, and sleep latency.
Brown et al. (1979)	(Double-blind study) *Nutrition Measures*: • 1 g of L-tryptophan or 3 g of L-tryptophan. *Sleep Measure*: • Sleep recordings.	18 female participants	• REM, slow-wave sleep, or wakefulness did not differ when comparing the 1 g, 3 g, or controlled doses of tryptophan. • Sleep latency was significantly reduced when 3 g of tryptophan was consumed.
Fernstrom (2012)	Review article.	N/A	• Review article focusing on the side effects of tryptophan supplementation as a psychopharmacologic agent to improve conditions such as mood and sleep.
Fernstrom (2013)	Review article.	N/A	• Linkages were described between tryptophan, large neutral amino acids, and their uptake into the brain as they convert into serotonin and catecholamines. • Dietary protein and amino acid mixtures are proposed as treatments for neurobehavioral and sleep conditions.
Hartmann and Spinweber (1979)	(Laboratory design) *Nutrition Measures*: • Compared doses of 1/4, 1/2, and 1 g of tryptophan with a placebo control. *Sleep Measure*: • Polysomnography.	15 normal male mild insomniacs (21–35 years of age)	• Significantly reduced sleep latency was reduced when participants received 1 g doses of L-tryptophan. • Consumption of 1/4 g doses of tryptophan led to a significant increase in deep sleep.

(Continued)

TABLE 25.2 (*Continued*)
High-Protein Diet

Reference	Study Design and Instrumentation	Sample Size	Results Related to Sleep Implications
Husain et al. (2004)	Nutrition Measure: • Atkin's diet plan. Sleep Measures: • Narcolepsy Symptom Status Questionnaire. • Epworth Sleepiness Scale. • Stanford Sleepiness Scale.	9 narcolepsy patients: • 8 men • 1 woman (36.7–58.5 years of age)	• Patients with narcolepsy experienced modest improvements in daytime sleepiness using a low-carbohydrate, ketogenic diet.
Landstrom et al. (2000)	*Nutrition Measures*: • High-carbohydrate/low-fat or high-fat/low-carbohydrate meals (10 meal/snack combinations). *Sleep Measures*: • Wakefulness rated on a 100 mm rating scale.	12 drivers; 6 day drivers and 6 night drivers	• No significant differences in wakefulness when comparing the fat, protein, and carbohydrate meals.
Lindseth et al. (2013)	(Repeated-measure, counterbalanced, crossover design) *Nutrition Measures*: • Controlled, high-protein, high-fat, and high-carbohydrate meals weighed for four treatment periods. *Sleep Measures*: • Actigraphs.	44 young adult participants (18–22 years of age)	• High-protein diets were associated with significantly fewer wake episodes.
Schneider-Helmert (1981)	(Double-blind design) *Nutritional Measures*: • Tryptophan supplements. *Sleep Measures*: • Polysomnography.	5 males and 3 females with chronic insomnia (mean age 38.4 years)	• Insomnia was significantly improved using interval therapy with tryptophan.
Soh and Walter (2011)	Review article.	N/A	• The benefits of consuming dietary tryptophan as a treatment for depressed patients are discussed.
Voderholzer et al. (1998)	(Double-blind, crossover) *Nutrition Measures*: • Low-protein diets (2 days). • 2–3 g tryptophan amino acid mixture. • Tryptophan controlled mixture. *Sleep Measures*: • Polysomnography.	12 healthy participants; 6 males and 6 females (23–55 years of age)	• Decreased rapid eye movement followed tryptophan depletion. • Sleep latency was not affected.

female American college students (18–25 years of age) to determine the impact of dietary fat intakes and body fat percentages on sleep quality and tiredness. Ten of nineteen participants kept a detailed record of their consumption of a high-carbohydrate, high-fat diet for 10 days; sleep decreased and daytime tiredness increased in individuals who had higher body fat percentages (Malone 2001).

The association between dietary factors and sleep quality was also examined in an investigation of 3129 Japanese, middle-aged, female workers who self-administered a diet-history questionnaire and responded to the Pittsburgh Sleep Quality Index; a low intake of vegetables and fish, the consumption of high-carbohydrate foods, and unhealthy eating habits were significantly related to poor sleep quality (Katagiri et al. 2014).

In a review article, the relationship of sleep loss and its impact on the body's ability to use glucose was described. For example in one study, within 1 week of sleeping 4 h/night, healthy, lean, fit individuals spiraled into a prediabetic state (Van Cauter et al. 2007). Consistent with this observation, low sleep efficiency correlated significantly with high serum glucose levels (Lindseth et al. 2013). In another study, eight Australian children (8–12 years old, four girls and four boys) were served either low- or high-glycemic-index drinks 1 h before bedtime for three nights and were monitored with polysomnography (Jalilolghadr et al. 2011). The results indicated that high-glycemic-index beverages correlated positively with non-REM sleep and total overnight arousals. The authors concluded that poorer sleep quality was a result of consuming large quantities of carbohydrates close to bedtime (Jalilolghadr et al. 2011).

Overall there is an interesting mix of research on high-carbohydrate diets and sleeping patterns, with contradicting results. For example Afaghi, O'Connor, and Chow conducted two studies 1 year apart that reached different conclusions; their 2007 study found that high-carbohydrate, high-glycemic-index meals led to shorter sleep latencies, while their 2008 study on the same topic suggested that low-carbohydrate meals shorten sleep latencies. Summaries of studies of carbohydrate-rich diets and their impact on sleep are shown in Table 25.3.

25.5 MICRONUTRIENTS: VITAMINS, MINERALS, AND SLEEP

The consumption of vitamins and minerals can also affect the quality and quantity of sleep in humans. Evidence suggests that lower levels of vitamin D consumption can lead to the development of sleep disorders (Shiue 2013). Data obtained from 4552 adults in the 2007–2008 National Health and Nutrition Examination Survey (NHANES) also linked increased vitamin D consumption with fewer wake episodes during sleep (Grandner et al. 2014b). In the same study, vitamins and minerals such as carotene, selenium, and calcium were correlated with difficulty in falling asleep. Salt and lycopene (a phytochemical found in tomatoes and other fruits and vegetables) were associated with difficulties in maintaining sleep; and nonrestorative sleep correlated independently with butanoic acid, calcium, vitamin C, and water. Finally, sleepiness independently correlated with theobromine (found in chocolate), potassium, and water (Grandner et al. 2014b).

Other vitamin and mineral intakes that had significant relationships with short sleep duration times were described in a 2013 study using the 2007–2008 NHANES data by Grandner et al. (2013). When adjusting for overall diet, decreased thiamin, folate, and folate equivalents were associated with very short (<5 h) sleep duration times. Again, after adjusting for overall diet, very short (<5 h) sleep times were associated with significantly decreased intake of phosphorus, magnesium, iron, zinc, and selenium as were long sleep (>9 h) duration times (Grandner et al. 2013).

McCarty et al. (2012) employed a sleep disruption symptoms scale and the Epworth Sleepiness Scale to determine if serum vitamin D levels correlated with excessive daytime sleepiness in 81 sleepy and nonsleepy, middle-aged participants. Excessive sleepiness inversely correlated with vitamin D consumption in patients not suffering from vitamin D deficiency. Data from black participants, but not white participants, with vitamin D deficiency were also associated with sleep problems. McCarty et al. concluded that vitamin D deficiency may have a mechanistic role in sleepiness and/or sleep disorders and recommended more research in this area.

TABLE 25.3
High-Carbohydrate Diet

Reference	Study Design and Instrumentation	Sample Size	Results Related to Sleep Implications
Afaghi et al. (2007)	*Nutrition Measures*: • Three standardized meals randomly received 1 week apart. *Sleep Measures*: • 2-week sleep diary polysomnography.	12 healthy Australian men (18–35 years of age)	• Significant reduction in the mean sleep onset latency with high-glucose-index meals versus low-glucose-index meals. • High-glucose index meal 4 h before bedtime showed significantly shortened sleep onset latency compared to the same meal 1 h before bedtime.
Afaghi et al. (2008)	(Repeated-measure design) *Nutrition Measures*: • Test meals. • Likert scales measured hunger and fullness. *Sleep Measures*: • Polysomnography.	14 healthy, nonobese men (good sleepers) (18–35 years of age)	• Very-low-carbohydrate diets promoted short-term increases in the percentage of slow-wave sleep, while leading to a reduction in the percentage of REM sleep compared to the controlled mixed diet.
Jalilolghadr et al. (2011)	*Nutrition Measures*: • Low- or high-glycemic-index (GI) drinks. *Sleep measures*: • Polysomnography.	8 Australian children (4 girls, 4 boys) (8–12 years of age)	• Both non-REM sleep and total arousal indices were greater with high-GI drink consumption 1 h before sleep. • Consuming a high quantity of carbohydrates just before bedtime led to frequent overnight arousals and diminished sleep quality.
Katagiri et al. (2014)	*Nutrition Measures*: • Self-administered diet history and eating habit questionnaires. *Sleep Measures*: • Pittsburgh Sleep Quality Index (PSQI)	3129 female Japanese workers (34–65 years of age)	• Poor sleep quality correlated positively with lower vegetable intakes and fish intakes and higher intakes of confectionary items and carbohydrates. • Poor sleep quality also correlated with energy drinks, sugar-sweetened beverages, skipping breakfast, and eating irregularly.
Lindseth et al. (2013)	(Repeated-measure, crossover design). *Nutrition Measures*: • Weighed-controlled, high-protein, high-fat, and high-carbohydrate meals. *Sleep Measures*: • Actigraphs.	44 American young adult participants (18–22 years of age)	• High-carbohydrate diets were associated with significantly shorter sleep latencies than controlled diets.

(Continued)

TABLE 25.3 (*Continued*)
High-Carbohydrate Diet

Reference	Study Design and Instrumentation	Sample Size	Results Related to Sleep Implications
Malone (2001)	*Nutrition Measures*: • Body fat percentages (bioelectrical impedance) (Phase I). • Daily food record (8 days) (Phase I). • Detailed food record (10 days) (Phase II). *Sleep Measures*: • 21-day sleep record and Likert Self-Reported Tiredness Scale (Phase I).	19 healthy female American college students (18–25 years of age)	• *Phase I*: No correlation between body fat percentages and sleep during the controlled, carbohydrate, fat, or protein diets. • *Phase II*: Both dietary fat and carbohydrates consistently decreased sleep and increased tiredness in high body fat percentage individuals.
Nehme et al. (2014)	*Nutrition Measures*: • 24 h dietary recall • Dietary interventions. • Week 1, no change; week 2, 20%–30% more carbohydrates; week 3, 30%–40% more protein. *Sleep Measures*: • Actigraphs.	54 male night security guards (25.3–36.3 years of age)	• Sleep duration was higher in obese workers compared with nonobese workers during the increased carbohydrate intervention. • Significant differences in sleepiness were also noted between the obese and nonobese groups.
Phillips et al. (1975)	(Experimental design) *Nutrition Measures*: • Normal balanced diet, high-carbohydrate/low-fat diet. • Low-carbohydrate/high-fat diet. *Sleep Measures*: • EEG sleep changes.	8 young healthy male participants	• Significantly less slow-wave sleep was found after consuming a high-carbohydrate/low-fat diet in comparison to the normal balanced diet or low-carbohydrate/high-fat diet. • High-carbohydrate/low-fat diets were associated with more REM sleep.
Van Cauter et al. (2007)	Review article.	N/A	• Experimental sleep restriction is associated with (a) alterations in glucose metabolism, (b) regulation of appetite, and (c) decreased energy expenditure. Evidence links short sleep with obesity and diabetes risk.

25.6 CAFFEINE, ALCOHOL, AND SLEEP

Research on alcohol consumption and sleep indicates that consuming alcohol to "self-medicate" impacts the amount of slow-wave sleep and REM sleep (Danel et al. 2001; Feige et al. 2006). In an investigation by Feige et al. (2006), a blood alcohol level of 0.1% led to a significant increase in slow-wave sleep and reduced REM sleep during the first half of the night. REM sleep increased after alcohol levels decreased to 0.03%. It was concluded that alcohol is an unsuitable hypnotic when consumed in great quantities over a period of days.

The neurologic stimulant, caffeine, was also found to disrupt sleep when consumed at bedtime; and the need for sleep decreased after caffeine consumption. Caffeine occurs in many common foods and beverages such as tea, coffee, and chocolate and thus is widely consumed (Nehlig et al. 1992). Caffeine has also been found to produce sleep disruption when taken just prior to going to bed. The effect of caffeine consumption on sleep was studied in a randomized, five-way, crossover investigation of 30 healthy British volunteers (Hindmarch et al. 2000). Sleep and activity were measured using the Leeds Sleep Evaluation Questionnaire, wrist actigraphy, and psychometric tests of critical flicker fusion, choice reaction time, and subjective sedation. Caffeinated beverages correlated positively with poorer sleep onset, sleep time, and sleep quality scores; however, repeated ingestion of caffeinated beverages helped sustain cognitive and psychomotor performance throughout the day and evening.

25.7 KILOCALORIES AND SLEEP

In a study of 12 healthy male participants who were given low- or high-kilocalorie liquid carbohydrate lunches over 4 days, thermogenesis was significantly greater after high-calorie meals, but the total minutes or stages of REM sleep did not differ between meal conditions, nor did sleep latency (Zammit et al. 1992). Postprandial sleep was thus associated with increased thermogenesis, which decreases both postprandial heat production and body temperature (Zammit et al. 1992). Finally, a rise in body temperature after food intake, also referred to as the thermic effect of food, positively correlated with high-energy food consumption and was found to influence sleep for up to 2 h after dietary intake (Driver et al. 1999). In another study, higher caloric intakes resulted in better sleep efficiency in a study of 44 young adults (Lindseth et al. 2013). In contrast, pilot study results demonstrated that a 1-week fasting period promoted the quality of sleep and resulted in decreased sleep arousals in nonobese participants (Michalsen et al. 2003).

Sleep disturbances are at the forefront of obesity research. Sleep deprivation is known to increase ghrelin, the hormone responsible for appetite, and to decrease leptin, the hormone responsible for satiety (Grandner et al. 2010, 2013, 2014b; Shi et al. 2008). This imbalance in hormone levels was found to increase cravings for high-satiety foods, such as pastries and potato chips, which tend to be rich in both fat and carbohydrates (Shi et al. 2008). Although energy expenditures may slightly increase after a lengthened period of wakefulness, physical activity often declines due to sleep-deprived fatigue (Grandner et al. 2014b; Shi et al. 2008). Therefore, sleep deprivation can yield to greater energy intake than energy expenditure, thus contributing to overweight and obesity conditions.

In the National Health Interview Survey, almost 30% of adults reported that they slept less than 6 h/night, even though 7–8 h of sleep is the recommended nightly amount for adults (Centers for Disease Control and Prevention 2014). Shorter sleep times have also been associated with higher energy intake in early childhood (Fisher et al. 2014). A sleep questionnaire for infants was used to measure the sleep duration of children at 16 months of age in more than 1300 families; at 21 months, parents recorded the macronutrients consumed per day with 3-day diaries. Children who slept less than 10 h/night were associated with an increased consumption of 50 kcal/day in comparison to children who slept 11–12 h/night (the advised sleep duration for children of this age) (Fisher et al. 2014). However, in turn, macronutrient consumption did not affect the children's sleep duration.

25.8 FLUID INTAKE AND SLEEP

In the Grandner et al. (2013) analysis of data from the 2007–2008 NHANES, increased difficulty in initiating and maintaining sleep was associated with the consumption of cow's milk, which contains the saturated fatty acid butanoic acid. In a subsequent study by Grandner et al. (2014b), dairy products were also associated with increased difficulty in falling asleep. In that study, nonrestorative sleep was associated independently with calcium, commonly found in milk products, and vitamin C, commonly found in fruit juices. Nutrients that were associated independently with sleepiness included water and potassium; both are commonly found in sports drinks.

A review article by Grandner et al. (2014a) discussed research concerning the consumption of energy drinks as a possible contributing factor to loss of sleep and shortened duration of sleep. Two groups seen as being particularly vulnerable to excessive energy drink consumption include people in lower socioeconomic classes and racial minorities (Grandner et al. 2014a).

The relationship between fluids and sleep was further illustrated in a study of sleep patterns in four young, adult Nigerian men who were randomly assigned to sedentary (baseline), cycling, aerobic exercise, or recovery conditions, with and without rehydration (Montmayeur et al. 1994). Polysomnography recorded for two consecutive nights in each condition suggested that a combined action of hyperthermia, water balance, and stress were needed to support slow-wave and REM sleep. Also, Grandner et al. (2014b) analyzed data from the 2007–2008 National Health and Nutrition Examination Survey (NHANES) data and found that nonrestorative sleep correlated independently with water intakes by the study participants. In addition, sleepiness had a statistical relationship with water intake (Grandner et al. 2014b).

25.9 IMPLICATIONS

According to several studies, attention to nutritional intake could be a key strategy for improving sleep (Centers for Disease Control and Prevention 2014; Ford et al. 2013; Grandner et al. 2014b; Jaussent et al. 2011; Lopresti et al. 2013; Shi et al. 2008). Some research has suggested that consuming certain dietary fats or high-glycemic-index diets has decreased sleep quality (Crispim et al. 2011; Grandner et al. 2010; Shi et al. 2008) and on average resulted in fewer hours of sleep per night. On the other hand, consumption of dietary fatty acids, certain LNNA, and complex carbohydrates resulted in longer sleep duration and better sleep quality. For example consuming a high-protein diet significantly reduced wake episodes compared with a controlled diet, and a high-carbohydrate diet significantly reduced sleep latency compared with a controlled diet (Afaghi et al. 2007; Lindseth et al. 2013). While increased caloric intake positively correlated with sleep efficiency (Lindseth et al. 2013), most studies have indicated that highglycemic-index diets result in frequent overnight arousals and diminished sleep quality.

According to a study of 5885 older men and women, adherence to a Mediterranean diet containing fewer saturated fatty acids and more PUFAs substantially decreased self-reported insomnia symptoms in both genders, with significant benefits experienced by female participants (Jaussent et al. 2011). Mediterranean diets are traditionally higher in both the monounsaturated fatty acids found in olive oil and the PUFAs found in fatty fish (Ford et al. 2013; Lopresti et al. 2013). In contrast, Western diets are higher in saturated and trans fatty acids, which are primarily found in red meat, fast food, and pastries.

Some research has suggested that consuming certain fatty acids decreased sleep quality (Crispim et al. 2011) and on average resulted in fewer hours of sleep per night (Grandner et al. 2010; Shi et al. 2008). Other studies rejected this trend and reported that saturated fatty acids actually improved sleep time and efficiency (Papandreou 2013). While omega-3 fatty acid (PUFA) intake resulted in better sleep (Grandner et al. 2013; Montgomery et al. 2014), hexadecanoic acid (a saturated fatty acid) was associated with increased difficulty in falling asleep and hexanoic acid (an unsaturated fatty acid) was associated with increased difficulty in maintaining sleep (Grandner et al. 2014b; Irmisch et al. 2007).

25.10 SUMMARY

In summary, the previous studies described in this chapter provide supporting evidence that specific nutrients in the diet may influence sleep quality. Grandner et al. (2014b) concluded that novel associations between sleep symptoms and diet metabolism may explain associations between sleep and cardiometabolic diseases. The implications of sleep deprivation may also promote the release of proinflammatory cytokines and tumor necrosis factors that could result in immunocompromised conditions (Boland and Alloy 2013; Lopresti et al. 2013). Research has shown that the benefits of diet to sleeping the recommended daily amount can be derived from consuming a range of complementary foods.

REFERENCES

Adam, K. and I. Oswald. One gram of L-tryptophan fails to alter the time taken to fall asleep. *Neuropharmacology* 18(12) (1979): 1025–1027.

Afaghi, A., H. O'Connor, and C.M. Chow. High-glycemic-index carbohydrate meals shorten sleep onset. *The American Journal of Clinical Nutrition* 85(2) (2007): 426–430.

Afaghi, A., H. O'Connor, and C.M. Chow. Acute effects of the very low carbohydrate diet on sleep indices. *Nutritional Neuroscience* 11(4) (2008): 146–154.

Altevogt, B.M. and H.R. Colten, eds. *Sleep Disorders and Sleep Deprivation: An Unmet Public Health Problem*. National Academies Press, Washington, DC (2006).

Aneja, A. and E. Tierney. Autism: The role of cholesterol in treatment. *International Review of Psychiatry* 20 (2) (2008): 165–170. doi: 10.1080/09540260801889062.

Boland, E.M. and L.B. Alloy. Sleep disturbance and cognitive deficits in bipolar disorder: Toward an integrated examination of disorder maintenance and functional impairment. *Clinical Psychology Review* 33(1) (2013): 33–44. doi:10.1016/j.cpr.2012.10.001.

Bravo, R., S. Matito, J. Cubero, S.D. Paredes, L. Franco, M. Rivero, A.B. Rodríguez, and C. Barriga. Tryptophan-enriched cereal intake improves nocturnal sleep, melatonin, serotonin, and total antioxidant capacity levels and mood in elderly humans. *Age* 35(4) (2013): 1277–1285.

Brown, C.C., N.J. Horrom, and A.M. Wagman. Effects of l-tryptophan on sleep onset insomniacs. *Waking & Sleeping* 3 (1979): 101–108.

Carskadon, M.A. and W.C. Dement. Normal human sleep: An overview. *Principles and Practice of Sleep Medicine* 4 (2000): 13–23.

Centers for Disease Control and Prevention (CDC). Insufficient sleep is a public health epidemic (2014). Retrieved from http://www.cdc.gov/features/dssleep/. Accessed on May 27, 2015.

Crispim, C.A., I.Z. Zimberg, B.G. dos Reis, R.M. Diniz, S. Tufik, and M.T. de Mello. Relationship between food intake and sleep pattern in healthy individuals. *Journal of Clinical Sleep Medicine: JCSM: Official Publication of the American Academy of Sleep Medicine* 7(6) (2011): 659–664.

Danel, T., C. Libersa, and Y. Touitou. The effect of alcohol consumption on the circadian control of human core body temperature is time dependent. *American Journal of Physiology-Regulatory, Integrative and Comparative Physiology* 281(1) (2001): R52–R55.

Driver, H.S., I. Shulman, F.C. Baker, and R. Buffenstein. Energy content of the evening meal alters nocturnal body temperature but not sleep. *Physiology & Behavior* 68(1) (1999): 17–23.

Ekstedt, M., T. Åkerstedt, and M. Söderström. Microarousals during sleep are associated with increased levels of lipids, cortisol, and blood pressure. *Psychosomatic Medicine* 66(6) (2004): 925–931.

Feige, B., H. Gann, R. Brueck, M. Hornyak, S. Litsch, F. Hohagen, and D. Riemann. Effects of alcohol on polysomnographically recorded sleep in healthy subjects. *Alcoholism: Clinical and Experimental Research* 30(9) (2006): 1527–1537.

Fernstrom, J.D. Effects and side effects associated with the non-nutritional use of tryptophan by humans. *The Journal of Nutrition* 142 (2012): 2236S–2244S.

Fernstrom, J.D. Large neutral amino acids: Dietary effects on brain neurochemistry and function. *Amino Acids* 45, 3 (2013): 419–430.

Fisher, A., L. McDonald, C.H.M. van Jaarsveld, C. Llewellyn, A. Fildes, S. Schrempft, and J. Wardle. Sleep and energy intake in early childhood. *International Journal of Obesity* 38 (2014): 926–929.

Ford, P.A., K. Jaceldo-Siegl, J.W. Lee, W. Youngberg, and S. Tonstad. Intake of Mediterranean foods associated with positive affect and low negative effect. *Journal of Psychosomatic Research* 74(2) (2013): 142–148. doi:10.1016/j.jpsychores.2012.11.002.

Gangwisch, J.E., D. Malaspina, L.A. Babiss, M.G. Opler, K. Posner, S. Shen, J.B. Turner, G.K. Zammit, and H.N. Ginsberg. Short sleep duration as a risk factor for hypercholesterolemia: Analyses of the National Longitudinal Study of Adolescent Health. *Sleep* 33(7) (2010): 956–961.

Grandner, M.A., N. Jackson, J.R. Gerstner, and K.L. Knutson. Dietary nutrients associated with short and long sleep duration. Data from a nationally representative sample. *Appetite* 64 (2013): 71–80. doi:10.1016/j.appet.2013.01.004.

Grandner, M.A., N. Jackson, J.R. Gerstner, and K.L. Knutson. Sleep symptoms associated with intake of specific dietary nutrients. *Journal of Sleep Research* 23(1) (2014b): 22–34. doi:10.1111/jsr.12084.

Grandner, M.A., K.L. Knutson, W. Troxel, L. Hale, G. Jean-Louis, and K.E. Miller. Implications of sleep and energy drink use for health disparities. *Nutrition Reviews* 72(S1) (2014a): 14–22.

Grandner, M.A., D.F. Kripke, N. Naidoo, and R.D. Langer. Relationships among dietary nutrients and subjective sleep, objective sleep, and napping in women. *Sleep Medicine* 11(2) (2010): 180–184. doi: 10.1016/j.sleep.2009.07.014.

Grimmett, A., and M.N. Sillence. Calmatives for the excitable horse: a review of L-tryptophan. *The Veterinary Journal* 170(1) (2005): 24–32.

Guyton, A.C. and J.E. Hall. *Human Physiology and Mechanisms of Disease*, 6th edn. Elsevier Health Sciences, Philadelphia, PA (1996).

Hartmann, E. and C.L. Spinweber. Sleep induced by L-tryptophan. Effect of dosages within the normal dietary intake. *The Journal of Nervous and Mental Disease* 167(8) (1979): 497–499.

Hindmarch, I., U. Rigney, N. Stanley, P. Quinlan, J. Rycroft, and J. Lane. A naturalistic investigation of the effects of day-long consumption of tea, coffee and water on alertness, sleep onset and sleep quality. *Psychopharmacology* 149(3) (2000): 203.

Husain, A.M., W.S. Yancy, S.T. Carwile, P.P. Miller, and E.C. Westman. Diet therapy for narcolepsy. *Neurology* 62(12) (2004): 2300–2302.

Huss, M., A. Völp, and M. Stauss-Grabo. Supplementation of polyunsaturated fatty acids, magnesium and zinc in children seeking medical advice for attention-deficit/hyperactivity problems-an observational cohort study. *Lipids in Health and Disease* 9(1) (2010): 105. doi: 10.1186/1476–511X-9–105.

Irmisch, G., D. Schläfke, W. Gierow, S. Herpertz, and J. Richter. Fatty acids and sleep in depressed inpatients. *Prostaglandins, Leukotrienes and Essential Fatty Acids* 76(1) (2007): 1–7. doi:10.1016/j.plefa.2006.09.001.

Jalilolghadr, S., A. Afaghi, H. O'Connor, and C.M. Chow. Effect of low and high glycaemic index drink on sleep pattern in children. *The Journal of the Pakistan Medical Association* 61(6) (2011): 533.

Jaussent, I., Y. Dauvilliers, M.-L. Ancelin, J.-F. Dartigues, B. Tavernier, J. Touchon, K. Ritchie, and A. Besset. Insomnia symptoms in older adults: Associated factors and gender differences. *The American Journal of Geriatric Psychiatry* 19(1) (2011): 88–97. doi:10.1097/JGP.0b013e3181e049b6.

Judge, M.P., X. Cong, O. Harel, A.B. Courville, and C.J. Lammi-Keefe. Maternal consumption of a DHA-containing functional food benefits infant sleep patterning: An early neurodevelopmental measure. *Early Human Development* 88(7) (2012): 531–537. doi:10.1016/j.earlhumdev.2011.12.016.

Katagiri, R., K. Asakura, S. Kobayashi, H. Suga, and S. Sasaki. Low intake of vegetables, high intake of confectionary, and unhealthy eating habits are associated with poor sleep quality among middle-aged female Japanese workers. *Journal of Occupational Health* 56 (2014): 359–368.

Landström, U., A. Knutsson, and M. Lennernäs. Field studies on the effects of food content on wakefulness. *Nutrition and Health* 14(4) (2000): 195–204.

Lindseth, G., P. Lindseth, and M. Thompson. Nutritional effects on sleep. *Western Journal of Nursing Research* 35, 4 (2013): 497–513.

Lopresti, A.L., S.D. Hood, and P.D. Drummond. A review of lifestyle factors that contribute to important pathways associated with major depression: Diet, sleep and exercise. *Journal of Affective Disorders* 148(1) (2013b): 12–27. doi:10.1016/j.jad.2013.01.014.

Malone, M. The effect of meal composition and body fat on sleep and tiredness. Paper 130(1) (2001). Retrieved on May 27, 2015 at http://digitalcommons.unf.edu/ojii_volumes/130.

Marino, M., Y. Li, M.N. Rueschman, J.W. Winkelman, J.M. Ellenbogen, J.M. Solet, H. Dulin, L.F. Berkman, and O.M. Buxton. Measuring sleep: Accuracy, sensitivity, and specificity of wrist actigraphy compared to polysomnography. *Sleep* 36(11) (2013): 1747.

Markus, C.R., L.M. Jonkman, J.H.C.M. Lammers, N.E.P. Deutz, M.H. Messer, and N. Rigtering. Evening intake of α-lactalbumin increases plasma tryptophan availability and improves morning alertness and brain measures of attention. *The American Journal of Clinical Nutrition* 81(5) (2005): 1026–1033.

McCarty, D.E., A. Reddy, Q. Keigley, P.Y. Kim, and A.A. Marino. Vitamin D, race, and excessive daytime sleepiness. *Journal of Clinical Sleep Medicine: JCSM: Official Publication of the American Academy of Sleep Medicine* 8(6) (2012): 693–697.

Michalsen, A., F. Schlegel, A. Rodenbeck, R. Lüdtke, G. Huether, H. Teschler, and G.J. Dobos. Effects of short-term modified fasting on sleep patterns and daytime vigilance in non-obese subjects: Results of a pilot study. *Annals of Nutrition and Metabolism* 47(5) (2003): 194–200.

Montgomery, P., J.R. Burton, R.P. Sewell, T.F. Spreckelsen, and A.J. Richardson. Fatty acids and sleep in UK children: Subjective and pilot objective sleep results from the DOLAB study—A randomized controlled trial. *Journal of Sleep Research* 23 (2014): 364–388.

Montmayeur, A., A. Buguet, H. Sollin, and J-R. Lacour. Exercise and sleep in four African sportsmen living in the Sahel. *International Journal of Sports Medicine* 15(1) (1994): 42–45.

National Sleep Foundation. 2009 Sleep in America Poll (2009). Retrieved from October 20, 2014, http://sleepfoundation.org/sites/default/files/2009%20POLL%20HIGHLIGHTS.pdf;http://sleepfoundation.org/sites/default/files/2009%20NSF%20POLL%20PRESS%20RELEASE.pdf.

Nehlig, A., J.-L. Daval, and G. Debry. Caffeine and the central nervous system: Mechanisms of action, biochemical, metabolic and psychostimulant effects. *Brain Research Reviews* 17(2) (1992): 139–170.

Nehme, P., E.C. Marqueze, M. Ulhôa, E. Moulatlet, M.A. Codarin, and C.R. Moreno. Effects of a carbohydrate-enriched night meal on sleepiness and sleep duration in night workers: A double-blind intervention. *Chronobiology International* 31(4) (2014): 453–460.

Papandreou, C. Gluteal adipose tissue fatty acids and sleep quality parameters in obese adults with OSAS. *Sleep and Breathing* 17(4) (2013): 1315–1317.

Phillips, F., A.H. Crisp, B. McGuinness, E.C. Kalucy, C.N. Chen, J. Koval, R.S. Kalucy, and J.H. Lacey. Isocaloric diet changes and electroencephalographic sleep. *The Lancet* 306(7938) (1975): 723–725.

Rontoyanni, V.G., S. Baic, and A.R. Cooper. Association between nocturnal sleep duration, body fatness, and dietary intake in Greek women. *Nutrition* 23(11) (2007): 773–777.

Santana, A.A., G.D. Pimentel, M. Romualdo, L.M. Oyama, R.V. Thomatieli Santos, R.A. Pinho, C.T. de Souza, B. Rodrigues, E.C. Caperuto, and F.S. Lira. Sleep duration in elderly obese patients correlated negatively with intake fatty. *Lipids in Health and Disease* 11(1) (2012): 99.

Schneider-Helmert, D. Interval therapy with L-tryptophan in severe chronic insomniacs. A predictive laboratory study. *International Pharmacopsychiatry* 16(3) (1980): 162–173.

Scorza, F.A., E.A. Cavalheiro, C.A. Scorza, J.C.F. Galduróz, S. Tufik, and M.L. Andersen. Sleep apnea and inflammation—Getting a good night's sleep with omega-3 supplementation. *Frontiers in Neurology* 4 (2013): 193.

Sharon, K. and Hirshkowitz, M. 2011. Monitoring and staging human sleep. In *Principles and practice of sleep medicine*. 5th ed. Edited by Kryger, M. H., Thomas R., and William C. D. (pp 1602–1609). St. Louis: Elsevier Saunders.

Shi, Z., M. McEvoy, J. Luu, and J. Attia. Dietary fat and sleep duration in Chinese men and women. *International Journal of Obesity* 32(12) (2008): 1835–1840. doi:10.1038/ijo.2008.191.

Shiue, I. Low vitamin D levels in adults with longer time to fall asleep: US NHANES, 2005–2006. *International Journal of Cardiology* 168(5) (2013): 5074–5075.

Soh, N.L. and G. Walter. Tryptophan and depression: Can diet alone be the answer? *Acta Neuropsychiatrica* 23(1) (2011): 3–11.

Urade, Y., and Hayaishi, O. Prostaglandin D_2 and sleep/wake regulation. *Sleep Medicine Reviews* 15(6) (2011): 411–418. doi:10.1016/j.smrv.2011.08.003.

Van Cauter, E., U. Holmbäck, K. Knutson, R. Leproult, A. Miller, A. Nedeltcheva, S. Pannain, P. Penev, E. Tasali, and K. Spiegel. Impact of sleep and sleep loss on neuroendocrine and metabolic function. *Hormone Research in Paediatrics* 67(Suppl. 1) (2007): 2–9.

Voderholzer, U., M. Hornyak, B. Thiel, C. Huwig-Poppe, A. Kiemen, A. König, J. Backhaus, D. Riemann, M. Berger, and F. Hohagen. Impact of experimentally induced serotonin deficiency by tryptophan depletion on sleep EEG in healthy subjects. *Neuropsychopharmacology: Official Publication of the American College of Neuropsychopharmacology* 18(2) (1998): 112–124.

Weiss, A., F. Xu, A. Storfer-Isser, A. Thomas, C.E. Ievers-Landis, and S. Redline. The association of sleep duration with adolescents' fat and carbohydrate consumption. *Sleep* 33(9) (2010): 1201–1209.

Werner, H., L. Molinari, C. Guyer, and O.G. Jenni. Agreement rates between actigraphy, diary, and questionnaire for children's sleep patterns. *Archives of Pediatrics & Adolescent Medicine* 162, 4 (2008): 350–358.

Yehuda, S., S. Rabinovitz-Shenkar, and R.L. Carasso. Effects of essential fatty acids in iron deficient and sleep-disturbed attention deficit hyperactivity disorder (ADHD) children. *European Journal of Clinical Nutrition* 65(10) (2011): 1167–1169. doi:10.1038/ejcn.2011.80.

Yehuda, S., S. Rabinovtz, R.L. Carasso, and D.I. Mostofsky. Essential fatty acids preparation (SR-3) improves Alzheimer's patient's quality of life. *International Journal of Neuroscience* 87(3–4) (1996): 141–149.

Zammit, G.K., S.H. Ackerman, R. Shindledecker, M. Fauci, and G.P. Smith. Postprandial sleep and thermogenesis in normal men. *Physiology & Behavior* 52(2) (1992): 251–259.

Section XIII

Wound Healing

26 Oral Supplementation of a Standardized Naturally Fermented Papaya Preparation May Correct Type 2 Diabetes Mellitus–Induced Reactive Oxygen Species Dysregulation

Ryan Dickerson and Sashwati Roy

CONTENTS

26.1 INTRODUCTION

The distinction between "good reactive oxygen species (ROS)" and "bad ROS" has recently been reported in regard to diabetes [14]. The harmful or "bad ROS," resulting in systemic oxidative stress, has widely been implicated in the etiology of type 2 diabetes mellitus (T2DM) [6]. In addition to weight loss and increased fiber intake, the incorporation of functional foods to reduce oxidative stress on the body has been suggested. Fermented papaya preparation (FPP) is a nutritional supplement that is made from yeast fermentation of ripe *Carica papaya* Linn that has been reported to be a potent antioxidant capable of relieving the burden of "bad ROS" [13]. It has also been reported that T2DM leukocytes are deficient in their ability to produce a *respiratory burst*, good ROS, in response to a stimulus [8,10]. Our lab has recently provided novel evidence that in addition to scavenging free radicals and reducing "bad ROS," oral supplementation of FPP to T2DM patients promotes the production of "good ROS" in the form of the bactericidal *respiratory burst* production of superoxide anion ($O_2^{\bullet-}$) [10].

26.2 FERMENTED PAPAYA PREPARATION

The production of FPP is carried out following strict international quality control regulations. Ripe, organic, nongenetically modified papayas grown in Hawaii are yeast biofermented using technologies that have received ISO 9001:2000 (international quality standard), ISO 14001:2004 (international environmental standard), and ISO 22000:2005 (international food safety standard) certifications by Osato International (Gifu, Japan). FPP is rich in carbohydrates and amino acids, and also contains free radical–scavenging residual phenolic or flavonoid compounds that have been shown to significantly reduce the rate of hemolysis and protein oxidation in the blood plasma of prediabetic individuals [13]. Other conditions associated with increased hemolysis of hemoglobin, such as paroxysmal nocturnal hemoglobinuria, thalassemia, and sickle cell disease, might also find benefit from the supplementation of FPP. In addition to reducing hemolysis, FPP has been shown to protect against free radical–induced single- and double-strand breaks in supercoiled plasmid DNA in vitro [3], suggesting that FPP may protect cells at the most basic level.

26.3 ROS: THE GOOD, THE BAD, AND THE UGLY

During innate immune response, leukocytes (neutrophils and monocytes) are stimulated to produce their characteristic *respiratory burst*, which produces superoxide anion ($O_2^{\bullet-}$) and derivative ROS, which are utilized for bactericidal purposes and cell signaling. This "good ROS" is produced by the leukocyte NADPH oxidase, which catalyzes the production of $O_2^{\bullet-}$ by the one-electron reduction of oxygen at the expense of NADPH, the electron donor [4,5]. It has also been reported that ROS generated by NADPH oxidase is essential for proper intracellular signaling [14]. Insulin resistance (IR), a major implication of T2DM, has also been shown to be attenuated by H_2O_2 in vivo [14]. Conversely, a major source of harmful ROS or "bad ROS" is leakage of $O_2^{\bullet-}$ from complex I and complex III of the electron transport chain during mitochondrial respiration. It is thought that oversaturation of the electron transport chain in the absence of ATP demand, associated with overfeeding, obesity, and T2DM, results in excess reducing equivalents (NADH and $FADH_2$) leading to overabundant $O_2^{\bullet-}$ generation [14]. The buildup of free radicals associated with nutrient overload (high-fat diet) has been linked to IR and mitochondrial damage. Conversion of $O_2^{\bullet-}$ to hydroxyl radical ($^{\bullet}OH$) and reactive metal complexes, via either iron-catalyzed Haber–Weiss reactions or superoxide anion-driven Fenton reaction, has been shown to induce oxidative damage to DNA [2]. Because T2DM is associated with both excess "bad ROS" and compromised "good ROS," our lab has been investigating the potential of the supplementation of FPP to ameliorate ROS-associated T2DM complications [9–11].

26.4 FPP IN DIABETIC WOUND HEALING

In 2010, it was estimated that chronic wounds affected ~6.5 million patients in the United States, resulting in over U.S. $25 billion spent in treatment costs. More than 23 million Americans (7.8% of the population) are currently diagnosed with T2DM, with an ever-increasing prevalence of the disease resultant from poor diet and sedentary lifestyle. It is estimated that almost one-quarter of all diabetic patients will develop diabetic foot ulcers [1]. It is no surprise that 67% of all lower-extremity amputation patients have been diagnosed with T2DM. There are various natural plant sources that are considered for the care of diabetes. The long history of safe human consumption of, and breadth of data associated with, FPP as an antioxidant implicates the supplementation of the standardized natural preparation to T2DM populations, which are known to have elevated oxidative stress. For our model, we used adult male obese *Lepr*db mice (db/db, 8–10-week age), which were group housed and allowed ad libitum access to food and water. Mice were divided randomly into FPP-supplemented and placebo-controlled groups. The FPP group mice were fed 0.2 g/kg body weight FPP, 5 days/week, for 8 weeks via oral gavage. Placebo group mice were administered by matching the amount of D-glucose in the same method. Blood glucose and lipid profiling were measured at the baseline (prior to supplementation), after 8 weeks of supplementation, then followed by an 8-week post supplementation. FPP significantly blunted blood glucose (~30% reduction) during the supplementation period. Triglycerides were significantly reduced in FPP-supplemented animals compared to placebo, as was total cholesterol and LDL. HDL, or *good cholesterol*, was increased significantly in FPP-treated animals [9].

To investigate wound-healing outcomes, anesthetized diabetic db/db and control nondiabetic db/+ mice were given two 6 mm full-thickness excisional wounds via skin punch biopsy equidistant from the midline on the dorsum and equidistant from the limbs. Wounds were allowed to heal by secondary intention. Photographs of the wound were taken, and open area was determined using WoundMatrix software (Chadds Ford, PA). Nondiabetic animals' wounds were ~70% closed 7 days post wounding. Unsupplemented diabetic mice wound area showed impaired wound closure. When diabetic mice were supplemented with FPP, the wound area 7 days post wounding was significantly smaller than that in the placebo group. In FPP-supplemented animals, increased expression of CD68 and VEGF suggests that FPP improved the recruitment of microphages to the wound site and provided a favorable microenvironment for angiogenesis. Wound infection is a major cause of concern in diabetic wounds. Professional phagocytic and immune-regulating macrophages are known to produce $O_2^{\bullet-}$ during their inducible *respiratory burst* via NADPH oxidase as a bactericidal agent in a wound microenvironment. In our study, FPP potently increased diabetic macrophage-inducible respiratory burst, as indicated by the measurement of $O_2^{\bullet-}$ [9].

Taken together, this 2010 work provided the first evidence that oral supplementation of FPP may benefit diabetic wound closure in a mouse model. It has been reported that alveolar macrophages from diabetic animals have a compromised respiratory burst [12]. Hyperglycemia is also known to inhibit the activity of NADPH oxidase [15]. The ability of FPP supplementation to preserve NADPH oxidase function and "good ROS" is a novel concept with the potential to translate into the ability for diabetics to mount a more efficient defense against wound infection, a noted problem in T2DM populations, allowing for improved wound outcomes [9].

26.5 FPP IN T2DM IMMUNE CELL FUNCTION

Impaired immune function, including leukocyte dysfunction, makes infection a major problem for the T2DM population. Of 1000 hospitalized patients enrolled in a comparative study, two-thirds of the T2DM patients screened suffered from bacteremia [7]. It is also previously reported that peripheral blood mononuclear cells (PBMCs) from T2DM individuals cannot mount a proper respiratory burst when stimulated [7]. Conclusions from our 2010 in vivo mouse work suggested that oral supplementation of FPP improved wound-healing outcomes in diabetic mice. One of the major actions of FPP we observed was a potent induction of ROS production via NADPH oxidase in supplemented animals. In this work, we aimed to determine the effect of FPP supplementation to T2DM PBMCs, which are the circulating blood precursor to the mature wound macrophages (MΦ) investigated previously [11].

In this work, we corroborate the literature observation that PBMCs from T2DM patients suffer from compromised inducible respiratory burst potential. To test the effect of FPP on PBMC ex vivo, we isolated PBMC from whole blood drawn from T2DM and non-T2DM patients. We supplemented the culture media of PBMC (3 mg FPP/mL), which were cultured in for 24 h. We stimulated respiratory burst from PBMC with phorbol 12-myristate 13-acetate (1 μg/mL, 30 min) and measured superoxide anion ($O_2^{\bullet-}$) production. Similar to our mouse study, FPP enhanced T2DM PBMC "good ROS" production in the respiratory burst. T2DM ROS production after FPP supplementation was rescued to near non-T2DM levels [11].

NADPH oxidase, the enzyme responsible for catalyzing the production of $O_2^{\bullet-}$, is an assembly of several protein subunits that require localization and assemblage on the cell membrane to function properly. Knowing that this enzyme's activity is affected in T2DM, we looked at the protein expression of the protein subunits of the NADPH oxidase complex via western blot. We discovered that two of the protein subunits differed significantly after FPP supplementation. First, p47phox, whose activity is modulated post translationally and is active in the phosphorylated state, showed significantly more phosphorylation after FPP supplementation. Second, Rac2-a Rho family GTPase required for the activation of the complex expression was significantly upregulated in

FPP-supplemented PBMC. We also looked at Rac2 mRNA expression via quantitative real-time PCR and observed similarly induced expression in FPP-supplemented PBMC. Comparing T2DM to non-T2DM PBMCs, we observed that T2DM cells had attenuated expression of Rac2 mRNA compared to the healthy donors. Most significantly, when we introduced FPP to T2DM PBMC ex vivo, Rac2 expression was rescued to non-T2DM levels [11].

Trying to understand the mechanism by which FPP is able to rescue Rac2 expression and therefore NADPH oxidase–mediated "good ROS" production, we contemplated the *Rac2* gene promoter, which contains several transcription factor binding sites. We showed the first evidence suggesting that FPP enhances the binding of the Sp1 transcription factor to the DNA promoter for *Rac2* in PBMC.

Curious about the dose dependency of FPP activity, we performed a dose titration identifying that even with as low as 10% (0.3 mg FPP/mL) of the dose we were standardly using (3.0 mg FPP/mL), we were able to measure significant Rac2 mRNA expression induction. Investigating the kinetics of FPP action, we looked at Rac2 mRNA expression from baseline (0 h) through 48 h. FPP was able to induce Rac2 in as short as 6 h and maintain steady expression from 6 to 24 h, before tapering back down to the baseline by 48 h suggesting that continual administration of FPP would be required for prolonged benefit of supplementation [11].

Having identified in 2010 the potential for orally supplemented FPP to induce "good ROS" in diabetic mouse wound MΦ and then in 2012 establishing that FPP was able to rescue "good ROS" production in human PBMC ex vivo, the need to continue the investigation in vivo in humans was warranted. In order to ethically start a large-scale human clinical trial, it was necessary to establish that the FPP, which is carbohydrate rich, is safe for T2DM individuals to consume in regard to their hyperglycemia levels. We set up a trial where T2DM patients would provide a blood sample at a baseline visit (0 week), begin supplementation, and return at 2 and 6 weeks before discontinuing supplementation and returning for washout analysis (7 and 8 weeks). Over the course of the supplementation period, there was no significant effect showing that FPP negatively affected fasting blood glucose or the long-term indicator of blood glucose–glycated hemoglobin (HbA1c). In addition, FPP showed no effect on total cholesterol levels. Taken together, we establish that FPP is indeed safe for T2DM patient consumption.

In the continued effort to establish the relationship of FPP in regard to "good ROS" and "bad ROS" levels, we measured inducible respiratory burst of the orally treated PBMC isolated from donor blood and excitingly observed results similar to our mouse model and ex vivo previous models; stimulated superoxide anion ($O_2^{\bullet -}$) production was more than double the baseline for each patient during FPP supplementation. To continue to establish the safety of oral supplementation of FPP in T2DM humans, we investigated "bad ROS" during supplementation by measuring the protein oxidation, via protein carbonyls, and lipid peroxidation, via 4-hydroxynonenal (4-HNE), and found no significant increase in "bad ROS" during the supplementation period.

In 2012, we observed that FPP significantly upregulated the phosphorylation of the p47phox subunit of NADPH oxidase, which may be required for the activation of the enzyme complex. Adenosine triphosphate (ATP), the energy currency of the cell, is required for phosphorylation reactions to proceed. Interestingly, we observed that human THP-1, monocytic model, cells supplemented in vitro with FPP had 75% higher cellular ATP levels than nonsupplemented cells. To control for potentially increased substrate availability in treated groups, due to FPP's large carbohydrate composition, we matched comparable D-glucose levels to the culture media and did not see an increase in ATP concentration, suggesting a glucose-independent upregulation of ATP during FPP supplementation.

NADPH is oxidized and is the electron donor in the conversion of O_2 to $O_2^{\bullet -}$ by the enzyme NADPH oxidase. The availability of NADPH might also be a consideration for the ability of FPP to rescue "good ROS" production during a respiratory burst. In this work, we report a minor increase in total NADP and a major increase in NADPH. The ratio of NADPH/total NADP dramatically shifts toward NADPH in FPP-treated THP-1 cells, suggesting an increased availability of the electron donor necessary for NADPH oxidase respiratory burst function.

The majority of ATP synthesis is accomplished during oxidative phosphorylation (oxyphos) along the electron transport chain in the mitochondria. Production of ATP relies on the pumping of protons outside of the mitochondrial membrane, establishing an electrochemical gradient, measured as mitochondrial membrane potential ($\Delta\psi m$). We measured the $\Delta\psi m$ of THP-1 cells supplemented with FPP, without FPP, and with matching glucose and observed a significant increase in $\Delta\psi m$ in FPP-supplemented cells. If the increased ATP concentration we observed was a result of increased mitochondrial oxyphos, one would expect increased mitochondrial respiration due to the needs for increased oxygen as a final electron acceptor during ATP synthesis. Using a Clark electrode, we measured mitochondrial oxygen consumption by comparing state IV and uncoupled state oxygen consumption rates in FPP-supplemented and control populations. FPP-supplemented cells had significantly increased oxygen consumption compared to nonsupplemented cells.

26.6 CONCLUSIONS

Taken together, the three recent publications from our group and the current existing literature show strong evidence that FPP taken orally may be a functional food able to benefit T2DM individuals (Figure 26.1). Systemic oxidative stress, "bad ROS," is a problem reported in various T2DM implications. Reports of FPP reducing DNA oxidation damage among a myriad of other works are encouraging in suggesting that FPP may relieve oxidative burden in T2DM patients. Our works suggest a pivotal role of FPP in the rescue of compromised "good ROS" in the form of inducible respiratory burst in innate immune cells. More efficient innate immune response in T2DM populations may be beneficial in a chronic wound situation. Now that FPP consumption has been shown

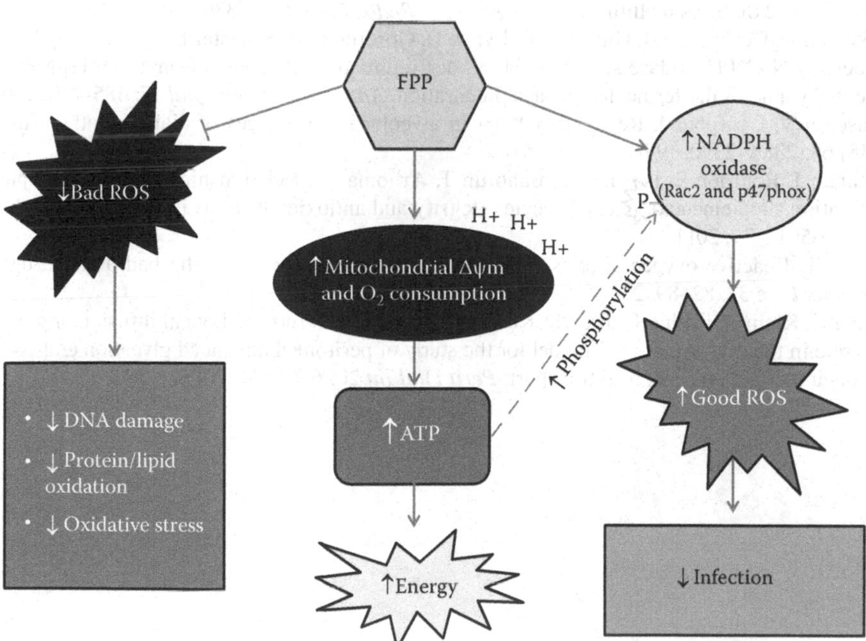

FIGURE 26.1 **(See color insert.)** FPP corrects T2DM-mediated aberrant ROS in innate immune cells. FPP's antioxidant properties combat harmful "bad" ROS, thereby reducing the negative effects of elevated oxidative stress (DNA damage, protein and lipid oxidation, etc.). FPP supplementation increases mitochondrial membrane potential leading to elevated ATP levels, which may be used in phosphorylation reactions to activate NADPH oxidase, rescuing compromised useful "good" ROS production via respiratory burst, reducing the infection.

to be safe for T2DM consumption, our group has future plans to investigate the supplementation of FPP to T2DM patients suffering from chronic wounds in regard to wound-healing outcomes.

REFERENCES

1. ADA. Direct and indirect costs of diabetes in the United States. http://www.diabetes.org/diabetes-basics/statistics/. Accessed on June 03, 2015.
2. Aruoma OI, Halliwell B, Gajewski E, Dizdaroglu M. Damage to the bases in DNA induced by hydrogen peroxide and ferric ion chelates. *J Biol Chem* 264: 20509–20512, 1989.
3. Aruoma OI, Hayashi Y, Marotta F, Mantello P, Rachmilewitz E, Montagnier L. Applications and bioefficacy of the functional food supplement fermented papaya preparation. *Toxicology* 278: 6–16, 2010.
4. Babior BM. Oxygen-dependent microbial killing by phagocytes (first of two parts). *N Engl J Med* 298: 659–668, 1978.
5. Babior BM. Oxygen-dependent microbial killing by phagocytes (second of two parts). *N Engl J Med* 298: 721–725, 1978.
6. Baynes JW. Role of oxidative stress in development of complications in diabetes. *Diabetes* 40: 405–412, 1991.
7. Carton JA, Maradona JA, Nuno FJ, Fernandez-Alvarez R, Perez-Gonzalez F, Asensi V. Diabetes mellitus and bacteraemia: A comparative study between diabetic and non-diabetic patients. *Eur J Med* 1: 281–287, 1992.
8. Chang FY, Shaio MF. Respiratory burst activity of monocytes from patients with non-insulin-dependent diabetes mellitus. *Diabetes Res Clin Pract* 29: 121–127, 1995.
9. Collard E, Roy S. Improved function of diabetic wound-site macrophages and accelerated wound closure in response to oral supplementation of a fermented papaya preparation. *Antioxid Redox Signal* 13: 599–606, 2010.
10. Dickerson R, Banerjee J, Rauckhorst A, Pfeiffer DR, Gordillo GM, Khanna S, Osei K, Roy S. Does oral supplementation of a fermented papaya preparation correct respiratory burst function of innate immune cells in type 2 diabetes mellitus patients? *Antioxid Redox Signal*, 22: 339–345, 2014.
11. Dickerson R, Deshpande B, Gnyawali U, Lynch D, Gordillo GM, Schuster D, Osei K, Roy S. Correction of aberrant NADPH oxidase activity in blood-derived mononuclear cells from type II diabetes mellitus patients by a naturally fermented papaya preparation. *Antioxid Redox Signal* 17: 485–491, 2012.
12. Mohsenin V, Latifpour J. Respiratory burst in alveolar macrophages of diabetic rats. *J Appl Physiol* (1985) 68: 2384–2390, 1990.
13. Somanah J, Bourdon E, Rondeau P, Bahorun T, Aruoma OI. Relationship between fermented papaya preparation supplementation, erythrocyte integrity and antioxidant status in pre-diabetics. *Food Chem Toxicol* 65: 12–17, 2014.
14. Tiganis T. Reactive oxygen species and insulin resistance: The good, the bad and the ugly. *Trends Pharmacol Sci* 32: 82–89, 2011.
15. Zeltzer E, Klein O, Rashid G, Katz D, Korzets Z, Bernheim J. Intraperitoneal infusion of glucose-based dialysate in the rat—An animal model for the study of peritoneal advanced glycation end-products formation and effect on peritoneal transport. *Perit Dial Int* 20: 656–661, 2000.

Section XIV

Hair and Skin Health

27 Herbal Treatment for Hair Loss and Alopecia
An Overview

Nattaya Lourith and Mayuree Kanlayavattanakul

CONTENTS

27.1 INTRODUCTION

Human hair plays an important role in social and sexual communications with pronounced differences between ages and sexes in addition to its protective function. Major hair types distributed on scalp and body are terminal and vellus hairs, whereas lanugo hair is prevalent on unborn baby. Vellus hair has less content of keratin and melanin than terminal hair. It is therefore smaller in diameter than the terminal one, which is greater than the vellus in these parameters. Hair undergoes cyclic periods of growth, which are anagen, catagen, and telogen. The longest phase is anagen, whose length varies on the type of species and body site. Baldness directly distresses self-confidence affecting the individual's quality of life that Caucasian men are largely affected. The significant psychosocial manifestation of hair loss is therefore worth a lot of expense for treatment.

Hair loss or alopecia is caused by several factors including insufficient diet. Major classifications of hair loss are androgenetic alopecia (AGA), telogen effluvium (TE), and alopecia areata (AA). AGA is the major problematic hair disorder ruled by male hormones, androgen, and interchangeably known as male pattern hair loss. This hair loss has a specific pattern on the scalp and is well defined in men and women. AGA is noticed as a slow transformation of large scalp terminal hair follicles to shorter, thinner, and less deep vellus hair with a much shorter anagen. Hamilton–Norwood hair loss pattern is widely used to discrete the severity of hair loss in men, in the meantime that Ludwig and Christmas tree patterns are differentiated in women associated with the Savin scale, which is a hair width measuring scale to determine hair loss. Hair loss with the shortening of anagen hair and extending the telogen phase, which is characterized by a lessen hair diameter and melanin content in hair shaft, is known as TE. AA is a hair disorder in which the loss of hair causes patches of baldness but with no scarring of the affected area. This hair disorder that can affect the entire of hair scalp becomes alopecia totalis or loss of all body hair (alopecia universalis). Causes of hair loss or alopecia could be molecularly explained upon the mechanism at various phases of hair cycle as discussed elsewhere in addition to the relating clinical instruments and testing procedures. However, those sessions are out of scope of this chapter that exclusively focuses on the active agents treating alopecia.

The treatment for hair loss needs a longer time to notify the improvement that is differing from other dermatological disorders. Oral and topical administrations of synthetic ingredients combating hair loss possess adverse reactions and more severely in some case due to drug interactions. Therefore, naturally derived compounds or herbal treatment for hair loss is preferred more among the consumers [1].

27.2 NUTRICOSMETICS AND HAIR

Botanical actives, minerals, and vitamins, for instance phytoestrogens, zinc, and vitamin B, are associated with hair growth and hair strength. These agents are therefore efficient to delay or inhibit hair loss with the anagen-prolonging and anagen-inducing activities, shortening telogen hair phase and also stimulating proliferation of hair follicle and sustaining the cell age as well. Topical applications of therapeutic agents against hair loss have been already summarized [1] and available for the readers upon this sort of treatment with more information about the causes of AGA.

Phytosterols, phytoestrogens, essential fatty acids, and terpenoids in plants prevent androgenetic-mediated diseases by free radical–scavenging activity, blocking the harmful effects of sex hormone reducing serum excretion/production [2]. In addition to zinc and biotin deficiency associated with hair loss, iron deficiency had been addressed in alopecia recently [3]. Therefore, adequate dietary supplementation is required for limiting hair loss with a sufficient activity promoting hair growth [1]. Furthermore, the importance of nutraceutical and functional food has currently hit the consumers' awareness upon health benefits [4].

Daily calorie intake less than 1000 kcal may lead to hair loss as inadequate protein intake. Low protein intake causes reddish, short, and dull telogen hair that results to TE, which is consequently similar to zinc deficiency. In addition, deficiency of niacin and iron also accumulates in diffuse hair loss [5]. Although there are several researches exhibiting in vitro activities of therapeutic agents against hair loss, clinical evaluation in human volunteers shows adverse results. Therefore, efficacy evaluation in the panelists is needed to ensure the efficacy of the actives. In addition, administration methods also influence the efficacy of the actives due to bioavailability and permeation. Recently, beauty from the inside out that is widely known as nutricosmetics is highly in focus. This trend especially meets the consumers' preference due to multifunctional nature of food or dietary intake [4] associated with aesthetic benefits for skin, hair, and nail [6]. This chapter therefore chiefly overviews the oral administration of herbs, which include botanical actives, minerals, and vitamins that are potential for hair loss prevention and treatment on the basis of scientific evidences as evaluated majorly in human volunteers, although some of the efficient herbal treatment is available only in an animal model, for example ginseng treatment. The readers will therefore optimize their choices upon food and/or dietary intake to maintain the delay of hair loss and/or stimulate hair growth as well.

27.3 HERBAL TREATMENT FOR HAIR LOSS

27.3.1 Botanical Treatment

27.3.1.1 Capsaicin and Isoflavone

These botanical-derived compounds that are found plenty *in Capsicum frutescens, Serenoa repens, Urtica dioica*, and *Cucurbita* spp. are efficient for hair loss combating [1]. Capsaicin 0.1 mg/kg/day that was subcutaneously injected in male C57BL/6 mice (6–8 weeks-old) for 4 weeks significantly ($p < 0.01$) increased insulin-like growth factor I (IGF-I) in skin higher than the controlled group. The activity was significantly ($p < 0.01$) enhanced in combination with isoflavone (0.22% w/w) pellet. The result was in harmony in terms of hair growth activity in animal model. Thereafter, clinical evaluation in human volunteer was conducted in 48 Japanese (25 males and 23 females) aged 9–58 years, of which 34 suffered from AGA, 13 from alopecia totalis, and 1 from AA. The randomized placebo-controlled trial orally had taken either the combination of capsaicin and isoflavone (6 and 75 mg/day) or placebo for 5 months. IGF-I level in serum was significantly ($p < 0.01$) increased, whereas that of the placebo was not. In addition, hair growth also was significantly ($p < 0.01$) greater (64.5%) in the capsaicin and isoflavone administration group than the placebo (11.8%) [7].

In addition to the actives from several herbs, single herb appraisals for hair loss treatment are included as the following.

27.3.1.1.1 *Glycine max*

Soy peptide, in particular soymetide-4, which is constructed with four amino acids isolated from trypsin digestion, was one of the herbal products sufficient to suppress alopecia [8]. It exhibited the ability to suppress hair loss induced by etoposide. Therefore, oral administration of soymethide-4 at 300 mg/kg for 8 days was conducted. Soymetide-4 with the sequence of amino acids of Met-Ile-Trp-Leu was superior over its other homologues with different amino acids replacing Trp, of which 100 mg/kg of the most active soymetide-4 showed the same results with 300 mg/kg of other soymetide-4 derivatives [9].

27.3.1.1.2 *Panax ginseng*

Cell regeneration herb, that is ginseng with anti-inflammatory and blood circulation effect, was also used for skin and scalp treatment limiting hair loss [10]. Potential of ginseng in hair regeneration was confirmed in cell proliferation improvement including an in vivo efficacy evaluation in animal at 1 mg/mL topical application on mice that showed comparable results to 5% minoxidil [11].

Further purification of ginseng active and clinical evaluation in human volunteers were performed consequently. Ginsenoside F2, a minor saponin of ginseng, significantly ($p < 0.01$) increased the proliferation of cell (in a dose-dependent manner) comparable to finasteride. Anagen induction of the natural active compound was further evaluated in 7-week-old C57BL/6 mice with telogen hair. Oral administration of ginsenoside F2 (0.2 and 2.5 mg/kg) for 56 days is compared with that of finasteride (0.5 mg/kg) in 0.5% of carboxymethyl cellulose. At an equal amount of ginseng and finasteride, hair density was greater in the natural treatment than the benchmark product (65% and 37%), and the density was enhanced to 98% in 2.5 mg/kg ginsenoside F2–administrated group. This was in harmony with the thickness of hair that ginseng was more superior over finasteride (25% and 13% in 2.5 and 0.5 mg/kg extract and 8% of finasteride 0.5 mg/kg). In addition, ginseng also significantly increased and reduced hair in anagen and telogen phases in a dose-dependent manner. Thus, anagen/telogen ratio of ginseng treatment was significantly ($p < 0.05$) higher than finasteride [12,13]. However, confirmatory result in human volunteers remains unrevealed.

27.3.1.1.3 *Serenoa repens*

Saw palmetto, a 5α-reductase inhibitor [14], is commercialized in Permixon®, which is a lipidosterolic extract containing high essential fatty acid content [15] with phytosterols, β-carotene, and tocopherols including β-sitosterol [16–18]. This phytotherapeutic agent for hair loss treatment is very popular in Europe [19,20] and found effective without any enhancer [21]. Although there was hepatotoxicity of saw palmetto reported in rat [22], its safety was later confirmed [23]. Alopecia treatment of saw palmetto was examined in human by an oral route. Standardized saw palmetto extract (200 mg) containing 85%–95% liposterolic acid was orally assigned to the volunteers in the form of softgel consisted of β-sitosterol (50 mg), lecithin (50 mg), inositol (100 mg), phosphatidyl choline (25 mg), niacin (15 mg), and biotin (100 μg). A randomized double-blind, placebo-controlled (soybean oil 540 mg) trial was conducted in 19 males aged 23–64 years facing hair loss in the vertex area of grade II vertex through grade VI vertex by the Hamilton–Norwood scale. The efficacy of a twice-daily application of the softgel by the volunteers with the study duration of 18–24.7 weeks was further evaluated by the investigator. The improvement in hair loss of the placebo-controlled group was only 11% , whereas it was 60% in the active-treated group. However, none of significant result was reported in the study due to the small sample size [24].

27.3.1.1.4 Kampo Medicine

Anti–hair loss efficacy of a kampo medicine, kamishoyosangoshimotsuto, was evaluated in 20 females for 24 weeks. The volunteers conducted an open-label study by orally taking 3.9 g of the traditional medicine 18 tablets a day. Six tablets were taken before or between meals three times a day. The herbal extract mixture significantly increased hair diameter ($p < 0.01$) and strength ($p < 0.05$) as well [25]. However, the ratio of each extract in this kampo medicine that is the mixture of Japanese angelica root (*Aralia elata*), peony root, *Poria sclerotium*, *Atractylodes lancea* rhizome, Bupleurum root, *Glycyrrhiza*, dry ginger, peppermint, moutan bark (*Paeonia moutan*), Gardenia fruit (*Gardenia jasminoides*), Cnidium rhizome (*Cnidium officinale*), Chinese cnidium rhizome (*C. monnieri*), and Rehmannia root (*Rehmannia glutinosa*) was not reported. Furthermore, the activity evaluation of each herb should be conducted to reveal the mechanism of the herb in promotion efficacy of hair growth.

27.3.2 Amino Acid Treatment

Regarding the fact that hair is compounded with keratin, which is constructed of amino acids, amino acids are therefore essential for good health condition of hair. In addition, those of soy actives are relied on soymethide-4 [9], which is amino acids, and this class of natural active is also contributed and used in combination with the botanical extract [24]. Amino acids themselves have also been evaluated on their efficacy against alopecia.

Dietary supplement containing gelatin, cysteine, methionine, Cu, and Zn was taken four pills per day by 24 volunteers aged 21–38 years who affected with AGA types III and IV according to the Hamilton–Norwood scale. This randomized double-blind, placebo-controlled trial was studied for 50 weeks. The amino acid active significantly ($p < 0.005$) increased hair number and mass 18% and 24% following 10 weeks of administration. The efficacy of oral supplement amino acid was better than topical application of saw palmetto lotion (17% and 20%). The result was pronounced at week 50 as the number and mass were significantly ($p < 0.005$) increased to 29% and 40% [26]. However, the content of active in each formulation was omitted. Therefore, discussion per the active activity remained unclear.

In addition to the earlier treatment, a mixture of lysine (1.5 g) and iron (72 mg) was supplemented for 6 months. The formulation was shown to significantly ($p < 0.0001$) reduce telogen hair (11.3% ± 1.0%) with an enhancement of serum ferritin (89 ± 11 μg/L) compared to the baseline in a clinical evaluation in 22 women [27].

Therefore, several dietary supplements claiming on hair rejuvenation and protection against alopecia are commercialized. Amino acids from shark and mollusk patented as AminoMar™ Marine Complex are marketed in the name of Viviscal®. One tablet of this dietary supplement with marine complex as the main ingredient (450 mg), composed with vitamin C from acerola, niacinamide, biotin, iron, zinc oxide, horsetail and millet seed extracts, and silicon dioxide, was clinically evaluated by means of randomized, double-blind controlled in comparison with fish extract. Male volunteers (20 persons/group) affected with alopecia on the basis of Hamilton–Norwood scale of III–V took two tablets of each product once a day for 6 months. Bald scalp biopsy at the baseline was compared with that at the end of the study. The Viviscal had showed both clinical and histological cure. The marine amino acids significantly ($p < 0.0001$) increased nonvellus hair (38%) over the fish extract (2%) [28].

Increase of hair growth by means of a randomized, placebo-controlled, double-blind study in 60 volunteers supplemented with Hairgain® for 6 months was reported. The volunteers who took two capsules (body weight <80 kg) or three capsules (body weight >80 kg) a day with one capsule with meal in the morning and one or two capsules in the evening had accelerated hair growth (32.4%) that was significantly ($p < 0.001$) better than the placebo [29]. Anti–hair loss efficacy of this commercial product is relied on the active ingredients, which are vitamin C (20 mg), tocopherol succinate (5 IU), niacinamide (20 mg), folic acid (200 mcg), vitamin B_{12} in the form of cyanocobalamin (3 mcg), biotin (200 mcg), calcium pantothenate (100 mg), iron in the form of fumarate (8 mg), iodine from kelp (100 mcg), magnesium oxide (25 mg), and zinc oxide (10 mg).

27.3.3 Mineral and Vitamin Treatment

In addition to zinc, iron, iodine, niacinamide, tocopherol, panthenol, and vitamin C that have been compounded in several nutricosmetics treating alopecia as addressed previously, single mineral also exhibits its potential for hair loss treatment.

Silicon is one of the important nutrients sustaining good condition of hair accumulating its efficacy against hair loss. The element (10 mg) in the form of choline-stabilized orthosilicic acid ($Si(OH)_4$), the prevalent form of silicon in physiological fluid, was orally administrated in 48 Caucasian females aged between 18 and 65 years with fine hair. The randomized, double-blind, placebo-controlled trial was conducted for 9 months taking the silicon capsule or placebo twice daily (morning and evening). Hair width was increased in the treated group due to the significant ($p < 0.05$) higher value of cross section compared to the baseline, whereas that of the placebo group was not changed. The thicker hair enhanced by Si was associated on tensile strength and elasticity of hair as well [30]. This positive effect of silicon intake may regulate by stimulating effect of orthosilicic acid in collagen synthesis [31] associated with biological benefit of choline. Stimulation of collagen in extracellular matrix where dermal papilla embedded therefore resulting in positive effect on hair follicle leading thicker hair shaft consequently.

Furthermore, synergistic effect of each active enhancing efficacy against hair loss is of important concept upon nutricosmetics design. Combinations of amino acids and vitamins are commercialized in Pantogar®. The capsule containing vitamin B_1 (60 mg), calcium pantothenate or vitamin B_5 (60 mg), vigar yeast or *Saccharomyces* medicinal extract (100 mg), cysteine (20 mg), keratin (20 mg), and *p*-aminobenzoic acid (20 mg) was studied in a randomized double-blind, placebo-controlled trial. Thirty female volunteers aged 25–65 years facing with TE were guided to take one capsule for three times a day with meals for 6 months, of which the placebo consisted with lactose, microcrystalline cellulose, and magnesium stearate was examined in parallel. Following 6 months of the study, anagen hair of the active treatment group was enhanced to 80.5% ± 5.3% significantly ($p < 0.003$) better than the placebo. Although hair number and density were not differed in both groups, hair shaft diameter of the active-treated group was better than the placebo (18.5 ± 4.3 and 16.9 ± 4.5 μm) [32].

27.4 CONCLUSIONS

There are several options for choosing the appraisal treatment methods against hair loss or alopecia. Dietary intake of multifunctional food or beverage containing active ingredients is one of the important methods. The efficiency of herbs including mineral and vitamins as evidenced in human volunteers is summarized and ready for the readers to design their nutricosmetics for hair loss protection and hair rejuvenation remedies. Moreover, eating behavior associating good condition of hair with natural actives as exemplified would protect the individual from hair loss. However, regulation of the nutricosmetics as used in terms of nutraceutical and functional food should be concerned to ensure the safety of the products, preventing or limiting adverse effects [4].

REFERENCES

1. Lourith N, Kanlayavattanakul M. Hair loss and herbs for treatment. *J Cosmet Sci* 2013; 12:210–222.
2. Park J, Shin DW, Ahn TY. Complementary and alternative medicine in men's health. *J Men Health* 2008; 5:303–313.
3. Olsen EA. Iron deficiency and hair loss: The jury is still out. *J Am Acad Dermatol* 2006; 54:903–906.

4. Debasis B. *Nutraceutical and Functional Food Regulations in the United States and Around the World*, 2nd edn. Elsevier: New York, 2014.
5. Finner AM. Nutrition and hair loss: Deficiencies and supplements. *Dermatol Clin* 2013; 31:167–172.
6. Taeymans J, Clarys P, Barel AO. Use of food supplements as nutricosmetics in health and fitness: A review. In: *Handbook of Cosmetic Science and Technology*, 4th edn., Barel AO, Paye M, Maibach HI (eds). CRC Press: Boca Raton, FL, 2014, pp. 583–596.
7. Harada N, Okajima K, Arai M, Kurihara H, Nakata N. Administration of capsaicin and isoflavone promotes hair growth by increasing insulin-like growth factor-I production in mice and in humans with alopecia. *Growth Horm IGF Res* 2007; 17:408–415.
8. Tsuruki T, Takahata K, Yoshikawa M. Anti-alopecia mechanisms of soymetide-4, an immunostimulating peptide derived from soy β-conglycini. *Peptides* 2005; 26:707–711.
9. Tsuruki T, Yoshikawa M. Design of soymetide-4 derivatives to potentiate the anti-alopecia effect. *Biosci Biotechnol Biochem* 2004; 68:1139–1141.
10. Kim SH, Jeong KS, Ryu SY, Kim TH. *Panax ginseng* prevents apoptosis in hair follicles and accelerates recovery of hair medullary cells in irradiated mice. *In Vivo* 1998; 12:219–222.
11. Park S, Shin W-S, Ho J. Fructus panax ginseng extract promotes hair regeneration in C57BL/6 mice. *J Ethnoparmacol* 2011; 138:340–344.
12. Shin HS, Park SY, Hwang ES, Lee DG, Song HG, Mavlonov GT, Yi TH. The inductive effect of ginsenoside F2 on hair growth by altering the WNT signal pathway in telogen mouse skin. *Eur J Pharmacol* 2014; 730:82–89.
13. Shin HS, Park SY, Hwang ES, Lee DG, Mavlonov GT, Yi TH. Ginsenoside F2 reduced hair loss by controlling apoptosis through the sterol regulatory element-binding protein cleavage activating protein and transforming growth factor-β pathways in a dihydrotestosterone-induced mouse model. *Biol Pharm Bull* 2014; 37:755–763.
14. Palin MF, Faguy M, LeHoux JG, Pelletier G. Inhibitory effects of *Serenoa repens* on the kinetic of pig prostatic microsomal 5α-reductase activity. *Endocrine* 1998; 9:65–69.
15. Raynaud JP, Cousse H, Marin PM. Inhibition of type 1 and type 2 5α-reductase activity by free fatty acids, active ingredients of Permixon®. *J Steroid Biochem Mol Biol* 2002; 82:233–239.
16. Shimada H, Tyler VE, McLaughlin JL. Biological active acylglycerides from the berries of saw palmetto (*Serenoa repens*). *J Nat Prod* 1997; 60:417–418.
17. Schantz MM, Bedner M, Long SE et al. Development of saw palmetto (*Serenoa repens*) fruit and extract standard reference materials. *Anal Bioanal Chem* 2008; 392:427–438.
18. Bedner M, Schantz MM, Sander LC, Sharpless KE. Development of liquid chromatographic methods for the determination of phytosterols in standard reference materials containing saw palmetto. *J Chromatogr A* 2008; 1192:74–80.
19. Madersbacher S, Ponholzer A, Berger I, Marszalek M. Medical management of BPH: Role of plant extracts. *Eur Assoc Urol* 2007; 5:197–205.
20. Debruyne F, Koch G, Boyle P et al. Comparison of a phytotherapeutic agent (Perximon) with an α-blocker (tamsulosin) in the treatment of benign prostatic hyperplasia: A 1 year randomised international study. *Eur Urol* 2002; 41:497–507.
21. Hizli F, Uygur MC. A prospective study of the efficacy of *Serenoa repens*, Tamsulosin and *Serenoa repens* plus Tamsulin treatment for patients with benign prostate hyperplasia. *Int Urol Nephrol* 2007; 39:879–886.
22. Singh YN, Devkota AK, Sneeden DC, Singh KK, Halaweish F. Hepatotoxicity potential of saw palmetto (*Serenoa repens*) in rats. *Phytomed* 2007; 14:204–208.
23. Avins AL, Bent S, Staccone SA, Badua E, Padula A, Goldberg H, Neuhaus J, Hudes E, Shinohara K, Kane C. A detailed safety assessment of a saw palmetto extract. *Comp Ther Med* 2008; 16:147–154.
24. Prager N, Bickett K, French N, Marcovici G. A randomized, double-blind, placebo-controlled trial to determine the effectiveness of botanically derived inhibitors of 5-α-reductase in the treatment of androgenetic alopecia. *J Alt Com Med* 2002; 8:143–152.
25. Ichihashi M, Yoshida I, Yamaguchi H, Tamashita K, Akiba T. KGS1 kamishoyosangoshimotsuto extract tablets improved skin condition and hair properties. *Anti-Aging Med* 2011; 8:15–22.
26. Morganti P, Fabrizi G, James B, Bruno C. Effect of gelatin-cystine and *Serenoa repens* extract on free radical level and hair growth. *J App Cosmetol* 1998; 16:57–64.
27. Rushton DH, Norris MJ, Dover R, Busuttil N. Causes of hair loss and the developments in hair rejuvenation. *Int J Cosmet Sci* 2002; 24:17–23.
28. Lassus A, Eskelinen E. A comparative study of a new food supplement, Viviscal®, with fish extract for the treatment of hereditary androgenic alopecia in young males. *J Int Med Res* 1992; 20:445–453.

29. Thom E. Efficacy and tolerability of Hairgain® in individuals with hair loss: A placebo-controlled, double-blind study. *J Int Med Res* 2001; 29:2–6.
30. Wickett RR, Kossmann, BA, Demeester N, Clarys P, Vanden Berghe D, Calomme M. Effect of oral intake of choline-stabilized orthosilicic acid on hair tensile strength and morphology in women with fine hair. *Arch Dermatol Res* 2007; 299:499–505.
31. Reffitt DM, Ogston N, Jugdaosingh R, Cheung HFJ, Evans BAJ, Thompson RPH, Powell JJ, Hampson GN. Orthosilicic acid (OSA) stimulates collagen type I synthesis and osteoblast differentiation in human osteoblast-like cells *in vitro*. *Bone* 2003; 32:127–135.
32. Lengg N, Heidecker B, Seifert B, Trüeb RM. Dietary supplement increases anagen hair rate in women with telogen effluvium: Results of a double-blind, placebo-controlled trial. *Therapy* 2007; 4:59–65.

28 Nutrition, Nutraceuticals, and Hair Growth

Mi-Ryung Kim and Jae-Suk Choi

CONTENTS

28.1 INTRODUCTION

Hair is one of the specific characteristics of mammals.[1] There are roughly 500 million hairs on our bodies, from small, fine unpigmented vellus hair to longer, thicker, pigmented terminal hair.[2] Among them, the longest and thickest terminal hair is scalp hair.

The main function of scalp hair is thermal protection of the head and neck from hot or cold environments, including the reduction of physical injury, protection against insect penetration and electromagnetic radiation, and provision of a sensory antenna to *feel* the environment.[3] A more important function of hair is its significant role in social communication as a sign of beauty and a contribution to an individual's identity, indicating its psychological and symbolic importance in social perspectives throughout human history. In particular, hair strongly influences whether a person is seen as physically attractive. In most human interactions, persons with hair problems, especially baldness, have been considered as being significantly older, less physically or socially attractive, weaker, duller, and less potent than their peers.[4–9] The consequences of such conditions can extend beyond personal isolation to extremes that include overt discrimination in, for example employment practices.

Hairs grow from follicles, which are invaginations of the superficial epithelium of the skin. On average, an adult scalp contains 100,000 follicles.[10] The maximum number of hair follicles (HFs) is present at birth. Thus, the area concentration of scalp HFs then decreases as the head enlarges; it has been estimated that the 700–750 follicles per cm^2 at birth decrease to ~318 per cm^2 in adult life.[11,12]

Normal hair loss from the scalp is ~50–60 hairs a day and has no noticeable effect on appearance, but excessive loss (>~100 hairs) will result in baldness (alopecia). This is common throughout the world and has been estimated to affect between 0.2% and 2% of the world's population.[13–15] Although it is viewed medically as a relatively minor dermatological condition, alopecia may have potentially great adverse impacts on a person's quality of life, based on the psychological and symbolic importance of hair.

Thus, it is not surprising that the demand for drugs that alter hair growth and appearance has resulted in a multibillion-dollar industry. About 300,000 products have claimed to help hair regrowth over the past several years. Great expectations are often associated with pharmaceutical hair loss management. However, as yet, few drugs that are effective for these purposes are available.[16]

Indeed, to date, only two U.S. Food and Drug Administration–approved pharmacotherapies, minoxidil and finasteride, are available for the treatment of alopecia. Topical minoxidil solution (Rogaine for men and women; OTC, Pharmacia Corp., Peapack, NJ) has been shown to stimulate new hair growth and to help prevent further hair loss in affected areas in both men and women with alopecia,[17,18] but the specific mechanism of action remains unclear. Finasteride (Propecia; Merck Co, Rahway, NJ) is a synthetic azosteroid, which is a potent and highly selective noncompetitive antagonist of 5α-reductase type 2. It binds irreversibly to the enzyme and inhibits the conversion of testosterone to dihydrotestosterone (DHT).[19]

Generally, minoxidil is well tolerated for long-term daily use. Side effects of minoxidil are uncommon, but skin irritation,[20,21] dizziness, tachycardia,[20] and contact dermatitis[22] have been described. Finasteride is also generally well tolerated, with few adverse effects being reported in the 5-year data. In the finasteride group, loss of libido was reported in 1.9% and erectile dysfunction in 1.4% in the first year. The placebo group reported the same events with frequencies of 1.3% and 0.6%, respectively. These events appeared to resolve on cessation of the treatment and, in some cases, during continued treatment.[23]

Both drugs were the result of serendipity, not of rational hair drug design. Thus, to search for more precise therapies for alopecia, the mechanisms of hair growth–promoting effects and new drugs or hair growth enhancers from natural origins need to be explored. Nutrition and nutraceuticals from natural sources have been used widely for hair growth promotion since ancient times in the Ayurveda, Chinese, and Unani systems of medicine. Natural products are popular and well accepted in the cosmetic and hair care industries.[24,25]

The contents of this chapter present important aspects concerning the mechanisms of hair growth as now understood and recent research on nutrition and nutraceuticals showing hair growth–promoting effects.

28.2 MECHANISM OF HAIR GROWTH

28.2.1 Structure of Hair Follicles

Hair grows from primary follicles in the hair root. Actively growing HFs penetrate the entire epidermis and dermis. HFs are structured with several concentric cylinders of epithelial cells, known as root sheaths, which surround the hair shaft.[26] At its base, the follicle contains specialized dermal cells in a ball shape, the dermal papilla, which plays a crucial part in the regulation of successive cycles of postnatal hair growth.[27] An actively growing follicle expands into the hair bulb and virtually encloses the dermal papilla, with capillary vessels supplying nutrients and oxygen.

In hair growth, signals from the mesenchymal dermal papilla are thought to instruct the adjacent epithelial stem cells to divide transiently.[28–31] Stem cells migrate to the base of the follicle, where they surround the dermal papilla, forming the hair matrix.[32,33] In response to further signals from the dermal papilla, matrix cells proliferate and begin the process of terminal differentiation, moving upward in the follicle and forming the hair shaft and inner root sheath (IRS),[28,32,33] the dimensions and curvature of which largely determine the shape of the hair. The outer root sheath (ORS) is continuous with the surface epidermis and enclosed by the glassy membrane. Cells in the ORS normally express an array of keratins, adhesion molecules, cytokines, and growth factor receptors.[34,35] They migrate out of the follicle and regenerate the epidermis. The bulge in the ORS consists of epithelial stem cells and serves as a reservoir for epidermal and sebaceous gland cells.[29,36] The entire follicle is surrounded by connective tissue, including fibroblasts, collagen, and elastic fibers.[37] Pigmentation of the hair results from the activity of melanocytes, which reside in the HF bulb and deposit pigment granules into the hair shaft as it forms.

The HF is also often referred to as the "pilosebaceous unit" due to the presence of one or more sebaceous glands within the follicle. These produce a waxy secretion that coats the hair under regulation by hormones, particularly androgens.[38]

28.2.2 Hair Growth Cycle

Hair is the cumulative physical result of a coordinated process of cellular proliferation and differentiation within an HF. The HF can regenerate itself through the cycle of growth (anagen), regression (catagen), rest (telogen), and shedding (exogen). This HF cycle is a complex process involving cell differentiation, epithelial–mesenchymal interactions, stem cell augmentation, pattern formation, apoptosis (programmed cell death), cell and organ growth cycles, and pigmentation.[39]

With the onset of the anagen stage, the formation of the new HF begins with the proliferation of secondary germ cells in the bulge.[29,31] A new HF base develops and grows into the bottom of the existing telogen follicle. Then, the new hair pushes up beside the existing one, which is then shed. The length of anagen varies with the species and at different sites of the body; it may also be influenced by circulating factors, such as androgens.

When the hair reaches its full length, the hair bulb begins to regress, and the hair base becomes a fully keratinized, expanded *club*, which anchors the fully grown hair in the skin. During this catagen stage, the condensed dermal papilla moves upward, coming to rest underneath the HF bulge, and HFs go through a highly controlled process of involution, reflecting the programmed cell death (apoptosis) of follicular keratinocytes. Follicular melanogenesis also ceases during this stage, and some follicular melanocytes also undergo apoptosis. If the dermal papilla fails to reach the bulge and does not interact with the stem cells of the bulge, the follicle stops cycling, and the hair is lost, resulting in permanent alopecia.

During the telogen stage, the hair shaft matures into a club hair, which is eventually shed from the follicle, typically during combing or washing. It is unclear whether shedding is an active regulated process or a passive event that occurs at the onset of the anagen stage, as the new hair grows in. At the end of the resting telogen phase, a new anagen phase begins as the secondary germ cells divide and move down into the dermis with the dermal papilla cells (DPCs).

The scalp hairs have a relatively long life cycle: the anagen stage ranges from 2 to 5 years, the catagen stage ranges from a few days to a few weeks, and the telogen stage typically lasts for 2–3 months. On average, some 90% or more of scalp hairs are in the anagen phase, compared with 5%–15% of scalp follicles in the telogen stage at any one time.

The signals for change from one phase to the next remain poorly understood, although it has been suggested that perhaps a mitotic inhibitor accumulates during the anagen phase and is then dispersed during the telogen phase.

28.2.3 Molecular Factors Controlling Hair Growth

The control factors that regulate the hair growth cycle may reside within the HF itself. It has been suggested that the initiation of a new growth phase and the subsequent downgrowth, proliferation, and differentiation of the follicle may require signaling between the dermal papilla and epithelial cells,[28] although the molecular signals for hair growth remain poorly understood.

The dermal papillae at the base of follicles may determine hair growth characteristics, especially the regulation of cell proliferation and differentiation of the HF matrix. There is substantial evidence from bioassays that cultured DPCs can secrete some cytokines, growth factors, and other, as yet unidentified bioactive molecules that influence growth in other DPCs, ORS cells, keratinocytes, and endothelial cells.[40]

At the onset of anagen, an unknown signal(s) that triggers the proliferation of secondary germ cells in the bulge may arise from near the dermal papilla. It has been reported that an antagonist of the estrogen receptor (ER) and parathyroid hormone–responsive protein promoted normal anagen onset in mice, but signal transducer and activator of transcription 3 (STAT 3) and estradiol prevented it. While not required for anagen onset, sonic hedgehog (SHH) is necessary for the subsequent events of anagen, inducing the proliferation of epithelial cells and downgrowth of the follicle into the dermis,[41,42] and ectopic expression of *shh* is capable of inducing the resting follicle to enter a growth phase.

As anagen proceeds, signals from the dermal papilla regulate the proliferation of hair matrix cells, whereas epithelial cells maintain the inductive properties of the dermal papilla. Two secreted molecules that have important roles in this process are insulin-like growth factor 1 (IGF-1) and fibroblast growth factor 7 (FGF-7). Both are produced by the dermal papilla, and their receptors are found predominantly in the overlying matrix cells. Mice that lack IGF-1 or its receptor have poorly developed HFs. IGF-1 maintains and increases follicle growth in vitro.[35,40] FGF-7 is expressed in the dermal papilla and has strong mitogenic effects on epithelial cells. Mice that lack FGF-7 have relatively normal HFs, but disruption of the receptor for FGF causes markedly reduced and aberrant HF formation.[43–47] Additionally, DPCs cultured in the presence of WNT protein maintain their inductive abilities over many rounds of culture, suggesting that the epithelial signal consists of one or more WNT family members.[48]

The cessation of the anagen stage is controlled by FGF-5, which is first expressed in the follicle just before the end of this stage.[49] Mice that lack FGF-5 have an extended anagen stage, resulting in the "angora" phenotype, with hair that is 50% longer than normal.[50] Even in these mice, the follicle still eventually enters the catagen stage, suggesting that other signaling pathways are also important for the induction of this stage. In contrast, overexpression of either of the antiapoptotic genes *Bcl-XL* or *Bcl-2* in the ORS decreases the duration of anagen, suggesting that the regulation of cell survival in the ORS might also play a role in the control of the hair growth cycle.[3]

Although it is known that catagen involves massive programmed cell death, the means by which this is achieved are poorly understood at the molecular level. Catagen has been suggested to occur as a consequence of decreased expression of anagen-maintaining factors, such as IGF-1, basic fibroblast growth factor (bFGF), and vascular endothelial growth factor (VEGF), and increased expression of cytokines promoting apoptosis, such as transforming growth factor β1 (TGF-β1), interleukin-1 alpha (IL-1α), and tumor necrosis factor alpha (TNFα).[35,51] In mice lacking the hairless (HR) protein, a putative transcription factor, the dermal papilla fails to move upward during catagen.[3] As a consequence, contact between the dermal papilla and stem cells in the bulge is lost, and subsequent hair growth cycles fail to occur. Mice lacking the retinoid X receptor-α (RXRα) and vitamin D receptor (VDR) in the epidermis also display separation of the proximal and distal portions of the HF and fail to initiate the first postnatal anagen.[52,53]

28.2.4 Hormonal Factors Controlling Hair Growth

The distribution of hair, as well as its type, growth rate, and follicular cycle, is mediated, at least in part, by complex hormonal regulatory mechanisms; however, they are not fully understood. Generally, it is known that the estrogen, thyroid hormone, glucocorticoids, retinoids, prolactin, and growth hormone are all involved in hair growth. Among them, the hormones with the strongest effects in modulating hair growth are the androgens. Androgens regulate vellus hair changing into terminal hair.[54] However, androgens also show different effects on the scalp, inducing the regression of HFs by turning terminal hairs into vellus ones later in life.

Testosterone, a major male androgen, is converted to 5α-DHT by 5α-reductase prior to binding with androgen receptor (AR) in the dermal papilla.[52,53,55] Based on the affinity of 5α-reductase for AR, DHT is fivefold more potent than testosterone.[56] DHT diffuses through the plasma membrane of the target cell and binds to the AR. The AR–DHT complex undergoes conformational changes, exposing DNA-binding sites, and then binds to specific hormone response elements in the DNA, regulating the expression of specific genes related to hair growth.[57] There are two separate isoenzymes of 5α-reductase (types I and II). Type I is predominantly in scalp skin, whereas type II has been specifically localized within the HF itself, in the innermost layer of the ORS and the prostate.[58–61]

Testosterone and DHT can circulate systemically to follicles or be manufactured locally in the follicle from circulating weak androgens, such as dehydroepiandrosterone (DHEA) and androstenediol, via complex enzyme-mediated processes involving specific dehydrogenase and reductase enzyme pathways. DHEA is potentially converted into testosterone, which is subsequently metabolized into DHT.[62] Some fraction of testosterone may also be oxidized to androstenedione. 3α-Hydroxysteroid dehydrogenase converts DHT to the less potent androstenediol. Another enzyme related to hair loss is aromatase, located in the other root sheath of HFs. Aromatase converts testosterone and androstenedione to the estrogens estradiol and estrone, respectively, which prolong the anagen stage.[63,64]

Androgens stimulate the production of growth factors and proteases; affect angiogenesis, basement membrane proteins, and cell metabolism; and appear to shorten the length of the anagen phase of growth. Each HF, regionally as well as locally, appears to be independently genetically regulated to respond to androgens. Increased levels of DHT shorten the hair cycle and progressively miniaturize scalp follicles, and this may be due to atherosclerotic processes blocking the microvasculature that nourishes the HFs.

28.3 HAIR LOSS

28.3.1 Alopecia

Hair loss is a natural daily phenomenon, but this ordinary shedding of hair cannot be the main cause of alopecia. Each strand of scalp hair is genetically programmed to a cycle that includes proliferation, involution, resting, and shedding. The normal head sheds 50–125 hairs (depending on gender) each day, but most of them will come back after a resting stage because the follicle itself is not damaged.[65] However, loss of more than 100 hairs per day will result in baldness (alopecia). "Baldness" can refer to general hair loss or androgenicalopecia (male pattern baldness). Other types of baldness include alopecia areata (AA), permanent alopecia, and telogen effluvium.

Androgenic alopecia (AGA) is the most common type of hair loss in humans; it is caused by the influence of androgens on HFs and by hereditary factors. In addition, because the volume of the dermal papilla determines the diameter of the hair shaft and may determine the duration of the anagen stage,[66,67] abnormalities of the dermal papilla may also underlie AGA. As this condition progresses, scalp hairs and their follicles become miniaturized progressively, and the terminal hair normally found on the scalp is replaced with vellus hairs, which are shorter, finer, and nonpigmented.[52] Because AGA involves a process of premature termination of anagen, associated with premature entry into catagen,[12] it is important to dissect the molecular controls of the anagen–catagen transformation of the hair cycle[63] and to block the conversion of testosterone to its more active metabolite, DHT. Nevertheless, HFs are still present and cycling, even in bald scalps; thus, AGA is often considered as potentially reversible.[66,68] While male pattern AGA is characterized by its typical frontal recession and thinning at the vertex, female pattern AGA is distinguished by the loss of hair primarily over the crown, with sparing of frontal hair.[69,70] AGA affects ~30% of men under the age of 30, more than 50% of men over the age of 50, and up to 70% of all males in later life.[71] AGA may also affect many women; 6% of women aged under 50 years are affected, increasing to 30%–40%

of women aged 70 years and over.[72] However, there is no consensus on whether hair loss is truly androgen dependent in women.

AA is an autoimmune disorder, causing patchy loss of hair on the scalp and/or body; extensive forms of the disorder are called alopecia areata totalis (hair loss over the entire scalp) and alopecia areata universalis (hair loss over the entire body). The presence of atopy and the onset in prepubertal children indicate poor prognosis for AA.[73] Prevalence in the general population is between 1% and 2%,[74] and it can occur at any age. Genetic, immunological, and neurological factors play a role in the origin of AA. Clinical features of AA include abrupt hair loss, hair shedding, scalp lesions, smooth spots on the scalp, and broken or short hairs that resemble an exclamation mark. AA is due to attack by lymphocytes on the cells of the anagen hair bulb.[75] As a result, anagen follicles enter a dystrophic catagen, and the hair shaft breaks off. Matrix keratinocytes, DPCs, and melanocytes have been suggested as possible targets of the immune attack. Such hair loss is potentially reversible, even after years without hair, confirming the nonscarring nature of the inflammatory process, which apparently spares the stem cell–rich bulge area.[76]

Permanent alopecia is caused by destruction of HFs as a result of inflammation, trauma, fibrosis, or unknown causes; examples include lichen planopilaris and discoid lupus erythematosus.

Telogen effluvium, another common form of alopecia, manifests as excessive shedding of hair. Follicles are stimulated to leave anagen and enter telogen prematurely resulting in an increased hair shedding at the end of telogen approximately 2–3 months later. It is common after a physiologic stress such as severe illness and with drug-induced hair loss. Several different mechanisms can cause telogen effluvium, but all result from the synchronous entry of many follicles into exogen.[77]

28.3.2 Factors Leading to Hair Loss

Beyond endogenous molecular and hormonal factors, including FGF, IGF, and DHT, hair loss is also affected by various other factors including psychoemotional stress, severe illness, chemotherapy, genetic predisposition, excessive sebum, cardiovascular diseases, advanced age, and seasonal changes.[78]

Stress has long been implicated as one of the causal factors involved in hair loss.[79–81] With respect to the connections between psychoemotional stress and hair loss, several levels of interactions can be distinguished: (1) acute or chronic stress as a primary inducer of telogen effluvium; (2) acute or chronic stress as an aggravating factor in a hair loss disorder whose primary pathogenesis is of endocrine, toxic, metabolic, or immunological nature (e.g. AGA, AA); and (3) stress as a secondary problem in response to prior hair loss.

Hair loss also can be caused by several medications, including those for blood pressure problems, diabetes, heart disease, and cholesterol. Any drug that affects the body's hormone balance can have a profound effect: these include the contraceptive pill, hormone replacement therapy, steroids, and acne medications. Additionally, excessive sebum may cause a high level of 5α-reductase and pore clogging and then malnutrition of the hair root.[82]

Hair loss shows seasonal and environmental variation. Scalp hair growth has been shown to peak in the spring and reach a nadir in the autumn. This may be influenced via the hypothalamus, responding to changes in sun exposure and ambient temperature.[83]

Normal hair growth also requires an adequate diet and nutrition. *Healthy-appearing* hair *is* indeed typically a sign of good general health, as well as good hair care practices. Most healthy individuals have adequate nutrients in their normal diet; however, many people do not have access to good nutrition, and others have medical illnesses that predispose them to nutritional deficiencies. This is often reflected in changes in scalp, and sometimes body and hair.[82] Many nutritional components and nutraceuticals have been suggested to have effects on hair growth; they are discussed in the next section.

28.4 NUTRITION AND HAIR GROWTH

The integrity of normal skin and hair function relies largely on adequate and balanced nutritional intake.[83] In particular, because HF cells have a high turnover, their active metabolism requires a good supply of nutrients and energy. Caloric deprivation or deficiency in several nutrients, such as proteins, minerals, essential fatty acids (EFAs), and vitamins, caused by inborn errors or reduced intake or uptake can lead to structural loss, although exact data are often lacking.[84] Hair nutrition is thus a vital part of any treatment regime. However, nutrition is a complex subject, and the effects of correct nutrition for hair are indirect and often slow to appear.

Vitamins are organic compounds that are required in small amounts for normal health, function, and growth. They are divided into those that are fat soluble (A, D, E, and K) and water soluble (B and C). Most are obtained from a regular mixed diet, and in addition, vitamin D can be synthesized in the skin in the presence of sunlight.[82] Vitamin C functions to help produce and maintain healthy collagen, the connective tissue type found within HFs. Vitamin C is also a strong antioxidant and protects both cells found within follicles and cells in nearby blood vessels.[84] The absence of the VDR leads to the development of alopecia. Vitamin E helps to maintain the integrity of cell membranes in HFs and acts as an antioxidant while promoting healthy hair. Pantothenic acid (vitamin B_5) gives hair flexibility, strength, and shine and helps prevent hair loss and graying. Vitamin B_6 helps prevent dandruff and can be found in cereals, egg yolk, and liver. Reduced levels of thiamine (vitamin B_1), riboflavin (vitamin B_2), niacin, and pantothenic acid can contribute to the undernourishment of HF cells. A decrease in folic acid may contribute to decreased HF cell division and growth. Folic acid is also essential for the maintenance of healthy methionine levels in the body. Biotin is a water-soluble vitamin that acts as an essential cofactor for four different carboxylases, each of which catalyzes an essential step in intermediary metabolism. Biotin deficiency has been reported to result in dermatitis and hair loss.[82]

Minerals are very important in enzyme action, electrolyte balance, nerve impulse transmission, muscle contraction, bone formation, and growth and development in the body. Mineral deficiencies such as zinc, copper, and iron are associated with several diseases that are sometimes due to a primary defect in trace mineral metabolism. Zinc and copper deficiencies have been reported to be prevalent in countries with low standards of living.[85] Zinc is essential for DNA and RNA production and in normal follicle cell division. Zinc is also responsible for helping to stabilize cell membrane structures and assists in the breakdown and removal of superoxide radicals. Zinc intake is generally low. Topical application of zinc has been shown to reduce hair loss activity of type II 5α-reductase. Copper is crucial for aminoxydases required for the oxidation of thiol groups to dithio-cross links, which are essential for keratin fiber strength. Additionally, suboptimal thyroid function, where iodine supports normal functioning, can also lead to abnormal hair growth. Iron works as a catalyst in many oxidations and reductions and may control DNA synthesis through the ribonuclease in dividing cells. Iron deficiency causes microcytic and hypochromic anemia. Even in the absence of anemia, diffuse hair loss and other skin symptoms can occur. Serum ferritin concentrations provide a good assessment of an individual's iron status. Serum ferritin concentrations may be a factor in female hair loss.[86]

EFA deficiency can also cause dermatitis and hair loss.[87,88] EFA deficiency is purely of dietary origin. EFA plays an important role in cell structure, barrier function, lipid synthesis, inflammation, and immunity. Omega-6 EFAs, derived from linoleic acid, and omega-3 EFAs, derived from α-linolenic acid, are involved in many physiologically important pathways.[83] Linolenic, linoleic, palmitoleic, oleic, myristoleic, and stearic acids are claimed on their 5α-reductase inhibitory effect.[89,90] Protein is the major component of the hair fiber. Thus, reduced protein uptake can impair hair growth, even before serum albumin levels are decreased.[91] The role of the essential amino acid L-lysine also appears to be important in hair loss.[92]

28.5 NUTRACEUTICALS AND HAIR GROWTH

28.5.1 Nutraceuticals from Plant Sources

To date, nutraceuticals posing efficiency in hair growth promoter and prevention of hair loss have been reported from various plant sources, including grains such as rice bran and wheat sprouts, fruits and vegetables like tomato, cauliflower mushrooms, rosary peas, and jujube seeds, and many traditional oriental herb medicines that have been used for centuries to treat hair loss. Various agents from plant sources associated with hair growth activity are summarized in Table 28.1.

Abrus precatorius, popularly known as rosary pea or crab's eye, is a slender, woody perennial climber reported to have antioxidant, antibacterial, cytotoxic, antidiabetic, antitubercular, and antiplasmodial activities. Sandhya et al. (2012)[93] evaluated the hair growth–promoting potential of an aqueous extract of *Abrus precatorius* leaf. The extract showed good hair growth–promoting activity at a dose of 300 mg per kg; it was comparable to that of 2% minoxidil.

Activation of the Wnt/β-catenin signaling pathway plays an important role in HF morphogenesis by stimulating bulge stem cells. In total, 800 natural product extracts were screened using a pTOP-Flash assay and a neural progenitor cell differentiation assay.[94] *Aconiti ciliare* tuber (ACT) extract was one of the most active materials in both assays. ACT extract activates the Wnt/β-catenin signaling pathway by enhancing β-catenin transcription and has the potential to promote the induction of hair growth via activation of the stem cell activity of the DPCs.

According to the results of Rho et al. (2005),[95] among 45 plant extracts tested, the extract of *Asiasari radix* showed the most potent hair growth stimulation in C57BL/6 and C3H mice experiments. Additionally, this extract markedly increased the protein synthesis in vibrissae follicle cultures and the proliferation of both HaCaT and human DP cells in vitro. Moreover, the *A. radix* extract induced the expression of VEGF in human DP cells cultured in vitro.

Chinese black tea extract (CBTE, *Camellia sinensis* fermented with *Aspergillus* sp.) promoted hair growth significantly after 2 weeks of topical application in shaved 6-week-old male C3H/He mice.[96] The hair growth–promoting effect of CBTE was potentiated synergistically by capsaicin, which has no effect on hair growth by itself. CBTE displayed an affinity for the ERα, with an IC_{50} value of 74.8 μg per mL.

Kumar et al. (2012)[97] screened 17 Thai plants used traditionally in hair treatment. *Carthamus tinctorius* L. was the most potent 5α-reductase inhibitor, with a finasteride equivalent 5α-reductase inhibitory activity (FEA) value of 24.30 ± 1.64 mg finasteride equivalent per 1 g crude extract. *Phyllanthus emblica* L. was the second most potent, with an FEA of 18.99 ± 0.40. *Rhinacanthus nasutus* (L.) Kurz. was the least potent inhibitor (FEA 10.69 ± 0.96). Thus, an ethanolic extract of *Carthamus tinctorius* was the most potent 5α-reductase inhibitor and hair growth promoter.

The florets of *Carthamus tinctorius* have been used traditionally for hair growth promotion. Junlatat and Sripanidkulchai (2014)[98] examined the potential of hydroxysafflor yellow A-rich *C. tinctorius* extract on hair growth both in vitro and in vivo. The extract promoted the proliferation of both DPCs and HaCaT and significantly stimulated hair growth–promoting genes, including VEGF and keratinocyte growth factor.

Lee et al. (2010)[99] examined the hair growth–promoting effects of *Chamaecyparis obtusa* oils in a male C57BL/6 mouse model. The essential oils of *C. obtuse* were divided into seven fractions for the treatment of HaCaT cells. VEGF transcripts were induced by fractions 6 and 7; however, TGF-β1 and KGF mRNA levels were unchanged by *C. obtusa* oils or fractions. Cuminol, eucarvone, and calamenene were common to these two subfractions, although the effects of these components were not determined individually in this research.

Park et al. (2013a)[100] also evaluated the hair growth effects of *Chamaecyparis obtusa* oil (CO) in C57BL/6 mice. They applied 100 μL 3% CO topically to the backs of C57BL/6 mice once per day, 6 days per week, for 4 weeks. Histological results showed that the HF number and depth and dermal

TABLE 28.1
Summary of the Hair Growth–Promoting Agents from Plant Origin

Species	Common Name	Part for Use	Extract or Active Component	Activity Test Model	References
Abrus precatorius	Rosary pea	Leaf	Aqueous extract	BALB/C mice	Sandhya et al. [93]
Aconiti ciliare			Aqueous extract	Wnt/β-catenin signaling pathway in bulge stem cells, C57BL/6 mice	Park et al. [94]
Asiasari radix		Dried root	Ethanol extract	C57BL/6 and C3H mice, vibrissae follicle cultures, HaCaT and human DP cells	Rho et al. [95]
Camellia sinensis	Chinese black tea	Fermented leaf	Propylene glycol/ethanol/distilled water (5:3:2) extract	6-week-old male C3H/He mice	Hou et al. [96]
Carthamus tinctorius	Safflower		Ethanol extract	5α-reductase, 57BL/6 mice	Kumar et al. [97]
Carthamus tinctorius	Safflower	Floret	Hydroxysafflor yellow A-rich *C. tinctorius* ethanol extract	Female C57BL/6 mice	Junlatat and Sripanidkulchai [98]
Chamaecyparis obtusa			Essential oil	Male C57BL/6 mice, HaCaT cells	Lee et al. [99]
Chamaecyparis obtusa			Essential oil	C57BL/6 mice	Park et al. [100]
Chamaecyparis obtusa			Essential oil	Alkaline phosphatase and γ-glutamyl transpeptidase	Park et al. [101]
Citrullus colocynthis	Colocynth	Fruit	Petroleum ether extract	Swiss albino mice	Dhanotia et al. [102]
Cornus officinalis		Fruits	Fermented with *Lactobacillus rhamnosus*	C57BL/6 mice	Park and Lee [103]
Crataegus pinnatifida		Dried fruit	Hot water extract	7-week-old C57BL/6 mice, human dermal papilla cells	Shin et al. [104]
Cuscuta reflexa			Petroleum ether extract	Albino mice 5α-reductase enzyme	Pandit et al. [105]
Eclipta alba	False daisy	Whole plant	Methanol extract	C57BL/6 mice	Datta et al. [106]

(Continued)

TABLE 28.1 (*Continued*)
Summary of the Hair Growth–Promoting Agents from Plant Origin

Species	Common Name	Part for Use	Extract or Active Component	Activity Test Model	References
Eclipta alba	False daisy		Petroleum ether extracts	Wistar strain male albino rats	Roy et al. [107]
Erica multiflora		Dried plant	70% ethanol extract	Human dermal papilla cells in vitro, male C3H/He mice dorsal skin in vivo	Kawano et al. [108]
Fructus panax ginseng		Root	95% ethanol extract	Human hair dermal papilla cells, C57BL/6 mice	Park et al. [109]
Ginkgo biloba		Leaves	70% ethanolic extract	Normal and high butter diet-pretreated C3H strain mice	Kubo et al. [110]
Ginseng radix	Red ginseng	Steamed and dried roots of *Panax ginseng*	70% methanol extract, ginsenoside-Rb1, 20(*S*)-ginsenoside-Rg3	Mice vibrissal follicles in organ culture	Matsuda et al. [111]
Ginseng radix	Red ginseng	Steamed and dried roots of *Panax ginseng*	0.003% Rg3 hair shampoo	Clinical study	Hyun et al. [112]
Ginseng radix	Red ginseng	Steamed and dried roots of *Panax ginseng*	Red ginseng itself	Clinical trial	Oh and Son [113]
Glycine max	Black soy bean	Seed	Boiled black bean itself	Orally administered in human	Lee and Kim [114]
Glycine max	Black soy bean	Seed	20% ethanol	NIH3T3 cells in vitro and C57BL/6 mice	Jeon et al. [115]
Hibiscus rosa-sinensis		Fresh leaves and flowers	Petroleum ether extract	Female Wistar albino rats	Adhirajan et al. [116]
Ishige sinicola	A kind of brown seaweed	Thallus	80% ethanol extract, octaphlorethol A	Female C57BL/6 mice, immortalized vibrissa dermal papilla cells	Kang et al. [117]
Lycopersicon esculentum	Tomato	Fruit	Semipurified lycopene Tween 80 solution	Female C57BL/6 mice	Choi et al. [118]
Opuntia ficusindica var. sarboten		Fruits	Fermented with *Lactobacillus rhamnosus*	C57BL/6 mice	Song et al. [119]

(*Continued*)

TABLE 28.1 (*Continued*)
Summary of the Hair Growth–Promoting Agents from Plant Origin

Species	Common Name	Part for Use	Extract or Active Component	Activity Test Model	References
Oryza sativa	Rice	Bran	Supercritical CO_2	Female C57BL/6 mice	Choi et al. [89]
Phyllanthus emblica			Ethanol extract	5α-reductase	Kumar et al. [97]
Pinelliae rhizoma			Chloroform fractions of 80% ethanol extract	C57BL/6N mice	Jeong et al. [120]
Pleuropterus cilinervis		Root	*Fermented with Lactobacillus rhamnosus*	C57BL/6 mice	Park and Lee [121]
Polygonum multiflorum		Dried, powdered leaves	Hot water extract	C57BL6/N mice	Park et al. [122]
Prunus Tomentosa	Nanking cherry		Total flavone	C57BL/6 mice	Zhang et al. [123]
Rosa multiflora		Root	Extracts	4-week-old male C57BL/6 mice	Kim et al. [124]
Rosmarinus officinalis	Rosemary		Essential oil	Male C57BL/6 mice	Kim and Kim [125]
Rosmarinus officinalis	Rosemary	Leaf	50% aqueous ethanol extract, 12-methoxycarnosic acid	C57BL/6NCrSlc mice	Murata et al. [126]
Rubus coreanum		Dried root	Extracts	C57BL/6 mice	Oh et al. [127]
Schisandra nigra			85% ethanol extract	Rat vibrissa follicles C57BL/6 mice	Kang et al. [128]
Sophora flavescens		Dried root	Methanol extract	C57BL/6, type II 5α-reductase	Rho et al. [129]
Sparassis crispa	Cauliflower mushroom	Mushroom	70% ethanol, ethyl acetate extract	C57BL/6 mice	Ryu et al. [130]
Thuja orientalis			Ethanol extract	Macrophage cell line RAW264.7, hair loss–induced DBA1J mice	Kim et al. [131]
Triticum aestivum	Wheat	Sprout	80% ethanol extract	Female C57BL/6 mice	Ryu et al. [132]
Vitex rotundifolia		Fruit	70% ethanol extract	C57BL/6 mice, human hair dermal papilla cells	Shin et al. [133]
Zizyphus jujuba	Jujube	Seed	Essential oil	BALB/C mice	Yoon et al. [134]

thickness in the MXD- and CO-treated groups were increased significantly ($p < 0.001$). Park et al. (2013b)[101] examined the mechanism of action of *Chamaecyparis obtusa* oil (3%) on hair growth in C57BL/6 mice. On the basis of effects on alkaline phosphatase (higher by 48%) and γ-glutamyl transpeptidase (higher by 254%) activity and the expression of IGF-1 (expression higher by 426%), VEGF (expression higher by 96%), and stem cell factor, it can be concluded that CO induced the proliferation and division of HF cells and maintained the anagen phase. Because EGF expression was decreased significantly, CO could delay the transition into the catagen phase.

Dhanotia et al.[102] evaluated the hair growth activity of the *Citrullus colocynthis* fruit in androgen-induced alopecia in Swiss albino mice. Petroleum ether extract of *C. colocynthis* was applied topically to assess its hair growth–promoting activity. The extract exhibited promising hair growth–promoting activity, as reflected in the follicular density, anagen/telogen ratio, and skin sections. The results of treatment with 2% and 5% petroleum ether extracts were comparable to the positive control, finasteride. The petroleum ether extract of *C. colocynthis* and its isolate may be useful in the treatment of androgen-induced alopecia.

After topical application of *Cornus officinalis*, fermented with *Lactobacillus rhamnosus* for 8 days, hair regrowth was observed in 6-week-old male C57BL/6 mice.[103]

Shin et al.[104] assessed the effects of *Crataegus pinnatifida* extract on hair growth using a mouse model and examined its mechanisms of action. *C. pinnatifida* extract promoted hair growth by inducing anagen phase, which might be mediated by the activation of cellular signaling that enhanced the survival of cultured hDPC and increased the ratio of Bcl-2 to Bax, which would protect against cell death.

Cuscuta reflexa was evaluated for hair growth activity in androgen-induced alopecia by Pandit et al.[105] in Swiss albino mice–induced alopecia by testosterone administration. Petroleum ether extract of *C. reflexa* exhibited promising hair growth–promoting activity as reflected by follicular density, anagen/telogen ratio, and skin sections. Inhibition of 5α-reductase activity by the extract and isolate suggested that the extract reversed androgen-induced alopecia by inhibiting the conversion of testosterone to DHT. The extract and an isolate, CR1, may be useful in the treatment of androgen-induced alopecia by inhibiting 5α-reductase.

Eclipta alba is a well-known Ayurvedic herb with purported claims of hair growth promotion. Roy et al.[106] evaluated petroleum ether and ethanol extract of *E. alba* for their effects in promoting hair growth in albino rats. Quantitative analysis of hair growth after treatment with petroleum ether extract (5%) showed a greater number of HFs in the anagen phase (69 ± 4) versus the control (47 ± 13).

Datta et al.[107] investigated the efficacy of methanol extract of *Eclipta alba* as a hair growth promoter in C57BL/6 mice. Activity was assessed by studying melanogenesis in resected skin, follicle count in the subcutis, skin thickness, and surrogate markers in vehicle control and extract-treated animals.

According to the results of Kawano et al.,[108] among plant extracts collected in Tunisia, *E. multiflora* extract promoted DPC growth and the cell cycle with high activity and induced hair growth in in vivo male C3H/He mice by the induction of anagen phase, from telogen phase.

Fructus panax ginseng (FPG) extract increased the proliferation of DPCs significantly in dose-dependent (1 and 10 mg per mL, 100 μL per day) and time-dependent manners.[109] FPG extract also enhanced Bcl-2 expression and decreased Bax expression, compared with the control ($p < 0.01$). Moreover, significant elongation of the anagen phase during the hair cycle after the application of FPG was evaluated by photographic and histological observations. FPG extract improved cell proliferation in human DPCs through antiapoptotic activation.

According to the results of Kubo et al.,[110] 70% ethanolic extract from leaves of *Ginkgo biloba* L. showed hair regrowth–promoting effects in C3H strain mice. *G. biloba* extract had inhibitory effects on blood platelet aggregation, thrombin activity, and fibrinolysis.

The hair growth–promoting effects of various types of *Ginseng radix* were evaluated with cultured mouse vibrissal HFs.[111] A 70% methanol extract from red ginseng (steamed and dried roots of *Panax ginseng* C.A. Meyer, one kind of Ginseng Radix) had superior activity to that of white ginseng (peeled and dried root of *P. ginseng*, another kind of Ginseng Radix) in a hair growth–promoting assay using mouse vibrissal follicles in organ culture. Of the major constituents of *P. ginseng*, ginsenoside-Rb1 (G-Rb_1) exhibited activity, but ginsenosides-Rgl (G-Rg_1) and -Ro (G-Ro) were ineffective. Additionally, 20(*S*)-ginsenoside-Rg3 (20(*S*)-G-Rg_3), formed in the processing of red ginseng from the crude root of *P. ginseng*, also showed hair growth–promoting activity.

Recently, the hair growth effects of red ginseng have been demonstrated in many in vitro experiments, but there have been few clinical studies. Hyun et al.[112] evaluated the efficacy of Rg3 shampoo containing 0.003% Rg3 extract from ginseng radix in preventing hair loss and promoting hair growth in a clinical study. After 8- and 16-week use of Rg3 shampoo, the results in the Rg3 shampoo group showed statistically significant improvements in the density, thickness, and growth rate of the hair. Results from clinicians and patients and the subjective satisfaction of patients also showed better responses for the group using the Rg3 shampoo.

AA is known to be caused by an immunological disorder, but the details are not fully understood. Oh and Son[113] studied the hair growth efficacy and safety of red ginseng (*Ginseng radix*) in AA, comparing a corticosteroid intralesional injection (ILI) alone patient group with an ILI + red ginseng patient group using a Folliscope 2.5 for 12 weeks.

The black soy bean (*Glycine max*), both when eaten and when applied topically, has significant hair growth–promoting effects. According to the results of Lee and Kim,[114] when 60 g of boiled black soy beans were administered orally to nine subjects (three men, six women) once per day for 3 months, among the two measured parts (thin and thick parts), hair thickness in the thin part showed a greater increase and, by gender, the hair thickness of the women showed a higher rate of increase than the men.

Jeon et al.[115] assessed the effect of black soybean (*Glycine max*) on hair growth. Specifically, they evaluated topical application and mitosis induction in DPCs and mitogenic effects on NIH3T3 cells in vitro. Significant stimulation of the DPCs and NIH3T3 cell proliferation were observed with black soybean treatment in a dose-dependent manner.

Petroleum ether extract of leaves and flowers of *Hibiscus rosa-sinensis* was evaluated for its potential in hair growth both in vivo and in vitro.[116] In vivo, 1% extract of leaves and flowers in liquid paraffin was applied topically over the shaved skin of albino rats and monitored and assessed for 30 days. The length of hair and the different cyclic phases of the HFs were determined at different time points. In vitro, HFs from albino rat neonates were isolated and cultured in DMEM supplemented with 0.01 mg per mL petroleum ether extract of leaves and flowers.

Kang et al.[117] evaluated the promoting effect of *Ishige sinicola*, an alga native to Jeju Island, Korea, on hair growth. When vibrissa follicles were cultured in the presence of *I. sinicola* extract for 21 days, the extract increased hair-fiber length. *I. sinicola* extract and octaphlorethol A, a component of *I. sinicola*, have the potential to treat alopecia via stimulating the proliferation of DPCs, in addition to the activation of the β-catenin pathway and 5α-reductase inhibition.

Choi et al.[118] evaluated the potential hair growth–promoting activity and expression of cell growth factors in *Lycopersicon esculentum* extracts using the dorsal skin of C57BL/6 mice. At week 4, isolated lycopene Tween 80 solution (LTS) and test hair tonic containing LTS (THT) exhibited hair growth–promoting potential, similar to that of 3% minoxidil, the positive control. Further, in the LTS group, significant increases in mRNA levels of VEGF, KGF, and IGF-1 were observed over the positive and negative controls. The increases in IGF-1 and the decrease in VEGF and TGF-β expression were significant for THT over the negative control. In a histological examination, in the THT group, the induction of the anagen stage of HFs was faster than that in the negative control.

Song et al.[119] evaluated the hair growth–promoting effects in mice of an essence manufactured with products fermented from *Opuntia ficusindica* var. sarboten fruits and *Lactobacillus rhamnosus*. In the mice, 0.1 mL essence was applied topically once daily for 8 days after shaving the fur on their backs; the treatment showed a more significant hair growth–promoting effect than did minoxidil. Furthermore, a histological evaluation showed that the essence containing fermented products increased the depth and size of the HFs markedly versus minoxidil.

The potential hair growth–promoting activity of rice (*Oryza sativa*) bran supercritical CO_2 extract (RB-SCE) and major components of RB-SCE—linoleic acid, policosanol, γ-oryzanol, and γ-tocotrienol—were evaluated in C57BL/6 mice.[89] RB-SCE showed hair growth–promoting potential similar in extent to 3% minoxidil; the HFs were induced to enter the anagen stage. The numbers of the HFs were also increased significantly. Additionally, mRNA levels of VEGF, IGF-1, and KGF were increased significantly, whereas that of TGF-β decreased in the RB-SCE-treated groups. Among the major components of RB-SCE, linoleic acid and γ-oryzanol strongly induced the formation of HFs, according to an examination of the histological morphology and mRNA expression levels in cell growth.

Jeong et al.[120] investigated the effects of fresh *Pinelliae rhizoma* extracts on hair growth activity in C57BL/6N mice over 16 days. In the *P. rhizoma* extract–treated group, a hair growth effect was observed over the whole skin area (100%) in all the normal mice whose hair had been clipped on the 16th day. In the *P. rhizoma* extract–treated group, HFs in the middle stage of anagen were observed, and the follicles had grown down to the subcutaneous tissue of the skin in all the mice on the 10th day. Treatment with the extract of fresh *P. rhizoma* increased the expression of TGF-β (146%), IGF (107%), and prolactin (115%) in the skin of normal C57BL/6N mice compared with the control group (=100%).

Pleuropterus cilinervis extracts and animal milk, fermented with *Lactobacillus rhamnosus*, were applied topically to the back skin of the C57BL/6 mice for 8 days.[121] At the end of the experiment, it was noted that hair regrowth in the experimental group, using gross and histological examinations, was higher than that in the positive control group.

Polygonum multiflorum has been used traditionally for treating patients suffering from baldness and hair loss in East Asia. Park et al.[122] investigated the hair growth–promoting activities of *P. multiflorum* and its mechanism of action. In *P. multiflorum* extract–treated C57BL6/N mice group, they observed increases in the number and size of HFs, which was considered evidence of anagen phase induction. Immunohistochemical analysis showed the earlier induction of β-catenin and SHH in the *P. multiflorum* extract–treated group versus the control group.

Nanking cherry (*Prunus tomentosa*) total flavone was assessed in C57BL/6 mouse phalacrosis models. The mean length of new hair was measured, and tissues of the phalacrosis zones were selected for pathological analysis. The results showed that *P. tomentosa* total flavone could prolong the hair growth cycle markedly, promoting hair growth and follicular maturation.[123]

Kim et al.[124] evaluated the hair growth–promoting effects of herbal products containing *Rosa multiflora* root extracts as a major component (RMHP). The RMHP group showed 100% hair growth, a significant stimulation of hair growth versus 80% in the negative control group using 4-week-old male C57BL/6 mice. Also, 37 patients were treated with RMHP, and the therapeutic effect was evaluated at 16 weeks. The results of clinical photointerpretation using a seven-point rating scale assessment showed that, after 16 weeks, clinical symptoms had improved significantly by 1.23 ± 0.05 ($p < 0.05$).

Kim and Kim[125] investigated the effects of rosemary (*Rosmarinus officinalis*) essential oil on hair growth in a shaving animal model of C57BL/6 mice. After a 4-week application, hair regrowth on the dorsal skin in the 3% rosemary oil–treated group (42%) and 3% minoxidil group (55%) was much faster than in the negative control group (3%) in gross observations. HF number, follicle depth, and dermal thickness in the treatment and positive control groups were significantly higher ($p < 0.05$) than in the negative control group in histological observations. Also, the numbers of mast cells in the dermis and hypodermis of the treatment and positive control groups were significantly lower ($p < 0.05$) than in the negative and vehicle control groups.

The hair growth–promoting effects of *Rosmarinus officinalis* were confirmed using a 50% aqueous ethanol extract.[126] Topical administration of *Rosmarinus officinalis* leaf extract (RO-ext, 2 mg per day/mouse) improved hair regrowth in C57BL/6NCrSlc mice. Testosterone 5α-reductase showed inhibitory activity of 82.4% and 94.6% at 200 and 500 mg per mL of RO-ext, respectively. As an active constituent in 5α-reductase inhibition, 12-methoxycarnosic acid was identified by activity-guided fractionation. Additionally, the extract of *R. officinalis* and 12-methoxycarnosic acid inhibited androgen-dependent proliferation of LNCaP cells by 64.5% and 66.7%, at 5 mg per mL and 5 mM, respectively.

Oh et al.[127] found that an extract of the dried root of *Rubus coreanum* had a hair growth–promoting effect. After topical application of these extracts to the back of C57BL/6 mice, an earlier conversion from telogen-to-anagen phase was induced. However, the effects of these materials on hair growth promotion were apparently not mediated through inhibition of 5α-reductase I or II activity, but through stimulation of HF cells and the expression of growth factors in the DPCs.

When rat vibrissa follicles were treated with 85% ethanol (EtOH) extract of *Schisandra nigra* (a plant native to Jeju Island, South Korea), the hair-fiber lengths of the vibrissa follicles increased significantly.[128] After topical application of the EtOH extract of *S. nigra* onto the back of C57BL/6 mice every other day, anagen progression of the hair shaft was induced. The extract increased both the expression of proliferating cell nuclear antigen in the bulb matrix region and the proliferation of immortalized vibrissa DPCs. When the vibrissa follicles in the anagen phase were treated with *S. nigra* extract for 7 days, the expression of TGF-β2 in the bulb matrix region was found to be lower than that of the control follicles that were expected to be in the anagen–catagen transition phase.

After topical application of *Sophora flavescens* extract onto the back of C57BL/6 mice, the earlier conversion of telogen-to-anagen was induced.[129] The growth of DPCs cultured in vitro, however, was unaffected by *S. flavescens* extract treatment. RT-PCR analysis showed that *S. flavescens* extract induced mRNA levels of growth factors, such as IGF-1 and KGF, in DPCs, suggesting that the effects of *S. flavescens* extract on hair growth may be mediated through the regulation of growth factors in DPCs. Additionally, the *S. flavescens* extract possessed potent inhibitory activity against type II 5α-reductase.

An edible and medicinal mushroom, *Sparassis crispa*, commonly called the "cauliflower mushroom," is known to be a nutritious food and source nutraceuticals due to its rich flavors and β-glucan content. Hair growth was stimulated in the *S. crispa* water extract test group compared with an ethyl acetate extract and 70% extract group, along with a positive control (3% minoxidil) and negative control, for 4 weeks in a hair-removed 5-week-old C57BL/6 mice model.[130]

Thuja orientalis extracts have been used as a hemostatic, roborant, and sedative in Oriental medicine. Kim et al.[131] investigated the inhibitory effects on the production of proinflammatory cytokines, such as IL-1β, IL-6, TNFα, and nitric oxide (NO) and the hair growth–promoting properties of *Thuja orientalis* extract (TOE) in the macrophage cell line RAW264.7 and hair loss-induced DBA1J mice. TOE (50–500 μg per mL) had no cytotoxic effect on nonstimulated cells, but the extract reduced the release of NO, IL-1β, IL-6, and TNF-α concentration dependently in RAW264.7 cells stimulated with lipopolysaccharide. Moreover, when TOE (500 μg per mL) was applied to DBA 1J/mice, hair growth was markedly promoted. These data suggest that TOE promoted hair growth in hair loss–induced model mice and that these properties may contribute to the anti–hair loss activity of *Thuja orientalis.*

Ryu et al.[132] evaluated the hair growth–promoting effects of wheat (*Triticum aestivum*) sprout extract with antioxidants in female C57BL/6 mouse. Specifically, 80% ethanol extract of wheat sprout was used with minoxidil (3%) as a positive control. After 4 weeks, observation with an optical microscope showed similar hair growth in the positive control and wheat sprout groups. The dermal tissue at 4 weeks after the C57BL/6 mouse had been treated with wheat sprout had started the transition to growth.

In the study of Shin et al. (2008),[133] C57BL/6 mice were treated topically on depilated dorsal skin with *Vitex rotundifolia* extract dissolved in 70% EtOH. The ratio of follicle number in anagen phase/total was increased. Also, treatment with *V. rotundifolia* extract on human hair dermal papilla cells induced more than 20% growth (proliferation) than in the control-treated group.

Essential oil from the seeds of jujube (*Zizyphus jujuba*) was applied at different concentrations (0.1%, 1%, and 10%) over the shaved skin on the backs of BALB/c mice, and they were monitored for 21 days.[134] After 21 days, mice treated with 1% and 10% oil showed a greater effect on the length of hair, measured at 9.96 and 10.02 mm, respectively, compared with the negative control (8.94 mm).

28.5.2 Nutraceuticals from Animal Sources

It has been reported that cow (*Bos taurus*) placenta extract,[135] red deer (*Cervus elaphus*) antler extract,[136] *Mylabris Phalerata*,[137] autologous platelet-rich plasma (PRP),[138] and *Selenarctos thibetanus* (bear) oil[139] have hair growth–promoting effects. A summary of hair growth–promoting agents from animal sources is presented in Table 28.2.

Zhang et al.[135] examined whether cow (*Bos taurus*) placenta extract could promote hair growth by elongating the hair shaft and increasing HF number. Results showed that placenta extract more efficiently accelerated cell division and growth factor expression, by raising the IGF-1 mRNA and protein level to increase HF size and hair length in a C57BL/6 mouse model.

To investigate and evaluate the effects of red deer (*Cervus elaphus*) antler extract on hair growth in a full-thickness wound healing model, Sprague Dawley rats were given incision wounds through the full thickness of their dorsal skin, and deer antler extract was applied for 40 days.[136] At post-injury days 16, 32, and 40, longer and more active new hair appeared around the healing wound of the antler-treated skin. Histological studies showed that the antler extract markedly increased the depth, size, and number of HFs. Expression of IGF-1 mRNA was detected by RT-PCR and real-time RT-PCR. The results showed that the expression of IGF-1 (days 16, 32, and 40) was obviously upregulated in antler extract–treated skin versus controls.

"Mylabris" is the dried body of Chinese blister beetles *Mylabris phalerata* and *M. cichorii*. Jo et al.[137] examined the effect of extracts and fractions, obtained from *M. phalerata* Pall. on hair growth activity of C57BL/6N mice after topical application to the skin. A hair growth effect from the extracts of *M. phalerata* Pall. (0.312%) was observed in 80% and 100% of mice, whose hair had been removed, after 13 and 20 days, respectively. A hair growth effect from the cantharidin fraction

TABLE 28.2
Summary of the Hair Growth–Promoting Agents from Animal Origin

Species	Common Name	Part for Use	Extract or Active Component	Activity Test Model	References
Bos taurus	Cow	Placenta	Crude extract	C57BL/6 mice	Zang et al. [135]
Cervus elaphus	Red deer	Antler	Acetone and a 2:1 chloroform–methanol mixture extract	Sprague Dawley rats	Yang et al. [136]
Mylabris Phalerata	Mylabris, the dried body of the Chinese blister beetle	Dried body	Crude extracts	C57BL/6N mice	Jo et al. [137]
Mus musculus		Autologous platelet-rich plasma	Plasma itself	C57BL/6 mice	Li et al. [138]
Selenarctos thibetanus	Bear		Oil	C57BL/6 mice	Shin et al. [139]

(0.5%) and water fraction (0.5%) of *M. phalerata* Pall. was observed in 100% of mice, whose hair had been clipped, after 24 days.

Autologous PRP has been tested during facelifts and hair transplantation to reduce swelling and pain and to increase hair density.[138] Activated PRP increased the proliferation of DPCs and stimulated extracellular signal-regulated kinase (ERK) and Akt signaling. FGF-7 and β-catenin, which are potent stimuli for hair growth, were upregulated in DPCs. The injection of mice with activated PRP induced a faster telogen-to-anagen transition than was seen in control mice.

Shin et al.[139] investigated the effects of *Selenarctos thibetanus* (bear) oil on hair growth in a depilated C57BL/6 mouse model. With topical treatment of the dorsal skin with 5% bear oil for 2 weeks, HFs showed accelerated hair regrowth versus the 2% bear oil group, minoxidil group, and 70% EtOH group. Additionally, hair density was increased in the group treated with bear oil; it markedly increased the depth and the size of the HFs in comparison with the groups treated with minoxidil and 70% EtOH.

28.5.3 Polyherbal Complex

For adequate hair growth promotion with fewer adverse effects, many in vitro and in vivo tests and human clinical trials have recommended combination therapy using two or more drugs. Such combination therapies, especially using polyherbal complexes based on traditional Oriental medicine, have shown therapeutic potential for hair growth promotion. Generally, the effect of a blend of several herbal extracts that are already known to have hair growth–promoting effects is more potent than each extract's effect alone. A summary of polyherbal complexes as hair growth–promoting agents is provided in Table 28.3.

According to a bibliographic study of Park et al.[140] on herbal medicines for alopecia in ancient Oriental medicinal literature, the most frequently used single herbs in the prescriptions were *Angelicae gigantis* Radix, Rehmanniae Radix Preparat, Cnidii Rhizoma, Glycyrrhizae Radix, Poria cocos Wolf, and Paeoniae Radix Alba. Herbs frequently used in prescriptions specifically for alopecia included Polygoni Multiflori Radix, Rehmanniae Radix, Cuscutae Semen, Bupleuri Radix, Scutellariae Radix, Viticis Fructus, and Aconiti Lateralis Preparata Radix.

Angelica gigas and *Glycyrrhiza uralensis* Oriental medicine complex extracts effectively stimulated hair growth in C57BL/6 mice and can be used practically for hair growth or the prevention of hair loss in humans.[141]

Kim et al.[142] investigated the hair regrowth–promoting effects of a mixture of water and alcohol extract from *Eclipta prostrata*, *Mori cortex radicis*, *Thuja orientalis folium*, and *Drynaria fortunei* in C3H/HeJ mice. The herbal extract used had a promoting effect on hair regrowth, possibly by increasing the activities of ALP and γ-GT and the expression of EGF and VEGF.

In Korean folk medicine, several herbs, such as *Glycyrrhizae Radix*, *Persicae Semen*, *Salviae Radix*, *Angelicae Gigantis* Radix, *Zanthoxyli Fructus*, *Ginseng Radix Alba*, *Cnidii Rhizoma*, and *Carthami Flos*, are known to enhance blood circulation and to have wound healing or anti-inflammatory effects. Choi et al.[143] found that a herbal mixture possessed significant hair cycle–converting activity, from the telogen phase to the anagen phase, in C3H mice. Furthermore, the mixture enhanced hair density in AGA subjects and inhibited steroid 5α-reductase activity.

Choi et al.[144] investigated the effect of Korean medicinal herbs, including hair tonic (MHT) and food (MF), on hair growth in a C57BL/6 mouse alopecia model. Not only the external appearance but also the hair density and hair thickness on the dorsal skin were increased more in the test (HT epidermal application + MF diet-treated group) group than in a negative control group at 21 days. Also, the expression of IGF-1 on dorsal skin was higher in the test group than in the negative control group.

Yikgeebohyul-tang is a representative prescription for the invigoration of vitality and nourishing of the blood. Hong et al.[145] investigated the effects of Yikgeebohyul-tang on hair regrowth and

TABLE 28.3
Summary of Polyherbal Complexes as Hair Growth–Promoting Agents

Common Name or Species	Extract or Active Component	Activity Test Model	References
Angelica gigas, Glycyrrhiza uralensis		C57BL/6 mice	Lee and Kim [141]
Eclipta prostrata, Mori cortex radicis, Thuja orientalis folium, Drynaria fortunei	The mixture of water and alcohol extract	C3H/HeJ mice	Kim et al. [142]
Glycyrrhizae Radix, Persicae Semen, Salviae Radix, Angelicae Gigantis Radix, *Zanthoxyli Fructus, Ginseng Radix Alba, Cnidii Rhizoma, Carthami Flos*	A mixture of their extracts	C3H mice	Choi et al. [143]
Hair tonic (*Morus alba, Platycladus orientalis, Sesamum indicum, Laminaria japonica, Undaria pinnatifida* = 3:3:1:2:2, MHT) and food (*Morus alba, Platycladus orientalis, Pinus densiflora, Sesamum indicum*, Lycium chinense, black bean, *Undaria pinnatifida*, red ginseng = 2:3:1:3:2:2, MF)		C57BL/6 mice	Choi et al. [144]
Yikgeebohyul-tang *Astragali Radix, Atractylodis Rhizoma Alba, Crataegi Fructus, Cyperi Rhizoma, Pinelliae Tuber, Citri Pericarpium, Hoelen, Massa Medicata Fermentata, Hordei Germinatus Fructus, Glycyrrhizae Radix, Magnoliae Cortex, Amomi Xanthioides Fructus, Angelicae Gigantis Radix, Paeoniae Radix, Rehmanniae Recens Radix, Ginseng Radix, Poria, Ophiopogonis Radix, Polygalae Radix, Cnidii Rhizoma, Saussureae Radix, Zingiberis Rhizoma Recens, Zipyphi Fructus*		C57BL/6 mice	Hong et al. [145]
Sophorae Radix, Panax ginseng, Salvia miltiorrhiza BUNGE		C57/BL6 mice	Hwang et al. [146]

(*Continued*)

TABLE 28.3 (*Continued*)
Summary of Polyherbal Complexes as Hair Growth–Promoting Agents

Common Name or Species	Extract or Active Component	Activity Test Model	References
Hwanggumgung® (HGG) Dipotassium Glycyrrhizinate, *Swertia pseudochinensis*, *Panax ginseng*		C57BL6 mice	Hue et al. [147]
Angelica gigas Nakai, *Psoralea corylifolia* Linne, *Biota orientalis* Endlilcher, *Eclipta prostrata* Linne, *Lycium chinense* Miller, *Rubus coreanus* Miquel, *Morus alba* Linne, *Rehmannia glutinosa Liboschitz var. purpurea* Makino, *Ligustrum lucidum* Aiton, *Polygonum multiflorum* Thunberg, *Sesamum indicum* Linne, *Sophora angustifolia* Siebold et Zuccarini, *Angelica dahurica* Bentham et Hooker, *Leonurus sibiricus* Linne, *Salvia miltiorrhiza* Bunge, *Prunus persica* Batsch, *Commiphora molmol* Engler, *Chrysanthemum indicum* Linne, *Boswellia carterii* Birdwood, *Panax ginseng* C. A. Meyer, *Cnidium officinale* Makino, *Albizia julibrissin* Durazzini, *Corydalis ternata* Nakai	Enzyme-modified (Viscozyme, Pectinex) Oriental medical prescriptions	5α-reductase, B16 melanoma cell	Im et al. [148]
Yonnyuniksoogobon-dan *Polygoni Mutiflori Radix, Lycii Radicis Cortex, Polia, Rehmanniae Radix, Rehmanniae Radix Preparat, Asparagi Radix, Liriopis Tuber, Lycii Fructus, Acori Graminei Rhizoma, Angelicae Acutiloba Radix, and Pini Folium)*		C57BL/6 mice	Jeong et al. [149]
DCS-HT® β-Sitosterol from black bean, *Mori cortex, Polygonum multiflorum* (3:1:1)		6-week-old male C57BL/6 mice	Lee and Hwang [150]

(*Continued*)

TABLE 28.3 (*Continued*)
Summary of Polyherbal Complexes as Hair Growth–Promoting Agents

Common Name or Species	Extract or Active Component	Activity Test Model	References
Angelica gigas Nakai, Psoralea corylifolia Linne, Biota orientalis Endlicher, Eclipta prostrata Linne, Rehmannia glutinosa Liboschitz var. purpurea Makino, Ligustrum lucidum Aiton, Polygonum multiflorum Thunberg, Sesamum indicum Linne, Sophora angustifolia Siebold et Zuccarini, Angelica dahurica Bentham et Hooker, Leonurus sibiricus Linne, Salvia miltiorrhiza Bunge, Prunus persica Batsch, Commiphora molmol Engler, Chrysanthemum indicum Linne, Boswellia carterii Birdwood, Panax ginseng C. A. Meyer, Cnidium officinale Makino, Albizia julibrissin Durazzini, Corydalis ternata Nakai		C57BL/6 mice	Lee et al. [151]
Mylabris phalerata Pall., *Drynariae Rhizoma*		C57BL/6N mice	Lee et al. [152]
Mylabris phalerata Pall., *Arisaematis* Rhizoma, *Pinelliae* Rhizoma Ternata		C57BL/6N mice	Chung et al. [153]
Emblica officinalis, Bacopa, monnieri, Trigonella foenumgraecum, Murraya koenigii	Herbal oil	Wistar albino rats	Purwal et al. [154]
Eclipta alba, Citrullus colocynthis, Tridax procumbens	Petroleum ether extract (3:1:2)	Wistar albino rats	Adhirajan et al. [155]
Cicer arietinum, Ocimum sanctum, Cyperus rotundus	1:2:3	Topically on shaved skin of rats	Rathi et al. [156]
Cuscuta reflexa (Roxb.), Citrullus colocynthis (Schrad.), Eclipta alba (Hassk.)	Petroleum ether extracts	Wistar albino rats	Roy et al. [157]
Trichosanthes cucumerina, Abrus precatorius	Aqueous extract	Wistar albino rats	Sandhya et al. [158]
Poria cocos, Thuja orientalis, Espinosilla, Lycium chinense, Coix lacrymajobi, Polygonum multiflorum	70% ethanol	Male C57BL/6 mice	Seo et al. [159]

(*Continued*)

TABLE 28.3 (*Continued*)
Summary of Polyherbal Complexes as Hair Growth–Promoting Agents

Common Name or Species	Extract or Active Component	Activity Test Model	References
Eclipta alba Hassk, Hibiscus rosa-sinensis, Nardostachys jatamansi	Hot coconut oil extract	Female Wistar albino rats	Thorat et al. [160]
Gamissanghwa-tang *Angelica gigas NAKAI, Rehmannia glutinosa Libosch, Paeonia lactiflora Pallas, Cnidium officinale Makino, Lycium chinense, Cuscuta chinensis Lamark, Rubus coreanus Miquel, Schisandra chinensis Baillon, Torilis japonica Houtt, Astragalus membranaceus Bung, Glycyrrhiza glabra* L., *Cinnamomum Cassia Blume*	Hot water extract	C57BL/6 mice, 5α-reductase type II	Yun et al. [161]

cytokine changes in a C57BL/6 mouse shaving model. The effects were related to EGF levels in hair roots, a decrease in serum IFN-γ, and an increase in serum IL-4.

Hwang et al.[146] investigated the effects of Monegy (a mix of *Sophorae* Radix, *Panax ginseng*, *Salvia miltiorrhiza* Bunge) on epilate-induced hair loss in the dorsal region of C57BL/6 mice and external structure of human hair. Confocal analysis showed the distribution of FITC-conjugated Monegy and penetration depth compared with the normal and control group. When Monegy was administered topically on a C57BL/6 mouse, it penetrated very well. The fluorescence intensity was increased up to 205- and 113-fold compared with the control group. Also, the area of fluorescence was increased by up to 255- and 127-fold compared with the control group.

Hue et al.[147] investigated the effects of Hwanggumgung (HGG, a hair care product composed of several plant extracts, including dicalcium glycyrrhizinate, *Swertia japonica*, and *Panax ginseng*) on hair regrowth in a C57BL/6 mouse shaving model with 0.15 mL per mouse applied each day for 21 days. The topical application of HGG in female mice promoted hair regrowth earlier and faster than in the control groups. In male mice, the topical application of HGG also accelerated hair growth compared with the controls. HGG promoted elongation of HFs compared with the controls in both female and male mice. Activities of alkaline phosphatase and γ-glutamyl transpeptidase, enzymes related to hair growth, increased significantly after treatment with HGG for 2 weeks in both female and male mice ($p < 0.05$).

Im et al.[148] investigated the effect of enzyme-modified (Viscozyme, Pectinex) Oriental medical prescriptions (23 herbal species) on hair growth and melanogenesis. Enzyme-modified Oriental medical prescriptions showed antioxidative effects and inhibitory effects on lipoxygenase, 5α-reductase activity, and melanogenic activity.

Jeong et al.[149] evaluated the hair growth–promoting effects of Yonnyuniksoogobon-dan (composed of 11 herbs, that is *Polygoni Mutiflori* Radix, *Lycii Radicis* Cortex, Polia, *Rehmanniae Radix*, *Rehmanniae Radix* Preparat, *Asparagi Radix*, Liriopis Tuber, Lycii Fructus, *Acori Graminei* Rhizoma, *Angelica Acutiloba* Radix, and Pini Folium) on shaved C57BL/6 mice. Yonnyuniksoogobon-dan had hair growth–promoting activity, and these effects were related to upregulation of EGF and VEFG expression and downregulation of TGF-β1 and iNOS expression in hair roots.

Lee and Hwang[150] evaluated the effects of DCS-HT (a hair care product including β-sitosterol from black beans, *Mori cortex*, and *Polygonum multiflorum* [3:1:1]) on hair growth in a C57BL/6 mouse alopecia model; it was applied to dorsal skin at 150 μL per mouse once each day for 21 days. Topical treatment with DCS hair tonic accelerated hair regrowth significantly faster than in the other groups ($p < 0.05$). ALP and γ-GT activities after 21 days were increased significantly in the DCS-HT group ($p < 0.01$). DCS hair tonic and 3% minoxidil also increased the expression of IGF-1 significantly in the skin of C57BL/6 mice ($p < 0.01$).

Lee et al.[151] developed a medicinal herbal complex extract (MHCE) using 23 herbs (Table 28.3). They examined the hair growth effect of MHCE in vitro and in vivo. Their results showed that MHCE increased the proliferation significantly in HFDPC (175% proliferation at 50 μg per mL), HaCaT cells (133% proliferation at 20 μg per mL), and NIH3T3 cells (120% proliferation at 50 μg per mL). MHCE also increased melanogenesis in B16F1 cells (154% melanin synthesis at 50 μg per mL). Moreover, MHCE showed potential for hair growth stimulation in C57BL/6 mice experiments (98% hair growth area in 4 weeks).

Hair growth effects of mixed extracts of *Mylabris phalerata* Pall. (5 mg per 100 mL) and *Drynariae Rhizoma* (1 g per 100 mL) were observed in 100% of mice in a spontaneous alopecia C57BL/6N mouse model in 15 days.[152] In the mixed extract–treated mice, VEGF, c-kit, and PKC-α were strongly stained in the IRS and ORS in the skin. Treatment with the mixed extract increased the expression of TGF-β, placental lactogen, and prolactin in the skin of normal C57BL/6N mice compared with the control group.

Chung et al.[153] assessed whether the topical application of trimix extracts of *Mylabris phalerata* Pall., *Arisaematis Rhizoma*, and *Pinelliae Rhizoma* Ternata resulted in the effects on hair growth activity in C57BL/6N mice. The experimental groups were group I (0.5 mg cantharidin, 1 g extract of *Pinelliae Rhizoma*, 2 g extract of *Arisaematis Rhizoma*/50 mL 50% EtOH), group II (1.5 mg cantharidin, 0.5 g extract of *P. Rhizoma*, 1 g extract of *A. Rhizoma*/50 mL 50% EtOH), and group III (2.5 mg cantharidin, 0.25 g extract of *P. Rhizoma*, 0.5 g extract of *A. Rhizoma*/50 mL 50% EtOH). PKC-α immunoreactivity in all the experimental groups showed mild staining in the epidermis and cutaneous trunci muscles versus the control group on day 12. On day 12, the expression of bFGF (138%, 119%, and 120%, respectively), VEGF (146%, 144%, and 133%, respectively), IGF-1 (165%, 141%, and 119%, respectively), and PLI (121%, 116%, and 123%, respectively) in the three experimental groups was increased versus the control group.

Purwal et al.[154] studied hair growth activity of formulations of *Emblica officinalis*, *Bacopa monnieri*, *Trigonella foenumgraecum*, and *Murraya koenigii*, in various concentrations, in the form of a herbal oil. Each herb was tested for its hair growth activity in a concentration range of 1%–10%, separately. The result revealed that the hair growth activity of each herb was proportional to the concentration. A formulation containing 7.5% of each herb showed excellent hair growth activity, with enlargement of follicular size and prolongation of the anagen phase.

In an evaluation of Indian herbal formulations, Adhirajan et al.[155] studied the hair growth activities of a mixture of petroleum ether extracts of *Eclipta alba*, colocynth, bitter apple, *Citrullus colocynthis*, and coat button, *Tridax procumbens*, in various concentrations in the form of a herbal cream and a herbal oil. At a ratio of *E. alba*/*C. colocynthis*/*T. procumbens* of 3:1:2, there was excellent hair growth activity, and they showed 35% more anagen HFs, while the reference drug, 2% minoxidil ethanolic solution, showed 20% more anagen HFs than the control. At a ratio of 1:2:3, they showed comparable activity to the standard.

Rathi et al.[156] sought to formulate and evaluate hair growth–promoting activity of three polyherbal formulations. Polyherbal formulations were prepared using extracts of *Cicer arietinum*, *Ocimum sanctum*, and *Cyperus rotundus* in various ratios to obtain the best formulation. The extract, incorporated into a cream, was applied topically on the shaved skin of rats, and a primary skin irritation test, hair growth initiation time, completion time, and hair length and diameter were recorded. The ratio of *C. arietinum*/*O. sanctum*/*C. rotundus* at 1:2:3 showed excellent hair growth activity, comparable to the positive control.

Cuscuta reflexa, *Citrullus colocynthis*, and *Eclipta alba* are commonly used herbs with hair growth–promoting properties. Roy et al.[157] prepared herbal formulations containing petroleum ether extracts of the three herbs in varying ratios and evaluated the formulations for hair growth–promoting activity using Wistar strain albino rats. Hair growth initiation time was reduced markedly, to one-third, on treatment with the prepared formulation compared with control animals. The time required for complete hair regrowth was also reduced by 32%. Quantitative analysis of the hair growth cycle after treatment with the formulations and minoxidil (2%) showed a greater number of HFs in the anagen phase than in the control.

Sandhya et al.[158] reported preclinical studies on a polyherbal phytocomplex hair growth–promoting cream incorporating aqueous extracts of *Trichosanthes cucumerina* and *Abrus precatorius*. Their studies showed that the formulated 2% polyherbal phytocomplex hair growth–promoting cream was an effective hair growth promoter in Wistar albino rats, and the results were comparable to those with minoxidil 2%. It was observed that the percentage of HFs in the anagen phase increased considerably.

Seo et al.[159] investigated the in vivo hair growth–promoting efficacies of six herbal extracts (obtained from *Poria cocos*, *Thuja orientalis*, *Espinosilla*, *Lycium chinense Mill*, *Coix lacryma-jobi*, and *Polygonum multiflorum Thunberg*) and monoolein cubosomal suspensions containing the extracts after they were applied daily on the backs of C57BL/6 male mice for 20 days (herbal extract concentration of 3% and cubosome concentration of 1%). Among them, *T. orientalis* extract, *P. multiflorum Thunberg* extract, and *Espinosilla* extract showed some hair growth–promoting efficacy. Cubosomes significantly enhanced the efficacies of the herbal extracts, and the cubosomal suspensions containing the extracts were as potent as minoxidil solution (2.4%) in propylene glycol/water/ethanol (20/30/50, v/v/v).

Eclipta alba, *Hibiscus rosa-sinensis*, and *Nardostachys jatamansi* is a well-known Ayurvedic herbal mixture with purported claims of hair growth promotion. According to the results of Thorat et al.,[160] a formulation of *E. alba* (10% w/v), *H. rosa-sinensis* (10% w/v), and *N. jatamansi* (5% w/v) in a herbal oil showed excellent hair growth activity, comparable with the standard (2% minoxidil ethanolic solution) in Wistar albino rats. Hair growth initiation time was reduced significantly, by half, on treatment with the oil, compared with the control animals. The time required for complete hair growth was also reduced significantly. Quantitative analysis of hair growth after treatment with the oil showed a greater number of HFs in the anagen phase (82) than in the control (52).

Yun et al.[161] found that Gamissanghwa-tang extracts had hair growth–promoting effects. After topical application of the test materials on the backs of CS7BL/6 mice, earlier conversion of telogen-to-anagen phase was induced. In experiments with a 5α-reductase-type II inhibition assay, Radix Paeoniae Alba and Semen Cuscutae showed effective potential to inhibit the activity of 5α-reductase type II. The hair growth index of the Gamissanghwa-tang extracts was ranked as 1.2 and that of *Fructus Rubi* was highest, at 1.8. However, none of the plant extracts tested had any effect on DNA proliferation in hair DPCs, as measured by [^{3}H]thymidine incorporation, the expression of growth factors, such as IGF-1, KGF, and hepatocyte growth factor (HGF), as estimated by RT-PCR, or protein synthesis in vibrissae HFs, as measured by [^{35}S] cysteine incorporation.

28.5.4 Single Compounds

Numerous bioactive single compounds have been investigated for potent hair growth–promoting effect in a few decades. A summary of these single compounds tested as hair growth–promoting agents is provided in Table 28.4.

Kim et al.[162] evaluated the effects of *Acanthopanax koreanum* and acankoreoside J from *A. koreanum* on the promotion of hair growth. When immortalized rat vibrissa DPCs were treated with the extract of *A. koreanum* leaves, cell proliferation increased significantly. Acankoreoside J, a lupane-triterpene of *A. koreanum*, has potential for promoting hair growth by promoting cell cycle

TABLE 28.4
Summary of Single Compounds as Hair Growth–Promoting Agents

Compound	Origin	Activity Test Model	Concentration	References
Acankoreoside J	*Acanthopanax koreanum*	Rat vibrissa dermal papilla	0.1, 1, 10 μM	Kim et al. [162]
Adiponectin		Dermal papilla cells	10 ng per mL to 5 μg per mL	Won et al. [163]
l-Ascorbic acid 2-phosphate		Dermal papilla cells C57BL/6 mice	0.25 mM 250 mM	Sung et al. [164]
l-Ascorbic acid 2-phosphate		Human hair follicles, mice		Kwack et al. [165]
Ascorbigen	*Brassica* vegetables	Human dermal papilla	0–1.25 mM	Wang et al. [166]
l-Carnitine–l-tartrate		Follicular keratinocytes in vitro	0.5–50 μM	Foitzik et al. [167]
Cyclosporine A		Mice vibrissae follicles	10^{-10} to 10^{-7} mol per L	Xu et al. [168]
Epigallocatechin-3-gallate (EGCG)	Green tea	Human dermal papilla cells	3, 30 and 300 nM	Kwon et al. [169]
Erythropoietin		Dermal papilla cells C57BL/6 mice	1, 10 unit per mL 10 Unit	Kang et al. [170]
Gallic acid ester of torachrysone-8-*O*-β-D-glucoside (1) and (*E*)-2,3,5,4′-tetrahydroxystilbene-2-*O*-β-D-xyloside (4), along with eight known compounds (2, 3, 5–10)	70% ethanol extract of *Polygonum multiflorum* roots	Dermal papilla cells	10 μM or 20 μM	Sun et al. [171]
Ginsenoside Ro and Rg3	*Panax ginseng* rhizome	Testosterone 5α-reductase, testosterone-treated C57BL/6 mice	5αR with IC50 values of 259.4 μM (Ro) and 86.1 μM (Rg3), Ro (0.2 mg per mice)	Murata et al. [172]
Ginsenoside Rg3		Dermal papilla cells		Shin et al. [173]
KF19418, a newly synthesized compound		C3H/HeN mice	1%	Shirai et al. [174]
Magnesium ascorbyl phosphate		Male mice	1%–10%	Shanmugam et al. [175]
4-*O*-methylhonokiol	*Magnolia officinalis*	Rat vibrissa follicles, C57BL/6 mice	3, 30, and 300 nM	Kim et al. [176]
α-Methyl spermidine		Human dermal papilla cells C57BL/6 mice	5 μM 5%	Fashe et al. [177]
Mycophenolic acid		Human dermal papilla cells		Kang et al. [178]

(*Continued*)

TABLE 28.4 (*Continued*)
Summary of Single Compounds as Hair Growth–Promoting Agents

Compound	Origin	Activity Test Model	Concentration	References
Platelet-derived growth factor isoforms		C3H mice		Tomita et al. [179]
7-phloroeckol	Marine brown algae, *Ecklonia cava*	Human dermal papilla cells and outer root sheath cells	0.1, 1, 10 μM	Bak et al. [180]
Polyamine		Cultured wool follicles		Hynd and Nancarrow [181]
Polyamines (spermidine, putrescine, and spermine)				Ramot et al. [182]
Proanthocyanidins		Hair follicle cells, C3H mice	3 μM 3%	Takahashi et al. [24]
Procyanidin oligomers		Hair epithelial cells C3H mice	3–30 μM 1%	Takahashi et al. [183]
Procyanidin b-2		Clinical trial	1%	Takahashi et al. [184]
Selenium at nanosize (nano-Se)		Cashmere goats	Fed with the basal diet with 0.5 mg per kg nano-Se	Wu et al. [185]
Sodium silicate		C57BL/6 mice	50%, 100% solution	Hue et al. [186]
Triiodothyronine		CD rats	3.8, 12.8 μg	Safer et al. [187]
Tripeptide–copper complex		Dermal papilla cells	10^{-12} to 10^{-9} M	Pyo et al. [188]

progression of the DPCs through an increase in nuclear β-catenin, along with the upregulation of cyclin D1, cyclin E, and CDK2, and downregulation of $p27^{kip1}$.

Leptin, another adipocyte hormone, has been proposed as a novel regulator of the hair growth cycle. Won et al.[163] evaluated the effect of adiponectin on HFs and demonstrated that normal human scalp HFs express adiponectin receptors. As HFs actively respond to adiponectin via receptors in DPCs in ex vivo organ culture and also in vitro, adiponectin seems to be a hair growth stimulator that promotes hair matrix keratinocyte proliferation. Thus, adiponectin receptor stimulation may be a potential clinical strategy for the promotion of hair growth. Additionally, it is possible that pathological alterations in the level of adiponectin or adiponectin receptors may affect normal hair growth.

L-Ascorbic acid 2-phosphate magnesium salt ("Asc 2-P"), a derivative of L-ascorbic acid (vitamin C), is more stable than ascorbic acid and is known to stimulate the growth of human dermal fibroblasts and osteoblast-like cells. Sung et al.[164] investigated the biological effects of Asc 2-P on hair. Asc 2-P at 0.25 mM stimulated the growth of DPCs. In contrast, there was no growth-stimulating effect on the ORS keratinocytes. Asc 2-P treatment resulted in significant elongation of hair shafts in isolated HFs in culture. P values of 0.012 and 0.025 were obtained for HFs exposed to 0.05 and 0.25 mM Asc 2-P, respectively. Asc 2-P at 250 mM induced an earlier telogen-to-anagen conversion than in the vehicle-treated group. Histology at necropsy also showed that mice treated with Asc 2-P and control mice showed anagen and telogen HF stages, respectively. Vitamin C or its derivatives may regulate mesenchymal–epithelial interactions in the follicle. Asc 2-P also promotes the elongation of hair shafts in cultured human HFs and induces hair growth in mice.[165] According to the results of Kwack et al.,[165] Asc 2-P-inducible IGF-1 from DPCs promotes proliferation of follicular keratinocytes and stimulates HF growth in vitro via PI3K.

Ascorbigen is a predominantly indole-derived compound from *Brassica* vegetables. Wang et al.[166] found that 1.25 mM ascorbigen induced a 1.2-fold increase in the growth of dermal follicle cells, but not keratinocytes. However, ascorbigen did not exert significant protective effects against chemotherapy-induced alopecia in a mouse model. These findings suggest that ascorbigen may not be able to counteract chemotherapy-induced alopecia and that further investigation of the therapeutic potential of ascorbigen in disease models is required.

The trimethylated amino acid L-carnitine plays a key role in the intramitochondrial transport of fatty acids for β-oxidation and thus serves important functions in energy metabolism. Foitzik et al.[167] tested the hypothesis that L-carnitine, a frequently used dietary supplement, may also stimulate hair growth by increasing energy supply to the rapidly proliferating and energy-consuming anagen hair matrix. At day 9, HFs treated with 5 μM or 0.5 μM of L-carnitine/L-tartrate showed a moderate, but significant, stimulation of hair shaft elongation compared with vehicle-treated controls. Also, CT prolonged the duration of anagen VI, downregulated apoptosis (as measured by a TUNEL assay) and upregulated proliferation (as measured by Ki67 immunohistology) of hair matrix keratinocytes ($p < 0.05$). By immunohistology, intrafollicular immunoreactivity for TGF-β2, a key catagen-promoting growth factor, was downregulated in the dermal papilla and TGF-βII receptor protein in the ORS and dermal papilla. As shown by a caspase activity assay, caspases 3 and 7, which are known to initiate apoptosis, were downregulated at days 2 and 4 after treatment of HFs with CT, compared with the vehicle-treated control, indicating that CT has an immediate protective effect on HFs against undergoing programmed cell death. These findings suggest that L-carnitine stimulates human scalp hair growth by upregulation of proliferation and downregulation of apoptosis in follicular keratinocytes in vitro.

Hypertrichosis is a common side effect of systemic cyclosporine A therapy. It has been shown previously that cyclosporine A induces anagen and inhibits catagen development in mice. Xu et al.[168] investigated the effects of cyclosporine A on hair shaft elongation, HF cell proliferation, apoptosis, and mRNA expression of selected growth factors using a mouse vibrissae organ culture model. In this model, cyclosporine A stimulated the hair growth of normal mouse vibrissae follicles by inhibiting catagen-like development and promoting matrix cell proliferation. In addition, cyclosporine A caused an increase in the expression of VEGF, HGF, and nerve growth factor, and inhibited follistatin expression. These findings may provide an explanation for the clinically observed effects of cyclosporine A on hair growth.

Green tea is a popular beverage worldwide, and its potential beneficial effects, such as anticancer and antioxidant properties, are believed to be mediated by epigallocatechin-3-gallate (EGCG), a major constituent of its polyphenols. Recently, it was reported that EGCG might be useful in the prevention or treatment of AGA by selectively inhibiting 5α-reductase activity. Kwon et al. (2007)[169] measured the effects of EGCG on hair growth in vitro to investigate its effect on human DPCs in vivo and in vitro. EGCG promoted hair growth in HF ex vivo culture and the proliferation of cultured DPCs. The growth stimulation of DPCs by EGCG in vitro may be mediated through the upregulation of phosphorylated Erk and Akt and by an increase in the ratio of Bcl-2/Bax. Similar results were obtained in in vivo dermal papillae of human scalps. Thus, EGCG apparently stimulates human hair growth through these dual pro-proliferative and anti-apoptotic effects on DPCs.

Recent studies have shown that erythropoietin (EPO)/erythropoietin receptor (EPOR) signaling exists in both human and mouse HFs. Kang et al.[170] investigated whether DPCs expressed functional EPOR and went on to investigate the effects of EPO on hair shaft growth in cultured human scalp HFs and hair growth in mice. Agarose beads containing EPO were implanted into the dorsal skin of C57BL/6 mice to examine the effects of EPO on hair growth in vivo. EPOR mRNA and protein were expressed in cultured human DPCs. EPOR signaling pathway mediators, such as EPOR and Akt, were phosphorylated by EPO in DPCs. EPO promoted the growth of DPCs and elongated hair shafts significantly with increased proliferation of matrix keratinocytes in cultured human HFs.

Additionally, EPO not only promoted anagen induction from telogen but also prolonged the anagen phase. Thus, EPO may modulate hair growth by stimulating DPCs that express functional EPOR.

Two new compounds, gallic acid ester of torachrysone-8-*O*-β-D-glucoside and (*E*)-2,3,5,4′-tetrahydroxystilbene-2-*O*-β-D-xyloside, along with eight known compounds were isolated from a 70% ethanol extract of *Polygonum multiflorum* roots. The structures were determined by ^{1}H and ^{13}C NMR, HMQC, and HMBC spectrometry. Extracts of *P. multiflorum* have been reported to promote hair growth in vivo. Sun et al.[171] evaluated the effects of isolated compounds from *P. multiflorum* in promoting hair growth using DPCs, which play an important role in hair growth. When DPCs were treated with the 10 compounds from *P. multiflorum*, gallic acid ester of torachrysone-8-*O*-β-D-glucoside, torachrysone-8-*O*-β-D-glucoside, (E)-2,3,5,4′-tetrahydroxystilbene-2-O-β-D-glucoside, (Z)-2,3,5,4′-tetrahydroxystilbene-2-*O*-β-D-glucoside, and emodin-8-*O*-β-D-glucopyranoside increased the proliferation of DPCs, compared with the control. Torachrysone-8-*O*-β-D-glucoside (10 and 20 μM) induced a greater increase in the proliferation of DPCs than minoxidil (10 μM). Additionally, treatment of vibrissa follicles with torachrysone-8-*O*-β-D-glucoside for 21 days increased hair-fiber length significantly.

Murata et al.[172] examined the properties of *Panax ginseng* C.A. Meyer, focusing on the effects of ginseng rhizome on hair regrowth in AGA. Extracts of red ginseng rhizome showed greater dose-dependent inhibitory effects against testosterone 5α-reductase (5αR) than extracts of the main root. Ginsenoside Ro, the predominant ginsenoside in the rhizome, and ginsenoside Rg3, a unique ginsenoside in red ginseng, showed inhibitory activity against 5αR with IC_{50} values of 259.4 and 86.1 μM, respectively. The rhizome of *P. japonicus*, which contains larger amounts of ginsenoside Ro, also inhibited 5α-reductase. Topical administration of extracts of red ginseng rhizomes (2 mg per mouse) and ginsenoside Ro (0.2 mg per mouse) to shaved skin inhibited hair regrowth suppression after shaving in testosterone-treated C57BL/6 mice.

Shin et al.[173] determined the effects of ginsenoside Rg3 on hair growth. Thymidine incorporation was determined to measure cell proliferation. Reverse transcription polymerase chain reaction showed dose-dependent increases in VEGF mRNA levels on treatment with Rg3. Immunohistochemical analysis showed that expression of VEGF was significantly upregulated by Rg3 in a dose-dependent manner in human DP cells and in mouse HFs. Additionally, CD8 and CD34 were upregulated by Rg3 in mouse HFs. Thus, Rg3 may increase hair growth through stimulation of HF stem cells, and it is a candidate molecule for use in hair growth products.

KF19418, a newly synthesized compound, stimulated the proliferation of cultured hair bulb cells from new born mice in a concentration-dependent manner below 10 μM.[174] In the culture system of whole skin pieces from 4-week-old C3H/HeN mice, KF19418 promoted HF elongation, as did minoxidil. After topical application of KF19418 or minoxidil for 2 weeks to the dorsal skin in a hair-clipped mouse alopecia model, KF19418 in 1% suspension accelerated hair regrowth at a rate comparable to 1% minoxidil solution.

Shanmugam et al.[175] evaluated the effects of methylsulfonylmethane on hair growth promotion of magnesium ascorbyl phosphate in the treatment of alopecia. Aqueous solutions of magnesium ascorbyl phosphate 7.5%, with or without methylsulfonylmethane 1%, 5%, or 10%, were prepared and applied onto the depilated back skin of male mice once per day for 20 days. The effects of methylsulfonylmethane on hair growth promotion of magnesium ascorbyl phosphate were dose-proportional to the concentration of methylsulfonylmethane, due to enhanced intradermal retention of magnesium ascorbyl phosphate in the presence of methylsulfonylmethane.

Kim et al.[176] investigated the effects of 4-O-methylhonokiol, an isolated neolignan from *Magnolia officinalis*, on the growth of hair. When rat vibrissa follicles were treated with 4-*O*-methylhonokiol at 3, 30, and 300 nM for 14 days, it significantly increased the lengths of hair fibers, by 142.9% ± 39.5% ($p < 0.05$) at 3 nM, 253.5% ± 43.1% ($p < 0.05$) at 30 nM, and 154.2% ± 25.9% at 300 nM, compared with the control group. The compound 4-*O*-methylhonokiol has the potential to promote hair growth via downregulation of TGF-β1 and TGF-β2, upregulation of PCNA, and by stimulating the proliferation of DPCs.

Recent studies using transgenic animals have revealed a key role for polyamines in the development and the growth of skin and hair follicles. The polyamine pool during the anagen phase is higher than in the telogen and catagen phases. Fashe et al.[177] used α-methylspermidine, a metabolically stable polyamine analogue, to artificially elevate the polyamine pool during telogen. This manipulation was sufficient to induce hair growth in telogen phase mice after 2 weeks of daily topical application. The application site was characterized by typical features of anagen, such as pigmentation, growing HFs, proliferation of follicular keratinocytes, and upregulation of β-catenin. The analogue penetrated the protective epidermal layer of the skin and could be detected in the dermis. The natural polyamines were partially replaced by the analogue at the application site. However, the combined pool of natural spermidine and α-methylspermidine exceeded the physiological spermidine pool in telogen phase skin.

Mycophenolic acid (MPA) acts as a cell cycle inhibitor that produces reversible noncompetitive blockade of the purine synthesis pathway enzyme, the type II isoform of inosine monophosphate dehydrogenase (IMPDH). The major target of MPA is lymphocytes, which contain abundant IMPDH. Among several kinds of hair loss disorders, lymphocytic cicatricial alopecia and AA are representative hair loss conditions induced by T lymphocyte attack on the HF. Recently, an in vitro study demonstrated that MPA affected cellular proliferation and upregulated the expression of some important genes. Kang et al.[178] assessed whether MPA has a direct effect in vitro. They also determined the effect of microneedles immediately around the HF. Human DPCs responded to MPA, as assessed by RT-PCR assays. MPA treatment increased the phosphorylation of ERK1/2 and β-catenin, and direct β-catenin pathway targets, such as Axin2 and Lef-1, were upregulated by MPA. These data suggest the activation of the β-catenin pathway by MPA.

It is known that platelet-derived growth factor (PDGF) receptors are expressed in HF epithelium. Tomita et al.[179] clarified the effects of PDGF-AA and PDGF-BB on the cyclical growth of HFs. PDGF-AA or -BB was injected into the dorsal skin of C3H mice during the second telogen phase, once daily, for 5 consecutive days, or PDGF-AA or PDGF-BB dissolved in hyaluronic acid was injected only once. To confirm the effects of different PDGF isoforms, anti-PDGF-AA antibodies or anti-PDGF-BB antibodies were injected immediately after each injection of PDGF-AA or PDGF-BB. Anti-PDGF antibodies were also injected into the skin of C3H mice during the second anagen phase, once daily, for 5 days. The expression of signaling molecules was studied in the skin where anagen phase had been induced by PDGF injection using real-time RT-PCR. Both PDGF-AA and PDGF-BB injection experiments immediately induced the anagen phase of the hair growth cycle at the injection sites. The induction of anagen was interfered with by the anti-PDGF antibody treatments. Real-time RT-PCR using RNA extracted from the PDGF-injected sites in skin samples showed upregulated expression of key HF differentiation-related signaling molecules: sonic hedgehog (Shh), Lef-1, and Wnt5a. These results indicate that both PDGF-AA and PDGF-BB are involved in the induction and maintenance of the anagen phase in the mouse hair cycle. Local application of PDGF-AA and PDGF-BB may be an effective treatment option for alopecia associated with early catagen induction and an elongated telogen phase.

7-Phloroeckol, a phloroglucinol derivative isolated from the marine brown algae, *Ecklonia cava*, has antioxidative, anti-inflammatory, and MMP-inhibitory activities. Bak et al.[180] evaluated the hair growth–promoting effects of 7-phloroeckol in human HFs. 7-Phloroeckol induced an increase in the proliferation of human DPCs and ORS cells. Additionally, hair shaft growth was measured using an HF organ culture system. 7-Phloroeckol resulted in the elongation of the hair shaft in cultured human HFs. 7-Phloroeckol induced IGF-1 mRNA expression and the protein concentration in human DPCs and conditioned media, respectively.

The activities of ornithine decarboxylase (ODC) and S-adenosylmethionine decarboxylase, two of the enzymes involved in the synthesis of the polyamines, were found to be high in follicle-rich homogenates of sheep skin and to be responsive to the nutritional state of the animal. Systemic provision of the inhibitor of ODC, α-difluoromethylornithine, markedly altered the length, diameter, and composition of the fiber, accompanied by an increase in the proportion of the fiber occupied by paracortical cells and an increase in the level of mRNA encoding a cysteine-rich family of keratin proteins. The growth of wool follicles cultured in media containing α-difluoromethylornithine was not inhibited, even at high concentrations. In contrast, low concentrations of methylglyoxal(bis)guanylhydrazone, an inhibitor of S-adenosylmethionine decarboxylase, completely inhibited fiber growth in cultured follicles. The addition of spermidine to the medium overcame this inhibition, but spermine had no effect. Further evidence that spermine is not required for normal follicle function was provided by incubating follicles with a specific inhibitor of spermine synthase, *n*-butyl-1,3-diaminopropane. This inhibitor, even at high concentrations, had no effect on fiber growth in vitro. Spermidine partially overcame the growth depression that occurred in follicles cultured in methionine-deficient media, suggesting that part of the requirement for methionine is for spermidine synthesis in the follicle. The polyamines, in general, and spermidine, in particular, play major roles in hair growth.[181] Polyamines (spermidine, putrescine, and spermine) are multifunctional cationic amines that are indispensable for cellular proliferation. Growing (anagen) HFs show the highest activity of ODC, the rate-limiting enzyme of polyamine biosynthesis, while inhibition of ODC, using, for example eflornithine, results in a decreased rate of excessive facial hair growth in vivo and inhibits human scalp hair growth in organ culture. In sheep, manipulation of dietary intake of polyamines also results in altered wool growth. Polyamine-containing nutraceuticals have therefore been proposed as promoters of human hair growth.[182]

Takahashi et al.[24] examined about 1000 kinds of plant extracts with a view to identifying growth-promoting activity with respect to HF cells. After an extensive search, they discovered that proanthocyanidins extracted from grape seeds promoted the proliferation of HF cells isolated from mice by ~230% relative to controls (=100%) and that proanthocyanidins possessed remarkable hair cycle–converting activity, from the telogen phase to the anagen phase in C3H mice in vivo test systems. The profile of the active fraction of the proanthocyanidins was determined by thiolytic degradation and tannase hydrolysis. They found that the constitutive monomers were epicatechin and catechin and that the degree of polymerization was 3.5.

The results of Takahashi et al.[183] showed that procyanidin dimer and trimer exhibited higher growth-promoting activity than the monomer. The maximum growth-promoting activity for hair epithelial cells with procyanidin B-2, an epicatechin dimer, reached about 300% (at 30 μM) relative to controls (=100%) in a 5-day culture. Optimum concentration of procyanidin C-1, an epicatechin trimer, was lower than that of procyanidin B-2; the maximum growth-promoting activity of procyanidin C-1 was about 220% (3 μM). No other flavonoid compounds examined exhibited higher proliferative activities than the procyanidins. In skin constituent cells, only epithelial cells, such as hair keratinocytes or epidermal keratinocytes, respond to procyanidin oligomers. Topical application of 1% procyanidin oligomers on shaven C3H mice in the telogen phase led to significant hair regeneration (procyanidin B-2, 69.6%, procyanidin B-3, 80.9%, procyanidin C-1, 78.3%) on the basis of the shaven area; application of vehicle only led to regeneration of 41.7%.

Procyanidin B-2 is a compound originally identified in apples that acts as a growth-promoting factor in murine hair epithelial cells. A double-blind clinical trial was performed for 4 months.[184] In the procyanidin B-2 group, 78.9% showed an increased mean value of hair diameter, whereas only 30.0% in the placebo group showed any increase ($p < 0.02$, Fisher's exact probability test). The increased ratio of hairs measuring more than 40 μm in diameter after 4 months of procyanidin B-2 treatment was significantly higher than that of the placebo controls ($p < 0.05$; two-sample *t*-test). The increase in the number of total hairs in the designated scalp area (0.25 cm^2) of procyanidin B-2 subjects after a 4-month trial was significantly greater than that of the placebo controls.

To investigate the effects of maternal and dietary selenium on antioxidant status and HF development in 110-day fetal skin from cashmere goats, 80 cashmere goats ($n = 80$) were divided randomly into two groups, C group (fed with the basal diet) and S group (fed with the basal diet with 0.5 mg per kg nano-Se).[185] Nano-Se was provided as a supplement from 30 days prior to gestation to fetal day 110. Maternal supplementation with nano-Se could influence antioxidant status in fetal skin; the resulting low ROS could upregulate IGF-1 and IGF-1R, improving fetal HF development and promoting fetal growth development.

The promoting effect of Na_2SiO_3 on hair regrowth was investigated using a C57BL/6 mouse animal model.[186] Na_2SiO_3 accelerated hair regrowth, compared with distilled water (DW). Elongation of HFs was observed clearly in the 50% and 100% Na_2SiO_3 groups. The activities of alkaline phosphatase and γ-glutamyl transpeptidase were not significantly increased in the Na_2SiO_3 groups, compared with DW. The expression of epidermal growth factor was significantly increased in the Na_2SiO_3 groups, compared with DW ($p < 0.05$). The expression of VEGF was not significantly changed by Na_2SiO_3 treatments. The expression of TGF-β1 was clearly decreased in the Na_2SiO_3 groups, compared with DW.

Safer et al.[187] investigated the direct effect of thyroid hormone on skin. Triiodothyronine (T_3) was applied topically, daily, in liposomes to SKH-1 HR mice for 7 days and to CD rats for 2 weeks. There was a dose-dependent increase in epidermal proliferation, dermal thickening, and hair growth in T_3-treated animals. Mice that received 3.8 μg of T_3 had 42% more hairs per mm^2 than controls ($p < 0.01$), hair length that was 1180% longer ($p < 0.001$), 49% greater epidermal ^3H-thymidine incorporation ($p < 0.01$), and 80% more 5-bromo-2′-deoxyuridine (BrdU)-stained cells ($p < 0.05$). Rats receiving 12.8 μg T_3 had 48% greater dermal thickness than controls ($p < 0.001$), 26% greater epidermal thickness ($p < 0.001$), 85% more hairs per mm^2 ($p < 0.005$), and 130% greater ^3H-thymidine incorporation into the epidermis ($p < 0.01$). Thus, topically applied thyroid hormone had dramatic effects on both skin and hair growth.

A tripeptide–copper complex, described as a growth factor for various kinds of differentiated cells, stimulated the proliferation of dermal fibroblasts and elevated the production of VEGF, but decreased the secretion of TGF-β1 by dermal fibroblasts. The effects of L-alanyl-L-histidyl-L-lysine-Cu^{2+} (AHK-Cu) on human hair growth ex vivo, and cultured DPCs were evaluated by Pyo et al. (2007).[188] AHK-Cu (10^{-12} to 10^{-9} M) stimulated the elongation of human HFs ex vivo and the proliferation of DPCs in vitro. Annexin V-fluorescein isothiocyanate/propidium iodide labeling and flow cytometric analysis showed that 10^{-9} M AHK-Cu reduced the number of apoptotic DPCs, but the decrease was not statistically significant. The ratio of Bcl-2/Bax was elevated, and the levels of the cleaved forms of caspase-3 and PARP were reduced by treatment with 10^{-9} M AHK-Cu. Specifically, AHK-Cu promoted the growth of human HFs, and this stimulatory effect may occur due to stimulation of the proliferation and the preclusion of apoptosis in DPCs.

28.6 CONCLUSIONS

The goal of this chapter was to provide an overview of nutrition and nutraceuticals with hair growth–promoting activity. The structure of the HF and mechanism of hair growth have been discussed to identify factors involved in the prevention of hair loss and promotion of good hair health. Balanced dietary supplementation and nutraceuticals from plant and animal sources that help to limit hair loss have also been discussed.

With the recent advances in our understanding of the mechanisms involved in the hair growth cycle, modern synthetic drugs have been found to show potential in promoting hair growth. Various clinical trials and studies have validated their use. However, despite their proven hair growth–promoting effects, therapy with synthetic drugs has become questionable due to their occasional lack of efficacy, poor safety, and incidence of side effects. From this viewpoint, proper nutrition and nutraceuticals from natural sources are reportedly more effective alternatives for hair growth than are synthetic drugs, although most hair growth–promotion studies involving nutraceuticals from natural sources are preliminary, and more scientific data are necessary to prove the activities of these agents. Accordingly, nutraceutical products must be standardized to ensure their efficacy, safety, stability, and usability (Lourith, 2013) through the careful and accurate characterization of the active chemical compounds, elucidation of the molecular mechanisms of their actions, performance of in vivo studies on proper animal models of hair loss, and, finally, analysis of their safety and effectiveness in clinical trials (Semalty, 2011).

REFERENCES

1. Young, J. Z. 1981. *The Life of the Vertebrates*, 3rd edn. Oxford University Press, Oxford, U.K.
2. Trancik, R. J. 2000. Hair growth enhancers. In *Cosmeceuticals: Drugs vs. Cosmetics* (P. Elsner and H. I. Maibach, eds). New York, NY: Marcel Dekker, Inc. pp. 57–72.
3. Stenn, K. S. and R. Paus. 2001. Control of hair follicle cycling. *Physiol. Rev.* 81:449–494.
4. Lawson, E. D. 1971. Hair color, personality, and the observer. *Psychol. Rep.* 28:311–3112.
5. Cash, T. F. 1990. Losing hair, losing points. The effects of male pattern baldness on impression formation. *J. Appl. Soc. Psychol.* 20:154–167.
6. Roll, S. and J. S. Verinis. 1971. Stereotypes of scalp and facial hair as measured by the semantic differential. *Psychol. Rep.* 28:975–980.
7. Cash, T. F. 1992. The psychological effects of androgenetic alopecia in men. *J. Am. Acad. Dermatol.* 26:926–931.
8. Franzoi, S. L., J. Anderson, and S. Frommelt. 1990. Individual differences in men's perceptions of and reactions to thinning hair. *J. Soc. Psychol.* 130:209–218.
9. Wells, P., T. Wilmoth, and R. J. H. Russell. 1995. Psychological correlates of hair loss in males. *Br. J. Psychol.* 86:337–344.
10. Orentreich, N. and N. P. Durr. 1982. Biology of scalp hair growth. *Clin. Plastic. Surg.* 9:197–205.
11. Whiting, D. A. 1996. Chronic telogen effluvium: Increased scalp hair shedding in middle-aged women. *J. Am. Acad. Dermatol.* 35:899–906.
12. Whiting, D. A. 1993. Diagnostic and predictive value of horizontal sections of scalp biopsy specimens in male androgenetic alopecia. *J. Am. Acad. Dermatol.* 28:755–763.
13. Bertolino, A. P. 2000. Alopecia areata: A clinical overview. *Postgrad Med. J.* 107:81–90.
14. Olsen, E. A. 1993. Androgenetic alopecia. In: Olsen E. A., *Disorders of Hair Growth: Diagnosis and Treatment*. New York: McGraw-Hill, pp. 257–287.
15. Madani, S. and J. Shapiro. 2000. Alopecia areata update. *J. Am. Acad. Dermatol.* 42:549–566.
16. Bandaranayake, I. and P. Mirmirani. 2004. Hair loss remedies—Separating fact from fiction. *Cutis* 73:107–114.
17. Olsen, E. A., F. E. Dunlap, T. Funicella, J. A. Koperski, J. M. Swinehart, E. H. Tschen, and R. J. Trancik. 2002. A randomized clinical trial of 5% topical minoxidil versus 2% topical minoxidil and placebo in the treatment of androgenetic alopecia in man. *J. Am. Acad. Dermatol.* 47:377–385.
18. Price, V. H. 1999. Treatment of hair loss. *N. Engl. J. Med.* 341:964–973.
19. Libecco, J. F. and W. F. Bergfeld. 2004. Finasteride in the treatment of alopecia. *Expert Opin. Pharmacother.* 5:933–940.
20. Shapiro, J. and V. H. Price. 1998. Hair regrowth: Therapeutic agents. *Dermatol. Ther.* 16:341–356.
21. Wilson, C., V. Walkden, S. Powell, S. Shaw, J. Wilkinson, and R. P. R. Dawber. 1991. Contact dermatitis in reaction to 2% topical minoxidil solution. *J. Am. Acad. Dermatol.* 24:643–646.
22. Friedman, E. S., P. M. Friedman, D. E. Cohen, and K. Washenik. 2002. Allergic contact dermatitis to topical minoxidil solution: etiology and treatment. *J. Am. Acad. Dermatol.* 46:309–312.
23. Tosti, A., B. M. Piraccini, and M. Soli. 2001. Evaluation of sexual function in subjects taking finasteride for the treatment of androgenetic alopecia. *J. Eur. Acad. Dermatol. Venereol.* 15:418–421.
24. Takahashi, T., T. Kamiya, and Y. Yokoo. 1998. Proanthocyanidins from grape seeds promote proliferation of mouse hair follicle cells in vitro and convert hair cycle *in vivo. Acta. Derm. Venereol.* 78:428–432.
25. Saraf, S., A. K., Pathak, and V. K. Dixit. 1991. Hair growth promoting activity of *Tridax procumbens. Fitoterapia.* 62:495–498.
26. Sperling, L. C. 1991. Hair anatomy for clinician. *J. Am. Acad. Dermatol.* 25:1–17.
27. Millar, S. E. Mechanisms regulating hair follicle development. *J. Invest. Dermatol.* 118:216–225.
28. Oliver, R. F. and C. A. Jahoda. 1988. Dermal epidermal interactions. *Clin. Dermatol.* 6:74–82.
29. Cotsarelis, G., T. T. Sun., and R. M. Lavker. 1990. Label-retaining cells reside in the bulge area of pilosebaceous unit: Implications for follicular stem cells, hair cycle, and skin carcinogenesis. *Cell* 61:1329–1337.
30. Wilson, C., G., Cotsarelis, and Z. G. Wei. 1994. Cells within the bulge region of mouse hair follicle transiently proliferate during early anagen: Heterogeneity and functional differences of various hair cycles. *Differentiation* 55:127–136.
31. Lyle, S., M. Christofidou-Solomidou, Y. Liu, D. E. Elder, S. Albelda, and G. Cotsarelis. 1998. The C8/144B monoclonal antibody recognizes cytokeratin 15 and defines the location of human hair follicle stem cells. *J. Cell. Sci.* 111:3179–3188.
32. Oshima, H., A. Rochat, C. Kedzia, K. Kobayashi, and Y. Barrandon. 2001. Morphogenesis and renewal of hair follicles from adult multipotent stem cells. *Cell* 104:233–245.

33. Taylor, G., M. S. Lehrer, P. J. Jensen, T. T. Sun, and R. M. Lavker. 2000. Involvement of follicular stem cells in forming not only the follicle but also the epidermis. *Cell* 102:451–461.
34. Chuong, C. M. 1998. *Molecular Basis of Epithelial Appendage Morphogenesis. Molecular Biology Intelligence Unit 1.* Austin, TX: R.G. Landes.
35. Danilenko, D. M., B. D. Ring., and G. F. Pierce. 1996. Growth factors and cytokines in hair follicle development and cycling: Recent insights from animal models and the potentials for clinical therapy. *Mol. Med. Today* 2:460–467.
36. Rochat, A., K. Kobayashi, and Y. Barrandon. 1994. Location of stem cells of human hair follicles by clonal analysis. *Cell* 76:1063–1073.
37. Whiting, D. A. 1998. Male pattern hair loss: Current understanding. *Int. J. Dermatol.* 37:561–566.
38. Ebling, F. J. G. and W. J. Cunliffe. 1992. Disorders of the sebaceous glands. In *Textbook of Dermatology*, 5th edn. (A. Rook, D. S. Wilkinson, F. J. G. Ebling, R. H. Champion, and J. L. Burton, eds.). Oxford, U.K.: *Blackwell Scientific Publications.* pp. 1699–1745.
39. Semalt, M., A., Semalt, G. P., Joshi, and M. S. M. Rawat. 2011. Hair growth and rejuvenation. *J. Dermatolog. Treat.* 22:123–132.
40. Stenn, K. S., N. J. Combates, and K. J. Eilertsen. 1996. Hair follicle growth controls. *J. Clin. Dermatol.* 14:543–558.
41. Sato, N., P. L. Leopold, and R. G. Crystal. 1999. Induction of the hair growth phase in postnatal mice by localized transient expression of Sonic hedgehog. *J. Clin. Invest.* 104:855–886.
42. Wang, L. C., Z.-Y. Liu, L. Gambardella, A. Delacour, R. Shapiro, J. Yang, I. Sizing, P. Rayhorn, E. A. Garber, C. D. Benjamin, K. P. Williams, F. R. Taylor, Y. Barrandon, L. Ling, and L. C. Burkly. 2000. Conditional disruption of Hedgehog signaling pathway defines its critical role in hair development and regeneration. *J. Invest. Dermatol.* 114:901–908.
43. McGowan, K. and P. A. Coulombe. 1998. The wound repair-associated keratins 6, 16, and 17: Insights into the role of intermediate filaments in specifying keratinocyte cytoarchitecture. *Subcell. Biochem.* 31:173–204.
44. Guo, L., L. Degenstein., and E. Fuchs. 1996. Keratinocyte growth factor is required for hair development but not for wound healing. *Genes Dev.*10:165–175.
45. Werner, S., H. Smola, and X. Liao. 1994. The function of KGF in morphogenesis of epithelium and reepithelialization of wounds. *Science* 266:819–822.
46. Millar, S. E. 1997. The role of patterning genes in epidermal differentiation. In *Cytoskeletal-Membrane Interactions and Signal Transduction* (Cowin, P. and M. W. Klymkowsky, eds). Austin, TX: Landes. pp. 87–102.
47. Hardy, M. H. 1992. The secret life of the hair follicle. *Trends Genet* 8:55–61.
48. Kishimoto, J., R. E. Burgeson, and B. A. Morgan. 2000. Wnt signaling maintains the hair-inducing activity of the dermal papilla. *Genes Dev* 14:1181–1185.
49. Rosenquist, T. A. and G. R. Martin. 1996. Fibroblast growth factor signaling in the hair growth cycle: Expression of the fibroblast growth factor receptor and ligand genes in the murine hair follicle. *Dev. Dyn.* 205:379–386.
50. Hebert, J. M., T. Rosenquist, J. Gotz, and G. R. Martin. 1994. FGF5 as a regulator of the hair growth cycle: evidence from targeted and spontaneous mutations. *Cell* 78:1017–1025.
51. Fujie, T., S. Katoh, H. Oura, Y. Urano, and S. Arase. 2001. The chemotactic effect of a dermal cell-derived factor on outer root sheath cells. *J. Dermatol. Sci.* 25:206–212.
52. Kaufman, K. D. 1996. Androgen metabolism as it affects hair growth in androgenetic alopecia. *Clin. Dermatol.* 14:697–711.
53. Sawaya, M. E. 1994. Biochemical mechanisms regulating human hair growth. *Skin Pharmacol. Physicol.* 7:5–7.
54. Botchkareva, N. V., G. Ahluwalia, and D. Shander. 2006. Apoptosis in the hair follicle. *J. Invest. Dermatol.* 126:258–264.
55. Jänne, O. A., J. J. Palvimo, P. Kallio, and M. Mehto. 1993. Androgen receptor and mechanism of androgen action. *Ann. Med.* 25:83–89.
56. Trüeb, R. M. 2005. Aging of hair. *J. Cosmet. Dermatol.* 4:60–72.
57. Trüeb, R. M. 2002. Molecular mechanisms of androgenetic alopecia. *Exp. Gerontol.* 37:981–990.
58. Thigpen, A. E., R. I. Silver, J. M. Guileyardo, M. L. Casey, J. D. McConnell, and D. W. Russell. 1993. Tissue distribution and ontogeny of steroid 5a-reductase isozyme expression. *J. Clin. Invest.* 92:903–910.
59. Sawaya, M. E. and V. H. Price. 1997. Different levels of 5a-reductase type I and II, aromatase and androgen receptor in hair follicles of women and men with androgenetic alopecia. *J. Invest. Dermatol.* 109:296–300.

60. Hibberts, N. A., A. E. Howell, and V. A. Randall, 1998. Balding hair follicle dermal papilla cells contain higher levels of androgen receptors than those from non balding scalp. *J. Endocrinol.* 156:59–65.
61. Ellis, J. A., M. Stebbing., and S. B. Harrap. 2001. Polymorphism of the androgen receptor gene is associated with male pattern baldness. *J. Invest. Dermatol.* 116:452–455.
62. Sawaya, M. E. and J. Shapiro. 2000. Androgenetic alopecia: New approved and unapproved treatments. *Dermatol. Clin.* 18:47–61.
63. Paus, R. and G. Cotsarelis. 1999. The biology of hair follicles. *N. Engl. J. Med.* 341:491–497.
64. Sawaya, M. E. and N. S. Penneys. 1991. Immunohistochemical distribution of aromatase and 3b-hydroxysteroid dehydrogenase in human hair follicle and sebaceous gland. *J. Cutan. Pathol.* 19:309–314.
65. Chumlea, W., T. Rhodes., C. Girman., A. Johnson-Levonas., F. Lilly., and R. Wu. 2004. Family history and risk of hair loss. *Dermatology* 209:33–39.
66. Dawber, R. 1997. *Diseases of the Hair and Scalp*, 3rd edn. Oxford, U.K.: Blackwell Science.
67. Jahoda, C. A. and A. J. Reynolds. 1996. Dermal-epidermal interactions: Adult follicle derived cell populations and hair growth. *J. Clin. Dermatol.* 14:573–583.
68. Olsen, E. A. 1994. Androgenetic alopecia. In *Disorders of Hair Growth: Diagnosis and Treatment* (E. A. Olsen, ed.). New York: McGraw-Hill, pp. 257–283.
69. Hamilton, J. B. 1942. Male hormone stimulation is a prerequisite and an incitant in common baldness. *Am. J. Anat.* 71:451–480.
70. Guarrera, M. and A. Rebora. 1996. Anagen hairs may fail to replace telogen hairs in early androgenic female alopecia. *Dermatology* 192:28–31.
71. Norwood, O. T. 1975. Male-pattern baldness. Classification and incidence. *South Med. J.* 68:1359–1370.
72. Norwood, O. T. 2001. Incidence of female androgenetic alopecia (female pattern alopecia). *Dermatol. Surg.* 27:53–54.
73. Muller, S. A. and R. K. Winkelmann. 1963. Alopecia areata: An evaluation of 736 patients. *Arch. Dermatol.* 88:290–297.
74. Safavi, K. H., S. A. Muller, V. J. Suman, A. N. Moshell, and L. J. Melton III. 1995. Incidence of alopecia areata in Olmsted County, Minnesota, 1975 through 1989. *Mayo Clin. Proc.* 70:628–633.
75. Gilhar, A., Y. Ullmann, T. Berkutzki, B. Assy, and R. S. Kalish. 1998. Autoimmune hair loss (alopecia areata) transferred by T lymphocytes to human scalp explants on SCID mice. *J. Clin. Invest.* 101:62–67.
76. Cotsarelis, G. and S. E. Millar. 2001. Towards a molecular understanding of hair loss and its treatment. *Trends Mol. Med.* 7:293–301.
77. Headington, J. T. 1993. Telogen effluvium. New concepts and review. *Arch. Dermatol.* 129:356–363.
78. Randall, V. A. 1994. Androgens and human hair growth. *Clin. Endocrinol.* 40:439–457.
79. Bosse, K. A. and U. Gieler. 1987. *Seelische Faktoren bei Haustkrankheiten: Beiträge zur psychosomatischen Dermatologie.* Bern, Switzerland: Verlag Hans Huber.
80. Paus, R. 2000. Stress, hair growth control and the neuro-endocrine immune connection. *Allergo. J.* 9:611–620.
81. Botchkarev, V. A. 2003. Stress and the hair follicle: Exploring the connections. *Am. J. Pathol.* 162:709–712.
82. Goldberg, L. J. and Y. Lenzy. 2010. Nutrition and hair. *Clin. Dermatol.* 28:412–419.
83. Rushton, D. H. 2002. Nutritional factors and hair loss. *Clin. Dermatol.* 27:396–404.
84. Finner, A. M. 2013. Nutrition and hair deficiencies and supplements. *Dermatol. Clin.* 31:167–172.
85. Weber, C. W., G. W. Nelson, M. V. de Vaquera, and P. B. Pearson. 1990. Trace elements in the hair of health and malnourished children. *J. Tropical Pediatrics* 36:230–234.
86. Rasheed, H., D. Mahgoub, R. Hegazy, M. El-Komy, R. Abdel Hay, M. A. Hamid, and E. Hamdy. 2013. Serum ferritin and vitamin d in female hair loss: Do they play a role? *Skin Pharmacol. Physiol.* 26:101–107.
87. Riella, M. C., J. W. Broviac, M. Wells, and B. H. Scribner. 1975. Essential fatty acid deficiency in human adults during total parenteral nutrition. *Ann. Intern. Med.* 83:786–789.
88. Skolnik, P., W. H. Eaglstein, and V. A. Zibouth. 1977. Essential fatty acid deficiency. *Arch. Dermatol.* 113:939–941.
89. Choi, J. S., M. H. Jeon., W. S. Moon., J. N. Moon., E. J. Cheon., J. W. Kim., S. K. Jung., Y. H. Ji., S. W. Son., and M. R. Kim. 2014. Hair growth promoting effect of *Oryza sativa* bran extract prepared by supercritical carbon dioxide fluid. *Biol. Pharm. Bull.* 37:44–53.
90. Raynaud, J. P., H. Cousse, and P. M. Marin. 2002. Inhibition of type 1 and type 2 5a-reductase activity by free fatty acids, active ingredients of Permixon. *J. Steroid Biochem. Mol. Biol.* 82:233–239.
91. Jordan, V. E. 1976. Protein status of the elderly as measured by dietary intake, hair tissue, and serum albumin. *Am. J. Clin. Nutr.* 29:522–528.

92. Rushton, D. H., I. D., Ramsay, K. C., James, M. J., Norris, and J. J. H. Gilkes. 1990. Biochemical and trichological characterisation of diffuse alopecia in women. *Br. J. Dermatol.* 123:187–197.
93. Sandhya, S., S. J., Chandra, and K. Vinod. 2012. Preclinical studies of a novel polyherbal phyto-complex hair growth promoting cream. *Asian Pac. J. Trop. Biomed.* 2:S296–S304.
94. Park, P. J., B. S. Moon, and S. H. Lee. 2012. Hair growth-promoting effect of *Aconiti ciliare* Tuber extract mediated by the activation of Wnt/β-catenin signaling. *Life Sci.* 91:935–943.
95. Rho, S. S., S. J., Park, S. L., Hwang, M. H., Lee, C. D., Kim, I. H., Lee, S. Y., Chang, and M. J. Rang. 2005. The hair growth promoting effect of *Asiasari radix* extract and its molecular regulation. *J. Dermatol. Sci.* 38:89–97.
96. Hou, I. C., Y. Oi, and H. Fujita. 2013. A hair growth-promoting effect of Chinese black tea extract in mice. *Biosci. Biotechnol. Biochem.* 77:1606–1607.
97. Kumar N., W. Rungseevijitprapa, N. Narkkhong, M. Suttajitd, and C. Chaiyasut. 2012. 5α-reductase inhibition and hair growth promotion of some Thai plants traditionally used for hair treatment. *J. Ethnopharmacol.* 139:765–771.
98. Junlatat, J. and B. Sripanidkulchai. 2014. Hair growth-promoting effect of *Carthamus tinctorius* floret extract. *Phytother. Res.* 28:1030–1036.
99. Lee, G. S., E. J. Hong, K. S. Gwak, M. J. Park, K. C. Choi, I. G. Choi, J. W. Jang, and E. B. Jeung. 2010. The essential oils of *Chamaecyparis obtusa* promote hair growth through the induction of vascular endothelial growth factor gene. *Fitoterapia* 81:17–24.
100. Park, Y. O., Y. C. Kim, and B. S. Chang. 2013a. Hair growth effect of *Chamaecyparis obtusa* oil in C57BL/6 mice. *J. Invest. Cosmetol.* 9:87–95.
101. Park, Y. O., S. E. Kim, and Y. C. Kim. 2013b. Action mechanism of *Chamaecyparis obtusa* oil on hair growth. *Toxicol. Res.* 29:241–247.
102. Dhanotia, R., N. S. Chauhan, D. K. Saraf, and V. K. Dixit. 2011. Effect of *Citrullus colocynthis* Schrad fruits on testosterone-induced alopecia. *Nat. Prod. Res.* 25:1432–1443.
103. Park, J. S. and J. S. Lee. 2011. The promoting effect of *Cornus officinalis* fermented with *Lactobacillus rhamnosus* on hair growth. *Kor. J. Pharmacogn.* 42:260–264.
104. Shin, H. S., J. M. Lee, S. Y. Park, J. E., Yang, J. H., Kim, and T. H. Yi. 2013. Hair growth activity of *Crataegus pinnatifida* on C57BL/6 mouse model. *Phytother. Res.* 27:1352–1357.
105. Pandit, S., N. S. Chauhan, and V. K. Dixit. 2008. Effect of *Cuscuta reflexa* Roxb on androgen-induced alopecia. *J. Cosmet. Dermatol.* 7:199–204.
106. Roy, R. K., M, Thakur, and V. K. Dixit. 2008. Hair growth promoting activity of *Eclipta alba* in male albino rats. *Arch. Dermatol. Res.* 300:357–364.
107. Datta, K., A. T. Singh, A. Mukherjee, B. Bhat, B. Rameshb, and A. C. Burman, 2009. *Eclipta alba* extract with potential for hair growth promoting activity. *J. Ethnopharmacol.* 124:450–456.
108. Kawano, M., J. Han, M. E. Kchouk, and H. Isoda. 2009. Hair growth regulation by the extract of aromatic plant *Erica multiflora*. *J. Nat. Med.* 63:335–339.
109. Park, S. J., W. S. Shin, and J. Y. Ho. 2011. *Fructus panax* ginseng extract promotes hair regeneration in C57BL/6 mice. *J. Ethnopharmacol.* 138:340–344.
110. Kubo, M., H. Matsuda, and R. Suzuki. 1993. Hair growth promoting effect of ethanolic extract from leaves of *Ginkgo biloba* L. (GBE) and their inhibitory effects on blood platelet aggregation. *Fragr. J.* 21:27–36.
111. Matsuda, H., M. Yamazaki, Y. Asanuma, and M. Kubo. 2003. Promotion of hair growth by ginseng radix on cultured mouse vibrissal hair follicles. *Phytother. Res.* 17:797–800.
112. Hyun, M. Y., J. M. Suk, S. W. Jung, J. O. Park, B. H. Kim, J. D. Jang, J. G. Joe, I. K. Yeo, B. J. Kim, and M. N. Kim. 2013. The efficacy of shampoo containing ginseng radix on preventing hair loss and promotion hair growth. *J. Soc. Cosmet. Sci. Korea* 39:187–194.
113. Oh, G. N. and S. W. Son. 2012. Efficacy of Korean red ginseng in the treatment of alopecia areata. *J. Ginseng Res.* 36:391–395.
114. Lee, C. S. and H. H. Kim. 2005. A study on the soybean effects for scalp hair treatment. *J. Beau. Tricho.* 1:77–90.
115. Jeon, H. Y., S. H. Kim, C. W. Kim, H. J. Shin, D. B. Seo, and S. J. Lee. 2011. Hair growth promoting effect of black soybean extract in vitro and *in vivo*. *Kor. J. Food Sci. Technol.*, 43:747–753.
116. Adhirajan, N., T. R. Kumar, N. Shanmugasundaram, and M. Babu. 2003. In vivo and in vitro evaluation of hair growth potential of *Hibiscus rosa-sinensis* Linn. *J. Ethnopharmacol.* 88:235–239.
117. Kang, J. I., E. J. Kim, M. K. Kim, Y. J. Jeon, S. M. Kang, Y. S. Koh, E. S. Yoo, and H. K. Kang. 2013. The promoting effect of *Ishige sinicola* on hair growth. *Mar. Drugs* 11:1783–1799.

118. Choi, J. S., S. K. Jung, M. H. Jeon, J. N. Moon, W. S. Moon, Y. H. Ji, I. S. Choi, and S. W. Son. 2013. The effects of *Lycopersicon esculentum* extract on hair growth and alopecia prevention. *J. Cosmet. Sci.* 64:429–443.
119. Song, J. H., J. S. Lee, and H. J. Choi. 2012. Hair growth promoting effect of essence manufactured with products fermented by *Lactobacillus rhamnosus* and Backryeoncho (*Opuntia ficusindica* var. *sarboten*) fruits in mice. *Food Sci. Biotechnol.* 21:1101–1104.
120. Jeong, I. K., H. Y. Jo, T. H. Kim, N. S. Kim, H. S. Jeong, and C. H. Lee. 2009. Experimental studies on the hair growth activity of extracts of *Pielliae phizoma* in spontaneous alopecia model and normal C57BL/6N mice. *Kor. J. Orient. Physiol. Pathol.* 23:84–92.
121. Park, J. S. and J. S. Lee. 2011. The promoting effect of *Pleuropterus cilinervis* extracts fermented with *Lactobacillus rhamnosus* on hair growth. *J. Microbiol. Biotechnol.* 39:345–349.
122. Park, H. J., Z. Nannan, and D. K. Park. 2011. Topical application of *Polygonum multiflorum* extract induces hair growth of resting hair follicles through upregulating Shh and β-catenin expression in C57BL/6 mice. *J. Ethnopharmacol.* 135:369–375.
123. Zhang, C., X. Chen, and B. Lin. 2011. Effect of *Prunus tomentosa* Thumb total flavone on hair growth. *Human Health and Biomedical Engineering (HHBE), 2011 International Conference*, Jilin, China, August 19–22, 2011, pp. 35–38.
124. Kim, J. H., S. K. Hong, S. J. Hwang, S. W. Son, and Y. S. Choi. 2012. The preclinical and clinical effects of herbal product containing *Rosa multiflora* root extracts as a main component on the hair growth promotion. *Kor. J. Med. Crop Sci.* 20:108–116.
125. Kim, M. H. and Y. C. Kim. 2010. The promoting effect of rosemary oil on hair growth by gross and histological observation in C57BL/6 mice. *J. Cosmetol. Sci.* 6:121–129.
126. Murata, K., K. Noguchi, M. Kondo, M. Onishi, N. Watanabe, K. Okamura, and H. Matsuda. 2013. Promotion of Hair Growth by *Rosmarinus officinalis* leaf extract. *Phytother. Res.* 27:212–217.
127. Oh, Y. S., M. S. Oh, and S. S. Roh. 2006. The experimental study on the effect of herbal extracts on hair growth and acnes. *J. Kor. Orient Med. Ophthalmol. Otolaryngol. Dermatol.* 19:34–54.
128. Kang, J. I., S. C. Kim, J. H. Hyun, J. H. Kang, D. B. Park, Y. J. Lee, E. S. Yoo, and H. K. Kang. 2009. Promotion effect of *Schisandra nigra* on the growth of hair. *Eur. J. Dermatol.* 19:119–125.
129. Roh, S. S., C. D. Kim, M. H. Lee, S. L. Hwang, M. J. Rang, and Y. K. Yoon. 2002. The hair growth promoting effect of *Sophora flavescens* extract and its molecular regulation. *J. Dermatol. Sci.* 30:43–49.
130. Ryu, E. M. and H. J. Shin. 2011. Hair growth effect of ethyl acetate and water fractions of *Sparassis crispa* extracts on hair-removed C57BL/6 mice. *Kor. J. Aesthet. Cosmetol.* 9:1–10.
131. Kim, Y. J., H. C. Chung, H. T. Chun, K. Y. Choi, Y. G. Yun, and S. I. Jang. 2004. Hair growth promoting effect of *Thuja orientalis* ethanol extracts on hair loss-induced DBA1J mice. *Kor. J. Orient. Physiol. Pathol.* 18:1471–1475.
132. Ryu, E. M., G. W. Seo, K. H. Kee, and H. J. Shin. 2013. Effect of ethanolic extract from wheat sprout on hair growth of C57BL/6 mouse. *Kor. J. Aesthet. Cosmetol.* 11:1051–1057.
133. Shin, H. S., K. J. Lee, and T. H. Yi. 2008. Effect of *Vitex rotundifolia* on hair regeneration: In vitro and in vivo study. *J. Beau. Tricho.* 5:1–5.
134. Yoon, J. I., S. M. Al-Reza, and S. C. Kang. 2010. Hair growth promoting effect of *Zizyphus jujuba* essential oil. *Food Chem. Toxicol.* 48:1350–1354.
135. Zhang, D. L., L. J. Gu, J. J. Li, Z. Li, C. Y. Wang, Z. Wang, L. Liu, M. R. Li, and C. K. Sung. 2011. Cow placenta extract promotes murine hair growth through enhancing the insulin-like growth factor-1. *Indian J. Dermatol.* 56:14–18.
136. Yang, Z. H., L. J. Gu, D. L. Zhang, Z. Li, J. J. Li, M. R. Lee, C.Y. Wang, Z. Wang, J. H. Cho, and C. K. Sung. 2012. Red deer antler extract accelerates hair growth by stimulating expression of insulin-like growth factor I in full-thickness wound healing rat model. *Asian Aust. J. Anim. Sci.* 25:708–716.
137. Jo, H. Y., T. H. Kim, H. Kim, H. S. Jeong, C. H. Lee, and K. G. Lee. 2008. Experimental studies on the hair growth activity of *Mylabris Phalerata* Pall. extracts and fractions in C57BL/6N mice. *Kor. J. Orient. Physiol. Pathol.* 22:357–364.
138. Li, Z. J., H. I. Choi, and D. K. Choi. 2012. Autologous platelet-rich plasma: A potential therapeutic tool for promoting hair growth. *Dermatol. Surg.* 38:1040–1046.
139. Shin, H. S., S. Y. Park, W. C. Lee, J. H. Shin, and T. H. Yi. 2011. Effect of *Selenarctos thibetanus* (bear oil) on hair growth promotion in C57BL/6 mice. *J. Invest. Cosmet.* 7:243–248.
140. Park, S. G., H. G. Jo, M. S. Yang, J.B. Choi, and S. J. Kim. 2010. Bibliographic study on herbal medicine for alopecia. *Kor. J. Oriential Physiol. Pathol.* 24:367–372.
141. Lee, J. S. and Y. C. Kim. 2010. The promoting effect of *Angelica gigas* Nakai and *Glycyrrhiza uralensis* Fischet oriental medicine complex extracts on hair growth. *J. Cosmetol. Sci.* 6:49–56.

142. Kim, J. D., J. J. Hue, and B. S. Kang. 2009. Effects of herbal extracts on hair growth in an animal model of C3H/HeJ mice. *Lab. Anim. Res.* 25:225–232.
143. Choi, E. Y., S. N. Park., and S. U. Park. 2003. Promoting effect of a mixture of 8 herbal extracts (SPELA 707) on hair growth. *Kor. J. physiol. Pharmacol.* 7:91–96.
144. Choi, H. M., S. J. Hwang., J. S. Lee., E. J. Do., M. Y. Kim, and M. R. Kim. 2011. Effects of hair tonic and food including Korean medicinal herbs on hair growth in an alopecia model of C57BL/6 Mice. *Kor. J. Herbol.* 26:119–124.
145. Hong, J. A., M. Y. Song, I. H. Choi, N. W. Sohn, and S. H. Chung. 2010. Effect of Yikgeebohyul-tang (Yìqìbǔxuè-tāng) on hair regrowth and cytokine changes on hair-removed C57BL/6 mice. *J. Kor. Ori. Med.* 31:138–152.
146. Hwang, C. W., J. W. Hwang, and S. T. Kim. 2010. The effect of hair growth and distribution by *Sophorae radix*, *Panax ginseng*, *Salvia miltiorrhiza* BUNGE water extracts. *J. Soc. Cosmet. Sci. Korea* 36:215–219.
147. Hue, J. J., L. Li., S. H. Lyu., I. J. Baek., J. M. Yon., S. Y. Nam., Y. W. Yun., S. Y. Hwang., J. T. Hong., and B. J. Lee. 2005. Effect of Hwanggumgung, a natural product, on hair growth promotion in C57BL6 mice. *Yakhak Hoeji* 49:518–526.
148. Im, K. R., M. J. Kim, and K. S. Yoon. 2011. Hair growth activity and melanogenic activity of oriental medical prescription. *J. Soc. Cosmet. Sci. Korea* 37:161–169.
149. Jeong, C. G., M. H. Park, J. W. Seong, H. S. Lee, S. K. Park, S. Y. Kim, Y. B. Kim, H. S. Jung, N. W. Sohn, and Y. J. Sohn. 2008. Immunohistochemical study on hair growth promoting effect of Yonnyuniksoogobon-dan. *J. Kor. Oriental. Med.*, 29:77–89.
150. Lee, H. S. and S. Y. Hwang. 2009. Effects of DCS® hair tonic on hair growth promotion in an alopecia model of C57BL/6 mice. *Kor. J. Aesthet. Cosmetol.* 7:131–141.
151. Lee, J. Y., K. R. Im, T. K. Jung, M. H. Lee, and K. S. Yoon. 2012. Medicinal herbal complex extract with potential for hair growth-promoting activity. *J. Soc. Cosmet. Sci. Korea* 38:277–287.
152. Lee, M. W., H. Y. Jo, T. H. Kim, N. S. Kim, H. S. Jeong, and C. H. Lee. 2008. Experimental studies on the hair growth activity of mixed extracts of *Mylabris phalerata* Pall. and *Drynariae rhizome* in spontaneous alopecia model and normal C57BL/6N mice. *Kor. J. Orient. Physiol. Pathol.* 22:778–790.
153. Chung, H. S., H. Y. Cho, and C. H. Lee. 2009. Experimental studies on the hair growth activity of trimix extracts of Mylabris Phalerata Pall., *Arisaematis Rhizoma* and *Pinelliae Rhizoma Ternata* in C57BL/6N mice. *Kor. J. Ori. Physiol. Pathol.* 23:1116–1124.
154. Purwal, L., S. P. B. N. Gupta, and S. M. Pande. 2008. Development and evaluation of herbal formulations for hair growth. *J. Chem.* 5:34–38.
155. Adhirajan, N., V. K. Dixit., and G. Chandrakasan. 2001. Development and evaluation of herbal formulations for hair growth. *Indian Drugs* 38:559–563.
156. Rathi, V., J. C. Rathi, and S. Tamizharasi. 2009. Development and evaluation of polyherbal formulations for hair growth potential. *Phcog. Res.* 1:234–237.
157. Roy, R. K., M. Thakur, and V. K. Dixit. 2007. Development and evaluation of polyherbal formulation for hair growth–promoting activity. *J. Cosmet. Dermatol.* 6:108–112.
158. Sandhya, S., J. Chandrasekhar, D. Banji, and K. R. Vinod. 2012. Potentiality of hair growth promoting activity of aqueous extract of *Abrus precatorius* Linn. on Wistar albino rats. *J. Natur. Remedi.* 12:1–11.
159. Seo, S. R., G. Kang, and J. W. Ha. 2013. In vivo hair growth-promoting efficacies of herbal extracts and their cubosomal suspensions. *J. Ind. Eng. Chem.* 19:1331–1339.
160. Thorat, R. M., V. M., Jadhav, and V. J. Kadam. 2009. Development and evaluation of polyherbal formulations for hair growth-promoting activity. *Int. J. Pharm. Tech. Res.* 1:1251–1254.
161. Yun, J. H., N. K. Kim, K. S. Lim, S. S. Roh, and C.Y. Hwang. 2004. Study on the effect of Gamissanghwatang and each medicinal plant extract for the hair growth of the mice using in vivo and in vitro test. *Kor. J. Ori. Med. Physiol. Pathol.* 18:561–570.
162. Kim, S. C., J. I. Kang, D. B. Park, Y. K. Lee, J. W. Hyun, Y. S. Koh, E. S. Yoo, J. A. Kim, Y. H. Kim, and H. K. Kang. 2012. Promotion effect of acankoreoside J, a lupane-triterpene in *Acanthopanax koreanum*, on hair growth. Arch. *Pharm. Res.* 35:1495–1503.
163. Won, C. H., H. G. Yoo, and K. Y. Park. 2012. Hair growth–promoting effects of adiponectin *in vitro*. *J. Invest. Dermatol.* 132:2849–2851.
164. Sung, Y. K., S.Y. Hwang, S.Y. Cha, S. R. Kim, S. Y. Park, M. K. Kim, and J. C. Kim. 2006. The hair growth promoting effect of ascorbic acid 2-phosphate, a long-acting vitamin C derivative. *J. Dermatol. Sci.* 41:150–152.
165. Kwack, M. H., S. H. Shin, S. R. Kim, S. U. Im, I. S. Han, M. K. Kim, J. C. Kim, and Y. K. Sung. 2009. L-Ascorbic acid 2-phosphate promotes elongation of hair shafts via the secretion of insulin-like growth factor-1 from dermal papilla cells through phosphatidylinositol 3-kinase. *British J. Dermatol.* 160:1157–1162.

166. Wang, C. H., H. S., Huang, N. T., Dai, M. J., Sheu, and D. M. Chang. 2013. Ascorbigen induces dermal papilla cell proliferation *in vitro*, but fails to modulate chemotherapy-induced alopecia *in vivo*. *Phytother. Res.* 27:1863–1867.
167. Foitzik, K., E. Hoting, T. Förster, P. Pertile, and R. Paus. 2007. L-Carnitine–L-tartrate promotes human hair growth *in vitro*. *Exp. Dermatol* 16:936–945.
168. Xu, W., W. Fan, and K. Yao. 2012. Cyclosporine. A stimulated hair growth from mouse vibrissae follicles in an organ culture model. *J. Biomed. Res.* 26:372–380.
169. Kwon, O. S., J. H. Han, H. G. Yoo, J. H. Chung, K. H. Cho, H. C. Eun, and K. H. Kim. 2007. Human hair growth enhancement in vitro by green tea epigallocatechin-3-gallate (EGCG). *Phytomedicine* 14:551–555.
170. Kang, B. M., S. H. Shin, M. H. Kwack, H. R. Shin, J. W. Oh, J. Kim, C. Moon, C. Moon, J. C. Kim, M. K. Kim, and Y. K. Sung. 2010. Erythropoietin promotes hair shaft growth in cultured human hair follicles and modulates hair growth in mice. *J. Dermatol. Sci.* 59:86–90.
171. Sun, Y. N., L. Cui, and W. Li. 2013. Promotion effect of constituents from the root of *Polygonum multiflorum* on hair growth. *Bioorg. Med. Chem. Lett.* 23:4801–4805.
172. Murata, K., F. Takeshita, K. Samukawa, T. Tani, and H. Matsuda. 2012. Effects of ginseng rhizome and ginsenoside Ro on testosterone 5α-reductase and hair re-growth in testosterone-treated mice. *Phytother. Res.* 26:48–53.
173. Shin, D. H., Y. J. Cha, K. E. Yang, I. S. Jang, C. G. Son, B. H. Kim, and J. M. Kim. 2014. Ginsenoside Rg3 up-regulates the expression of vascular endothelial growth factor in human dermal papilla cells and mouse hair follicles. *Phytother. Res.* 28:1088–1095.
174. Shirai, A., J. Ikeda, S. Kawashima, T. Tamaokia, and T. Kamiya. 2001. KF19418, a new compound for hair growth promotion in vitro and in vivo mouse models. *J. Dermatol. Sci.* 25:213–218.
175. Shanmugam, S, R. Baskaran, S. Nagayya-Sriraman, C. S. Yong, H. G. Choi, J. S. Woo, and B. K. Yoo. 2009. The effect of methylsulfonylmethane on hair growth promotion of magnesium ascorbyl phosphate for the treatment of alopecia. *Biomol. Ther.* 17:241–248.
176. Kim, S. C., J. I. Kang, M. K. Kim, H. J. Boo, D. B. Park, Y. K. Lee, J. H. Kang, E. S. Yoo, Y. H. Kim, and H. K. Kang. 2011. The hair growth promoting effect of 4-O-methylhonokiol. *Eur. J. Dermatol.* 21:1012–1013.
177. Fashe, T. M., T. A. Keinänen, N. A. Grigorenko, A. R. Khomutov, J. Jänne, L. Alhonen, and M. Pietila. 2010. Cutaneous application of a-methyl spermidine activates the growth of resting hair follicles in mice. *Amino Acids* 38:583–590.
178. Kang, H., J. E. Kim, K. H. Jeong, and Y. M. Park. 2014. Direct hair growth promoting effects of mycophenolic acid. *J. Am. Acad. Dermatol.* 70:AB90.
179. Tomita, Y., M. Akiyama, and H. Shimizu. 2006. PDGF isoforms induce and maintain anagen phase of murine hair follicles. *J. Dermatol. Sci.* 43:105–115.
180. Bak, S. S., Y. K. Sung, and S. K. Kim. 2014. 7-Phloroeckol promotes hair growth on human follicles *in vitro*. *Naunyn Schmiedebergs Arch. Pharmacol.* 387:789–793.
181. Hynd, P. I. and M. J. Nancarrow. 1996. Inhibition of polyamine synthesis alters hair follicle function and fiber composition. *J. Invest. Dermatol.* 106:249–253.
182. Ramot, Y., M. Pietilä, G. Giuliani, F. Rinaldi, L. Alhonen, and R. Paus. 2010. Polyamines and hair: A couple in search of perfection. *Exp. Dermatol.* 19:784–790.
183. Takahashi, T., T. Kamiya, A. Hasegawa, and Y. Yokoo. 1999. Procyanidin oligomers selectively and intensively promote proliferation of mouse hair epithelial cells in vitro and activate hair follicle growth *in vivo*. *J. Invest. Dermatol.* 112:310–316.
184. Takahashi, T., A. Kamimura, Y. Yokoo, S. Honda, and Y. Watanabe. 2001. The first clinical trial of topical application of procyanidin b-2 to investigate its potential as a hair growing agent. *Phytother. Res.* 15:331–336.
185. Wu, X., J. Yao, Z. Yang, W. Yue, Y. Ren, C. Zhang, X. Liu, H. Wang, X. Zhao, S. Yuan, Q. Wang, L. Shi, and L. Shi. 2011. Improved fetal hair follicle development by maternal supplement of selenium at nano size (Nano-Se). *Livest. Sci.* 142:270–275.
186. Hue, J. J., B. K. Jo, and B. S. Kang. 2010. Effect of sodium silicate on hair growth in C57BL/6 mice. *Lab. Anim. Res.* 26:55–62.
187. Safer J. D., L. M. Fraser, S. Ray, and M. F. Holick. 2001. Topical triiodothyronine stimulates epidermal proliferation, dermal thickening, and hair growth in mice and rats. *Thyroid* 11:717–724.
188. Pyo, H. K., H. G. Yoo, C. H. Won, S. H. Lee, Y. J. Kang, H. C. Eun, K. H. Cho, and K. H. Kim. 2007. The effect of tripeptide-copper complex on human hair growth *in vitro*. *Arch. Pharm. Res.* 30:834–839.

29 Herbal Treatment for Skin Wrinkle

An Overview

Mayuree Kanlayavattanakul and Nattaya Lourith

CONTENTS

29.1 INTRODUCTION

When an individual ages, the turnover rate of epidermal cells slows down and the vascular network between epidermal cells and the skin elastic fibers and fluids is poorer. In addition, these cells are decreased resulting in reduction of skin thickness [1,2].

Skin aging is caused by several factors that damage cell membranes and components, including lipids, proteins, and DNA. Reactive molecules with unpaired electrons or free radicals initiate cellular damage known as intrinsic, chronologic, and extrinsic aging. Natural cellular metabolism generates free radicals in a self-defense mechanism and efficiently scavenges these species and neutralizes the radicals; however, these are decreased with age [2]. Dermal damage is also induced by UV exposure at the shorter wavelengths (UVB) that are absorbed by the epidermis prior to irradiation of keratinocytes. During that time, longer wavelengths (UVA) penetrate the skin and interact with epidermal and dermal cells. Proteolytic enzyme activities are propagated resulting in degradation of collagen and elastin fibers that include glycosaminoglycans (GAGs), hyaluronan, chondroitin, keratin, dermatan, and heparin. The matrix metalloproteinases (MMPs) are degradation enzymes of the extracellular matrix (ECM), which include collagen, elastin, and GAGs. These enzymes with 28 members (MMP-1 to MMP-28) are functioned and accelerated by age and radicals, including inflammatory mediators as well [3]. Therefore, deactivation, inhibition, or suppression of MMP in addition to stimulation of synthase are regarded as the leading strategy in the management of skin aging [4–8]. In addition, cellular damage results in inflammatory mediators and generation of free radicals and worsens intrinsic aging in turn, as well as in the induction of MMP activation [1].

Therefore, prevention of radicals damaged by antioxidative molecules and nonenzymatic antioxidants terminate the radicals, protecting against radical generations and increasing self-defense mechanisms with a limitation of radical generations [8], are contributing to antiaging products and have been extensively commercialized. In particular, herbal products as they are thought to be milder, safer, and healthier are the main source of interests in treating skin wrinkles and protection against aging [9].

29.2 NUTRICOSMETICS AND SKIN

Physiology of skin is precisely related with the dietary intake as higher intake of vegetable, fish, legumes, and olive oil reveals a significant ($p < 0.0001$) minimal of skin wrinkles [10]. The importance of dietary is therefore emerging with the latest technical term known as nutraceuticals including nutricosmetics. This term refers to food and dietary supplements that enhance aesthetic condition decelerating aging of skin and youthfulness of skin improvement [11–16]. Recently, this trend has interestingly hit the consumers' preference and has been largely approved in many countries, legislation [17]. Although several herbs, minerals, and vitamins are respected as the potential actives for treating wrinkles of skin delaying aging as evidenced on the basis of clinical evaluation in human subjects by oral administration, these have sparely been reported. In addition, most of the herbs, minerals, vitamins, and fatty acids are recommended at the daily allowance. This chapter, therefore, emphasizes those of *in vivo* evaluations monitored by the devices relating to skin texture and elasticity. Those of *in vitro*, cell culture, or *ex vivo* and animal studies are excluded as well as those of dermatologist scoring as there might be some of variation that makes it difficult for validation between different studies. Technical information according to the assessment instruments is out of the scope of this chapter that exclusively informs upon active, dose, and duration of dietary uptake for skin aging combat, of which probiotics and prebiotics are excluded.

29.3 HERBAL ACTIVES FOR SKIN WRINKLE TREATMENT

Although there are several herbs in complementary and alternative medicine (CAM) claimed upon potentials against aging, clinical evidence on the basis of skin wrinkle reduction and skin firmness improvement is limited. Therefore, evidence-based antiaging herbs are listed as follows.

Aloe vera drink was daily consumed at a higher (3600 mg gel/day) and lower (1200 mg gel/day) doses with the same volume proportion (120 mL) in a double-blind randomized study in 30 Korean women aged 49–74 years for 90 days. Facial wrinkles were monitored using a skin replica and analyzed by Visiometer® SV 600 (CK). Skin elasticity was examined in parallel with Cutometer® MPA 580 (CK). Roughness of the facial wrinkles was significantly ($p < 0.05$) reduced at the higher-dose gel exhibited by each parameter, whereas average roughness of the lower dose was not changed. Although skin elasticity was improved in the higher gel group, that of lower dose was significantly ($p < 0.05$) enhanced with a clearer result [18]. However, the authors did not discuss the difference in results from different instrumental evaluations.

In addition, a combination of actives was found to be extensively used to treat skin aging. A 6-month randomized double-blind, placebo-controlled study was undertaken in postmenopausal Caucasians female volunteers aged between 45 and 65 years. Following 28 days of washout period, 38 subjects were orally given two tablets of the active twice a day. During that time, the placebo was taken by 42 volunteers. During the 6 months of study, the volunteers were controlled with the same usage of moisturizer and cleanser. The tablet (Imedeen Prime Renewal™, Feerosan A/S, Denmark) containing 350 mg of soy extract (10% soy isoflavones), 210 mg of fish protein polysaccharides, 62.4 mg of white tea extract (*Camellia sinensis*, 40% polyphenols), 27.5 mg of grape (*Vitis vinifera*) seed extract, 28.8 mg of tomato (*Lycopersicum aesculentum*) extract, 60 mg of sodium ascorbate (99%), 10 mg of tocopheryl acetate, 5 mg of zinc gluconate, and 100 mg of chamomile (*Matricaria recutita*) extract was orally taken in the morning and the evening (two tablets, each time). Assessments were conducted on forehead, periocular, and perioral wrinkles, mottled pigmentation, laxity, sagging, under eye dark circles, and overall appearance using a photo evaluation and ultrasound measurement. The active group was significantly improved as examined by photo ($p < 0.05$) and the ultrasound measurement ($p < 0.0001$) [19]. Photoaged skin was found to be improved as examined in a randomized placebo-controlled clinical trial in 111 Caucasian subjects aged 35–50 years for 12 months. Wrinkles in the crow's feet area were significantly improved ($p = 0.015$) on the basis of a visual assessment with a reduction of transepidermal water loss or TEWL ($p < 0.05$) and enhancement of skin smoothness as well, as determined by skin replica [20].

French maritime pine bark (*Pinus pinaster*), the rich source of pycnogenol, was combined in a dietary tablet. The tablet containing pycnogenol (10 mg), vitamins C and E (30 and 5 mg), a mixture of hydrolyzed collagen and GAGs from salmon (50 mg), selenium (25 μg), zinc gluconate (7.5 mg), extracts of horsetail (40 mg), blueberry (15 mg), and tomato that were claimed to be composed with 34 mg of β- and γ-carotene, lycopene, and lutein was a randomized double-blind, placebo-controlled drug orally administrated twice a day by 58 female volunteers aged 45–75 years. Elasticity of skin was examined following 6 weeks of supplementation and was found significantly increased ($p = 0.04$, 9%) more than the placebo. The study was further continued until 12 weeks and reassessed upon skin benefits using PRIMOS® (GF Messtechnik). Those of placebo were greater in skin roughness (6%), which is significantly ($p = 0.02$) higher than the verum group that remained unchanged [21].

A cocoa beverage containing 328.5 mg of total flavonols was consumed daily by 12 female volunteers aged between 18 and 65 years for 12 weeks in a comparison with the placebo group receiving 26.8 mg flavonol cocoa. The maximum epicatechin and catechin gained in the test group were 61.1 and 20.4 mg, whereas those in the placebo were 6.6 and 1.6 mg/day, respectively. This randomized double-blind, placebo-controlled trial was examined upon skin benefits of the functional drink at the baseline, 6 and 12 weeks. Sensitivity toward UV irradiation was conducted in terms of minimal erythemal dose (MED) on dorsal skin exposed with a blue-light solar simulator. MED or redness of skin was detected by Minolta CR 300 chromameter. MED of the high-flavonol cocoa group was significantly increased with a reduction of erythema as exhibited by the chromametry a-value following 6 and 12 weeks of treatment ($p = 0.001$ and 0.012), whereas that of the placebo was not differed. In addition, the blood flow in cutaneous (1 mm) was enhanced in the treated group in similar to the subcutaneous (7–8 mm) tissues. The flow was significantly increased ($p < 0.05$) following 6 and 12 weeks, whereas the placebo remained unchanged. To strengthen the benefits of flavonol cocoa in skin wrinkle prevention, structure and texture of skin were additionally examined in addition to photoprotection. Density and thickness of skin were significantly ($p < 0.05$) increased as exhibited by the ultrasound technique (Dermascan® C, Cortex) following 6 and 12 weeks of supplementation. Hydration of skin (Corneometer® CM 825, CK) was significantly enhanced at week 12 in harmony with a reduction of TEWL as examined by Tewameter® TM 300 (CK). Moisturizing of skin is in concert with skin texture. Skin roughness and scaling monitored by Visioscan were significantly improved at the end of study. Skin wrinkle and smoothness improved, though not significantly [22]. The skin benefits of chocolate eating were additionally confirmed in 30 subjects who were orally supplemented with 20 g of chocolate containing either 600 mg minimum of flavonols or less than 30 mg of flavonols. Following 12 weeks of supplementation, the high-flavonol group significantly ($p = 0.005$) improved in MED, whereas that of placebo remained unchanged [23].

Green tea extract with 250 mg polyphenols (70% catechins) and 99.5% caffeine free in a capsule was randomly taken twice daily in a comparison with placebo by 56 healthy females aged between 25 and 75 years for 2 years. The improvement of the subjects' photoaged skin was tracked by Visia® (Canfield Imaging Systems). Overall solar damage of the green tea group was significantly ($p = 0.02$) reduced following 6 months of study in similar to erythema ($p = 0.05$), which is highly achieved after 2 years ($p = 0.00$). However, histological assessments in terms of dermal collagen and elastin showed none of any difference between placebo and treated groups [24].

29.3.1 Carotenoids

In addition to the aforementioned botanical and herbal extracts, carotenoid is another class of actives that gained large credits in treating and preventing cutaneous aging. Major carotenoids in human epidermis and dermis are carotenes, lycopenes, phytoenes, phytofluenes, xanthophylls, luteins, zeaxanthins, and cryptoxanthins. On the basis of light protection capacity, they are majorly presented in the target site of a photoaged skin.

A mixture of carotenoids derived from *Brassica oleracea* convar. *acephala* var. *sabellica* or curly kale, sea buckthorn (*Hippophae rhamnoides*), and olive oils, containing lutein (2200 μg), β-carotin (1000 μg), α-carotin (50 μg), lycopin (400 μg), zeaxanthin (700 μg), and cryptoxanthin (100 μg) commercializing with the trade name of Lutexskin™ (Bioactive Food GmbH, Germany), was daily supplemented in 24 volunteers aged between 22 and 66 years for 8 weeks. Antioxidant for skin was increased (48%, $p = 0.045$) after 8 weeks as monitored by a noninvasive EPR spectroscopy that is in accord with a significant (34%, $p < 0.01$) reduction of radical formation irradiated by VIS/NIR. Skin protection capability was enhanced as evidenced by a significant ($p < 0.05$) greater content of skin lipid, particularly ceramide [25].

A comparative study upon the combination of carotenoids in terms of lycopene (6 mg) and a mixture of lycopene and lutein (3 mg, each) at the same dose of β-carotene (3 mg), α-tocopherol (4.8 mg), and selenium (75 μg) on skin texture was conducted. A randomized double-blind, placebo-controlled study was conducted in 39 volunteers aged 18–65 years that were split into three groups and assigned to supplement daily for 12 weeks with the aforementioned antioxidants or placebo. Skin density and thickness were significantly ($p < 0.005$) improved in both groups of carotenoids taken as monitored by Dermascan C, of which results with lycopene showed more increased density of skin, whereas that of lycopene and lutein showed a greater achievement upon skin thickness. Visioscan was additionally used to track the relief of roughness and scaliness of skin. Both of the tested carotenoid formula significantly reduced scaling of skin ($p < 0.05$). The combination of lycopene and lutein was highly effective (–57.99%) than the lycopene formula (–44.22%). That was in accord with treatment of roughness as the combination of carotenoids is more effective (–37.78%) than the lycopene (–32.71%). Thus, skin wrinkle treatment using carotenoids, although at the same content, should better encompassed with a mixture of carotenoids to enhance the efficacy as exhibited [26].

Astaxanthin 4 mg was daily supplemented by 49 healthy American women enrolled in a single-blind, placebo-controlled study. The dietary supplement containing 2 mg astaxanthin (Astavita®) in the form of a softgel capsule was supplemented every breakfast and dinner in a comparison with the placebo for 6 weeks. Skin improvement was examined by a questionnaire, skin inspection by dermatologist, Dermal Phase Meter® 9003 (Nova), and Dermalab (Cortex). Satisfaction of the enrolled volunteers on the improvement of skin dryness, moisture content, roughness, elasticity, and wrinkle was significantly higher in the test group. More than 50% of the subjects had reported improvements of all parameters. During that time, the dermatologist scored insignificant reduction of dryness but significant ($p < 0.05$) improvement of wrinkle and elasticity, of which skin hydration was significantly better, in similar to elasticity as exhibited by the instruments that are highly pronounced following the last 3 weeks of application [27].

A mixture of lutein (5 mg) and zeaxanthin (0.3 mg) in the form of oral soft gelatin capsule (20% FloralGLO® Lutein in Safflower oil) was a randomized double-blind, placebo-controlled supplement given in the morning and in the evening with meals for 12 weeks. The study was conducted in 20 healthy women aged 25–50 years with a requested restriction upon diet with less than 0.5 mg of β-carotene with a wash out period of 15 days. Skin lipid was claimed to have significantly increased ($p < 0.05$) in the lutein/zeaxanthin group and coined with a protection of skin lipid peroxidation. Furthermore, MED was significantly reduced with an improvement of skin elasticity as shown by Dermaflex (Cortex) [28].

Furthermore, skin roughness was significantly ($p < 0.01$) correlated (–0.843) with cutaneous lycopene as studied in 20 human volunteers aged between 40 and 50 years using PRIMO® 4.0 (GF Messtechnik) and Raman spectroscopy, respectively [29].

29.3.2 Polysaccharides

These important actives derived from plant, animal, and marine products majorly contribute in dietary supplements treating aging as they were used as minor actives in combinations with plants [19,21]. In addition, they are implied as the main actives and assessed upon their antiaging supplement. A complex of polysaccharides that are chitin/hyaluronic acid (1.4 mg in butylene glycol) and β-glucan (1.6 mg) containing melatonin and vitamin E (1.6 mg, each) in capsule was orally administrated twice daily (morning and evening) with meals for 12 weeks by 70 women aged 22–45 years who enrolled in a randomized, double-blind, placebo-controlled study. Skin elasticity examined by Dermaflex A was found significantly ($p < 0.05$) achieved from the baseline at each point of interval (4, 8, and 12 weeks). The improvement was highest at the end of study [30].

29.4 MINERALS FOR SKIN WRINKLE TREATMENT

Silicon in the form of bioavailable choline-stabilized orthrosilicic acid was investigated in a randomized double-blind, placebo-controlled study in 50 healthy Caucasian females with photoaged skin. Oral administration of Si (10 mg/day) for 20 weeks was followed by the examination in terms of skin roughness using Reviscometer® MPA 5 (CK). The shear propagation time in the active group was significantly decreased ($p < 0.05$) conferring an isotropy of the skin with the reduction of skin roughness ($p < 0.05$) [31]. In addition, zinc gluconate and selenium were also evidenced in skin firmness enhancement [20,21,26].

29.5 VITAMINS AND ESSENTIAL FATTY ACIDS FOR SKIN WRINKLE TREATMENT

Vitamins are the second most commonly known actives combating skin aging, particularly vitamins C and E [21,26,30] that are widely used in the forms of sodium ascorbate and tocopheryl acetate [20] due to their bioavailability. In addition, the mixture of vitamins and fatty acids is also applied due to their synergistic effects. Oral administration of higher vitamin C and linoleic acid with the lower intake of fats and carbohydrates is associated in the youthfulness of skin that brings better skin appearance with lower wrinkles and senile dryness of skin as examined in 4025 middle-aged American women [32].

In addition to the aforesaid dietary supplement, beverage and softgel capsule containing isoflavone, lycopene, vitamins C and E, and essential fatty acids from fish oil were orally taken. A randomized double-blind, placebo-controlled study was conducted in 159 postmenopausal women that were divided into three groups taking placebo, high-active, and low-active drinks and capsules, separately. Following 14 weeks of supplementation, plasma levels of actives revealed the effective absorption into teh bloodstream that is significantly ($p < 0.05$) higher than the placebo group. Skin texture was further evaluated by means of wrinkle replica collection at the crow's foot area of both sides of the face. Skin roughness (PRIMOS) of the high-active tested group was significantly ($p < 0.005$) improved and better than the low-active one that significantly ($p < 0.01$) reduced wrinkle in a comparison with placebo. However, skin firmness and elasticity as examined by Cutomerter CM 825 on the inner and outer forearms showed no improvement. Skin collagen was significantly ($p < 0.05$) enhanced in the high-active group as examined by skin biopsy analysis. However, the quantity of elastin was remained [33].

A combination of marine proteins (350 mg); α-lipoic acid (100 mg); vitamins C (90 mg), E (18 mg), B3 (18 mg), and B5 (8 mg); the extracts of red clover (8%, 62 mg), tomato (5% lycopene, 40 mg), pine bark (95%, 30 mg), and soy (40%, 12 mg); and minerals (zinc 12 mg and copper 2 mg) in the form of tablets was taken twice daily (morning and evening) by 44 females who enrolled the study in a comparison with placebo. The volunteers taken this dietary product (DermaVite™, Biovite, United Kingdom) for 6 months were found significantly ($p < 0.05$) improved in skin thickness and elasticity as exhibited by Dermascan A and Dermaflex. A self-evaluation by the volunteers pointed out the significant ($p < 0.05$) improvement against skin aging following 4 months of enrollment. The results were exacerbated at the end of a 6-month study ($p < 0.001$) [34].

A capsule of 180 mg polyunsaturated fatty acids of omega-3, 8 mg topopherols, 18 mg flavonoids, and 6 mg carotenes with total lipids of 308 mg, combined with protein (220 mg), which is commercialized as Estime® (Swiss Pharmaceutical Industries SA), was a randomized double-blind placebo-controlled supplement given daily in 39 female volunteers for 4 months. Skin density was significantly ($p < 0.001$) increased (48%) following 3 months and slightly enhanced ($p < 0.01$) at the end of the study (12%) as examined by Dermascan C. The result was in accord with skin thickness that significantly increased ($p < 0.001$) following 3 and 4 months of evaluation (20% and 15%) [35].

29.6 CONCLUSIONS

Aging of skin is caused by several factors of which those of antioxidative herbs are regarded as the main actives for treatment. Dietary products encompassing actives are currently presented in several forms to fit the lifestyle of the consumers nowadays. In addition, synergistic effects strengthening the capability of the antiaging products by using a mixture of actives are gaining higher preferences as evidenced by the clinical evaluations. Therefore, the readers have the flexibility to choose herbal actives, vitamins, minerals, and fatty acids as well, with the variety forms in either beverage, tablet, or capsule. In addition, selection of vegetable, meat, and oil enriching with the actives combating aging is encouraged to be opted in cuisine. However, stability of the actives in each dosage forms and bioavailability following ingestion should be the major concerns including safety, for instance interaction with the uptaking medicine and also the influence upon different immunological conditions of the individual. Therefore, regulation upon these sorts of supplementary products should be ensured.

REFERENCES

1. Bennett MF, Robinson MK, Baron ED, Cooper KD. Skin immune systems and inflammations: Protector of the skin or promoter of aging? *J Invest Dermatol Sym Proc* 2008;13:15–19.
2. Naylor EC, Watson REB, Sherratt MJ. Molecular aspects of skin ageing. *Maturitas* 2011;69:249–256.
3. Gupta A, Kaur CD, Jangdey M, Saraf S. Matrix metalloproteinase enzymes and their naturally derived inhibitors: novel targets in photocarcinoma therapy. *Ageing Res Rev* 2014;13:65–74.
4. Chen LL, Wang SQ. From the bottle to the skin: challenges in evaluating antioxidants. *Photodermatol Photoimmunol Photomed* 2012;28:228–234.
5. Masaki H. Role of antioxidants in the skin: Anti-aging effects. *J Dermatol Sci* 2010;58:85–90.
6. Nichols JA, Katiyar SK. Skin photoprotection by natural polyphenols: Anti-inflammatory, antioxidant and DNA repair mechanism. *Arch Dermatol Res* 2010;302:71–83.
7. Nolan BV, Levender MM, Davis SA, Feneran AN, Fleischer AB Jr, Feldman SR. Trends in the use of topical over the counter products in the management of dermatologic disease in the United States. *Dermatol Online J* 2012;18:1.
8. Shah H, Mahajan SR. Photoaging: New insights into its stimulators, complications, biochemical changes and therapeutic interventions. *Biomed Aging Phathol* 2013;3:161–169.
9. Bruce S. Cosmeceuticals for the attenuation of extrinsic and intrinsic dermal aging. *J Drugs Dermatol* 2008;7:s17–s22.
10. Purba M, Kouris-Blazos A, Wattanapenpaiboon N, Lukito W, Rotehnberg EM, Steen BC, Wahlqvist ML. Skin wrinkling: Can food make a difference? *J Am Coll Nutr* 2001;20:71–80.
11. Ryan AS, Goldsmith LA. Nutrition and the skin. *Clin Dermatol* 1996;14:389–406.
12. Dattner AM. Nutritional dermatology. *Clin Dermatol* 1999;17:57–64.
13. Rona C, Berardesca E. Aging skin and food supplements: The myth and the truth. *Clin Dermatol* 2008;26:641–647.
14. Draelos ZD. Nutrition and enhancing youthful-appearing skin. *Clin Dermatol* 2010;28:400–408.
15. Lakdawala N, Babalola O 3rd, Fedeles F, McCusker M, Ricketts J, Whitaker-Worth D, Grant-Kels JM. The role of nutrition in dermatologic diseases: Facts and controversies. *Clin Dermatol* 2013;31:677–700.
16. Draelos ZD. Aging skin: The role of diet: Facts and controversies. *Clin Dermatol* 2013;31:701–706.
17. Bagchi D. *Nutraceutical and Functional Food Regulations in the United States and Around the World* (2nd edn.). San Diego, CA: Elsevier, 2014.
18. Cho S, Lee S, Lee MJ, Lee DH, Won CH, Kim SM, Chung JH. Dietary *Aloe vera* supplementation improves facial wrinkles and elasticity and its increases the type I procollagen gene expression in human skin *in vivo*. *Ann Dermatol* 2009;21:6–11.

19. Skovgaard GRL, Jensen AS, Sigler ML. Effect of a novel dietary supplement on skin aging in post-menopausal women. *Eur J Clin Nutr* 2006;60:1201–1206.
20. Kieffer ME, Efsen J. Imedeen® in the treatment of photoaged skin: An efficacy and safety trial over 12 months. *J Eur Acad Dermatol Venereol* 1998;11:129–136.
21. Segger D, Schönlau F. Supplementation with Evelle® improves skin smoothness and elasticity in a double-blind, placebo-controlled study with 62 women. *J Dermatol Treat* 2004;15:222–226.
22. Heinrich U, Neukam K, Tronnier H, Sies H, Stahl W. Long-term ingestion of high flavonol cocoa provides photoprotection against UV-induced erytherma and improved skin condition in women. *J Nutr* 2006;136:1565–1569.
23. Williams S, Tamburic S, Lally C. Eating chocolate can significantly protect the skin from UV light. *J Cosmet Dermatol* 2009;8:169–173.
24. Janjau R, Munoz C, Gorell E, Rehmus W, Egbert B, Kern D, Chang ALS. A two-year, double-lind, randomized placebo-controlled trial of oral green tea polyphenols on the long-term clinical and histologic appearance of photoaging skin. *Dermatol Surg* 2009;35:1057–1065.
25. Meinke MC, Friedrich A, Tscherch K, Haag SF, Darvin ME, Vollert H, Groth N, Lademann J, Rohn S. Influence of dietary carotenoids on radical scavenging capacity of the skin and skin lipids. *Eur J Pharm Biopharm* 2013;84:365–373.
26. Heinrich U, Tronnier H, Stahl W, Béjot M, Maurette J-M. Antioxidant supplements improve parameters related to skin structure in humans. *Skin Pharmacol Physiol* 2006;19:224–231.
27. Yamashita E. The effects of a dietary supplement containing astaxanthin on skin condition. *Carotenoid Sci* 2006;10:91–95.
28. Palombo P, Fabrizi G, Ruocco V, Ruocco E, Fluhr J, Roberts R, Morganti P. Beneficial long-term effects of combined oral/topical antioxidant treatment with the carotenoids lutein and zeaxanthin on human skin: a double-blind, placebo-controlled study. *Skin Pharmacol Physiol* 2007;20:199–210.
29. Darvin M, Patzelt A, Gehse S, Schanzer S, Benderoth C, Sterry W, Lademann J. Cutaneous concentration of lycopene correlates significantly with the roughness of the skin. *Eur J Pharm Biopharm* 2008;69:943–947.
30. Morganti P, Fabrizi G, Palombo P, Palombo M, Guarneri F, Cardillo A, Morganti G. New chitin complexes and their anti-aging activity from inside out. *J Nutr Health Aging* 2012;16:242–245.
31. Barel A, Calomme M, Timchenko A, De Paepe K, Demeester N, Rogiers V, Clarys P, Vanden Berghe D. Effect of oral intake of choline-stabilized orthosilicic acid on skin, nails and hair in women with photodamaged skin. *Arch Dermatol Res* 2005;297:147–153.
32. Cosgrove MC, Franco OH, Granger SP, Murray PG, Mayes AE. Dietary nutrient intakes and skin-aging appearance among middle-aged American women. *Am J Clin Nutr* 2007;86:1225–1231.
33. Jenkins G, Wainwright LJ, Holland R, Barrett KE, Casey J. Wrinkle reduction in post-menopausal women consuming a novel oral supplement: A double-blind placebo-controlled randomized study. *Int J Cosmet Sci* 2014;36:22–31.
34. Thom E. A randomized, double-blind, placebo-controlled study on the clinical efficacy of oral treatment with DermaVite™ on ageing symptoms of the skin. *J Int Med Res* 2005;33:267–272.
35. Béguin A. A novel micronutrient supplement in skin aging: A randomized placebo-controlled double-blind study. *J Cosmet Dermatol* 2005;4:277–284.

Section XV

Fertility and Sexual Health

30 Nutraceuticals and Male Fertility

A Review

Michelle Lightfoot, Muhannad Alsyouf, and Edmund Y. Ko

CONTENTS

ABBREVIATIONS

CAM: Complementary and alternative medicine
cAMP: Cyclic adenosine monophosphate
CI: Confidence interval
CoQ10: Coenzyme Q10
ETC: Electron transport chain
LAC: L-acetyl carnitine
LC: L-carnitine
MDA: Malondialdehyde
NAC: *N*-acetyl-cysteine
OAT: Oligoasthenoteratozoospermia
OR: Odds ratio
PUFA: Polyunsaturated fatty acids
RCT: Randomized controlled trial
RDA: Recommended dietary allowance
ROS: Reactive oxygen species
SOD: Superoxide dismutase
TUNEL: Terminal deoxyribonucleotidyl transferase-mediated dUTP nick-end labeling (assay)
VDR: Vitamin D receptor
WMD: Weighted mean difference

30.1 INTRODUCTION

Infertility or subfertility is a common condition occurring in 15%–20% of couples attempting to conceive. Of these, a male factor is found to be solely or partially responsible in approximately 50% of cases.[1,2] Numerous underlying etiologies have been implicated in male factor infertility, including anatomic abnormalities, genetic disorders, hormonal alterations, and infectious causes. However, despite a full workup, 30–40% of men are diagnosed with idiopathic infertility.[3,4] This can result in the need for assistive reproductive technologies to achieve pregnancy and may be associated with a significant financial burden, as infertility treatments are typically not covered by insurance in the United States.[5]

As with many other medical conditions, the use of complementary and alternative medicine (CAM) has become increasingly popular with couples experiencing infertility. Explanations for this increase include widespread availability, comparatively low cost, and a desire for more "holistic" or "natural" treatments.[6] In the context of infertility, CAM may include interventions such as acupuncture and mind–body–spirit counseling, as well as a variety of herbal supplements and dietary changes. Despite the popularity of CAM treatments, research has been hampered by a lack of standardization, paucity of well-designed randomized controlled trials (RCT), and inconsistent reporting of pregnancy and live birth rates.[2,7]

The term "nutraceutical" was first coined in 1989 and refers to "a food (or part of a food) that provides medical or health benefits, including the prevention and/or treatment of a disease."[8] Plant-based by-products, supplements, vitamins, and minerals are thus classified as nutraceuticals when used for the purposes of disease prevention or treatment.[2]

This review begins with an overview of oxidative stress and antioxidant activity, which is the primary mechanism through which nutraceuticals are thought to exert their effects on fertility parameters. We then discuss the role of diet and obesity in male infertility treatment, followed by an examination of individual nutraceuticals.

30.2 OXIDATIVE STRESS

Reactive oxygen species (ROS) are chemically and biologically active molecules that are formed as by-products of oxygen metabolism (Figure 30.1).[9,10] Although ROS are necessary for multiple phases of normal spermatogenesis including capacitation, acrosomal reaction, and fertilization,[11] elevated levels of ROS may be detrimental to semen quality. Excess production of ROS, known as oxidative stress, may be induced by a variety of stimuli including infection, inflammation, strenuous exercise, trauma, tobacco exposure, chemotherapeutic agents, varicoceles, cryptorchidism, and exogenous heat exposure to the testicles (sauna, hot tub, laptop computers).[12–14] Endogenous ROS are produced primarily by leukocytes and immature spermatozoa. Teratozoospermic forms produce higher levels of oxidants compared to morphologically normal sperm.[15] ROS are also produced physiologically in response to bacterial and chemical stimuli.[16]

Spermatozoa are susceptible to oxidative damage for a number of reasons. First, plasma membranes of sperm contain a large number of polyunsaturated fatty acids, compounds that are intrinsically vulnerable to oxidative stress.[17] Second, the majority of the cells' cytoplasm is removed during spermatogenesis along with cytoplasmic enzymes such as catalase and glutathione peroxidase, which normally serve to scavenge free radicals.[16] Third, high levels of ROS are associated both with sperm DNA damage[10] and decreased ability to repair such damage.[18] Damaged sperm in turn produce more ROS, thereby perpetuating this cycle.

30.3 ANTIOXIDANTS

To counterbalance the negative effects of oxidative stress, the body uses antioxidants to buffer free radicals and protect cells against oxidative damage.[19] This physiological state of equilibrium can be disrupted by excess ROS production, decreased clearance, or a combination of both factors. Antioxidants can be classified as enzymatic and nonenzymatic. Enzymatic antioxidants are produced endogenously and include superoxide dismutase, catalase, and glutathione peroxidase. Nonenzymatic antioxidants include vitamins C and E, carotenoids, carnitine, taurine, hypotaurine, and glutathione.[20]

Antioxidants can be obtained from dietary intake of various fruits, vegetables, nuts, legumes, herbs, meat, and dairy products. Alternatively, oral supplements can provide physiologic or supraphysiologic doses. Increased consumption of antioxidants may potentially improve sperm DNA integrity and semen quality.[21] Conversely, low intake and total body concentration of antioxidants has been associated with poor semen quality.[22]

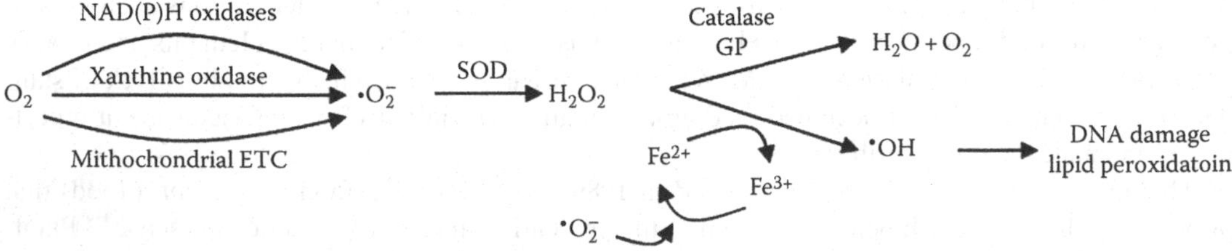

FIGURE 30.1 Overview of ROS formation and elimination. Superoxide radicals are produced from cellular redox reactions by way of NAD(P)H or xanthine oxidases, or compounds in the mitochondrial electron transport chain (ETC). Superoxide dismutase (SOD) transforms superoxide anions into hydrogen peroxide, which may then be broken down into water and oxygen by glutathione peroxidase (GP) or catalase. Alternatively, some transition metals can donate an electron to hydrogen peroxide to form hydroxyl radicals. The oxidized metal ions are then reduced by superoxide anions, perpetuating the formation of free radicals. ROS can then cause cellular DNA damage and lipid peroxidation. (Adapted from Valko, M. et al., *Int. J. Biochem. Cell Biol.*, 39, 44, 2007.)

30.4 DIET AND OBESITY

Several studies have evaluated the association between weight and male factor fertility parameters. A recent meta-analysis found that the prevalence of oligozoospermia or azoospermia increased with BMI. Compared to normal-weight men, low sperm counts were more common in overweight (OR 1.11, CI 1.01–1.21), obese (OR 1.28, CI 1.06–1.55), and morbidly obese men (OR 2.04, CI 1.59–2.62).[23] Similarly, semen quality and reproductive hormone levels were found to be associated with BMI in young Danish men undergoing physical exams for military service. Men with a BMI >25 kg/m^2 had a reduction in total sperm count of 23.9% when compared to men with BMI between 20 and 25. Additionally, men with low BMI (<20 kg/m^2) exhibited a total sperm count that was 36.4% lower than the normal-weight group. The underweight and overweight groups also showed a reduction in sperm concentration, although semen volume and proportion of mobile spermatozoa had no association with BMI.[24] Among a cohort of men who were primarily overweight or obese (82%) and sedentary (58% reporting exercise <1 time/week), a negative linear decline in ejaculate volume and total sperm count was seen with increasing waist circumference. However, semen concentration, sperm motility, morphology, and DNA fragmentation index did not correlate with waist circumference or BMI.[25] Conversely, another meta-analysis did not find a relationship between BMI and semen parameters.[26]

Despite a trend toward impaired semen quality in overweight and obese men, the data on pregnancy outcomes are mixed. A prospective observational study of couples attempting to conceive found that although several individual semen parameters were associated with fecundity on univariate analysis, no characteristics were strongly associated with pregnancy outcomes after multivariable regression; however, increasing male age and increasing female (but not male) BMI were associated with longer time to pregnancy.[27] Conversely, loss of abdominal fat through lifestyle modification was seen to significantly decrease the rate of sperm DNA fragmentation and improve metabolic and hormonal profiles in one small case series. Furthermore, superoxide dismutase levels increased with weight loss, and all spouses became pregnant and carried the pregnancies to term.[28]

Potential mechanisms to explain the effects of obesity on abnormal semen parameters and infertility include alterations in hormonal profiles (decreased androgens and inhibin B, increased estrogens), induction of sleep apnea, and higher scrotal temperatures.[29,30] In an intriguing mouse study, Fullston et al. reported that alterations in sperm parameters in mice that were fed high-fat diets persisted even into the second generation of progeny. This occurred despite the offspring being fed conventional diets and having normal weights and testosterone levels.[31] Further research into this topic may reveal surprising results about the long-term impact of obesity on male fertility.

Independent of BMI, diet has also been studied as a factor in male infertility. Diets high in saturated fat have been associated with alterations in semen quality, with one study showing that men in the highest quartile of saturated fat intake had 41% lower sperm counts than those in the lowest quartile.[32] In another study, men aged 18–22 who adhered to a "Prudent" diet (high intake of fish, chicken, vegetables, fruits, whole grains, and legumes) had higher proportions of motile sperm than those who followed a "Western" diet (high intake of red meat, processed foods, pizza, refined grains, high-energy drinks, and sweets). However, no associations with sperm concentration or morphology were noted.[33] Case–control studies have shown that the risk of asthenozoospermia is elevated for men with the highest intake of sweets and processed meats and lowest in those with high intakes of fruits and vegetables, poultry, seafood, and skim milk.[34,35]

The data on alcohol consumption and fertility appear mixed: although some studies have reported impaired spermatogenesis in moderate and heavy drinkers[36] and lower success rates of IVF for men who consume alcohol,[37] other studies have found no association.[38,39]

The factors that affect semen parameters may differ from those that influence pregnancy and live birth rates. A study of male patients undergoing cycles of ICSI showed that BMI and alcohol consumption were negatively correlated with sperm concentration. BMI, alcohol consumption, and smoking were negatively correlated with sperm motility, while fruit and cereal consumption showed a positive correlation. Fertilization rates were likewise negatively influenced by alcohol and coffee consumption, and implantation rates were negatively influenced by red meat consumption, being on a weight loss diet, and female BMI. Pregnancy rates were negatively affected by the consumption of red meat and being on a weight loss diet.[40]

This highlights one of the major limitations associated with studies of nutraceuticals in the treatment of male infertility. Although the primary goal for couples undergoing fertility treatment is a successful pregnancy and live birth, very few studies of nutritional supplements use these as outcome variables. Instead, a variety of semen parameters are typically reported as surrogate outcomes; these may or may not correlate with the desired pregnancy outcomes.

30.5 REVIEW OF NUTRACEUTICALS

Nutraceuticals are commonly thought to be safe and have a generally favorable side effect profile. However, no medication or supplement is without risks, and side effects may be encountered when these substances are consumed in excess beyond the recommended daily allowance. Furthermore, these items are not regulated by the U.S. Food and Drug Administration.[7] Table 30.1 summarizes the natural dietary sources, recommended dietary allowance (RDA), tolerable upper limit, and toxicity with excess intake for each nutraceutical discussed later.[41]

30.5.1 Arginine

30.5.1.1 Mechanism of Action

Arginine, a conditionally essential amino acid, is a precursor of nitric oxide via nitric oxide synthase. As a ROS, nitric oxide is utilized for signal transduction during sperm capacitation.[42] Arginine also serves as a precursor for several polyamines that are thought to function in sperm motility.[43]

30.5.1.2 Evidence for Benefit

Early studies in which arginine was administered in doses up to 4 g/day reported improvements in sperm motility and concentration.[44–46] One placebo-controlled, crossover RCT assessed the effects of the combination supplement Prelox (L-arginine and pycnogenol, an antioxidant) on various semen parameters. They reported improvements in semen volume, sperm concentration, and motility in the treatment group.[47] However, the relative effects from each supplement were not examined independently.

30.5.1.3 Evidence against Benefit

A double-blind, placebo-controlled crossover trial of oligozoospermic men showed no difference in conception rates or semen quality after supplementation with arginine for 12 weeks.[48] Vasopressin, a neurohypophysial hormone derived from arginine, was recently studied in a mouse model. In this study, vasopressin was associated with a detrimental effect on fertilization, sperm function, and embryonic development.[49]

30.5.1.4 Conclusion

Published data on the effects of arginine in male infertility are contradictory, and arginine supplementation has not been well studied.

30.5.2 Carnitines

30.5.2.1 Mechanism of Action

L-carnitine (LC) and L-acetyl carnitine (LAC) are quaternary amine compounds derived from the amino acids lysine and methionine. Physiologically, they transport long-chain fatty acids into the mitochondria for intracellular metabolism. Carnitines act as antioxidants, serve as an energy source for spermatozoa, and assist in sperm maturation and motility.[50,51]

TABLE 30.1
Dietary Sources, Recommended Intake, and Toxicity of Individual Nutraceuticals

Nutraceutical	Dietary Sources	RDA[a]	Tolerable Upper Limit[a]	Potential Toxicity with Excess Intake
Arginine	Nuts, seeds, brown rice, raisins, coconut, cereals	NE, but dietary intake is usually 2–6 g	NE	GI distress, hypotension, renal insufficiency, increased bleeding risk, elevated glucose
Carnitines	Red meat, milk, poultry	NE	NE; toxicity reported at 4 g/day	GI distress, "fishy" body odor, muscle weakness, seizures
Cobalamin (vitamin B12)	Fish, meat, poultry, eggs, milk, fortified cereals	2.4 µg	NE	NE
Coenzyme Q10	Endogenously produced	NE	NE	Mild GI intolerance
Folic acid	Leafy green vegetables, fruits and fruit juices, nuts, beans, dairy, meat and poultry, seafood, grains; fortified cereal and grain products	400 µg[b]	1000 µg (from synthetic forms only); NE for natural foods	Possible acceleration of preneoplastic lesions, possible masking of anemia or cognitive symptoms from concurrent B12 deficiency
Glutathione	NE	NE	~3 g	NE
Lycopene	Tomato	NE	NE	GI distress, alteration of skin color
Omega fatty acids	Fish, organ meats, leafy green vegetables, nuts, vegetable oils (canola, soy, flaxseed)	1.1–1.6 g (ALA), 11–17 g (LA)[c]	NE	GI distress, increased bleeding risk with anticoagulant medication
Pentoxyfylline	NE	NE	NE	NE
Phytoestrogens	Soy products, tofu, cereals, walnuts, berries, apples, ginseng, soy-based infant formulas	NE	NE	NE
Selenium	Seafood, meat, bread, grains, eggs, Brazil nuts	55 µg	400 µg	GI distress, respiratory distress, myocardial infarction, hair loss, tremors, garlic odor on breath, facial flushing, tremors, muscle tenderness
Vitamin A	Fish oils, milk, eggs, leafy green vegetables, orange and yellow vegetables, tomato, fortified cereals	900 µg	3000 µg	Dizziness, nausea, increased intracranial pressure, skin irritation, joint/bone pain, liver toxicity, possible increased risk of lung cancer or cardiovascular mortality
Vitamin C	Raw fruits (citrus, kiwifruit, strawberries) and vegetables (bell peppers, broccoli, Brussels sprouts, cabbage)	90 mg	2000 mg	GI distress, possible risk of nephrolithiasis from conversion to oxalate

(*Continued*)

TABLE 30.1 (*Continued*)
Dietary Sources, Recommended Intake, and Toxicity of Individual Nutraceuticals

Nutraceutical	Dietary Sources	RDA[a]	Tolerable Upper Limit[a]	Potential Toxicity with Excess Intake
Vitamin E	Nuts, seeds, vegetable oils, green leafy vegetables, fortified cereals	15 mg (22.4 IU)	1000 mg (1500 IU)	Bleeding complications, hemorrhagic stroke
Zinc	Red meat, poultry, beans, nuts, whole grains, fortified cereals, dairy	11 mg	40 mg	GI distress, loss of appetite, headaches, altered iron function

ALA, alpha-linolenic acid (omega-3 fatty acid); LA, linolenic acid (omega-6 fatty acid); NE, not established; GI, gastrointestinal.

[a] When available, values are reported for reproductive age males.

[b] 400 µg from natural food sources = 240 µg from fortified foods or dietary supplements.

[c] Adequate intake (level assumed to ensure adequate nutrition).

30.5.2.2 Evidence for Benefit

Carnitines are among the most well-studied nutraceuticals for male infertility. Studies have shown that infertile men have lower seminal LC concentrations than their fertile counterparts, with the lowest levels seen in azoospermic men. LC levels were positively correlated with sperm concentration, sperm motility, and vitality.[52,53] Supplementation with LC and/or LAC has also been tested in several RCTs. Lenzi et al. randomized patients to combination therapy (LC 2 g/day + LAC 1 g/day) versus placebo. After 6 months, patients in the therapy group had improvements in forward motile sperm compared to patients receiving placebo. Patients with the lowest numbers of motile sperm exhibited the greatest improvement in motility parameters. Although a spontaneous pregnancy rate of 15% was achieved in the therapy group (compared to 0% in the placebo group), analysis of the patients who achieved fertility showed no improvement in semen parameters throughout the trial period.[51]

In a similar study, Balercia et al. reported an improvement in sperm motility after 6 months of therapy with LAC (3 g/day) and LC+LAC (2 g + 3 g/day) compared to placebo. Combination therapy was also associated with improvements in straight progressive velocity after 3 months, and patients who received LAC showed improvements in total oxyradical scavenging capacity compared to placebo or LC alone. However, pregnancy rates were identical in patients who received placebo or carnitine supplementation (20% in each group).[54]

Zhou conducted a systematic review and meta-analysis of 9 RCTs involving 862 patients. In the pooled analysis, carnitines were associated with an increase in weighted mean difference (WMD) of total sperm motility (WMD 7.4%, 95% CI 1.7–13.1, $p = 0.01$), forward sperm motility (WMD 11.8%, 95% CI 0.5–23.2, $p = 0.04$), and decrease in atypical sperm forms (WMD −5.7%, 95% CI −7.8 to −3.6, $p < 0.0001$). In addition, carnitines were associated with an increase in pregnancy rates (OR 4.1%, 95% CI 2.1–8.1, $p < 0.0001$) compared to placebo. A Cochrane review of antioxidants in male subfertility also found an improvement in pregnancy rates with LC (OR 5.1%, 95% CI 1.5–17.1, $p = 0.009$) or LC + LAC (OR 4.5%, 95% CI 1.8–11.4, $p = 0.002$) versus placebo.[55] Other studies have reported an increase in sperm vitality, motility, semen volume, and total sperm count with carnitine supplementation.[56,57]

More recently, Banihani et al. studied the effects of the addition of LC to cryopreservation medium on sperm characteristics of infertile men. When compared to semen samples preserved with a standard cryopreservation medium, the addition of LC improved sperm motility and vitality ($p < 0.05$). However, no effect on sperm DNA oxidation levels were seen.[58]

30.5.2.3 Evidence against Benefit

A small RCT by Sigman et al. randomized infertile men with sperm motility of 10%–50% to placebo versus carnitine (LC 2 g/day + LAC 1 g/day). After 24 weeks of therapy, no increase in sperm motility or total motile sperm counts was seen.[59] Although the 2011 Cochrane review showed an overall increase in pregnancy rates with carnitine supplementation, there was conflicting evidence on the effects of LC and LAC on individual semen parameters. With regards to overall sperm motility, LC was superior to placebo at 3, 6, and 9 months. However, LAC improved sperm motility only at 6 months and LC + LAC did not show an improvement at any time point. LC was associated with an improvement in sperm concentration with 3 months of supplementation, but no improvement was seen at 6 or 9 months with LC, LAC, or LC + LAC.[55] Another RCT not included in the Cochrane review also found that supplementation with LC (1 g/day) for 12 weeks did not improve semen volume, sperm concentration, percent motile sperm, or percent morphologically normal sperm.[60]

30.5.2.4 Conclusion

Carnitine supplementation (LC ± LAC) may lead to improvements in pregnancy rates, although reported confidence intervals remain wide. The optimal agent and duration of supplementation have not been well established, and the evidence on the effects on individual semen parameters has been conflicting.

30.5.3 Coenzyme Q10

30.5.3.1 Mechanism of Action

Coenzyme Q10 (CoQ10) is a molecule found in mitochondria that plays a critical role in the production of adenosine triphosphate via the electron transport chain, which may have implications for sperm motility.[61] It also serves as a lipid-soluble antioxidant, potentially contributing to the overall seminal antioxidant buffering capacity given the high levels of ubiquinol (the reduced form of CoQ10) in sperm.[62]

30.5.3.2 Evidence for Benefit

Levels of seminal CoQ10 have been correlated with sperm count and motility,[63] while the ratio of ubiquinol to ubiquinone (the oxidized form of CoQ10) in seminal fluid has been shown to be inversely related to oxidative stress and abnormal sperm morphology.[64]

Two RCTs utilizing CoQ10 were summarized in a 2011 Cochrane review.[55,65,66] This review demonstrated an improvement in sperm motility at 6 months, which was not sustained at 9 months. There was also a modest improvement in sperm concentration at 9 months; however, these results were based almost entirely on a single trial.[65]

A more recent meta-analysis, which also included a third RCT that was published after the Cochrane review, similarly reported improvements in seminal plasma CoQ10 levels with supplementation and improvements in sperm concentration and motility.[67,68] This RCT showed increases in the levels of catalase and superoxide dismutase in men with idiopathic oligoasthenoteratozoospermia (OAT). Seminal CoQ10 level was positively correlated with normal sperm morphology.[69]

A recent nonrandomized study included patients with idiopathic OAT and infertility after 2 years of unprotected intercourse. Supplementation with vitamin C, vitamin E, and CoQ10 was found to improve sperm concentration and motility at 3 and 6 months compared to baseline. In addition, a 28.4% pregnancy rate was reported (9.5% spontaneous, 18.9% assisted), although previous attempts using ART were not reported.[70] With multiple supplements, however, it is difficult to attribute semen analysis improvements and pregnancy rates to CoQ10 alone.

30.5.3.3 Evidence against Benefit

The Cochrane review did not demonstrate an improvement in pregnancy rates (OR 2.2, CI 0.5–8.8) or sperm concentration at 6 months. The most recent RCT did not report pregnancy rates, and no improvement in sperm concentration or motility was seen in this trial.[69]

30.5.3.4 Conclusion

Supplementation with CoQ10 appears to improve several markers of oxidative stress. However, studies have shown conflicting effects on sperm concentration and motility, and the impact on pregnancy rates is not well defined.

30.5.4 Folic Acid

30.5.4.1 Mechanism of Action

Naturally occurring folate (vitamin B_9) and its synthetic version folic acid are required for purine and pyrimidine production. It is therefore essential for DNA synthesis and normal cell function, including spermatogenesis.[16] Folate also serves as a scavenger of free radicals via creation of methyl donor compounds.[71] Mandatory fortification of enriched cereal-grain products with folic acid was implemented in the United States in 1998, which has led to significant increases in folate intake across all age groups.[72]

30.5.4.2 Evidence for Benefit

Men in the >75th percentile of folate intake (722 μg/day) were shown in one study to have 20%–30% lower incidence of sperm aneuploidy (disomy X, disomy 21, sex nullisomy, and aggregate aneuploidy) compared to men with lower intake.[21] An inverse relationship has been demonstrated between seminal plasma folate and DNA fragmentation in fertile men.[73] Another study observed a lower dietary intake of folate among infertile men compared to fertile controls. It also demonstrated that folate intake positively correlated with sperm motility.[74]

Two double–blind, placebo-controlled RCTs have evaluated the effects of combined folic acid and zinc supplementation on sperm characteristics of subfertile men. Wong et al. demonstrated a 74% increase in total sperm count along with a 4% increase in abnormal sperm ($p < 0.01$),[75] while Ebisch et al. showed that supplementation significantly increased sperm concentration from a median of 7.0 to 8.0 million/mL after 26 weeks.[76]

30.5.4.3 Evidence against Benefit

In 1978, Landau et al. reported one of the first trials of folic acid supplementation in both normo- and oligospermic men. They failed to show any improvement in sperm count, motility, or sperm DNA content. It is important to note that this intervention used higher folic acid doses (10 mg three times/day) for a shorter duration (30 days) than the later RCTs (5 mg daily for 26 weeks)[75,76] and did not include zinc combination therapy.[77] Other studies have failed to show an improvement in sperm concentration with folic acid supplementation in men with OAT,[78] and a lack of association between polymorphisms in the folate metabolism pathway and reduced sperm counts in infertile men.[79] Importantly, no study of folic acid supplementation reported pregnancy rates as an outcome variable.

30.5.4.4 Conclusion

The currently available evidence has not demonstrated a reliable improvement in semen characteristics or fertility with folic acid supplementation.

30.5.5 Glutathione

30.5.5.1 Mechanism of Action

Glutathione is produced in the liver and functions as an endogenous reducing agent against toxic xenobiotics (i.e. carcinogens, drugs, pollutants).[80] It is part of an antioxidant scavenger system that participates in the recycling of reactive oxygen species. Sperm cells are highly susceptible to ROS-induced damage, particularly during maturation and capacitance.[81]

30.5.5.2 Evidence for Benefit

In a prospective, placebo-controlled, double-blinded, crossover study, intramuscular injection of 600 mg glutathione every other day in 20 infertile men with abnormal semen analyses significantly improved sperm motility.[82] Glutathione supplementation, in combination with vitamins C and E, has also been associated with improved sperm count and decreased DNA fragmentation, although it remains to be determined whether this association is attributable to glutathione alone or the synergistic effect of the combined agents.[83]

30.5.5.3 Evidence against Benefit

Dietary glutathione supplementation is unable to raise circulating levels to a clinically adequate extent due to its poor oral bioavailability. The subsequent need for intramuscular or intravenous injection to achieve satisfactory clinical levels limit its use as a dietary supplement.[84]

30.5.5.4 Conclusion

Supplementation with glutathione appears to improve sperm motility; however, the impact on conception rates has yet to be determined. Poor oral absorption remains a limiting factor for its use as a supplement.

30.5.6 Lycopene

30.5.6.1 Mechanism of Action

Lycopene is a potent antioxidant that can be found concentrated in the adrenal glands, breasts, liver, prostate, and testes.[85] Apart from its antioxidative properties, it also acts as an immunomodulator, anti-inflammatory agent, and proapoptotic and cell growth inhibitor.[86]

30.5.6.2 Evidence for Benefit

In vitro studies suggest a protective role of lycopene supplementation against oxidative DNA damage in sperm.[87] Gupta and Kumar reported that men receiving 2000 mg of lycopene twice daily had significant median increases in sperm concentration, motility, and morphology.[88] In a prospective study, Filipcikova and colleagues reported that 51% of 43 infertile couples were able to conceive successfully (either spontaneously or after in vitro fertilization) after 3 months of supplementation with lycopene.[89] A recent placebo-controlled, crossover RCT assessed the effect of lycopene supplementation on seminal biomarkers of oxidative stress. The study reported a significant decrease in the seminal concentration of the biomarker and concluded that this may in part explain the improvement in fertility rates observed after lycopene supplementation.[90]

30.5.6.3 Evidence against Benefit

There is currently a lack of evidence of a negative impact of lycopene supplementation on male reproductive health.

30.5.6.4 Conclusion

Current studies demonstrate promising evidence of lycopene supplementation and its effect on seminal parameters in infertile males. There is a need for larger well-designed RCTs to delineate the clinical significance of this supplement as well as optimal dosing regimens.

30.5.7 Omega Fatty Acids (Polyunsaturated Fatty Acids)

30.5.7.1 Mechanism of Action

Fatty acids are classified into saturated, monounsaturated and polyunsaturated. The polyunsaturated fatty acids (PUFA) omega-3 and omega-6 are nutritionally essential since they cannot be synthesized intrinsically. Fatty acids are a major constituent of the lipid bilayer, a component of the cell membrane that contributes to the structure of spermatozoa. The concentration of long chain fatty acids have been shown to significantly correlate with normal sperm morphology and function.[91] The antioxidant properties of PUFAs also play a role in sperm function.

30.5.7.2 Evidence for Benefit

Most of the research regarding omega fatty acids has highlighted the cardiovascular health benefit of this supplement. People known to have cardiovascular heart disease are encouraged to consume at least 1 g of omega-3 fatty acids per day, as recommended by the America Heart Association, to reduce the risk of cardiovascular disease mortality.[92]

PUFA supplementation has been demonstrated to have a beneficial effect on seminal parameters. A study comparing human immature germ cells to mature spermatozoa reported a significantly higher fatty acid cell membrane concentration in the latter. The study concluded that the concentration of long chain fatty acids in the sperm membrane is correlated with sperm motility and function.[91] Supplementation with PUFAs can improve sperm count, motility, and morphology in addition to improving semen antioxidant activity.[93–95] A double-blinded, placebo-controlled, RCT demonstrated similar findings. The study randomized 238 patients to 1.84 g of omega-3 fatty acids or placebo daily for 32 weeks and showed a significant improvement in sperm cell total count and concentration in the omega-3 group ($p < 0.05$).[94]

30.5.7.3 Evidence against Benefit

A prospective study comparing 82 infertile to 78 age matched fertile men demonstrated a significant positive correlation between blood plasma and spermatozoa omega-3 fatty acid concentration and sperm concentration, motility, and morphology ($p < 0.05$). However, there was a negative correlation between omega-6 fatty acid of spermatozoa and sperm count, motility, and morphology ($p < 0.001$). The authors concluded that a diet rich in omega-6 fatty acids and poor in omega-3 fatty acids contributes to poor semen quality and sperm function.[93]

30.5.7.4 Conclusion

Omega fatty acids are generally safe, inexpensive, and have demonstrated a beneficial impact on spermatic function in human studies.[93] More research into individual fatty acids and their effect on sperm function is needed, as the currently available literature is conflicting. In addition, patients on antiplatelet or anticoagulation therapy should be cautioned about the increasing risk of bleeding with concurrent fish oil supplementation.[92,96]

30.5.8 Pentoxyfylline

30.5.8.1 Mechanism of Action

Pentoxyfylline, a methylxanthine derivative, functions in the sperm to inhibit the enzyme phosphodiesterase thereby increasing spermatic cyclic adenosine monophosphate (cAMP). cAMP controls sperm capacitation and motility and regulates the acrosomal reaction. [97–99] Pentoxyfylline has also been shown to exhibit antioxidant properties.[100]

30.5.8.2 Evidence for Benefit

A recent double-blind placebo-controlled study randomized 254 infertile men to 400 mg twice daily oral pentoxyfylline therapy or placebo. A significant increase in sperm concentration ($26.4 \pm 4.6 \times 10^6$/mL vs. $16.2 \pm 3.4 \times 10^6$/mL), sperm motility (35.8% ± 4.2% vs. 26.4% ± 2.4%), and sperm with normal morphology (25.4% ± 4.3% vs. 17.4% ± 4.20%) was reported in the pentoxyfylline group when compared with baseline ($p = 0.001$). In addition, no serious adverse events were noted in the study, although mild–moderate adverse events were significantly higher in the pentoxyfylline group (nausea, vomiting, dyspepsia, headache, and diarrhea).[101]

30.5.8.3 Evidence against Benefit

Spermatozoa contain several different phosphodiesterase subtypes, and the regulation of cAMP is therefore largely dependent on the target action and localization of phosphodiesterase inhibitors.[102] This may partly explain the findings of studies that did not show a beneficial impact of pentoxyfylline supplementation on sperm function.[103,104]

30.5.8.4 Conclusion

The interest in this supplement for the treatment for male infertility showed a decline in the late 1990s.[105] Although one recent RCT suggested a benefit on several sperm parameters, the impact on pregnancy outcomes and the optimal dosing remain unknown.

30.5.9 Phytoestrogens (Isoflavones)

30.5.9.1 Mechanism of Action

Phytoestrogens are plant-derived estrogens most notably found in soy products, tofu, cereals, walnuts, berries, apples, ginseng, soy-based infant formulas, as well as many vegetables.[106,107] Phytoestrogens are able to bind and activate estrogen receptors in the human body allowing them to replicate the biological actions that are produced by physiological estrogens.[108] This mechanism of action has led to their description as endocrine disrupting agents. Phytoestrogen exposure may also interfere with the androgen receptor pathway and affect the end stages of spermatogenesis.[109] In vitro studies have reported that phytoestrogens can alter the function of enzymes involved in steroid biosynthesis (aromatase and 5α-reductase).[110] Phytoestrogens may also interfere with the androgen–estrogen balance by displacing testosterone and 17β estradiol from their binding sites on sex hormone binding globulins,[111] ultimately altering the free "active" fraction of these sex hormones.

30.5.9.2 Evidence for Benefit

The potential therapeutic benefits of soy products for the prevention of obesity, diabetes mellitus,[112,113] osteoporosis,[114] cardiovascular disease,[115] and hormone-dependent cancers (e.g. breast cancer)[116] have garnered much research interest. Conversely, to our knowledge, there is a lack of evidence supporting the beneficial role of phytoestrogens for male infertility.

30.5.9.3 Evidence against Benefit

In animal models, exposure to phytoestrogens in utero or in the early postnatal period resulted in multiple reproductive derangements in the adult life. Although the results were not replicated across all the studies, a decrease in testicular size,[117] spermatogenesis,[117,118] testosterone,[119] and diydrotestosterone[120,121] was noted in the groups exposed to phytoestrogens.

In humans, there are very few clinical studies designed to evaluate the effect of phytoestrogens or phytoestrogen-containing products (soy) on reproductive parameters in males. The currently available human studies have shown contradictory results. Mitchell et al. evaluated the effect of daily 40 mg phytoestrogen containing tablets taken by 14 men aged 18–35 years over 2 months with no significant reproductive history. The study found no change in post-supplement testosterone concentration, sperm concentration, count, motility, or ejaculate volume.[122]

In a cross-sectional study, Chavarro et al. collected information about dietary intake of soy foods from 99 men and found a negative correlation between soy food intake and sperm concentration but no association with sperm motility, morphology, or ejaculate volume.[123] In another cross-sectional study, Nagata et al. showed that total and free testosterone concentrations were inversely correlated with soy product intake in 69 Japanese men, although these correlations were only borderline significant.[124] Both of these studies were observational and depended on nonvalidated self-administered questionnaires to estimate the amounts of soy intake.

Nagata et al. performed a follow-up study that randomized 35 men into a group consuming 400 mL of soymilk compared to a control group for 8 weeks. The results of his follow-up study did not reflect his previous study findings as there was no difference in total and free testosterone or sex hormone binding globulin levels between the two groups.[125]

In a randomized crossover dietary intervention study, Habito et al. studied 42 men placed on either a 150 g lean meat diet or a 290 g tofu diet for 4 weeks. Tofu intake resulted in significantly higher sex hormone binding globulin (8.8%, $p = 0.01$) and a lower testosterone to estradiol ratio ($p = 0.049$).[126]

Soy protein–based milk infant formulas account for almost 20% of the formula market in the United States.[127] With millions of infants being fed soy formulas, a major concern is whether phytoestrogen exposure during infancy causes any reproductive effects in this critical developmental period. Sharpe et al. found a decrease in neonatal testosterone levels in Marmoset monkeys fed with soymilk at 6 weeks of age.[128] However, no adverse reproductive outcomes were reported in the adult population.[129] A retrospective human study by Strom and colleagues assessed the effects of soy formula consumption during infancy on adult reproductive outcomes and found no difference in the onset of puberty or reproductive functions when compared to a group consuming milk-based formula.[130] However, hormone levels and reproductive outcomes were not directly measured in this study.

30.5.9.4 Conclusion

Phytoestrogens might in principle interfere with the male reproductive system due to their estrogen receptor effect and effects on androgen receptor pathways. The lack of consistency in human and animal studies may be explained by the differences in study design, small sample size, and variations in outcome assessment methods. More robust research is needed to elucidate the clinical effect of this compound on fertility. For now, and based on theoretical risk, phytoestrogen intake and supplementation should not be encouraged for infertile males.

30.5.10 Selenium

30.5.10.1 Mechanism of Action

Selenium is an essential trace element that is integral to the structure of many selenoproteins. As a part of glutathione peroxidase, it has a significant role in the reduction of antioxidant enzymes.[131,132] It also has an important role in maintaining testicular development, spermatogenesis, and sperm function, such as motility and capacitation.[133–135]

30.5.10.2 Evidence for Benefit

Like many antioxidants, selenium has been shown to improve several spermatic parameters (sperm count, motility, and morphology).[136,137] Deficiency in seminal selenium has been found to decrease sperm count, resulting in abnormal sperm morphology and lower sperm motility.[138–140]

Multiple studies have examined the effect of selenium's combination with other supplements on sperm motility. Safarinejad studied the individual effects of selenium and *N*-acetyl-cysteine (NAC) as well as in combination on male fertility in a prospective, double-blind, placebo-controlled trial. After 26 weeks of therapy, groups receiving selenium, NAC, and combination therapy demonstrated significant increases over baseline ($p < 0.05$) in mean total sperm count, sperm concentration, ejaculate volume, and WHO morphology. Selenium and combination therapy groups also showed improvement in sperm motility. The combination of selenium and NAC showed the best overall improvement compared to individual agent therapy suggesting an additive effect with simultaneous intake.[137]

Other studies have demonstrated the positive impact of selenium supplementation on sperm motility. In a single-arm prospective study, 690 asthenoteratospermic men received 200 μg of selenium and 400 IU of vitamin E daily for 14 weeks. At the conclusion of the study, a significant increase in sperm motility over baseline was observed ($p \leq 0.005$) and pregnancy occurred in 10.8% of cases.[141] However, the absence of a control group to compare pregnancy outcomes was a major limitation of this study. Another prospective study demonstrated similar findings. Men with OAT receiving 210 μg selenium and 400 mg vitamin E for 3 months had an 8% increase in sperm motility ($p < 0.05$) and an 8% decrease in spermatic lipid peroxidation, ($p < 0.05$).[142] Similarly a prospective, double-blind, placebo-controlled randomized trial by Scott et al. demonstrated a 12.9% increase in sperm motility in asthenozoospermic men treated with selenium therapy alone or in combination with other vitamins ($p = 0.023$). In the 3-month period, treatment groups reported five pregnancies resulting in live births (11%) while no pregnancies occurred in the placebo group. [143]

30.5.10.3 Evidence against Benefit

In a prospective, randomized blinded study, Hawkes and Turek studied the effect of a controlled diet containing high or low selenium on 11 men for 17 weeks.[144] At week 13, subjects in the high selenium diet group had a 32% average decrease in the fraction of motile sperm ($p \leq 0.05$). However, by week 17 the fraction of motile sperm was only 17% lower than baseline. The small sample size of the study ($n = 11$) must be considered as a limitation when interpreting the findings.

A noncontrolled study with selenium only supplementation demonstrated increases in serum and seminal selenium levels above baseline, but did not demonstrate change in spermatozoal characteristics (sperm count, motility, or morphology).[145] This result may highlight the need for selenium to be taken in conjunction with other antioxidants to attain the synergistic effects. Additionally, it is worth noting that not all studies that showed a positive effect on spermatic parameters were able to demonstrate this impact on their entire cohort. In Moslemi and Tavanbakhsh's study, 36.6% (253 cases) did not show any response to a combination of selenium and vitamin E after 14 weeks of treatment.[141] This finding was also noted in the study by Scott et al.[143]

30.5.10.4 Conclusion

Selenium may have a positive and synergistic effect on male infertility when used with other supplements. However, a minority of men may not show improvement in sperm parameters with selenium.

30.5.11 Vitamin A

30.5.11.1 Mechanism of Action

Vitamin A and its derivatives are collectively called retinoids or carotenoids and are a constituent of visual pigments (retinal).[146] Vitamin A is lipophilic and is readily stored in the body. It is essential for maintaining the mucous membranes of the skin, gastrointestinal tract, and genitourinary tract. Vitamin A may also have antioxidant properties, although the exact mechanism is unknown.[147]

30.5.11.2 Evidence for Benefit

In animal models, vitamin A deficiency resulted in decreased spermatogenesis and decrease in the integrity of Sertoli cell tight junctions, thereby compromising the blood–testis barrier.[148,149] Combination therapy studies involving vitamin A in combination with other supplements (vitamins C and E, selenium, NAC, and zinc) have demonstrated positive effects on sperm motility and count ($p < 0.05$).[143,150]

30.5.11.3 Evidence against Benefit

The studies that have documented the positive effects of vitamin A on seminal parameters have done so in combination therapy, thus improvements in seminal parameters may be attributed to the synergistic effect of multiple supplements. The effect of vitamin A therapy alone on male infertility is difficult to delineate due to the lack of vitamin A only studies. Supplementation beyond daily dietary intake can result in accumulation of toxic levels.[151]

30.5.11.4 Conclusion

Consuming adequate amounts of vitamin A–rich foods to maintain important physiological processes within the body is recommended. However, there is insufficient evidence to recommend additional supplementation above daily dietary intake to improve male fertility on the basis of current available studies.

30.5.12 Vitamin C

30.5.12.1 Mechanism of Action

Also known as ascorbic acid, vitamin C is a water-soluble vitamin that functions as a key cofactor for many hydroxylation and amidation processes.[152] It is utilized in the synthesis of collagen, proteoglycans, and components of the intercellular matrix. Vitamin C is also an electron donor (antioxidant)[153] that plays a role in the recycling of oxidized vitamin E.[12]

30.5.12.2 Evidence for Benefit

Vitamin C can be found in high concentrations within seminal plasma.[154] It has a role in protecting sperm and sperm DNA from oxidative damage by neutralizing ROS.[155] Vitamin C supplementation has shown a positive correlation with improvements in seminal qualities. Adequate seminal concentrations have been shown to reduce sperm DNA damage and fragmentation.[22,155,156] By using the terminal deoxyribonucleotidyl transferase-mediated dUTP nick-end labeling (TUNEL) assay to assess sperm DNA damage, Greco et al. demonstrated a reduction in the percentage of DNA fragmented spermatozoa after 2 months of treatment with vitamin C and E ($p < 0.001$).[155]

Combinations of vitamin C with other vitamins and antioxidants (β-carotene, vitamin E, zinc) have shown a synergistic improvement in sperm motility and concentration. In smokers, daily vitamin C supplementation with 200 mg or higher has shown significant improvement in sperm motility, viability, and count from baseline ($p < 0.05$).[157] In addition, the study reported a significant correlation between the serum and seminal plasma vitamin C levels and sperm quality improvement.

30.5.12.3 Evidence against Benefit

It is difficult to discern the effects of vitamin C on spermatic function as many of the studies demonstrating positive findings used concurrent supplementation with other vitamins or antioxidants. Therefore, any improvements in spermatic parameters may be attributed to a synergistic or confounding effect of multiple agents. Conversely, a randomized, placebo-controlled, double-blind study demonstrated no benefit of concurrent vitamin C (1000 mg) and vitamin E (800 mg) supplementation on semen parameters or pregnancy rates of infertile men over a 56-day period.[158]

30.5.12.4 Conclusion

Vitamin C may have positive effects on certain semen parameters; however, the impact on pregnancy rates has not been studied. Prospective, controlled, clinical trials on single-agent vitamin C supplementation are needed to assess the true effect of this vitamin on sperm parameters.

30.5.13 Vitamin D

30.5.13.1 Mechanism of Action

Vitamin D is a fat-soluble vitamin and a steroid hormone. Body stores of vitamin D consist mostly of sunlight-induced production in the skin while a small portion is derived from diet or supplements. Vitamin D receptors (VDRs) located in various tissues are responsible for the physiologic actions of vitamin D.[159] In the reproductive system, VDRs have been localized in the head and midpiece of the human sperm, epididymis, seminal vesicle, and prostate.[160–162] VDRs function by influencing multiple biologic pathways including gene transcription, second messenger systems, and calcium homeostasis.[163–165]

30.5.13.2 Evidence for Benefit

Animal models have demonstrated the impact of vitamin D deficiency on reproductive health. Vitamin D deficient male rats demonstrated a 45% decrease in successful mating and a 73% decrease in fertility compared to vitamin D replete males.[166]

Several cross-sectional studies have considered the association between vitamin D intake and semen quality. Bloomberg, Jensen et al. evaluated 300 men from the general population and found a positive correlation between serum levels of vitamin D ($1{,}25(OH)_2D_3$) and sperm motility ($p < 0.05$).[167] Additionally, men with vitamin D less than 25 nM had less motility ($p = 0.027$) and morphologically normal spermatozoa ($p = 0.044$) compared to men with vitamin D levels greater than 75 nM. The European Male Ageing Study, evaluating 3369 men aged 40–79 years old, demonstrated a significant association between vitamin D deficiency with compensated and secondary hypogonadism (relative risk ratio = [1.52; $p = 0.03$] and [1.16; $p = 0.05$]; respectively).[168]

A recent randomized, placebo-controlled study evaluated the effect of vitamin D supplementation on testosterone levels in healthy overweight men undergoing a weight reduction program.[169] Subjects were randomized into either an 83 μg daily vitamin D supplement group or placebo for 1 year. A significant increase in total testosterone, bioavailable testosterone, and free testosterone levels was observed in the interventional arm when compared to the placebo group and baseline.

30.5.13.3 Evidence against Benefit

Another cross-sectional study of 307 men demonstrated lower median sperm count (94 million vs. 137 million; $p = 0.05$) and percentage of morphologically normal sperm (5.0% vs. 6.5%; $p = 0.05$) at higher vitamin D levels compared with men with lower vitamin D levels.[170] However, after adjusting for multiple confounding factors, these associations were no longer observed.

Like all fat-soluble vitamins, vitamin D has the potential for toxicity if supplemented in excessive amounts.[171] Moreover, sunlight exposure is the most important determinant of vitamin D levels and may negate the need for supplementation beyond the normal dietary intake in healthy populations.

30.5.13.4 Conclusion

Promising associations between vitamin D and male fertility have been demonstrated in the observational setting. As is the case for many nutraceuticals, well-designed RCTs that can replicate these observational results are needed.

30.5.14 Vitamin E

30.5.14.1 Mechanism of Action

A fat-soluble vitamin and a member of the tocopherol family, vitamin E is a well-known potent antioxidant that inhibits free radical–mediated damage to cell membranes, prevents lipid peroxidation, and exhibits synergistic actions with other antioxidants.[172,173] Many of the functions of vitamin E can be attributed to its ability to act as a chain-breaking compound against pathological ROS reactions.[174]

30.5.14.2 Evidence for Benefit

Vitamin E exhibits its protective effect by preventing the cell membrane of sperm from oxidative damage.[175] Additionally, vitamin E is effective in reducing seminal ROS in infertile men.[19,176] A retrospective study on healthy fertile men who were asked to complete a dietary survey and seminal analysis demonstrated a positive correlation between increased dietary intake of vitamin E (and other antioxidants) and improvement in spermatic function.[177] Particularly, those with higher intake of antioxidants had a higher sperm concentration of 84 million/mL and 5% greater sperm motility ($p < 0.05$). Another prospective study assessed pregnancy outcomes after daily supplements of vitamin E, vitamin C, and coenzyme Q. At the end of follow-up, 48 (28.4%) pregnancies occurred, 16 (9.5%) of which were achieved spontaneously.[70]

Several RCTs have studied the effect of vitamin E in male infertility. Suleiman et al. demonstrated a decrease in lipid peroxidation ($p < 0.001$) and improvement in sperm motility by 17.8% ($p < 0.001$) in infertile men receiving 300 mg of vitamin E for 6 months.[178] Additionally, 21% of infertile couples achieved pregnancy in the supplement group compared to none in the placebo group ($p < 0.001$). Similar improvements in motility and decrease in lipid peroxidation were replicated by Keskes-Ammar and colleagues using combination therapy of vitamin E (400 mg) and selenium (225 μg).[142] Another study of combination therapy with 1000 mg of vitamin E and 500 mg of vitamin C demonstrated a decrease in DNA fragmentation rates from 22.1 to 9.1 with antioxidant treatment, as assessed by the TUNEL assay ($p < 0.001$).[155] In a double-blinded, randomized controlled, crossover trial by Kessopoulou et al, intake of 600 mg of vitamin E for 3 months demonstrated an improvement in spermatozoa zona binding ($p = 0.004$).[176] However, no changes in other seminal parameters or ROS levels were observed when compared to placebo.

30.5.14.3 Evidence against Benefit

In one randomized, placebo-controlled, double-blinded study, high oral dose with vitamin E (800 mg) and vitamin C (1000 mg) for 56 days did not improve seminal parameters in infertile men or pregnancy outcomes.[158] Also, vitamin E supplementation does not come without risk. Although no consistent adverse effects were seen in subjects taking up to 2000 mg/day of vitamin E,[179] recent studies showed an increase risk of cardiovascular events at doses higher than 400 IU/day, particularly heart failure and all-cause mortality.[180] Moreover, vitamin E increases antiplatelet effect and bleeding risk in doses higher than 800 IU/day and also affects the function of anticoagulant medications.[181,182]

30.5.14.4 Conclusion

Considerable literature supports improvements in sperm motility, seminal ROS, and DNA fragmentation rates with vitamin E supplementation. The effects of vitamin E alone are difficult to identify because of possible synergistic interactions as most studies used multiple antioxidant supplements.

30.5.15 Zinc

30.5.15.1 Mechanism of Action

Zinc serves as a cofactor in many enzymatic functions including protein synthesis and DNA transcription. It also possesses antiapoptotic and antioxidant properties, in part as a component of copper/zinc superoxide dismutase.[183] High concentrations of zinc are found in the male reproductive tract, especially the prostate, and are involved in a variety of processes including testicular development and steroidogenesis, acrosome reaction, sperm chromatin stabilization, and testosterone synthesis.[16]

30.5.15.2 Evidence for Benefit

One trial with a total of 45 asthenozoospermic men (≥40% immotile sperm) compared a control group to groups undergoing supplementation with zinc, zinc + vitamin E, or zinc + vitamin E + vitamin C for 3 months. Although no differences were found between the three supplement groups, the treatment groups receiving any zinc supplementation demonstrated an improvement in sperm motility and fertilizing capacity compared to controls.[184] Another trial randomized infertile men to 3 months of zinc therapy (250 mg twice daily) or no therapy; patients were also followed for an additional 12 months after supplementation. Patients receiving zinc exhibited an improvement in sperm count, progressive motility, sperm membrane integrity, and a reduction in nonmotile spermatozoa. In addition, partners of men receiving zinc supplementation had higher pregnancy (22.5% vs. 4.3%, $p = 0.04$) and live birth rates (16.3% with two additional pregnancies ongoing at the time of publication vs. 4.3%, $p = 0.05$).[185] In a more recent trial, 3 months of zinc supplementation (440 mg/day) was associated with improvements in seminal volume, progressive sperm motility, and total normal sperm count in infertile men.[186]

30.5.15.3 Evidence against Benefit

Colagar et al. reviewed a number of publications regarding zinc and male infertility. Although their study did find a positive relationship between seminal zinc levels and sperm count, normal morphology and fertility status, they noted that other studies have not found a consistent relationship between zinc levels and fertility status or sperm parameters.[183] A double-blind RCT randomized men to 26 weeks of supplementation with placebo, folic acid, zinc, or folic acid + zinc. No difference in baseline zinc concentration in blood or seminal plasma was noted between fertile and infertile men. Although a significant increase in sperm concentration and total normal sperm count was seen in the combination group (folic acid + zinc), no change in these variables was seen with zinc supplementation alone.[75] Of note, zinc supplementation was only 66 mg/day, which is significantly lower than the doses used other trials (440–500 mg/day).

30.5.15.4 Conclusion

The available data, although limited, seem to suggest a benefit for zinc supplementation on a number of semen parameters as well as pregnancy and live birth rates.

30.6 DISCUSSION

For many infertile men, no anatomically or medically correctable cause of infertility is found on evaluation.[187] Faced with the high cost of assisted reproductive technologies—which may easily run into the tens of thousands of dollars in the United States—many men use empiric treatments such as nutraceuticals for infertility. Although the exact prevalence of nutraceutical use for treatment of male infertility is unknown, the use of complementary and alternative medicine has become more accepted in recent years. In 2007, data from the National Health Interview Survey revealed that more than one in six Americans had used a nonvitamin, nonmineral natural product in the past 12 months.[188]

Despite an abundance of studies investigating the use of nutritional supplements, their results must be interpreted with caution. First, there is a lack of standard dosing and administration schedule for most supplements reviewed in this chapter. Second, relatively few prospective double-blind, placebo-controlled RCTs exist. Even well-designed studies are often of short duration (6 months or less of supplement administration) and report a variety of outcome variables, a factor that may limit the conclusions that can be drawn from meta-analyses and reviews. Many trials also do not report other factors that may influence infertility such as dietary patterns, BMI, alcohol intake, or specific partner data. Third, most trials have been designed to study the effects of a single nutraceutical on fertility outcomes. This may not reflect real-world usage, as men may employ multiple treatments simultaneously. Although an exhaustive review of all combination therapies—including either multiple different nutraceuticals or nutraceuticals in combination with more traditional therapies for infertility—is beyond the scope of this text, the reader is referred to two RCTs that showed a combined improvement in pregnancy rates (OR 4.0, CI 1.4–11.3) with supplementation of multiple nutraceuticals.[150,189] Fourth, although the ultimate goal of infertility treatment is the successful delivery of an infant, few studies report pregnancy and live birth rates. Instead, a variety of semen parameters have been reported as surrogate endpoints, which may not necessarily correlate with fertility outcomes.[190]

Despite these shortcomings, several reviews have suggested an overall benefit to antioxidant therapy in male infertility treatment. A 2010 review by Ross et al. reported the results of 17 RCTs including 1665 men who were treated with a variety of antioxidants. A majority of studies (14/17 trials) reported an improvement in semen parameters and/or pregnancy rates compared to placebo or no treatment. Of the nine trials reporting spontaneous pregnancy rates, antioxidant therapy was associated with a significant improvement compared to controls (19% vs. 3% pregnancy rates; OR 7.9, CI 3.9–16.1). One additional study reported a higher viable pregnancy rate after ICSI in men who received a combination antioxidant supplement (38% vs. 16%, $p = 0.046$). However, heterogeneity in the reported RCTs precluded a meta-analysis of the data, and several trials did not include data on fertility status of the female partners.[19]

More recently, an exhaustive 2011 review by the Cochrane Collaboration summarized the results of 34 trials involving 2876 couples. Although only three trials reported live birth rates (two trials of vitamin E vs. placebo, one trial of zinc vs. no treatment), antioxidant therapy was found to have a statistically significant benefit (pooled OR 4.85, 95% CI 1.92–12.24; $p = 0.008$). The live birth rate was 15.5% (18/116) in the treatment group compared to 2.0% (2/98) in the control arm. In the 15 trials that reported pregnancy rates, antioxidant use was associated with a similar improvement compared to control (pooled OR 4.18, 95% CI 2.65–6.59; $p < 0.001$). Pregnancy rates were 15.9% (82/515) in the treatment arm and 3.1% (14/449) in the control arm. Trials of antioxidants that reported pregnancy rates included carnitines, coenzyme Q10, pentoxifylline, magnesium, vitamin E, vitamin C, zinc, and a combination supplement. In addition, no difference in the miscarriage rate was seen (pooled OR 7.24, 95% CI 0.14–364.94; $p = 0.32$). However, not enough information was available to perform head-to-head comparisons between different antioxidants or between different doses of the same antioxidant. There was also significant heterogeneity in the reporting of sperm motility at 3, 6, or 9 months and sperm concentration at 6 months. This limits the conclusions that can be drawn about the effects of antioxidants on specific semen parameters. Only seven trials reported side effects of the interventions; these were primarily gastrointestinal (nausea, gastroesophageal reflux, constipation, and diarrhea) and were not different between antioxidant and control groups (pooled OR 1.63, 95% CI 0.48–5.58; $p = 0.44$).[55]

30.7 SUMMARY

Numerous studies have investigated the effects of nutraceuticals on male subfertility. When used at doses that do not exceed the tolerable upper limits, most nutraceuticals appear to have an acceptable side effect profile and are likely less costly than traditional assisted reproductive techniques. Although many trials have shown improvements in sperm parameters with supplementation, the data on pregnancy and live birth outcomes are less robust. This precludes any definitive recommendations on the use of specific nutraceuticals, doses, or duration of supplementation for the treatment of male subfertility. However, meeting the recommended daily allowance of nutraceuticals through a well-balanced diet is encouraged.

REFERENCES

1. B. R. Winters and T. J. Walsh, *Urologic Clinics of North America*, 2014, 41, 195–204.
2. E. Y. Ko and E. S. Sabanegh, *Urologic Clinics of North America*, 2014, 41, 181–193.
3. A. Jungwirth, A. Giwercman, H. Tournaye, T. Diemer, Z. Kopa, G. Dohle, C. Krausz, and I. European association of urology working group on male, *European Urology*, 2012, 62, 324–332.
4. H. Elzeiny, C. Garrett, M. Toledo, K. Stern, J. McBain, and H. W. Baker, *The Australian & New Zealand Journal of Obstetrics & Gynaecology*, 2014, 54, 156–161, DOI: 10.1111/ajo.12168.
5. M. C. Lindgren and L. S. Ross, *Urologic Clinics of North America*, 2014, 41, 205–211.
6. E. K. Kalra, *AAPS PharmSci*, 2003, 5, E25.
7. N. A. Clark, M. Will, M. B. Moravek, and S. Fisseha, *International Journal of Gynecology and Obstetrics*, 2013, 122, 202–206.
8. V. Brower, *Nature Biotechnology*, 1998, 16, 728–731.
9. M. Valko, D. Leibfritz, J. Moncol, M. T. Cronin, M. Mazur, and J. Telser, *International Journal of Biochemistry & Cell Biology*, 2007, 39, 44–84.
10. A. Agarwal, R. A. Saleh, and M. A. Bedaiwy, *Fertility and Sterility*, 2003, 79, 829–843.
11. J. F. Griveau and D. Le Lannou, *International Journal of Andrology*, 1997, 20, 61–69.
12. J. C. Kefer, A. Agarwal, and E. Sabanegh, *International Journal of Urology: Official Journal of the Japanese Urological Association*, 2009, 16, 449–457.
13. Y. Sheynkin, R. Welliver, A. Winer, F. Hajimirzaee, H. Ahn, and K. Lee, *Fertility and Sterility*, 2011, 95, 647–651.

14. A. Jung and H. C. Schuppe, *Andrologia*, 2007, 39, 203–215.
15. R. Henkel, E. Kierspel, T. Stalf, C. Mehnert, R. Menkveld, H. R. Tinneberg, W. B. Schill, and T. F. Kruger, *Fertility and Sterility*, 2005, 83, 635–642.
16. I. M. Ebisch, C. M. Thomas, W. H. Peters, D. D. Braat, and R. P. Steegers-Theunissen, *Human Reproduction Update*, 2007, 13, 163–174.
17. M. A. Ghaffari and M. Rostami, *Journal of Reproduction & Infertility*, 2012, 13, 81–87.
18. T. C. Ryan, G. J. Weil, P. E. Newburger, R. Haugland, and E. R. Simons, *Journal of Immunological Methods*, 1990, 130, 223–233.
19. C. Ross, A. Morriss, M. Khairy, Y. Khalaf, P. Braude, A. Coomarasamy, and T. El-Toukhy, *Reproductive Biomedicine Online*, 2010, 20, 711–723.
20. P. S. Agarwal, S. A. Prabhakaran, and Sikka SC, *AUA Update Series*, 2007, 26, 1–12.
21. S. S. Young, B. Eskenazi, F. M. Marchetti, G. Block, and A. J. Wyrobek, *Human Reproduction*, 2008, 23, 1014–1022.
22. J. Mendiola, A. M. Torres-Cantero, J. Vioque, J. M. Moreno-Grau, J. Ten, M. Roca, S. Moreno-Grau, and R. Bernabeu, *Fertility and Sterility*, 2010, 93, 1128–1133.
23. N. Sermondade, C. Faure, L. Fezeu, A. G. Shayeb, J. P. Bonde, T. K. Jensen, M. Van Wely et al., *Human Reproduction Update*, 2013, 19, 221–231.
24. T. K. Jensen, A. M. Andersson, N. Jorgensen, A. G. Andersen, E. Carlsen, J. H. Petersen, and N. E. Skakkebaek, *Fertility and Sterility*, 2004, 82, 863–870.
25. M. L. Eisenberg, S. Kim, Z. Chen, R. Sundaram, E. F. Schisterman, and G. M. Buck Louis, *Human Reproduction*, 2014, 29, 193–200.
26. A. A. MacDonald, G. P. Herbison, M. Showell, and C. M. Farquhar, *Human Reproduction Update*, 2010, 16, 293–311.
27. G. M. Buck Louis, R. Sundaram, E. F. Schisterman, A. Sweeney, C. D. Lynch, S. Kim, J. M. Maisog, R. Gore-Langton, M. L. Eisenberg, and Z. Chen, *Fertility and Sterility*, 2014, 101, 453–462.
28. C. Faure, C. Dupont, M. A. Baraibar, R. Ladouce, I. Cedrin-Durnerin, J. P. Wolf, and R. Levy, *PLoS One*, 2014, 9, e86300.
29. S. S. Du Plessis, S. Cabler, D. A. McAlister, E. Sabanegh, and A. Agarwal, *Nature Reviews Urology*, 2010, 7, 153–161.
30. A. O. Hammoud, A. W. Meikle, L. O. Reis, M. Gibson, C. M. Peterson, and D. T. Carrell, *Seminars in Reproductive Medicine*, 2012, 30, 486–495.
31. T. Fullston, N. O. Palmer, J. A. Owens, M. Mitchell, H. W. Bakos, and M. Lane, *Human Reproduction*, 2012, 27, 1391–1400.
32. T. K. Jensen, B. L. Heitmann, M. B. Jensen, T. I. Halldorsson, A. M. Andersson, N. E. Skakkebaek, U. N. Joensen et al, *The American Journal of Clinical Nutrition*, 2013, 97, 411–418.
33. A. J. Gaskins, D. S. Colaci, J. Mendiola, S. H. Swan, and J. E. Chavarro, *Human Reproduction*, 2012, 27, 2899–2907.
34. G. Eslamian, N. Amirjannati, B. Rashidkhani, M. R. Sadeghi, and A. Hekmatdoost, *Human Reproduction*, 2012, 27, 3328–3336.
35. J. Mendiola, A. M. Torres-Cantero, J. M. Moreno-Grau, J. Ten, M. Roca, S. Moreno-Grau, and R. Bernabeu, *Fertility and Sterility*, 2009, 91, 812–818.
36. J. Pajarinen, V. Savolainen, M. Perola, A. Penttila, and P. J. Karhunen, *International Journal of Andrology*, 1996, 19, 314–322.
37. H. Klonoff-Cohen, P. Lam-Kruglick, and C. Gonzalez, *Fertility and Sterility*, 2003, 79, 330–339.
38. S. La Vignera, R. A. Condorelli, G. Balercia, E. Vicari, and A. E. Calogero, *Asian Journal Of Andrology*, 2013, 15, 221–225.
39. J. Olsen, F. Bolumar, J. Boldsen, and L. Bisanti, *Alcoholism-Clinical and Experimental Research*, 1997, 21, 206–212.
40. D. P. Braga, G. Halpern, C. Figueira Rde, A. S. Setti, A. Iaconelli, Jr., and E. Borges, Jr., *Fertility and Sterility*, 2012, 97, 53–59.
41. Office of Dietary Supplements, Dietary supplement fact sheets, http://ods.od.nih.gov/factsheets/list-all/, Accessed March 26, 2014.
42. J. Thundathil, E. de Lamirande, and C. Gagnon, *Biology of Reproduction*, 2003, 68, 1291–1298.
43. S. Sinclair, *Alternative Medicine Review*, 2000, 5, 28–38.
44. A. Schachter, J. A. Goldman, and Z. Zukerman, *The Journal of Urology*, 1973, 110, 311–313.
45. D. De Aloysio, R. Mantuano, M. Mauloni, and G. Nicoletti, *Acta Europaea Fertilitatis*, 1982, 13, 133–167.
46. J. Tanimura, *Bulletin of the Osaka Medical School*, 1967, 13, 84–89.

47. R. Stanislavov, V. Nikolova, and P. Rohdewald, *Phytotherapy Research*, 2009, 23, 297–302.
48. J. P. Pryor, J. P. Blandy, P. Evans, D. M. Chaput De Saintonge, and M. Usherwood, *British Journal of Urology*, 1978, 50, 47–50.
49. W. S. Kwon, Y. J. Park, Y. H. Kim, Y. A. You, I. C. Kim, and M. G. Pang, *PLoS One*, 2013, 8, e54192.
50. X. Zhou, F. Liu, and S. Zhai, *Asia Pacific Journal of Clinical Nutrition*, 2007, 16(Suppl 1), 383–390.
51. A. Lenzi, P. Sgro, P. Salacone, D. Paoli, B. Gilio, F. Lombardo, M. Santulli, A. Agarwal, and L. Gandini, *Fertility and Sterility*, 2004, 81, 1578–1584.
52. S. D. Ahmed, K. A. Karira, and J. S. Ahsan, *Journal of Pakistan Medical Association*, 2011, 61, 732–736.
53. K. Li, W. Li, Y. F. Huang, and X. J. Shang, *Zhonghua Nan Ke Xue*, 2007, 13, 143–146.
54. G. Balercia, F. Regoli, T. Armeni, A. Koverech, F. Mantero, and M. Boscaro, *Fertility and Sterility*, 2005, 84, 662–671.
55. M. G. Showell, J. Brown, A. Yazdani, M. T. Stankiewicz, and R. J. Hart, *The Cochrane Database of Systematic Reviews*, 2011, 19, CD007411, DOI: 10.1002/14651858.CD007411.pub2.
56. H. J. Cheng and T. Chen, *Zhonghua Nan Ke Xue*, 2008, 14, 149–151.
57. M. Moradi, A. Moradi, M. Alemi, H. Ahmadnia, H. Abdi, A. Ahmadi, and S. Bazargan-Hejazi, *Journal of Urology*, 2010, 7, 188–193.
58. S. Banihani, A. Agarwal, R. Sharma, and M. Bayachou, *Andrologia*, 2013, 46, 637–641.
59. M. Sigman, S. Glass, J. Campagnone, and J. L. Pryor, *Fertility and Sterility*, 2006, 85, 1409–1414.
60. F. Dimitriadis, S. Tsambalas, P. Tsounapi, H. Kawamura, E. Vlachopoulou, N. Haliasos, S. Gratsias et al., *BJU International*, 2010, 106, 1181–1185.
61. L. Ernster and P. Forsmark-Andree, *Clinical Investigation*, 1993, 71, S60–S65.
62. A. Mancini, L. De Marinis, G. P. Littarru, and G. Balercia, *BioFactors*, 2005, 25, 165–174.
63. A. Mancini, L. De Marinis, A. Oradei, M. E. Hallgass, G. Conte, D. Pozza, and G. P. Littarru, *Journal of Andrology*, 1994, 15, 591–594.
64. A. Mancini and G. Balercia, *BioFactors*, 2011, 37, 374–380.
65. M. R. Safarinejad, *The Journal of Urology*, 2009, 182, 237–248.
66. G. Balercia, E. Buldreghini, A. Vignini, L. Tiano, F. Paggi, S. Amoroso, G. Ricciardo-Lamonica, M. Boscaro, A. Lenzi, and G. Littarru, *Fertility and Sterility*, 2009, 91, 1785–1792.
67. R. Lafuente, M. Gonzalez-Comadran, I. Sola, G. Lopez, M. Brassesco, R. Carreras, and M. A. Checa, *Journal of Assisted Reproduction and Genetics*, 2013, 30, 1147–1156.
68. A. Nadjarzadeh, M. R. Sadeghi, N. Amirjannati, M. R. Vafa, S. A. Motevalian, M. R. Gohari, M. A. Akhondi, P. Yavari, and F. Shidfar, *Journal of Endocrinological Investigation*, 2011, 34, e224–e228.
69. A. Nadjarzadeh, F. Shidfar, N. Amirjannati, M. R. Vafa, S. A. Motevalian, M. R. Gohari, S. A. Nazeri Kakhki, M. M. Akhondi, and M. R. Sadeghi, *Andrologia*, 2014, 46, 177–183.
70. Y. Kobori, S. Ota, R. Sato, H. Yagi, S. Soh, G. Arai, and H. Okada, *Archivio italiano di urologia, andrologia: organo ufficiale [di] Societa italiana di ecografia urologica e nefrologica/Associazione ricerche in urologia*, 2014, 86, 1–4.
71. R. Joshi, S. Adhikari, B. S. Patro, S. Chattopadhyay, and T. Mukherjee, *Free Radical Biology & Medicine*, 2001, 30, 1390–1399.
72. M. Dietrich, C. J. Brown, and G. Block, *Journal of the American College of Nutrition*, 2005, 24, 266–274.
73. J. C. Boxmeer, M. Smit, E. Utomo, J. C. Romijn, M. J. Eijkemans, J. Lindemans, J. S. Laven, N. S. Macklon, E. A. Steegers, and R. P. Steegers-Theunissen, *Fertility and Sterility*, 2009, 92, 548–556.
74. A. Nadjarzadeh, A. Mehrsai, E. Mostafavi, M. R. Gohari, and F. Shidfar, *Medical Journal of the Islamic Republic of Iran*, 2013, 27, 204–209.
75. W. Y. Wong, H. M. Merkus, C. M. Thomas, R. Menkveld, G. A. Zielhuis, and R. P. Steegers-Theunissen, *Fertility and Sterility*, 2002, 77, 491–498.
76. I. M. Ebisch, F. H. Pierik, F. H. De Jong, C. M. Thomas, and R. P. Steegers-Theunissen, *International Journal of Andrology*, 2006, 29, 339–345.
77. B. Landau, R. Singer, T. Klein, and E. Segenreich, *Experientia*, 1978, 34, 1301–1302.
78. M. Raigani, B. Yaghmaei, N. Amirjannti, N. Lakpour, M. M. Akhondi, H. Zeraati, M. Hajihosseinal, and M. R. Sadeghi, *Andrologia*, 2013, 46, 956–962.
79. C. Ravel, S. Chantot-Bastaraud, C. Chalmey, L. Barreiro, I. Aknin-Seifer, J. Pfeffer, I. Berthaut et al., *PloS one*, 2009, 4, e6540.
80. A. Pompella, A. Visvikis, A. Paolicchi, V. De Tata, and A. F. Casini, *Biochemical Pharmacology*, 2003, 66, 1499–1503.
81. J. R. Drevet, *Molecular and Cellular Endocrinology*, 2006, 250, 70–79.

82. A. Lenzi, F. Culasso, L. Gandini, F. Lombardo, and F. Dondero, *Human Reproduction*, 1993, 8, 1657–1662.
83. H. Kodama, R. Yamaguchi, J. Fukuda, H. Kasai, and T. Tanaka, *Fertility and Sterility*, 1997, 68, 519–524.
84. A. Witschi, S. Reddy, B. Stofer, and B. H. Lauterburg, *European Journal of Clinical Pharmacology*, 1992, 43, 667–669.
85. A. V. Rao and L. G. Rao, *Pharmacological Research: The Official Journal of the Italian Pharmacological Society*, 2007, 55, 207–216.
86. K. Wertz, *Nutrition and Cancer*, 2009, 61, 775–783.
87. A. Zini, M. San Gabriel, and J. Libman, *Fertility and Sterility*, 2010, 94, 1033–1036.
88. N. P. Gupta and R. Kumar, *International Urology and Nephrology*, 2002, 34, 369–372.
89. R. Filipcikova, I. Oborna, J. Brezinova, J. Novotny, G. Wojewodka, J. B. De Sanctis, L. Radova, M. Hajduch, and D. Radzioch, *Biomedical Papers of the Medical Faculty of the University Palacky, Olomouc, Czechoslovakia*, (2013: e-publishing) 2015, 159, 77–82.
90. I. Oborna, K. Malickova, H. Fingerova, J. Brezinova, P. Horka, J. Novotny, H. Bryndova, R. Filipcikova, and M. Svobodova, *American Journal of Reproductive Immunology*, 2011, 66, 179–184.
91. A. Lenzi, L. Gandini, V. Maresca, R. Rago, P. Sgro, F. Dondero, and M. Picardo, *Molecular Human Reproduction*, 2000, 6, 226–231.
92. E. J. Chan and L. Cho, *Cleveland Clinic Journal of Medicine*, 2009, 76, 245–251.
93. M. R. Safarinejad, S. Y. Hosseini, F. Dadkhah, and M. A. Asgari, *Clinical Nutrition*, 2010, 29, 100–105.
94. M. R. Safarinejad, *Andrologia*, 2011, 43, 38–47.
95. J. A. Attaman, T. L. Toth, J. Furtado, H. Campos, R. Hauser, and J. E. Chavarro, *Human Reproduction*, 2012, 27, 1466–1474.
96. M. S. Buckley, A. D. Goff, and W. E. Knapp, *The Annals of Pharmacotherapy*, 2004, 38, 50–52.
97. P. E. Visconti, G. D. Moore, J. L. Bailey, P. Leclerc, S. A. Connors, D. Pan, P. Olds-Clarke, and G. S. Kopf, *Development*, 1995, 121, 1139–1150.
98. P. Leclerc, E. de Lamirande, and C. Gagnon, *Biology of Reproduction*, 1996, 55, 684–692.
99. C. J. De Jonge, H. L. Han, H. Lawrie, S. R. Mack, and L. J. Zaneveld, *The Journal of Experimental Zoology*, 1991, 258, 113–125.
100. V. B. Bhat and K. M. Madyastha, *Biochemical and Biophysical Research Communications*, 2001, 288, 1212–1217.
101. M. R. Safarinejad, *International Urology and Nephrology*, 2011, 43, 315–328.
102. L. Lefievre, E. de Lamirande, and C. Gagnon, *Biology of Reproduction*, 2002, 67, 423–430.
103. P. Terriou, E. Hans, C. Giorgetti, J. L. Spach, J. Salzmann, V. Urrutia, and R. Roulier, *Journal of Assisted Reproduction and Genetics*, 2000, 17, 194–199.
104. B. Faka, M. Api, C. Ficicioglu, A. Gurbuz, and O. Oral, *Acta Europaea Fertilitatis*, 1994, 25, 351–353.
105. S. J. Publicover and C. L. Barratt, *Molecular Human Reproduction*, 2011, 17, 453–456.
106. A. Giwercman, *Current Opinion in Urology*, 2011, 21, 519–526.
107. C. R. Cederroth, C. Zimmermann, and S. Nef, *Molecular and Cellular Endocrinology*, 2012, 355, 192–200.
108. G. G. Kuiper, J. G. Lemmen, B. Carlsson, J. C. Corton, S. H. Safe, P. T. van der Saag, B. van der Burg, and J. A. Gustafsson, *Endocrinology*, 1998, 139, 4252–4263.
109. C. R. Cederroth, J. Auger, C. Zimmermann, F. Eustache, and S. Nef, *International Journal of Andrology*, 2010, 33, 304–316.
110. K. Almstrup, M. F. Fernandez, J. H. Petersen, N. Olea, N. E. Skakkebaek, and H. Leffers, *Environmental Health Perspectives*, 2002, 110, 743–748.
111. H. Adlercreutz, Y. Mousavi, J. Clark, K. Hockerstedt, E. Hamalainen, K. Wahala, T. Makela, and T. Hase, *The Journal of Steroid Biochemistry and Molecular Biology*, 1992, 41, 331–337.
112. S. J. Bhathena and M. T. Velasquez, *The American Journal of Clinical Nutrition*, 2002, 76, 1191–1201.
113. M. T. Velasquez and S. J. Bhathena, *International Journal of Medical Sciences*, 2007, 4, 72–82.
114. S. S. Chiang and T. M. Pan, *Applied Microbiology and Biotechnology*, 2013, 97, 1489–1500.
115. F. M. Sacks, A. Lichtenstein, L. Van Horn, W. Harris, P. Kris-Etherton, M. Winston, and American Heart Association Nutrition Committee, *Circulation*, 2006, 113, 1034–1044.
116. C. C. Douglas, S. A. Johnson, and B. H. Arjmandi, *Anti-Cancer Agents in Medicinal Chemistry*, 2013, 13, 1178–1187.
117. N. Atanassova, C. McKinnell, K. J. Turner, M. Walker, J. S. Fisher, M. Morley, M. R. Millar, N. P. Groome, and R. M. Sharpe, *Endocrinology*, 2000, 141, 3898–3907.
118. C. R. Cederroth, C. Zimmermann, J. L. Beny, O. Schaad, C. Combepine, P. Descombes, D. R. Doerge, F. P. Pralong, J. D. Vassalli, and S. Nef, *Molecular and Cellular Endocrinology*, 2010, 321, 152–160.

119. A. B. Wisniewski, S. L. Klein, Y. Lakshmanan, and J. P. Gearhart, *The Journal of Urology*, 2003, 169, 1582–1586.
120. M. A. Yi, H. M. Son, J. S. Lee, C. S. Kwon, J. K. Lim, Y. K. Yeo, Y. S. Park, and J. S. Kim, *Nutrition and Cancer*, 2002, 42, 206–210.
121. L. Q. Cai, J. Cai, W. Wu, and Y. S. Zhu, *The Journal of Urology*, 2011, 186, 1489–1496.
122. J. H. Mitchell, E. Cawood, D. Kinniburgh, A. Provan, A. R. Collins, and D. S. Irvine, *Clinical Science*, 2001, 100, 613–618.
123. J. E. Chavarro, T. L. Toth, S. M. Sadio, and R. Hauser, *Human Reproduction*, 2008, 23, 2584–2590.
124. C. Nagata, S. Inaba, N. Kawakami, T. Kakizoe, and H. Shimizu, *Nutrition and Cancer*, 2000, 36, 14–18.
125. C. Nagata, N. Takatsuka, H. Shimizu, H. Hayashi, T. Akamatsu, and K. Murase, *Cancer Epidemiology, Biomarkers & Prevention: A Publication of the American Association for Cancer Research, Cosponsored by the American Society of Preventive Oncology*, 2001, 10, 179–184.
126. R. C. Habito, J. Montalto, E. Leslie, and M. J. Ball, *The British Journal of Nutrition*, 2000, 84, 557–563.
127. J. Bhatia, F. Greer, and American Academy of Pediatrics Committee on Nutrition, *Pediatrics*, 2008, 121, 1062–1068.
128. R. M. Sharpe, B. Martin, K. Morris, I. Greig, C. McKinnell, A. S. McNeilly, and M. Walker, *Human Reproduction*, 2002, 17, 1692–1703.
129. K. A. Tan, M. Walker, K. Morris, I. Greig, J. I. Mason, and R. M. Sharpe, *Human Reproduction*, 2006, 21, 896–904.
130. B. L. Strom, R. Schinnar, E. E. Ziegler, K. T. Barnhart, M. D. Sammel, G. A. Macones, V. A. Stallings, J. M. Drulis, S. E. Nelson, and S. A. Hanson, *JAMA*, 2001, 286, 807–814.
131. J. T. Rotruck, A. L. Pope, H. E. Ganther, A. B. Swanson, D. G. Hafeman, and W. G. Hoekstra, *Science*, 1973, 179, 588–590.
132. R. F. Burk, K. E. Hill, and A. K. Motley, *The Journal of Nutrition*, 2003, 133, 1517S-1520S.
133. F. Ursini, S. Heim, M. Kiess, M. Maiorino, A. Roveri, J. Wissing, and L. Flohe, *Science*, 1999, 285, 1393–1396.
134. K. M. Brown and J. R. Arthur, *Public Health Nutrition*, 2001, 4, 593–599.
135. C. Boitani and R. Puglisi, *Advances in Experimental Medicine and Biology*, 2008, 636, 65–73.
136. D. Vezina, F. Mauffette, K. D. Roberts, and G. Bleau, *Biological Trace Element Research*, 1996, 53, 65–83.
137. M. R. Safarinejad and S. Safarinejad, *The Journal of Urology*, 2009, 181, 741–751.
138. T. Watanabe and A. Endo, *Mutation Research*, 1991, 262, 93–99.
139. J. Marin-Guzman, D. C. Mahan, and J. L. Pate, *Journal of Animal Science*, 2000, 78, 1537–1543.
140. M. I. Camejo, L. Abdala, G. Vivas-Acevedo, R. Lozano-Hernandez, M. Angeli-Greaves, and E. D. Greaves, *Biological Trace Element Research*, 2011, 143, 1247–1254.
141. M. K. Moslemi and S. Tavanbakhsh, *International Journal of General Medicine*, 2011, 4, 99–104.
142. L. Keskes-Ammar, N. Feki-Chakroun, T. Rebai, Z. Sahnoun, H. Ghozzi, S. Hammami, K. Zghal, H. Fki, J. Damak, and A. Bahloul, *Archives of Andrology*, 2003, 49, 83–94.
143. R. Scott, A. MacPherson, R. W. Yates, B. Hussain, and J. Dixon, *British Journal of Urology*, 1998, 82, 76–80.
144. W. C. Hawkes and P. J. Turek, *Journal of Andrology*, 2001, 22, 764–772.
145. K. Iwanier and B. A. Zachara, *Journal of Andrology*, 1995, 16, 441–447.
146. M. Zhong, R. Kawaguchi, M. Kassai, and H. Sun, *Nutrients*, 2012, 4, 2069–2096.
147. A. Kamal-Eldin and L. A. Appelqvist, *Lipids*, 1996, 31, 671–701.
148. S. S. Chung and D. J. Wolgemuth, *Cytogenetic and Genome Research*, 2004, 105, 189–202.
149. A. Morales and J. C. Cavicchia, *Tissue & Cell*, 2002, 34, 349–355.
150. G. Paradiso Galatioto, G. L. Gravina, G. Angelozzi, A. Sacchetti, P. F. Innominato, G. Pace, G. Ranieri, and C. Vicentini, *World Journal of Urology*, 2008, 26, 97–102.
151. L. Ovesen, *Drugs*, 1984, 27, 148–170.
152. C. L. Linster and E. Van Schaftingen, *The FEBS Journal*, 2007, 274, 1–22.
153. S. J. Padayatty, A. Katz, Y. Wang, P. Eck, O. Kwon, J. H. Lee, S. Chen et al., *Journal of the American College of Nutrition*, 2003, 22, 18–35.
154. E. B. Dawson, W. A. Harris, W. E. Rankin, L. A. Charpentier, and W. J. McGanity, *Annals of the New York Academy of Sciences*, 1987, 498, 312–323.
155. E. Greco, M. Iacobelli, L. Rienzi, F. Ubaldi, S. Ferrero, and J. Tesarik, *Journal of Andrology*, 2005, 26, 349–353.
156. A. H. Colagar and E. T. Marzony, *Journal of Clinical Biochemistry and Nutrition*, 2009, 45, 144–149.
157. E. B. Dawson, W. A. Harris, M. C. Teter, and L. C. Powell, *Fertility and Sterility*, 1992, 58, 1034–1039.

158. C. Rolf, T. G. Cooper, C. H. Yeung, and E. Nieschlag, *Human Reproduction*, 1999, 14, 1028–1033.
159. M. F. Holick, *The New England Journal of Medicine*, 2007, 357, 266–281.
160. S. T. Corbett, O. Hill, and A. K. Nangia, *Urology*, 2006, 68, 1345–1349.
161. S. Aquila, C. Guido, I. Perrotta, S. Tripepi, A. Nastro, and S. Ando, *Journal of Anatomy*, 2008, 213, 555–564.
162. M. Blomberg Jensen, J. E. Nielsen, A. Jorgensen, E. Rajpert-De Meyts, D. M. Kristensen, N. Jorgensen, N. E. Skakkebaek, A. Juul, and H. Leffers, *Human Reproduction*, 2010, 25, 1303–1311.
163. G. Jones, S. A. Strugnell, and H. F. DeLuca, *Physiological Reviews*, 1998, 78, 1193–1231.
164. R. Bouillon, G. Carmeliet, L. Verlinden, E. van Etten, A. Verstuyf, H. F. Luderer, L. Lieben, C. Mathieu, and M. Demay, *Endocrine Reviews*, 2008, 29, 726–776.
165. T. I. Ellison, D. R. Dowd, and P. N. MacDonald, *Molecular Endocrinology*, 2005, 19, 2309–2319.
166. G. G. Kwiecinski, G. I. Petrie, and H. F. DeLuca, *The Journal of Nutrition*, 1989, 119, 741–744.
167. M. Blomberg Jensen, P. J. Bjerrum, T. E. Jessen, J. E. Nielsen, U. N. Joensen, I. A. Olesen, J. H. Petersen, A. Juul, S. Dissing, and N. Jorgensen, *Human Reproduction*, 2011, 26, 1307–1317.
168. D. M. Lee, A. Tajar, S. R. Pye, S. Boonen, D. Vanderschueren, R. Bouillon, T. W. O'Neill et al, *European Journal of Endocrinology/European Federation of Endocrine Societies*, 2012, 166, 77–85.
169. S. Pilz, S. Frisch, H. Koertke, J. Kuhn, J. Dreier, B. Obermayer-Pietsch, E. Wehr, and A. Zittermann, *Hormone and Metabolic Research = Hormon- und Stoffwechselforschung = Hormones et Metabolisme*, 2011, 43, 223–225.
170. C. H. Ramlau-Hansen, U. K. Moeller, J. P. Bonde, J. Olsen, and A. M. Thulstrup, *Fertility and Sterility*, 2011, 95, 1000–1004.
171. F. Alshahrani and N. Aljohani, *Nutrients*, 2013, 5, 3605–3616.
172. J. R. Palamanda and J. P. Kehrer, *Lipids*, 1993, 28, 427–431.
173. R. Brigelius-Flohe and M. G. Traber, *FASEB Journal: Official Publication of the Federation of American Societies for Experimental Biology*, 1999, 13, 1145–1155.
174. K. U. Ingold, A. C. Webb, D. Witter, G. W. Burton, T. A. Metcalfe, and D. P. Muller, *Archives of Biochemistry and Biophysics*, 1987, 259, 224–225.
175. C. Mora-Esteves and D. Shin, *Seminars in Reproductive Medicine*, 2013, 31, 293–300.
176. E. Kessopoulou, H. J. Powers, K. K. Sharma, M. J. Pearson, J. M. Russell, I. D. Cooke, and C. L. Barratt, *Fertility and Sterility*, 1995, 64, 825–831.
177. B. Eskenazi, S. A. Kidd, A. R. Marks, E. Sloter, G. Block, and A. J. Wyrobek, *Human Reproduction*, 2005, 20, 1006–1012.
178. S. A. Suleiman, M. E. Ali, Z. M. Zaki, E. M. el-Malik, and M. A. Nasr, *Journal of Andrology*, 1996, 17, 530–537.
179. A. Bendich, *Annals of the New York Academy of Sciences*, 1992, 669, 300–310; discussion 311–302.
180. E. Lonn, J. Bosch, S. Yusuf, P. Sheridan, J. Pogue, J. M. Arnold, C. Ross et al., *JAMA*, 2005, 293, 1338–1347.
181. P. Weber, A. Bendich, and L. J. Machlin, *Nutrition*, 1997, 13, 450–460.
182. S. A. Mousa, *Methods in Molecular Biology*, 2010, 663, 229–240.
183. A. H. Colagar, E. T. Marzony, and M. J. Chaichi, *Nutrition Research*, 2009, 29, 82–88.
184. A. E. Omu, M. K. Al-Azemi, E. O. Kehinde, J. T. Anim, M. A. Oriowo, and T. C. Mathew, *Medical Principles and Practice: International Journal of the Kuwait University, Health Science Centre*, 2008, 17, 108–116.
185. A. E. Omu, H. Dashti, and S. Al-Othman, *European Journal of Obstetrics, Gynecology, and Reproductive Biology*, 1998, 79, 179–184.
186. M. H. Hadwan, L. A. Almashhedy, and A. R. Alsalman, *Reproductive Biology and Endocrinology: RB&E*, 2014, 12, 1.
187. B. Urman and O. Oktem, *Seminars in Reproductive Medicine*, 2014, 32, 245–252.
188. P. M. Barnes, B. Bloom, and R. L. Nahin, *National Health Statistics Reports*, 2008, 10, 1–23.
189. K. Tremellen, G. Miari, D. Froiland, and J. Thompson, *The Australian & New Zealand Journal of Obstetrics & Gynaecology*, 2007, 47, 216–221.
190. C. De Jonge, *Fertility and Sterility*, 2012, 97, 260–266.

31 Sexual Dysfunctions and Nutraceutical Therapy

An Examination of Human Research

Gene Bruno

CONTENTS

INTRODUCTION

Although there are a range of sexual dysfunctions, the focus of this chapter is the examination of strictly human research in which specific nutraceuticals have shown promise in the treatment of specific sexual dysfunctions, including erectile dysfunction (ED), hypogonadism/low T, low estradiol, and sexual dissatisfaction.

31.1 PREVALENCE OF SEXUAL DYSFUNCTIONS

A 2006 study in the *Journal of Sexual Medicine* (Lewis et al. 2006) reported that in an effort to provide recommendations and guidelines concerning epidemiology and risk factors for sexual dysfunctions in men and women, an international consultation in collaboration with the major urology and sexual medicine associations assembled over 200 multidisciplinary experts from 60 countries into 17 committees. Results showed that the prevalence of sexual dysfunction increases as men and women age. Approximately, 40%–45% of adult women and 20%–30% of adult men had at least one manifest sexual dysfunction. The study also found that the incidence rate for ED was 25–30 cases per thousand person-years and increases with age.

In a 1999 analysis of data from the National Health and Social Life Survey, including a national probability sample of 1749 women and 1410 men aged 18–59 years, the risk of experiencing sexual dysfunction as well as negative concomitant outcomes was assessed (Laumann et al. 1999). The results showed the prevalence of sexual dysfunction in 43% of women and 31% of men and was found to be more likely among women and men with poor physical and emotional health. Differences were also seen with various demographic characteristics, including age and educational attainment. Not surprisingly, sexual dysfunction was highly associated with negative experiences in sexual relationships and overall well-being.

More recently, Kingsberg and Rezaee (2013) conducted a literature review that, in part, examined the epidemiology of low sexual desire/hypoactive sexual desire disorder (HSDD). They found a high prevalence of low sexual desire (43%) and close to a 10% prevalence of HSDD.

31.2 D-ASPARTIC ACID

Potential application(s): Hypogonadism/low testosterone (T)

31.2.1 Background

An endogenous amino acid, D-aspartic acid, is found in the nervous and endocrine tissues of many other animals, including humans (D'Aniello 2007). D-Aspartic acid occurs at very high concentrations in the pituitary, testis, ovary, pineal, and adrenal glands and has also been found in Leydig cells in rat testis fluid, and in epididymal spermatozoa. Results from *in vitro* research have demonstrated that D-aspartic acid is capable of inducing the synthesis and release of testosterone and progesterone from the gonads (D'Aniello et al. 2005).

31.2.2 Clinical Research

To investigate the effect of this D-aspartic acid on the release of luteinizing hormone (LH) and testosterone (T), a placebo-controlled trial (Topo et al. 2009) was conducted in which healthy male volunteers (aged 27–37 years) (experimental group n = 23, placebo group n = 20) consumed 3.12 g L-aspartic as sodium D-aspartate (with vitamin B6, folic acid, and vitamin B12) in 10 mL of water or fruit juice, every morning at breakfast for 12 consecutive days or a placebo solution with sodium chloride. Blood samples were taken in the morning between 9:30 and 10:30 a.m. (when serum oscillations of LH and testosterone are at their minimum value before treatment), 6 and 12 days after treatment, and 3 days after suspension of the treatment. The results were that after 12 days of D-aspartic acid treatment, 87% of participants had significantly increased blood concentrations of LH (33.3% increase, $P < 0.0001$). There was no significant LH in the placebo group. Likewise, 87% of participants using D-aspartic acid had a 42% increase in serum testosterone concentrations (from a mean of 4.5 ± 0.6 to 6.4 ± 0.8 ng/mL, $P < 0.0082$).

31.2.3 Adverse Reactions/Drug Interactions

There are no reported adverse reactions or drug interactions associated with D-aspartic acid supplementation (Natural Medicines Comprehensive Database 2014).

31.2.4 Comments

While the increase in LH and T resulting from D-aspartic acid supplementation is significant, the study does not reveal the amount of vitamin B6, folic acid, and vitamin B12 that were included in the solution. This solution is marketed in Italy under the name DADAVIT®, but a quick internet search did not reveal that this product is readily available for purchase. In any case, additional human clinical research is necessary to corroborate the results of this single study.

31.3 FENUGREEK

Potential application(s):

Hypogonadism/low T (male)
Low estradiol (female)
Sexual satisfaction (male and female)
Sexual arousal (female)

31.3.1 Background

In Ayurveda, fenugreek (*Trigonella foenum-graecum*) is called methika and its seeds have been used as medicine for the treatment of wounds, abscesses, arthritis, bronchitis, and digestive disorders. In traditional Chinese medicine, fenugreek is used as a treatment for kidney disorders affecting the male reproductive tract. More recent studies have examined the potential benefit of fenugreek for the treatment of atherosclerosis, constipation, diabetes, hypercholesterolemia, and hypertriglyceridemia (Yadav et al. 2011). In addition, a few different human clinical studies have examined the effects of different, proprietary fenugreek seed extracts on testosterone levels and other aspects of human performance.

31.3.2 Clinical Research

Testofen® (Gencor Nutrients) is a fenugreek seed extract standardized to 50% Fenuside™, a proprietary term used to describe phytochemical constituents, which include furostanol saponins, and steroidal saponins. Libifem™ (Gencor Nutrients) is the exact same fenugreek seed extract, but marketed to women. Testosurge™ (Biotech, India) is a fenugreek seed extract standardized for 80% grecunin, a compound whose name does not appear in the literature.

31.3.2.1 Testofen Study 1

An 8-week, prospective, double-blind, randomized, placebo-controlled study (Unpublished 2008) was conducted to determine the effect of Testofen on safety, anabolic activity, blood testosterone, immune function, body composition, creatinine, prolactin, and muscle mass variation during 8 weeks of intense resistance exercise. The participants were 60 healthy males, aged 18–35, and trained at least for a period of 1 month for resistance exercise. Twice daily, the Active group received a tablet, which provided 300 mg Testofen brand fenugreek extract powder. Assessment was performed via standard blood hematology and biochemistry variables, vital signs, and anthropometric methods. The results were as follows:

- *Blood urea nitrogen (BUN)*: BUN can be a measure of nitrogen uptake and retention, signifying anabolic activity. A decrease in BUN signifies anabolic activity. The Testofen group demonstrated significant anabolic activity as evidenced by BUN reduction ($P < 0.05$) compared to placebo.
- *Free T*: Although free testosterone increases in both groups, the Testofen group's increase was double of that in the placebo group's (percentage change 96% Testofen, 48% placebo). After adjusting for plasma changes, it acquires a significant value ($P < 0.05$). Thus, the Testofen group showed significant increase with respect to baseline ($P < 0.0001$) and with respect to placebo ($P < 0.05$).
- *Immunity*: Intense and chronic exercise often leads to impairment of immunity. The Testofen group experienced an increase in lymphocytes with respect to baseline. The placebo group experienced a significant decrease with respect to baseline ($P < 0.02$). If we look at the percentage change, Testofen had a significant increase in lymphocytes with respect to placebo ($P < 0.03$), demonstrating that Testofen not only compensated the loss of immunity significantly compared to placebo but has also increased immunity.
- *Creatinine*: Serum creatinine indicates the level of degradation of creatine from muscle tissues in normal subjects having good kidney function. Serum creatinine has decreased significantly in both Testofen and placebo groups, signifying that creatine uptake and recycle in muscle are increased by exercise. However, Testofen group showed a percentage decrease of 16.66 compared to placebo of 4.99 ($P < 0.02$). This confirms that Testofen exerts a beneficial effect on creatine uptake and recycle in muscle cells over and above physical workout.
- *Body fat*: Testofen has shown a significant ($P = 0.003$) decrease in body fat compared to baseline. This decrease was seen in the triceps, thigh, and chest. While the placebo group also saw a decrease in body fat, the percentage changes were not significant.

31.3.2.2 Testofen Study 2

A double-blind, randomized, placebo-controlled study (Steels et al. 2011) was conducted to assess the effectiveness of Testofen on sexual function (libido), as well as its effects on general health, muscle mass, energy, sleep, and mood. The safety and tolerability of Testofen was also evaluated. The participants were healthy heterosexual males aged between 21 and 50 years of age. Initially, 60 participants were enrolled in the trial. There were 6 withdrawals from the study (3 from the Active group and 3 from the placebo group), so the analysis was completed on the remaining 54 participants. Twice daily, the Active group received a tablet, which provided 300 mg Testofen brand fenugreek extract powder, 225 mg magnesium aspartate equivalent to 16.875 mg magnesium, 78.75 mg zinc amino acid chelate 20% equivalent to 15 mg zinc, and 6.80 mg pyridoxine HCL equivalent to 4.94 mg vitamin B6. To determine the effectiveness of Testofen on sexual function, performance, and satisfaction, the validated quantitative Derogatis Interview for Sexual Functioning (DISF-SR) (Male) was used. The DISF-SR consists of a total of 21 questions divided into 4 domains that ask about different aspects of sexual experiences: sexual fantasies, kinds of sexual arousal, nature of sexual experiences, and quality of orgasm. The intergroup difference between active and placebo was calculated at week 3 and week 6. A statistically significant intergroup difference was found at week 6 ($P = 0.004$), supporting the hypothesis that Testofen improves libido in healthy adult males. Improvements in the various domains of sexual function were noted (Figure 31.1):

In addition, statistically significant improvements were also found in performance, muscle, strength, energy, and stamina.

Muscle and strength: There were also higher ratings in muscle mass with 63.0% (17 of 27) reporting greater satisfaction with muscle (6.0–6.9, $P < 0.001$). This was also accompanied by higher ratings in strength in 66.7% (18 of 27) with an average change of 6.1–7.1 ($P < 0.001$). There was no change observed in the placebo group in either muscle mass or strength.

Energy and stamina: In the Active group, 77.8% (21 of 27) also reported a higher rating in energy levels. The average change was (5.7–7.5, $P < 0.001$). There was less noticeable changes in the area of stamina, with 51.2% (13 of 27) reporting a higher rating, with the average change of 6.1–7.3 ($P < 0.001$). There was no change observed in the placebo group in these parameters.

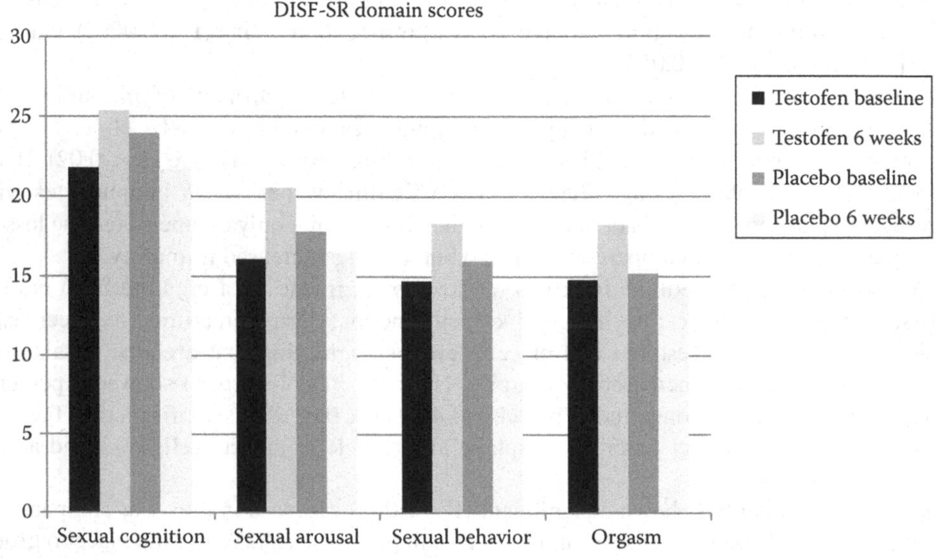

FIGURE 31.1 Improvements in various domains of sexual function with Testofen.

31.3.2.3 Libifem

A short-term, phase III, single site, double-blind, randomized, placebo-controlled study (Rao et al. 2012) was conducted on 80 healthy menstruating women (aged 21–49) in stable relationships, to evaluate the effect of 300 mg Libifem twice daily over 2 menstrual cycles (starting in follicular phase) on sexual function, hormonal profile, and metabolism. The DISF-SR and FSFI self-administered questionnaires at baseline, 4 weeks, and 8 weeks to measure sexual functioning. The sex hormone profile and specific markers of metabolism were measured at baseline and 8 weeks. Results were that DISF-SR and the FSFI questionnaires showed a significant increase in sexual functioning in those participants in the Libifem group after 8 weeks. This included significant increases in the subanalysis of the 5 domains of the DISF-SR at week 4 and week 8: sexual cognition/fantasy, sexual arousal, sexual experience, orgasm, and sexual drive/relationship. The placebo group showed no difference in the DISF-SR domain scores except for a significant increase in sexual drive/relationship at week 8 of treatment (Figure 31.2).

There was also a significant change in the domains of the FSFI in the Libifem group, primarily arousal at week 8, but no significant change in the placebo group.

After 8 weeks estradiol, it increased from 202.9 to 327.2 pmol/L in the Libifem group with no significant differences in the placebo group. There was a significant ($P < 0.05$) intergroup difference between Libifem group and placebo group at 8 weeks. The levels of free testosterone increased and SHBG decreased in the Libifem group and the opposite effect was observed in the placebo group, but these changes were not significant.

31.3.2.4 Testosurge

A double-blind, placebo-controlled study (Wilborn et al. 2010) examined the effects of a once daily 500 mg dose of Testosurge (TS, N = 17, 21 ± 2.8 years) or placebo (PL, N = 13, 21 ± 3 years) on strength, body composition, and hormonal profiles in 30 resistance-trained men for 8 weeks. Participants participated in a 4-day per week resistance-training program. At weeks 0, 4, and 8, body composition, 1-repetition-maximum (1RM) bench press and leg press, muscle endurance, anaerobic power, and hormonal profiles were assessed. Results showed significant group × time interaction effects for:

- Percent body fat (TS: −1.77% ± 1.52%, PL: −0.55% ± 1.72%; P = 0.048)
- Total testosterone (TS: 0.97 ± 2.67 ng/mL, PL: −2.10 ± 3.75 ng/mL; P = 0.018)
- Bioavailable testosterone (TS: 1.32 ± 3.45 ng/mL, PL: −1.69 ± 3.94 ng/mL; P = 0.049)

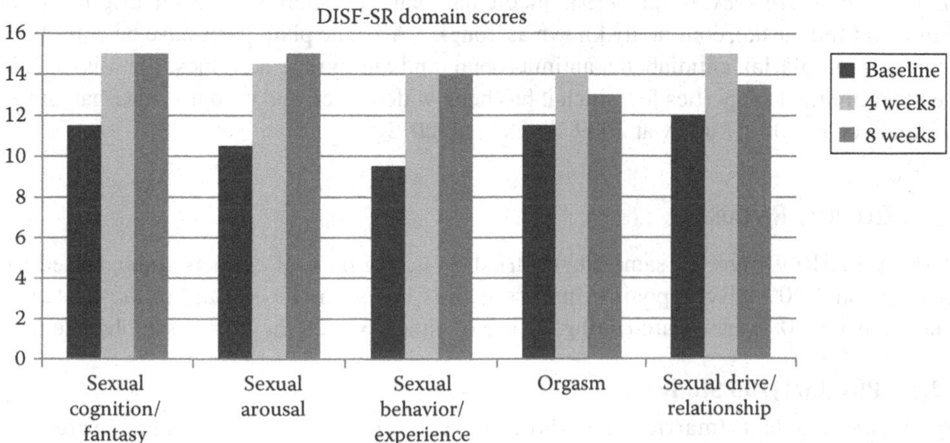

FIGURE 31.2 Increases in the subanalysis of the five domains of the DISF-SR at week 4 and week 8 with Libifem.

In addition, there were significant main effects for time ($P \leq 0.05$) for bench- and leg-press 1RM, lean body mass, and estradiol. There were no significant changes for Wingate peak or mean power, total body weight, dihydrotestosterone, hemodynamic variables, or clinical safety data.

31.3.3 Adverse Reactions/Drug Interactions

Reported adverse reactions and drug interactions are generally associated with the consumption of fenugreek seeds (Natural Medicines Comprehensive Database 2014), not extracts such as Testofen, Libifem, or Testosurge. In a previously cited study (Unpublished 2008), Testofen was very well tolerated by all subjects in 8 weeks, with normal safety parameters associated with blood biochemistry, kidney function, liver function, and immune function. Allergic reaction to fenugreek may result in symptoms including nasal congestion, hoarseness, persistent coughing, wheezing, facial angioedema, and shock (Patil et al. 1997).

31.3.4 Comments

The fact that SHBG levels decreased in the Libifem study (albeit not to a statistically significant level) suggests that this is the mechanism of action by which Testofen was shown to increase free T levels.

According to Wilborn et al. (2010), Testosurge is purported to inhibit aromatase and 5-α reductase activity. However, their study did not measure these activities directly; so at this point, it cannot be definitively stated that these are the mechanisms of action for this particular extract. Additional research would help to better define this issue.

31.4 EURYCOMA LONGIFOLIA

Potential application(s):

Hypgonadism/Low T (male)
Sexual satisfaction (male and female)

31.4.1 Background

Eurycoma longifolia Jack is an herbal medicinal plant of southeast Asian origin (Malaysia, Thailand, and Indonesia), commonly known as Tongkat Ali. The plant parts have been traditionally used for its antimalarial, antidiabetic, antimicrobial, and antipyretic activities, but it is its aphrodisiac/sexual stimulant properties for which it has been widely used and recognized (Bhat and Karim 2010, Handa et al. 2006, Ramawat 2009, Singh et al. 2012).

31.4.2 Clinical Research

Physta™ and LJ100™ are the same freeze-dried *E. longifolia* root extracts standardized to 22% eurypeptides and 40% glycosaponins. In Europe, it is known as Physta and in the United States, it is known as LJ100. Any research citing the use of either extract, therefore, is applicable to both.

31.4.2.1 Physta/LJ100 Study 1

Thirty human volunteers (married men whose age ranges between 31 and 52 years) were recruited in a 3-week, randomized open trial (Tambi and Saad 2000). Subjects received 100 mg daily of LJ100. At baseline, 1 week, and 3 weeks, peripheral venous blood sample was collected from volunteers to evaluate their total testosterone hormone, DHEA sulfate (DHEA), and sex hormone–binding globulin (SHBG) levels; and the volunteers filled out two questionnaires: (1) a validated Sexual Health Inventory Questionnaires (SHIQ) and (2) the Partial Androgen Deficiency in Aging Men (PADAM) Score Questionnaires. Results showed that DHEA levels gradually increased from 26% after 1 week to 47% after 3 weeks. SHBG levels decreased in 36% of the cases after one week, and 66% after 3 weeks. The free testosterone index (FTI is calculated as a percentage of the total testosterone against SHBG) escalated in 39% of the subjects after 1 week to 73% after 3 weeks. Analysis of the SHIQ demonstrated that 62% of the cases had either increased or maximum scores after consuming LJ100. Another 24% showed reduction while 14% of the cases showed no change in the score. Analysis of the PADAM score demonstrated that 82% of the cases showed a decrease in the total score. There was 91% improvement of sexual component of PADAM score, 73% improvement in physical component, and 82% improvement of psychological component of PADAM Score. The vasomotor score showed improvement in 50% of the subjects.

31.4.2.2 Physta/LJ100 Study 2

In an open label, clinical trial (Unpublished n.d.), saliva testosterone tests were conducted on 9 individuals 26–52 years of age. Five of the volunteers were athletes, while four of the volunteers did not exercise on a regular basis. All volunteers received 100 mg of LJ100 twice daily, once in the morning and once in the evening for 10 days. The data are an average of three different studies at different times. Results show that the mean increase in testosterone for all subjects was 71.55%. The mean increase in athletes only was 90.52%, while the mean increase for nonathletes only was 47.83%. Following are the data in the pre- and posttreatment blood levels of testosterone for each volunteer (Table 31.1).

31.4.2.3 Physta/LJ100 Study 3

A placebo-controlled study (Talbott et al. 2006) was conducted to determine the effects of Physta on testosterone and cortisol levels during intense endurance exercise. Male subjects (N = 30) were recruited from a 24 h mountain biking event and asked to provide a saliva sample before and after each lap for measurement of cortisol and testosterone by enzyme immunoassay. Subjects consumed 100 mg of Physta (N = 15) or a placebo (N = 15) approximately 30 min prior performing 4 laps (14.91 miles/lap) and providing 8 saliva samples over a 24 h period. Results showed that, compared to placebo, cortisol levels were 32.3% lower and testosterone levels were 16.4% higher with Physta (Table 31.2):

Researchers concluded that Physta may help promote an overall *anabolic* hormonal state during intense endurance exercise.

TABLE 31.1
Pre- and Post-Treatment Blood Levels of Testosterone with Physta

Volunteer	Age	Pretreatment ng/dL Blood	After Treatment ng/dL Blood Increase	%
1	26	860 = 30	1650 = 50	91.86
2	28	580 = 30	985 = 35	69.83
3	35	875 = 40	1576 = 60	80.11
4	24	950 = 45	2210 = 55	132.63
5	29	755 = 30	1345 = 35	78.15
6	48	650 = 20	875 = 30	34.62
7	52	450 = 25	765 = 35	70.00
8	50	585 = 25	875 = 35	49.57
9	42	350 = 30	480 = 35	37.14

TABLE 31.2
Differences in Cortisol and Testosterone Levels with Physta

	Physta	Placebo	Significance between Groups
Cortisol	0.552 + 0.665 µg/dL	0.816 + 0.775 µg/dL	P < 0.05
Testosterone	86.72 + 40.90 pg/mL	72.47 + 33.77 pg/mL	P < 0.05

31.4.2.4 Physta/LJ100 Study 4

A double-blind, placebo-controlled human clinical trial (Tambi 2009) was conducted in which 20 male volunteers of various health conditions from the ages of 38–58 were randomly given 200, 400, or 600 mg* Physta or placebo daily for 2 months. The results were that all three dosage levels resulted in elevated SHIM scores and showed improvements in sexual desire and performance. Likewise, the AMS score showed improvement in sexual, physical, psychology, and vasomotor domains for the majority of volunteers. Testosterone and DHEAS levels showed high normal levels when compared to baseline. Diabetic volunteers showed an improved level of blood glucose. The cortisol levels were fluctuating, suggesting the extract modulates the release of cortisol. The majority of volunteers had high normal levels of thyroxin and IGF-1 compared to the placebo group. There were no changes to the tumor markers, liver function, renal function, blood profile and lipid profile, though the majority showed elevation of HDL.

31.4.2.5 Physta/LJ100 Study 5

This study (Tambi and Imran 2010) investigated the effect of treatment with 200 mg/day Physta on male fertility with regard to higher semen volumes, sperm concentrations, the percentage of normal sperm morphology, and sperm motility in 75 male partners of subfertile couples with idiopathic infertility. Follow-up semen analyses were performed every 3 months for 9 months. Results showed that the mean sperm motility at the first cycle of treatment was significantly increased from baseline ($P = 0.037$), and increases from baseline in the mean sperm concentration (65.5%, $P = 0.007$) and sperm with normal morphology (94.9%, $P = 0.007$) occurred in the third cycle. Additionally, there were 11 (14.7%) spontaneous pregnancies during this time, 6 of which were achieved at completion of the first cycle of treatment and 5 of which were achieved at completion of 2 cycles of treatment.

31.4.2.6 Physta/LJ100 Study 6

A 12-week randomized, double-blind, placebo-controlled, parallel group study (Ismail et al. 2012) was conducted to investigate the efficacy of 300 mg/day Physta versus placebo in 109 men (30–55 years). Primary endpoints were quality of live (SF-36 questionnaire) and sexual well-being (International Index of Erectile Function (IIEF) and sexual health questionnaires (SHQ), seminal fluid analysis (SFA), fat mass and safety profiles, the changes of which were compared using repeated measures ANOVA analysis. Results showed that the Physta group experienced significant improvements in the domain physical functioning (SF-36) from baseline to week 12 compared to placebo ($P = 0.006$) and in between group at week 12 ($P = 0.028$). The Physta group also showed higher scores in the overall erectile function domain in IIEF ($P < 0.001$), sexual libido (14% by week 12), SFA: with sperm motility at 44.4%, and semen volume at 18.2% at the end of treatment. Furthermore, subjects with BMI ≥ 25 kg/m^2 significantly improved in fat mass lost ($P = 0.008$). All safety parameters were comparable to placebo.

* This was a poster presentation form the Proceedings of the Third Asia-Pacific Forum on Andrology, published in *Asian Journal of Andrology*. Since the abstract lacked some data about which doses were associated with efficacy, the author was contacted and provided the information that efficacy was achieved at all three dosage levels.

31.4.2.7 Physta/LJ100 Study 7

In an open-label trial (Tambi et al. 2012), 76 of 320 patients suffering from late-onset hypogonadism (LOH) were given 200 mg of Physta for 1 month. Patients were assessed using The Ageing Males' Symptoms (AMS) standardized rating scale and serum testosterone concentrations. Results show that treatment of LOH patients with Physta significantly ($P < 0.0001$) improved the AMS score as well as the serum testosterone concentration. While before treatment, only 10.5% of the patients did not show any complaint according to the AMS scale and 35.5% had normal testosterone levels, after the completed treatment, 71.7% and 90.8% of the patients showed normal values, respectively. The researchers concluded that Physta appears to be useful as a supplement in overcoming the symptoms of LOH and for the management of hypogonadism.

31.4.2.8 Physta/LJ100 Study 8

In a randomized, placebo-controlled trial (Talbott et al. 2013), researchers assessed stress hormones and mood state in 63 subjects (32 men and 31 women) screened for moderate stress and supplemented with 200 mg/day Physta or placebo (PL) for 4weeks. Significant improvements ($P < 0.05$) were found in the Physta group for tension (−11%), anger (−12%), and confusion (−15%). Stress hormone profile (salivary cortisol and testosterone) was significantly improved ($P < 0.05$) by Physta supplementation, with reduced cortisol exposure (−16%, $P < 0.05$) and increased testosterone status (+37%, $P < 0.05$).* Researchers concluded that daily supplementation of Physta may be an effective approach to shielding the body from the detrimental effects of "modern" chronic stress, which may include general day-to-day stress, as well as the stress of dieting, sleep deprivation, and exercise training.

31.4.2.9 Physta/LJ100 Study 9

A pilot study (Henkel et al. 2014) investigated the ergogenic effects of 200 mg Physta, twice daily, in 13 physically active male and 12 physically active female seniors (57–72 years) for 5 weeks. Blood chemistry included standard hematological parameters, total and free testosterone, DHEA, cortisol, insulin-like growth factor-1, SHBG, blood urea nitrogen, and creatine kinase (as parameters of kidney function and muscle damage, respectively). Muscle strength was determined by a simple handgrip test. Results showed that hemoglobin, testosterone, and DHEA concentrations, and the ratio of total testosterone/cortisol and muscle force remained significantly lower in female seniors than in male seniors. Hematocrit and erythrocyte count increased slightly in male seniors but were significantly higher than in female seniors. Treatment resulted in increases in total testosterone, free testosterone, and muscular force (Table 31.3):

The increase in free testosterone in women is thought to be due to the significant decline in sex hormone–binding globulin concentrations. The study affirms the ergogenic benefit of Physta through enhanced muscle strength.

31.4.2.10 Physta/LJ100 Study 10

A 12-week, double-blind, placebo-controlled, parallel-group study (Udani et al. 2014) was conducted to examine the efficacy of a combination of Physta (200 mg/day) and *Polygonum minus*

TABLE 31.3
Increases in Total Testosterone, Free Testosterone and Muscular Force with Physta

	Total Testosterone	Free Testosterone	Muscular Force (Handgrip Test)
Men	+0.58 ng/mL (P = 0.0090)	+3.18 pg/mL (P = 0.0005)	+7.64 kg (P = 0.0375)
Women	+0.14 ng/mL (P = 0.0098)	+0.61 pg/mL (P = 0.0032)	+4.06 (n.s.)

* A weakness of this study was that the percentage increase in testosterone was not identified by gender, but rather provided as the mean of both genders combined. However, personal communication with one of the study authors suggest that the greater increase in testosterone was seen in women.

TABLE 31.4
Improvements in Scores for EHS, SHIM, and AMS with Physta

	Baseline (Mean ± SE)		6 Weeks (Mean ± SE)		12 Weeks (Mean ± SE)	
	Active	**Placebo**	**Active**	**Placebo**	**Active**	**Placebo**
Erectile Dysfunction Inventory of Treatment Satisfaction (EDITS)	n/a	n/a	52.56 ± 6.80	68.59 ± 8.03	74.68 ± 8.98	78.53 ± 9.89
Erection Hardness Scale (EHS)	2.54 ± 0.22	2.14 ± 0.23	2.95 ± 0.22[d]	2.68 ± 0.15	3.54 ± 0.11[b,c]	2.87 ± 0.27
Sexual Health Inventory for Men (SHIM)	15.77 ± 1.32	12.36 ± 1.45	16.92 ± 1.46	14.21 ± 1.26	19.85 ± 1.21[a,c]	14.29 ± 1.81
Aging Male Symptom (AMS) scale	25.85 ± 2.02	29.43 ± 2.25	23.31 ± 1.54[d]	24.71 ± 1.79[c]	20.85 ± 1.10[b,c]	26.00 ± 2.78

[a] $P < 0.005$ versus placebo.
[b] $P < 0.05$ versus placebo.
[c] $P < 0.005$ versus baseline.
[d] $P < 0.05$ versus baseline.

(100 mg/day), an antioxidant, compared to placebo, on sexual performance and well-being in 26 men, aged 40–65 (Active group = 12, placebo group = 14). The following validated questionnaires were used to evaluate erectile function, satisfaction with intervention, sexual intercourse performance, erectile hardness, mood, and overall quality of life: the Erectile Dysfunction Inventory of Treatment Satisfaction (EDITS) questionnaire, the Sexual Intercourse Assessment (SIA) diary, the Erection Hardness Scale (EHS) scale, the Sexual Health Inventory for Men (SHIM) questionnaire, the Aging Males Symptom (AMS) score, and the International Index of Erectile Function (IIEF-5). Results indicated significant improvements in scores for EHS, SHIM, and AMS (Table 31.4):

Regarding sexual intercourse assessment at 12 weeks, significant improvements versus placebo included the following:

- Foreplay preceding attempted intercourse and erection rating during sexual intercourse attempt ($P < 0.05$)
- Ability to achieve some erection, ability to achieve vaginal insertion, erection long enough for successful intercourse, satisfaction with sexual experience ($P < 0.0005$)

Laboratory evaluations, including liver and kidney function testing, showed no clinically significant abnormality. Researchers concluded that supplementation for 12 weeks with Physta and *P. minus* was well tolerated and more effective than placebo in enhancing sexual performance in healthy volunteers.

31.4.3 Adverse Reactions/Drug Interactions

In the previously cited research, no adverse reactions were reported. There are no reported drug interactions associated with *E. longifolia Jack* supplementation (Natural Medicines Comprehensive Database 2014).

31.4.4 Comments

While various dose ranges were used in human research on Physta/LJ100, 200 mg/day was used in 6 out of the 10 studies cited. Consequently, when used clinically, 200 mg/day is the dose likely to yield beneficial results.

According to Effendy et al. (2012), *E. longifolia Jack's* mechanism of action is effectuated by its eurypeptides, which exert their effects on the biosynthesis of various androgens, the stimulation of dihydroepiandosterone (which initiate the conversion of androstenedione and androstenediol to testosterone and estrogen, respectively), and which may also reduce SHBG to subsequently increase free testosterone levels.

31.5 YOHIMBINE

Potential application(s)

ED
SSRI-induced sexual dysfunction (male)
Orgasmic dysfunction (male)
Sexual arousal disorder (female)

31.5.1 Background

The bark of the yohimbe tree (*Pausinystalia johimbe*, syn. *Pausinystalia yohimbe*) has long been valued as an aphrodisiac in West Africa (Betz et al. 1995). It is the alkaloid yohimbine, typically derived from yohimbe bark, which provides the predominant pharmacological activity as an antagonist of alpha-2-adrenoceptors and which has been used for about 90 years as a treatment for male and female sexual difficulties (Riley 1994). In addition, yohimbine has monoamine oxidase (MOA)-inhibiting, calcium channel–blocking, and peripheral serotonin receptor–blocking activities (Leung and Foster 1996). Yohimbine's effect is likely mediated through genital blood vessel dilation, nerve impulse transmission to genital tissue, and increased reflex excitability in the sacral region of the spinal cord (Kunellius et al. 1997, Leung and Foster 1996, Montorsi et al. 1994). Although yohimbe bark extracts standardized for yohimbine content are available, it should be noted that the human research cited in the following text was conducted using synthetic yohimbine, typically as yohimbine hydrochloride. In studies 8 and 9 cited in the following text, L-arginine was used in combination with yohimbine. L-Arginine alone is addressed separately in this chapter.

31.5.2 Clinical Research

31.5.2.1 Yohimbine Study 1

In this double-blind, crossover, placebo-controlled study (Riley et al. 1989), 70 men with erectile inadequacy of mixed etiology were given 5.4 mg yohimbine hydrochloride 3 times daily or placebo. Efficacy data were presented on 61 of 70 men recruited to the trial. The results were that yohimbine was associated with a significant improvement in the quality of stimulated erections and was generally well tolerated.

31.5.2.2 Yohimbine Study 2

In some instances, SSRI medications have been reported to induce sexual dysfunction. Research (Jacobsen 1992) was undertaken to examine percentages of patients experiencing different types of sexual dysfunction after successful antidepressant treatment with standard doses of fluoxetine. Fifty-four (34%) of 160 outpatients reported sexual dysfunction after successful treatment with fluoxetine, including decreased libido and decreased sexual response. Nine of those patients participated in a follow-up, open trial of yohimbine (5.4 mg t.i.d.) as a potential treatment for fluoxetine-induced sexual dysfunction. Eight of nine patients reported improvement in sexual function. Five patients reported side effects.

31.5.2.3 Yohimbine Study 3

In an open clinical trial (Hollander and McCarley 1992), yohimbine (2.7–16.2 mg/day) was given on a p.r.n. basis to six patients who suffered sexual side effects after treatment with SSRI medications. Results were that five of the six patients experienced improved sexual functioning. The one patient who did not experience therapeutic effects had failed to comply with yohimbine treatment. Side effects included excessive sweating, increased anxiety, and a wound-up feeling in some patients.

31.5.2.4 Yohimbine Study 4

In this double-blind placebo-controlled study (Mann et al. 1996), 31 male patients (25–64 years) underwent extensive clinical, urological, and psychiatric diagnoses and were classified into an organic and a nonorganic subgroups. Patients were randomly assigned to a placebo or a yohimbine group (15 mg/day) for a treatment period of 7 weeks, following a 1-week placebo run-in period. Results were as follows: global assessment of erectile function applying the Clinical Global Impression (CGI) scale revealed a therapeutic effect in the subgroup of nonorganic patients, with a significantly greater improvement in the yohimbine group compared to the placebo group ($P < 0.05$). No superiority of yohimbine compared to placebo was found in the organic patients.

31.5.2.5 Yohimbine Study 5

Researchers conducted systematic review and meta-analysis (Ernst and Pittler 1998) of all randomized, placebo-controlled trials of yohimbine monotherapy for ED to determine its therapeutic efficacy, with a secondary aim to evaluate the safety of yohimbine. The results were that seven trials fit the predefined inclusion criteria. The doses used in the seven trials were described as follows: 18 mg (2 studies), 16.2 mg (2 studies), 15 mg (2 studies), and 30 mg (1 study). Overall methodological quality of these studies was considered satisfactory, and yohimbine was deemed superior to placebo in the treatment of ED (odds ratio 3.85, 95% confidence interval 6.67–2.22). Serious adverse reactions were infrequent and reversible. The researchers concluded that the benefit of yohimbine medication for ED seems to outweigh its risks, and yohimbine should be considered a reasonable therapeutic option for ED as initial pharmacological intervention.

31.5.2.6 Yohimbine Study 6

In this dose-escalation trial (Guay et al. 2002), 18 men (aged 40–80 years) with ED were given 5.4 mg yohimbine HCl three times daily for 4 weeks. Florida Sexual History Questionnaire, blood tests, nocturnal penile tumescence, and rigidity testing were completed at baseline and again at 4 weeks. The dose was increased to 10.8 mg three times daily for an additional 4 weeks with the same questionnaire and tests completed. Of the 18 men, 9 (50%) were successful in completing intercourse in more than 75% of attempts. Mean tip rigidity activity unit score of the responders was significantly higher than that of the nonresponders with the 5.4 mg dose ($P = 0.011$). For responders, a significant increase in the questionnaire total score was observed from baseline to the time the 5.4 mg dose was administered. The yohimbine responders were men with less severe ED as manifested by improved increased rigidity on RigiScan testing, higher Florida SHQ scores, and slightly higher levels of serum testosterone.

31.5.2.7 Yohimbine Study 7

In an open-label trial (Adeniyi et al. 2007), 29 men with orgasmic dysfunction of different etiology were treated with 20 mg/day yohimbine to assess the outcome. Patients were then allowed to increase the dose at home under more favorable circumstances. The results were that 16 men managed to reach orgasm and were able to ejaculate either during masturbation or sexual intercourse. Three additional men achieved orgasm, but only with the additional stimulation of a vibrator. Two have subsequently fathered children (one set of twins), and another three men were also cured. Side effects were not sufficient to cause the men to cease treatment.

31.5.3 Adverse Reactions/Drug Interactions

Reported adverse effects associated with oral supplementation with yohimbe bark or yohimbine include stomach upset, tachycardia, anxiety or agitation, hypertension, flushing, profuse sweating (diaphoresis), tremor, chest pain, chills or shivering, tachypnea, mydriasis, and altered mental status or behavior (Kearney et al. 2010). Yohimbe/yohimbine should not be taken with MAO inhibitors, since it can result in additive effects (Leung and Foster 1996, McGuffin et al. 1997).

31.5.4 Comments

Yohimbine has an established history for the treatment of ED. Reported adverse effects were not found to be sufficient to cause the men to cease treatment in previously cited studies.

31.6 VITAMIN D

Potential application(s): Hypogonadism/low T (male)

31.6.1 Background

Outright vitamin D deficiency is present in up to 41.6% of the U.S. population (Forrest and Stuhldreher 2011), while vitamin D insufficiency (i.e. lacking sufficient vitamin D) is present in up to 77% of the population (Ginde et al. 2009). It has long been known that severe vitamin D deficiency has serious consequences for bone health (Holick 2003), but other research indicates that lesser degrees of vitamin D deficiency are common and increase the risk of osteoporosis and other health problems (Heaney 2003, Zittermann 2003).

Germane to the topic of this chapter, research has demonstrated that hypogonadism is sometimes associated with vitamin D deficiency (Lee et al. 2012). Likewise, other research has demonstrated that lower plasma levels of vitamin D are associated with lower testosterone levels, while higher levels of vitamin D are associated with higher testosterone levels (Nimptsch et al. 2012, Wehr et al. 2010)

31.6.2 Clinical Research

31.6.2.1 Vitamin D Study 1

After being analyzed for testosterone levels, 54 healthy overweight men undergoing a weight reduction program participated in a randomized controlled trial (Pilz et al. 2011) in which they received either 83 mcg (3332 IU) vitamin D daily for 1 year (n = 31) or placebo (n = 23). Initial 25(OH)D concentrations were in the deficiency range (<50 nmol/L) and testosterone values were at the lower end of the reference range (9.09–55.28 nmol/L for males aged 20–49 years) in both groups. As expected, mean circulating 25(OH)D concentrations increased significantly in the vitamin D group, but remained almost constant in the placebo group. Results also showed that compared to baseline values, the vitamin D supplemented group experienced a significant increase in total testosterone, bioactive testosterone, and free testosterone (Table 31.5):

By contrast, there was no significant change in any testosterone measure in the placebo group. Searchers concluded that vitamin D supplementation might increase testosterone levels.

TABLE 31.5
Increases in Total Testosterone, Bioactive Testosterone and Free Testosterone with Vitamin D Supplementation

	Baseline (nmol/L)	Post (nmol/L)	Significance
Total testosterone	10.7 ± 3.9	13.4 ± 4.7	P < 0.001
Bioactive testosterone	5.21 ± 1.87	6.25 ± 2.01	P = 0.001
Free testosterone	0.222 ± 0.080	0.267 ± 0.087	P = 0.001

31.6.2.2 Vitamin D Study 2

The relationship between vitamin D and testosterone in men was examined in a cross-sectional population based study (n = 282) with pooled data from three randomized clinical trials (RCTs) with weight reduction, insulin sensitivity, and depression scores as endpoints, and one testosterone RCT (n = 37) in subjects with low serum testosterone (<11.0 nmol/L) and with body composition as endpoint.

In the cross-sectional study, serum 25(OH)D and androgens were measured at baseline and after 6–12 months of supplementation with vitamin D 20,000—40,000 IU per week versus placebo, and at baseline and after 1 year treatment with testosterone undecanoate 1,000 mg or placebo injections (at baseline and after 6, 16, 28, and 40 weeks) in the testosterone RCT (n = 37). Results were that in the cross-sectional study, serum 25(OH)D was found to be a significant and positive predictor of serum testosterone. In subjects without significant vitamin D deficiency, there is no increase in serum testosterone after high-dose vitamin D supplementation. Similarly, in subjects with moderately low serum testosterone levels, substitution with testosterone does not increase serum 25(OH) D (Jorde et al. 2013).

31.6.3 Adverse Reactions/Drug Interactions

Vitamin D has been safely used in a wide range of doses (Cava and Javier 2007, Diamond et al. 2005, Food and Nutrition Board 1999), and is well tolerated. Research suggests that vitamin D toxicity (hypervitaminosis D) is very unlikely in healthy people at intake levels lower than 10,000 IU/day (Heaney et al. 2003, Vieth 1999, Vieth et al. 2001). However, the Food and Nutrition Board of the Institute of Medicine (1999) conservatively set a tolerable upper intake level of 4000 IU/day for all adults.

Vitamin D stimulates a protein, which may bind and transport aluminum, therefore increasing aluminum absorption (Adler and Berlyne 1985, Moon 1994). This mechanism may contribute to increased aluminum levels and toxicity in people using aluminum-containing phosphate binders chronically, such as those with renal failure (Adler and Berlyne 1985, Demontis et al. 1986, 1989).

Clinical research shows that taking vitamin D–containing products (Therapeutic-M, Goldline Laboratories and Oyster shell calcium with vitamin D, Major Pharmaceuticals) significantly reduces levels of atorvastatin and its active metabolites—although total cholesterol, low-density lipoprotein (LDL), and high-density lipoprotein (HDL) cholesterol levels did not substantially change (Schwartz 2009). It should be noted that the products researched contained other nutrients besides vitamin D.

31.6.4 Comments

Those data seem to indicate that men with low T and vitamin D deficiency may experience an increase in T levels with vitamin D supplementation. Conversely, men with normal vitamin D levels are not likely to experience an increase in T. Nevertheless, given the prevalence of vitamin D deficiency and insufficiency, and the relative safety and low cost of vitamin D, supplementation may be a worthwhile consideration for patients with low T.

31.7 DHEA

Potential application(s):

Hypogonadism/Low T (male)
ED
Sexual satisfaction (male and female)
Sexual arousal (female)

31.7.1 Background

Produced in the adrenal glands and testes, dehydroepiandrosterone or dehydroepiandrostenedione (DHEA) has been referred to as both a "weak hormone" and a "prohormone." It is a weak hormone: it has a much lower affinity for the androgen receptor than testosterone (Nussey and Whitehead 2001), and it is prohormone: it is transformed into testosterone and/or estrogens in a cell-specific manner in a large series of peripheral target tissues (Labrie et al. 2005). In females, adrenal-derived testosterone is important in maintaining normal pubic and axillary hair, and after the menopause, DHEA may also be an important source of estradiol once converted peripherally. However, plasma DHEA decreases about 80% between ages 25 and 75 years (Weiss et al. 2011), and DHEA secretion is already decreased by a mean of 60% at the time of menopause (Labrie 2010).

DHEA-S is the blood marker for measuring DHEA. In a study involving 348 male patients, DHEA-S levels were significantly lower in the men with aging male symptoms (e.g. decrease in sexual desire/libido), and the DHEA-S was significantly lower in men with sexual dysfunction (Basar et al. 2005). In another study of 442 male subjects, serum levels of DHEA-S in patients with ED were lower than in healthy volunteers until 60 years of age (Reiter et al. 2000). An additional study with 53 patients found that ED is associated with a lower level of serum DHEA-S (Vakina et al. 2003).

31.7.2 Clinical Research

31.7.2.1 DHEA Study 1

A prospective study (Reiter et al. 2001) was conducted on ED patients with different organic letiologies. The study patients comprised 27 patients (group 1) with hypertension, 24 patients (group 2) with diabetes mellitus, 6 patients with neurological disorders (group 3), and 28 patients (group 4) with no organic etiology. All were treated with 50 mg DHEA for 6 months. The effectiveness was assessed by using the responses to questions about frequency of penetration and maintenance of erections after penetration within the 15-question IIEF. DHEA treatment was associated with statistically significantly higher mean scores compared to baseline values for questions in the IIEF in groups 1 and 4 after a period of 24 weeks. The researchers concluded that oral DHEA treatment may be of benefit to patients with ED who have hypertension or to patients with ED without organic etiology.

31.7.2.2 DHEA Study 2

In a prospective, double-blind, randomized, placebo-controlled study (Reiter et al. 1999), 40 ED patients were randomly divided into 2 groups of 20 patients each. Group 1 was treated with an oral dose of 50 mg DHEA and group 2 with a placebo one time a day for 6 months. The IIEF was used to rate the success of this therapy. The results were DHEA treatment was associated with higher mean scores for all five domains of the IIEF, including the ability to achieve or maintain an erection sufficient for satisfactory sexual performance. The researchers concluded that oral DHEA treatment may be of benefit in the treatment of ED.

31.7.2.3 DHEA Study 3

Two hundred and eighty healthy individuals (women and men 60–79 years old) were given DHEA, 50 mg, or placebo, orally, daily for a year in a double-blind, placebo-controlled study (Baulieu et al. 2000). Besides the reestablishment of a "young" concentration of DHEA-S, a small increase of testosterone and estradiol was noted, particularly in women, and may be involved in the significantly demonstrated physiological-clinical manifestations here reported. A significant increase in most libido parameters was also found in women >70 years old. The authors concluded that 50 mg/day DHEA administration over 1 year normalized some effects of aging, but does not create "supermen/superwomen" (doping).

31.7.2.4 DHEA Study 4

In a double-blind study (Arlt et al. 1999), 24 women with adrenal insufficiency randomly received 50 mg of DHEA orally each morning for 4 months and placebo daily for 4 months, with a 1-month washout period. The results were that treatment with DHEA raised the initially low serum concentrations of DHEA, DHEA-S, androstenedione, and testosterone into the normal range. As compared with placebo, DHEA significantly increased the frequency of sexual thoughts ($P = 0.006$), sexual interest ($P = 0.002$), and satisfaction with both mental and physical aspects of sexuality ($P = 0.009$ and $P = 0.02$, respectively). DHEA also significantly improved overall well-being as well as scores for depression and anxiety. For the global severity index, the mean change from baseline was -0.18 ± 0.29 after 4 months of DHEA therapy, as compared with 0.03 ± 0.29 after 4 months of placebo ($P = 0.02$).

31.7.2.5 DHEA Study 5

In a prospective 6-month trial (Villareal et al. 2000), 10 women and 8 men (aged 73 ± 1 years) received 50 mg DHEA daily. Control subjects were 10 women and 8 men (aged 74 ± 1 years). The results were that bone mineral density (BMD) of the total body and lumbar spine increased ($P \leq 0.05$), fat mass decreased ($P < 0.01$), and fat-free mass increased ($P \leq 0.05$) in response to DHEA replacement. DHEA replacement also resulted in significant increases ($P \leq 0.05$) in total serum testosterone concentrations (from 10.7 ± 1.2 to 15.6 ± 1.8 nmol/L in the men and from 2.1 ± 0.2 to 4.5 ± 0.4 nmol/L in the women).

31.7.3 Adverse Reactions/Drug Interactions

The advantage of DHEA over other androgenic compounds is that it is converted into androgens and/or estrogens only in the specific target tissues that possess the appropriate physiological enzymatic machinery. This limits the action of the sex steroids to those tissues possessing the tissue-specific profile of expression of the genes responsible for their formation, thereby leaving other tissues unaffected and minimizing the potential side effects observed with androgens or estrogens administered systemically (Labrie et al. 2003). Furthermore, in the aforementioned Baulieu et al. (2000) study, subjects were orally supplemented with 50 mg/day DHEA or placebo for a year with no potentially harmful accumulation of DHEA-S and active steroids recorded. In addition, a number of biological indices confirmed the lack of harmful consequences of this 50 mg/day DHEA administration.

DHEA and DHEA-S inhibited platelet aggregation in human and *in vitro* research (Bertoni et al. 2012, Jesse et al. 1995). Consequently, there is theoretical concern that DHEA might increase the risk of bleeding when used with antiplatelet or anticoagulant drugs. Nevertheless, there have been no reports of this interaction in humans. In addition, the use of a selective serotonin reuptake inhibitor (SSRI) with DHEA in a human case report (Dean 2000) increased the risk of mania, again leading to a theoretical concern that DHEA might increase the risk of psychiatric adverse events when used with antidepressants.

31.7.4 Comments

Despite its role as a weak hormone and a prohormone, supplementation with DHEA appears to be relatively safe and effective. While it always makes sense to assess patients' DHEA-S levels prior to beginning supplementation, it is particularly important in populations younger than 40 years of age who are more likely to have higher endogenous secretion of DHEA.

31.8 L-ARGININE

Potential application(s): ED

31.8.1 Background

L-Arginine is a semiessential amino acid, since its rate of synthesis does not increase to compensate for depletion or inadequate supply (Castillo et al. 1993, 1994), thereby consigning dietary intake as the primary contributor of L-arginine levels since. While involved in numerous areas of human biochemistry, including ammonia detoxification, hormone secretion, and immune modulation, L-arginine is best known for its effects on the vascular system. Specifically, L-arginine is metabolized via the enzyme nitric oxide synthase into nitric oxide (NO). NO causes blood vasodilation (Appleton 2002). Consequently, through its role as an NO precursor, L-arginine offers many benefits for cardiovascular health, as well as for erectile function (Peters and Noble 1996, Wang et al. 1996). The oral bioavailability of L-arginine is 68% and it has an elimination half-life of approximately 80 min (Bode-Boger et al. 1998).

31.8.2 Clinical Research

31.8.2.1 L-Arginine Study 1

To determine the effect of 6 weeks of high-dose 5 g/day orally administered L-arginine, a prospective randomized, double-blind placebo-controlled study (Chen et al. 1999) was conducted in 50 men with organic ED. In addition to a sexual function questionnaire and a sexual activity diary, all participants underwent a complete physical examination, including an assessment of bulbocavernosus reflex and penile hemodynamics. Also plasma and urine nitrite and nitrate (designated NO) were determined at the end of the placebo run-in period, and after 3 and 6 weeks. The results were that 9 of 29 (31%) patients taking L-arginine and 2 of 17 controls reported a significant subjective improvement in sexual function. All objective variables assessed remained unchanged. All nine patients treated with L-arginine and who had subjectively improved sexual performance (responders) had an initially low urinary NO, and this level had doubled at the end of the study.

31.8.2.2 L-Arginine Study 2

In a placebo-controlled, crossover trial published in the *International Journal of Impotence Research* (Zorgniotti and Lizza 1994), 15 impotent men were treated with 2.8 g L-arginine per day for 2 weeks. Subjects were either responders or nonresponders (i.e. those with low NO were responders). Six of the 15 men (40%) were responders, and experienced significant improvements in sexual function, including improvement in erections. None of the placebo grouped experienced improvements of any kind. In general, lower doses of L-arginine alone do not seem to be effective for ED. For example in one study (Klotz et al. 1999), 1500 mg L-arginine daily was ineffective in treating men with mixed-type impotence. However, when L-arginine is combined with certain other nutraceuticals, lower doses may be effective. See Section 31.10.

31.8.3 Adverse Reactions/Drug Interactions

Orally, L-arginine can cause abdominal pain and bloating, diarrhea, and gout, although this occurred with relatively high dosage ranges (e.g. 12.6 g/day, 30 g/day) (Brittenden et al. 1994, Rector et al. 1996).

Since L-arginine increases nitric oxide, which promotes vasodilation, supplementation has resulted in blood pressure reduction in some hypertensive individuals (Dong et al. 2011, Huynh and Tayek 2002, Nagaya et al. 2001). Combining L-arginine with some hypertensive drugs may have additive blood pressure–lowering effects (Cheng and Balwin 2001, Komers et al. 2000, Stokes et al. 2003).

31.8.4 Comments

While L-arginine certainly appears to have efficacy in promoting NO with subsequent vasodilation and improvements in ED in some individuals, the evidence suggests that better results may be obtained when combined with other nutraceuticals. See Section 31.10.

31.9 L-CITRULLINE

Potential application(s): ED

31.9.1 Background

L-citrulline is a nonessential amino acid (Schwedhelm et al. 2008) obtained from food such as watermelon, containing 0.7–3.6 mg/g of fruit (Mandel et al. 2005), and is also synthesized in the intestinal mucosa and liver (Mandel et al. 2005, Schwedhelm et al. 2008). It is a potent hydroxyl radical scavenger and much more effective precursor of arginine and nitric oxide than arginine itself (Schwedhelm et al. 2008).

31.9.2 Clinical Research

In a single-blind, placebo-controlled study (Cormio et al. 2011), 24 men (mean age 56.5 ± 9.8 years) with mild ED received oral supplementation with a placebo for 1 month and 1.5 g/day L-citrulline for another month to test the efficacy and safety of oral L-citrullines in improving erection hardness. The erection hardness score, number of intercourses per month, treatment satisfaction, and adverse events were recorded. All patients completed the study with no adverse events. Results demonstrated that 50% of men taking the L-citrulline experienced improvement in the erection hardness score from 3 (mild ED) to 4 (normal erectile function) ($P < 0.01$). By contrast, 8.3% of men taking the placebo had the same improvement. In addition, the mean number of intercourses per month increased from 1.37 ± 0.93 at baseline to 2.3 ± 1.37 at the end of the treatment phase ($P < 0.01$). At the end of the placebo phase, the increase was nonsignificant. All patients reporting erection hardness score improvement from 3 to 4 reported being very satisfied. The researchers concluded that L-citrulline supplementation has been proved to be safe and psychologically well accepted by patients, at least in the short term.

31.9.3 Adverse Reactions/Drug Interactions

There are no reported adverse reactions associated with L-citrulline supplementation (Natural Medicines Comprehensive Database 2014). Since L-citrulline is converted to L-arginine, which can cause vasodilation (Osowska et al. 2004, Romero et al. 2006), there is a theoretical concern that when used together with nitrates or phosphodiesterase-5 inhibitors, it might increase the chance of hypotension. However, these drug interactions have not yet been reported.

31.9.4 Comments

The previously cited clinical study suggests that L-citrulline has the potential to be a promising nutraceutical for the treatment of ED. Nevertheless, additional studies should be conducted before L-citrulline is routinely used for this purpose.

31.10 L-ARGININE WITH OTHER NUTRACEUTICALS

Potential application(s):

ED
Hypogonadism/Low T (male, w/pycnogenol)

31.10.1 Background

One of the nutraceuticals to be discussed for use in combination with L-arginine is pycnogenol, a proprietary extract from the bark of the French maritime pine tree (Grosse Duweller and Rohdewald 2000). While pycnogenol contains a number of compounds, its naturally occurring oligomeric pro-anthocyanidins (OPC) have been identified as particularly active (Grosse Duweller and Rohdewald 2000, Packer et al. 1999). A large body of research on pycnogenol has demonstrated efficacy for a number of health conditions, including a pilot study (Durackova et al. 2003) in which 120 mg/day pycnogenol was found to have a beneficial effect on the treatment of ED.

31.10.2 Clinical Research

31.10.2.1 L-Arginine + Yohimbine Study 1

A randomized, double-blind, placebo-controlled, three-way crossover study (Meston and Worcel 2002) examined the effects of the yohimbine and L-arginine (a nitric oxide-precursor) on subjective and physiological sexual arousal in postmenopausal 24 women with female sexual arousal disorder. Subjects participated in three treatment sessions in which self-report and physiological (vaginal photoplethysmograph) sexual responses to erotic stimuli were measured approximately 30, 60, and 90 min following treatment with either L-arginine glutamate (6 g) plus yohimbine HCl (6 mg), yohimbine alone (6 mg), or placebo. Results demonstrated that the combined oral administration of L-arginine glutamate and yohimbine substantially increased vaginal pulse amplitude responses to the erotic film at 60 min post administration compared with placebo.

31.10.2.2 L-Arginine + Yohimbine Study 2

This randomized, double-blind, placebo-controlled, three-way crossover study (Lebret et al. 2002) examined the safety and efficacy of 6g L-arginine glutamate + 6 mg of yohimbine hydrochloride, compared to 6 mg yohimbine hydrochloride alone and placebo, for the treatment of ED when administered orally, 1–2 h before intended sexual intercourse. Change in the erectile function domain score of the IIEF was the primary endpoint. Results at the end of each treatment period for the erectile function domain scores were

- L-arginine + yohimbine: 17.2 ± 7.17
- Yohimbine: 15.4 ± 6.49
- Placebo: 14.1 ± 6.56

The difference between L-arginine + yohimbine and placebo was statistically significant ($P = 0.006$). Those patients with mild-to-moderate ED had a better erectile function domain response to treatment than those with scores 14 and below. Assessment of efficacy by investigators and patients showed significant improvement with L-arginine + yohimbine over placebo. Researchers concluded that on-demand oral administration of L-arginine + yohimbine is effective in improving erectile function in patients with mild-to-moderate ED, and appears to be a promising addition to first-line therapy for ED.

31.10.2.3 L-Arginine + Pycnogenol Study 1

In a 3-month trial (Stanislavov and Nikolova 2003), 40 mean (aged 25–45 years) with ED were initially treated with 1700 mg of L-arginine daily (as L-arginine aspartate) for 1 month. The result was that only 5% of the men achieved normal erectile function. During the second month, 80 mg of pycnogenol extract daily was added. The result was that 80% of the men reported normal erections. During the third month, pycnogenol extract was increased to 120 mg daily. The result was that 92.5% of the men experienced a normal erection. The authors concluded that oral administration of L-arginine in combination with pycnogenol extract caused a significant improvement in sexual function in men with ED, without any side effects.

31.10.2.4 L-Arginine + Pycnogenol Study 2

In a randomly allocated, double-blind, placebo-controlled, crossover design trial (Stanislavov et al. 2008), 50 patients with mild-to-moderate ED were treated for 1 month with placebo or a combination of L-arginine aspartate and 80 mg pycnogenol extract. The IIEF was used to quantify changes in sexual function (with IIEF scores of > 25 defined as normal). Testosterone levels and endothelial NO synthase (e-NOS) were monitored along with routine clinical chemistry. At the conclusion of the treatment period, men treated with L-arginine and pycnogenol extract reported restored erectile function to normal (improved IIEF scores from 11–17 to 26–30), while the men on the placebo did not report significant improvement in erectile function. On average, it took approximately 5 days for the combination of L-arginine and pycnogenol extract to improve erectile function. In addition, intercourse frequency doubled. Significant improvements in orgasmic function, sexual desire, and intercourse were also reported in the treatment group. Furthermore, e-NOS in spermatozoa and testosterone levels in blood increased significantly. Cholesterol levels and blood pressure were lowered. No unwanted effects were reported.

31.10.2.5 L-Arginine + Pycnogenol Study 3

In this double-blind, placebo-controlled study (Ledda et al. 2010), researchers assessed the effects of a formulation of pycnogenol extract and L-arginine aspartate in 124 patients (aged 30–50 years) with moderate ED over an investigational period of 6 months. The IIEF was used to quantify changes in sexual function. The results showed statistically significant benefits of L-arginine + pycnogenol over placebo for the erectile domain of the IIEF (questions 1–5 plus 15) and testosterone ($P < 0.05$ for both) (Table 31.6):

The researchers concluded that L-arginine + pycnogenol is effective for improving erectile function and may continue to improve the longer the therapy is used.

TABLE 31.6
Increases in the Erectile Domain of the IIEF and Testosterone with l-Arginine + Pycnogenol over Placebo

	L-Arginine + Pycnogenol			Placebo		
	Baseline	3 Months	6 Months	Baseline	3 Months	6 Months
IIEF (erectile domain) score	15.2	25.2	27.1	15.1	19.1	19.0
Testosterone (nmol/L)	15.9		18.9	16.9		17.3

31.10.2.6 L-Arginine + Pycnogenol Study 4

An 8-week, double-blind, placebo-controlled, parallel group study (Aoki et al. 2012) examined the effect of Pycnogenol® 60 mg/day, L-arginine 690 mg/day, and aspartic acid 552 mg/day or placebo in Japanese patients with mild-to-moderate ED. Subjects were assessed using the five-item erectile domain (IIEF-5), blood biochemistry, urinalysis, and salivary testosterone measurements. The results were that supplementation improved the total score of the IIEF-5, including a marked improvement in "hardness of erection" and "satisfaction with sexual intercourse." Additionally, the supplement group experienced a decrease in blood pressure, aspartate transaminase, and γ-glutamyl transpeptidase (γ-GTP), as well as a slight increase in salivary testosterone. No adverse reactions were observed during the study period.

31.10.3 Adverse Reactions/Drug Interactions

Since adverse reactions and drug interactions for L-arginine and yohimbine have been addressed previously in this chapter, only pycnogenol will be addressed here. Orally, pycnogenol seems to be well tolerated (Natural Medicines Comprehensive Database 2014). Theoretically, pycnogenol may interfere with immunosuppressant therapy because of its immunostimulating activity (Liu et al. 1998, Rice-Evans and Packer 1998), although this has not been demonstrated in clinical research.

31.10.4 Comments

Research suggests that greater efficacy may be obtained when L-arginine is combined with yohimbine or pycnogenol, rather than administered alone.

31.11 SAW PALMETTO + ASTAXANTHIN

Potential application(s): ED

Hypogonadism/Low T (male, w/pycnogenol)

31.11.1 Background

Saw palmetto (*Serenoa repens*) is a small palm tree native to the North American East Coast, from South Carolina to Florida, and west to Texas. Native Americans used its berries as both a food and a medicine.

The clinical efficacy of the saw palmetto extract in mitigating the urological disorders associated with benign prostate hyperplasia (BPH) and its good tolerability is well documented by many clinical studies, carried out on patients suffering from mild-to-moderate BPH (Gerber 2000, Mantovani 2010, Wilt et al. 1998). In vitro research suggests that a possible mechanism of action by which saw palmetto exerts its effects is through the noncompetitive inhibition of 5 alpha-reductase types 1 and 2, preventing the conversion of testosterone to dihydrotestosterone (DHT) (Levin and Das 2000)—although some in vivo research indicated that this inhibition may not be significant (Marks and Tyler 1999). In addition, in vivo research suggests that saw palmetto may reduce estradiol (Di Silverio et al. 1992).

Astaxanthin is a carotenoid derived from the microalgae *Haematococcus pluvialis* and is found in foods such as salmon, trout, shrimp, and lobster (Goodwin 1986, Kobayashi et al. 1997). Structurally similar to beta-carotene (Yuan et al. 2011), astaxanthin has tremendous antioxidant activity (Miki 1991). In vitro research (Anderson 2005) has demonstrated that a combination of saw palmetto and astaxanthin demonstrated a 20% greater inhibition of 5 alpha-reductase than saw palmetto extract alone in vitro. Commercially, this combination is known as Re-Settin® (Triarco Industries), although it has also gone by the names MyTosterone™ and Alphastat®).

31.11.2 Clinical Research

31.11.2.1 Saw Palmetto + Astaxanthin Study 1

In a 14-day, open-label clinical study (Angwafor and Anderson 2008), 42 healthy males aged 37–70 years were divided into two groups of 21, and dosed with either 800 mg/day or 2000 mg/day of Re-Settin. Blood samples were collected on days 0, 3, 7, and 14 and assayed for T, DHT, and estradiol.

The results were presented, although far more detail about the results were presented in an unpublished report (Anonymous 2007), which provided all of the data for the published study. In the group taking 800 mg/day, total T concentrations increased 61%, DHT levels decreased by 16% in 14 days. There were no changes in E. The group taking 2000 mg/day experienced a 38% increase in total T concentrations, a 27% decrease in DHT, and a 9% decrease in E in 14 days. With the exception of no changes in E in the 800 mg/day group, all of the changes were statistically significant.

31.11.2.2 Saw Palmetto + Astaxanthin Study 2

A prospective single-blind, randomized, placebo-controlled clinical trial (Anderson 2014) was conducted with 20 healthy, sedentary men between the ages of 21 and 70, randomized into either an 800 mg/day or 1200 mg/day Resettin® or placebo. After a 14-day treatment period, there was a 14-day washout period. After the wash-out period, participants were crossed over within their respective group for 14 days. Results showed that 800 mg/day Resettin significantly reduced baseline-subtracted serum DHT levels in comparison to the placebo control group ($P < 0.05$), and 1200 mg/day Resettin significantly reduced baseline-subtracted serum DHT and E2 levels in comparison to the placebo control group ($P < 0.05$). In addition, 1200 mg/day Resettin increased serum testosterone levels 38% in comparison to placebo, but the effect did not reach statistical significance.

31.11.3 Adverse Reactions/Drug Interactions

Orally, the adverse effects of saw palmetto are generally mild and comparable to placebo (Natural Medicines Comprehensive Database 2014). Since saw palmetto has been reported to prolong bleeding time (Cheema et al. 2001), theoretically, it might increase the risk of bleeding when used with anticoagulant/antiplatelet drugs although this has not been demonstrated in human research. There are no reported adverse reactions or drug interactions with astaxanthin placebo (Natural Medicines Comprehensive Database 2014).

31.11.4 Comments

The research on Resettin is limited by the fact that the Angwafor and Anderson study (2008) had no placebo group, and the Anderson study (2014) may have been too small ($n = 12$) to detect any significant increase in T. Further controlled research should be conducted on Resettin using a larger study population.

31.12 SHILAJIT

Potential application(s): Hypogonadism/Low T (male)

31.12.1 Background

Shilajit is a pale-brown to blackish-brown exudate secreted from sedimentary rocks, largely in the Himalayas, composed of rock humus, rock minerals, and organic substances that have been compressed by layers of rock mixed with marine organisms and microbial metabolites (Ghosal 1994).

Said to carry the healing power of these great mountains (David and Vasant, 2001), shilajit is an important drug of the Ayurvedic materia medica and is used extensively by Ayurvedic physicians for a variety of conditions, including the management of male reproductive disorders (Sharma 1998).

31.12.2 Clinical Research

31.12.2.1 Shilajit Study 1

A 90-day clinical trial (Biswas et al. 2010) was conducted to examine the effects of 100 mg shilajit twice daily in 28 infertile, oligospermic male patients. Total semenogram (sperm analysis) and serum testosterone, luteinizing hormone, and follicle-stimulating hormone were measured before and at the end of the treatment. In addition, malondialdehyde (MDA), a marker for oxidative stress, content of semen, and biochemical parameters for safety were also evaluated. Results showed significant ($P < 0.001$) improvement in various parameters, including 37.6% increase spermia (sperm mobility), 61.4% increase in total sperm count, 12.4%–17.4% increase in motility (after different time intervals), and 18.9% increase in normal sperm count. There was also a significant 18.7% decrease of semen MDA content and a significant 23.5% increase in serum testosterone ($P < 0.001$), and 9.4% increase in FSH ($P < 0.05$) levels. Hepatic and renal profiles indicated that shilajit is safe.

31.12.2.2 Shilajit Study 2

A 90-day, randomized, double-blind, placebo-controlled clinical study (Pandit et al. 2014) evaluated the effects of 250 mg/twice daily PrimaVie® Purified Shilajit or placebo on male androgenic hormones in 98 healthy male volunteers between 45 and 55 years. On days 0 (baseline), 30, 60, and 90 total and free testosterones, LH, FSH, and DHEAs were measured from fasting blood of each volunteer. Results showed that the PrimaVie treated group experienced an increase of testosterone levels on days 30 (6.82%), 60 (3.09%), and 90 (20.45%, $P < 0.05$) compared to baseline. By contrast, there was a decreasing trend of testosterone levels in the placebo group ($P < 0.05$). Testosterone levels in the PrimaVie group were significantly better those of the placebo group at day 90 ($P < 0.05$). Levels of free testosterone in the PrimaVie group significantly increased by 19.14% ($P < 0.05$), which was significantly higher than the placebo group ($P < 0.05$). In addition, FSH levels significantly increased ($P < 0.004$) in the PrimaVie group, which was significantly better than the placebo group on day 90. Also, DHEAs increased by 31.35% on day 90 in the PrimaVie group, which was significantly higher than baseline or the placebo group ($P < 0.05$).

31.12.3 Adverse Reactions/Drug Interactions

The safety of shilajit is well documented based on animal and human studies (Stohs 2014). Currently, there does not appear to be any relevant data on drug interactions with shilajit.

31.12.4 Comments

Despite the fact that the two studies summarized earlier were conducted on oligospermic and healthy male populations using 200 and 500 mg shilajit daily, the increase in T levels was markedly similar: 23.5% and 20.45%, respectively. This similarity suggests the potential for a greater likelihood of efficacy in different populations.

31.13 ASHWAGANDHA

Potential application(s): Hypogonadism/Low T (male)

31.13.1 Background

A small, woody shrub found growing in Africa, the Mediterranean, and India, the root of ashwagandha (*Withania somnifera*) has been used in Ayurvedic medicine (Anonymous 2004) for over 3000 years, and was described by Dioscorides (78 AD) in his book "Kitab-ul-Hashaish" (Uddin et al. 2012). The therapeutic actions of ashwagandha have been said to include tonic, aphrodisiac, narcotic, diuretic, anthelmintic, astringent, anti-inflammatory, sedative, alterative, thermogenic, and stimulant (Singh et al. 2011, Uddin et al. 2012). In the literature, steroidal lactones known as withanolides have been discussed as important active compounds in ashwagandha (Uddin et al. 2012), although a full spectrum extract (KSM-66®, Ixoreal Biomed Inc.) has also demonstrated significant efficacy in human clinical research (Ambiye et al. 2013, Sachin 2014).

31.13.2 Clinical Research

31.13.2.1 Ashwagandha Study 1

A 90-day, two-arm, double-blind, randomized, placebo-controlled, parallel-group study (Ambiye et al. 2013) was conducted to evaluate the effects of Ashwagandha root extract (KSM-66 ashwagandha, 675 mg/day in three doses, $n = 21$) or placebo ($n = 25$) on spermatogenic activity and serum hormone levels in 46 patients with oligospermia. Semen parameters and serum hormone levels were estimated at the end of 90-day treatment. Results showed that there was a 167% increase in sperm count ($P < 0.0001$), 53% increase in semen volume ($P < 0.0001$), and 57% increase in sperm motility ($P < 0.0001$) on day 90 from baseline. The improvement in these parameters was minimal in the placebo-treated group. Furthermore, a significantly greater improvement and regulation were observed in serum hormone levels with the ashwagandha treatment as compared to the placebo. Serum testosterone increased significantly by 17% (from 4.45 ± 1.41 to 5.22 ± 1.39 ng/mL; $P < 0.01$) and LH by 34% (from 3.97 ± 1.21 to 5.31 ± 1.33 mIU/mL; $P < 0.02$), following treatment with ashwagandha root extract, as compared to the baseline (Day 0) values of these parameters.

31.13.2.2 Ashwagandha Study 2

An 8-week randomized, prospective, double-blind, placebo-controlled clinical study (Sachin 2014) was conducted to examine the effects of the KSM-66 ashwagandha root extract (one 300 mg capsule, twice daily) or placebo on muscle strength and endurance, size and recovery, testosterone, and body fat in 50 healthy and physically active males (18–45 years of age, $n = 25$ for each group) with little experience in resistance training. Creatine kinase (CK) was assessed as a biomarker of recovery from muscle injury. Following baseline measurements, subjects underwent resistance training for 8 weeks; thereafter, measurements of the specific parameters were repeated at the end of week 8 (completion of study). The results were that both muscle strength (bench press) and muscle size (arm) increased significantly in the ashwagandha group as compared to the placebo group ($P < 0.001$ and $P < 0.05$, respectively). There was also a significant increase of 15% in the concentration of total serum testosterone in the Ashwagandha group at week 8 of the study period as compared to the corresponding baseline value ($P < 0.05$). The increase was significant also as compared to the Placebo group ($P < 0.01$). In addition, the expected increase in CK between 24 and 48 h following exercise was significantly lower in the ashwagandha group compared to placebo ($P < 0.05$), and the reduction in body fat percentage was significantly greater in the ashwagandha group compared to placebo ($P < 0.05$).

31.13.2.3 Ashwagandha Study 3

A prospective study (Ahmad et al. 2010) was conducted to investigate the impact of 5 g/day ashwagandha root powder on semen profile, oxidative biomarkers, and reproductive hormone levels. Seventy-five normal healthy fertile men (control subjects) and 75 infertile men undergoing infertility screening were the subjects. Measurements of the following were taken before and after the

TABLE 31.7
Ashwagandha Improves Hormonal Parameters in Infertile Men

Group	LH	T	FSH	PRL
Normozoospermic	+14.3%[a]	+14.7%[a]	–5.3%[a]	–4%[c]
Oligozoospermic	+48.8%[a]	+40.7%[a]	–19.4%[a]	–17.2%[a]
Asthenozoospermic	+40.6%[a]	+21%[a]	–8.3%[a]	–7.6%[a]

[a] $P < 0.01$ compared to baseline.
[b] $P < 0.05$ compared to baseline.
[c] Not statistically significant.

treatment: seminal plasma biochemical parameters, antioxidant vitamins, and serum testosterone (T), luteinizing hormone (LH), follicle-stimulating hormone (FSH), and prolactin (PRL) levels. Results showed that ashwagandha inhibited lipid peroxidation and protein carbonyl content and improved sperm count and motility. Treatment of infertile men recovered the seminal plasma levels of antioxidant enzymes and vitamins A, C, and E and corrected fructose. Moreover, treatment also significantly improved hormonal parameters (Table 31.7):

31.13.2.4 Ashwagandha Study 4

A 3-month, controlled study (Mahdi et al. 2011) was conducted to examine the role of stress in male infertility, and to test the effect of ashwagandha root powder (5 g/day) on stress and the treatment of normozoospermic male infertility (n = 60). Subjects included normozoospermic heavy smokers (n = 20), normozoospermics under psychological stress (n = 20), and normozoospermics with infertility of unknown etiology (n = 20). Normozoospermic fertile men (n = 60) were used as controls. Measuring various biochemical and stress parameters before and after treatment suggested a definite role of stress in male infertility and the ability of ashwagandha to treat stress-related infertility. In normozoospermics with infertility of unknown etiology, normozoospermic cigarette smokers, and normozoospermics under psychological stress, the following points were noted:

- Sperm concentration was increased by 17%, 20%, and 36%, respectively.
- Motility of spermatozoa increased by 9%, 10%, and 13%, respectively.
- Semen liquefaction time decreased by 19%, 20%, and 34%, respectively.
- Cortisol levels significantly decreased by 11%, 28%, and 32%, respectively.
- Testosterone levels improved by 13%, 10%, and 22%, respectively.
- Luteinizing hormone levels improved by 5%, 14%, and 22%, respectively.

Likewise, treatment resulted in a decrease in stress and improved the level of antioxidants in a significant number of individuals. The treatment also resulted in pregnancy in the partners of 14% of the patients.

31.13.3 Adverse Reactions/Drug Interactions

Ashwagandha appears to be well tolerated, although large doses exceeding 6 g may result gastrointestinal upset, diarrhea, and vomiting secondary to irritation of the mucous and serous membranes (Upton 2000). With regard to drug interactions, there is some evidence that ashwagandha might have an additive effect with diazepam and clonazepam (Upton 2000), and might decrease immunosuppression caused by cyclophosphamide (Davis and Kuttan 1998, 2000).

31.13.4 Comments

There may be equivalency between 675 mg of KSM-66 ashwagandha root extract and 5 g of root powder (the amounts used the aforementioned following studies). The rational is that the amount of withanolides found in commercial ashwagandha root ranges between 0.38% and 0.76% based upon whether the plant is harvested during its vegetative, flowering, or seed phenostage (Kumar et al. 2001), which would yield 26–38 mg total withanolides. Correspondingly, KSM-66 ashwagandha root extract provides >5% total withanolides, so 675 mg would provide at least 33.75 mg of withanolides.

REFERENCES

Adeniyi, A.A., Brindley, G.S., Pryor, J.P., and Ralph, D.J. Yohimbine in the treatment of orgasmic dysfunction. *Asian J Androl* 2007;9:403–407.

Ahmad, M.K., Mahdi, A.A., Shukla, K.K., Islam, N., Rajender, S., Madhukar, D., Shankhwar, S.N., and Ahmad, S. *Withania somnifera* improves semen quality by regulating reproductive hormone levels and oxidative stress in seminal plasma of infertile males. *Fertil Steril* 2010;94:989–996.

Ambiye, V.R., Langade, D., Dongre, S., Aptikar, P., Kulkarni, M., and Dongre, A. Clinical evaluation of the spermatogenic activity of the root extract of ashwagandha (*Withania somnifera*) in oligospermic males: A pilot study. *Evid Based Complement Alternat Med* 2013;571420:6.

Anderson, M.L. A preliminary investigation of the enzymatic inhibition of 5alpha-reduction and growth of prostatic carcinoma cell line LNCap-FGC by natural astaxanthin and Saw Palmetto lipid extract in vitro. *J Herb Pharmacother* 2005;5:17–26.

Anderson, M.L. Evaluation of Resettin® on serum hormone levels in sedentary males. *JISSN* 2014;11:43.

Angwafor III, F. and Anderson, M.L. An open label, dose response study to determine the effect of a dietary supplement on dihydrotestosterone, testosterone and estradiol levels in healthy males. *JISSN* 2008;5:12.

Anonymous. Final Clinical Report on Alphastat. Laboratory of Nutrition & Nutritional Biochemistry, Department of Biochemistry, University of Yaounde I, Cameroon. October 2007.

Anonymous. Monograph. *Withania somnifera*. *Altern Med Rev* 2004;9:211–214.

Aoki, H., Nagao, J., Ueda, T., Strong, J.M., Schonlau, F., Yu-Jing, S., Lu, Y., and Horie, S. Clinical assessment of a supplement of Pycnogenol® and L-arginine in Japanese patients with mild to moderate erectile dysfunction. *Phytother Res* 2012;26:204–207.

Appleton, J. Arginine: Clinical potential of a semi-essential amino. *Altern Med Rev* 2002;7(6):512–522.

Arlt, W., Callies, F., van Vlijmen, J.C., Koehler, I., Reincke, M., Bidlingmaier, M., Huebler, D., Oettel, M., Ernst, M., Schulte, H.M., and Allolio, B. Dehydroepiandrosterone replacement in women with adrenal insufficiency. *N Engl J Med* 1999;341:1013–1020.

Basar, M.M., Aydin, G., Mert, H.C., Keles, I., Caglayan, O., Orkun, S, and Batislam, E. Relationship between serum sex steroids and Aging Male Symptoms score and International Index of Erectile Function. *Urology* 2005;66:597–601.

Baulieu, E.E., Thomas, G., Legrain, S. et al. Dehydroepiandrosterone (DHEA), DHEA sulfate, and aging: Contribution of the DHEAge Study to a sociobiomedical issue. *Proc Natl Acad Sci USA* 2000;97:4279–4284.

Bertoni, A., Rastoldo, A., Sarasso, C., Di Vito C., Sampietro, S., Nalin, M., Bagarotti, A., and Sinigaglia, F. Dehydroepiandrosterone-sulfate inhibits thrombin-induced platelet aggregation. *Steroids* 2012;77(3):260–268.

Betz, J.M., White, K.D., and der Marderosian, A.H. Gas chromatographic determination of yohimbine in commercial yohimbe products. *J AOAC Int* 1995;78:1189–1194.

Bhat, R. and Karim, A.A. Tongkat Ali (*Eurycoma longifolia* Jack): A review on its ethnobotany and pharmacological importance. *Fitoterapia* 2010;81:669–679.

Biswas, T.K., Pandit, S., Mondal, S., Biswas, S.K., Jana, U., Ghosh, T., Tripathi, P.C., Debnath, P.K., Auddy, R.G., and Auddy, B. Clinical evaluation of spermatogenic activity of processed Shilajit in oligospermia. *Andrologia* 2010;42:48–56.

Bode-Boger, S.M., Boger, R.H., Galland, A., Tsikas, D., and Frölich J.C. L-Arginine-induced vasodilation in healthy humans: Pharmacokinetic–pharmacodynamic relationship. *Br J Clin Pharmacol* 1998;46:489–497.

Brittenden, J., Park, K.G., Heys, S.D., Ross, C., Ashby, J., Ah-See, A.K., and Eremin, O. L-Arginine stimulates host defenses in patients with breast cancer. *Surgery* 1994;115:205–212.

Castillo, L., Chapman, T.E., Sanchez, M., Yu, Y.M., Burke, J.F., Ajami, A.M., Vogt, J., and Young, V.R. Plasma arginine and citrulline kinetics in adults given adequate and arginine-free diets. *Proc Natl Acad Sci USA* 1993;90:7749–7753.

Castillo, L., Ajami, A., Branch, S. et al. Plasma arginine kinetics in adult man: Response to an arginine-free diet. *Metabolism* 1994;43:114–122.

Cava, R.C. and Javier, A.N. Vitamin D deficiency [editorial]. *N Engl J Med* 2007;357:1981.

Cheema, P., El-Mefty, O., and Jazieh, A.R. Intraoperative haemorrhage associated with the use of extract of Saw Palmetto herb: A case report and review of literature. *J Intern Med* 2001;250:167–169.

Chen, J., Wollman, Y., Chernichovsky, T., Iaina, A., Sofer, M., and Matzkin, H. Effect of oral administration of high-dose nitric oxide donor L-arginine in men with organic erectile dysfunction: Results of a double-blind, randomized, placebo-controlled study. *BJU Int* 1999;83:269–273.

Cheng, J.W. and Balwin, S.N. L-Arginine in the management of cardiovascular diseases. *Ann Pharmacother* 2001;35:755–764.

Cormio L., De Siati, M., Lorusso, F. Z., Mirabella, L., Sanguedolce, F., and Carrieri, G. Oral L-Citrulline supplementation improves erection hardness in men with mild erectile dysfunction. *Urology* 2011;77:119–122.

D'Aniello, A. D-Aspartic acid: An endogenous amino acid with an important neuroendocrine role. *Brain Res Rev* 2007;53:215–234.

D'Aniello, G., Ronsini, S., Guida, F., Spinell, P., and D'Aniello, A. Occurrence of D-aspartic acid in human seminal plasma and spermatozoa: Possible role in reproduction. *Fertil Steril* 2005;84:1444–1449.

David, F. and Vasant, L. 2001. *The Yoga of Herbs*. Twin Lakes, WI: Lotus Press.

Davis, L. and Kuttan, G. Effect of *Withania somnifera* on cyclophosphamide-induced urotoxicity. *Cancer Lett* 2000;148:9–17.

Davis, L. and Kuttan G. Suppressive effect of cyclophosphamide-induced toxicity by *Withania somnifera* extract in mice. *J Ethnopharmacol* 1998;62:209–214.

Dean, C.E. Prasterone (DHEA) and mania. *Ann Pharmacother* 2000;34:1419–1422.

Demontis, R., Leflon, A., Fournier, A., Tahiri, Y., Herve, M., Moriniere, P., Abdull-Massih, Z., Atik, H., Belbrik, S., and Renaud, H. 1 alpha(OH) vitamin D3 increases plasma aluminum in hemodialyzed patients taking AI(OH)3. *Clin Nephrol* 1986;26:146–149.

Demontis, R., Reissi, D., Noel, C., Boudailliez, B., Westeel, P.F., Leflon, P., Brasseur, J., Coevoet, B., and Fournier, A. Indirect clinical evidence that 1alphaOH vitamin D3 increases the intestinal absorption of aluminum. *Clin Nephrol* 1989;31:123–127.

Diamond, T.H., Ho, K.W., Rohl, P.G., and Meerkin, M. Annual intramuscular injection of a megadose of cholecalciferol for treatment of vitamin D deficiency: Efficacy and safety data. *Med J Aust* 2005;183:10–12.

Di Silverio, F., D'Eramo, G., Lubrano, C., Flammia, G.P., Sciarra, A., Palma, E., Caponera, M., and Sciarra, F. Evidence that *Serenoa repens* extract displays an antiestrogenic activity in prostatic tissue of benign prostatic hypertrophy patients. *Eur Urol* 1992;21(4):309–314.

Dong, J. Y., Qin, L. Q., Zhang, Z., Zhao, Y., Wang, J., Arigoni, F., and Zhang, W. Effect of oral L-arginine supplementation on blood pressure: A meta-analysis of randomized, double-blind, placebo-controlled trials. *Am Heart J* 2011;162:959–965.

Durackova, Z., Trebaticky, B., Novotny, V., Žitňanová, I., and Breza, J. Lipid metabolism and erectile function improvement by Pycnogenol, extract from the bark of *Pinus pinaster* in patients suffering from erectile dysfunction-a pilot study. *Nutr Res* 2003;23:1189–1198.

Effendy, N.M., Mohamed, N., Muhammad, N., Mohamad, I.S., and Shuid, A.N. *Eurycoma longifolia*: Medicinal plant in the prevention and treatment of male osteoporosis due to androgen deficiency. *Evid Based Complement Alternat Med* 2012;Article ID 125761:9pp.

Ernst, E. and Pittler, M.H. Yohimbine for erectile dysfunction: A systematic review and meta-analysis of randomized clinical trials. *J Urol* 1998;159:433–436.

Food and Nutrition Board, Institute of Medicine. 1999. *Dietary Reference Intakes for Calcium, Phosphorus, Magnesium, Vitamin D, and Fluoride*. Washington, DC: National Academy Press.

Forrest, K.Y. and Stuhldreher, W.L. Prevalence and correlates of vitamin D deficiency in US adults. *Nutr Res* 2011;31:48–54.

Gerber, G.S. Saw palmetto for the treatment of men with lower urinary tract symptoms. *J Urol* 2000;163:1408–1412.

Ghosal, S. The aroma principles of Gomutra and Karpuragandha Shilajit. *Indian J Indg Med* 1994;11:11–14.

Ginde, A.A., Liu, M.C., and Camargo Jr, C.A. Demographic differences and trends of vitamin D insufficiency in the US population, 1988–2004. *Arch Intern Med* 2009;169:626–632.

Goodwin, T.W. Metabolism, nutrition, and function of carotenoids. *Annu Rev Nutr* 1986;6:273–297.

Grosse Duweler, K. and Rohdewald, P. Urinary metabolites of French maritime pycnogenol extract in humans. *Pharmazie* 2000;55:364–368.

Guay, A.T., Spark, R.F., Jacobson, J., Murray, F.T., and Geisser, M.E. Yohimbine treatment of organic erectile dysfunction in a dose-escalation trial. *Int J Impot Res* 2002;14:25–31.

Handa, S.S., Rakesh, D.D., and Vasisht, K. 2006. *Compendium of Medicinal and Aromatic Plants—Volume II: Asia.* Trieste, Italy: ICS-UNIDO.

Heaney, R.P. Long-latency deficiency disease: Insights from calcium and vitamin D. *Am J Clin Nutr* 2003;78:912–919.

Heaney, R.P., Davies, K.M., Chen, T.C., Holick, M.F., and Barger-Lux, M.J. Human serum 25-hydroxycholecalciferol response to extended oral dosing with cholecalciferol. *Am J Clin Nutr* 2003;77:204–210.

Henkel, R.R., Wang, R., Bassett, S.H., Chen T., Liu, N., Zhu, Y., and Tambi, M.I. Tongkat ali as a potential herbal supplement for physically active male and female seniors—A pilot study. *Phytother Res* 2014;28:544–550.

Holick, M.F. Vitamin D: A millenium perspective. *J Cell Biochem* 2003;88:296–307.

Hollander, E. and McCarley, A. Yohimbine treatment of sexual side effects induced by serotonin reuptake blockers. *J Clin Psychiatry* 1992;53:207–209.

Huynh, N.T. and Tayek, J.A. Oral arginine reduces systemic blood pressure in type 2 diabetes: Its potential role in nitric oxide generation. *J Am Coll Nutr* 2002;21:422–427.

Ismail, S.B., Mohammad, W.M.Z.W., George, A., Hussain, N.H.N., Kamal, Z.M.M., and Liske, E. Randomized clinical trial on the use of PHYSTA freeze-dried water extract of *Eurycoma longifolia* for the improvement of quality of life and sexual well-being in men. *Evid Based Complement Alternat Med* 2012;Article ID 429268:10pp.

Jacobsen, F.M. Fluoxetine-induced sexual dysfunction and an open trial of yohimbine. *J Clin Psychiatry* 1992;53:119–122.

Jesse, R.L., Loesser, K., Eich, D.M., Qian, Y.Z., Hess, M.L., and Nestler, J.E. Dehydroepiandrosterone inhibits human platelet aggregation in vitro and in vivo. *Ann NY Acad Sci* 1995;774:281–290.

Jorde, R., Grimnes, G., Hutchinson, M.S., Kjærgaard, M., Kamycheva, E., and Svartberg, J. Supplementation with vitamin D does not increase serum testosterone levels in healthy males. *Horm Metab Res* 2013;45:675–681.

Kearney, T., Tu, N., and Haller, C. Adverse drug events associated with yohimbine-containing products: A retrospective review of the California Poison Control System reported cases. *Ann Pharmacother* 2010;44:1022–1029.

Kingsberg, S.A. and Rezaee, R.L. Hypoactive sexual desire in women. *Menopause* 2013;20:1284-1300.

Klotz, T., Mathers, M.J., Braun, M., Bloch, W., and Engelmann, U. Effectiveness of oral L-arginine in first-line treatment of erectile dysfunction in a controlled crossover study. *Urol Int* 1999;63:220–223.

Kobayashi, M., Kakizono, T., Nishio, N., Nagai, S., Kurimura, Y., and Tsuji, Y. Antioxidant role of astaxanthin in the green alga Haematococcus pluvialis. *Appl Microbiol Biotechnol* 1997;48:351–356.

Komers, R., Komersova, K., Kazdova, L., Ruzickova, J., and Pelikanova, T. Effect of ACE inhibition and angiotensin AT1 receptor blockade on renal and blood pressure response to L-arginine in humans. *J Hypertens* 2000;18:51–59.

Kumar, A., Kaul, B.L., and Verma, H.K. Phenological observations on root yield and chemical composition in different morphotypes of *Withania somnifera. JMAPS* 2001;23:21–23.

Kunellius, P., Hakkinen, J., and Lukkarinen, O. Is high-dose yohimbine hydrochloride effective in the treatment of mixed-type impotence? A prospective, randomized, controlled, double-blind crossover study. *Urology* 1997;49:441–444.

Labrie, F., Luu-The, V., Labrie, C., Bélanger, A., Simard, J., Lin, S.X., and Pelletier, G. Endocrine and intracrine sources of androgens in women: Inhibition of breast cancer and other roles of androgens and their precursor dehydroepiandrosterone. *Endocr Rev* 2003;24:152–182.

Labrie, F., Luu-The, V., Bélanger, A., Lin, S.X., Simard, J., Pelletier, G., and Labrie, C. Is dehydroepiandrosterone a hormone? *J Endocrinol* 2005;187:169–196.

Labrie, F. DHEA, important source of sex steroids in men and even more in women. *Prog Brain Res* 2010;182:97–148.

Laumann, E.O., Paik, A., and Rosen, R.C. Sexual dysfunction in the United States: Prevalence and predictors. *JAMA* 1999;281:537–544.

Lebret, T., Hervé, J.M., Gorny, P., Worcel, M., and Botto, H. Efficacy and safety of a novel combination of L-arginine glutamate and yohimbine hydrochloride: A new oral therapy for erectile dysfunction. *Eur Urol* 2002;41:608–613.

Ledda, A., Belcaro, G., Cesarone, M.R., Dugall, M., and Schönlau, F. Investigation of a complex plant extract for mild to moderate erectile dysfunction in a randomized, double-blind, placebo-controlled, parallel-arm study. *BJU Int* 2010;106:1030–1033.

Lee, D.M., Tajar, A., Pye, S.R. et al., EMAS study group. Association of hypogonadism with vitamin D status: The European Male Ageing Study. *Eur J Endocrinol* 2012;166:77–85.

Leung, A.Y. and Foster, S. 1996. *Encyclopedia of Common Natural Ingredients Used in Food, Drugs and Cosmetics*, 2nd edn. New York: John Wiley & Sons.

Lewis, R.W., Fugl-Meyer, K.S., Bosch, R., Fugl-Meyer, A.R., Laumann, E.O., Lizza, E., and Martin-Morales, A. Epidemiology/risk factors of sexual dysfunction. *J Sex Med* 2004;1:35–39.

Levin, R.M. and Das, A.K. A scientific basis for the therapeutic effects of *Pygeum africanum* and *Serenoa repens*. *Urol Res* 2000;28:201–209.

Liu, F.J., Zhang, Y.X., and Lau, B.H. Pycnogenol enhances immune and haemopoietic functions in senescence-accelerated mice. *Cell Mol Life Sci* 1998;54:1168–1172.

Mahdi, A.A., Shukla, K.K., Ahmad, M.K., Rajender, S., Shankhwar, S.N., Singh, V., and Dalela, D. *Withania somnifera* improves semen quality in stress-related male fertility. *Evid Based Complement Alternat Med* 2011;576962:9.

Mandel, H., Levy, N., Izkovitch, S., and Korman, S.H. Elevated plasma citrulline and arginine due to consumption of *Citrullus vulgaris* (watermelon). *J Inherit Metab Dis* 2005;28:467–472.

Mann, K., Klingler, T., Noe, S., Röshchke, J., Müller, S., and Benkert, O. Effects of yohimbine on sexual experiences and nocturnal penile tumescence and rigidity in erectile dysfunction. *Arch Sex Behav* 1996;25:1–16.

Mantovani, F. *Serenoa repens* in benign prostatic hypertrophy: Analysis of 2 Italian studies. *Minerva Urol Nefrol* 2010;62:335–340.

Marks, L.S. and Tyler, V.E. Saw palmetto extract: Newest (and oldest) treatment alternative for men with symptomatic benign prostatic hyperplasia. *Urology* 1999;53:457–461.

McGuffin, M., Hobbs, C., Upton, R., and Goldberg, A. (eds.). 1997. *American Herbal Products Association's Botanical Safety Handbook*. Boca Raton, FL: CRC Press, LLC.

Meston, C.M. and Worcel, M. The effects of yohimbine plus L-arginine glutamate on sexual arousal in postmenopausal women with sexual arousal disorder. *Arch Sex Behav* 2002;31:323–332.

Miki, W. Biological functions and activities of animal Carotenoids. *Pure Appl Chem* 1991;63:141–146.

Montorsi, F., Strambi, L.F., Guazzoni, G., Galli, L., Barbieri, L., Rigatti, P., Pizzini, G., and Miani, A. Effect of yohimbine-trazodone on psychogenic impotence: A randomized, double-blind, placebo-controlled study. *Urology* 1994;44:732–736.

Moon, J. The role of vitamin D in toxic metal absorption. *J Am Coll Nutr* 1994;13:559–564.

Adler, A.J. and Berlyne, G.M. Duodenal aluminum absorption in the rat: Effect of vitamin D. *Am J Physiol* 1985;249:G209–G213.

Nagaya, N., Uematsu, M., Oya, H., Sato, N., Sakamaki, F., Kyotani, S., Ueno, K., Nakanishi, N., Yamagishi, M., and Miyatake, K. Short-term oral administration of L-arginine improves hemodynamics and exercise capacity in patients with precapillary pulmonary hypertension. *Am J Respir Crit Care Med* 2001;163:887–891.

Natural Medicines Comprehensive Database. 2014. Therapeutic Research Faculty. Stockton, CA. http://naturaldatabase.therapeuticresearch.com. Accessed August 5, 2014.

Nimptsch, K., Platz, E.A., Willett, W.C., and Giovannucci, E. Association between plasma 25-OH vitamin D and testosterone levels in men. *Clin Endocrinol (Oxf)* 2012;77:106–112.

Nussey, S. and Whitehead, S. 2001. *Endocrinology: An Integrated Approach*. London, U.K.: BIOS Scientific Publishers.

Osowska, S., Moinard, C., Neveux, N., Loï, C., and Cynober, L. Citrulline increases arginine pools and restores nitrogen balance after massive intestinal resection. *Gut* 2004;53:1781–1786.

Packer, L., Midori, H., and Toshikazu, Y. (eds.). 1999. *Antioxidant Food Supplements in Human Health*. San Diego, CA: Academic Press.

Pandit, S., Biswas, S., Jana, U., Kumar De, R., and Chandan S. Clinical evaluation of purified shilajit on testosterone levels in healthy volunteers. Research Unit, J. B. Roy State Ayurvedic Medical College and Hospital, Department of Health and Family Welfare, Government of West Bengal, Kolkata, India. Under the West Bengal University of Health Sciences, submitted for publication, 2014:16pp.

Patil, S.P., Niphadkar, P.V., and Bapat, M.M. Allergy to fenugreek (*Trigonella foenum graecum*). *Ann Allergy Asthma Immunol* 1997;78:297–300.

Peters, H. and Noble, N.A. Dietary L-arginine in renal disease. *Semin Nephrol* 1996;16:567–575.

Pilz, S., Frisch, S., Koertke, H., Kuhn, J., Dreier, J., Obermayer-Pietsch, B., Wehr, E., and Zittermann, A. Effect of vitamin D supplementation on testosterone levels in men. *Horm Metab Res* 2011 March;43(3):223–225.

Ramawat, K.G. (ed.). 2009. *Herbal Drugs: Ethnomedicine to Modern Medicine*. Heidelberg, Germany: Springer-Verlag.

Rao, A., Steels, E., Beccaria, G., and Vitetta, L. Influence of Libifem, a specialized extract of *Trigonella foenum-graecum* (Fenugreek) on sexual function, hormones and metabolism is healthy menstruating women, in a randomized placebo controlled study. Unpublished. Gencor Nutrients, Anaheim, CA, 2012:18pp.

Rector, T.S., Bank, A.J., Mullen, K.A., Tschumperlin, L.K., Sih, R., Pillai, K., and Kubo, S.H. Randomized, double-blind, placebo-controlled study of supplemental oral L-arginine in patients with heart failure. *Circulation* 1996;93:2135–2141.

Reiter, W.J., Pycha, A., Schatzl, G., Pokorny, A., Gruber, D.M., Huber, J.C., and Marberger M. Dehydroepiandrosterone in the treatment of erectile dysfunction: A prospective, double-blind, randomized, placebo-controlled study. *Urology* 1999;53:590–594.

Reiter, W.J., Pycha, A., Schatzl, G., Klingler, H.C., Märk, I., Auterith, A., and Marberger, M. Serum dehydroepiandrosterone sulfate concentrations in men with erectile dysfunction. *Urology* 2000;55(5):755–758.

Reiter, W.J., Schatzl, G., Märk, I., Zeiner, A., Pycha, A., and Marberger, M. Dehydroepiandrosterone in the treatment of erectile dysfunction in patients with different organic etiologies. *Urol Res* 2001;29:278–281.

Rice-Evans, C.A. and Packer, L. (eds.). 1998. *Flavonoids in Health and Disease*. New York: Marcel Dekker, Inc.

Riley, A.J., Goodman, R.E., Kellet, J.M., and Orr. R. Double blind trial of yohimbine hydrochloride in the treatment of erection inadequacy. *Sex Marital Ther* 1989; 4:17–26.

Riley, A.J. Yohimbine in the treatment of erectile disorder. *Br J Clin Pract* 1994;48:133–136.

Romero, M.J., Platt, D.H., Caldwell, R.B., and Caldwell, R.W. Therapeutic use of citrulline in cardiovascular disease. *Cardiovasc Drug Rev* 2006;24:275–290.

Sachin, W. Effects of Ashwagandha Root Extract (*Withania somnifera*) on Muscle Strength, Size and Recovery, Testosterone, and Body Fat in Healthy Adults. Unpublished; 2014:25pp.

Schwartz, J.B. Effects of vitamin D supplementation in atorvastatin-treated patients: A new drug interaction with an unexpected consequence. *Clin Pharmacol Ther* 2009;85:198–203.

Schwedhelm, E., Maas, R., Freese, R., Jung, D., Lukacs, Z., Jambrecina, A., Spickler, W., Schulze, F., and Böger, R.H. Pharmacokinetic and pharmacodynamic properties of oral L-citrulline and L-arginine: Impact on nitric oxide metabolism. *Br J Clin Pharmacol* 2008;65:51–59.

Sharma, P.V. 1998. *Charaka Samhita. Chowkhambha Orientalia Chikitsasthana, Varanasi, Karaprchitiya RasayanaPada*, 4th edn., Vol. 2. Varanasi, India: Chowkhambha Orientlia Chikitsasthana.

Singh, N., Bhalla, M., de Jager, P., and Gilca, M. An overview on Ashwagandha: A rasayana (Rejuvenator) of ayurveda. *Afr J Tradit Complement Altern Med* 2011;8:208–213.

Singh, R., Singh, S., Jeyabalan, G., and Ali, A. An overview on traditional medicinal plants as aphrodisiac agent. *J Pharmacogn Phytochem* 2012;1:43–56.

Stanislavov, R. and Nikolova, V. Treatment of erectile dysfunction with pycnogenol and L-arginine. *J Sex Marital Ther* 2003;29:207–213.

Stanislavov, R., Nikolova, V., and Rohdewald, P. Improvement of erectile function with Prelox: A randomized, double-blind, placebo-controlled, crossover trial. *Int J Impot Res* 2008;20:173–180.

Steels, E., Rao, A., and Vitetta, L. Physiological aspects of male libido enhanced by standardized *Trigonella foenum-graecum* extract and mineral formulation. *Phytother Res* 2011; 25:1294–1300.

Stohs, S.J. Safety and efficacy of shilajit (mumie, moomiyo). *Phytother Res* 2014;28:475–479.

Stokes, G.S., Barin, E.S., Gilfillan, K.L., and Kaesemeyer, W.H. Interactions of L-arginine, isosorbide mononitrate, and angiotensin II inhibitors on arterial pulse wave. *Am J Hypertens* 2003;16:719–724.

Tambi, M.I.M. and Saad, J.M. Water-soluble extract of *Eurycoma longifolia* Jack soluble extract as a potential natural energizer for healthy aging men. Unpublished. Specialist Reproductive Research Center, National Population & Family Development Board, Ministry of Women & Family Development, Malaysia. 2000:9pp.

Tambi, M.I. Nutrients and botanicals for optimizing men's health. Examining the evidence for *Eurycoma longifolia* longjack, the Malaysian Ginseng in men's health. *Asian J Androl* 2009;11:37–38.

Tambi, M.I. and Imran, M.K. *Eurycoma longifolia* Jack in managing idiopathic male infertility. *Asian J Androl* 2010;12:376–380.

Talbott, S., Talbott, J., Negrete, J., Jones, M., Nichols, M., and Roza, J. Poster 32: Effect of *Eurycoma longifolia* extract on anabolic balance during endurance exercise. *JISSN* 2006;3:S32.

Talbott, S.M., Talbott, J.A., George, A., and Pugh, M. Effect of Tongkat Ali on stress hormones and psychological mood state in moderately stressed subjects. *JISSN* 2013;10:28.

Tambi, M.I., Imran, M.K., and Henkel, R.R. Standardised water-soluble extract of *Eurycoma longifolia*, Tongkat ali, as testosterone booster for managing men with late-onset hypogonadism? *Andrologia* 2012;44:226–230.

Topo, E., Soricelli, A., D'Aniello, A., Ronsini, S., and D'Aniello, G. The role and molecular mechanism of D-aspartic acid in the release and synthesis of LH and testosterone in humans and rats. *Reprod Biol Endocrinol* 2009;7:120.

Udani, J.K., George, A.A., Musthapa, M., Pakdaman, M.N., and Abas, A. Effects of a proprietary freeze-dried water extract of *Eurycoma longifolia* (Physta) and *Polygonum minus* on sexual performance and well-being in men: A randomized, double-blind, placebo-controlled study. *Evid Based Complement Alternat Med* 2014; Article ID 179529:10pp.

Uddin, Q., Samiulla, L., Singh, V.K., and Jamil, S.S. Phytochemical and pharmacological profile of *Withania somnifera* Dunal: A review. *JAPS* 2012;2:170–175.

Unpublished. 2008. Human clinical trial report: Effect of Testofen® on safety, anabolic activity and factors affecting exercise physiology. Gencor Nutrients, Anaheim, CA: 11pp.

Unpublished. n.d. LJ100® Saliva Testosterone Test. HP Ingredients. Bandenton, PL. http://www.hpingredients.com/lj100_human_clinical_research.htm (accessed August 24, 2012).

Upton, R. (ed.). 2000. *Ashwagandha Root (Withania somnifera): Analytical, Quality Control, and Therapeutic Monograph*. Santa Cruz, CA: American Herbal Pharmacopoeia.

Vakina, T.N., Shutov, A.M., Shalina, S.V., Zinov'eva, E.G., and Kiselev, I.P. Dehydroepiandrosterone and sexual function in men with chronic prostatitis. *Urologiia* 2003;1:49–52.

Villareal, D.T., Holloszy, J.O., and Kohrt, W.M. Effects of DHEA replacement on bone mineral density and body composition in elderly women and men. *Clin Endocrinol (Oxf)* 2000;53:561–568.

Vieth, R. Vitamin D supplementation, 25-hydroxyvitamin D concentrations, and safety. *Am J Clin Nutr* 1999;69:842–856.

Vieth, R., Chan, P.C., and MacFarlane, G.D. Efficacy and safety of vitamin D3 intake exceeding the lowest observed adverse effect level. *Am J Clin Nutr* 2001;73:288–294.

Wang, R., Ghahary, A., Shen, Y.J., Scott, P.G., and Tredget, E.E. Human dermal fibroblasts produce nitric oxide and express both constitutive and inducible nitric oxide synthase isoforms. *J Invest Dermatol* 1996;106:419–427.

Wehr, E., Pilz, S., Boehm, B.O., März, W., and Obermayer-Pietsch. B. Association of vitamin D status with serum androgen levels in men. *Clin Endocrinol (Oxf)* 2010;73:243–248.

Weiss, E.P., Villareal, D.T., Fontana, L., Han, D.-H., and Holloszy, J.O. Dehydroepiandrosterone (DHEA) replacement decreases insulin resistance and lowers inflammatory cytokines in aging humans. *Aging* 2011;3:533–542.

Wilborn, C., Taylor, L., Poole, C., Foster, C., Willoughby, D., and Kreider, R. Effects of a purported aromatase and 5α-reductase inhibitor on hormone profiles in college-age men. *Int J Sport Nutr Exerc Metab* 2010 20:457–465.

Wilt, T.J., Ishani, A., Stark, G., MacDonald, R., Lau, J., and Mulrow, C. Saw palmetto extracts for treatment of benign prostatic hyperplasia: A systematic review. *JAMA* 1998;280:1604–1609.

Yadav, R., Tiwari, R., Chowdhary, P., and Pradhan, C.H. Pharmocognostical monograph of *Trigonella feonum*-graecum seeds. *Int J Pharm Pharm Sci* 2011;3:442–445.

Yuan, J.-P., Peng, J., Yin, K., and Wang, J.-H. Potential health-promoting effects of astaxanthin: A high-value carotenoid mostly from microalgae. *Mol Nutr Food Res* 2011;55:150–165.

Zittermann, A. Vitamin D in preventive medicine: Are we ignoring the evidence? *Br J Nutr* 2003;89:552–572.

Zorgniotti, A.W. and Lizza, E.F. Effect of large doses of the nitric oxide precursor, L-arginine, on erectile dysfunction. *Int J Impot Res* 1994;6:33–35.

Section XVI

Cosmeceuticals

32 Nutraceuticals in Cosmeceuticals

Palma Ann Marone

CONTENTS

32.1 INTRODUCTION

The increasing importance of healthy lifestyles in the industrialized world has resulted in increased longevity and a concomitant burgeoning growth of antiaging and personal care products across all age groups. Two pharmaceutical action-derived blended terms combine to claim benefit for health and potential medical benefit: cosmeceutical and nutraceutical. Cosmeceuticals (lotions, creams, etc.), a term attributed to Albert Kligman in 1984 (Kligman, 2005), includes the topical application of biologically active components such as antioxidants, enzymes, proteins, and botanicals, while the term "nutraceuticals" includes the oral ingestion of similarly acting functional foods, supplements, oils, beverages, and botanicals, also for potential health benefit. These terms have been further specialized to include cosmeceuticals as topical products, while nutricosmetics are those ingested internally for improved appearance. Recent global markets forecast that the U.S. $35 billion cosmeceutical industry, the fastest-growing segment in the cosmetics and personal care industry, is expected to grow over 7% during 2013–2018*, while the global nutraceuticals market will reach an estimated U.S. $207 billion by 2016, and the clinical nutrition market is set to reach U.S. $10.7 billion. Even as the United States, the European Union, and Japan are the prominent current markets, the rise of the middle class; the increased disposable income in emerging countries like China, India, Brazil, and Russia; and the desire for natural solutions all will fuel even greater growth and the need for culturally diverse products. Similarly, as functional food and cosmetic use

* Cosmeceuticals market to 2018—Technological Advances and Consumer Awareness Boost Commercial Potential for Innovative and Premium Priced Products, GBI Research, January 2013.

has progressed, so has the need to identify potential adverse factors that threaten the safety and quality of these products. This chapter details the current status of nutricosmeceuticals and, by extension, their potential direction and possible concerns with respect to their nutritional/efficacy and safety properties.

32.2 REGULATORY AGENCIES GOVERNING FOOD SAFETY AND COSMETICS

32.2.1 International

Following concern for food safety that began in the United States in the late 1800s and culminated in the 1906 Food and Drugs Act, numerous adaptations, revisions, and harmonizations in cooperation with the international community have served to safeguard the food supply. Today, with lead initiatives for the global food management safety system implemented by the International Organization for Standardization (ISO) (ISO 22000; FSSC 22000) used by its member countries to certify quality measures for manufacturing and processing under the original 1995 Hazard Analysis Critical Control Point (HACCP) regulations and the World Health Organization (WHO) and the Food and Agriculture Organization of the United Nations (FAO) joint Codex Alimentarius Commission for adopting internationally recognized guidelines for food production and safety (FAO/WHO, 2003), many countries now have harmonized standards for their own national food safety legislation (Magnuson et al., 2013).

The International Food Safety Authorities Network (INFOSAN), working with FAO/WHO, includes a 181-country network conferencing under Pan-American and Pan-European as well as Asia-Pacific regions. International consortia and commissions such as the European Food Safety Authority (EFSA), the Joint FAO/WHO Expert Committee on Food Additives (JECFA), the European Action on Latin America Functional Foods (EULAFF), and others along with the Office of Economic Cooperative and Development (OECD) now coordinate efforts to harmonize global food safety guidelines.

While more individualized under the various governmental entities in countries around the world, the manufacture and sale of cosmetics are similar globally in the common goal of safety and truth in labeling. Updated and amended versions of the original European Union (EU) Cosmetics Directive (76/768/EEC) of 1976 (European Commission, 1976, 2012a) protect consumers and safeguards all cosmetic products in the European market for safety (https://www.cosmeticseurope.eu/safety-and-science-cosmetics-europe/rules-and-regulations/the-eu-legislation.html). In addition, the Scientific Committee on Consumer Safety (SCCS) provides guidance on the testing and safety evaluation of cosmetic substances in Europe for harmonized compliance with cosmetic EU legislation (SCCS, 2012). In Japan, the second largest market after the United States, cosmetics are divided into quasidrugs and cosmetics, regulated by the Minister of Health, Labor, and Welfare (MHLW) governed under The Pharmaceutical Affairs Act (PAA) and further regulated as fragrance, soaps, and makeup cosmetics. In Brazil (Law # 6.360, September 23, 1976), perfumes, cosmetics, toiletries, and medicines, food, and consumer products are registered under the Brazilian Sanitary Vigilance Agency (ANVISA) of the Ministry of Health. Similar to that in the United States , the China Food and Drug Administration (CFDA) regulates the sale and manufacture of cosmetic products in China.

32.2.2 United States

Over a century has passed since physician and chemist Harvey Wiley, prompted by safety concerns over chemical preservatives in marketed food, advocated for the passage of the Food and Drugs Act of 1906. Increasing concerns calling for the standardization of food and consumer products, leading to the establishment of the Food and Drug Administration (FDA) in 1933, subsequently resulted in the passage of the Food, Drug, and Cosmetic Act (1938), extending regulatory control for the first time to cosmetics and consumer products. Amendments and revisions have followed over time, chief among them is the Delaney Clause of 1950 prohibiting known carcinogens from being added to the food supply. Today, the FDA's Center for Food Safety and Applied Nutrition (CFSAN) remains responsible for safe, sanitary, and properly labeled food and cosmetics. In cooperation with the Environmental Protection Agency (EPA) in control of clean water and air for the regulation of pesticides and antimicrobial agents, the FDA monitors residues in food and cosmetics. Similarly, with other consumer protection agencies and the federal departments of transportation, agriculture, health, and human services and justice, comprehensive coordination of various activities serves to ensure adequate safety. More recently, the Food Safety Modernization Act, incepted on 2011, was implemented to enforce food safety standards by the FDA for manufacturers producing, packaging, and distributing food both within the United States and from other countries through premarket approval of any substance expected to become a component of food unless determined as Generally Recognized as Safe (GRAS) by scientific experts. For cosmetics, the FDA recognizes categories, drugs, cosmetics, and soaps but, except for color additives in the cosmetic product, does not require premarket approval of its ingredients. Cosmetics are defined as "articles intended to be rubbed, poured, sprinkled, or sprayed on, introduced into, or otherwise applied to the human body… for cleansing, beautifying, promoting attractiveness, or altering the appearance" [FD&C Act, sec. 201(i)] and apart from drugs as "articles intended for use in the diagnosis, cure, mitigation, treatment, or prevention of disease" and "articles (other than food) intended to affect the structure or any function of the body of man or other animals" [FD&C Act, sec. 201(g)(1)]. Here, the agency monitors safety through inspections, surveys, voluntary industry registration, consumer reports, and the Cosmetic Ingredient Review (CIR) expert panel, an independent, industry-funded panel of medical and scientific experts that meets quarterly to assess the safety of cosmetic ingredients based on data in the published literature (*International Journal of Toxicology*) and trade.

The United States' FDA's Redbook II and the Organization of Economic Cooperative and Development (OECD) for member countries provide standardized health guidelines for safety testing of food additives, which are applicable to human food as well as pet food. While there are no standardized guidelines governing the generalized safety testing of cosmetics in the United States, the FDA has consistently advised cosmetic manufacturers to employ whatever testing is appropriate and effective for substantiating the safety of their products. And similar to food, it remains the responsibility of the manufacturer to substantiate the safety of both ingredients and finished cosmetic products prior to marketing. In recognition of the close association of cosmetics and food, the FDA most recently has issued regulation on the safety of nanomaterials (FDA, 2012a, 2014). The EU, having actively prohibited animal testing, does consider in vitro testing under accepted and verified methods. Most recently, harmonization through the International Cooperation on Cosmetics Regulation (ICCR), an international group of regulatory authorities from Canada, the European Union, Japan, and the United States, met (June 4, 2014) to promote regulatory alignment and maximize consumer protection. Reported current topics include nanomaterials (Schellauff, 2012; Nasir, 2014) and impurities in cosmetics and alternatives to animal testing, under revision of the EU Cosmetics Directive (76/768/EEC), as of March 11, 2013.

Generally, guidelines governing the safety of nutraceuticals and functional foods also apply to ingested nutricosmetics, while topical formulations as cosmetics are less well defined and may vary across international borders.

32.3 CLASSIFICATION OF COSMECEUTICALS AND NUTRICOSMETICS

Growth of the natural skin care industry has progressed as the fastest of the personal care sector for nearly 10 years. The appearance of the skin is influenced by many factors (genetic, environmental, and hormonal) including nutrition. These products are governed and are the potential target of alteration by the same physicosensory properties, marketing strategies, and assessments as traditional functional foods. Herbals may be screened for their antioxidant capacity (Kim et al., 2007; Tsai and Hantash, 2008; Mishra et al., 2011), while traditional in vitro testing for skin irritation, sensitization, dermal photoirritation/sensitization, mutagenicity/genotoxicity, skin penetration/permeation, and phototoxicity testing, most often using epidermal skin models, is recommended and performed as an alternative to in vivo testing (FDA, 2012a; European Commission, 2013). The current regulatory status of quality and safety for essential foods is greater and more rigorous than for cosmetics, which, at present, are viewed more as luxury. Most importantly, as the world market has and continues to grow, standards for cosmeceuticals and nutricosmetics are fast becoming of paramount interest as the subject of regulatory scrutiny and regulation.

32.4 NUTRITIONAL, EFFICACY, AND QUALITY

32.4.1 Sensory Properties

Today's consumers are becoming very discerning and knowledgeable about their food and cosmetics and are more demanding than ever for safe products of good value and high sensory quality. The importance of sensory analysis will often contribute significantly to product success in the market. In vitro assessment of cosmetics and food sensory quality assumes greater significance where in vivo assessment is not practical and serves as a complement to information provided by sensory panels. Similarly, altered appearances, textures, and colors, and for foods, flavors, and aromas, occurring naturally from inadequate/prolonged storage or as a result of processing and manufacture, may cause undesirable effects. An excellent detailed guide to the principles and practices of sensory evaluation and instrumental assessment, considered beyond the scope of this chapter, is provided by Kilcast (2013) and Lawless and Heymann (2010). Their work analyzed the texture, viscosity, and appearance as well as flavor in the processing of meats, poultry and fish, baked goods, crisp products, dairy products, and beverages (wine, beer, juices) in human food preferences and consumption of foods with respect to cosmetic health effect.

32.4.1.1 Physical and Chemical Characteristics

32.4.1.1.1 Appearance and Texture

While largely determined in vivo by sensory panels, the appearance of foods and cosmetics, fundamentally tied to the texture of their solids, can ultimately be determined by and broken down to cellular structure and composition. The appeal of beverages for cosmetic purposes also depends upon their density and mouth feel. Relating the physical properties of a food/beverage or cosmetic microstructure to its overall acceptability is now being assessed to greater sensitivity (below 100 μm) through microscopy, magnetic resonance imaging, computer vision, porosimetry, infrared spectroscopy, and x-ray tomography/scattering mechanical techniques, principal component analysis (PCA) as well as the traditional usages of rheology for food viscosity for a number of food products (Garcia-Ramos et al., 2005; Salvatore and Chisvert, 2007; Norton et al., 2011; Ghosh and Chattopadhyay, 2012; Pico, 2012; Alander et al., 2013; Herremans et al., 2013; Moravkova and Filip, 2013). This is coordinate with the development of nanomaterials and their increasingly common use in food/cosmetic design and packaging (Risvi et al., 2010; Sekhon, 2010; FDA, 2012a, 2014; Pico, 2012; Raj et al., 2012; Panagiotou and Fisher, 2013; Nasir, 2014). It has been clear for some time that a certain and complex relationship exists between food structure and digestibility for carbohydrates (Bjorck et al., 1994; Mishra et al., 2012), determinants for glycemic, moisture, and hydrolytic properties; for proteins (Owusu-Apenten, 2002; de Jongh and Broersen, 2012) in the form of secondary amino acid structure and potential determinants of allergenicity; and pro/prebiotics (Soccol et al., 2010) for immunity, most prominently. It is expected that the same relationship holds for ingested nutriceuticals and topical cosmetics. There are data available on the physical properties of foods and, to a much lesser extent cosmetics, but the relationship to microstructure and overall appeal is less well known and is the subject of current study. Furthermore, the physiologic bioavailability of bioactive ingredients in functional foods contributes significantly to the health and well-being of the individual (Wang and Bohn, 2012).

Ingested nutriceuticals have been more extensively studied, and recent research has focused on the relationship of chewing sounds to crunchiness and crispness of foods. In the new field of neurogastronomy, Charles Spence, the University of Oxford, has used audio recording, human psychophysics, functional magnetic resonance imaging, electroencephalography, and transcranial magnetic stimulation to test the influence of sound on consumers' perceptions of foods in vivo (Marmelstein, 2013). Acoustic energy analyzers with sensitive electronics, filters, and microphones are now being introduced into existing texture analyzers to generate sound profiles for evaluation of new formulations and processes, packaging, and shelf-life. Tribometers, instruments used to measure the lubricating ability (moisture content) of food materials to reduce friction (against the tongue), are being used to generate an acoustic signal, and acoustic tribology technology is a recent award winner in the Institute of Food Technologists 2013 Food Expo Innovation competition for the Nizo Corporation. It would not be difficult to foresee similar applications of such instrumentation in the cosmetics of skin care in the near future.

For cosmetics and nutricosmetics, the added dimension and interest, focusing on perception, sensation, neuromarketing, and the emotional impact evaluation of a product, have attracted new and widespread attention. Recent programs (Cosmetics and Sensory, The Program of Sensory, Tours, France, June 23–24, 2014), as well as studies on these topics, apart from anecdotal and traditional awareness, are just beginning to be formally recognized and are expected to grow and become more scientifically based in the near future.

32.4.1.1.2 *Flavors and Colorants in Nutriceuticals*

Flavor, either natural or synthetic, remains the single most important factor in consumer (functional) food choice and appeal, followed closely by color. In the United States, the Expert Panel of the Flavor and Extract Manufacturers Association (FEMA) evaluates new flavorings for GRAS determination under the authority of the 1958 Federal Food, Drug, and Cosmetics Act (Hallagan and Hall, 1995, 2009; Harman et al., 2013; Marnett et al., 2013). Interestingly, like texture and appearance, the structure of the food matrix also has an important role in the flavor release. Further, food aroma and the ability to isolate aromas are closely tied to flavor perception and food appeal and marketability. The widespread use of electronic noses and tongues, gas chromatography–olfactometry (GC–O) often combined with mass spectroscopy, is designed to mimic the mammalian nose to integrate and recognize patterns of preference for design of foodstuffs (Baldwin et al., 2011; Falasconi et al., 2012). The sensitivity of these systems may have the ability to reveal the perception of taste from thermal sensors alone (chemesthesis), a quality some sensitive individuals possess (Green et al., 2005). Some flavoring manufacturers have adapted high-throughput screening techniques to identify molecules that interact with and enhance taste cells, often with the goal of developing fresh natural combinations of existing tastes and flavors. Results may include "tricking" the tongue through the use of nearby chemoreceptors by changing the size and shape of salt crystals, or triggering capsaicin receptors from spicy pepper flavoring in close proximity, for example (Gravitz, 2012).

Color in food has traditionally been measured using computer vision digital imaging models. Quantitative capture of the pixels on the surface of food has the advantage of simplicity and low cost although lighting, angle of observation, and equipment standardization may be disadvantages (Yam and Papadakis, 2004). More sensitive methods may include the use of spectrophotometers and colorimeters to provide accurate quantitative measures. Color has the added significance to carry with it the potential to impart a preconceived flavor, particularly for beverages: yellow for tart lemon, red/blue for berry, and green for lime. When the two are incongruous, flavor identity is often compromised; a brown color is often associated with a poor-quality food. Further, intensity of color may influence taste perception with strong, deep colors as more appealing than lighter, weak ones (Spence et al., 2010; Esquivel, 2013).

Any substance added to impart color to the food is a color additive. Under the Federal Food, Drug, and Cosmetic Act (FFDCA) (Chapter VII, section 721), color additives (FDA, 2012b), except for coal tar hair dyes, are subject to FDA approval before they may be used in food, drugs, or cosmetics, or in medical devices that come in contact with the bodies of people or animals for a significant period of time. Under 21 CFR 70.3(g), a material that otherwise meets the definition of color additive can be exempt from that definition on the basis that it is used or intended to be used solely for a purpose or purposes other than coloring, as long as the material is used in a way that any color imparted is clearly unimportant insofar as the appearance, value, marketability, or consumer acceptability is concerned. Any color additive in food is deemed unsafe unless its use is either permitted by regulation or exempt by regulation. Cosmetic color additives are specifically regulated under 21 CFR 73-Subpart C. Unlike the definition for food additive, there is no GRAS exemption for color additives. Any food that contains an unsafe color additive is adulterated under section 402(c) of the FFDCA. The most recent changes to functional food labeling by the FDA includes a proposed requirement for declaring added sugars and increased prominence and specification of calories and serving sizes, as well as new cosmetic labeling guidelines (http://www.fda.gov/downloads/Cosmetics/Labeling/UCM391202.pdf).

32.4.1.2 Processing, Preservation, and Packaging of Functional Foods and Cosmeceuticals

Processing and packaging of functional foods and cosmetic products has a significant capacity to influence its sensory appeal and, depending on the method and type, may cause unwelcome changes in color and/or taste and aroma and by way of changes to its microstructure through leachability (Wang and Bohn, 2012). Ideally, product processing and packaging strives to preserve the natural ingredients in raw materials to the greatest extent possible while maintaining an inert barrier. Processing has traditionally included thermal and nonthermal treatments used to prepare, enhance (Maillard reaction), or preserve (sterilize) solid and liquid food products. These treatments often resulted in a loss of ingredient bioactivity. Newer methods of processing technologies, such as microencapsulation, have proven useful in minimizing microstructural modifications. Microencapsulation provides the advantage of protection of core ingredients from degradation or reaction while offering the option of controlled release (Sultanbawa, 2011; Wang and Bohn, 2012). Encapsulation and combined nanocapabilities have stimulated newer technologies in advanced delivery systems aside from the traditional pills and creams. Fast-melting oral strips and the use of biopolymers for enhanced bioavailability, biodegradability, biostability, safety, nonantigenicity, and nutritive value at low cost are just a few of the delivery areas now being explored and developed (Hu and Huang, 2013).

Increasingly, functional food and cosmetic packaging must meet longer shelf life and adhere to international safety and quality standards. An active barrier, including the addition of antimicrobial coatings in the form of bioactive packaging, will protect against product spoilage (water and water vapor, oil and grease, oxygen and aroma) and influence visual appeal (clear vs. opaque) at the same time, reflecting on brand image. Similarly, synergies in flavors have been used to maximize antimicrobial properties (Sultanbawa, 2011). Most recently, the use of mild heat stress combined with a low concentration of preservatives provides a safe, high-quality food. These techniques include nonthermal processing, high-pressure processing, and pulsed electric field active packaging. The growing use of nanotechnology in food packaging has resulted in new safety, environmental, and regulatory guidance in the United States and Europe (Duncan, 2011; EFSA, 2011; European Commission, 2012b; FDA, 2012a, 2014; OECD, 2010, 2012).

32.4.2 Functional Responses, Safety, and Efficacy of Nutritional Cosmeceuticals

With the burgeoning interest in natural therapies, numerous scientific reviews are presently available on the health benefits and modalities of nutraceuticals and functional foods. However, scientific determination and reporting of the benefits of nutritional cosmeceuticals, used both as ingested (nutricosmetic) and/or topical (cosmeceutical) elixirs, is still in its infancy. The market has reflected these trends: Sales for more traditional topical formulations under the purview of dermatology have seen much greater growth than those for nutricosmetics, probably owing to, as yet, lacking or inconclusive evidence of efficacy for the latter. Nonetheless, consumers are discovering the potential for beauty from within as a balanced diet provides the foundation for extrinsic and extrinsic processes. Indeed, many of the beauty ingredients traditionally used for only one type of application are now being rediscovered and repurposed for dual external, topical- and internal, ingestible-capable functions as common modes of action for nutricosmeceuticals are determined. Similarly, greater uses of diversified products from various nontraditional sources are penetrating into mainstream usage. Examples include marine nutritional cosmeceuticals, including algal and seaweed species, for their potential as antioxidants, anti-inflammatory, antitumorigenic, antidiabetic, antiallergic, and antihypertensive effects, among others (Thomas and Kim, 2013; Kim, 2014); plant-derived stem cells rich in polyphytols from grape, lilac, and Swiss apple, and used for bioregenerative purposes, interact with and influence melanocytes, hair growth, growth factors, and others to form emulsions for topical or injectable treatments (Dahl, 2014). While the market use of topical cosmeceuticals are largely directed at antiaging purposes, natural botanical and vitamin treatments are used for skin ailments such as purpura, hyperpigmentation, and various dermatitis-related maladies.

32.4.2.1 Cosmeceutical Classifications

Pursuits for the fountain of youth have been ongoing since time immemorial. The greatest ease of use and market share of these age-defying products is directed to topically administered skin elixirs, often seeking to replace the natural components of skin lost with age, termed intrinsic aging and resulting in thinner, weaker, less elastic skin. While administered to the epidermal layer, many of these products penetrate into the lower levels of skin, the dermis, to deliver nutrients to the structural foundation of the skin to restore skin's youthful appearance. Most of these products are antioxidants derived from botanicals, since these organisms must thrive under conditions of ultraviolet light, nature's most prolific source of free radicals. In relation, natural skin whitening agents, such as grape and safflower seed, aloe vera, and licorice, with active ingredients vitamin C (ascorbic acid), nicatinamide, hydroquinone, and flavonoids (quercetin), applied either topically or ingested (pomegranate rich in ellagic acid), act at various levels of melanocyte production or cell transport, through modulation of the enzyme, tyrosinase, which controls melanogenesis (Smit et al., 2009; Renden et al., 2014).

32.4.2.1.1 Antioxidants and Collagens

One mode of action of these products is their antioxidant properties at the cellular level. Oxidative stress and the resultant free radicals produced are considered the effects of environmental toxins, stress, unhealthy diet, illness, and ultraviolet light. Topical agents such as carotenoids (beta-carotene, astaxanthin), lycopene, vitamin C alone and in combination with vitamin E, selenium, CoQ10, and pycnogenol facilitate their free radical scavenger activity to promote moisture and elasticity retention of the skin (Olivo, 2014). Vitamin E in the deeper levels of the stratum corneum protects cell membranes from lipid peroxidation by free radicals resulting from UV exposure where it is most effective in combination with stabilizing vitamin C. Vitamin E does not appear to be an effective treatment for the reduction of visible signs of photoaging when used alone (Jacob et al., 2012).

While topically applied carotenoids, vitamin E (α-tocophorol), glutathione, and selenium have improved the appearance of UV-induced skin aging superficially, other topically applied agents, such as Vitamin C, promote the synthesis of collagen, glycosaminoglycans, and glycoproteins, which themselves support the deeper dermal connective tissue to improve skin elasticity to reduce fine lines and wrinkles (Farris, 2014b). Vitamin C works uses this mechanism. Collagen itself has also been used in support of nail and hair health along with biotin (Vitamin B7), which works through its enzymatic function associated with the formation of keratin. Ingredient silica also works to strengthen hair and nails by increasing collagen production to support the structural foundation of the skin.

Among the best known derivatives for building collagen support is Vitamin A. The biologically active tretinoin passes through the epidermis to act on nuclear receptors, increasing the production of procollagen types II and III to modulate genes for epidermal proliferation and differentiation (Jacob et al., 2012). These genes include retinoic acid–binding protein 2, CRABP2, and heparin-binding epidermal growth factor–like growth factor [HBEGF] (Varani et al., 1994, 2000; Elder et al., 1996; Singh and Griffiths, 2006). In a dual role, tretinoin also reduces collagen degradation by inhibiting matrix metalloproteinases (Varani et al., 2000). Pycnogenol selectively binds collagen and elastin as well as aids in the production of endothelial nitric oxide to improve dermal blood flow and hydration. Coffeeberry, with its rich supply of polyphenols, acts to enhance collagen production through its stimulatory effects on fibroblasts (Stallings and Lupo, 2009). In many prepared formulations, a combination of agents, such as the addition of lutein, zeanxanthin, and vitamin A, can augment skin hydration. Similarly, hyaluronic acid, a natural epidermal component of youthful skin, as well as aloe vera, a natural humectant, attracting moisture and holding it in the skin, topically applied binds large quantities of water to support skin elasticity and smoothness (Del'balo et al., 2006).

32.4.2.1.2 Anti-Inflammatories

In addition to their antioxidant capacities, topical formulations may also act as anti-inflammatory agents by limiting carcinogen-induced reactive oxygen species. These include soys, teas, chamomile, coffees, and oatmeal (Stallings, 2009; Pazyar, 2012; Emer and Waldorf, 2014; Houston and Kimball, 2014). Soy extracts with their active components of isoflavones and phytoestrogens have been used to treat skin changes associated with postmenopause, particularly hyperpigmentation where topical formulations appear to promote skin lightening. Generalized effects include increased skin elasticity, reduced oil production, and skin moisturization. Topical estrogens have been noted to promote collagen synthesis and augment skin thickness.

Teas (white, black, and green), particularly green teas, containing phenols and flavonoids, have their various antiaging effects grounded in reducing inflammation and promoting scavenging of free radicals. They have been used as sunscreens for their photoprotective effects as well as in wound healing for their ability to promote keratinocyte cell differentiation as well as to suppress melanoma cell growth in culture. Aside from synthetic physical sunblocks, zinc oxide and titanium dioxide among them, epigallocatechin gallate, the active ingredient in teas and caffeine, has shown promise in its ability to promote apoptosis of photo-induced carcinoma cells in humans and mice (Stalling and Lupo, 2009). In addition, terpenoids, flavonoids, and hydroxycoumarins as the active ingredients of chamomile are considered beneficial in the treatment of contact dermatitis and conjunctivitis. It too diminishes the effects of photodamage while promoting elasticity through its natural moisturizing properties. Although incompletely explored scientifically, the avenanthramide phenolic compounds present in oats and oatmeal also have shown promise for its role in skin photoprotection against ultraviolet rays. By decreasing arachidonic acid, cytosolic phospholipase A2, and tumor necrosis factor-alpha (TNF-alpha), oatmeal extract has demonstrated the ability to inhibit nuclear factor kappa B (NF-kappa B) in keratinocytes and the release of proinflammatory cytokines and histamine, critical processes in the pathophysiology of inflammatory dermatoses. It is these pro-inflammatory cytokines, aberrant transcription factors, and matrix enzymes, including the enzyme MMP-1, which cleaves collagen type 1, the primary form of collagen within the dermal extracellular matrix, which are responsible for degradation of the dermal support structure of the skin following UVA and UVB radiation exposure (Decker, 2013). Nicotinamide (Vitamin B3) and curcumin have been shown to selectively protect against UVA radiation, a property not inherent in most sunscreens, and acts through anti-inflammatory ability to inhibit leukocyte peroxidase and ornithine decarboxylase activity, respectively. Through its ability to stimulate synthesis of sphingolipids, ceramides, free fatty acids, cholesterol, and collagen, nicotinamide is effective in promoting skin moisturization and wrinkle reduction (Korac and Khambholja, 2011; Muszalska et al., 2013; Berson et al., 2014), one method of which appears to be through the differentiation of keratinocytes via genetically controlled transcription processes (Jacob et al., 2012).

32.4.2.2 Nutricosmetics

Topical botanical compounds and the active ingredients of which they are composed can also be applied to various functional food applications. Nutricosmetics for the dual purpose of nutrition and beauty from the inside-out are rapidly becoming a favored choice of savvy consumers. Fresh fruits and vegetables containing vitamins, collagens, carotenoids, flavonoids, and others acting as antioxidants, anti-inflammatories, and supports for skin, immunity, and cardiac and digestive health have long been the staple of a balanced diet and active lifestyle. With more emphasis on locally grown produce, the increased availability and use of these nonprocessed dietary "basics" has afforded a greater awareness of the essential vitamins and minerals of how they work to maximize outward appearance and inner well-being. Anthocyanins, proanthocyanidins, and carotenoids, the natural deep colorants in fruits (acai, pomegranate, blueberries, grapes, etc.) and vegetables (carrots, tomatoes, eggplant, asparagus, etc.), are examples of well-known key components in antioxidant protection and antiscavenging behavior. Enhancement of hair, skin, nail, and eye health has been reported with lutein, zeaxanthin, lycopene and reservatrol, as among the more well-known nutritional ingredients (Del'balo et al., 2006; Farris, 2014a). Resveratrol, the active polyphenol ingredient in red wine, helps to prevent damage to blood vessels, reduces atherosclerotic plaque accumulation from low-density lipoprotein cholesterol, and prevents blood clots (Farris, 2014a). Ingestion of coffee and green teas has been associated with the upregulation of tumor suppressor genes (Huang et al., 2011; Al-Ansari and Aboussekhra, 2014). Lesser known oral and topical supplements include rosemary, olive oil, lavender, mushrooms, and those of exotic countries native to Africa and Asia such as shea, argan, cocoa, mangosteen, and baobob, as just a few examples. If a daily healthy lifestyle is also a component of appearance, the reduction of daily stressors and the endogenous production of cortisol is also an important consideration for optimum well-being. Integral to stress management and cortisol lowering is promotion of restful sleep. Sleep aids may reduce cortisol while promoting the production of growth hormone, an anabolic steroid normally produced during sleep, which declines with age. Similarly, dehydroepiandrosterone (DHEA), an endogenous steroid hormone, functioning as a metabolic intermediate in sex hormone production that declines with age, has been marketed as an oral dietary supplement for its purported anticancer, antiaging (photoprotective), and immunomodulatory capabilities.

32.5 TARGETED POPULATIONS

Topical formulations, generally those focusing on protective/antiaging capacities and specifically targeting the skin as largest affected organ and consumer market, are designed for use in all ages of life. These are easily applied and are most available worldwide as natural botanicals although little distinction needs be made between natural and synthetic ingredients.

Specific preferences for nutricosmetics parallel those for functional foods for taste, fortification, and digestibility and are specifically targeted to include the sensitive populations of children, medical disorders, and the elderly. Textured (soft) and taste-specific foods are employed in weanlings and the elderly, while satiety-enhancing food products are used in obese populations (Rolls, 1999; Mojet et al., 2004; Ghavidel, 2011; Van Kleef et al., 2012). Further, the use of prebiotics and probiotics and the numerous attempts to mimic the composition in breastmilk in infancy has the capability to imprint the intestinal flora in childhood and later life (Forssten et al., 2011). In addition, cultural preferences play a role in food selection in all ages (Eertmans et al., 2001) as well as special needs populations of women of childbearing age, adolescents, athletes, and military personnel (IFT, 2005). The potential vulnerability of these groups and the general population for age-defying schemes emphasize the importance of regulatory controls and standards of product manufacture and production. In the United States and worldwide, undesirable effects of nutritional cosmeceutical use arise as the result of naturally occurring and/or contamination/adulteration or processing changes caused by either the desire for financial gain or due to carelessness of regulatory controls and/or lack in proper hygienic conditions of processing, storing, transportation, and marketing.

Undesirable product formulations may include the presence of environmental, pesticide and heavy metal residues, microbiologic and animal contamination, and intentional ingredient replacement (adulteration), thus giving rise to allergic and/or systemic toxic reactions associated with unregulated products.

32.6 FUTURE CONSIDERATIONS

With the continuing importance on youthful appearance, longevity, and healthy lifestyle, it is expected that the market for nutritional cosmeceuticals will continue to grow at an accelerated pace. New and continuing formulations combining active ingredients are continuing to be developed for the mass market, as competition drives prices for what was once a luxury populace is now becoming a mainstream essential. The availability and prominent usage of these products will, in turn, accelerate the need for safety and authenticity grounded in sound science as consumers engage physicians and researchers. Innovative, more effective delivery systems combined with ingredients from nontraditional sources will continue to be developed. Consumer awareness is both advised and encouraged as technologies advance toward the merging of drugs and nutricosmeceuticals coordinate with increased worldwide regulatory and harmonized guidance.

REFERENCES

Alander JT, Bochko V, Martinkauppi B, Saranwong S, Mantere T. (2013). A review of optical nondestructive visual and near-infrared methods for food quality and safety. *Int J Spectrosc.* 2013:1–36. Available at: http://dx.Doi.org/10.1155/2013/341402, accessed on line December 3, 2013.

Al-Ansari MM, Aboussekhra A. (2014). Caffeine mediates sustained inactivation of breast cancer-associated myofibroblasts via up-regulation of tumor suppressor genes. *PLOS One.* 9:1–9.

Baldwin EA, Bai G, Plotto A, Dea S. (2011). Electronic noses and tongues: Applications for the food and pharmaceutical industries. *Sensors.* 11:4744–4766. doi: 10.3390/s110504744.

Berson DS, Oblong JE, Osborne R, Hakozaki T, Johnson MB, Bissett DL. (2014). Niacinamide: A topical vitamin with wide-ranging skin appearance benefits, Chapter 10. In: *Cosmeceuticals and Cosmetic Practice*, P.K. Farris, ed. Wiley-Blackwell, Oxford, U.K., pp. 103–112. ISBN: 978-1-118-38480-0.

Bjork I, Granfeldt Y, Liljeberg H, Tovar J, Asp NG. (1994). Food properties affecting the digestion and absorption of carbohydrates. *Am J Clin Nutr.* 59:699S–705S.

Dahl MV. (2014). Stem cell cosmeceuticals In: *Cosmeceuticals and Cosmetic Practice*, P.K. Farris, ed. Wiley-Blackwell, Oxford, U.K., pp. 192–199. ISBN: 978-1-118-38480-0.

de Jongh HHJ, Broersen K. (2012). Application potential of food protein modification. In: *Advances in Chemical Engineering*, Z. Nawaz, ed. InTech. Available at: http://www.intechopen.com/books/advances-in-chemical-engineering/chemical-engineering-of-proteinsto-provide-a-toolbox-to-study-functional-properties-of-proteins, accessed on line December 3, 2013.

Decker KJ. (2013). Cosmeceutical ingredients: Natural approaches. Nutritional Outlook, April 18, 2013. http://www.nutritionaloutlook.com/article/cosmeceutical-ingredients-natural-approaches-4-12727, accessed on-line 14, 2014.

Del'balo S, Gaspar L, Campos P. (2006). Moisturizing effect of cosmetic formulations containing aloe vera extract in different concentrations assessed by skin bioengineering techniques. *Skin Res Technnol.* 12:241–246.

Duncan TV. (2011). Applications of nanotechnology in food packaging and food safety: Barrier materials, antimicrobials and sensors. *J Coll Interf Sci.* 363:1–24.

Eertmans A, Baeyens F, Van den Bergh O. (2001). Food likes and their relative importance in human eating behavior: A review and preliminary suggestions for health promotion. *Health Educ Res.* 16:443–456.

Elder JT, Kaplan A, Cromie MA, Kang S, Voorhees JJ. (1996). Retinoid induction of CRABP II mRNA in human dermal fibroblasts: use as a retinoid bioassay. *J Invest Dermatol.* 106:517–521.

Emer J, Waldorf HA. (2014). Soy and oatmeal-based cosmeceuticals, Chapter 13. In: *Cosmeceuticals and Cosmetic Practice*, P.K. Farris, ed. Wiley-Blackwell, Oxford, U.K., pp. 133–141. ISBN: 978-1-118-38480-0.

Esquivel T. (November/December 2013). Trends in RTD beverages. *Food Prod Des.* 32–40.

European Commission (1976). Council directive of 27 July 1976 on the approximation of the laws of the Member States relating to cosmetic products (76/768/EEC) (OJ L 262, 27.9.1976, p. 169), pp. 1–129, http://www.emergogroup.com/sites/default/files/file/cosmetics_directive_76-768-eec_0.pdf, accessed on line July 17, 2014.

European Commission. (2012a). The SCCS's notes of guidance for the testing of cosmetic substances and their safety evaluation, 8th revision. Scientific Committee on Consumer Safety, SCCS/1501/12, https://www.cosmeticseurope.eu/safety-and-science-cosmetics-europe/rules-and-regulations/the-eu-legislation.html. Accessed on December 13, 2014.

European Commission. (2012b). Guidance on the safety assessment of nanomaterials in cosmetics. Scientific Committee on Consumer Safety, SCCS/1484/12.

European Commission. (2013). Full EU ban on animal testing for cosmetics enters into force. Press Release. Reference: IP/13/210, Brussels, Belgium, March 11, 2013 (Online). Available at: http://europa.eu/rapid/press-release_IP-13–210_en.htm, accessed on May 27, 2014.

European Food Safety Authority (EFSA). (2011). Guidance on the risk assessment of the application of nanoscience and nanotechnologies in the food and feed chain. *EFSA J.* 9:2140. doi: 10.2903/j.efsa.2011.2140.

Falasconi M, Concina I, Gobbi E, Sberveglieri V, Pulvirenti A, Sberveglieri G. (2012). Review article: Electronic nose for microbiological quality control of food products. *Int J Electrochem.* 2012:1–12. Article ID 715kioxi63. Doi.org/10.1155/2012/715763, accessed on line December 3, 2013.

FAO/WHO (World Health Organization/Food and Agriculture Organization of the United Nations). (2003). FAO/WHO Report of the fourth session of the codex ad hoc intergovernmental task force on foods derived from biotechnology. JOINT FAO/WHO Food Standards Programme Code Alimentarius Commission. Twenty-sixth Session, Rome, Italy, June 30–July 7, 2003. Yokohama, Japan, March 11–14, 2003, ftp://ftp.fao.org/docrep/fao/meeting/006/y9220e.pdf, accessed on line October 2, 2013.

Farris PK. (2014a). Resveratrol and synthetic surtuin activators, Chapter 16. In: *Cosmeceuticals and Cosmetic Practice*, P.K. Farris, ed. Wiley-Blackwell, Oxford, U.K., pp. 165–172. ISBN: 978-1-118-38480-0.

Farris PK. (2014b). Skin aging, glycation and glycation inhibitors, Chapter 17. In: *Cosmeceuticals and Cosmetic Practice*, P.K. Farris, ed. Wiley-Blackwell, Oxford, U.K., pp. 173–183. ISBN: 978-1-118-38480-0.

FDA (Food and Drug Administration). (2012a). Draft Guidance for Industry. Safety of nanomaterials in cosmetic products. http://www.fda.gov/downloads/Cosmetics/GuidanceComplianceRegulatoryInformation/GuidanceDocuments/UCM300932.pdf, accessed on line December 4, 2013.

FDA. (2012b). Draft Guidance for Industry: Assessing the effects of significant manufacturing process changes, including emerging technologies on the safety and regulatory status of food ingredients and food contact substances, including food ingredients that are color additives. http://www.fda.gov/Food/GuidanceRegulation/GuidanceDocumentsRegulatoryInformation/IngredientsAdditivesGRASPackaging/ucm300661.htm, accessed on line December 4, 2013.

FDA. (2014). Guidance for Industry. Safety of nanomaterials in cosmetic products. U.S. Department of Health and Human Services Food and Drug Administration, Center for Food Safety and Applied Nutrition, http://www.fda.gov/downloads/Cosmetics/Labeling/UCM391202.pdf. Accessed on June 2014.

Forssten SD, Lahtinen SJ, Ouwehand AC. (2011). The intestinal microbiota and probiotics. In: *Probiotic Bacteria and Enteric Infections*, J.J. Malago, J.F.J.G. Koninkx, and R. Marinsek-Logar, eds. Springer, New York, pp. 41–63.

García-Ramos FJ, Valero C, Homer I, Ortiz-Cañavate J, Ruiz-Altisent M. (2005). Non-destructive fruit firmness sensors: A review. *Sp J Agric Res.* 3:61–73.

Ghavidel RA, Davoodi MG. (2011). Processing and assessment of quality characteristics of composite baby foods. *World Acad Sci Eng Technol.* 59:2041–2043.

Ghosh D, Chattopadhyay P. (2012). Application of principal component analysis (PCA) as a sensory assessment tool for fermented food products. *J Food Sci Technol (Mys).* 49:328–334.

Gravitz L. (2012). Food science: Taste bud hackers. *Nature.* 486:S14–S15. doi: 10.1038/486S14a, http://www.nature.com/nature/journal/v486/n7403_supp/full/486S14a.html, accessed on line December 3, 2013.

Green BG, Alvarez-Reeves M, George P, Akirav C. (2005). Chemesthesis and taste: Evidence of independent processing of sensation intensity. *Physiol Behav.* 86:526–37.

Hallagan JB, Hall RL. (1995). FEMA GRAS—A GRAS assessment program for flavor ingredients. *Regul Toxicol Pharmacol.* 21:422–430.

Hallagan JB, Hall RL. (2009). Under the conditions of intended use-new developments in the FEMA GRAS program and the safety assessment of flavor ingredients. *Food Chem Toxicol.* 47:267–278.

Harman CL, Hallagan JB. (November 2013). FEMA Science Committee Sensory Data Task Force. Sensory testing for flavorings with modifying properties. *Food Technol.* 44–47.

Herremans E, Bongaers E, Estrade P, Gondek E, Hertog M, Jakubczyk E, Nguyen Do Trong N et al. (2013). Microstructure–texture relationships of aerated sugar gels: Novel measurement techniques for analysis and control. *Innov Food Sci Emerg Technol.* 18:202–211.

Houston N, Kimball AB. (2014). Green tea extract, Chapter 12. In: *Cosmeceuticals and Cosmetic Practice*, P.K. Farris, ed. Wiley-Blackwell, Oxford, U.K., pp. 122–132. ISBN: 978-1-118-38480-0.

Hu B, Huang Q. (2013). Biopolymer based nano-delivery systems for enhancing bioavailability of nutraceuticals. *Chin J Poly Sci.* 31:1190–1203.

Huang J, Plass C, Gerhauser C. (2011). Cancer chemoprevention by targeting the epigenome. *Curr Drug Targets.* 12:1–32.

Institute of Food Technologists (IFT). (2005). Expert Report. *Functional Foods: Opportunities and Challenges.* IFT Foundation, Chicago, IL.

Jacob L, Baker C, Farris P. (2012). Vitamin-Based Cosmeceuticals. *Cosmet Dermatol.* 25:405–410.

Kilcast D. (2013). *Instrumental Assessment of Food Sensory Quality: A Practical Guide.* Wood Head Publishing Series in Food Science, Technology and Nutrition No. 253. Woodhead Publishing Ltd., Cambridge, U.K.

Kim SK. (2014). Marine cosmeceuticals. *J Cosmet Dermatol.* 13:56–67.

Kim SS, Hyun CG, Lee J, Lim, J, Kim JY, Park D. (2007). In vitro screening of jeju medicinal plants for cosmeceutical materials. *J Appl Biol Chem.* 50:215–220.

Kligman A. (2005). The future of cosmeceuticals: An interview with Albert Kligman, MD, PhD. Interview by Zoe Diana Draelos. *Dermatol Surg.* 31:890–891.

Korac RR, Khambholja KM. (2011). Potential of herbs in skin protection from ultraviolet radiation. *Pharmacogn Rev.* 5:164–173.

Lawless HT, Heymann H. (2010). *Sensory Evaluation of Food. Principles and Practices*, 2nd edn. Springer, New York. doi: 10.1007/978-1-4419-6488-5.

Magnuson B, Munro I, Abbot P, Baldwin N, Lopez-Garcia R, Ly K, McGirr L, Roberts A, Socolovsky S. (2013). Review of the regulation and safety assessment of food substances in various countries and jurisdictions. *Food Addit Contam A.* 30:1147–1220. http://dx.doi.org/10.1080/19440049.2013.795293, accessed on line January 7, 2014.

Marmelstein NH. (2013). Not the sound of silence. *Food Technol.* 12(13):84–88.

Marnett LJ, Cohen SM, Fukushima S, Gooderham NJ, Hecht SS, Rietjens IMCM, Smith RL et al. (August 2013). GRAS flavoring substances. *Food Technol.* 38–56.

Mishra AK, Mishra A, Chattopadhyay P. (2011). Herbal cosmeceuticals for photoprotection from ultraviolet B radiation: A review. *Trop J Pharm Res.* 10:351–360. doi: 10.4314/tjpr.v10i3.7.

Mishra S, Hardacre A, Monro J. (2012). Food structure and carbohydrate digestibility. In: *Carbohydrates- Comprehensive Studies on Glycobiology and Glycotechnology*, C. Fa Chang, ed. InTech. doi: 10.5772/51969, ISBN: 978-953-51-0864-1. Available at: http://www.intechopen.com/books/carbohydrates-comprehensive-studies-on-glycobiology-and-glycotechnology/food-structure-and-carbohydrate-digestibility, accessed on line December 3, 2013.

Mojet J, Heidema JJ, Christ-Hazelhof E. (2004). Effect of concentration on taste–taste interactions in foods for elderly and young subjects. *Chem Sens.* 29:671–681.

Moravkova T, Filip P. (2013). The Influence of emulsifier on rheological and sensory properties of cosmetic lotions. *Adv Mater Sci Eng.* 2013:1–7. http://dx.doi.org/10.1155/2013/168503.

Muszalska I, Kiaszewicz K, Kson D, Sobczak A. (2013). Determination of nicotinamide (vitamin B3) in cosmetic products using differential spectrophotometry and liquid chromatography (HPLC). *J Anal Chem.* 68:1007–1013.

Nasir A. (2014). Nanopharmaceuticals and nanocosmeceuticals, Chapter 5. In: *Cosmeceuticals and Cosmetic Practice*, P.K. Farris, ed. Wiley-Blackwell, New York, pp. 45–54. ISBN: 978-1-118-38483-1.

Norton IT, Spyropoulos F, Cox P, eds. (2011). *Practical Food Rheology: An Interpretive Approach.* Wiley-Blackwell, New York. ISBN: 978-1-4051-9978-0.

OECD (Office of Economic Cooperative Development). (2010). Guidance manual for the testing of manufactured nanomaterials: OECD's sponsorship programme; first revision. *Environment Directorate Joint Meeting of the Chemicals Committee and the Working Party on Chemicals, Pesticides and Biotechnology.* ENV/JM/MONO(2009)20/REV. Available at: http://search.oecd.org/officialdocuments/displaydocumentpdf/?cote=env/jm/mono(2009)20/rev&doclanguage=en, accessed on line October 4, 2013.

OECD. (2012). Guidance on sample preparation and dosimetry for the safety testing of manufactured nanomaterials. Series on the Safety of Manufactured Nanomaterials, No. 36 JT03332780, ENV/JM/MONO(2012)40.

Olivo L. (2014). Beauty built naturally. *Nutraceutical World*, June 2014, pp. 41–46.

Owusu-Apenten RK. (2002). Protein digestibility-corrected amino acid scores. In: *Food Protein Analysis: Quantitative Effects on Processing*. Marcel Dekker, Inc., New York, pp. 411–416.

Panagiotou T, Fisher RJ. (2013). Producing micron- and nano-size formulations for functional foods applications. *Funct Foods Health Dis*. 3:274–289.

Pazyar N, Yaghoobi R, Kazerouni A, Feily A. (2012). Oatmeal in dermatology: A review. *Ind J Derm Ven Lep*. 78:142–145.

Pico Y., ed. (2012). *Chemical Analysis of Food*. Elsevier, Waltham, MA. ISBN: 978-0-12-384862-8.

Raj S, Jose S, Sumud US, Subitha M. (2012). Review article: Nanotechnology in cosmetics: Opportunities and challenges. *J Pharm Bioanal Sci*. 4:186–193. doi: 10.4103/0975-7406.99016.

Renden MI, Vazquez Y, Micciantuono S. (2014). Cosmeceutical skin lighteners, Chapter 22. In: *Cosmeceuticals and Cosmetic Practice*, P.K. Farris, ed. Wiley-Blackwell, New York, pp. 218–225. ISBN: 978-1-118-38483-1.

Rizvi SSH, Moraru CI, Bouwmeester H, Klampers FWH. (2010). Nanotechnology and food safety. In: *Ensuring Global Food Safety: Exploring Global Harmonization*, C. Boisrobert, S. Oh, A. Stjaponovic, H. Lelieveld, eds. Academic Press, London, U.K., pp. 263–279.

Rolls BJ. (1999). Do chemosensory changes influence food intake in the elderly? *Physiol Behav*. 66:193–197.

Salvatore A, Chisvert A., eds. (2007). *Analysis of Cosmetic Products*. Elsevier, Oxford, U.K. ISBN-13: 978-0-444-52260-3.

Schellauf F. (2012). The nano-specific regulatory requirements for cosmetic products—Learnings from the implementation of the nano-notification. *Commission Workshop on Second Regulatory Review on Nanomaterials*, Cosmetic Europe, January 30, 2012.

Sekhon BS. (2010). Food nanotechnology—An overview. *Nanotech Sci Appl*. 3:1–15. Accessed on line December 5, 2013.

Singh M, Griffiths CE. (2006).The use of retinoids in the treatment of photoaging. *Dermatol Ther*. 19:297–305.

Smit N, Vicanova J, Pavel S. (2009). The hunt for natural skin whitening agents. *Int J Mol Sci*. 10:5326–5349. doi: 10.3390/ijms10125326.

Soccol CR, Vandenberghe LPS, Spier MR, Medeiros ABP, Yamaguishi CT, Lindner JDD, Pandey A, Thomaz-Soccol V. (2010). The potential of probiotics: A review. *Food Technol Biotechnol*. 48:413–434.

Spence C, Levitan CA, Shankar MU, Zampini M. (2010). Does food color influence taste and flavor perception in humans? *Chem Percept*. 3:68–84. doi: 10.1007/s12078-010-9067z. http://www.researchgate.net/publication/225762625_Does_Food_Color_Influence_Taste_and_Flavor_Perception_in_Humans, accessed on line December 3, 2013.

Stallings AF, Lupo MP. (2009). Practical uses of botanicals in skin care. *J Clin Aesthet Derm*. 2:36–40.

Sultanbawa Y. (2011). Plant antimicrobials in food applications: Minireview. In: *Science against Microbial Pathogens: Communicating Current Research and Technological Advances*, A. Méndez-Vilas, ed. Formatex Research Center, Badajoz, Spain, pp. 1084–1093.

Thomas NV, Kim SK. (2013). Beneficial effects of marine algal compounds in cosmeceuticals. *Mar Drugs*. 11:146–164.

Tsai TC, Hantash BM. (2008). Cosmeceutical agents: A comprehensive review of the literature. *Clin Med Derm*. 1:1–20.

Van Kleef E, Van Trijp JCM, Van den Borne JJGC, Zondervan C. (2012). Successful development of satiety enhancing food products: Towards a multidisciplinary agenda of research challenges. *Crit Rev Food Sci Nutr*. 52:611–628.

Varani J, Perone P, Griffiths CEM, Inman DR, Fligiel SEG, Voorhees JJ. (1994). All-trans retinoic acid (RA) stimulates events in organ-cultured human skin that underlie repair. Adult skin from sun-protected and sun-exposed sites responds in an identical manner to RA while neonatal foreskin responds differently. *J Clin Invest*. 94:1747–1756.

Varani J, Warner RL, Gharaee-Kermani M, Phan SH, Kang S, Chung JH, Wang A, Datta SC, Fisher GJ, Voorhees JJ. (2000). Vitamin A antagonizes decreased cell growth and elevated collagen-degrading matrix metalloproteinases and stimulates collagen accumulation in naturally aged human skin. *J Invest Dermatol*. 114:480–486.

Wang L, Bohn T. (2012). Health-promoting food ingredients and functional food processing technology. In: *Nutrition, Well-Being and Health*, J. Bouayed, ed. Intech, University Campus STeP Ri, Rijeka, Croatia.

Yam KL, Papadakis SE. (2004). A simple digital imaging method for measuring and analyzing color of food surfaces. *J Food Eng*. 61:137–142.

Section XVII

Exercise and Physical Health

33 Nutrition, Functional Foods, and Exercise

A Review

Wataru Aoi and Yuji Naito

CONTENTS

33.1 INTRODUCTION

Appropriate nutrition is necessary for athletes to maintain or improve exercise performance. Correct intake of nutrients is critically important for improving endurance, and building muscle, conditioning, and recovery from fatigue after exercise. The recommended daily allowance for nutrients increases as volume and intensity of exercise increase. Thus, athletes need to eat a well-balanced basic diet and supplement with those components that are difficult to obtain in sufficient quantities from a normal diet. Previously, it has been argued that optimal timing and combination of macronutrient intake can improve sporting performance (Figure 33.1). Several natural food components have also been shown to exert physiological effects, with some considered useful (when ingested at high doses or continuously) at improving athletic performance or avoiding the disturbance of homeostasis caused by strenuous exercise. Such food components with physiological actions have been called "functional foods"; the effects of such foods have been scientifically investigated. Thus far, some functional foods have been shown to have constant beneficial influence on the physiological changes that occur during exercise (Table 33.1).

33.2 REPLENISHMENT OF WATER

Water is the major constituent of our human body, and it plays an essential role in body fluid circulation, chemical reactions in energy metabolism, and excretion of waste products. In particular, the role for maintenance of body temperature is important during exercise. When the body temperature rises with elevating energy metabolism due to physical activity, sweating occurs in order to radiate heat, leading to loss of a large amount of water and electrolytes, such as sodium contained in body fluid. This loss of body fluid impairs thermoregulation and blood circulation, which leads to a decline in various physiological functions and can result in health problems, such as heat exhaustion and heat stroke. Therefore, to maintain homeostasis and avoid disorder, replenishment of water and electrolytes is necessary before and during or after exercise (American College of Sports Medicine et al. 2007). Individuals should drink 1.5 L of fluid per 1 kg of body weight lost (due to water loss from exercise-induced sweating) to achieve rapid and complete recovery from dehydration. The general

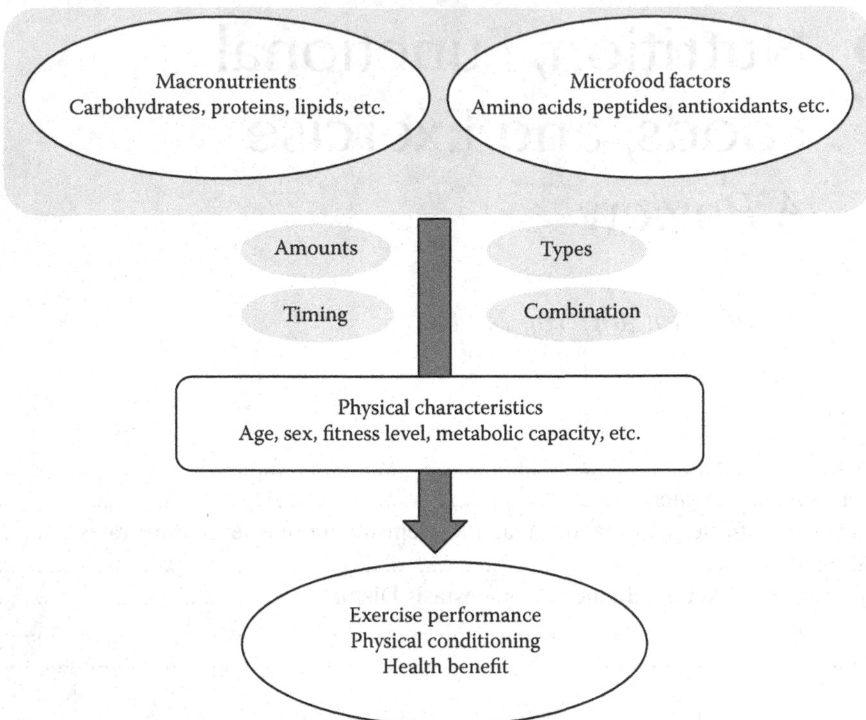

FIGURE 33.1 Dietary strategy for improvement of exercise performance and fitness. Exercise training improves physical performance, in that it builds muscle and enhances endurance. In addition, daily exercise is also important for prevention of lifestyle diseases and maintenance of fitness with age. To obtain the effect efficiently, we need to consider the amounts, types of nutrients, optimal timing, and combination of both macronutrients and microfood factors.

TABLE 33.1
Potential Functions of Microfood Factors in Exercise

Function	Food Factor
Metabolic improvement	Carnitine, astaxanthin, catechin, α-lipoic acid, and caffeine
Blood flow improvement	Inorganic nitrate, arginine, and citrulline
Protein synthesis	Protein, branched-chain amino acids, creatine, β-HMB, glutamine, and vitamin D
Suppression of exercise-induced stress	
Oxidative damage	Vitamins C and E, carotenoids, and polyphenols
Muscle soreness	Branched-chain amino acids and peptides
Immunosuppression	Carbohydrates, vitamins C and E, glutamine, and probiotics

recommendation is to drink an isotonic or slightly hypotonic beverage that contains electrolytes, such as sodium, potassium, and chloride, at concentrations close to those in body fluids (Castellani et al. 1998). In contrast, replenishment of water alone is not recommended for maintaining homeostasis of body fluid in prolonged exercise that produces high sweat rates. Drinking water alone during prolonged exercise frequently leads to hyponatremia and a decrease in the osmotic pressure of body fluids, which inhibits release of antidiuretic hormone, resulting in suppressed water intake and increased urine output (Takamata et al. 1994). During prolonged exercise lasting longer than 90 min, one should drink a fluid containing electrolytes and carbohydrate to sustain carbohydrate oxidation and physical activity (Latzka and Montain 1999). Alternative methods to maintain body fluid have been suggested, such as glycerol loading. This method prevents high temperatures and dehydration during exercise because glycerol acts as an osmolyte in body fluid, leading to an elevated plasma osmolality (Robergs 1998). Thus, water reabsorption in the kidney increases and urine excretion decreases. Oral administration of 1.0–1.2 g glycerol/kg body weight with water transiently results in an increase of 300–700 mL body fluid (Riedesel 1998, Robergs 1998). It remains controversial whether hyperhydration with additional fluids in the extra- and intracellular space before exercise can provide a performance advantage; however, several studies have reported that glycerol loading seems to improve endurance performance compared with placebo (Lyons 1990, Anderson 2001).

33.3 IMPROVEMENT OF ENERGY METABOLISM AND REPLENISHMENT OF ENERGY SUBSTRATES

Energy consumed in muscle during exercise is mainly supplied by carbohydrates and lipids. Lipids are supplied by meals, and also by adipose tissues; however, carbohydrates must be acquired from meals before exercise because very little carbohydrate is stored as glycogen in the liver and muscle tissue. During prolonged exercise, glycogen, an energy substrate for muscle contraction, is gradually depleted, making it difficult to continue exercise. Therefore, it is considered that an effective way to improve endurance is to increase the glycogen stores in skeletal muscle. When tissue glycogen is depleted, glycogen synthetase activity is transiently elevated, so it is possible to increase glycogen storage by carbohydrate intake at that time (Hulyman and Nilsson 1971, Forgac 1980). As a representative method, it has been known that glycogen storage for a competition can be improved by eating low carbohydrate foods for 3 days, starting from 6 days prior to competition, and high carbohydrate foods for the next 3 days, resulting in the storage of 1.5 times more glycogen than usual (Evans and Hughes 1985). Additional intake of citrate, which has an inhibitory action on glycolysis, with high carbohydrate food, can be expected to accelerate glycogen storage through inhibition of glycolysis (Saito et al. 1983, 1994, Saito and Suzuki 1986).

When exercise continues for a long time, taking carbohydrates immediately before or during the event is also effective for maintaining performance. Under such conditions, it is beneficial to consume monosaccharides or oligosaccharides, because these are rapidly absorbed and transported to the peripheral tissues after ingestion. On the other hand, carbohydrates inhibit degradation of another energy substrate, body fat, by stimulating insulin secretion, which prevents fat oxidation in muscle tissue through inhibition of lipoprotein lipase activity (Kiens et al. 1989). This leads to impairment of energy production through lipid metabolism, and to acceleration of glycolysis as another energy production pathway. As a result, use of muscular glycogen will increase, and intramuscular pH will decrease due to increased lactic acid production, which may lead to impairment of muscular contraction. Therefore, it has been suggested that intake of other carbohydrates, such as fructose and dextrin, would be better for improving endurance because these carbohydrates stimulate less insulin secretion than monosaccharides and oligosaccharides, and thus are unlikely to inhibit lipolysis (Mitsuzono et al. 1995).

The timing of carbohydrate intake before exercise affects substrate utilization during exercise. A major opinion on efficient timing is to consume a carbohydrate supplement (beverage or bar/snack) 30 min before exercise because plasma insulin reaches a peak approximately 30 min after ingestion of carbohydrates and thereafter gradually decreases to the basal level. Regarding intake of a whole meal before exercise, several organizations, including the American Dietetic Association, the Dietitians of Canada, and the American College of Sports Medicine, have encouraged the consumption of a substantial meal 2–4 h before exercise for athletes (Rodriguez et al. 2009). However, these guidelines for carbohydrate intake depend on individual physical characteristics, such as insulin sensitivity (Sasaki et al. 2014).

In contrast to utilization of carbohydrates, which reduces muscular pH and decreases glycogen storage, a large amount of energy can be continuously obtained via aerobic metabolism when lipids are the primary energy source. Therefore, elevation of lipid utilization in skeletal muscle has major effects on both aerobic endurance and body fat accumulation. In general, the ratio of energy substrates depends on exercise intensity, a habit of exercise, and the level of physical performance. Additionally, the potential effects of several food factors on lipid metabolism in exercise have been investigated; some of them accelerate lipid utilization through (1) catabolism of adipose tissue, (2) accelerated entry of fatty acids into mitochondria, and (3) increased mitochondrial biogenesis.

A rate-limiting step of lipid metabolism in myocyte is entry of long chain fatty acids into mitochondria. Carnitine is essential for the transport of long-chain fatty acids across the mitochondrial membrane associated with carnitine parmitoyltransferase (CPT), and it acts to promote the β-oxidation of fatty acids (Cerretelli and Marconi 1990, Brass 2000). Carnitine supplementation is expected to activate lipid metabolism in skeletal muscles, and to also achieve sparing of glycogen. Among persons who are performing aerobic training, some authors have reported that an intake of 2–4 g of carnitine before exercise, or on a daily basis, increased the maximum oxygen consumption (an aerobic threshold) and inhibited lactate accumulation after exercise (Marconi et al. 1985, Vecchiet et al. 1990). CPT I, located on the mitochondrial outer membrane, plays an important role in the entry of fatty acids. We found that a novel antioxidant, astaxanthin, limits the oxidative modification of CPT I by hexanoyl lysine (HEL), a good marker for oxidative modification by oxidized ω–6 fatty acids, with elevating CPT I activity during exercise, which caused acceleration of body fat reduction by exercise training and prevention of fatigue (Ikeuchi et al. 2006, Aoi et al. 2008, Earnest et al. 2011). In addition, levels of peroxisome proliferator-activated receptor gamma coactivator 1-alpha (PGC-1α), and its downstream proteins, were significantly elevated in astaxanthin-fed mice compared with mice fed a normal diet (Liu et al. 2014). Astaxanthin intake resulted in a PGC-1α elevation in skeletal muscle, which can lead to acceleration of lipid utilization through activation of mitochondrial aerobic metabolism. Other food compounds that have antioxidative capacities have also been identified. Catechin, one of the polyphenols found in Japanese green tea, accelerates utilization of fatty acid as a source of energy production in skeletal muscle during exercise (Murase et al. 2006). It has been indicated that the effect of catechin is related to enhancement of β-oxidation activity and the level of fatty acid translocase/CD36 mRNA in the muscle. Another antioxidant, α-lipoic acid, improves glucose transport activity in skeletal muscle. Intake of α-lipoic acid combined with endurance exercise training further accelerates glucose uptake and insulin signal pathway compared with training alone (Henriksen 2006). Caffeine is another compound that can affect energy metabolism. Caffeine inhibits phosphodiesterase by promoting catecholamine release and increasing hormone-sensitive lipase activity, leading to an increase of circulating free fatty acids and further improvement of endurance (Ryu et al. 2001).

It has been suggested that supplementation of factors with improving circulation could affect energy metabolism during exercise. As a typical example, inorganic nitrate has been shown to reduce oxygen uptake during prolonged exercise, which leads to enhancement of muscle contractile efficiency (Bailey et al. 2009, Cermak et al. 2012). Nitric oxide plays an important role in circulation functions in the body regulating vasodilatation and blood flow. Thus, it may support oxygen delivery to exercising muscle. Other compounds such as arginine and citrulline that induce production of nitric oxide, also have the potential effect (Takeda et al. 2011, Yavuz et al. 2014).

33.4 BUILDING MUSCLE

Muscle strength is generally proportional to the cross-sectional area of muscle; thus, it is necessary to increase muscle bulk to enhance strength. Protein is a major composition of muscle cells. To obtain muscle bulk, it is important to increase the protein content by modulating protein metabolism. Namely, muscle bulk and strength can be increased by accelerating protein synthesis or by preventing protein degradation in muscle cells. Resistance exercise is known as an essential method to increase muscle bulk because it enhances secretion of growth hormone and various growth factors, which lead to promotion of protein synthesis and muscular enlargement compared with aerobic exercise. In order to accelerate the effect of resistance exercise, it is important to maintain the muscular pool and blood levels of amino acids that are substrates for synthesis of muscle proteins. For this purpose, dietary protein intake must increase to maintain a positive nitrogen balance. The daily recommended protein intake is generally estimated as 1.2–1.7 g/kg for endurance training and 1.6–1.7 g/kg for strength training under conditions in which energy intake is adequate (Lemon 1998). However, it is actually difficult to maintain such a high intake of protein from the diet, so protein supplements can be useful. A wide variety of raw materials are utilized for production of powdered protein supplements; products derived from soy beans or eggs and further derived from whey separated from lactoprotein are commercially available. All these products contain essential amino acids in a well-balanced ratio, and the amino acid score is 100 for many of these products. In particular, whey protein is believed to be an ideal source for building muscles since this type of protein is well digested and is easily absorbed, resulting in a rapid increase in the blood level of amino acids (Boirie et al. 1997, Ha and Zemal 2003). In addition, branched-chain amino acids are abundant in whey protein (de Wit 1998, Ha and Zemal 2003).

Intake of amino acids or peptides also benefits the supply of protein substrate for muscle. Free amino acids and peptides do not need to be digested, and rapid absorption can be expected. In addition to being used as substrates for synthesis of muscle protein, amino acids also have a variety of physiological effects. Researchers have focused on the role of branched-chain amino acids (e.g. valine, leucine, and isoleucine) in muscle building because contents of these amino acids are known to be relatively high in muscle proteins. Many amino acids are metabolized in the liver, but branched-chain amino acids are metabolized through special processes in the muscles (Harper et al. 1984). Branched-chain amino acids are metabolized in the muscles and utilized as energy substrates, and their oxidation is enhanced during exercise by activation of branched-chain-α-keto acid dehydrogenase (Shimomura et al. 2004). These branched-chain amino acids can modulate protein metabolism in the muscles by promoting synthesis and inhibiting the degradation of protein (Buse and Reid 1975, Tischler et al. 1982, Casperson et al. 2012). Glutamine has also been reported to promote muscle growth by inhibiting protein degradation (Antonio and Street 1999). It is the most abundant free amino acid in muscle tissue and its intake leads to an increase of myocyte volume, resulting in stimulation of muscle growth. Glutamine is also found at relatively high concentrations in many other human tissues and has an important homeostatic role. Therefore, during catabolic states such as exercise, glutamine is released from skeletal muscle into the plasma to be utilized for maintenance of glutamine levels in other tissues (Castell 2003). Uptake of amino acids into myocytes is accelerated by insulin, so it is believed that amino acids can be more effectively utilized for synthesis of body proteins when taken simultaneously with carbohydrates.

Supplementation with creatine is popular for enhancement of muscle power. The human body contains more than 100 g of creatine and almost all of it is stored in skeletal muscle as creatine phosphate, which produces adenosine triphosphate during the process of degradation to creatine. Because creatine metabolism occurs under anaerobic conditions, improvement of anaerobic metabolism and strength can be expected from increasing the stores of creatine. Moreover, creatine stimulates water retention and protein synthesis (Balsom et al. 1994, 1995). It has been reported that intake of 3 g/day or more creatine increases the intramuscular content of creatine phosphate and improves endurance, especially during activities with high power output, such as short distance running, resistance exercise, and muscle strength (Kreider et al. 1998, Terjung et al. 2000). In addition, it has been reported that intake of creatine accelerates the increase in muscle bulk and muscle strength during resistance exercise (Vandenburghe et al. 1997, Volec et al. 1999).

β-Hydroxy-β-methylbutyrate (βHMB) is a metabolite of the branched-chain amino acid leucine. It increases muscle mass by inhibiting degradation of protein via an influence on the metabolism of branched-chain amino acids. A meta-analysis of studies conducted between 1967 and 2001 supported the use of βHMB to augment lean body mass and strength when performing resistance exercise (Nissen and Sharp 2003). It has been shown that intake of 3.0 g/day βHMB for at least 4 weeks achieved a greater increase in lean body mass or power compared with the intake of placebo (Alon et al. 2002). In addition, supplementation of vitamin D is effective to improve strength, which would be involved in protein synthesis (Tomlinson et al. 2014).

Muscle loss leads to a decrease in muscle strength. Age-related muscle, loss, known as sarcopenia, contributes to various health problems, reduced quality of life, and increased healthcare expenditures. Because skeletal muscle is the primary consumer of energy in the body, the loss of muscle mass decreases energy metabolism, resulting in body fat accumulation and increased risk of metabolic disease. Muscle atrophy occurs via several factors, including apoptosis and decrease of differentiation capacity of satellite cells, as well as from protein loss caused by decreased protein synthesis and increased protein degradation. The cross-sectional area of a quadriceps muscle after a 12-week resistance training program is increased more immediately after exercise than 2 h later in older men (Esmarck et al. 2001). Additionally, muscle protein synthesis can be promoted by intake of protein combined with carbohydrates via the actions of insulin to accelerate increases in muscle mass and strength (Borsheim et al. 2004).

Oxidative stress in the muscle increases with age due to the increased production of reactive oxygen species (ROS) combined with a decrease in antioxidant capacity of the muscle. Such oxidative stress acts as a regulator of metabolism, apoptosis, and inflammation, leading to muscle loss and metabolic dysfunction. Several food factors that have antioxidant effects have been suggested to prevent muscle atrophy in animal and cell culture experiments (Hemdan et al. 2009, Ogawa et al. 2013, Wang et al. 2014); however, it is still controversial whether they can be useful in our daily life.

33.5 MAINTENANCE OF EXERCISE-INDUCED HOMEOSTASIS DISTURBANCE

Intense or unaccustomed exercise induces various excess stress, such as oxidative damage, muscle pain, and immune depression. Exercise leads to production of ROS mainly via the mitochondrial electron transport chain in muscle cells, endothelial xanthin oxidase, and nicotinamide adenine dinucleotide phosphate oxidase in phagocytes. Exercise-induced ROS oxidize several targets, such as proteins, lipids, and DNA in skeletal muscle, heart, and liver, which may be a causative pathway to health disorder. Previous studies have demonstrated that dietary supplementation with antioxidants, such as vitamin E, vitamin C, and carotenoids, can decrease oxidative damage induced by intense exercise (Kanter et al. 1993, Aoi et al. 2004). In addition, several compounds such as branched-chain amino acids and peptides, attenuate muscle soreness induced by intense exercise (Shimomura et al. 2004) although the mechanism is unclear. In contrast, recent studies reported that high dose of supplemental vitamin C and vitamin E cancelled many exercise-induced benefits, such as improvement of insulin sensitivity, blood pressure, and endurance capacity (Gomez-Cabrera et al. 2008, Ristow et al. 2009). These effects are caused by suppression of the expression of redox-sensitive proteins including PGC-1α, AMP-activated kinase, and superoxide dismutase-2 (Gomez-Cabrera et al. 2008, Ristow et al. 2009). Therefore, the benefit of dietary intake of antioxidants during exercise therapy for treating and preventing diseases and for training to improve athletic performance is debatable. In contrast, some antioxidants increase energy metabolism and insulin sensitivity induced by exercise through elevation of the level and activity of key modulators (Saengsirisuwan et al. 2004, Murase et al. 2006, Aoi et al. 2008, Wu et al. 2012). This effect may be responsible for the specific actions of each compound, and physical properties such as sex, age, and individual performance (Higashida et al. 2011, Abadi et al. 2013, Draeger et al. 2014).

Moderate intensity and regular exercise enhances immunocompetence and decreases circulating levels of inflammatory cytokines and oxidative stress and also enhances the function of immune cells in the resting state. Several studies have reported that moderate-intensity exercise reduces the incidence of upper respiratory tract infection (URTI), the most useful index of immune function. In contrast, strenuous exercise increases the production of inflammatory cytokines in muscle tissues and causes delayed-onset muscle damage. Therefore, persons performing strenuous or unaccustomed exercise are exposed to the risk of impaired immunocompetence. Intake of carbohydrates during prolonged exercise at submaximal intensity attenuates the increase of plasma cortisol and cytokine levels after exercise, which could lead to the inhibition of immunosuppression (Nehlsen-Cannarella et al. 1997, Gleeson et al. 2004). Antioxidants such as vitamin C and vitamin

E have actions that promote immunity. These vitamins are essential for T cell differentiation and for maintenance of T cell function (Moriguchi and Muraga 2000, Peake 2003). However, there is limited evidence about the effects of vitamins supplementation on immune function in relation to exercise. Glutamine is an important energy source for lymphocytes, macrophages, and neutrophils, and is also an essential amino acid for the differentiation and growth of these cells (Castell 2003). Glutamine is utilized by leukocytes, the gut mucosa, and bone marrow stem cells, and the plasma concentration of glutamine is decreased with prolonged exercise, which can suppress immune function (Mackinnon and Hooper 1996, Kargotich et al. 2005). Thus, dietary glutamine supplements may be beneficial in maintaining plasma glutamine concentrations and preventing immune suppression following prolonged exercise. Exercise also induces mechanical changes in gastrointestinal barrier function, depending on intensity of exercise. Exercise increases gastrointestinal permeability through several mechanisms related to reduced blood flow and hyperthermia in the gut. Recently, benefits of probiotics, such as the most common strains belonging to the *Lactobacilli* and *Bifidobacteria* genera, have been examined (Kekkonen et al. 2007, Gleeson et al. 2012, Cox et al. 2010, West et al. 2011); however, few studies have focused on athletes.

33.6 CONCLUSION

Active life is necessary to maintain and promote health, which cannot be substituted by diet. However, to accelerate the benefits of exercise or prevent the negative effects of exercise, intake of appropriate nutrition should be considered. Recent research has investigated the effects of functional foods on sporting performance; however, the efficacy of many of them is still controversial. The effectiveness of the components could differ according to gender, between individuals, and with the mode of ingestion. Thus, the optimum method of intake, the quantity and quality of foods to be ingested, and the timing of their intake need to be established in accordance with the purpose of using each food or food component after understanding the physiological changes induced by exercise. In the future, guidelines for the use and evaluation of athletic functional foods should be established on the basis of clear scientific evidence related to the individual foods.

REFERENCES

Abadi, A., Crane, J.D., Ogborn, D. et al. 2013. Supplementation with α-lipoic acid, CoQ10, and vitamin E augments running performance and mitochondrial function in female mice. *PLoS One* 8:e60722.

Alon, T., Bagchi, D., and Preuss, H.G. 2002. Supplementing with beta-hydroxy-beta-methylbutyrate (HMB) to build and maintain muscle mass: A review. *Res Commun Mol Pathol Pharmacol* 111:139–151.

American College of Sports Medicine, Sawka, M.N., Burke, L.M. et al. 2007. Exercise and fluid replacement. *Med Sci Sports Exerc* 39:377–390.

Anderson, M.J. 2001. Effect of glycerol-induced hyperhydration on thermoregulation and metabolism during exercise in heat. *Int J Sport Nutr Exerc Metab* 11:315–333.

Antonio, J. and Street, C. 1999. Glutamine: A potentially useful supplement for athletes. *Can J Appl Physiol* 24:1–14.

Aoi, W., Naito, Y., Takanami, Y. et al. 2004. Oxidative stress and delayed-onset muscle damage after exercise. *Free Radic Biol Med* 37:480–487.

Aoi, W., Naito, Y., Takanami, Y. et al. 2008. Astaxanthin improves muscle lipid metabolism in exercise via inhibitory effect of oxidative CPT I modification. *Biochem Biophys Res Commun* 366:892–897.

Bailey, S.J., Winyard, P., Vanhatalo, A. et al. 2009. Dietary nitrate supplementation reduces the O_2 cost of low-intensity exercise and enhances tolerance to high-intensity exercise in humans. *J Appl Physiol* 107:1144–1155.

Balsom, P., Soderlund, K., and Ekblom, B. 1994. Creatine in humans with special references to creatine supplementation. *Sports Med* 18:268–280.

Balsom, P., Soderlund, K., Shodin, B., and Ekblom, B. 1995. Skeletal muscle metabolism during short duration high-intensity exercise: Influence of creatine supplementation. *Acta Physiol Scand* 1154:303–310.

Boirie, Y., Dangin, M., Gachon, P., Vasson, M.P., Maubois, J.L., and Beaufrere, B. 1997. Slow and fast dietary proteins differently modulate postprandial protein accretion. *Proc Natl Acad Sci USA* 94:14930–14935.

Borsheim, E., Aarsland, A., and Wolfe, R.R. 2004. Effect of an amino acid, protein, and carbohydrate mixture on net muscle protein balance after resistance exercise. *Int J Sport Nutr Exerc Metab* 14:255–271.

Brass, E.P. 2000. Supplemental carnitine and exercise. *Am J Clin Nutr* 72:618S–623S.

Buse, M.G. and Reid, S.S. 1975. Leusine: A possible regulator of protein turnover in muscle. *J Clin Invest* 56:1250–1261.

Casperson, S.L., Sheffield-Moore, M., Hewlings, S.J., and Paddon-Jones, D. 2012. Leucine supplementation chronically improves muscle protein synthesis in older adults consuming the RDA for protein. *Clin Nutr* 31:512–519.

Castell, L.M. 2003. Glutamine supplementation in vitro and in vivo, in exercise and in immunodepression. *Sports Med* 33:323–345.

Castellani, J.W., Maresh, C.M., Armstrong, L.E. et al. 1998. Endocrine responses during exercise-heat stress: Effects of prior isotonic and hypotonic intravenous rehydration. *Eur J Appl Physiol Occup Physiol* 77:242–248.

Cermak, N.M., Gibala, M.J., and van Loon, L.J. 2012. Nitrate supplementation's improvement of 10-km time-trial performance in trained cyclists. *Int J Sport Nutr Exerc Metab* 22:64–71.

Cerretelli, P. and Marconi, C. 1990. L-carnitine supplementation in humans. The effects on physical performance. *Int J Sports Med* 11:1–14.

Cox, A.J., Pyne, D.B., Saunders, P.U., and Fricker, P.A. 2010. Oral administration of the probiotic *Lactobacillus fermentum* VRI-003 and mucosal immunity in endurance athletes. *Br J Sports Med* 44:222–226.

de Wit, J.N. 1998. Marschell Rhone-Poulenc Award Lecture. Nutritional and functional characteristics of whey proteins in food products. *J Dairy Sci* 81:597–608.

Draeger, C.L., Naves, A., Marques, N. et al. 2014. Controversies of antioxidant vitamins supplementation in exercise: Ergogenic or ergolytic effects in humans? *J Int Soc Sports Nutr* 11:4.

Earnest, C.P., Lupo, M., White, K.M., and Church, T.S. 2011. Effect of astaxanthin on cycling time trial performance. *Int J Sports Med* 32:882–888.

Esmarck, B., Andersen, J.L., Olsen, S., Richter, E.A., Mizuno, M., and Kjaer, M. 2001. Timing of postexercise protein intake is important for muscle hypertrophy with resistance training in elderly humans. *J Physiol* 535:301–311.

Evans, W.J. and Hughes, V.A. 1985. Dietary carbohydrates and endurance exercise. *Am J Clin Nutr* 41:1146–1154.

Forgac, M.T. 1980. Carbohydrate loading—A review. *J Appl Physiol* 48:624–629.

Gleeson, M., Bishop, N.C., Oliveira, M., McCauley, T., Tauler, P., and Lawrence, C. 2012. Effects of a *Lactobacillus salivarius* probiotic intervention on infection, cold symptom duration and severity, and mucosal immunity in endurance athletes. *Int J Sport Nutr Exerc Metab* 22:235–242.

Gleeson, M., Nieman, D.C., and Pederson, B.K. 2004. Exercise, nutrition and immune function. *J Sports Sci* 22:115–125.

Gomez-Cabrera, M.C., Domenech, E., Romagnoli, M. et al. 2008. Oral administration of vitamin C decreases muscle mitochondrial biogenesis and hampers training-induced adaptations in endurance performance. *Am J Clin Nutr* 87:142–149.

Ha, E. and Zemal, M.B. 2003. Functional properties of whey, whey components, and essential amino acids: Mechanisms underlying health benefits for active people (review). *J Nutr Biochem* 14:251–258.

Harper, A.E., Miller, R.H., and Block, K.P. 1984. Branched-chain amino acid metabolism. *J Nutr* 4:409–454.

Hemdan, D.I., Hirasaka, K., Nakao, R. et al. 2009. Polyphenols prevent clinorotation-induced expression of atrogenes in mouse C2C12 skeletal myotubes. *J Med Invest* 56:26–32.

Henriksen, E.J. 2006. Exercise training and the antioxidant alpha-lipoic acid in the treatment of insulin resistance and type 2 diabetes. *Free Radic Biol Med* 40:3–12.

Higashida, K., Kim, S.H., Higuchi, M., Holloszy, J.O., and Han, D.H. 2011. Normal adaptations to exercise despite protection against oxidative stress. *Am J Physiol Endocrinol Metab* 301, E779–E784.

Hulyman, E. and Nilsson, L.H. 1971. Liver glycogen in men. Effect of different diets and muscular exercise. In: *Advances in Experimental Medicine and Biology. Muscle Metabolism During Exercise*, Vol. 2. Pernow, B. and Saltin, B., eds., Plenum Press, New York, pp. 143–151.

Ikeuchi, M., Koyama, T., Takahashi, J., and Yazawa, K. 2006. Effects of astaxanthin supplementation on exercise-induced fatigue in mice. *Biol Pharm Bull* 29:2106–2110.

Kanter, M.M., Nolte, L.A., and Holloszy, J.O. 1993. Effects of an antioxidant vitamin mixture on lipid peroxidation at rest and postexercise. *J Appl Physiol* 74:965–969.

Kargotich, S., Goodman, C., Dawson, B., Morton, A.R., Keast, D., and Joske, D.J. 2005. Plasma glutamine responses to high-intensity exercise before and after endurance training. *Res Sports Med* 13:287–300.

Kekkonen, R.A., Vasankari, T.J., Vuorimaa, T., Haahtela, T., Julkunen, I., and Korpela, R. 2007. The effect of probiotics on respiratory infections and gastrointestinal symptoms during training in marathon runners. *Int J Sport Nutr Exerc Metab* 17:352–363.

Kiens, B., Lithell, H., Mikines, K.J., and Richter, E.A. 1989. Effects of insulin and exercise on muscle lipoprotein lipase activity in man and its relation to insulin action. *J Clin Invest* 84:1124–1129.

Kreider, R., Ferreira, M., Wilson, M. et al. 1998. Effects of creatine supplementation on body composition, strength and sprint performance. *Med Sci Sport Exerc* 30:73–82.

Latzka, W.A. and Montain, S.J. 1999 Water and electrolyte requirements for exercise. *Clin Sports Med* 18:513–524.

Lemon, P.W. 1998. Effects of exercise on dietary protein requirements. *Int J Sport Nutr* 8:426–447.

Liu, P.H., Aoi, W., Takami, M. et al. 2014. The astaxanthin-induced improvement in lipid metabolism during exercise is mediated by a PGC-1α increase in skeletal muscle. *J Clin Biochem Nutr* 54:86–89.

Lyons, T.P. 1990. Effects of glycerol-induced hyperhydration prior to exercise in the heat on sweating and core temperature. *Med Sci Sports Exerc* 22:477–483.

Mackinnon, L.T. and Hooper, S.L. 1996. Plasma glutamine and upper respiratory tract infection during intensified training in swimmers. *Med Sci Sports Exerc* 28:285–290.

Marconi, C., Sessi, G., Carpinelli, A., and Cerretelli, P. 1985. Effects of L-carnitine loading on the aerobic and anaerobic performance of endurance athletes. *Eur J Appl Physiol* 10:169–174.

Mitsuzono, R., Okamura, K., Igaki, K., Iwanaga, K., and Sakurai, M. 1995. Effects of fructose ingestion on carbohydrate and lipid metabolism during prolonged exercise in distance runners. *Appl Human Sci* 14:125–131.

Moriguchi, S. and Muraga, M. 2000. Vitamin E and immunity. *Vitam Horm* 59:305–336.

Murase, T., Haramizu, S., Shimotoyodome, A., Tokimitsu, I., and Hase, T. 2006. Green tea extract improves running endurance in mice by stimulating lipid utilization during exercise. *Am J Physiol Regul Integr Comp Physiol* 290:R1550–R1556.

Nehlsen-Cannarella, S.L., Fagoaga, O.R., Nieman, D.C. et al. 1997. Carbohydrate and the cytokine response to 2.5 h of running. *J Appl Physiol* 82:1662–1667.

Nissen, S. and Sharp, R. 2003. Effect of dietary supplements on lean mass and strength gains with resistance exercise: A meta-analysis. *J Appl Physiol* 94:651–659.

Ogawa, M., Kariya, Y., Kitakaze, T. et al. 2013. The preventive effect of β-carotene on denervation-induced soleus muscle atrophy in mice. *Br J Nutr* 109:1349–1358.

Peake, J.M. 2003. Vitamin C: Effects of exercise and requirements with training. *Int J Sport Nutr Exerc Metab* 13:125–151.

Riedesel, M.L. 1998. Hyperhtdration with glycerol solutions. *J Appl Physiol* 63:2262–2268.

Ristow, M., Zarse, K., Oberbach, A. et al. 2009. Antioxidants prevent health-promoting effects of physical exercise in humans. *Proc Natl Acad Sci USA* 106:8665–8670.

Robergs, R.A. 1998. Glycerol: Biochemistry, pharmacokinetics and clinical and practical applications. *Sports Med* 26:145–167.

Rodriguez, N.R., Di Marco, N.M., and Langley, S. 2009. American College of Sports Medicine position stand. Nutrition and athletic performance. *Med Sci Sports Exerc* 41:709–731.

Ryu, S., Choi, S.K., Joung, S.S. et al. 2001. Caffeine as a lipolytic food component increases endurance performance in rats and athletes. *J Nutr Sci Vitaminol* (*Tokyo*) 47:139–146.

Saengsirisuwan, V., Perez, F.R., Sloniger, J.A., Maier, T., and Henriksen, E.J. 2004. Interactions of exercise training and alpha-lipoic acid on insulin signaling in skeletal muscle of obese Zucker rats. *Am J Physiol Endocrinol Metab* 287:E529–E536.

Saito, A., Tasaki, Y., Tagami, K., and Suzuki, M. 1994. Muscle glycogen repletion and pre-exercise glycogen content: Effect of carbohydrate loading in rats previously fed a high fat diet. *Eur J Appl Physiol* 68:483–488.

Saito, S. and Suzuki, M. 1986. Nutritional design for repletion of liver and muscle glycogen during endurance exercise without inhibiting lipolysis. *J Nutr Sci Vitaminol* 32:343–353.

Saito, S., Yoshitake, Y., and Suzuki, M. 1983. Enhanced glycogen repletion in liver and skeletal muscle with citrate orally fed after exhaustive treadmill running and swimming. *J Nutr Sci Vitaminol* 29:45–52.

Sasaki, S., Nakae, S., Ebine, N., Aoi, W., Higashi, A., and Ishii, K. 2014. The effect of the timing of meal intake on energy metabolism during moderate exercise. *J Nutr Sci Vitaminol* (Tokyo) 60:28–34.

Shimomura, Y., Murakami, T., Nakai, N., Nagasaki, M., and Harris, R.A. 2004. Exercise promotes BCAA catabolism: Effects of BCAA supplementation on skeletal muscle during exercise. *J Nutr* 134:1583S–1587S.

Takamata, A., Mack, G.W., Gillen, C.M., and Nadel, E.R. 1994. Sodium appetite, thirst, and body fluid regulation in humans during rehydration without sodium replacement. *Am J Physiol* 266:R1493–R1502.

Takeda, K., Machida, M., Kohara, A., Omi, N., and Takemasa, T. 2011. Effects of citrulline supplementation on fatigue and exercise performance in mice. *J Nutr Sci Vitaminol (Tokyo)* 57:246–250.

Terjung, R.L., Clarkson, P., Eichner, E.R. et al. 2000. The physiological and health effects of oral creatine supplementation. *Med Sci Sports Exerc* 32:706–717.

Tischler, M.E., Desautels, M., and Goldberg, A.L. 1982. Does leucine, leucyl-tRNA, or some metabolite of leucine regulate protein synthesis and degradation in skeletal and cardiac muscle. *J Biol Chem* 257:1613–1621.

Tomlinson, P.B., Joseph, C., and Angioi, M. 2014. Effects of vitamin D supplementation on upper and lower body muscle strength levels in healthy individuals. A systematic review with meta-analysis. *J Sci Med Sport*, pii: S1440-2440(14)00163-7.

Vandenburghe, K., Goris, M., Van Hecke, P., Van Leemputte, M., Vangerven, L., and Hespel, P. 1997. Long-term creatine intake is beneficial to muscle performance during resistance-training. *J Appl Physiol* 83:2055–2063.

Vecchiet, L., Di Lisa, F., Pieralisi, G. et al. 1990. Influence of L-carnitine administration on maximal physical exercise. *Eur J Appl Physiol* 61:486–490.

Volec, J.S., Duncan, N.D., Mazzetti, S.A. et al. 1999. Performance and muscle fiber adaptations to creatine supplementation and heavy resistance exercise. *Med Sci Sport Exerc* 31:1147–1156.

Wang, D.T., Yin, Y., Yang, Y.J. et al. 2014. Resveratrol prevents TNF-α-induced muscle atrophy via regulation of Akt/mTOR/FoxO1 signaling in C2C12 myotubes. *Int Immunopharmacol* 19:206–213.

West, N.P., Pyne, D.B., Cripps, A.W. et al. 2011. *Lactobacillus fermentum* (PCC®) supplementation and gastrointestinal and respiratory-tract illness symptoms: A randomised control trial in athletes. *Nutr J* 10:30.

Wu, J., Gao, W., Wei, J., Yang, J., Pu, L., and Guo, C. 2012. Quercetin alters energy metabolism in swimming mice. *Appl Physiol Nutr Metab* 37:912–922.

Yavuz, H.U., Turnagol, H., and Demirel, A.H. 2014. Pre-exercise arginine supplementation increases time to exhaustion in elite male wrestlers. *Biol Sport* 31:187–191.

Section XVIII

Sickle Cell Anemia

34 Nutraceuticals in the Management of Sickle Cell Anemia

Ngozi Awa Imaga

CONTENTS

34.1 INTRODUCTION

Sickle cell disorder or sickle cell disease (SCD) is a group of hereditary illnesses affecting the red cell hemoglobin. Various types of these disorders exist including sickle thalassemia and sickle cell anemia (SCA; HbSS), also known as drepanocytosis. Parents who possess heterozygous genotypes (HbAS) are sickle cell carriers, and their offspring have a one in four chance of having a homozygous sickle genotype (HbSS) or a homozygous normal genotype (HbAA).[1,2]

In our daily diets, there are food substances we take that are rich in antioxidants and other nutritional components that help boost the immune system and ward off diseases. SCA is a genetic disease, and so dietary supplements cannot stop the manifestation of the disorder, but a well-nourished and supplemented SCD individual can be spared the severity of the disease and go about life without the crisis episodes inherent in the disorder.

There are several compounds such as amino acids that prevent sickling by affecting the erythrocyte membrane, causing an increase in the cell volume of the erythrocyte and thus reducing the intracellular hemoglobin concentration below its minimum gelling concentration.[3]

Presently, first-line clinical management of SCA includes the use of hydroxyurea, folic acid, and amino acid supplementation (as nutritional supplements), penicillin prophylaxis (helps prevent infection), and antimalarial prophylaxis (helps prevent malarial attack), for example Paludrine™ in varying doses in childhood, adulthood, and pregnancy. The faulty "S" gene is not eradicated in treatment, rather the condition is managed, and the synthesis of red blood cells is induced to stabilize the patient's hemoglobin level.[4]

Antisickling properties of amino acids have been recognized much earlier; of all the amino acids reported, phenylalanine was shown to be most active. The mode of transport and possible mechanism of action of some amino acid benzyl esters, for example L-phenylalanine benzyl ester (Phe-Bz), an aromatic compound and an antisickling agent, was found to be effective at a low concentration and is therefore a potential therapeutic agent for the treatment of sickle cell disease.[5]

Multivitamin supplements, proper diet, and calorie and protein intake are other ways to boost the immune system and extend the life span of the SCD individual.

A scope of work on antisickling agents with the focus on nutrition found that the concentrations of ascorbic acid and alpha-tocopherol were significantly depressed, while that of retinol was slightly reduced in subjects tested. The depletion in the levels of the antioxidant vitamins A, C, and E may account for some of the observed manifestations of SCA, such as increased susceptibility to infection and hemolysis.[6] Vitamin B_{12} levels have been observed to be diminished in patients with severe sickle cell disease. Patients with low vitamin B_{12} achieved a significant symptomatic improvement when treated with vitamin B_{12}, 1 mg intramuscularly weekly for 12 weeks. It was concluded that many patients with severe sickle cell disease may suffer from unrecognized vitamin B_{12} deficiency.[7]

34.2 ANTISICKLING PHYTOCHEMICALS

Phytomedicines and naturally occurring antisickling agents like Niprisan[R] with *Piper guineense*, *Pterocapus osun*, *Eugenia caryophyllus*, and *Sorghum bicolor* as components, Ciklavit[R] (*Cajanus cajan* as base), hydroxybenzoic acids, aqueous extracts of *Zanthoxylum zanthoxyloide* roots, Ajawaron HF[R] complex with *Cissus populnea* as main component, aqueous and alcoholic extracts of *Terminalia catappa* leaves, and *Carica papaya* unripe fruit and dried leaf extracts are also used in SCD management.[3,8]

Aqueous and ethanolic extracts of several phytomedicines have been evaluated for significant in vitro antisickling activity. Recent studies[5] support the claims of the traditional healers and suggest a possible correlation between the phytochemical composition of these plants and their uses in traditional medicine. *Z. zanthoxyloides* has shown drepanocyte (sickling) reversibility, appreciable increase in hemoglobin gelling time, and improved rheological properties of drepanocytary blood.

34.3 ANTIOXIDANTS

Antioxidants are literarily known as "scavengers" or "moppers" of free radicals in an organic entity. They scavenge for free radicals and, consequently, are a very special group of nutritional supplements. The term antioxidant (also "antioxygen") was originally used to refer specifically to a chemical that prevented the consumption of oxygen. In the late nineteenth and early twentieth centuries, extensive study was devoted to the uses of antioxidants in important industrial processes, such as the prevention of metal corrosion, the vulcanization of rubber, and the polymerization of fuels in the fueling of internal combustion engines. However, early research on the role of antioxidants focused on their use in preventing the oxidation of unsaturated fats, which causes rancidity. Then, antioxidant activity could be measured simply, by placing the fat in a closed container with oxygen and measuring the rate of oxygen consumption. Yet, it was the identification of β-carotene (precursor of vitamin A), vitamin C (ascorbic acid), and vitamin E (α-tocopherol) as antioxidants that revolutionized the field and led to the realization of the importance of antioxidants in the biochemistry of living organisms.

Antioxidants and their mechanisms of action were first explored when it was recognized that a substance with antioxidative activity is likely to be one that is itself readily oxidized. Further research into how vitamin E prevents the process of lipid peroxidation led to the identification of antioxidants as reducing agents that prevent oxidative reactions, often by scavenging reactive oxygen species before they can damage cells.

Among the numerous antioxidants available, flavonoids are naturally occurring phenolic compounds in plants. In fact, the majority of antioxidants, both natural and synthetic, are phenolic compounds. Vitamin C, beta-carotene, and vitamin E are all powerful natural antioxidants. Other natural antioxidants, which have been less well characterized, are the flavonoids and anthocyanins. These are all phenols, and several thousand different structural variants are found in nature. It has been estimated that the total intake of these compounds in the typical diet is close to 1000 mg/day, dwarfing the antioxidant content of antioxidant vitamins in the typical diet. Due to their remarkable importance, antioxidants have been the focus of considerable research, and the antioxidant properties of several plants in vivo and in vitro have been shown to be of great advantage to nutrition today.

For sickle cell disease (SCD), the study of antioxidants especially in various antisickling agents is of great importance because different antisickling agents have different degrees of effect. Antioxidants (scavengers of free radicals) are believed to be major components of these antisickling agents that add to their potential. Thus, it is believed that the higher the antioxidant property of an antisickling agent, the higher its possible antisickling effect, as this enables to reduce oxidative stress that contributes to sickle cell crisis.[8]

Antioxidants are found mostly in fruits (antioxidant vitamins) and vegetables. Diets rich in vitamins A, C, and E, and the selenium and zinc metals, will go a long way toward fortifying the SCD individual and prevent crisis.

Research on antioxidant status and susceptibility of sickled erythrocytes to oxidative and osmotic stress has been reported using a range of diluted saline–phosphate buffer in a typical osmotic fragility test to determine osmotic stress/membrane integrity and AAPH (a peroxyl radical generator) to induce hemolysis with oxygenated and deoxygenated RBCs for oxidative stress analysis. It was discovered that though there are differences in the antioxidant status between sickled and normal RBCs, these differences did not appear to be responsible for the observed difference in susceptibility to oxidative or osmotic stress–induced hemolysis.

34.4 NUTRITIONAL SUPPLEMENTATION

Oral magnesium supplementation reduces the number of dense erythrocytes and improves the erythrocyte membrane transport abnormalities of patients with sickle cell disease. Children with SCD are reported to demonstrate or exhibit normal serum magnesium level with accompanying hyperphosphatemia and hypocalcemia. They have also been observed to have decreased height and weight when compared with their peers. Although exact reasons for poor growth were not established, increased calorie and protein needs and deficiencies in zinc, folic acid, and vitamins A, C, and E were adduced to be the factors responsible. It has been suggested that the nutrient intake of patients with sickle cell disease is often inadequate, and a study suggests that education of patients with SCD should focus on the following:

- Specific nutrient needs, with proper distribution of dietary intake among the food groups
- Ways to provide nutritious meals on a limited income
- Methods for increasing calorie and protein intake

Patients with SCD that have adequate vitamin B_6 and B_{12} status, but elevated plasma homocysteine levels with indicated suboptimal folate status, especially pediatric sickle cell patients, may benefit from folate supplementation to reduce their high risk for endothelial damage.

A potential nutritional approach for the molecular disease SCD found that from both in vitro and pilot clinical trials, a *cocktail* of aged garlic extract, vitamin C, and vitamin E proved beneficial to patients. Ascorbic acid is important in SCA because significant oxidative stress occurs in the disease, and its role as an antioxidant is very beneficial.

Ascorbate levels in red blood cells and urine in patients with SCA have been analyzed, and the following points were reported[4]:

1. Ascorbate is present in sickled red blood cell (SRBC), most likely due to ascorbate recycling, despite increased free-radical generation.
2. There is increase in renal excretion, which may contribute to the low plasma levels of ascorbate.
3. The presence of ample ascorbate in SRBCs and decreased plasma ascorbate suggests that ascorbate movement across the SRBC membrane may be different from normal red blood cell.

The effect of vitamin C on arterial blood pressure, irreversibly sickled cells (ISCs), and osmotic fragility in sickle cell anemic subjects also suggests a potential benefit of vitamin C supplementation to SCA subjects because vitamins A, C, and E supplementation was shown to decrease arterial blood pressure, % ISCs, and mean corpuscular hemoglobin concentration but increased Hb (hemoglobin) and packed cell volume.

34.5 CURRENT TRENDS IN THE USE OF NUTRACEUTICALS FOR SICKLE CELL ANEMIA MANAGEMENT

It is acknowledged worldwide that traditional medicine can be explored and exploited to be used alongside synthetic pharmaceutical products for enhanced health management. Due to the high mortality rate of sickle cell patients, especially in children, and since chemotherapy has its adverse effects, there is need for rational drug development that must embrace not only synthetic drugs but also natural products (nutraceuticals/phytomedicines/herbal drugs), naturally occurring antisickling agents that can be obtained from our vast forest resources and can be used to effectively manage the sickle cell patient and treat the anemic condition accompanying this disorder.

Ciklavit® is a plant extract preparation available for the management of the SCA condition. It contains primarily extracts of the plant *C. Cajan*, proteins (essential amino acids), vitamins such as vitamin C (ascorbic acid), and minerals such as zinc. Ciklavit (*C. cajan* extract) has been reported to have antisickling properties and to improve the well-being of sicklers. The study also revealed that the antisickling effect of Ciklavit may not probably be through nitric oxide generation or arginase inhibition, since there were no appreciable changes in these parameters. Earlier reports of the antisickling constituents of *C. cajan* suggested cajaminose[3], phenylalanine, and hydroxybenzoic acid. Phytochemical studies on the aqueous extract confirm the presence of phenylalanine and several other amino acids and phenolic compounds and tannins. The antisickling properties of amino acids in in vitro studies have been recognized much earlier. Of all the amino acids reported, L-phenylalanine, found to have antigelling effects, was shown to be most active. The role played by other components in Ciklavit (besides *C. cajan*) is basically nutritional. Blood levels of several vitamins and minerals are often low in individuals with sickle cell disease, including vitamin A and carotenoids, vitamin B_6, vitamin C, vitamin E, magnesium, and zinc. These deficiencies cause a significant depreciation in blood antioxidant status in these patients, and the resulting oxidative stress may precipitate vasoclusion-related acute chest syndrome. Studies indicate that vitamin–mineral supplements of certain nutrients (vitamins C and E, zinc, magnesium) or treatment with a combination of high-dose antioxidants can reduce the percentage of ISCs. Zinc sulfate appears to help reduce red blood cell dehydration. Important studies indicate that it helps prevent sickle cell crises and reduce pain and life-threatening complications. A study on children with sickle cell suggested that supplements may help improve growth and weight gain. It may also boost the immune system and help protect against bacterial infections. Zinc deficiency is a common nutritional problem in sickle cell disease, so supplements may be important. Magnesium protects against potassium and water loss in sickle cells. In view of these findings, it can be concluded that Ciklavit may cause a reduction in bone pains (painful crises) and may ameliorate the adverse effect of SCA on the liver. It is also suggested that one of the antisickling effects or mechanisms of action of Ciklavit may involve the induction of fetal hemoglobin production. Ciklavit may therefore be a promising option for the treatment and management of SCA.

REFERENCES

1. F. H. Bunn, Pathogenesis and treatment of sickle cell disease, *The New England Journal of Medicine*, 337, 762–769, 1997.
2. M. H. Steinberg, Sickle cell disease, *Hematology*, 1, 35, 2004.

3. M. M. Iwu, A. O. Igboko, H. Onwubiko, and U. E. Ndu, Antisickling properties of *Cajanus cajan*: Effect on hemoglobin gelation and oxygen affinity, *Planta Medica*, 24, 431–432, 1986.
4. M. P. Westerman, Y. Zhang, J. P. McConnell, P. A. Chezick, R. Neelam, S. Freels, L. S. Feldman et al., Ascorbate levels in red blood cells and urine in patients with sickle cell anemia, *American Journal of Hematology*, 65(2), 174–175, 2000.
5. C. T. A. Acquaye, J. D. Young, and J. C. Ellory, Mode of transport and possible mechanisms of action of L-phenylalanine benzyl ester as an anti-sickling agent, *Biochimica et Biophysica Acta*, 693(2), 407–416, 1982.
6. E. U. Essien, Plasma levels of retinol, ascorbic acid, and alphatocopherol in sickle cell anaemia, *Central African Journal of Medicine*, 41(2), 48–50, 1995.
7. A. K. Al-Momen, Diminished vitamin B12 levels in patients with severe sickle cell disease, *Journal of Internal Medicine*, 237(6), 551–555, 1995.
8. N. O. A. Imaga, G. O. Gbenle, V. I. Okochi, S. O. Akanbi, S. O. Edeoghon, V. Oigbochie, M. O. Kehinde, and S. B. Bamiro, Antisickling property of *Carica papaya* leaf extract, *African Journal of Biochemistry Research*, 3(4), 102–106, 2009.

Section XIX

Role of Probiotics in Gastrointestinal and Dental Health

35 Health Benefits of Human Probiont *Lactobacillus plantarum*

Satish Kumar Ramraj and Arul Venkatesan

CONTENTS

35.1 BACKGROUND

Lactobacillus plantarum is among the most prominent lactic acid bacterium (LAB), which has one of the largest genomes of LAB [1]. Due to this, it can express various genes that provide this species with a high ability to customized to varying external conditions, and also it can attach to different substrates [2]. *Lb. plantarum* has been isolated from a wide array of sources including fermented foods all over the world [3], and, many strains, have been proposed to confer benefits on human health, being considered potential probiotics [4,5]. These human benefits include treatment and prevention of enteric infections and post-antibiotic syndromes, acute infectious diarrhea, prevention of antibiotic-associated diarrhea, inflammatory bowel disease (IBD), colorectal cancer (CRC), and treatment of irritable bowel syndrome. *Lb. plantarum* is also reported to be active against entero-pathogens such as *Listeria monocytogenes*, *L. innocuo*, *Staphylococcus aureus*, and influenza virus. Its beneficial role in various diseases is discussed in detail in the following sections.

The *Lb. plantarum* genome has yielded information on how this bacterium may have adapted to growth in diverse environments such as fermented foods, plants, and the human GIT [2]. The flexible and adaptive behavior is reflected by the relatively large number of regulatory and transport functions, including 25 complete PTS sugar transport systems. Consistent with the classification of *Lb. plantarum* as a facultative heterofermentative LAB, the genome also encodes all enzymes required for the glycolysis and phosphoketolase pathways, all of which appear to belong to the class of potentially highly expressed genes in this organism. *Lb. plantarum* encodes a large pyruvate-dissipating potential, emphasizing its fermentative capacity. As a result of this, *Lb. plantarum* is isolated from numerous traditional fermented foods. Table 35.1 describes the traditional fermented foods from which *Lb. plantarum* was isolated and some strains were screened for probiotic attributes. Many researchers have reported *Lb. plantarum* as efficient probiont by examining its attributes in specific conditions such as survival in acidic pH condition, bile salt tolerance, cholesterol assimilation, intestinal epithelial surface adherence, pathogen inhibition, etc. [6]. Some researchers have gone further than just examining probiotic attribute of *Lb. plantarum* by studying its role in human health benefits including certain disorders, disease such as cancer, and indirect benefits such as immunomodulation. These health benefits are discussed and also we had done a literature survey to find out the possible mechanism of *Lb. plantarum* for its probiotic action related to human health.

35.2 BENEFECIAL ROLE OF *Lactobacillus plantarum* IN HUMAN HEALTH CONDITIONS

35.2.1 Inflammatory Bowel Disease

IBD comprises a collection of disorders that mainly include Crohn's disease and ulcerative colitis. These disorders cause abdominal pain, vomiting, diarrhea, and gastrointestinal (GI) inflammation [7]. To date, no effective therapy has been developed and patients may have a reduced quality of life even under proper management. It has been shown that factors related to IBD include acquired factors (e.g. smoking and diet), pathogens, genetic factors, and irregular immune system [8]. Over the past decades, the homeostatic functions of microflora on host GI tract have attracted much attention because growing numbers of clinical studies have suggested that probiotics exhibited anti-inflammatory effects on IBD patients [9,10]. Arseneau et al. [11] suggested that innate immune responses play an equally significant, even more primary character compared with adaptive immune responses in IBD initiation and progression due to the observation that probiotics elicit anti-inflammatory effects in the GI tract by means of mucosal innate immune system stimulation, instead of suppression. Studies have shown that some strains of *Lb. plantarum* attenuate inflammation induced by *Shigella flexneri* peptidoglycan by inhibiting nuclear factor kappa-light chain-enhancer of activated B cells (NF-κB), inactivating mitogen-activated protein kinase (MAPK), and reducing NOD2 mRNA expression, as well as protein levels, the actions that in turn lead to a decrease in pro-inflammatory cytokine secretion [12]. Moreover, van Baarlen et al. [13,14] demonstrated that even dead *Lb. plantarum* can exert beneficial functions protecting the host against the enormous array of commensal bacteria in the gut via epithelial crosstalk of mucosal interface microbiota. *Lb. plantarum* MYL26 inhibited inflammation in Caco-2 cells through regulation of gene expressions of TOLLIP, SOCS1, SOCS3, and IκBα, rather than SHIP-1 and IRAK-3 [15]. *Lb. plantarum* 299v (*Lb. plantarum* 299v) (DSM 9843) is a probiotic strain able to reside in the human colonic mucosa in vivo due to a specific mechanism of mannose adhesion [16]. *Lb. plantarum* 299v (DSM 9843) also increases the amount of carboxylic acid, particularly acetic and propionic acids, in the stools of healthy volunteers [17]. The strain has shown antibacterial activity against several potential pathogenic agents such as *L. monocytogenes*, *Escherichia coli*, *Yersinia enterolytica*, *Enterobacter cloacae*, and *Enterococcus faecalis* [18]. *Lb. plantarum* 299v (DSM 9843) also has beneficial immunomodulatory activity *via* an increased interleukin-10 synthesis and secretion in macrophages and T-cells derived from the inflamed colon. A 4-wk treatment with *Lb. plantarum* 299v (DSM 9843) provided effective symptom relief, particularly of abdominal pain and bloating, in IBS patients [19].

35.2.2 Protection against Influenza Virus

Lb. plantarum DK119 (DK119) isolated from the fermented Korean cabbage food was used as a probiotic to determine its antiviral effects on influenza virus [20]. DK119 intranasal or oral administration

TABLE 35.1
***Lb. plantarum* Isolated from Traditional Fermented Foods**

Fermented Food	Usual Composition/Ingredients	Country of Origin/Usage	References
Kallappam	Boiled or raw rice, coconut toddy	India	[6]
Pozol	Fermented maize dough	Mexico	[66]
Enjera	Tef or other cereals	Ethiopia	[67]
Kishk	Wheat	Egypt	[67]
Ogi	Maize, sorghum, or millet	Nigeria	[67]
Uji	Maize, sorghum, millet or cassava flour	Kenya, Uganda, Tanzania	[67]
Bussa	Maize, sorghum, malt	Kenya	[67]
Tapuy	Rice, glutinous rice	Philippines	[67]
Bhaturu or Indigenous bread	Wheat and starter material *Khameer/Malera*	India	[68]
Curd (*Dahi, Thayir*)	Milk	India	[69]
Chhurpi or Durkha or churapi	Yak milk is preferred for making this cheese although any other fresh milk may be used	India	[70]
Koumiss	Fresh mare or camel milk	China	[71]
Kurdish cheese	Cow milk	Iran	[72]
Kule Naoto	Cow milk	Kenya	[73]
Gundruk	Leaves of mustard/radish/cauliflower	India	[74]
Sinki	Radish root	India	[74]
Sauerkraut or Sauerkohi	Cabbage	India	[75]
Soibum or Soijim	Bamboo shoots	India	[76]
Soidon	Bamboo shoots	India	[77]
Hiring	Bamboo shoots	India	[74,77]
Ekung	Bamboo shoots	India	[74]
Eup	Bamboo shoots	India	[77]
Mesu	Bamboo shoots	India	[77]
Khalpi	Cucumber	India	[78]
Goyang	Wild plant magane-saag (*Cardamine macrophylla* Willd.) leaves	India	[77]
Inziangsang	Mustard leaves	India	[77]
Kanji	Carrot or beet root, rice, mustard	India	[79]
Paocai	Cabbage, carrot, cucumber, radish and bamboo shoot	Taiwan	[80]
Gari	Cassava root	West Africa	[81]
cassava sour starch	Cassava	Colombia	[82]
Beja, Santarém, Ladoeiro	Fermented olive	Portugal	[83]
dongchimi, kimchi	Cabbage	Korea	[84]
Dhamuoi	Cabbage	Vietnam	[67]
Dakguadong	Mustard leaf	Thailand	[67]
Ngari	*Puntius sophore* ('Phoubu') Fish	India	[85]
Hentak	*Esomus danricus* (fish), petioles of *Alocasia macrorhiza*	India	[85]
Tungtap	*Danio* sp. (fish)	India	[85]
Yak kargyong	Meat of yak	India	[86]
Faak kargyong	Meat of pig	India	[86]
Suka Ko Masu	Red meat of buffalo or goat	India	[86]
salsiccia and *soppressata*	Meat sausages	Southern Italy	[87]
som-fak	Fish, rice, garlic and banana leaves	Thailand	[88]
Sikhae	Sea-water fish	Korea	[67]

(Continued)

TABLE 35.1 (*Continued*)
***Lb. plantarum* Isolated from Traditional Fermented Foods**

Fermented Food	Usual Composition/Ingredients	Country of Origin/Usage	References
Narezushi	Sea-water fish	Japan	[67]
Pla-ra	Fresh-water fish	Thailand	[67]
Nham	Pork	Thailand	[67]
Sai-krok-prieo	Pork	Thailand	[67]
Kinema	Soybeans	India	[74]
Tungrymbai	Soybeans	India	[77]
Wadi	Black gram and oil	India	[89]
Wari	Black bean and soybean	India	[90]
Masyaura	Blackgram or greengram, *Colocosia* tuber, ashgourd or radish	India	[91]
Stinky tofu	Soybeans	China	[92]
Dochi	black beans	Taiwan	[93]
Mungbean starch	Mungbean	China, Thailand, Korea, Japan	[67]

conferred 100% protection against subsequent lethal infection with influenza A viruses, prevented significant weight loss, and lowered lung viral loads in a mouse model. The antiviral protective efficacy was observed in a dose- and route-dependent manner of DK119 administration. Mice that were treated with DK119 showed high levels of cytokines IL-12 and IFN-c in bronchoalveolar lavage fluids, and a low degree of inflammation upon infection with influenza virus. Depletion of alveolar macrophage cells in lungs and bronchoalveolar lavages completely abrogated the DK119-mediated protection. Modulating host innate immunity of dendritic and macrophage cells, and cytokine production pattern appeared to be possible mechanisms by which DK119 exhibited antiviral effects on influenza virus infection [20]. In another study, daily intragastric administrations during 10 days before and 10 days after viral challenge (100 PFU of influenza virus H1N1 strain A Puerto Rico/8/1934 [A/PR8/34]/mouse) of *Lb. plantarum* CNRZ1997, one potentially proinflammatory probiotic strain, led to a significant improvement in mouse health by reducing weight loss, alleviating clinical symptoms, and inhibiting significantly virus proliferation in lungs [21].

35.2.3 Toxic Shock Syndrome

Toxic shock syndrome (TSS) is a systemic disease with a sudden onset of fever, hypotension, erythema, desquamation, and multisystem involvement that leads to fatality in 5% of cases [22,23]. The etiological agent in nearly all menstrual TSS (mTSS) cases and approximately half of nonmenstrual TSS cases is *S. aureus* strains producing one or more superantigenic toxins, primarily toxic shock syndrome toxin 1 (TSST-1) and staphylococcal enterotoxin (SE) B or C [24,25]. *Lactobacillus* species are a predominant member of the vaginal microflora and are critical in maintaining an acidic vaginal environment thought to contribute to the prevention of a number of urogenital diseases. However, during menstruation the pH of the vaginal environment increases to neutrality, a pH conducive for *S. aureus* proliferation and the production of toxic shock syndrome toxin 1 (TSST-1) in susceptible women. Coculture assays using buffered mGTS showed that lysostaphin expressed from *Lb. plantarum* WCFS1 reduced the growth of TSST-1-producing strains of *S. aureus* under neutral-pH conditions [26].

35.2.4 Obstructive Jaundice

The mechanisms of *Lb. plantarum* action on gut barrier in preoperative and postoperative experimental obstructive jaundice in rats were investigated [27]. *Lb. plantarum* administration substantially restored gut barrier, decreased enterocyte apoptosis, improved intestinal oxidative stress, promoted the activity and expression of protein kinase, and particularly enhanced the expression and phosphorylation of TJ proteins in the experimental obstructive. The protective effect of *Lb. plantarum* was more prominent after internal biliary drainage. This study concluded that *Lb. plantarum* can decrease intestinal epithelial cell apoptosis, reduce oxidative stress, and prevent TJ disruption in biliary obstruction by activating the PKC pathway [27].

35.2.5 Prevention of Hyperlipidemia

Salaj et al. [28] evaluated the effects of the different probiotic strains, *Lb. plantarum* LS/07 and *Lb. plantarum* Biocenol LP96, on lipid metabolism and body weight in rats fed a high-fat diet. Compared with the high-fat diet group, the results showed that *Lb. plantarum* LS/07 reduced serum cholesterol and low density lipoprotein (LDL) cholesterol, but *Lb. plantarum* Biocenol LP96 decreased triglycerides and very low density lipoprotein (VLDL), while there was no change in the serum high density lipoprotein (HDL) level and liver lipids. Both probiotic strains lowered total bile acids in serum. Wang et al. [29] studied that *Lb. plantarum* CAI6 and *Lb. plantarum* SC4 may protect against cardiovascular disease by lipid metabolism regulation and Nrf2-induced antioxidative defense in hyperlipidemic mice. Park et al. [30] studied that diet-induced obese mice treated with probiotics *Lb. plantarum* KY1032 showed reduced body weight gain and fat accumulation as well as lowered plasma insulin, leptin, total cholesterol, and liver toxicity biomarkers. Gut microbiota species were shared among the experimental groups despite the different diets and treatments. The diversity of the gut microbiota and its composition were significantly altered in the diet-induced obese mice and after probiotic treatment. Transcriptional changes in adipose tissue and the liver were observed. In adipose tissue, proinflammatory genes (TNF-a, IL6, IL1b, and MCP1) were downregulated in mice receiving probiotic treatment. In the liver, fatty acid oxidation–related genes (PGC1a, CPT1, CPT2, and ACOX1) were upregulated in mice receiving probiotic treatment.

35.2.6 Typhoid

Enteric fever is a global health problem, and rapidly developing resistance to various drugs makes the situation more alarming. The potential use of *Lb. plantarum* to control typhoid fever represents a promising approach, as it may exert protective actions through various mechanisms. Abdel-Daim et al. [31] studied the probiotic potential and antagonistic activities of 32 *Lactobacillus* isolates against *Salmonella typhi*. The antimicrobial activity of cell free supernatants of *Lactobacillus* isolates, interference of *Lb. plantarum* isolates with the *Salmonella adherence* and invasion, cytoprotective effect of *Lb. plantarum* isolates, and possibility of concurrent use of tested *Lactobacillus* isolates and antibiotics were evaluated by testing their susceptibilities to antimicrobial agents, and their oxygen tolerance was also examined. The results revealed that 12 *Lb. plantarum* isolates could protect against *S. typhi* infection through interference with both its growth and its virulence properties, such as adherence, invasion, and cytotoxicity.

35.2.7 Colorectal Cancer

Probiotic bacteria are increasingly being shown to be capable of influencing GI disease and disorders including CRC [32]. CRC is one of the leading causes of cancer death both in men and women [33]. Prognosis for advanced CRC is poor [34], and hence prevention is required to control the incidence of disease. Epidemiological studies show that diet plays a role in the etiology of most large bowel cancers, implying that it is potentially preventable disease. Many studies confirm the involvement of the exogenous microflora in the onset of colon cancer. This makes it reasonable to think that changing the intestinal microflora could influence tumor development. Satish Kumar et al. [35] studied the relationship between antioxidant and anticancer properties of probiotic bacterium strain

Lb. plantarum AS1 (AS1) in colon cancer induced by 1,2-dimethylhydrazine (DMH). AS1 was supplemented either before initiation or during initiation and selection/promotion phases of colon carcinogenesis and was found to be effective in altering lipid peroxidation and antioxidant enzyme activities and marker enzymes to a statistically significant level measured either in the colon and in the plasma. These alterations inclined toward normal in a time-dependent manner on AS1 supplementation. The mean tumor volume diameter and total number of tumors were found to be statistically decreased in AS1 pre- and post-treated rats. The in vitro antioxidant assay shows that AS1 has promising antioxidant property. Asha and Gayathri [36] concluded from their study that administration of *L. fermentum*, *Lb. plantarum* or vincristine decreased the incidence in the colon of aberrant crypt foci (ACF), and combined treatment achieved a level of inhibition of 90%.

35.2.8 Gastroenteritis

Gatroenteritis is caused by infection of enteropathogens such as *Vibrio parahaemolyticus*, *L. monocytogenes*, *E. coli*, etc. Many of the probiotic bacteria are lactic acid bacteria and are useful in the treatment for dysfunctions with disturbed intestinal microflora and abnormal gut permeability [37]. Successful probiotic bacteria are usually able to colonize the intestine, at least temporarily, by adhering to the intestinal mucosa [38]. *Lb. plantarum* AS1 was isolated from South Indian fermented food Kallappam batter [6]. It showed antibacterial activity against various enteropathogens. *Lb. plantarum* AS1 was assessed for in vitro probiotic characteristics such as bile tolerance, artificial gastric juice tolerance, and cholesterol reduction and in vivo safety assessment in Wistar rats [6]. Satish Kumar et al. [39] studied *Lb. plantarum* AS1 inhibitory activity against enteropathogen *V. parahaemolyticus*. *Lb. plantarum* AS1 was incubated with HT-29 adenocarcinoma cell line to assess its adhesion potency and examined for its inhibitory effect on the cell attachment by an enterovirulent bacterium *V. parahaemolyticus*. *Lb. plantarum* AS1 attached firmly to HT-29 cells as revealed by scanning electron microscopy and bacterial adhesion assay. *Lb. plantarum* AS1 significantly reduced *V. parahaemolyticus* attached to HT-29 cells by competition, exclusion, and displacement mode. *Lb. plantarum* AS1 adhered to human intestinal cells via mechanisms that involved different combinations of carbohydrate and protein factors on the bacteria and eukaryotic cell surface.

35.3 POSSIBLE MECHANISM OF PROBIOTIC ACTION OF *Lactobacillus plantarum*

35.3.1 Adherence Mechanism in *Lactobacillus plantarum*

Several genes encoding proteins involved in metabolizing various carbon sources were identified in *Lb. plantarum*, including a ribose permease, a ribokinase, and two di- and polysaccharide hydrolyzing enzymes [40,41]. Real-time quantitative RT-PCR confirmed that the *Lb. plantarum* ribokinase is expressed along the murine GIT [42]. The transcription of an important indicator for active fermentation, *ldhL*, was induced more than twofold in the cecum and colon [42]. Mutational analysis of the cellobiose PTS (lp_1164), ribose transport protein, and ribokinase (lp_3559-lp_3660) confirmed the key role of the cellobiose PTS in the functionality of *Lb. plantarum* WCFS1 in the murine GIT [43). In a competition experiment, the relative abundance of the _lp1164 mutant was 100- to 1000-fold lower than that of the wild-type control strain after passage through the GIT. Bron et al. identified nine genes that are involved in the acquisition of nonsugars, including factors involved in the uptake and synthesis of amino acids, nucleotides, cofactors, and vitamins [40]. In *L. monocytogenes*, proline metabolism is induced under high-osmolarity conditions [44], such as those present in the small intestine and colon. Under conditions of osmotic stress, lactobacilli have systems for accumulating specific solutes that do not interfere with the physiology of the cell, such as the accumulation of glycine betaine, carnitine, proline, and glutamate [45].

An elegant approach has been followed to identify the mannose-specific adhesin in *Lb. plantarum* WCFS1 [46]. First, a genome-wide microarray-based genotyping of *Lb. plantarum* strains was performed to select WCFS1 genes whose presence or absence in the different strains was significantly correlated with the presence or absence, respectively, of the yeast agglutination phenotype observed for the same strains (gene-trait matching). This yeast agglutination capacity was previously shown to be related to the mannose-specific adherence of *Lb. plantarum* to human intestinal epithelial cells [47]. This resulted in four candidate genes that showed a 100% gene-trait match, including two SDPs (lp_0373 and lp_1229). To validate the role of SDPs for mannose-specific adhesion, a sortase-lacking mutant (*srtA*) was constructed. This *srtA* mutant was not able to agglutinate yeast cells. Subsequently, knockout mutants were constructed for lp_0373 and lp_1229. The deletion of lp_1229 completely abolished the agglutination capacity. Moreover, the overexpression of lp_1229 resulted in a slight but significant enhancement of this capacity. Overall, those researchers concluded that lp_1229 encodes the mannose-specific adhesin of *Lb. plantarum* WCFS1 and renamed the gene *msa*. It encodes a large surface protein (_1,000 residues) with characteristic multidomain structure, including the mucus-binding domains described later. In *Lb. plantarum* WCFS1, two SDPs were identified (lp_0800 and lp_2940) as being induced in the murine GIT [40]. Quantitative RT-PCR study showed that they are induced primarily in the small intestine [42]. lp_0800 was induced along the length of the small intestine, while lp_2940 was most active at the distal end of the small intestine and in the cecum. Subsequent mutational analyses showed that the persistence capacity of the lp_2940 knockout mutant was 100–1000-fold decreased in the murine GIT, while the colonization dynamics of an lp_1403 knockout were not significantly different from those of the wild type [43]. This lp_1403 protein is a putative secreted cell surface protein of *Lb. plantarum*, for which the expression has also been shown to be induced in the murine GIT [40] and, more specifically, in the small intestine [42].

35.3.2 Extracellular Polysaccharide

Extracellular Polysaccharide (EPSs) generally play a role in nonspecific interactions of lactobacilli with abiotic and biotic surfaces by contributing to the cell surface physicochemical properties. EPSs have also been shown to have an indirect effect on adhesion by shielding other cell surface adhesins. EPSs can promote intercellular interactions and the formation of microcolonies, although this step also depends on many other intrinsic and environmental factors. In *Lb. plantarum* WCFS1, an *agr*-like 2CRS regulatory system, encoded by *lamBDCA*, which regulates EPS production and adherence, was identified [48]. An RR-deficient *lamA* mutant showed reduced biofilm formation on glass substrates. Global transcription analysis of the wild type and the RR *lamA* mutant showed that LamA is involved in the regulation of the expression of genes encoding surface polysaccharides, cell membrane proteins, and sugar utilization proteins, indicating that this system has a key role in the regulation of cell surface properties.

35.3.3 Bacteriocins

Bacteriocins are biologically active proteins or protein complexes that display a bactericidal mode of action toward usually closely related species. *Lb. plantarum* is isolated from various sources but more prominently from fermented food products. Todorov et al. [49], isolated *Lb. plantarum* AMA-K from naturally fermented milk and characterized its bacteriocin AMA-K. Bacteriocin production is stimulated by the presence of *Listeria innocua*. *Lb. plantarum* AMA-K grows in milk and produces only 800 AU/mL after 24 h. Similarly, bacteriocin ST8KF produced by a *kefir* isolate *Lb. plantarum* ST8KF was characterized by Powell et al. [50]. Bac ST8KF was heat resistant (121°C for 20 min), and showed bacteriostatic mode of activity. Leal et al. [51], studied bacteriocin production and competitiveness of *Lb. plantarum* LPC010 in olive juice broth. Todorov et al. [49], for the first time isolated bacteriocinogenic *Lb. plantarum* ST16Pa from papaya (*Carica papaya*). It was active against *Pseudomonas*, *Streptococcus*, *Staphylococcus*, and *Listeria* spp. In another report, *Lb. plantarum* NCIM 2084 was attempted to grow in a simple glucose broth to produce bacteriocin. Its bacteriocin Plantaricin LP84 exhibited a bactericidal and lytic effect against *Bacillus cereus* F4810 and *E. coli* D21 [52]. A bacteriocin produced by *Lb. plantarum* ATCC8014 showed inhibition of *S. aureus*, *E. coli*, *L. innocuo*, and *P. aeruginosa* [53]. Hata et al. [54] characterized Plantaricin ASM1 from *Lb. plantarum* A-1. It showed stability in a wide pH range, heat and finally concluded as potential food bio-preservative. Xie et al. [55] reported an antilisterial Pediocin LB-B1 produced by *Lb. plantarum* LB-B1, isolated from *Koumiss*, a fermented dairy product from China.

35.3.4 Competitive Exclusion

There is some evidence that probiotics could use the same attachment site so that the pathogen is in competition for binding to the host mucosal interface and thereby could be inhibited from invading the mucosal layer. This antipathogenic mechanism is known as competitive exclusion and generally requires that the probiotic lactobacilli are administered in a preventive setup, as the displacement of a pathogen by a *Lactobacillus* strain is usually not observed. One putative competitive exclusion factor is the mannose specific adhesin Msa of *Lb. plantarum* [46]. Its identification allows detailed studies with deletion and overproduction strains to identify strains that effectively exclude pathogens containing type 1 fimbriae. Mack et al. demonstrated that a spontaneous and noncharacterized *adh* mutant of the probiotic strain *Lb. plantarum* 299v, but which is suggested to be affected in the *msa* gene, showed 10 times less adherence to HT-29 epithelial cells and was not able to inhibit the adherence of enteropathogenic *E. coli*, in contrast to the wild type [56].

35.3.5 Immunomodulation

Probiotics can be used to stimulate or regulate epithelial and immune cells of the intestinal mucosa and generate beneficial mucosal immunomodulatory effects. Intestinal epithelium cells (IECs) actively participate in immune reactions. Together with IECs, dendritic cells (DCs) and macrophages continuously sense the environment and coordinate various defenses for the protection of mucosal tissues. Innate defenses include the production of antimicrobial compounds (defensins and nitric oxide, etc.) and the secretion of chemokines such as IL-8 that recruit neutrophils, that is phagocytes that are capable of ingesting microorganisms or particles. In addition, many adaptive immune responses against commensal, probiotic, and pathogenic bacteria are mediated in mucosal lymphoid follicles that are distributed throughout the GIT and are referred to as the gut-associated lymphoid tissue (GALT) [57]. DCs are the most important antigen-presenting cells in the mucosa. Particularly, the modulation of DC function and induction of regulatory T cells are increasingly gaining attention as important mechanisms of probiotic action [58]. Herias et al. [59] have studied the effect of the probiotic strain *Lb. plantarum* 299v on the immune functions of gnotobiotic rats. One group of germ-free rats was colonized with the type 1–fimbriated *E. coli* O6:K13:H1 and another group with the same *E. coli* strain together with *Lb. plantarum* 299v. One and five weeks after colonization, bacterial numbers were determined in the contents of the small intestine, caecum and mesenteric lymph nodes. Small intestinal sections were examined for CD8, CD4, CD25 (IL-2R a-chain), IgA and MHC class II cells, and mitogen-induced spleen cell proliferation was determined. Immunoglobulin levels and *E. coli*–specific antibodies were measured in serum. Rats given *Lb. plantarum* in addition to *E. coli* showed lower counts of *E. coli* in the small intestine and caecum 1 week after colonization compared with the group colonized with *E. coli* alone, but similar levels after 5 weeks. Rats colonized with *Lb. plantarum, E. coli* had significantly higher total serum IgA levels and marginally higher IgM and IgA antibody levels against *E. coli* than those colonized with *E. coli* alone. They also showed a significantly increased density of CD25 cells in the lamina propria and displayed a decreased proliferative spleen cell response after stimulation with concanavalin A or *E. coli* 1 week after colonization. *Lb. plantarum* colonization competes with *E. coli* for intestinal colonization and can influence intestinal and systemic immunity.

Modulation of the immune system is one of the most plausible mechanisms underlying the beneficial effects of probiotic bacteria on human health. Presently, the specific probiotic cell products responsible for immunomodulation are largely unknown. The genetic and phenotypic diversity of strains of the *Lb. plantarum* species were investigated to identify genes of *Lb. plantarum* with the potential to influence the amounts of cytokines interleukin 10 (IL-10) and IL-12 and the ratio of IL-10/IL-12 produced by peripheral blood mononuclear cells (PBMCs) [60]. A total of 42 *Lb. plantarum* strains isolated from diverse environmental and human sources were evaluated for their capacity to stimulate cytokine production in PBMCs. The *Lb. plantarum* strains induced the secretion of the anti-inflammatory cytokine IL-10 over an average 14-fold range and secretion of the proinflammatory cytokine IL-12 over an average 16-fold range. Comparisons of the strain-specific cytokine responses of PBMCs to comparative genome hybridization profiles obtained with *Lb. plantarum* WCFS1 DNA microarrays (also termed gene-trait matching) resulted in the identification of six candidate genetic loci with immunomodulatory capacities. These loci included genes encoding an *N*-acetyl-glucosamine/galactosamine phosphotransferase system, the LamBDCA quorum sensing system, and components of the plantaricin (bacteriocin) biosynthesis and transport pathway. Deletion of these genes in *Lb. plantarum* WCFS1 resulted in growth phase–dependent changes in the PBMC IL-10 and IL-12 cytokine profiles compared with wild-type cells.

In another study, gene loci in the model probiotic organism *Lb. plantarum* WCFS1 that modulate the immune response of host DCs was identified [61]. The amounts of IL-10 and IL-12 secreted by DCs after stimulation with 42 individual *Lb. plantarum* strains were measured and correlated with the strain-specific genomic composition using comparative genome hybridization and the Random Forest algorithm. This in silico "gene-trait matching" approach led to the identification of eight candidate genes in the *Lb. plantarum* genome that might modulate the DC cytokine response to *Lb. plantarum.* Six of these genes were involved in bacteriocin production or secretion, one encoded a bile salt hydrolase and one encoded a transcription regulator of which the exact function is unknown. Subsequently, gene deletions mutants were constructed in *Lb. plantarum* WCFS1 and compared to the wild-type strain in DC stimulation assays. All three bacteriocin mutants as well as the transcription regulator (lp_2991) had the predicted effect on cytokine production confirming their immunomodulatory effect on the DC response to *Lb. plantarum*. Transcriptome analysis and qPCR data showed that transcript level of gtcA3, which is predicted to be involved in glycosylation of cell wall teichoic acids, was substantially increased in the lp_2991 deletion mutant (44- and 29-fold, respectively).

35.3.6 Peptidoglycan Hydrolases

Lb. plantarum is able to interact with receptors of the immune system in the GI tract through Peptidoglycan hydrolase PGH-dependent processes such as autolysis and/or cell wall turnover that release muramyl-peptides or PGH fragments themselves [62]. In *Lb. plantarum* WCFS1, the analysis of its genome sequence has revealed the presence of 16 putative PGHs (carboxypeptidases are excluded), including 12 candidates displaying similarity with well-characterized PGHs, 3 hypothetical (lytic) transglycosylases containing a WY domain, and a pseudogene (acm3, three fragments) [63]. PGH activity of Acm2 and LytH (putative *N*-acetylmuramoyl-L-alanine amidase) could be modulated through *O*-acetylation of glycan chains of *Lb. plantarum* PG. MurNAc *O*-acetylation triggers LytH activity, whereas GlcNAc *O*-acetylation inhibits Acm2 activity [64]. Rolain et al. [65] investigated the functional role of the 12 more probable candidates of the PGH complement of *Lb. plantarum* WCFS1 by a systematic gene deletion strategy. Characterization of mutant cell morphology, growth, and autolytic behavior, in a range of conditions showed that 4 PGHs (Acm2, Lys2, LytA, and LytH) play important roles either in the cell cycle or in the autolysis process of *Lb. plantarum.* The putative *N*-acetylglucosaminidase Acm2 is the major autolysin of *Lb. plantarum* and that the putative γ-*D*-glutaminyl-meso-diaminopimelate muropeptidase LytA is a major morphogenic determinant in *Lb. plantarum.*

35.4 SUMMARY

In summary, *Lb. plantarum* strains have been isolated from various sources. Isolation from fermented foods in particular is very acceptable source for human use purpose. Many strains of *Lb. plantarum* have shown appreciable probiotic attributes, select strains were employed further for examining their efficacy in treating or preventing human diseases in in vitro and in vivo models. Human disorders such as IBD, TSS, obstructive jaundice, and typhoid were successfully treated either in in vitro or in vivo clinical studies. Further, human disease such as influenza virus infection, hyperlipidemia, CRC, and gastroenteritis could be prevented by *Lb. plantarum* to a significant level when tested alone or in combinatorial therapy. The mechanism by which human probiont *Lb. plantarum* prevent or treat the disease seems to include immunomodulation, EPS, bacteriocin, competitive exclusion, peptidoglycan hydrolases and various genes involved in adherence mechanism. We conclude from our literature survey on human health benefits of *Lb. plantarum* that it is a significant human probiont with great future potential in human health, more research on possible human clinical study would facilitate much deeper insight into beneficial effects of *Lb. plantarum*.

REFERENCES

1. Chevallier B, Hubert JC, Kammerer B. Determination of chromosome size and number of rrn loci in *Lactobacillus plantarum* by pulsed-field gel electrophoresis. *FEMS Microbiology Letters* 1994;120(1–2):51–56.
2. Kleerebezem M, Boekhorst J, van Kranenburg R, Molenaar D, Kuipers OP, Leer R et al. Complete genome sequence of *Lactobacillus plantarum* WCFS1. *Proceedings of the National Academy of Sciences of the United States of America* 2003;100(4):1990–1995.
3. Tallon R, Arias S, Bressollier P, Urdaci MC. Strain- and matrix-dependent adhesion of *Lactobacillus plantarum* is mediated by proteinaceous bacterial compounds. *Journal of Applied Microbiology* 2007;102(2):442–451.
4. de Vries MC, Vaughanb EE, Kleerebezem M, de Vos WM. *Lactobacillus plantarum*—Survival, functional and potential probiotic properties in the human intestinal tract. *International Dairy Journal* 2006;16:1018–1028.
5. Molin G. Probiotics in foods not containing milk or milk constituents, with special reference to *Lactobacillus plantarum* 299v. *The American Journal of Clinical Nutrition* 2001;73(2 Suppl.):380S–385S.
6. Satish Kumar R, Raghu varman D, Kanmani P, Yuvaraj N, Paari KA, Pattukumar V, Arul V. Isolation, characterization and identification of a potential probiont from South Indian fermented foods (Kallappam, Koozh and Mor Kuzhambu) and its use as biopreservative. *Probiotics and Antimicrobial Proteins* 2010;2:145–151.
7. Sorensen GV, Erichsen R, Svaerke C, Farkas DK, Sorensen HT. Risk of cancer in patients with inflammatory bowel disease and venous thromboembolism: A nationwide cohort study. *Inflammatory Bowel Diseases* 2012;18(10):1859–1863.
8. Baumgart DC, Sandborn WJ. Inflammatory bowel disease: Clinical aspects and established and evolving therapies. *Lancet* 2007;369(9573):1641–1657.
9. Parkes GC, Sanderson JD, Whelan K. Treating irritable bowel syndrome with probiotics: The evidence. *The Proceedings of the Nutrition Society* 2010;69(2):187–194.
10. McFarland LV, Dublin S. Meta-analysis of probiotics for the treatment of irritable bowel syndrome. *World Journal of Gastroenterology* 2008;14(17):2650–2661.
11. Arseneau KO, Tamagawa H, Pizarro TT, Cominelli F. Innate and adaptive immune responses related to IBD pathogenesis. *Current Gastroenterology Reports* 2007;9(6):508–512.
12. Kim HG, Lee SY, Kim NR, Lee HY, Ko MY, Jung BJ et al. *Lactobacillus plantarum* lipoteichoic acid down-regulated *Shigella flexneri* peptidoglycan-induced inflammation. *Molecular Immunology* 2011;48(4):382–391.
13. van Baarlen P, Troost FJ, van Hemert S, van der Meer C, de Vos WM, de Groot PJ et al. Differential NF-kappaB pathways induction by *Lactobacillus plantarum* in the duodenum of healthy humans correlating with immune tolerance. *Proceedings of the National Academy of Sciences of the United States of America* 2009;106(7):2371–2376.

14. Wells JM, Rossi O, Meijerink M, van Baarlen P. Epithelial crosstalk at the microbiota-mucosal interface. *Proceedings of the National Academy of Sciences of the United States of America* 2011;108 Suppl. 1:4607–4614.
15. Chiu YH, Lu YC, Ou CC, Lin SL, Tsai CC, Huang CT et al. *Lactobacillus plantarum* MYL26 induces endotoxin tolerance phenotype in Caco-2 cells. *BMC Microbiology* 2013;13:190.
16. Li CY, Lin HC, Lai CH, Lu JJ, Wu SF, Fang SH. Immunomodulatory effects of lactobacillus and Bifidobacterium on both murine and human mitogen-activated T cells. *International Archives of Allergy and Immunology* 2011;156(2):128–136.
17. Loguercio C, Federico A, Tuccillo C, Terracciano F, D'Auria MV, De Simone C et al. Beneficial effects of a probiotic VSL#3 on parameters of liver dysfunction in chronic liver diseases. *Journal of Clinical Gastroenterology* 2005;39(6):540–543.
18. Trebichavsky I, Rada V, Splichalova A, Splichal I. Cross-talk of human gut with bifidobacteria. *Nutrition Reviews* 2009;67(2):77–82.
19. Ducrotte P, Sawant P, Jayanthi V. Clinical trial: *Lactobacillus plantarum* 299v (DSM 9843) improves symptoms of irritable bowel syndrome. *World Journal of Gastroenterology* 2012;18(30):4012–4018.
20. Park MK, Ngo V, Kwon YM, Lee YT, Yoo S, Cho YH et al. *Lactobacillus plantarum* DK119 as a probiotic confers protection against influenza virus by modulating innate immunity. *PLoS ONE* 2013;8(10):e75368.
21. Kechaou N, Chain F, Gratadoux JJ, Blugeon S, Bertho N, Chevalier C et al. Identification of one novel candidate probiotic *Lactobacillus plantarum* strain active against influenza virus infection in mice by a large-scale screening. *Applied and Environmental Microbiology* 2013;79(5):1491–1499.
22. Parsonnet J, Goering RV, Hansmann MA, Jones MB, Ohtagaki K, Davis CC et al. Prevalence of toxic shock syndrome toxin 1 (TSST-1)-producing strains of *Staphylococcus aureus* and antibody to TSST-1 among healthy Japanese women. *Journal of Clinical Microbiology* 2008;46(8):2731–2738.
23. Todd J, Fishaut M, Kapral F, Welch T. Toxic-shock syndrome associated with phage-group-I Staphylococci. *Lancet* 1978;2(8100):1116–1118.
24. Bergdoll MS, Crass BA, Reiser RF, Robbins RN, Davis JP. A new staphylococcal enterotoxin, enterotoxin F, associated with toxic-shock-syndrome *Staphylococcus aureus* isolates. *Lancet* 1981;1(8228):1017–1021.
25. Dinges MM, Orwin PM, Schlievert PM. Exotoxins of *Staphylococcus aureus*. *Clinical Microbiology Reviews* 2000;13(1):16–34, table of contents.
26. Liu H, Gao Y, Yu LR, Jones RC, Elkins CA, Hart ME. Inhibition of *Staphylococcus aureus* by lysostaphin-expressing *Lactobacillus plantarum* WCFS1 in a modified genital tract secretion medium. *Applied and Environmental Microbiology* 2011;77(24):8500–8508.
27. Zhou YK, Qin HL, Zhang M, Shen TY, Chen HQ, Ma YL et al. Effects of *Lactobacillus plantarum* on gut barrier function in experimental obstructive jaundice. *World Journal of Gastroenterology* 2012;18(30):3977–3991.
28. Salaj R, Stofilova J, Soltesova A, Hertelyova Z, Hijova E, Bertkova I et al. The effects of two *Lactobacillus plantarum* strains on rat lipid metabolism receiving a high fat diet. *The Scientific World Journal* 2013;2013:135142.
29. Wang LX, Liu K, Gao DW, Hao JK. Protective effects of two *Lactobacillus plantarum* strains in hyperlipidemic mice. *World Journal of Gastroenterology* 2013;19(20):3150–3156.
30. Park DY, Ahn YT, Park SH, Huh CS, Yoo SR, Yu R et al. Supplementation of *Lactobacillus curvatus* HY7601 and *Lactobacillus plantarum* KY1032 in diet-induced obese mice is associated with gut microbial changes and reduction in obesity. *PLoS ONE* 2013;8(3):e59470.
31. Abdel-Daim A, Hassouna N, Hafez M, Ashor MS, Aboulwafa MM. Antagonistic activity of Lactobacillus isolates against *Salmonella typhi* in vitro. *BioMed Research International* 2013;2013:680605.
32. Guarner F, Malagelada JR. Gut flora in health and disease. *Lancet* 2003;361(9356):512–519.
33. Greenlee RT, Murray T, Bolden S, Wingo PA. Cancer statistics, 2000. *CA: A Cancer Journal for Clinicians* 2000;50(1):7–33.
34. Sant M, Capocaccia R, Verdecchia A, Gatta G, Micheli A, Mariotto A et al. Comparisons of colon-cancer survival among European countries: The Eurocare Study. *International Journal of Cancer [Journal international du cancer]* 1995;63(1):43–48.
35. Satish Kumar R, Kanmani P, Yuvaraj N, Paari KA, Pattukumar V, Thirunavukkarasu C et al. *Lactobacillus plantarum* AS1 isolated from south Indian fermented food Kallappam suppress 1,2-dimethyl hydrazine (DMH)-induced colorectal cancer in male Wistar rats. *Applied Biochemistry and Biotechnology* 2012;166(3):620–631.

36. Asha, Gayathri D. Synergistic impact of *Lactobacillus fermentum*, *Lactobacillus plantarum* and vincristine on 1,2-dimethylhydrazine-induced colorectal carcinogenesis in mice. *Experimental and Therapeutic Medicine* 2012;3(6):1049–1054.
37. Lee YK, Salminen, S. The coming of age of probiotics. *Trends in Food Science & Technology* 1995;6:241–244.
38. Lee YK, Puong KY, Ouwehand AC, Salminen S. Displacement of bacterial pathogens from mucus and Caco-2 cell surface by lactobacilli. *Journal of Medical Microbiology* 2003;52(Pt 10):925–930.
39. Satish Kumar R, Kanmani P, Yuvaraj N, Paari KA, Pattukumar V, Arul V. *Lactobacillus plantarum* AS1 binds to cultured human intestinal cell line HT-29 and inhibits cell attachment by enterovirulent bacterium *Vibrio parahaemolyticus*. *Letters in Applied Microbiology* 2011;53(4):481–487.
40. Bron PA, Grangette C, Mercenier A, de Vos WM, Kleerebezem M. Identification of *Lactobacillus plantarum* genes that are induced in the gastrointestinal tract of mice. *Journal of Bacteriology* 2004;186(17):5721–5729.
41. Lebeer S, Vanderleyden J, De Keersmaecker SC. Genes and molecules of lactobacilli supporting probiotic action. *Microbiology and Molecular Biology Reviews* 2008;72(4):728–764, Table of Contents.
42. Marco ML, Bongers RS, de Vos WM, Kleerebezem M. Spatial and temporal expression of *Lactobacillus plantarum* genes in the gastrointestinal tracts of mice. *Applied and Environmental Microbiology* 2007;73(1):124–132.
43. Bron PA, Meijer M, Bongers RS, de Vos WM, Kleerebezem M. Dynamics of competitive population abundance of *Lactobacillus plantarum* ivi gene mutants in faecal samples after passage through the gastrointestinal tract of mice. *Journal of Applied Microbiology* 2007;103(5):1424–1434.
44. Sleator RD, Clifford T, Hill C. Gut osmolarity: A key environmental cue initiating the gastrointestinal phase of *Listeria monocytogenes* infection? *Medical Hypotheses* 2007;69(5):1090–1092.
45. De Angelis M, Gobbetti M. Environmental stress responses in Lactobacillus: A review. *Proteomics* 2004;4(1):106–122.
46. Pretzer G, Snel J, Molenaar D, Wiersma A, Bron PA, Lambert J et al. Biodiversity-based identification and functional characterization of the mannose-specific adhesin of *Lactobacillus plantarum*. *Journal of Bacteriology* 2005;187(17):6128–6136.
47. Adlerberth I, Ahrne S, Johansson ML, Molin G, Hanson LA, Wold AE. A mannose-specific adherence mechanism in *Lactobacillus plantarum* conferring binding to the human colonic cell line HT-29. *Applied and Environmental Microbiology* 1996;62(7):2244–2251.
48. Sturme MH, Nakayama J, Molenaar D, Murakami Y, Kunugi R, Fujii T et al. An agr-like two-component regulatory system in *Lactobacillus plantarum* is involved in production of a novel cyclic peptide and regulation of adherence. *Journal of Bacteriology*. 2005;187(15):5224–5235.
49. Todorov SD, Nyati H, Meincken M, Dicks LMT. Partial characterization of bacteriocin AMA-K, produced by *Lactobacillus plantarum* AMA-K isolated from naturally fermented milk from Zimbabwe. *Food Control* 2007;18:656–664.
50. Powell JE, Witthuhn RC, Todorov SD, Dicks LMT. Characterization of bacteriocin ST8KF produced by a kefir isolate *Lactobacillus plantarum* ST8KF. *International Dairy Journal* 2007;17:190–198.
51. Leal MV, Baras M, Ruiz-Barba JL, Floriano B, Jimenez-Diaz R. Bacteriocin production and competitiveness of *Lactobacillus plantarum* LPCO10 in olive juice broth, a culture medium obtained from olives. *International Journal of Food Microbiology* 1998;43(1–2):129–134.
52. Suma K, Misra MC, Varadaraj MC. Plantaricin LP84, a broad spectrum heat-stable bacteriocin of *Lactobacillus plantarum* NCIM 2084 produced in a simple glucose broth medium. *International Journal of Food Microbiology* 1998;40(1–2):17–25.
53. Leroy F, De Vuyst, L. Bacteriocin production by *Enterococcus faecium* RZS C5 is cell density limited and occurs in the very early phase. *International Journal of Food Microbiology*. 2002;72(1–2):155–164.
54. Hata T, Tanaka R, Ohmomo S. Isolation and characterization of Plantaricin ASM1: A new bacteriocin produced by *Lactobacillus plantarum* A-1. *International Journal of Food Microbiology*. 2010;137:94–99.
55. Xie Y, An H, Hao Y, Qin Q, Huang Y, Luo Y, Zhang L. Characterization of an anti-Listeria bacteriocin produced by *Lactobacillus plantarum* LB-B1 isolated from koumiss, a traditionally fermented dairy product from China. *Food Control* 2011;22:1027–1031.
56. Mack DR, Ahrne S, Hyde L, Wei S, Hollingsworth MA. Extracellular MUC3 mucin secretion follows adherence of Lactobacillus strains to intestinal epithelial cells in vitro. *Gut* 2003;52(6):827–833.
57. Artis D. Epithelial-cell recognition of commensal bacteria and maintenance of immune homeostasis in the gut. *Nature Reviews Immunology* 2008;8(6):411–420.

58. Boirivant M, Strober W. The mechanism of action of probiotics. *Current Opinion in Gastroenterology* 2007;23(6):679–692.
59. Herias MV, Hessle C, Telemo E, Midtvedt T, Hanson LA, Wold AE. Immunomodulatory effects of *Lactobacillus plantarum* colonizing the intestine of gnotobiotic rats. *Clinical and Experimental Immunology* 1999;116(2):283–290.
60. van Hemert S, Meijerink M, Molenaar D, Bron PA, de Vos P, Kleerebezem M et al. Identification of *Lactobacillus plantarum* genes modulating the cytokine response of human peripheral blood mononuclear cells. *BMC Microbiology* 2010;10:293.
61. Meijerink M, van Hemert S, Taverne N, Wels M, de Vos P, Bron PA et al. Identification of genetic loci in *Lactobacillus plantarum* that modulate the immune response of dendritic cells using comparative genome hybridization. *PLoS ONE* 2010;5(5):e10632.
62. Bron PA, van Baarlen P, Kleerebezem M. Emerging molecular insights into the interaction between probiotics and the host intestinal mucosa. *Nature Reviews Microbiology* 2012;10:66–78.
63. Kleerebezem M, Hols P, Bernard E, Rolain T, Zhou M, Siezen RJ et al. The extracellular biology of the lactobacilli. *FEMS Microbiology Reviews* 2010;34(2):199–230.
64. Bernard E, Rolain T, Courtin P, Guillot A, Langella P, Hols P et al. Characterization of O-acetylation of N-acetylglucosamine: A novel structural variation of bacterial peptidoglycan. *The Journal of Biological Chemistry* 2011;286(27):23950–23958.
65. Rolain T, Bernard E, Courtin P, Bron PA, Kleerebezem M, Chapot-Chartier MP et al. Identification of key peptidoglycan hydrolases for morphogenesis, autolysis, and peptidoglycan composition of *Lactobacillus plantarum* WCFS1. *Microbial Cell Factories* 2012;11:137.
66. Ampe F, ben Omar N, Moizan C, Wacher C, Guyot JP. Polyphasic study of the spatial distribution of microorganisms in Mexican pozol, a fermented maize dough, demonstrates the need for cultivation-independent methods to investigate traditional fermentations. *Applied and Environmental Microbiology* 1999;65(12):5464–5473.
67. Lee C. Lactic acid fermented foods and their benefits in Asia. *Food Control.* 1997;10(6):259–260.
68. Kanwar SS, Gupta MK, Katoch C, Kumar R, Kanwar P. Traditional fermented foods of Lahaul and Spiti area of Himachal Pradesh. *Indian Journal of Traditional Knowledge* 2007;6(1):42–45.
69. Patil MM, Ajay P, Anand T, Ramana KV. Isolation and characterization of lactic acid bacteria from curd and cucumber. *Indian Journal of Biotechnology* 2010;9:166–172.
70. Prashant TS, Singh R, Gupta SC, Arora DK, Joshi BK, Kumar D. Phenotypic and genotypic characterization of lactobacilli from Churpi cheese. *Dairy Science and Technology* 2009; 89:531–540.
71. Liu S, Han Y, Zhou Z. Lactic acid bacteria in traditional fermented Chinese foods. *Food Research International* 2011;44:643–651.
72. Hashemi SMB, Shahidi F, Mortazavi SA, Milani E, Eshaghi Z. Potentially probiotic Lactobacillus strains from traditional kurdish cheese. *Probiotics and Antimicrobial Proteins* 2014;6:22–31.
73. Mathara JM, Schillinger U, Kutima PM, Mbugua SK, Guigas C, Franz C, Holzapfel WH. Functional properties of *Lactobacillus plantarum* strains isolated from Maasai traditional fermented milk products in Kenya. *Current Microbiology* 2008;56:315–321.
74. Singh A, Singh RK, Sureja AK. Cultural significance and diversities of ethnic foods of Northeast India. *Indian Journal of Traditional Knowledge* 2007;6(1):79–94.
75. Steinkraus KH. *Handbook of Indigenous Fermented Foods.* New York: Marcel Dekke; 1996.
76. Jeyaram K, Singh TA, Romi W, Devi AR, Singh WM, Dayanithi H et al. Traditional fermented foods of Manipur. *Indian Journal of Traditional Knowledge* 2009;8(1):115–121.
77. Tamang B, Tamang JP. Traditional knowledge of biopreservation of perishable vegetables and bamboo shoots in Northeast India as food resources. *Indian Journal of Traditional Knowledge* 2009;8(1):89–95.
78. Tamang JP, editor. Lactic acid bacteria in traditional food fermentation. *Fermentation Biotechnology—Industrial perspectives Proceedings of the Symposium*, All India Biotech Association and Department of Biotechnology, Government of India, New Delhi, India; 1998.
79. Kingston JJ, Radhika M, Roshini PT, Raksha MA, Murali HS, Batra HV. Molecular characterization of lactic acid bacteria recovered from natural fermentation of beet root and carrot Kanji. *Indian Journal of Microbiology* 2010;50:292–298.
80. Chang SM, Tsai C, Wee WC, Yan TR. Isolation and functional study of potentially probiotic Lactobacilli from Taiwan traditional paocai. *African Journal of Microbiology Research* 2013;7(8):683–691.
81. Kostinek M, Specht I, Edward VA, Schillinger U, Hertel C, Holzapfel WH, Franz CMAP. Diversity and technological properties of predominant lactic acid bacteria from fermented cassava used for the preparation of Gari, a traditional African food. *Systematic and Applied Microbiology* 2005;28:527–540.

82. Omar NB, Ampe F, Raimbault M, Guyot JP, Tailliez P. Molecular diversity of lactic acid bacteria from cassava sour starch (Colombia). *Systematic and Applied Microbiology* 2000;23:285–291.
83. Peres CM, Alves M, Hernandez-Mendoza A, Moreira L, Silva S, Bronze MR, Vilas-Boas L, Peres C, Malcata FX. Novel isolates of lactobacilli from fermented Portuguese olive as potential probiotics. *Food Science and Technology* 2014;59(1):234–246.
84. Lim SM, Im DS. Screening and characterization of probiotic lactic acid bacteria isolated from Korean fermented foods. *Journal of Microbiology and Biotechnology* 2009;19(2):178–186.
85. Thapa N, Pal J, Tamang JP. Microbial diversity in ngari, hentak and tungtap, fermented fish products of North East India. *World Journal of Microbiology and Biotechnology* 2004;20:599–607.
86. Rai AK, Tamang JP, Palni U. Microbiological studies of ethnic meat products of the Eastern Himalayas. *Meat Science*. 2010;85(3):560–567.
87. Bonomo MG, Ricciardi A, Zotta T, Parente E, Salzano G. Molecular and technological characterization of lactic acid bacteria from traditional fermented sausages of Basilicata region (Southern Italy). *Meat Science* 2008;80(4):1238–1248.
88. Paludan-Muller C, Huss HH, Gram L. Characterization of lactic acid bacteria isolated from a Thai low-salt fermented fish product and the role of garlic as substrate for fermentation. *International Journal of Food Microbiology* 1999;46(3):219–229.
89. Aidoo KE, Nout MJ, Sarkar PK. Occurrence and function of yeasts in Asian indigenous fermented foods. *FEMS Yeast Research* 2006;6(1):30–39.
90. Kulkarni SG, Manan J, Agarwal MD, Shukla IC. Studies on physico-chemical composition, packaging and storage of black gram and green gram Wari prepared in Uttar Pradesh. *Journal of Food Science and Technology* 1997;34(2):119–122.
91. Dahal NR, Karki TB, Swamylingappa B, Li Q, Gu G. Traditional foods and beverages of Nepal—A review. *Food Reviews International* 2005;21:1–25.
92. Chao SH, Tomii Y, Watanabe K, Tsai YC. Diversity of lactic acid bacteria in fermented brines used to make stinky tofu. *International Journal of Food Microbiology* 2008;123(1–2):134–141.
93. Chen YS, Yanagida F, Hsu JS. Isolation and characterization of lactic acid bacteria from suan-tsai (fermented mustard), a traditional fermented food in Taiwan. *Journal of Applied Microbiology*. 2006;101(1):125–130.

36 Probiotics in Functional Gastrointestinal Disorders in Children
Therapy and Prevention

Flavia Indrio, Giuseppe Riezzo, and Antonio Di Mauro

CONTENTS

INTRODUCTION

Probiotics, as defined by the FAO and the WHO in a joint consensus document, are live microorganisms that confer a health benefit on the host when administered in adequate amounts. Probiotics have been studied in the treatment and prevention of many gastrointestinal and nongastrointestinal diseases and their role in promoting health is now supported by many double-blind placebo-controlled human trials. Probiotics show convincing evidence in different fields as follows:

- Prevention of respiratory tract infections
- Prevention and therapy of allergy
- Treatment and prevention of gastrointestinal infections and antibiotic-associated diarrhea
- Treatment of Inflammatory bowel disease
- Prevention and treatment of Functional gastrointestinal disorders (FGIDs)

In order to understand the mechanisms by which probiotics are involved in the maintenance of intestinal microbiota and, as consequence, are useful in confer a health benefits, the concepts of intestinal barrier function and dysbiosis, immunology system, and gut–brain axis have to be introduced prior to describe the role of probiotics in specific diseases.

36.1 MICROBIOTA AND GASTROINTESTINAL HEALTH

The gastrointestinal tract and organisms within its lumen constitute an ecologic unit, where all of the components are important and depend upon each other. The huge surface area of the intestinal mucosa is constantly exposed to antigenic stimulation. Specific immunological and nonimmunological mechanisms are fundamental in oral tolerance, influencing the interaction between intestinal mucosa, gut-associated lymphoid tissue (GALT), and antigens, with suppression of the immune responses against both food proteins and the host's own intestinal microbiota.

The intestinal mucosa with its intestinal microflora represents a stable barrier for protecting the host and providing normal gastrointestinal function. In fact, the gut barrier is able to prevent luminal pathogens and harmful elements from entering into the internal milieu and yet promoting digestion transforming food into simpler components that can be absorbed and used to produce energy for cellular function [1].

Regarding the immunology system, the gastrointestinal tract has the most extensive lymphoid system of the human body: the GALT is formed by inductive (Peyer's patches) and effector sites (intraepithelial cells and lamina propria), which has defense and immunomodulatory functions.

GALT, dealing with intestinal microflora, prevents potentially harmful intestinal antigens from reaching the systemic circulation and induces systemic tolerance against luminal antigens by a process that involves polymeric immunoglobulin A (IgA) secretion and the induction of regulatory T cells. Antigen-presenting cells (APC) efficiently take up and transport a variety of microorganisms and present antigen. Recognition of antigens by APC triggers a family pattern of recognition receptor (TLRs) which changes cell phenotype and function, directing immune responses by activating signaling events leading to elevated expression cytokines and chemokines that recruit and regulate the immune and inflammatory cells, which in turn either initiate or enhance host immune responses [2].

Gut–brain interactions are well-known mechanisms for the guidance of intestinal function in both healthy and diseased conditions. The brain can alter the microbiota through modulation of intestinal secretion, permeability, and motility, removing excessive bacteria from the lumen and preventing bacterial overgrowth [3]. Signaling molecules released into the gut lumen from cells in the lamina propria that are under the control of the central nervous system (CNS) can result in changes in gastrointestinal motility and secretion as well as intestinal permeability, thus altering the gastrointestinal environment in which the bacteria reside [4]. Microbiota communicates and modulates the gut–brain axis through different mechanism such as an endocrine route, an immune route, and finally a neuronal route (Figure 36.1). Through the release of bacterial substances, microbiota

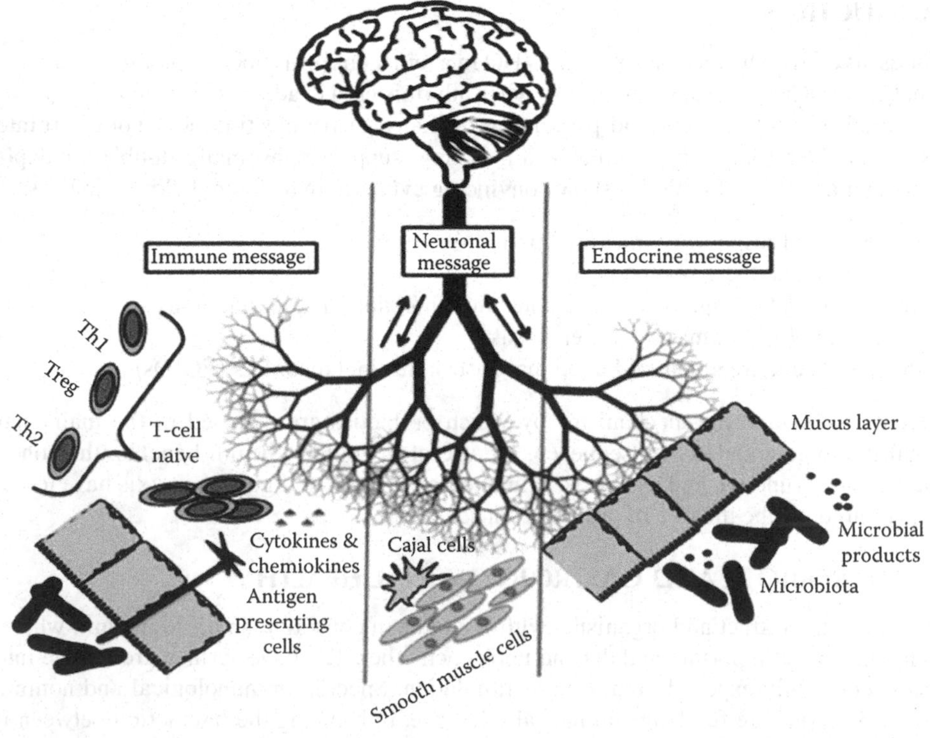

FIGURE 36.1 Gut brain axis.

has a direct interaction with mucosal cell, stimulating production of intestinal neuroendocrine factors. Through recognition of Pathogen-Associated Molecular Patterns (PAMPs) by toll-like receptors, microbiota can modulate expression of factors, such as cytokines and chemokines, that recruit and change the phenotype and function of immune and inflammatory cells. Through a direct contact to neuronal endings, microbiota can increase the expression of GABA receptors, by inducing expression of opioid and cannabinoid receptors in intestinal epithelial cells.

36.2 PROBIOTICS AND GASTROINTESTINAL DISEASE

Recently, the composition of intestinal microbiota is found to influence the pathogenesis of functional gastrointestinal diseases. In fact, there is growing evidence that an aberrant gut microbiota, specially an inadequate amount of lactobacilli and an increased concentration of coliforms, might influence the pathogenesis of functional diseases, with influence on immunity and sensorimotor networks [5,6]. A microbial imbalance compared to the normal healthy state results in alterations of bacterial metabolism as well as in the excessive growth of potentially pathogenic microorganisms in a process called dysbiosis, with the release of toxic products that play a critical role in the development of many chronic disorders.

FGIDs refer to an alteration in the way the body works, characterized by chronic or recurrent symptoms often result from a maladaptive behavioral reaction to interior or exterior stimuli. In term newborns, the structures that influence intestinal motility have already reached full maturity [7], but intestinal colonization by microbiota promoted the development of a neuroimmune interaction in the GALT [8], which play a crucial role in forming motility and sensitivity network [9].

During early life, microbiota affects functions of the gut–brain axis with repercussion on pain sensitivity, response to stress, and behavior [10]. An early alteration of the gut–brain axis has been thought to lead to the development of long-term visceral hypersensitivity and cognitive hypervigilance [11,12]. When either the normal microflora or the epithelial cells are disturbed by triggers such as dietary modifications, stress, antibiotic use, and several other environmental factor as chemicals or radiation, defects in the barrier mechanisms become evident. Altered permeability further facilitates the invasion of pathogens, foreign antigens, and other harmful substances [13].

There are many studies that target probiotic therapy for FGIDs such as colic [14], regurgitation [15], and constipation [16]. Taking into consideration the possible pathophysiological mechanism of FIGDs, such as gastrointestinal dysmotility, visceral hypersensitivity, impairment of intestinal permeability, imbalance of intestinal microbiota, and immune function, we can speculate that probiotics supplementation may be beneficial in regularizing of one or more of the above mechanisms [17,18]. All these factors have been suggested as crucial for development of FGIDs and the manipulation of the microbiota through probiotic supplementation is an important and expanding field in the prevention and management of these diseases. Probiotic might play an important role in maintaining gut homeostasis by modulating intestinal barrier function, immunity, motility, and influencing the gut–brain interaction (Table 36.1). Gut microbiota may modulate the sensation to pain, and some probiotics may inhibit hypersensitivity and perhaps intestinal permeability [19].

TABLE 36.1
The Postulated Mechanisms of Action of Probiotics

Inhibition of pathogenic bacteria through competitive action and direct antimicrobial activity
Improvement of the barrier function of the epithelium
Regulation of GI motility and permeability
Positive effect on visceral hypersensitivity and modulation of gut–brain axis

36.2.1 Infant Colic

Colic is not a serious condition since babies with colic continue to eat and gain weight, despite the crying [20]. The main problem with the condition is the stress and anxiety it creates at home, especially if it is your first child. Colic usually affects babies in the first few weeks of their lives but generally goes after about 4 months. Crying can be intense and furious and it may last for several hours a day over a few weeks. Although crying can occur at any time, it usually gets worse in the late afternoon and evening, and can affect your baby's sleep. According to Rome criteria, infant colic ranges from birth to 4 months of age and includes paroxysms of irritability and fussing/crying without cause, No failure to thrive. The episodes last 3 or more h/day for at least 3 days/week for at least 1 week.

The cause of colic is not known but is likely to be multifactorial. So, we can summarize the etiologies of infant colic as gastrointestinal and nongastrointestinal ones. Painful wind may contribute to colic, but there is little evidence to prove that it is linked to digestive problems [21]. Another theory is that the babies are intolerant to certain substances such as lactose passed on through breastfeeding and formula milk [22]. The hypothesis states that infantile colic is a pain syndrome and the excessive crying leads to aerophagia and abdominal discomfort. The pain comes from sucking the bottle or the nipple. Feeding for the infant is a heavy workload for the masticatory muscles. The tiny digastricus muscle moves the hyoid bone, takes part in opening the mouth and retrusion of the mandible, and assists in moving the tongue upward, forward, and backwards. In the adult population, pain from this muscle is well documented. The hypothesis explains the crying as being due to muscular pain at first, later on pain from the origins and insertions of the muscle. Then with increased muscular strength and development the pain fades away [23]. However, evidence to support this is limited. Another possible cause may be your baby's behavior and temperament.

The pathophysiology of FGIDs is multifactorial, involving esophageal and gastrointestinal motility and enteric nervous system abnormalities. Gastrointestinal motility develops during infancy and early childhood and may be influenced by various factors, including maturation, dietary and postural habits, arousal state, ongoing illnesses, congenital anomalies, and effects of medical or surgical interventions. It is possible that esophageal motility is involved because it regulates the movement of a bolus during swallowing. To date, there is no much evidence of esophageal defense mechanisms against GER in children, although data exist from adult studies [24,25]. With regard to alteration in gastric motility, gastric distension and impaired fundic relaxation as a result of disturbed gastric motility might play a role even if a recent paper has not demonstrated a correlation between gastric emptying time and esophageal gastric exposure [26]. The enlarged fasting antral area could trigger the gastric distension and consequently provoke symptoms. Furthermore, recent data on infants with cow's milk allergy showed a close link between gastrointestinal symptoms, gastroesophageal reflux, and gastric emptying time [27].

Although the available data fail to provide insight into the exact triggers of infantile colic, these do allow for the hypothesis that certain infants are predisposed to dietary protein intolerance and disturbed gut motility, such as visceral hypersensitivity/hyperalgesia, in the first few weeks of life. These processes lead to distress and altered perceptions, where normal stimuli (i.e. intestinal distension) are misinterpreted as painful events [28]. In addition, recent finding shows that ghrelin and motilin concentrations are higher in infants with colic than in controls, supporting an organicistic etiopathogenesis of this disorder. Furthermore, the role of ghrelin on gastrointestinal motility may open new doors to better understand the etiology of infantile colic [29].

The composition of intestinal microbiota, specially an inadequate amount of lactobacilli and an increased concentration of coliforms, might influence the pathogenesis of infantile colic. Probiotics promoted maturation and the development of a functioning motility network, but in older infants the structures that regulate intestinal motility have already reached full maturity [30]. So, the neuroimmune interaction is still the main interpretation of the possible effect of probiotics in the mechanism of intestinal motility [31,32]. As well is very widely reported in literature the action of probiotics with the GALT [33,34]. The coordinated interplay among these apparatus is fundamental for the appropriate function of the gut.

36.2.2 Infant Regurgitation

Uncomplicated regurgitation in otherwise healthy infants is not a disease. It consists of milk flow from mouth during or after feeding. Regurgitation is distinguished from vomiting, which is defined by a central nervous system reflex involving both autonomic and skeletal muscles in which gastric contents are forcefully expelled through the mouth because of coordinated movements of the small bowel, stomach, esophagus, and diaphragm. When the latter causes or contributes to tissue damage or inflammation (e.g. esophagitis, obstructive apnea, reactive airway disease, pulmonary aspiration, or failure to thrive), it is called gastroesophageal reflux disease (GERD). GERD is sometimes wrongly diagnosed in healthy infants with troublesome but harmless symptoms of "physiological" gastroesophageal reflux (GER). This has led to increasing, potentially inappropriate, use of acid-reducing drugs.

GER occurs in healthy infants and can be considered physiological process. Fifty percent of all infants 0–3 months regurgitate at least once a day, but the percentage drops to 5% in infants 10–12 months old. Prematurity, developmental delay, and congenital abnormalities of the oropharynx, chest, lungs, central nervous system, or gastrointestinal tract are considered risk factors for GERD. The presence of a systemic condition (i.e. milk allergy) may be considered in the case of eczema; an abnormal neurological exam needs further investigation. According to Rome criteria, it is characterized by regurgitation 2 or more times/day for 3 or more weeks but no retching, hematemesis, aspiration, apnea, failure to thrive, feeding or swallowing difficulties, or abnormal posturing.

Common causes include overfeeding, air swallowed during feeding, crying, or coughing; physical exam is normal and weight gain is adequate. History and physical exam are diagnostic, and conservative therapy is recommended. GERD refers to infants with regurgitation and vomiting associated with poor weight gain, respiratory symptoms, and esophagitis. Reflux episodes occur most often during transient relaxations of the lower esophageal sphincter unaccompanied by swallowing, which permit gastric content to flow into the esophagus. A minor proportion of reflux episodes occur when the lower esophageal sphincter fails to increase pressure during a sudden increase in intraabdominal pressure or when lower esophageal sphincter resting pressure is chronically reduced. Alterations in several protective mechanisms allow physiologic reflux to become gastroesophageal reflux disease; diagnostic approach is both clinical and instrumental; radiological series are useful to exclude anatomic abnormalities; pH-testing evaluates the quantity, frequency, and duration of the acid reflux episodes; and endoscopy and biopsy are performed in the case of esophagitis.

Uncomplicated GER can present with recurrent vomiting or regurgitation without any other symptoms and is usually managed by educating, reassuring, and guiding the parent without other intervention. Thickened feeds are helpful in reducing the symptoms of GER. Elevating the head of the crib in the supine position does not have any effect. Metoclopramide may have some benefit in comparison to placebo in the symptomatic treatment for GER, but that must be weighed against possible side effects [35]. Proton Pump Inhibitors (PPIs) are the most effective pharmacologic agents available for the treatment of children with GERD. In the pediatric practice, only omeprazole, lansoprazole, and esomeprazole are available over the first year of life. The empiric use in infants with nonspecific symptoms (excessive crying, regurgitation, feeding refusal, and chronic cough) is frequent without randomized controlled study [36].

36.3 PROBIOTICS AS THERAPEUTIC STRATEGY

Studies on probiotic or prebiotic formulas have demonstrated a healthy benefit in both term [37] and in preterm newborns [38]. Regurgitation and infant colic might benefit from prebiotics and probiotic administration [39] since they have shown their safety and tolerance in full-term infants [40] and the ability to promote a regression of GI symptoms without adverse growth or behavioral effects [41].

The reduction in crying time in colicky newborns fed with breast milk added with probiotics has been report recently by Savino et al. [42] and confirmed by other authors [45]. The benefit of supplementation with *Lactobacillus reuteri* has been recently reported in infants and experimental data suggest that the effect of probiotics may be related to the influence on immune response, gut motility, and pain transmission and perception [43]. In the case of infant, colic probiotics can inhibit colonic peristaltic activity and may stimulate tonic activity directly and or indirectly via short chain fatty acids (SCFA) that are able to modify colonic motility via the involving of GI hormones as polypeptide YY [44]. The studies on the postinfectious enteric muscle dysfunction have shown that the state of persistent dysfunction of the neuromuscular tissues is maintained by the production of mediators such as TGF beta and prostaglandin E2 by intestinal muscle layers themselves [45]. The interstitial cells of Cajal (ICC) network, the pacemaker of GI electrical activity, also could be damaged by inflammation and such alteration may explain motor abnormality as supported by Wang et al. [46]. Probiotics can restore muscle function after GI infection and modulate the mechanism influencing multiple proteins and other components of excitation–contraction coupling [47]. The same mechanism could be involved in functional disease as result of the so-called minimal inflammation state.

With regard to regurgitation in infants, alteration in gastric motility and its interplay with gastric distension and impaired fundic relaxation as a result of disturbed gastric motility might play a role in acid reflux to the esophagus. The action of probiotics on upper gastrointestinal motility could be explained in several ways. Volume and chemical characteristics of meals in the gut have been supposed to induce vagal signal affecting gastric emptying [48]. The fiber content was associated with a significant increase in gastric antral motility with respect to other diets [49]. Bacteria metabolites such as SCFA may stimulate smooth muscle [50]. Transient lower esophageal sphincter relaxations (TLESRs) seem to be triggered by gastric distension via activation of the stretch receptor in the stomach [51,52]. In addition, the rate of gastric emptying actually did not affect the number of reflux episodes, but slower emptying results in a less acidic refluxate. Some studies suggest that acid exposure may be reduced in the case of delayed gastric emptying [53]. A significant increase in the gastric emptying rate in the *L. reuteri*-supplemented infants was found. Reduced episodes of regurgitation linked with an increased gastric emptying rate and reduced fasting antral area were seen in formula-fed preterm supplemented with *L. reuteri* ATCC 55730 [54]. Furthermore, recent data on infants with cow's milk allergy showed a close link between gastrointestinal symptoms, gastroesophageal reflux, and gastric emptying time [55]. This findings on infants confirmed that regurgitation can be related to impaired accommodation and antral dysfunction.

36.4 CONCLUSION

A probiotic supplementation may represent a new strategy for preventing FGIDs, during early life: it could determine a beneficial colonization, improving intestinal permeability, and visceral sensitivity. Several trials showed that daily administration of probiotic early in life is effective in the prevention of infantile colic, regurgitation, and functional constipation in the first 3 months of life. It is also intriguing to speculate whether an early manipulation of the microbiota could have a preventive role against the later development of pain-related FGIDs in childhood. However, several questions remain unanswered, such as the optimal dose, the role of combination therapy, strain-specific activity, stability within gastrointestinal tract, possible development of antibiotic resistance, and the duration of therapy. The inconsistencies between the studies underline the need to look at each probiotic product separately for specific conditions, symptoms, and patient populations.

REFERENCES

1. Lu L, Walker WA. Pathologic and physiologic interactions of bacteria with the gastrointestinal epithelium. *Am J Clin Nutr.* 2001;73:1124S–1130S.
2. Mason KL, Huffnagle GB, Noverr MC, Kao JY. Overview of gut immunology. *Adv Exp Med Biol.* 2008;635:1–14.
3. Heijtz RD, Wang S, Anuar F et al. Normal gut microbiota modulates brain development and behavior. *Proc Natl Acad Sci USA.* 2011;108:3047–3052.

4. Diamond B, Huerta PT, Tracey K et al. It takes guts to grow a brain: Increasing evidence of the important role of the intestinal microflora in neuro- and immune-modulatory functions during development and adulthood. *Bioessays.* 2011;33:588–912.
5. Di Mauro A, Neu J, Riezzo G, Raimondi F, Martinelli D, Francavilla R, Indrio F. Gastrointestinal function development and microbiota. *Ital J Pediatr.* February 24, 2013;39:15. doi: 10.1186/1824-7288-39-15.
6. Di Mauro A, Neu J, Riezzo G et al. Gastrointestinal function development and microbiota. *Ital J Pediatr.* 2013;39:15.
7. Faussone-Pellegrini M, Vannucchi MG, Alaggio R, Faussone-Pellegrini MS, Vannucchi MG, Alaggio R, Strojna A, Midrio P. Morphology of interstitial cells of Cajal of the human ileum from foetal to neonatal life. *Cell Mol Med.* 2007;11:482–494.
8. Wood JD. Enteric neuro-immunophysiology and pathophysiology. *Gastroenterology.* 2004;127:635–657.
9. Rhee SH, Pothoulakis C, Mayer EA. Principles and clinical implications of the brain-gut-enteric microbiota axis. *Nat Rev Gastroenterol Hepatol.* 2009;6:306–314.
10. Indrio F, Riezzo G, Raimondi F, Di Mauro A, Francavilla R. Microbiota involvement in the gut-brain axis. *J Pediatr Gastroenterol Nutr.* December 2013;57(Suppl 1):S11–S15.
11. Collins SM, Surette M, Bercik P. The interplay between the intestinal microbiota and the brain. *Nat Rev Microbiol.* 2012;10(11):735–742. doi:10.1038/nrmicro2876.
12. Cryan JF, Dinan TG. Mind-altering microorganisms: The impact of the gut microbiota on brain and behaviour. *Nat Rev Neurosci.* 2012;13(10):701–712.
13. Cryan JF, O'Mahony SM. The microbiome-gut-brain axis: From bowel to behavior. *Neurogastroenterol Motil.* 2011;23:187–192.
14. Szajewska H, Gyrczuk E, Horvath A. *Lactobacillus reuteri* DSM 17938 for the management of infantile colic in breastfed infants: A randomized, double-blind, placebo-controlled trial. *J Pediatr.* 2013;162(2):257–262.
15. Indrio F, Riezzo G, Raimondi F et al. *Lactobacillus reuteri* accelerates gastric emptying and improves regurgitation in infants. *Eur J Clin Invest.* 2011;41(4):417–422.
16. Coccorullo P, Strisciuglio C, Martinelli M, Miele E, Greco L, Staiano A. *Lactobacillus reuteri* (DSM 17938) in infants with functional chronic constipation: A double-blind, randomized, placebo-controlled study. *J Pediatr.* 2010;157(4):598–602.
17. Chumpitazi BP, Shulman RJ. Five probiotic drops a day to keep infantile colic away? *JAMA Pediatr.* 2014;168(3):204–205.
18. Thomas CM, Versalovic J. Probiotics-host communication: Modulation of signaling pathways in the intestine. *Gut Microbes.* 2010;1(3):148–163.
19. Ahrne S, Hagslatt ML. Effect of lactobacilli on paracellular permeability in the gut. *Nutrients.* 2011;3:104–117.
20. Garrison MM, Christakis DA. Early childhood colic: Colic, child development, and poisoning prevention: A systematic review of interventions for infant colic. *Pediatrics.* 2000;106:S184–S190.
21. Cohen-Silver J, Ratnapalan S. Management of infantile colic: A review. *Clin Pediatr (Phil).* 2009;48:14–17.
22. Hill DJ, Roy N, Heine RG, Hosking CS, Francis DE, Brown J, Sperrs B, Sadowsky J, Carlin JB. Effect of a low-allergen maternal diet on colic among breastfed infants: A randomised, controlled trial. *Pediatrics.* 2005;116:e709–e715.
23. Gudmundsson G. Infantile colic: Is a pain syndrome. *Med Hypotheses.* 2010;75:528–529.
24. Shaker R, Lang IM. Reflex mediated airway protective mechanisms against retrograde aspiration. *Am J Med.* 1997;103(Suppl 5):64S–73S.
25. Shaker R. Airway protective mechanisms: Current concepts. *Dysphagia.* 1995;10:216–227.
26. Emerenziani S, Sifrim D. Gastroesophageal reflux and gastric emptying, revisited. *Curr Gastroenterol Rep.* 2005;7:190–195.
27. Ravelli AM, Tobanelli P, Volpi S, Ugazio AG. Vomiting and gastric motility in infants with cow's milk allergy. *J Pediatr Gastroenterol Nutr.* 2001;32:59–64.
28. Gupta SK. Update on infantile colic and management options. *Curr Opin Invest Drugs.* 2007;8:921–926.
29. Savino F, Grassino EC, Guidi C, Oggero R, Silvestro L, Miniero R. Ghrelin and motilin concentration in colicky infants. *Acta Paediatr.* 2006;95:738–741.
30. Faussone-Pellegrini M, Vannucchi MG, Alaggio R, Faussone-Pellegrini MS, Vannucchi MG, Alaggio R, Strojna A, Midrio P. Morphology of interstitial cells of Cajal of the human ileum from foetal to neonatal life. *Cell Mol Med.* 2007;11:482–494.
31. Wood JD. Enteric neuro-immunophysiology and pathophysiology. *Gastroenterology.* 2004;127:635–657.

32. Saavedra Y, Vergara P. Hypersensitivity to ovalbumin induces chronic intestinal dysmotility and increase the number of intestinal mast cells. *Neurogastroenterol Motil.* 2005;17:112–122.
33. Ruiz PA, Hoffmann M, Szcesny S, Blaut M, Haller D. Innate mechanisms for *Bifidobacterium lactis* to activate transient pro-inflammatory host responses in intestinal epithelial cells after the colonization of germ-free rats. *Immunology.* 2005;115:441–450.
34. Hölttä V, Klemetti P, Sipponen T, Westerholm-Ormio M, Kociubinski G, Salo H, Räsänen L, Kolho KL, Färkkilä M, Savilahti E, Vaarala O. IL-23/IL-17 immunity as a hallmark of Crohn's disease. *Inflamm Bowel Dis.* 2008;14:1175–1184.
35. Craig WR, Hanlon-Dearman A, Sinclair C, Taback SP, Moffatt M. Withdrawn: Metoclopramide, thickened feedings, and positioning for gastro-oesophageal reflux in children under two years. *Cochrane Database Syst Rev.* 2010;12:CD003502.
36. Romano C, Chiaro A, Comito D, Loddo I, Ferrau V. Proton pump inhibitors in pediatrics: Evaluation of efficacy in GERD therapy. *Curr Clin Pharmacol.* 2011;6:41–47.
37. Kullen MJ, Bettler J. The delivery of probiotics and prebiotics to infants. *Curr Pharm Des.* 2005;11:55–74.
38. Millar M, Wilks M, Costelle K. Probiotics for preterm infants? *Arch Dis Child Fetal Neonatal Ed.* 2003;88:F354–F358
39. Marteau PR, de Vrese M, Vellier CJ, Cellier CJ, Schrezenmeir J. Protection from gastrointestinal diseases with the use of probiotics. *Am J Clin Nutr.* 2001;73:S430–S436.
40. Weizman Z, Alsheikh A. Safety and tolerance of a prebiotic formula in early infancy comparing two probiotic agents: A pilot study. *J Am Coll Nutr.* 2006;25:415–419.
41. Indrio F, Riezzo G, Bisceglia M, Cavallo L, Francavilla R. The effects of probiotics on feeding tolerance, bowel habits and gastrointestinal motility in preterm newborns. *J Pediatr.* 2008;152:801–806.
42. Savino F, Pelle E, Palumeri E, Oggero R, Miniero R. *Lactobacillus reuteri* (American Type Culture Collection Strain 55730) versus simethicone in the treatment of infantile colic: A prospective randomized study. *Pediatrics.* 2007 January;119(1):e124–e130.
43. Ma X, Mao YK, Wang B et al. *Lactobacillus reuteri* ingestion prevents hyperexcitability of colonic DRG neurons induced by noxious stimuli. *Am J Physiol Gastrointest Liver Physiol.* 2009 April;296(4):G868–G875.
44. Voortman T, Hendriks HF, Witkamp RF, Wortelboer HM. Effects of long- and short-chain fatty acids on the release of gastrointestinal hormones using an ex vivo porcine intestinal tissue model. *J Agric Food Chem.* 2012;60:9035–9042.
45. Guerrini S, Barbara G, Stanghellini V, De PF, Corinaldesi R, Moses PL, Sharkey KA, Mawe GM. Inflammatory neuropathies of the enteric nervous system. *Gastroenterology.* 2004;26:1872–1883.
46. Wang XY, Berezin I, Mikkelsen HB, Der T, Bercick P, Collins SM, Huzinga JD. Pathology of interstitial cells of Cajal in relation to inflammation revealed by ultrastructure but not immunochemistry. *Am J Pathol.* 2002;160:1529–1540.
47. Verdue E, Bergonzelli G, Bercik P et al. *Lactobacillus paracaseii* normalizes postinfective dysmotility in vivo—Potential mechanism involved. *JPGN* 2006; 32:E96.
48. Schwartz GJ, Moran TH. Duodenal nutrient exposure elicits nutrient-specific gut motility and vagal afferent signals in rats. *Am J Physiol.* 1998;274:R1236–R1242.
49. Bouin M, Savoye G, Maillot C, Hellot MF, Guedon C, Denis P, Ducotte P. How do fiber-supplemented formulas affect antroduodenal motility during enteral nutrition? A comparative study between mixed and insoluble fibers. *Am J Clin Nutr.* 2000;72:1040–1046.
50. McManus CM, Michel KE, Simon DM, Washabau RJ. Effect of short chain fatty acids on contraction of smooth muscle in the canine colon. *Am J Vet Res.* 2002;63:295–300.
51. Massey BT, Simuncak C, LeCapitaine-Dana NJ, Pudur S. Transient lower esophageal sphincter relaxations do not result from passive opening of the cardia by gastric distention. *Gastroenterology.* 2006;130:89–95.
52. Penagini R, Carmagnola S, Cantu P, Allocca M, Bianchi PA. Mechanoreceptors of the proximal stomach: Role in triggering transient lower esophageal sphincter relaxation. *Gastroenterology.* 2004;126:49–56.
53. Herculano JR Jr, Troncon LE, Aprile LR et al. Diminished retention of food in the proximal stomach correlates with increased acidic reflux in patients with gastroesophageal reflux disease and dyspeptic symptoms. *Dig Dis Sci.* 2004;49:750–756.
54. Indrio F, Riezzo G, Raimondi F, Bisceglia M, Cavallo L, Francavilla R. *Lactobacillus reuteri* accelerates gastric emptying and improve regurgitation in infants. *Eur J Clin Invest.* 2011;41:417–422.
55. Ravelli AM, Tobanelli P, Volpi S, Ugazio AG. Vomiting and gastric motility in infants with cow's milk allergy. *J Pediatr Gastroenterol Nutr.* 2001;32:59–64.

37 Probiotics and Dental Health
An Overview

Maria Grazia Cagetti, Fabio Cocco, and Guglielmo Campus

CONTENTS

37.1 DENTAL CARIES: A BACTERIAL DISEASE

Dental caries still remains one of the most common chronic and multifactorial diseases worldwide, although a decline of the prevalence has been recorded in Western countries (Campus et al., 2007, 2009; Marja-Leena et al., 2008; Selwitz et al., 2007). It is the most common cause of tooth loss and pain in the oral cavity (Edelstein, 2006). The disease is the result over time of the interaction among cariogenic microorganisms, a diet rich in fermentable carbohydrates and host factors, like as saliva secretion rate and buffering capacity (Selwitz et al., 2007). A frequent intake of fermentable carbohydrates resulted in significant production of acid. The extent of the pH drop and the longevity of that fall are heavily regulated by saliva.

The acid production near the tooth structures causes the demineralization of enamel and dentin and subsequently may evolve in the development of cavitation. In the early stages, the caries lesion ("white spot") can be stopped or reversed, but if unfavorable environmental conditions persist and/or appropriate preventive methods are not applied, the lesion proceeds until destruction of the tooth structure leading to dysfunctions of the masticatory apparatus, pain, and systemic odontogenic infections.

The oral ecosystem is an extremely diverse, dynamic, and unique system with a characteristic feature being the instability of its ecological conditions (Marsh, 2005). The regular consumption of fermentable sugars can lead to an environment that favors aciduric species as cariogenic bacteria, reducing the biofilm diversity and resulting in a further plaque pH decrease. In conditions of low pH, cariogenic microorganisms multiply efficiently and take over the dominant position in the biofilm, producing weak acids (lactic, formic, acetic, and propionic acids). High caries risk status is characterized by increasing numbers of highly acid-tolerant and acidogenic bacteria in dental plaque (Lingström et al., 2000). The cariogenic potential of microorganisms is directly related to the consumption of carbohydrates, particularly of sucrose. *Streptococcus mutans* was considered for years the bacterial agent able to start enamel demineralization, first step of the carious lesion (Tanzer et al., 2001). Nowadays, its role is believed not dominant as it was previously assumed; nevertheless, there is an agreement that the microorganism has the highest cariogenic potential (He and Shi, 2009). The concept of a complex dental caries–associated microbiota has received significant attention in recent years and the predominance of *Lactobacillus*, *Actinomyces* species and nonmutans streptococci group in carious lesions confirms this hypothesis (Struzycka, 2014).

The environment of the oral cavity is constantly transformed with age, and thus the oral microbiome changes as well. During the first months of life, bacteria colonize mucosal surfaces, but with the eruption of the teeth, the hard tissues are also colonized by several microorganisms (Tweman et al., 2000).

Saliva plays a major role in protecting the teeth, owing to its cleaning actions as well as its acid neutralizing, antisolubility, and antimicrobial properties (Gupta et al., 2013). Saliva contains many antibacterial, antiviral, and antifungal agents, such as lysozyme, lactoferrin, lactoperoxidase, and other protein components as mucins and immunoglobulin A, G, and M (Van Nieuw Amerongen et al., 2004). Otherwise, saliva also contains proline-rich glycoproteins, which act as receptors for oral bacteria to strongly link the acquired pellicle that covers the tooth surface (Marsh, 2005) and it is the major source of nutrients for microorganisms also; its content in peptides and carbohydrates influences the quality and quantity of microorganisms of the oral biofilm (Nasidze et al., 2009).

37.2 DENTAL CARIES PREVENTION: TRADITIONAL AND INNOVATIVE STRATEGIES

Traditionally, caries preventive measures are based on oral health education, sweeteners intake reduction or replacement with no cariogenic sugar, enhancing host resistance primary with the use of topical fluoride products, dental sealants, and cariogenic bacteria reduction using antibacterial agents as chlorhexidine (Milgrom et al., 2012; Petersen and Lennon, 2004). The use of antibacterial agents in order to reduce cariogenic microflora, however, is not fully effective since a complete eradication of caries-associated microorganisms has proved to be difficult and almost impossible to obtain (Zero, 2006).

An advocated approach to prevent dental caries is through an effective vaccine. Traditionally, vaccine immunization should take place prior to infection. Given the apparent pattern of cariogenic microorganisms' colonization and the association of these bacteria with caries lesion development, immunization should begin early in childhood. If bacterial colonization of the dental biofilm is complete after eruption of primary dentition and if it is possible, through immunization, to prevent cariogenic bacteria colonization prior to this period, the benefit of this immunization might last in time, saving the permanent dentition also. Thus, a successful vaccination directed against *S. mutans* can go a long way in improving the caries status of subjects with a high caries risk.

There is a great promise in the implantation of benign oral microbial strains capable of successfully competing with *S. mutans* (replacement therapy), but few human trials have been performed to date.

Bacteriotherapy is the term used when a harmless strain is implanted in the host's microflora to maintain or restore a natural microbiome by interference and/or inhibition of other microorganisms, especially pathogens (Twetman, 2012; Twetman and Keller, 2012). This could lead to alternative ways of fighting infectious diseases with less harmful side effects.

Inside and outside biofilms from the body play an important role in health maintenance. This is true for both gastrointestinal health and oral health. Frequent ecological shifts in the microbiota allow pathogens to colonize the environment and to became manifest themselves causing disease. In the oral cavity, the microbiota contributes actively to maintaining hard and soft tissues health. Regarding enamel and dentine health, a frequent consumption of fermentable sugars can lead to an environment that favors aciduric species (e.g. mutans streptococci and lactobacilli), reducing the biofilm diversity and resulting in hard tissues demineralization.

Although the beneficial effects of probiotics on health are known from early 1900, the mechanisms of action are still not fully understood. Nevertheless, local (direct) as well as systemic (indirect) effects are recognized. In oral cavity, the local effects include a temporarily alteration of the composition and metabolism of the biofilm, while the systemic ones a regulation of the immune response.

37.3 PROBIOTICS IN CARIES PREVENTION

37.3.1 How Probiotics Work

The inhibition of pathogens in the dental plaque is linked to several mechanisms: production of antimicrobial substances, competing for nutrients, and competing for adhesion. Co-aggregation is an important factor in biofilm formation (Kolenbrander et al., 2006). Several other factors can influence bacterial adhesion like coating or modification of saliva pellicle (Haukioja et al., 2008a).

Probiotics are able to modify the environment of the biofilm toward a less acidogenic plaque (Campus et al., 2014; Kreth et al., 2005). Many different *Lactobacilli* strains showed the ability to inhibit the growth of *S. mutans*, but the effect is linked to the specific strain, sequence of colonization, and growth mode. Still today the exact sequence of how probiotics influence the growth of *S. mutans* is unknown. In 2011, several orally derived lactobacilli strains with the ability to inhibit the growth of cariogenic bacteria were described (Teanpaisan et al., 2011). A certain number of probiotic showed to be able to produce bacteriocine or similar substances and usually the effect is pH dependent. *Lactobacillus brevis* CD2 is a functional *Lactobacillus* strain with peculiar biochemical features, essentially related to the activity of arginine deiminase (Linsalata et al., 2004). This enzyme catalyzes arginine and affects the biosynthesis of polyamines (putrescine, spermidine, and spermine). Polyamines are polycations found in high concentrations in both normal and neoplastic cells. In the presence of glycerol, *Lactobacillus reuteri* is able to produce reuterin that has a wide antimicrobial activity (Talarico et al., 1990).

In vitro, *L. reuteri* strain has been shown to inhibit the growth of *S. mutans* (Hasslöf et al., 2010; Nikawa et al., 2004). In addition, the strain seems to be not able to increase the acidogenity of dental plaque (Marttinen et al., 2012). One probiotic strain the *Lactobacillus salivarius* has been shown to be cariogenic in rats (Matsumoto et al., 2005); however, the calcium release from hydroxyapatite caused by the probiotic was negligible compared to the release caused by *S. mutans* (Nikawa et al., 2004). Nevertheless, two probiotic *L. reuteri* strains, ATCC PTA 5289 and ATCC 55730, differed in their adhesion, biofilm formation, and arginine metabolism in vitro (Jalasvuori et al., 2012).

Lactococcus lactis, a probiotic extensively used in the dairy industry, was tested as an antagonist of *S. mutans*, and the feasibility of the application of the probiotic for the inhibition of the cariogenic microorganism in the oral cavity was evaluated (Tong et al., 2012). The study showed that *L. lactis* could antagonize the cariogenic bacterium and effectively colonized the surface of tooth enamel, producing lower demineralization of hard tissue than that caused by *S. mutans*.

Tanzer et al. (2010) observed that rats inoculated with *S. mutans* and fed with a diet with *Lactobacillus paracasei* showed a reduced number of *S. mutans* and less caries lesions with respect to rats not given lactobacilli (Tanzer et al., 2010).

37.3.2 Probiotics Use in Caries Prevention: A Contradiction?

Probiotics, mostly lactobacilli or bifidobacteria, are aciduric and acidogenic as well as the oral microorganisms involved in caries process. Therefore, their use in caries prevention could seem a contradiction. The scientific evidence from all studies that have administered probiotics in order to obtain a potential effect on oral health have found a positive effect and not a negative one. Some strains of *Lactobacillus* and *Bifidobacterium* including *Lactobacillus rhamnosus* and *B. lactis* BB-12 are not able to metabolize sucrose unlike what cariogenic bacteria do, and this can explain their lower pathogenicity for caries (Haukioja et al., 2008b). Lactic acid production in suspensions of dental plaque and probiotic lactobacilli has shown to be strain dependant and influenced by the type of sugar tested (Keller and Twetman, 2012). While strains of *Lactobacillus plantarum* produced acids at a rapid rate, *L. reuteri* was generally less active in the presence of glucose, lactose, and sucrose (Hedberg et al., 2008). In conclusion, the capacity to produce acid from dietary sugars varies significantly among the different probiotic strains. These findings suggest that the choice of the probiotic strain in caries prevention should be carefully considered in order to maximize the positive effects on oral health and minimize the potential adverse ones.

Since the initial stages of caries are related to the huge presence of different cariogenic microorganisms other than lactobacilli (Chhour et al., 2005), the reduction of these microorganisms produced by probiotics administration decreases the risk to development of the disease (Keller and Twetman, 2012).

37.3.3 Clinical Studies

Clinical evaluations of probiotic bacteria that are naturally specific to the mouth are poor. Probiotic strains administered for oral care are microorganisms mainly used to obtain gastrointestinal benefits, so they could not be ideal for the unique ecological oral environment. The effects of probiotics seem to be strain specific and the same strains may also have different effects on different individuals. The effect of probiotics on dental caries and its related risk factors has been evaluated in several experimental studies (for a list, see Cagetti et al., 2013) using different strains: *L. rhamnosus* GG, *Lactobacillus casei*, *L. reuteri*, *L. plantarum*, *L. brevis* CD2, *Bifidobacterium* spp., etc., were proposed and used to obtain caries incidence reduction, mutans streptococci and lactobacilli count reduction, plaque pH control, and root caries lesions reversal (Tables 37.1 through 37.3). The sample sizes were generally small or medium, and the majority of the investigations were short term (between 10 and 42 days). Different vehicles for the administration and different dosage of probiotics were proposed. The optimal dose for caries prevention is yet to be clarified. Up to now, the adopted dose regimens have been based on gastrointestinal dose standards.

Dairy products supplemented with probiotics are a natural means of oral administration and easily adopted in dietary regime for adults and children. However, specifically formulated devices with slow release of the microbial strain might be needed in order to produce benefits for oral health.

Another uncertain aspect of the probiotic use is whether the probiotics species are really able to colonize the oral *habitat*, and how the prolongation of the microbial shift is induced (Rao et al., 2012). It is well established for probiotics in the gastrointestinal tract that they usually colonize for a short time only (Ravn et al., 2012). Therefore, a prolonged administration of the probiotics bacteria seems to be mandatory to improve the benefits of the treatment.

The safety of administration of probiotic must be considered; generally the use of probiotic is absolute safe. The use of probiotic strains in gastrointestinal health promotion is considered safe and no side effects were observed (Saavedra et al., 2004). No adverse effects have been reported in either animal models or in humans (Laleman et al., 2014). Some strains used as probiotics for oral health also have been isolated from infections as endocarditis (Cannon et al., 2005), but this isolation was a quite rare phenomenon.

TABLE 37.1
Studies with Caries Risk Factors as Outcome (Children)

Reference Study Design	Subjects (Age)	Strain (Concentration)	Groups	Delivery System/ Treatment Duration	Follow-Up	Outcome(s)	Results
Hasslöf et al. (2013)	174 children (9 years)	*L. paracasei* F19 (10^8 CFU/mL)	A: Probiotics B: Placebo	Cereals once a day/9 months	9 years	MS and Lb in saliva	×
Taipale et al. (2013)	94 children (4 years)	*B. lactis* BB-12 (5×10^9 CFU/lozenge)	A: Probiotics B: Xylitol C: Sorbitol	Lozenges in slow-release pacifier or spoon twice daily/2 years	4 years	MS in plaque and Lb and yeasts in mucosa/teeth (plate culturing)	×
Burton et al. (2013)	100 children (5–10 years)	*S. salivarius* M18 (3.6×10^9 CFU/lozenge)	A: Probiotics B: Placebo	Lozenges twice a day/3 months	7 months	MS, *Candida* Lb and *S. salivarius* in saliva	×
Campus et al. (2014)	191 children (6–8 years)	*L. brevis* CD2 (2×10^9 CFU/g)	A: Probiotics B: Placebo	Lozenges twice a day/6 weeks	8 weeks	MS in saliva and plaque pH (plate culturing)	✓
Juneja et al. (2012)	40 children (12–15 years)	*L. rhamnosus* hct 70 (2.34×10^9 CFU/day)	A: Milk B: Milk + probiotics	Milk twice daily/3 weeks	6 weeks	MS in saliva (chair-side tests)	×
Taipale et al. (2012)	106 infants (1 month)	*B. lactis* BB-12 (5×10^9 CFU/lozenge)	A: Probiotics B: Xylitol C: Sorbitol	Lozenges in slow-release pacifier or spoon twice daily/2 years	2 years	MS in plaque and Lb and yeasts in mucosa/teeth (plate culturing)	✓
Singh et al. (2011) Crossover	40 children (12–14 years)	*B. lactis* Bb-12, *Lactobacillus acidophilus* La-5 (10^6 CFU/g)	A: Ice cream B: Ice cream/probiotics	Ice cream/10 days	10 days	MS and Lb in saliva (chair-side tests)	✓

(*Continued*)

TABLE 37.1 (*Continued*)
Studies with Caries Risk Factors as Outcome (Children)

Reference Study Design	Subjects (Age)	Strain (Concentration)	Groups	Delivery System/ Treatment Duration	Follow-Up	Outcome(s)	Results
Aminabadi et al. (2011)	105 children (6–12 years)	*L. rhamnosus* GG (2×10^8 CFU/g)	A: Chlorhexidine B: Probiotic C: Chlorhexidine/probiotic	Yogurt/3 weeks (chlorhexidine mouthrinse 2 weeks)	5 weeks	MS in saliva (plate culturing)	✓
Jindal et al. (2011)	150 children (7–14 years)	*L. rhamnosus*, *B. longum*, *S. cereviasae*, *B. coagulans* (1.25×10^{12} CFU/g)	A: Placebo B: Probiotics	Powders (dissolved in water and used as mouthrinse)/14 days	2 weeks	MS in saliva (plate culturing)	✓
Lexner et al. (2010)	18 adolescents (13–17 years)	*L. rhamnosus* LB21 (10^7 CFU/mL)	A: Probiotics B: Placebo	Milk once daily/2 weeks	2 weeks	MS and Lb in saliva (plate culturing)	×
Cildir et al. (2009) Crossover study	24 adolescents (12–16 years)	*B. animalis* subsp. *lactis* DN 173010 (2×10^8 CFU/g)	A: Probiotic B: Placebo	Yogurt once daily/2 weeks	2 weeks	MS and Lb in saliva (chair-side tests)	✓
Stecksén-Blicks et al. (2009)	248 children (1–4 years)	*L. rhamnosus* LB21 (10^7 CFU/mL)	A: Probiotics + fluoride B: Placebo	Milk/21 months	21 months	MS and Lb in plaque (plate culturing)	×
Näse et al. (2001)	594 children (1–6 years)	*L. rhamnosus* GG ($5–10 \times 10^5$ CFU/mL)	A: Milk + probiotics B: Milk	Milk five daily/7 months	7 months	MS in plaque and saliva (chair-side tests)	✓

×, no statistically significant differences between probiotics and placebo; ✓, statistically significant differences: efficacy in the probiotic group; ♯, statistically significant differences: efficacy in the placebo group.

TABLE 37.2
Studies with Caries Risk Factors as Outcome (Adults)

Reference Study Design	Subjects (Age)	Strain (Concentration)	Groups	Delivery System/ Treatment Duration	Follow-Up	Outcome(s)	Results
Marttinen et al. (2012) Crossover study	13 adults (mean age 25 years)	*L. rhamnosus* GG or *L. reuteri* (2 × 10^6/lozenges)	A: *L rhamnosus* B: *L. reuteri*	Lozenges twice a day/2 weeks	2 weeks	Plaque acidogenicity, MS and Lb in plaque (plate culturing)	×
Keller and Twetman (2012) Crossover study	18 adults (mean age 26 years)	*L. reuteri* 2 strains (10^8 CFU/lozenges)	A: Probiotics B: Placebo	Lozenges three times a day/2 weeks	2 weeks	MS and Lb in saliva Lactatic acid production	×
Keller et al. (2012)	62 adults (mean age 23 years)	*L. reuteri* 2 strains (10^8 CFU/lozenges)	A: Probiotics B: Placebo	Lozenges twice daily/6 weeks	12 weeks	Salivary MS after full-mouth disinfection (chair-side tests)	×
Petersson et al. (2011)	160 adults (58–84 years)	*L. rhamnosus* LB21 (10^7 CFU/mL)	A: Placebo B: Fluoride probiotic C: Probiotic D: Fluoride	Milk once daily/15 months	15 months	MS and Lb in saliva (chair-side tests) and plaque (plate culturing)	×
Chuang et al. (2011)	80 adults (20–26 years)	*L. paracasei* GMNL-33 (3 × 10^8 CFU/g)	A: Probiotics B: Xylitol	Lozenges 3 times day/2 weeks	4 weeks	MS and Lb in saliva	✓
Caglar et al. (2008b) Crossover study	24 adults (mean age 20 years)	*B. lactis* Bb-12 (10^7 CFU/g)	A: Probiotic B: Placebo	Ice cream once daily/10 days	10 days	MS and Lb in saliva (chair-side tests)	✓
Caglar et al. (2008a)	20 women (20 years)	*L. reuteri* (1.1 × 10^8 CFU/lozenge)	A: Probiotic B: Placebo	Lozenge once daily/10 days	10 days	MS and Lb in saliva (chair-side tests)	✓
Caglar et al. (2007)	80 adults (21–24 years)	*Lactobacilli reuteri* (10^8 CFU/g)	A: Probiotic B: Xylitol C: Probiotic + xylitol D: Placebo	Chewing gums three times daily/3 weeks	3 weeks	MS and Lb in saliva (chair-side tests)	✓

(*Continued*)

TABLE 37.2 (*Continued*)
Studies with Caries Risk Factors as Outcome (Adults)

Reference Study Design	Subjects (Age)	Strain (Concentration)	Groups	Delivery System/ Treatment Duration	Follow-Up	Outcome(s)	Results
Caglar et al. (2006)	120 adults (21–24 years)	*L. reuteri* (10^8 CFU/lozenge/straw)	A: Water/probiotic B: Placebo water/ lozenge C: Lozenge/probiotic	Water or lozenge once daily/3 weeks	4 weeks	MS and Lb in saliva (chair-side tests)	✓
Caglar et al. (2005) Crossover study	26 adults (21–24 years)	*B. lactis* DN-173010 (7×10^7 CFU/g)	A: Probiotic B: Placebo	Yogurt once daily/2 weeks	2 weeks	MS and Lb in saliva (chair-side tests)	✓
Montalto et al. (2004)	35 adults (23–37 years)	*Lactobacillus sporogens, bifidum, bulgaricus, termophilus, acidophilus, casei, rhamnosus* (1.88×10^9 CFU/day)	A: Probiotics capsules B: Liquid probiotics C: Placebo	Liquid and capsule/45 days	45 days	MS and Lb in saliva (chair-side tests)	✓
Ahola et al. (2002)	74 young adults (18–35 years)	*L. rhamnosus* GG (1.9×10^7/g), *L. rhamnosus* LC 705 (1.2×10^7 CFU/g)	A: Probiotics B: Placebo	Cheese five daily/3 weeks	6 weeks	MS, Lb, and yeasts in saliva (chair-side tests) and buffer capacity (Dentobuff strip)	✓

×, no statistically significant differences between probiotics and placebo; ✓, statistically significant differences: efficacy in the probiotic group; ♯, statistically significant differences: efficacy in the placebo group

TABLE 37.3
Studies with Caries Lesion Development as Outcome.

Reference	Subjects	Strain (Concentration)	Groups	Delivery System/ Treatment Duration	Follow-Up	Outcome(s)	Results
Hasslöf et al. (2013)	179 children (9 years)	*L. paracasei* F19 (10^8 CFU/mL)	A: Probiotics B: Placebo	Cereals once a day/9 months	9 years	Caries increment in deciduous and permanent dentition	×
Taipale et al. (2013)	94 children (4 years)	*B. lactis* BB-12 (5×10^9 CFU/lozenge)	A: Probiotics B: Xylitol C: Sorbitol	Lozenges in slow-release pacifier or spoon twice daily/2 years	4 years	Caries increment in deciduous dentition	×
Petersson et al. (2011)	160 adults (58–84 years)	*L. rhamnosus* LB21 (10^7 CFU/mL)	A: Placebo B: Fluoride and probiotic C: Probiotic D: Fluoride	Milk once daily/15 months	15 months	Root Caries Index (RCI) and Electric Resistance Measurements (ERM)	✓
Stecksén-Blicks et al. (2009)	248 children (1–4 years)	*L. rhamnosus* LB21 (10^7 CFU/mL)	A: Probiotics + fluoride B: Placebo	Milk once daily/21 months	21 months	Caries increment (dmfs index)	✓

×, no statistically significant differences between probiotics and placebo; ✓, statistically significant differences: efficacy in the probiotic group; ♯, statistically significant differences: efficacy in the placebo group.

37.4 PROBIOTICS AND CARIES PREVENTION IN CHILDREN AND ADOLESCENTS

The majority of the studies use several caries-related risk factors as outcomes (Table 37.1); only few studies use the clinical outcome like the caries increment as outcome (Table 37.3).

One study was performed to verify the effect of the early administration of probiotics (*Bifidobacterium animalis lactis* BB-12) on the oral colonization of *mutans* streptococci in infants (Taipale et al., 2012). Subjects received probiotic bacteria, xylitol, or sorbitol (polyol 100–300 mg) from the age of 1–2 months to the age of 2 years, twice a day. The *mutans* streptococci concentration in plaque of the mothers at the start of the study was high and similar in all subjects. At the end of the probiotic administration, children showed a rather low *mutans* streptococci colonization percentage, with a statistically significant difference among groups. Two years later, no differences were observed in *mutans* streptococci level and the occurrence of caries lesions in primary dentition among the three groups (Taipale et al., 2013).

The effect of milk containing *L. rhamnosus* on *mutans* streptococci counts was evaluated in two short- and two long-term studies. In the short-term studies (Juneja and Kakade, 2012; Lexner et al., 2010), the effect of milk containing *L. rhamnosus* (hct 70 or LB21) for few weeks was registered in small groups of adolescents. The difference in posttreatment regarding *mutans* streptococci counts between test and control group was not statistically significant, while the difference in follow-up was highly significant (Juneja and Kakade, 2012). No statistically significant differences in *mutans* streptococci were recorded in subjects who received milk with probiotic compared to subjects using milk without probiotics (Lexner et al., 2010). In two long-term studies (Näse et al., 2001; Stecksén-Blicks et al., 2009), *L. rhamnosus* was administered for several months (7 and 21 months). Statistically significant reductions in *mutans* streptococci counts were recorded with *L. rhamnosus* GG, ATCC use (Näse et al., 2001), while no statistically significant changes were observed in subjects receiving *L. rhamnosus* LB21 (Stecksén-Blicks et al., 2009).

A significant decrease in *mutans* streptococci counts immediately after the administration of yogurt containing *L. rhamnosus* GG for 3 weeks was evaluated (Aminabadi et al., 2011), but recolonization was described during the five consecutive weeks. Pretreatment with chlorhexidine produced a statistically significant reduction in salivary *mutans* streptococci counts that enhances during the five consecutive weeks. In a double-blind, crossover study on healthy adolescents undergoing orthodontic treatment, a statistically significant reduction of *mutans* streptococci was recorded after the daily consumption of yogurt containing *B. animalis lactis* DN-173010 (Cildir et al., 2009).

The effect of lozenges containing *L. brevis* CD2 administered for 6 weeks was evaluated in high-caries-risk children (Campus et al., 2014). A statistically significant reduction of the cariogenic microorganism was recorded. In another randomized double-blind, placebo-controlled study on caries-active children, lozenges containing *Streptococcus salivarius* strain M18 were administered for 3 months. Changes in plaque scores and salivary levels of *S. salivarius*, *S. mutans*, lactobacilli, β-hemolytic streptococci, and *Candida* species were evaluated (Burton et al., 2013). At treatment end, the plaque scores were significantly lower in children from the probiotics group, but no differences between the probiotic and placebo groups in counts of cariogenic microorganisms were recorded, except for the *S. salivarius* M18 that appeared to colonize children from the probiotic group.

One study used two powders as probiotic vehicle in children, containing one *L. rhamnosus*, *Bifidobacterium longum*, and *Saccharomyces cereviasae* and the second one *Bacillus coagulans* and compared them to a placebo powder (Jindal et al., 2011). Data analysis showed a statistically significant reduction in *mutans* streptococci counts in both probiotics groups.

The long-term effect of *L. paracasei* F19 (LF19), administered through cereals from 4 to 13 months of age, on mutans streptococci and lactobacilli in a group of children was recently investigated (Hasslöf et al., 2013). At the follow-up evaluation, cariogenic bacteria levels differed significantly between the probiotic and placebo groups.

Some of the studies reported earlier (Cildir et al., 2009; Lexner et al., 2010; Singh et al., 2011; Stecksén-Blicks et al., 2009; Taipale et al., 2012) investigated the effect of the probiotics strain on *Lactobacilli* level also. No study demonstrated a statistically significant change. Moreover, the effect of probiotic on oral yeasts was not demonstrated (Taipale et al., 2012). Otherwise, the effect on plaque acidogenicity resulted significantly in subjects that have used probiotic through lozenges (Campus et al., 2014). Only three studies evaluated the probiotic effect on caries lesion development (Hasslöf et al., 2013; Stecksén-Blicks et al., 2009; Taipale et al., 2013). A statistically significant difference in caries increment was recorded in subjects who received probiotic just in one of the studies (Stecksén-Blicks et al., 2009).

37.5 PROBIOTICS AND CARIES PREVENTION IN ADULTS

All but one study (Petersson et al., 2011) reported results based on caries risk factors (Tables 37.2 and 37.3). Several studies performed by the same research group and investigating the effect of several probiotic strains (*Bifidobacterium lactis* Bb-12, *L. reuteri* ATCC 55730 and ATCC PTA 5289, *Bifidobacterium* DN-173010) on salivary *mutans* streptococci concentration demonstrated a significant decrease of the cariogenic microorganism (Caglar et al., 2005, 2006, 2007, 2008a,b). Even if no statistically significant differences in *mutans* streptococci counts were found immediately after consumption of cheese containing *L. rhamnosus* GG and *L. rhamnosus* LC 705, the reduction became significant 3 weeks after the interruption of the administration (Ahola et al., 2002).

Conversely, some short- (2 weeks administration) and one long-term studies (15 months administration) did not reveal any effect of probiotics on *mutans* streptococci counts using *L. rhamnosus* or *L. reuteri* (Chuang et al., 2011; Keller et al., 2012; Marttinen et al., 2012; Petersson et al., 2011). Same results were obtained utilizing several strains of *Lactobacillus* spp. in liquid and capsules in adults (Montalto et al., 2004). The effect of the probiotics strain on lactobacilli level in saliva and/or plaque was also studied in nine investigations among those reported earlier, but only one study demonstrated a statistically significant change of these microorganisms (Ahola et al., 2002).

Finally, the effect of probiotics on plaque acidogenicity and buffer capacity was also evaluated, but no significant changes of the two parameters were found (Ahola et al., 2002; Chuang et al., 2011; Keller and Twetman, 2012; Marttinen et al., 2012).

37.6 CONCLUSIONS

Today probiotics are not considered a drug, and they are administered without regulation and licensing demands as pharmaceutical drugs do. In addition, a high number of different products are available on the market, but the scientific evidence of their benefits on health is still scarce. In the literature are present studies with laboratory assays, animal studies, and human clinical studies. The clinical trials (see Cagetti et al., 2013) gave contrasting but encouraging results, but the evidence is still not high. Most clinical trials available in literature had a small sample size and reported caries risk factors as intermediate or surrogate endpoints, which limited the conclusions about the real efficacy of probiotics administration in caries lesion prevention. The majority of the clinical studies used the salivary levels of *S. mutans* as a surrogate endpoint for caries development, but this strain is not the only one involved in the caries process.

A continuous regular almost daily intake is probably required to obtain benefits in health requiring a constant compliance by the patients. However, all products considered effective in caries prevention (i.e. fluoride and chlorhexidine) require a high frequency of use, so a possible way of probiotics administration could be to insert them in daily-used preventive products like toothpaste.

Various mechanisms of action for probiotic efficacy are reported in the literature, some of which are not fully understood. Several local and systemic effects are described, modifying oral microflora; however, probiotic bacteria seem to be not able to colonize oral cavity permanently, and this aspect reduces their benefits on time.

REFERENCES

Ahola, A.J., Yli-Knuuttila, H., Suomalainen, T. et al. 2002. Short-term consumption of probiotic-containing cheese and its effect on dental caries risk factors. *Arch. Oral Biol.* 47:799–804.

Aminabadi, N.A., Erfanparast, L., Ebrahimi, A., Oskouei, S.G. 2011. Effect of chlorhexidine pretreatment on the stability of salivary lactobacilli probiotic in six- to twelve-year-old children a randomized controlled trial. *Caries Res.* 45:148–154.

Burton, J.P., Drummond, B.K., Chilcott, C.N. et al. 2013. Influence of the probiotic *Streptococcus salivarius* strain M18 on indices of dental health in children: A randomized double-blind, placebo-controlled trial. *J. Med. Microbiol.* 62:875–884.

Cagetti, M.G., Mastroberardino, S., Milia, E., Cocco, F., Lingström, P., Campus, G. 2013. The use of probiotic strains in caries prevention: A systematic review. *Nutrients* 5:2530–2550.

Caglar, E., Cildir, S.K., Ergeneli, S., Sandalli, N., Twetman, S. 2006. Salivary mutans streptococci and lactobacilli levels after ingestion of the probiotic bacterium *Lactobacillus reuteri* ATCC 55730 by straws or tablets. *Acta Odontol. Scand.* 64:314–318.

Caglar, E., Kavaloglu, S.C., Kuscu, O.O., Sandalli, N., Holgerson, P.L., Twetman, S. 2007. Effect of chewing gums containing xylitol or probiotic bacteria on salivary mutans streptococci and lactobacilli. *Clin. Oral. Invest.* 11:425–429.

Caglar, E., Kuscu, O.O., Cildir, S.K., Kuvvetli, S.S., Sandalli, N. 2008a. A probiotic lozenge administered medical device and its effect on salivary mutans streptococci and lactobacilli. *Int. J. Paediatr. Dent.* 18:35–39.

Caglar, E., Kuscu, O.O., Selvi-Kuvvetli, S., Kavaloglu-Cildir, S., Sandalli, N., Twetman, S. 2008b. Short-term effect of ice-cream containing *Bifidobacterium lactis* Bb-12 on the number of salivary mutans streptococci and lactobacilli. *Acta Odontol. Scand.* 66:154–158.

Caglar, E., Sandalli, N., Twetman, S., Kavaloglu, S., Ergeneli, S., Selvi, S. 2005. Effect of yogurt with *Bifidobacterium* DN-173 010 on salivary mutans streptococci and lactobacilli in young adults. *Acta Odontol. Scand.* 63:317–320.

Campus, G., Cocco, F., Carta, G. et al. 2014. Effect of a daily dose of *Lactobacillus brevis* CD2 lozenges in high caries risk schoolchildren. *Clin. Oral. Invest.* 18:555–561.

Campus, G., Solinas, G., Cagetti, M.G. et al. 2007. National pathfinder survey of 12-year-old children's oral health in Italy. *Caries Res.* 41:512–517.

Campus, G., Solinas, G., Strohmenger, L. et al. 2009. Collaborating Study Group. National pathfinder survey on children's oral health in Italy: Pattern and severity of caries disease in 4-year-olds. *Caries Res.* 43:155–162.

Cannon, J.P., Lee, T.A., Bolanos, J.T., Danziger, L.H. 2005. Pathogenic relevance of *Lactobacillus*: A retrospective review of over 200 cases. *Eur. J. Clin. Microbiol. Infect. Dis.* 24:31–40.

Chhour, K.L., Nadkarni, M.A., Byun, R., Martin, E., Jacques, N.A., Hunter, N. 2005. Molecular analysis of microbial diversity in advanced caries. *J. Clin. Microbiol.* 43:843–849.

Chuang, L.C., Huang, C.S., Ou-Yang, L.W., Lin, S.Y. 2011. Probiotic *Lactobacillus paracasei* effect on cariogenic bacterial flora. *Clin. Oral. Invest.* 15:471–476.

Cildir, S.K., Germec, D., Sandalli, N. et al. 2009. Reduction of salivary mutans streptococci in orthodontic patients during daily consumption of yoghurt containing probiotic bacteria. *Eur. J. Orthodont.* 31:407–411.

Edelstein, B. 2006. The dental caries pandemic and disparities problem. *BMC Oral Health* 15(Suppl. 1):S2. http://www.biomedcentral.com/1472-6831/6/S1/S2. Accessed 24 September 2014.

Gupta, P., Gupta, N., Pawar, A.P., Birajdar, S.S., Natt, A.S., Singh, H.P. 2013. Role of sugar and sugar substitutes in dental caries: A review. *ISRN Dent.* 29:519421. http://www.hindawi.com/journals/isrn/2013/519421/.

Hasslöf, P., Hedberg, M., Twetman, S., Stecksen-Blicks, C. 2010. Growth inhibition of oral mutans streptococci and candida by commercial probiotic lactobacilli—An in vitro study. *BMC Oral Health* 10:18.

Hasslöf, P., West, C.E., Videhult, F.K., Brandelius, C., Stecksén-Blicks, C. 2013. Early intervention with probiotic *Lactobacillus paracasei* F19 has no long-term effect on caries experience. *Caries Res.* 47:559–565.

Haukioja, A., Loimaranta, V., Tenovuo, J. 2008a. Probiotic bacteria affect the composition of salivary pellicle and streptococcal adhesion in vitro. *Oral Microbiol. Immunol.* 23:336–343.

Haukioja, A., Söderling, E., Tenovuo, J. 2008b. Acid production from sugars and sugar alcohols by probiotic lactobacilli and bifidobacteria in vitro. *Caries Res.* 42:449–453.

He, X.S. and Shi, W.Y. 2009. Oral microbiology: past, present and future. *Int. J. Oral Sci.*1:46–58.

Hedberg, M., Hasslöf, P., Sjöström, I., Twetman, S., Stecksén-Blicks, C. 2008. Sugar fermentation in probiotic bacteria—An in vitro study. *Oral Microbiol. Immunol.* 23:482–485.

Jalasvuori, H., Haukioja, A., Tenovuo, J. 2012. Probiotic *Lactobacillus reuteri* strains ATCC PTA 5289 and ATCC 55730 differ in their cariogenic properties in vitro. *Arch. Oral Biol.* 57:1633–1638.

Jindal, G., Pandey, R.K., Agarwal, J., Singh, M. 2011. A comparative evaluation of probiotics on salivary mutans streptococci counts in Indian children. *Eur. Arch. Paediatr. Dent.* 12:211–215.

Juneja, A., Kakade, A. 2012. Evaluating the effect of probiotic containing milk on salivary mutans streptococci levels. *J. Clin. Pediatr. Dent.* 37:9–14.

Keller, M.K., Hasslöf, P., Dahlén, G., Stecksén-Blicks, C., Twetman, S. 2012. Probiotic supplements (*Lactobacillus reuteri* DSM 17938 and ATCC PTA 5289) do not affect regrowth of mutans streptococci after full-mouth disinfection with chlorhexidine: A randomized controlled multicenter trial. *Caries Res.* 46:140–146.

Keller, M.K., Twetman, S. 2012. Acid production in dental plaque after exposure to probiotic bacteria. *BMC Oral Health* 24(12):44. http://www.biomedcentral.com/1472-6831/12/44. Accessed 23 September 2014.

Kolenbrander, P.E., Palmer, R.J. Jr., Rickard, A.H., Jakubovics, N.S., Chalmers, N.I., Diaz, P.I. 2006. Bacterial interactions and successions during plaque development. *Periodontology* 42:47–79.

Kreth, J., Merritt, J., Shi, W., Qi, F. 2005. Competition and coexistence between *Streptococcus mutans* and *Streptococcus sanguinis* in the dental biofilm. *J. Bacteriol.* 187:7193–7203.

Laleman, I., Detailleur, V., Slot, D.E., Slomka, V., Quirynen, M., Teughels, W. 2014. Probiotics reduce mutans streptococci counts in humans: A systematic review and meta-analysis. *Clin. Oral Invest.* 18:1539–1552.

Lexner, M.O., Blomqvist, S., Dahlén, G., Twetman, S. 2010. Microbiological profiles in saliva and supragingival plaque from caries-active adolescents before and after a short-term daily intake of milk supplemented with probiotic bacteria—A pilot study. *Oral Health Prev. Dent.* 8:383–388.

Lingström, P., van Ruyven, F.O., van Houte, J., Kent, R. 2000. The pH of dental plaque in its relation to early enamel caries and dental plaque flora in humans. *J. Dent. Res.* 79:770–777.

Linsalata, M., Russo, F., Berloco, P. et al. 2004. The influence of *Lactobacillus brevis* on ornithine decarboxylase activity and polyamine profiles in *Helicobacter pylori*-infected gastric mucosa. *Helicobacter* 9:165–172.

Marja-Leena, M., Paivi, R., Sirkka, J., Ansa, O., Matti, S. 2008. Childhood caries is still in force: A 15-year follow-up. *Acta Odontol. Scand.* 66:189–192.

Marsh, P.D. 2005. Dental plaque biological significance of a biofilm and community life style. *J. Clin. Periodontol.* 32:7–15.

Matsumoto, M., Tsuji, M,, Sasaki, H. et al. 2005. Cariogenicity of the probiotic bacterium Lactobacillus salivarius in rats. *Caries Res.* 39:479–483.

Marttinen, A., Haukioja, A., Karjalainen, S. et al. 2012. Short-term consumption of probiotic lactobacilli has no effect on acid production of supragingival plaque. *Clin. Oral Invest.* 16:797–803.

Milgrom, P., Söderling, E.M., Nelson, S., Chi, D.L., Nakai, Y. 2012. Clinical evidence for polyol efficacy. *Adv. Dent. Res.* 24:112–116.

Montalto, M., Vastola, M., Marigo, L. et al. 2004. Probiotic treatment increases salivary counts of lactobacilli: A double-blind, randomized, controlled study. *Digestion* 69:53–56.

Näse, L., Hatakka, K., Savilahti, E. et al. 2001. Effect of long-term consumption of a probiotic bacterium, *Lactobacillus rhamnosus* GG, in milk on dental caries and caries risk in children. *Caries Res.* 35:412–420.

Nasidze, I., Li, J., Quinque, D., Tang, K., Stoneking, M., 2009. Global diversity in the human salivary microbiome. *Genome Res.* 19:636–643.

Nikawa, H, Makihira, S., Fukushima, H. et al. 2004. *Lactobacillus reuteri* in bovine milk fermented decreases the oral carriage of mutans streptococci. *Int. J. Food Microbiol.* 95:219–223.

Petersen, P.E., Lennon, M.A. 2004. Effective use of fluorides for the prevention of dental caries in the 21st century: The WHO approach. *Community Dent. Oral Epidemiol.* 32:319–321.

Petersson, L.G., Magnusson, K., Hakestam, U., Baigi, A., Twetman, S. 2011. Reversal of primary root caries lesions after daily intake of milk supplemented with fluoride and probiotic lactobacilli in older adults. *Acta Odontol. Scand.* 69:321–327.

Rao, Y., Lingamneni, B., Reddy, D. 2012. Probiotics in oral health—A review. *J. N.J. Dent. Assoc.* 83:28–32.

Ravn, I., Dige, I., Meyer, R.L., Nyvad, B. 2012. Colonization of the oral cavity by probiotic bacteria. *Caries Res.* 46:107–112.

Saavedra, J.M., Abi-Hanna, A., Moore, N., Yolken, R.H. 2004. Long-term consumption of infant formulas containing live probiotic bacteria: Tolerance and safety. *Am. J. Clin. Nutr.* 79:261–267.

Selwitz, R.H., Ismail, A.I., Pitts, N.B. 2007. Dental caries. *Lancet* 369:51–59.

Singh, R.P., Damle, S.G., Chawla, A. 2011. Salivary mutans streptococci and lactobacilli modulations in young children on consumption of probiotic ice-cream containing *Bifidobacterium lactis* Bb12 and *Lactobacillus acidophilus* La5. *Acta Odontol. Scand.* 69:389–394.

Stecksén-Blicks, C., Sjöström, I., Twetman, S. 2009. Effect of long-term consumption of milk supplemented with probiotic lactobacilli and fluoride on dental caries and general health in preschool children: A cluster-randomized study. *Caries Res.* 43:374–381.

Struzycka, I. 2014. The oral microbiome in dental caries. *Pol. J. Microbiol.* 63:127–135.

Taipale, T., Pienihäkkinen, K., Alanen, P., Jokela, J., Söderling, E., 2013. Administration of *Bifidobacterium animalis* subsp. *lactis* BB-12 in early childhood: A post-trial effect on caries occurrence at four years of age. *Caries Res.* 47:364–372.

Taipale, T., Pienihäkkinen, K., Salminen, S., Jokela, J., Söderling, E. 2012. *Bifidobacterium animalis* subsp. *lactis* BB-12 administration in early childhood: A randomized clinical trial of effects on oral colonization by mutans streptococci and the probiotic. *Caries Res.* 46:69–77.

Talarico, T.L., Axelsson, L.T., Novotny, J., Fiuzat, M., Dobrogosz, W.J. 1990. Utilization of glycerol as a hydrogen acceptor by *Lactobacillus reuteri*: Purification of 1,3-propanediol: NAD oxidoreductase. *Appl. Environ. Microbiol.* 56:943–948.

Tanzer, J.M., Livingston, J., Thompson, A.M. 2001. The micro- biology of primary dental caries in humans. *J. Dent. Educ.* 65:128–137.

Tanzer, J.M., Thompson, A., Lang, C. et al. 2010. Caries inhibition by and safety of *Lactobacillus paracasei* DSMZ16671. *J. Dent. Res.* 89:921–926.

Teanpaisan, R., Piwat, S., Dahlén, G. 2011. Inhibitory effect of oral Lactobacillus against oral pathogens. *Lett. Appl. Microbiol.* 53:452–459.

Tong, Z., Zhou, L., Li, J., Kuang, R., Lin, Y., Ni, L. 2012. An in vitro investigation of *Lactococcus lactis* antagonizing cariogenic bacterium *Streptococcus mutans*. *Arch. Oral Biol.* 57:376–382.

Twetman, S. 2012. Are we ready for caries prevention through bacteriotherapy? *Braz. Oral Res.* 26:64–70.

Twetman, S., Keller, M.K. 2012. Probiotics for caries prevention and control. *Adv. Dent. Res.* 24:98–102.

Van Nieuw Amerongen, A., Wolscher, J.G., Veerman, E.C. 2004. Salivary proteins: Protective and diagnostic value in cariology. *Caries Res.* 38:247–253.

Zero, D.T. 2006. Dentifrices, mouthwashes and remineralization/caries arrestment strategies. *BMC Oral Health* 6, S9. http://www.biomedcentral.com/1472-6831/6/S1/S9. Accessed 26 September 2014.

38 Antimicrobial Properties of Wild Oregano Extracts
A Compilation and Review of Current Research

Cassim Igram

CONTENTS

38.1 INTRODUCTION

In nature, plants have a wide range of protective powers that guard them from being harmed and/or destroyed. One such protective power is the aromatic or essential oils. Without aromatic oils, plants would be readily attacked and destroyed by pests, bacteria, viruses, fungi, and so on. In fact, without such oils or other protective agents, there would be no healthy or living plants left on this planet. That is because germs would routinely attack any plants devoid of protective mechanisms or that are depleted in this regard, disabling and ultimately destroying them.

The essential oils are a kind of "plant blood" that circulate within the plants like human blood within the veins and arteries. They are more than merely blood-like, though. They are the plants' circulating antiseptic and anti-inflammatory compounds. Antiseptics are antimicrobial compounds that kill germs. This includes those pathogens that cause diseases, including those that cause plant diseases.

These oils are aromatic complexes. Because they are aromatic, they can be readily harvested. This harvesting is largely done through steam distillation, where the compounds are driven off in an oil phase, then condensed through the appropriate methodology into distilled oils.

It has been long known that essential oils have therapeutic properties. Yet, in medical circles what has received little attention is the fact that a number of such oils are decided germicides. A germicide is a substance that has a broad spectrum of activity against a wide range of germs: bacterial, viral, fungal, and even parasitic. If nontoxic, any such substance would have immense utility in the treatment of disease. This is particularly important considering the toxicity of antibiotics as well as the immense increase in the incidence of infectious disease by antibiotic-resistant germs.

The most germicidal of all aromatic oils are those derived from spices. This makes sense since for centuries spices have been used as food. Logs from ship journals of eighteenth century America-bound ships demonstrate the link. On the long journeys from Europe, these logs note how perishable food was preserved from decay through the addition of cinnamon and cloves, both of which are relatively potent antiseptics.

The distilled oils are significantly more germicidal than the whole spices. Upon distillation, 100 lb of spice may yield a mere pound of essential oil. These spice oils are acrid, containing a wide range of exceedingly aromatic compounds and are also surely volatile. When taken orally, they are exceptionally pungent and thus combining them with carrier oils would be an essential methodology. Through emulsification in such carrier oils like extra virgin olive oil, they are rendered entirely safe for human consumption.

Premier of such distilled, germicidal spice oils is oil of wild oregano. This has been demonstrated by a number of scientific studies, including work done at America's most prominent universities such as Cornell University and Georgetown University. At Cornell University in a compendium evaluation of all aromatic spices, oregano was among the most potent in bactericidal activity. Other spices that possessed significant actions against the tested pathogens include onion and garlic as well as allspice. Each of these spices proved to be bactericidal against all pathogens tested. The distilled oils, of course, are far more bactericidal than the mere spices. At Georgetown University in a comparative evaluation, oils of wild oregano, wild sage, cumin, and cinnamon were found to be the most potent of all essential oils tested in bacteria-killing actions.

What makes essential oils so novel is the fact that certain complexes are capable of killing the full range of germs that are primary initiators of infectious diseases. In contrast to drugs, the essential spice oils do not discriminate. Rather, they kill the entire litany of pathogenic bacteria that are the primary causes of disease.

While essential oil chemistry and therapeutics have been a popular study for decades, what has been neglected is the investigation of spice oils as a field of study. Consider these oils: spices are edible. They are consumed by billions of people daily. Therefore, their oils are edible and would have a high profile of safety, higher than other plant oils. One of the most heavily researched spice oils in modern times is oil of wild oregano. Oregano is one of the most common food additives known. A cursory review in any supermarket will demonstrate that as a spice/herb oregano is found in hundreds of foods. Even the distilled oil is used in food, for instance, in some brands of pizza and spaghetti sauce.

So, is oregano oil a food? or, a medicine? Actually, it is both. The medicinal properties are based upon the wide spectrum of capacities of this oil. This is largely as a result of its germ-killing powers but also due to the fact that it is a potent antioxidant, anti-inflammatory agent, and antipain complex. It is also antitussive capable of halting or suppressing cough, while absorbing mucolytic, meaning capable of splitting apart and dissolving thick mucus.

This versatility may well be a surprise to people to the point of skepticism. How could mere oregano be that diverse as well as potent? Moreover, how could it actually be used medicinally, acting as if it is a drug? So, let us review the scientific studies to determine precisely what has been discovered.

Much of the most preeminent research has been done by our group at Washington DC's Georgetown University. In that pioneering work, it was confirmed that oregano oil, the wild-type, mountain-grown, is a medicinal agent on par with some of the most potent antimicrobial drugs known. In some cases, it acted superior to such drugs. The type of wild oregano oil used in this study was a blend of various high-mountain, wild species of extracted oils known as Oreganol P73.

38.2 ORIGANUM OIL'S ACTION AGAINST *CANDIDA ALBICANS*

In these pioneering studies, lab mice were infected with alternatively pathogenic *Candida albicans* and penicillin-resistant bacteria. The wild oregano oil in an organic extra virgin olive oil emulsion was compared in its actions to antifungal drugs, that is, mycostatin (Nystatin) and amphotericin B, and vancomycin, alternatively. The mice were infected by oral gavage and then treated with either the drugs or oregano oil, using extra virgin olive oil as the control. In both cases, the oregano oil complex worked equally well as the drugs in saving the mices' lives but had an additive benefit. It was less toxic to the mices' internal organs than the drugs. In the antifungal trial, 36 of 36 amphotericin-B mice survived, while 35 of 36 wild oregano oil–treated mice prevailed. In contrast, all of the mice treated with olive oil only ultimately died.[1]

It would seem that, though not statistically significant, the drugs were slightly better. However, upon further observation the amphotericin-B mice developed toxicity as manifested by matted and unhealthy coats of hair, while the animals were also sluggish. No such toxicity was observed in the oregano oil–treated mice. This caused the investigators to conclude that, in fact, the wild oregano oil is a superior antimicrobial agent for the treatment of such infections versus potent antibiotic drugs.[1]

The Georgetown work was truly the benchmark experimental model, delving into arenas never before pursued. Prior to the study, one of us (myself) said the oregano oil *will* work. It *will* kill the fungi and bacteria within animal tissue and could perform well equally with the drugs. That is, its role within the plant is to prevent the overgrowth and/or invasion of fungi and bacteria, as well as viruses, within the roots, leaves, flowers, and stems. The essential oil, trapped among other oils, courses within the plant structure, its fibrous veins and arteries, if you will, serving precisely the purpose of antisepsis.

38.3 ESSENTIAL OILS AS A COMPLEX

Essential oils are aromatic complexes found within the leaves, stems, flowers, and roots of medicinal plants. These complexes consist of a variety of chemicals, including esters, long- and short-chain alcohols, and phenolic compounds. Such compounds have known medicinal properties, including anti-inflammatory, antipain, antipyretic, antitussive, antifungal, antiseptic, antispasmodic, and antiparasitic actions.

The interest here is largely in the antibacterial, antiviral, antifungal properties of such oils. These oils exist in the plants largely for that purpose, that is to protect them from being attacked by pathogens: fungi, yeasts, bacteria, viruses, and more. In some respect, the essential oils are the plant's blood, flowing through every vein-like structure to ensure protection against plant pathogens.

When extracted, these essential oils offer such protective properties to humans as deliberate antimicrobial agents. It is, though, more than mere protection. Essential oils are therapeutic in the treatment of many diseases, including heart disease, cancer, diabetes, arthritis, lupus, neurological disorders, and fibromyalgia.

Regarding wild oregano, there is a significant history of ancient use. According to Anadolu University's Chen Basher, the first recorded history of the use of an aromatic plant medicinally dates some 50,000 years ago in Iraq. There, a grave was discovered and within it was an apparent woman of nobility who had a pouch of an aromatic herb around her neck. This actually proved to be wild oregano.

Consider, too, the ancient Greeks. They called this plant *oroganos*, meaning the "delight" or "pleasure" of the mountains. Thus, they realized its essential nature for human health. This authority maintained by wild oregano is proven by the discovery of an ancient Grecian shipwreck off the coast of Chios in the Aegean Sea. Incredibly, the cargo of the shipwreck was mainly olive oil flavored with wild oregano. Moreover, rather than a mere food additive it was used medicinally as a therapeutic rub.

It was the aromatic herb that the Greeks had packed into those amphora. Today, investigators are discovering the fact that both whole, crude herb, and distilled oil are medicinal. According to a study published in *Herba Polinica*, wild oregano has a unique capacity to bolster immune function. Of some 33 herbs tested, only oregano caused a significant increase in white blood cell, as determined by an increase in interferon production.[2]

In the early literature, 1500s through 1700s, there was mention of the greatness of wild oregano, as well as similar antiseptic spices, such as wild sage, cumin, cinnamon, and wild bay leaf. Then, British and Irish herbalists gave significant mention of these spices, describing them as indispensable medicines. Here, the spices and their extracts were held as cures for a wide range of disorders, including diarrhea, stomach conditions, earaches, colds, flu, rhinitis, and infected wounds. In ancient Rome, cinnamon, a powerful antiseptic and preservative, was purchased for an equal weight of gold. Moreover, early British herbalists, including Culpeper, Salmon, and Gerard, gave much praise to wild oregano for its effectiveness against infectious diseases, particularly head colds, lung infections, digestive disorders, and earaches.[3,4,6]

Culpeper's seventh-century writings alone demonstrate the real power of this spice medicine. Despite the huge number of herbs mentioned, he states that wild oregano *reigns supreme in a number of illnesses*. The illnesses for which oregano is the top natural medicine, Culpeper says, include food poisoning (sour stomach), head congestion/colds, cough (and, therefore lung infections) intestinal disorders, stomachache, tuberculosis, hepatitis, and ear disorders.[3] Salmon, who wrote in the 1500s, agreed, essentially saying that there is for numerous illnesses no natural medicine superior to wild oregano and that the oil in particular is a categorical cure for head and neck disorders, including colds and earaches.[6]

In the early 1900s in the United States, there were a number of books published on natural medicines. In these books, a variety of therapies were described. Virtually all the prescribed therapies were natural, although, admittedly, some of the natural substances, such as mercurial and arsenical compounds, are themselves poisonous. Yet, what is most revealing is the titles that were used to describe these treatments. In the *Library of Health*, published in the 1920s, there is an entire section entitled "Curative Medicine." Curiously, this was written before the establishment of drug monopolies by the petrochemical cartel. The naturalistic cures that are described included essential oils, boric acid, hot baths, roots, and herbs.

While it had been known since antiquity that wild oregano and its distilled oil were lifesaving, it has been only more recently that modern civilization has realized this. Research on its medicinal powers began in the early twentieth century. In 1910, it was W. H. Martindale who determined the ultimate power of this spice oil extract. After extensive research, he stated, categorically, that "the essential oil of oregano is the most powerful plant-derived antiseptic known." It was Martindale who first showed that oregano oil is *26 times more potent than synthetic phenol*, then known as carbolic acid. No drug or even any category of drugs can match such antiseptic power.[5]

In 1918, Cavell of the Pasteur Institute studied a number of essential oils regarding their abilities to sterilize septic water. She inoculated water from septic tanks with beef broth, dramatically increasing microbial growth. Then various essential oils were added. Oregano oil, she determined, was so powerful that in a mere 1/10th of a percent concentration, that is 1/1000, sterilized septic water. Once again, there is no medication known that can match such immense germicidal power, and surely none that can do so without significant side effects.

Despite such dramatic results in the initial decades of the twentieth century, oregano oil was rarely used. This may be due in part to the fact that interest in essential oils as germicides was dramatically displaced as a result of the discovery of antibiotics. Ultimately the research was revived. In 1977, Belaniche, while investigating a number of natural compounds, gave oregano oil the highest marks. The researcher regarding its germ-killing powers in comparison to all antiseptic oils said, "oregano is the best of the best." Furthermore, regarding oregano oil and similar spice oils according to the world-renown French physician Jean Valnet, M.D., working in the 1970s and 1980s, spice-based essential oils "proved to be *many times more effective at killing pathogenic microorganisms than antibiotics*." Clearly, "many times more" is a significant statement, proven by the extensive clinical work of this physician. Valnet routinely prescribed spice oils and found them to be effective in a wide range of conditions, including lung disease, cardiovascular disease, arthritis, kidney disease, infectious diseases of the respiratory tract, as well as skin and intestinal disorders.[13]

38.4 ANTIVIRAL ACTIVITY OF ORIGANUM OIL AGAINST THE MOST DEADLY VIRUSES OF THE TWENTY-FIRST CENTURY

In addition to its potent actions against bacteria and yeasts, wild oregano has significant potency against viruses. In most instances, it destroys these pathogens categorically. This is particularly true of the steam-distilled oil. This oil possesses this destructive effect whether used topically or internally. Viruses known to be killed by the oil of wild oregano include herpes viruses, hepatitis viruses, the cold virus, the flu virus, Newcastle virus, and respiratory syncytial virus. According to English investigators, the oil is even capable of inhibiting the growth of HIV/AIDS viruses.

Studies proved that the antiviral powers of the wild oil of oregano are exceptional, far exceeding anything in the drug armamentarium. In a study using the original wild Mediterranean brand (Oreganol P73) in an extra virgin olive oil base done by Microbiotest, the oil was found to decimate both cold and flu viruses. This was an *in vitro* study, meaning it was done inside the cells. In this instance, the viruses were used to infect chicken embryo cells, the latter being incubated at the appropriate temperatures to speed viral growth.

Initially, the human corona virus, a common cause of colds, was evaluated. Per milliliter of material some 5.5 million viruses were detected. After treatment with a small amount, that is .01% of the oil, only a mere 4000 or so viruses were detected. This is a 99.9% kill. What is more, this occurred in a mere 20 min. A combination of oils of wild oregano and sage, along with cumin and cinnamon oil, desiccated into a powder achieved an even more dramatic effect. Here, in 20 min a 100% kill was achieved. This desiccated spice extract is available in capsule form as a combination of the dried essential oils of wild oregano and sage plus cumin and cinnamon. It is also available as an oil complex emulsified in extra virgin olive oil.[7]

The same was achieved with the flu virus, although this agent proved more resistant. With oil of wild oregano treatment, it took a 1% solution to achieve in 20 min a 99.7% kill. And an even more vigorous kill was achieved by the multiple spice combination. A variant of bird flu was also tested. The bird flu viruses are extremely powerful as well as resistant. Here, for a 99.7% kill a 25% solution of the oil of wild oregano was required.[7]

This antiviral capacity was also confirmed by work done in British Columbia. Here, the antiinfluenza virus activity of a number of oil of oregano preparations was investigated. "All…oregano oils showed significant antiviral activity…" The investigators determined that the extra virgin olive oil, as a carrier, also exhibited antiviral powers.[14]

As an anti-influenza agent, a number of other investigators have demonstrated similar actions.[9] Additionally, Gilling and cohorts have shown that the oil completely inactivates the murine norovirus, acting with its destructive actions "directly on the viral capsid and subsequently on the RNA." In this regard, it essentially dissolves both the capsid and RNA.[8]

38.5 PROVEN ANTIFUNGAL ACTIVITIES OF ORIGANUM OIL

Whether in animals or humans it is in the war against fungal disorders where the wild oregano is exceptional. This is related to the nature of fungal infections. These infections are chronic. They are also deep-seated. In other words, they are well entrenched in the body. Fungi can penetrate virtually any tissue. Here, they cause tissue invasion and thus great inflammation. This ultimately leads to disease. There is need for a substance, which can be consumed regularly and in relatively large quantities to eradicate such infections. In this regard, wild oregano is supreme.

Preliminary studies demonstrate that spice oils obliterate fungi, even from the internal organs and surely from the bloodstream. This is based largely on studies in test tubes and Petri dishes. Yet, as mentioned previously animal studies have also confirmed this. So have a multitude of human cases.

It is not easy to eradicate fungi from the body. There are drugs that do so; however, each of these has a significant degree of toxicity. Yet, the naturally occurring wild spice oil, that is oil of wild oregano, has this capacity. It destroys the fungi directly, plus it prevents these organisms from becoming reestablished within the body.

With the majority of drugs, the fungus, after being killed or diminished, ultimately returns, and the infection is reestablished. This is why the oregano oil, along with the desiccated multiple spice extract, is so valuable. It tends to destroy the fungus permanently. It can also be taken routinely, that is, preventively in daily doses once such destruction is achieved. As a maintenance, it can even be taken on a daily basis, to prevent fungal recurrence. In addition, it has the versatility of being both a topical and an internal agent.

Fungi have the capacity for deep tissue invasion. The purpose of such invasion is to maintain a permanent presence in the tissues. These fungi are not easy to dislodge. To ultimately destroy any deep-seated infestation requires persistent treatment, largely through the use of a nontoxic approach. This is where spice oils are ideal as they exhibit no known toxicity when taken for prolonged periods.

38.6 ORIGANUM OIL'S MECHANISM OF ACTION

A. Rao has observed from a review of the literature that the active ingredients of oil of wild oregano, terpenoid phenols, exhibit "potent antifungal activity," this being due to a variety of mechanisms.[12] The effect was noted when taken internally, applied topically, or when used directly on the mucous membranes. Regarding the latter, oregano oil has been found effective in the treatment of denture-induced candidal stomatitis. It was found that the active ingredients of the oil were "very active" against the oral form of this yeast. In sheep, a mixture of essential oils including oil of oregano was found effective against ringworm.

Internally through a test involving broth cultures and microdilution method, wild oregano oil (origanum oil) was found to "completely inhibit the growth of C. albicans…." In a study published in *Obesity and Surgery*, it was found that "both the germination and the mycelial growth of C. albicans" were fully "inhibited" by the oregano oil as well as its key active ingredient, carvacrol.

The investigators did a repeat of the original Georgetown work, infecting mice in an experimental murine systemic candidiasis model. The daily administration of the oregano oil in an olive oil base for 30 days resulted in an 80% survival with no fungus found residually in the kidneys, that is no renal burden. Like the Georgetown authors, these investigators led by M. Sokovic found that oregano oil as a complex was superior to the mere active ingredient, carvacrol, alone. Noted the investigators, "similar results were obtained with carvacrol. However, mice fed origanum oil (as the unaltered, natural complex) exhibited cosmetically better clinical appearance compared to those cured with carvacrol." This led the researchers to conclude that wild oregano oil should be examined for "efficacy" in "systemic and superficial fungal infections" and even for other "pathogenic manifestations, including malignancy."

Even so, the real power of the wild oregano is easy to realize. It is a capacity that no drug can match. This is the power of the destruction not only of bacteria but also of the actual cold and flu viruses. This is a destruction that has been confirmed by scientific studies. The first hint of the mechanism behind its extensive antiviral powers was determined by Siddiqui and colleagues publishing in *Medical Science Research*. Here, it was found that the wild oregano oil destroyed a variety of cold and flu viruses, as well as herpes-like viruses. In fact, noted the researchers, the viruses were "disintegrated" by the oil.[15]

38.7 BACTERICIDAL PROPERTIES OF ORIGANUM EXTRACTS

Wild oregano oil shows promise in the treatment of bacterial infections that are often resistant to standard antibiotics. In the *Journal Ancient Science of Life*, 2013, the investigators evaluated the powers of oregano oil with the drug ciprofloxacin as a combined therapy, in this case against the pathogen that causes typhoid fever, *Salmonella typhi*. The study showed that "not only the formulation using O. vulgare and ciprofloxacin can overcome multidrug resistance but will also reduce the toxic effects" of the drug.[17] Again in the *Journal of Food Science* 2011, it was determined, that oregano oil had a "notable inhibitory effect" in this case "against 10…strains of Klebsiella pneumoniae."[18]

A rather thorough study performed by Sokovic and his group demonstrated the degree of broad spectrum action of wild oregano oil. Here, it was determined that the oil inhibited the growth of a number of rather resistant bacteria, as follows:

Pseudomonas
Proteus
Salmonella, including *S. typhi*
Staph[16]

This was confirmed by Turkish investigators Sarac and Ugur, who found that the oil dramatically inhibited the growth of a wide range of gram-positive and gram-negative bacteria. Preuss and cohorts also showed a similar action with wild oregano oil inhibiting the growth *in vitro* of *Klebsiella*, *Staph*, *Escherichia coli*, *Campylobacter pylori*, and *Mycobacterium terrae*.[10,11]

38.8 CONCLUSIONS

The full spectrum of research currently available clearly establishes the medicinal properties and therapeutic application for origanum oil. Human studies are needed to confirm the compelling findings of animal and *in vitro* investigations. It is hoped that clinical trials will be forthcoming regarding the obviously potent germicidal properties of origanum oil, which will demonstrate definitely the value of this oil in the treatment of human infectious diseases.

REFERENCES

1. Manohar, V., Ingram, C., Gray, J.K., Talpur, N.A., Echard, B.W., Bagchi, D., and H.G. Preuss, 2001. Antifungal activities of origanum oil against Candida albicans. *Mol. Cell. Biochem.* 228:111–117.
2. Skwavek, T., 1994. Plant inducers of interfurons. *Herba Polinica.* 40: 42–49.
3. Culpeper, N. 1652. *The English Physitian: Or an Astrologo-Physical Discourse of the Vulgar herbs of this Nation.* London, U.K.: Peter Cole.
4. Gerard, J. 1975. *The Herbal or General History of Plants: The Complete 1633 Edition as Revised and Enlarged by Thomas Johnson.* New York: Dover.
5. Martindale, W.H. 1932. *The Extra Pharmacopœia.* Martindale and Westcott. Vol. I, 20th ed. (27s. 6d. net) London, U.K.:H. K. Lewis & Co., Ltd.
6. Salmon, W. 1693. *The Compleat English Physician.* London, U.K.: Mathew Gilliflower.
7. Ijaz, M.K., Chen, Z., Raja, S.S., Suchmann, D.B., Royt, P.W., Ingram, C., Gray, J.K., and G. Paolilli, 2004. Antiviral and virucidal activities of oreganol P73-based spice extracts against human coronavirus in vitro. *Antiviral Research.* 62(2):A75. *The Seventh International Conference on Antiviral Research*, Tucson, AZ.
8. Gilling, D.H., Kitajima, M., Torrey, J.R., and K.R. Bright, 2014. Antiviral efficacy and mechanism of action of oregano essential oil and its primary component carvacrol against murine norovirus. *J. Appl. Microbiol.* 116:1149–1163.
9. Vimalanathan, S. and J. Hudson, 2012. Anti-influenza virus activities of commercial oregano oils and their carriers. *J. Appl. Pharm. Sci.* 2:214–218.
10. Preuss, H.G., Echard, B., Enig, M., Brook, I., and T.B. Elliott, 2005. Minimum inhibitory concentrations of herbal essential oils and monolaurin for gram-positive and gram-negative bacteria. *Mol. Cell. Biochem.* 272:29–34.
11. Preuss, H.G., Echard, B., Dadgar, A., Talpur, N., Manohar, V., Enig, M., Bagchi, D., and C. Ingram, 2005. Effects of essential oils and monolaurin on *Staphylococcus aureus*: In vitro and in vivo studies. *Toxicol. Mech. Methods* 15:279–285.
12. Rao, A., Zhang, Y., Muend, S., and R. Rao, 2010. Mechanism of antifungal activity of terpenoid phenols resembles calcium stress and inhibition of the TOR pathway. *Antimicrob. Agents Chemother.* 54:5062–5069.

13. Valnet, 1983. *Herbal Medicine: Treatment of Diseases in Plants.* ed. The Pocket Book No 7889. Paris, France.
14. Vimalanathan, S., and J. Hudson, 2012. Anti-influenza virus activities of commercial oregano oils and their carriers. *J. Appl. Pharm. Sci.* 07:214–218.
15. Siddiqui, Y.M. et al., 1996. Effect of essential oils on the enveloped viruses: Antiviral activity of oregano oils on herpes simplex virus type I and Newcastle disease virus. *Med. Sci. Res.* 24:185–186.
16. Soković, M., Glamočlija, J., Petar, D., Brkić, D., Leo, J., and L.D. van Griensven, 2010. Antibacterial effects of the essential oils of commonly consumed medicinal herbs using an in vitro model. *Molecules* 15:7532–7546.
17. Bharti, V., Vasudeva, N., Sharma, S., and J.S. Duhan, 2013. Antibacterial activities of *Origanum vulgare* alone and in combination with different antimicrobials against clinical isolates of *Salmonella typhi*. *Anc. Sci. Life* 32:212–216.
18. Orhan, I.E., Ozcelik, B., Kan, Y., and M. Kartal, 2011. Inhibitory effects of various essential oils and individual components against extended-spectrum beta-lactamase (ESBL) produced by *Klebsiella pneumoniae* and their chemical compositions. *J. Food Sci.* 76:538–546.

39 Nutraceuticals from Microalgae

Faisal Alsenani, Faruq Ahmed, and Peer M. Schenk

CONTENTS

39.1 INTRODUCTION

Nutraceuticals have been defined as food or food products that can simultaneously provide nutrition and pharmaceutical benefits to the body such as prevention and treatment of diseases (Borowitzka 2013). According to the US Institute of Medicine, this includes "any substance that is a food or part of a food which provides medicinal or health benefits including the prevention and treatment of disease, beyond the traditional nutrients it contains" (Burja and Radianingtyas 2008). They have also been termed as food supplements by the US Food and Drug Administration. Another synonymous term used is functional foods that have been defined as "products derived from natural sources, whose consumption is likely to benefit human health and enhance performance" (Burja and Radianingtyas 2008). This may include the fortification of conventional food to increase its nutritional or health benefit. Nutraceuticals can be either a whole food product (e.g. seaweed) or dietary supplements where the nutraceutical compound(s) may be concentrated to provide the claimed health benefits (e.g. *Haematococcus* in powder or tablet form or astaxanthin extract).

Neutraceuticals are increasingly becoming attractive for the biotechnology industry because of the fact that their market involves not only human beings but also animals, including pets. Microalgae have received a lot of attention in the scientific community and biotechnology industry due to the revelation that many microalgal strains are very good sources of various nutraceuticals, such as omega 3 and omega 6 fatty acids and carotenoids (Figure 39.1). The use of microalgal biomass is particularly attractive based on the advantages that microalgae are highly productive on arable and nonarable land, thus potentially avoiding competition with food production. They can also adapt to varying environmental conditions by producing secondary metabolites, and they can also be used to purify and take up nutrients from wastewater (Ahmed et al. 2014). Health benefits of algal nutraceuticals include promotion of healthy bones and teeth, weight reduction, cholesterol

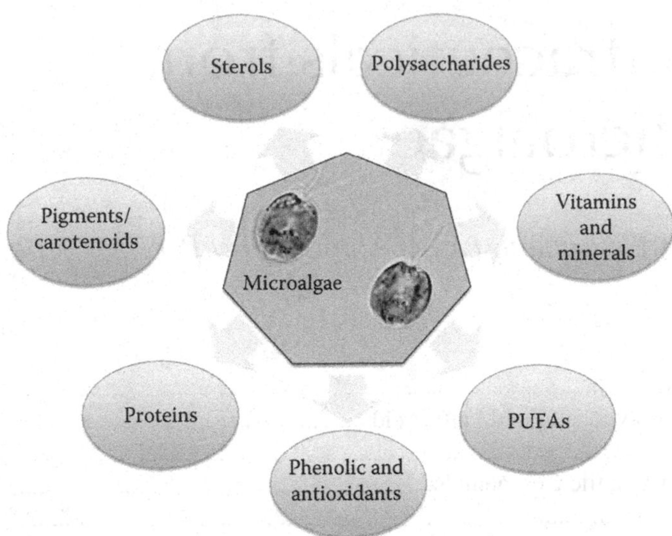

FIGURE 39.1 **(See color insert.)** An overview of nutraceuticals used from microalgae.

reduction, disease resistance, improved immune system and brain development, healthier gut and digestive system, blood pressure control and reduction, heart health, antioxidant, antiviral, and anticancer properties (Venugopal 2009).

In this chapter, we will give a brief overview of the different nutraceutical compounds currently reported as available from microalgae, their beneficial effects, and their potential in the biotechnology industry.

39.2 LONG CHAIN POLYUNSATURATED FATTY ACIDS

The long chain polyunsaturated fatty acids (PUFA) are defined as the fatty acids containing more than 18 carbon atoms and at least one double bond in their molecular structures. Examples are arachidonic acid (AA), linolenic acid, eicosapentaenoic acid (EPA), docosapentaenoic acid (DPA), and docosahexaenoic acid (DHA). These compounds are essential for human and animal nutrition and therefore have to be ingested from other sources of food as they are not produced in their bodies. These fatty acids are receiving increased attention due to the revelations that they are essential for normal brain development and cardiovascular health. They are also recognized to have antioxidant, anti-inflammatory, antimicrobial, and antiviral activities, and can reduce or prevent rheumatoid arthritis, atherosclerosis, arrhythmias, and chronic obstructive pulmonary diseases, several carcinomas, reduce symptoms in asthma patients, fight against manic-depressive illness, protect against chronic obstructive pulmonary diseases, alleviate symptoms of cystic fibrosis, prevent relapses in patients with Crohn's disease, provide bone health, and improve brain functions in children (Venugopal 2009; Stengel et al. 2011). Being an important component of tissues in the brain, nervous system, and eye, DHA (22:6 omega-3) and arachidonic acid (ARA omega-6) play very important roles in the development of infants and growing children (Venugopal 2009). Supplementation of diets with fatty acids was found to affect behavior of children, especially the ones with attention-deficit hyperactivity disorder (ADHD) (Venugopal 2009). However, it was reported that omega-6 could have a negative effect on human health and increase the risk of cardiovascular disease when consumed over the recommended dose, as this would cause a change in the omega-3/omega-6 ratio in the body (Simopoulos 2002).

Several microalgal strains have been reported as excellent producers of various PUFAs (Table 39.1) and can be very useful substitutes for fish oil, thus reducing pressure on already depleting fish stocks. *Phaeodactylum tricornutum* contains around 30%–45% PUFAs of which

TABLE 39.1
Microalgae-Derived Nutraceuticals, Sources, Health Benefits, and Companies Currently Commercializing Them

Functional Compounds	Sources	Health Benefits	Companies
Carotenoids Astaxanthin β-carotene Lutein Cantaxanthin Violaxanthin	*Dunaliella salina* *Haematococcus pluvialis* *Chlorella vulgaris* *Chlorella pyrenoidosa* *Chlorella ellipsoidea*	Antioxidant, immunomodulation, retinal degradation, muscular dystrophy, and cancer prevention	Cyanotech, Algatechnologies, Mera Pharmaceuticals, AstaReal AB, Jingzhou Natural Astaxanthin Inc. (Astaxanthin) BASF, Nikken Shohonsha Co. (β-carotene) Taiwan Chlorella Manufacturing and Co. Cognis Nutrition and Health (Germany)
Polyunsaturated fatty acids EPA DHA Oleic acid Linolenic acid Palmitoleic acid	*Crypthecodinium cohnii* *Phaeodactyllum tricornutum* *Monodus subterraneus* *Porphyridium cruentum* *H. pluvialis* *D. salina*	Antioxidant, antimicrobial activity Reduce risks of certain heart diseases	DSM Nutritional Products Inc. Hainan Simai Enterprising Ltd (China) Earthrise Farms and stretches (USA) Myanmar Spirulina Factory (Myanmar)
Proteins Phycobiliproteins	*S. platensis* *Porphyridium* spp.	Immunomodulation, anticancer, hepatoprotective, anti-inflammatory, antioxidant activity	Earthrise Nutritionals, Cyanotech, RBC Life Sciences (USA), DIC Lifetec (Japan), Green Valley, Sanatur Spirulina (Germany)
Polysaccharides Sulfated polysaccharides Insoluble fiber	*C. pyrenoidosa* *Porphyridium* spp. *C. vulgaris*	Antiviral, antitumor, antihyperlipidemia, anticoagulant, reduce total and LDL-cholesterol	
Vitamins Tocopherols	*Porphyridium* spp. *S. platensis*	Antioxidant activity	
Phenolic compounds	*S. platensis*	Antioxidant activity	
Volatile compounds	*S. platensis*	Antimicrobial activity	
Neophytadiene, phytol and others	*D. salina* *Phormidium*		
Phytosterols	*Dunaliella tertiolecta* *Dunaliella salina* *Karlodinium* spp. *Peridinium aciculiferum* *Polarella glacialis* *Scrippsiella hangoei* *Takayama* spp. *Lotharella amoeboformis* *Neochloris oleabundans*	Reduce LDL-cholesterol accumulation Anti-inflammatory, antiatherogenic, neuromodulatory activity	
Minerals	*Chlorella vulgaris* *Sochrisis galbana* *Spirulina platensis*	Growth and development Promote health and nutrition	

EPA accounts for 20%–40% of total fatty acids (Ramírez-Fajardo et al. 2007). Other useful sources of EPA are the yellow green alga *Monodus subterraneus* (producing 20%–37% of total fatty acids; Cohen, 1999), *Porphyridium cruentum*, *Chaetoceros calcitrans*, and *Nannochloropsis* spp. (producing around 24% of total fatty acids; Borowitzka 2013). Useful producers of DHA include *Crypthecodinium cohnii* (up to 39% of total fatty acids; Borowitzka 2013), *Isochrysis galbana*, and *Pavlova salina* (Guedes et al. 2011a; Custódio et al. 2014). *Crypthecodinium cohnii* is already commercially used as a source of DHA by DSM Nutritional Products Inc. (DHASCO®; Table 39.1). *Dunaliella salina* has been reported as a good source of, linolenic, and oleic acids constituting up to 85% of total fatty acids (Herrero et al. 2006). *Spirulina platensis* has been reported as a good source of γ-linolenic acid, lauric, palmitoleic, and oleic acids and DHA (Yukino et al. 2005; Mendiola et al. 2007). Although *Porphyridium cruentum* contains a small portion of lipids in its biomass (6.5%), a major proportion of the lipids constitute palmitic acid, arachidonic acid, EPA, and linoleic acid (Stengel et al. 2011). Additionally, lipid extracts from the microlaga *Nostoc commune* have been found useful in the treatment of cancer, viruses, burns, and chronic fatigue; however, the fatty acid compounds responsible for these activities are yet to be identified (Rasmussen et al. 2008).

39.3 PIGMENTS

Algal pigments are categorized into chlorophylls a, b, and c, phycobili pigments, and carotenoids (Stengel et al. 2011). Among them, the commercially sought after pigment groups are carotenoids and phycobilins with applications in various industries. Carotenoids are powerful antioxidants and provide photoprotection to the cells. However, recent discoveries in medicinal applications of various carotenoids have made them highly attractive to the biotechnology industries. Different algae-derived carotenoids have different protective functions against cancer, for example lutein, zeaxanthin, and β-carotene prevent premenopausal breast cancer, while cryptoxanthin and α-carotene prevent cervical cancer (Stengel et al. 2011). Moreover, fucoxanthin (available at high quantities in brown algae and diatoms) has antiobesity and anticancer activities (Maeda et al. 2005). Phycobilin pigments, such as phycocyanin, phycoerythrin, and allophycocyanin, are only produced in algae belonging to the groups cyanobacteria (*Spirulina* or *Arthrospira*), red algae (*Porphyridium*, *Rhodella*, *Galdieria*), cryptophyta, and glaucophyta (Borowitzka 2013) and have been known to have antioxidant, anti-inflammatory, and anticancer properties (Stengel et al. 2011). *Spirulina*, an excellent source of c-phycocyanin, is already approved as food and is commercially produced and marketed in different parts of the world (Table 39.1).

Among the different microalgae, two species, *Dunaliella salina* and *Haematococcus pluvialis*, are well known to accumulate β-carotene (up to 14% dry weight) and astaxanthin (2%–3% dry weight), respectively, under stress conditions (Ibañez and Cifuentes 2013). Astaxanthin is one of the carotenoids currently commercially produced from the freshwater microalga *H. pluvialis* by several companies (Table 39.1). This carotenoid is well known to have powerful antioxidant and anti-inflammatory activities capable of preventing or reducing protein degradation, macular degeneration, rheumatoid arthritis, cardiovascular diseases, neurodegenerative diseases such as Parkinson's, and cancers (Hudek et al. 2014). *D. salina* is the highest producer of carotenoids among all sources, including fruits, vegetables, and spices and therefore this strain of microalgae is currently commercially exploited for β-carotene in several countries (Table 39.1). Several other microalgae, such as *Muriellopsis* sp., *Scenedesmus almeriensis*, *Auxenochlorella* (*Chlorella*) *protothecoides*, *Chlorella zofigiensis* (high lutein producer), *Scenedesmus komareckii*, *D. salina* aplanospores (high cantaxanthin producer), *D. salina* mutants (high zeaxanthin producer), *Botryococcus braunii* (high echinenone producer), *Phaeodactyllum tricornutum* (high fucoxanthin producer), and specific metabolic inhibitor-treated *D. salina* (phytoene and phytofluene producer), have also been identified as high carotenoid producers. However, they have not been considered for commercialization yet due to the high cost of downstream processing for extraction and purification of these carotenoids (Borowitzka 2013).

Several strains of *Chlorella* are reported as good sources of lutein, α-carotene, β-carotene, violaxanthin, antheraxanthin, zeaxanthin, and astaxanthin. Studies on the carotenoid extracts of *Chlorella ellipsoidea* and *C. vulgaris* exhibited antiproliferative activity of human colon cancer cells, making them useful food for the prevention of certain cancers (Cha et al. 2008). Additionally, *Chlorella* extracts containing lutein and β-carotene reportedly caused prevention of macular degeneration and cognitive impairment in transgenic mice (Nakashima et al. 2009). Furthermore, the cyanobacterium *Synechococcus* and the microalgae *Nannochloropsis gaditana* have been reported as good sources of β-carotene, zeaxanthin, violaxanthin and vaucheriaxanthin, and chlorophyll a (Macías-Sánchez et al. 2007). Chlorophyll is reported to have antimutagenic, anticarcinogenic, and antioxidant activities (Tumolo and Lanfer-Marquez 2012).

39.4 PHENOLIC AND VOLATILE COMPOUNDS

Phenolic compounds are produced as secondary metabolites as a response to stress, and therefore they are involved in the chemical protective mechanism of cells. These compounds are mostly involved in the protective activities against biotic factors and stress, such as grazing and UV radiation, bacteria settlement, or other fouling organisms or metal contamination (Stengel et al. 2011). Phenolic compounds form groups of phytochemicals that have high biological functions, such as antioxidant, anti-inflammatory, and antimicrobial activities. Various preclinical and epidemiological studies have reported that phenolics can slow the progression of certain cancers and reduce the risks of cardiovascular disease, neurodegenerative diseases, and diabetes (Kim et al. 2009).

Among the different microalgal species studied so far, *Nostoc ellipsosporum*, *Nostoc piscinale*, *Chlorella protothecoides*, *Chlorella vulgaris*, *Anabaena cylindrica*, *Tolypothrix tenuis*, *Chlorella pyrenoidosa*, and *Chlamydomonas nivalis* (Li et al. 2007; Hajimahmoodi et al. 2010) have total phenolic contents that are similar to or higher than several popular fruits and vegetables such as kale, shallots, oriental plum, cashews, apples, and strawberries (Ismail et al. 2004; Hassimotto et al. 2005; Lin and Tang 2007). *Spirulina* has been reported as a good source of heptadecane and tetradecane, the volatile compounds known to have antibacterial capacity (Ozdemir et al. 2004). *D. salina* is reported to have volatile compounds such as β-cyclocitral, α- and β-ionone, neophytadiene, and phytol that have antimicrobial activity (Herrero et al. 2006). Moreover, *Synechocystis* sp. have been noted as a source of pentadecane (Plaza et al. 2010).

39.5 STEROLS

Sterols have become well known for their ability to reduce LDL-cholesterol and promote cardiovascular health. Moreover, sterols have been reported to be involved in anti-inflammatory and antiatherogenicity, anticancer, and antioxidative activities and can provide protection against nervous system disorders, such as autoimmune encephalomyelitis, amyotrophic lateral sclerosis, or Alzheimer's disease. Currently, pine tall oil and soy deodorized distillates are used as sources of sterols by the biotechnology industry, and these sterols are used as food additives or dietary supplements. Microalgae can produce a vast range of sterol compounds, such as brassicasterol, sitosterol, and stigmasterol, and the contents can be manipulated by changes in growth medium. Recent studies have suggested promising quantities of sterols in two microalgal strains, *Dunaliella tertiolecta* and *D. salina*, and these sterol compounds were found to have in vivo neuromodulatory activity (Francavilla et al. 2012). More studies are being conducted by our group to identify more promising strains that could provide alternatives to the current industrial sources.

39.6 PROTEINS

Microalgae have the potential to become an alternative protein source due to the fact that several strains such as *Chlorella*, *Spirulina*, *Scenedesmus*, *Dunaliella*, *Micractinium*, *Oscillatoria*, *Chlamydomonas*, and *Euglena* contain proteins of high quantities (more than 50% of dry weight) and qualities (Becker

2007). The presence of essential amino acids, such as lysine, leucine, isoleucine, and valine (comprising 35% of essential amino acids in muscle proteins of humans), contributes to the high quality of microalgal proteins, making them highly suitable for use as direct supplements (both for animal and human consumption) or as nutraceuticals (Dewapriya and Kim 2014). Studies have suggested that feeding of defatted *H. pluvialis* as a supplement to shrimps resulted in healthier animals than the commercial diet–fed controls (Ju et al. 2012). Moreover, in an algal biorefinery concept, the biomass left after oil extraction could be a cheap source of bioactive protein and could be very useful in recovering the high production costs of microalgal biofuels (Dewapriya and Kim 2014). Besides that, cyanobacteria, such as *S. platensis* and *Porphyridium* spp. contain phycobiliproteins, a group of proteins involved in photosynthesis (Stengel et al. 2011). Pigments such as phycobilin and phycoerythrin are associated with these proteins, and these compounds have been found to have hepatoprotective, anti-inflammatory, immunomodulating, anticancer, and antioxidant properties (Stengel et al. 2011).

Another area of usefulness of microalgal protein is bioactive peptides that are defined as 2–20 amino acids long protein fragments that generally remain dormant within the parent protein molecule but can be activated by hydrolysis to exert hormone-like effects on physiological processes of the human body (Himaya et al. 2012). Bioactive peptides are reported to have antioxidant, anticancer, antihypertensive, immunomodulatory, antimicrobial, and cholesterol-lowering effects (Agyei and Danquah 2011). Peptides purified from *C. vulgaris* have been reported to have noteworthy protective effects on DNA and preventative effects on oxidative damage of cells and therefore have been attributed to prevent diseases such as atherosclerosis, coronary heart disease, and cancer (Sheih et al. 2009). Besides *Chlorella*, *S. platensis*, *Navicula incerta*, and *Pavlova lutheri* have huge potential to generate bioactive peptides with therapeutic value. For example, *P. lutheri* biomass was recently successfully microbially fermented to generate small peptides with high antioxidant activity (Ryu et al. 2012). Additionally, peptides activated from *Chlamydomonas* sp. and *N. incerta* exhibited suppression of *Helicobacter pylori*–induced carcinogenesis and protection against ethanol-induced hepatotoxicity, respectively (Kang et al. 2012; Himaya et al. 2013).

Development of therapeutic protein from marine microalgae is another area of huge potential for production of low-cost, high-yield recombinant proteins. The discovery of the ability of *Chlamydomonas reinhardtii* to fold protein correctly and assemble very complex proteins more easily than many bacteria and yeasts has led to the production of several high-quality recombinant proteins at very low cost. This microalga also has the added advantage that it can be grown even in contaminated medium without compromising the characteristics of the desired recombinant proteins (Mayfield et al. 2007). The different recombinant proteins that could potentially be expressed in *C. reinhardtii* include HSV8-lsc and HSV8-scFv, a human IgA antiherpes monoclonal antibody, human tumor necrosis factor–related apoptosis-inducing ligand (TRAIL), human glutamic acid decarboxylase 65 (hGAD65), key autoantigen in type I diabetes, which is also an important marker for the prediction and diagnosis of type I diabetes, etc. (see Gong et al. 2011 for details). Moreover, *P. tricornutum* has been successfully used to express monoclonal human IgG antibody against the hepatitis B surface protein and the relevant antigen (Hempel et al. 2011).

39.7 VITAMINS

Microalgae have the ability to produce necessary vitamins, such as vitamin A, B family vitamins, C, D, E, and H. For example, 9%–18% of the dry weight of *Chlorella* may contain minerals, dietary fibers, and vitamins, especially vitamin B12 (Shim et al. 2008). The cyanobacterium *Spirulina* is also considered a good source of vitamin B12. However, vitamin B12 from *Chlorella* has been reported to have better bioavailability than that of *Spirulina* (Belay et al. 1993; Watanabe et al. 2002). The microalga *Porphyridium cruentum* has been reported as a good source of tocopherols or vitamin E (55.2 μg/g dry weight of α-tocopherol and 51.3 μg/g dry weight γ-tocopherol; Durmaz et al. 2007). Vitamin E is well known to protect membrane lipids from oxidative damage and also prevents diseases such as coronary diseases, atherosclerosis, and multiple sclerosis (Johnson 2000).

39.8 POLYSACCHARIDES

Polysaccharides from some microalgae have been reported to have antioxidant, antitumor, antihyperlipidemia, and anticoagulant activities (Plaza et al. 2009). For example, *C. pyrenoidosa* polysaccharides contain galactose, mannose, arabinose, xylose, ribose, fucose, and rhamnose and could be useful for the generation of drugs (Plaza et al. 2009). Another example is *Phorphiridium* spp., which contain sulphated polysaccharides composed of xylose, glucose, galactose, mannose, methylated galactose, and pentose. These polysaccharides reportedly showed significant antiviral activity against herpes simplex virus (type 1 and 2), both in vitro and in vivo (Huheihel et al. 2002). Moreover, nostoflan, a polysaccharide from *Nostoc flagelliforme* has been found to have antiviral activity against herpes simplex virus type a (HSV-1), HSV-2, human cytomegalovirus, and influenza A virus (Kanekiyo et al. 2005).

39.9 MINERALS

Microalgae have the ability to accumulate trace elements, but very few studies have been conducted on the mineral content of microalgae. Minerals have important functions and either are incorporated into compounds or remain in elemental form, such as zinc, calcium, phosphorus, magnesium, potassium, sodium, chlorine, sulfur, iron, cobalt, copper, iodine, molybdenum, manganese, fluorine, and selenium (Nose 1972). The studies by Tokuşoglu and Üunal (2003) and Fabregas and Herrero (1986) reported significant quantities of zinc, phosphorus, sodium, iron, potassium, manganese, magnesium, and calcium in *D. tertiolecta, Isochrisis galbana, Tetraselmis suecica, C. vulgaris, Sochrisis galbana, S. platensis*, and *Chlorella stigmatophora*.

In general, the mineral content of microalgae is adequate to fulfill the recommended daily intake for adults. According to Dietary Reference Intakes (DRIs), the recommended daily intake for calcium (Ca) is 1300 mg/day for adults, 800 mg/day for children up to 8 years old, and 270 mg/day for infants from 7 to 12 months (Office of Dietary Supplements). As a result, a daily intake of approximately 92 g of *I. galbana* is adequate to meet Ca requirements for an adult (Tokuşoglu and Üunal 2003).

The daily recommended intake for another essential mineral, zinc (Zn), is 8–11 mg/day for 9 year olds to adults, 5 mg/day for children aged 4–8 years, and 2–3 mg/day for children aged under 4. Based on such recommendations, daily consumption of *Tetraselmis suecica* at 2 g, 3.5 g, and 6 g will be sufficient for age groups under 4, 4–8 years, and 9 year olds to adults, respectively. A daily intake of 8 g of *Tetraselmis suecica* will also be sufficient to fulfill daily recommended intake of Zn for pregnant and lactating women (Tokuşoglu and Üunal 2003).

Similarly, the consumption of 40 g of *C. vulgaris* will meet the DRIs for phosphorus (P) for an adult because the recommended daily intake is 700 mg/day for adults, 500 mg/day for children, and 275 mg/day for infants (Tokuşoglu and Üunal 2003). Daily consumption of 142 g of *S. platensis* entirely meets the potassium (K) needs for adults and 42.5 g for infants. Alternatively, 37 g of *C. vulgaris* will meet the requirement for an adult (DRIs: 2000 mg/day for adults, 1600 mg/day for children, and 500 mg/day for infants). Approximately, 47 and 60 g of *I. galbana* will meet the DRIs for magnesium (Mg) for adult females and males, respectively (DRIs: 320 and 420 mg/day), while 11 g will fulfill the needs of infants (DRIs: 75 mg/day; Tokuşoglu and Üunal, 2003).

In addition, iron (Fe) content of the examined microalgae was adequate for the recommended daily consumption for adults. Daily intake of approximately 10.5 g of *S. platensis*, about 4.5 g of *I. galbana*, and 4 g of *C. vulgaris* fulfills the DRIs for iron for adult males, children, and infants (10 mg/day; Tokuşoglu and Üunal 2003). Around 6.6 mg/day of *I. galbana*, 5.8 mg/day of *C. vulgaris*, and 15.7 mg/day of *S. platensis* meet the DRIs of iron for adult females (15 mg/day). For selenium (Se) intake, about 6.86 g of *I. galbana* meet the RDIs of adult males (70 µg), while a 58.3 g/day of *S. platensis* and 100 g/day of *C. vulgaris* fulfill the DRIs for Se for adult males (DRIs: 55 µg/day for adult females, 30 µg/day for children, and 15 µg/day for infants). For manganese (Mn), approximately 52.7 mg/day of *I. galbana* fulfills the DRIs for adults and children (Tokuşoglu and Üunal 2003).

39.10 MICROALGAE AS BIOFACTORIES FOR PHARMACEUTICAL AND THERAPEUTIC APPLICATIONS

As mentioned previously in the protein section, the development of techniques for chloroplast and nuclear transformation especially in *C. reinhardtii* has led to the development of human therapeutics, antibodies, and immunotoxins (Guarnieri and Pienkos 2014). One such exciting area of application is the development of oral vaccines. Using microalgae to develop vaccines has many benefits that outweigh the others. As these are plant-based vaccines, the vaccine antigens are protected from proteolytic degradation and minimize the antigen purification process (Specht et al. 2010; Gregory et al. 2013). Advances have been demonstrated in this area through generation of single-chain antibodies that can target glycoprotein D of the herpes simplex virus and the production of a chimeric protein consisting of a mucosal adjuvant (CtxB) and a malaria transmission-blocking vaccine candidate (Pfs25) (Guarnieri and Pienkos 2014). Further success was demonstrated when production of IgG and IgA antibodies was induced through oral vaccination. Moreover, production of anticancer immunotoxin that can bind and reduce the viability of b-cell lymphoma has also been reported recently (Tran et al. 2013).

39.11 MICROALGAE AS ADDITIVES TO COSMETIC PRODUCTS

In the cosmetic industry, *Chlorella* and *Spirulina* are the predominant ones. They are used in skin products such as antiaging and anti-irritant preparation. For example, an extract rich of protein from *Spirulina* can repair the signs of skin aging and *Chlorella* extracts can stimulate collagen synthesis (Spolaore et al. 2006). Moreover, *Nannochloropsis* and *D. salina* produce compounds that have excellent skin tightening properties and stimulate cell proliferation (Stolz and Obermayer 2005; Spolaore et al. 2006).

39.12 MICROALGAE AS FOOD

Microalgae and cyanobacteria have been used as food for many centuries in some parts of the world, for example China and Mexico. Although microalgae have been mostly used as feed in aquaculture of crustaceans, molluscs, and finfish for many decades, the discovery of nutritional values of many microalgal strains led to the development of microalgae as food (e.g. *Spirulina* and *Chlorella* powder) and dietary supplement (e.g. astaxanthin from *H. pluvialis* and β-carotene from *D. salina*) industries. Currently, *Spirulina* and *Chlorella* are approved as food by the EU and FDA, the United States, and are commercially available for human consumption in different forms, such as powder, tablets, and capsules. They are also incorporated in beverages, biscuits, and candy bars (Spolaore et al. 2006). These different forms are marketed by companies, such as Synergy (Australia; product names: spirulina premium® and chlorella premium) and Cyanotech (USA; product name: spirulina Pacifica®). One key issue for addition of other microalgae to this list is the compliance with food regulatory requirements. The key criterion is that they need to have a "history of safe use" in order to be considered as food grade strains. The history of safe use has been defined as "significant human consumption of food over several generations and in a large genetically diverse population for which there exist adequate toxicological and allergenicity data to provide reasonable certainty that no harm will result from the consumption of the food" (Bourdichon et al. 2012). Moreover, scientific approaches required for identification of safe microalgae for food processing have been outlined that involve analyses of undesirable properties, opportunistic infections, toxic metabolites, virulence factors, and abiotic resistance (Bourdichon et al. 2012).

In addition to the regulatory requirements, there are other limiting factors for making microalgae an alternative food source. This includes the unacceptance of many consumers of the green color and fishy aroma of various microalgal strains. Some decades old studies suggested that consumers preferred when *Chlorella* powder was concealed in other green foods, such as spinach noodles or mint ice cream (Morimura and Tamiya 1954).

39.13 CONCLUSION AND FUTURE DIRECTION OF RESEARCH

Although many compounds of high biological value and their health benefits have already been discovered as outlined in this chapter, microalgae still remain one of the most unexplored groups of organisms in the world, as around 97% of marine microalgal compounds are yet to be isolated and characterized (Guedes et al. 2011b). This lack of information emphasizes the need for more research in the area of bioprospecting that involves isolation, identification, and growth optimization of new and locally available microalgal strains. This can lead to the discovery of novel metabolites with various health benefits or discovery of high-producing strains that can reduce the cost of producing nutraceuticals.

One key area of further research is the complete genome sequencing of high nutraceutical–producing microalgae. Although *C. reinhardtii* and 30 other organellar and whole algal genomes have reportedly been sequenced (Guarnieri and Pienkos 2014), more information on whole genome sequences is necessary to understand and characterize the genes and enzymes involved in the production of nutraceuticals and the mechanisms that trigger the production of these metabolites, such as nutrient deprivation, biotic and abiotic stress, etc. The sequence information and an understanding of trigger mechanisms can help in the genetic transformation and manipulation of microalgal strains to induce the high-level production of target compounds.

It is well known that the design and construction of bioreactors and dewatering and harvesting of microalgal biomass's and extraction and purification of target nutraceutical compounds present the major costs of microalgae production plants. In recent years, due to high focus of producing renewable energy from microalgae, major advancements have been made in these areas. However, more research with the aim of constructing bioreactors or open pond systems made of inexpensive and environmentally friendly materials and development of less energy demanding and inexpensive harvesting and extraction techniques is required.

Nutraceuticals harness and concentrate nutritious algal components to produce positive health effects when they are consumed. Microalgae have been included in many nutritional studies worldwide, and more nutritional benefits are likely to be discovered with increased human use. Undoubtedly, their potential for treating and preventing many types of diseases—in particular, cardiovascular conditions, viral infections, and cancers—will continue to create interest and fuel investigations into their value for human health. Moreover, more intensive research on identifying phenolic and volatile compounds from microalgae would give more health benefits to humans. Additionally, more detailed information about simple phenolic and volatile compounds and their aldehydes obtained from microalgae are required since this information was not identified till now due to the complexity of their isolation leading to low amounts and the need for advanced analytical techniques.

Since the global fish stocks are declining and are not a sustainable source of PUFAs (omega-3), microalgae have been used as an alternative source for PUFAs. However, very few species are used for the production. Thus, more in-depth investigation studies and continued isolation and screening are required.

Despite the high amount of protein in microalgae, the dried form has not attracted consumers as a food or food substitute. Some of the major difficulties are the fishy smell and dark green color, which limit their use and their combination with the traditional food. Therefore, the market of microalgae is restricted nowadays to health food products and functional foods. There is some research to overcome these difficulties, like covering its smell or taste by using microencapsulation techniques to combine it with food, but further investigations are required to deploy the benefits of the nutritious protein from microalgae and to overcome these obstacles.

Microalgae have been used for centuries to provide nourishment to humans, and only recently they have become much more widely cultured and harvested. Their role in providing health benefits and nutrition will continue to expand. As interests and investment in microalgae continue to grow in various parts of the world, these tiny biofactories might bring about revolutionary changes in the energy, pharmaceutical, cosmetics, and food industries in the coming years.

REFERENCES

Agyei, D. and Danquah, M. K. (2011) Industrial-scale manufacturing of pharmaceutical grade bioactive peptides. *Biotechnology Advances* **29**, 272–277.

Ahmed, F., Fanning, K., Netzel, M., Turner, W., Li, Y., and Schenk, P. M. (2014) Profiling of carotenoids and antioxidant capacity of microalgae from subtropical coastal and brackish waters. *Food Chemistry* **165**, 300–306.

Becker, E. W. (2007) Micro-algae as a source of protein. *Biotechnology Advances* **25**, 207–210.

Belay, A., Ota, Y., Miyakawa, K., and Shimamatsu, H. (1993) Current knowledge on potential health benefits of *Spirulina*. *Journal of Applied Phycology* **5**, 235–241.

Borowitzka, M. A. (2013) High-value products from microalgae-their development and commercialisation. *Journal of Applied Phycology* **25**, 443–756.

Bourdichon, F., Berger, B., Casaregola, S., Farrokh, C., Frisvad, J., Gerds, M. et al. (2012) Safety demonstration of microbial food cultures (MFC) in fermented food products. *Bulletin of the International Dairy Federation* **455**, 1–62.

Burja, A. M. and Radianingtyas, H. (2008) Nutraceuticals and functional foods from marine microbes: An introduction to a diverse group of natural products isolated from marine macroalgae, microalgae, bacteria, fungi, and cyanobacteria. In: *Marine Nutraceuticals and Functional Foods*. (eds. C. J. Barrow and F. Shahidi), CRC Press, Boca Raton, FL, pp. 367–403.

Cha, K. H., Koo, S. Y., and Lee, D. U. (2008) Antiproliferative effects of carotenoids extracts from *Chlorella ellipsoidea* and *Chlorella vulgaris* on human colon cancer cells. *Journal of Agricultural Food Chemistry* **56**, 10521–10526.

Chochois, V., Dauvillée, D., Beyly, A., Tolleter, D., Cuiné, S., Timpano, H., Ball, S., Cournac, L., and Peltier, G. (2009) Hydrogen production in *Chlamydomonas*: Photosystem II-dependent and independent pathways differ in their requirement for starch metabolism. *Plant Physiology* **151**, 631–640.

Cohen, Z., Ed. (1999) Monodus subterraneus. In: *Chemicals from Microalgae*. CRC Press, New York, pp. 25–41.

Custódio, L., Soares, F., Pereira, H., Barreira, L., Vizetto-Duarte, C., Rodrigues, M. J., Rauter, M. A., Albericio, F., Varela, J. (2014) Fatty acid composition and biological activities of *Isochrysis galbana* T-ISO, *Tetraselmis* sp. and *Scenedesmus* sp.: possible application in the pharmaceutical and functional food industries. *Journal of Applied Phycology* **26(1)**, 151–161.

Dewapriya, P. and Kim, S. K. (2014) Marine microorganisms: An emerging avenue in modern nutraceuticals and functional foods. *Food Research International* **56**, 115–125.

Durmaz, Y., Monteiro, M., Bandarra, N., Gokpinar, S., and Isik, O. (2007) The effect of low temperature on fatty acid composition and tocopherols of the red microalga, *Porphyridium cruentum*. *Journal of Applied Phycology* **19**, 223–227.

Fabregas, J. and Herrero, C. (1986) Marine microalgae as a potential source of minerals in fish diets. *Aquaculture* **51**, 237–243.

Francavilla, M., Colaianna, M., Zotti, M. G., Morgese, M., Trotta, P., Tucci, P., Schiavone, S., Cuomo, V., and Trabace, L. (2012) Extraction, characterization and in vivo neuromodulatory activity of phytosterols from microalga Dunaliella tertiolecta. *Current Medicinal Chemistry* **19(18)**, 3058–3067.

Gong, Y., Hu, H., Gao, Y., Xu, X., and Gao, H. (2011) Microalgae as platforms for production of recombinant proteins and valuable compounds: Progress and prospects. *Journal of Industrial Microbiology and Biotechnology* **38(12)**, 1879–1890.

Gregory, J. A., Topol, A. B., Doerner, D. Z., and Mayfield, S. (2013) Alga-produced cholera toxin-pfs25 fusion proteins as oral vaccines. *Applied and Environmental Microbiology* **79(13)**, 3917–3925.

Guarnieri, M. T. and Pienkos, P. T. (2014) Algal omics: Unlocking bioproduct diversity in algae cell factories. *Photosynthesis Research* **123(3)**, 1–9.

Guedes, A., Amaro, H. M., and Malcata, F. X. (2011b) Microalgae as sources of high added-value compounds—A brief review of recent work. *Biotechnology Progress* **27(3)**, 597–613.

Guedes, A. C., Amaro, H. M., Barbosa, C. R., Pereira, R. D., and Malcata, F. X. (2011a) Fatty acid composition of several wild microalgae and cyanobacteria, with a focus on eicosapentaenoic, docosahexaenoic and α-linolenic acids for eventual dietary uses. *Food Research International* **44**, 2721–2729.

Hajimahmoodi, M., Faramarzi, M. A., Mohammadi, N., Soltani, N., Oveisi, M. R., and Nafissi-Varcheh, N. (2010) Evaluation of antioxidant properties and total phenolic contents of some strains of microalgae. *Journal of Applied Phycology* **22(1)**, 43–50.

Hassimotto, N. M. A., Genovese, M. I., and Lajolo, F. M. (2005) Antioxidant activity of dietary fruits, vegetables, and commercial frozen fruit pulps. *Journal of Agricultural and Food Chemistry* **53(8)**, 2928–2935.

Hempel, F., Lau, J., Klingl, A., and Maier, U. G. (2011) Algae as protein factories: Expression of a human antibody and the respective antigen in the diatom *Phaeodactylum tricornutum*. *PLoS One* **6(12)**, 1–7.

Herrero, M., Ibáñez, E., Cifuentes, A., Reglero, G., and Santoyo, S. (2006) *Dunaliella salina* microalga pressurized extracts as potential antimicrobials. *Journal of Food Protection* **69**, 2471–2477.

Himaya, S. W. A., Dewapriya, P., and Kim, S. K. (2013) EGFR tyrosine kinase inhibitory peptide attenuate Helicobacter pylori-mediated hyper-proliferation in AGS enteric epithelial cells. *Toxicology and Applied Pharmacology* **269(3)**, 205–214.

Himaya, S. W. A., Ngo, D. H., Ryu, B., and Kim, S. K. (2012) An active peptide purified from gastrointestinal enzyme hydrolysate of Pacific cod skin gelatin attenuates angiotensin-1 converting enzyme (ACE) activity and cellular oxidative stress. *Food Chemistry* **132**, 1872–1882.

Hudek, K., Davis, L. C., Ibbini, J., and Erickson, L. (2014) Commercial products from algae. In: *Algal Biorefineries*. (eds. R. Bajpai, A. Prokop, and M. Zappi), Springer, Dordrecht, the Netherlands, pp. 275–295.

Huheihel, M., Ishanu, V., Tal, J., and Arad, S. M. (2002) Activity of *Porphyridium* sp. polysaccharide against herpes simplex viruses in vitro and *in vivo*. *Journal of Biochemical and Biophysical Methods* **50**, 189–200.

Ibañez, E. and Cifuentes, A. (2013) Benefits of using algae as natural sources of functional ingredients. *Journal of the Science of Food and Agriculture* **93(4)**, 703–709.

Ismail, A., Marjan, Z. M., and Foong, C. W. (2004) Total antioxidant activity and phenolic content in selected vegetables. *Food Chemistry* **87(4)**, 581–586.

Johnson, S. (2000) The possible role of gradual accumulation of copper, cadmium, lead and iron and gradual depletion of zinc, magnesium, selenium, vitamins B2, B6, D, and E and essential fatty acids in multiple sclerosis. *Medical Hypotheses* **55(3)**, 239–241.

Ju, Z. Y., Deng, D. F., and Dominy, W. (2012) A defatted microalgae (*Haematococcus pluvialis*) meal as a protein ingredient to partially replace fishmeal in diets of Pacific white shrimp (*Litopenaeus vannamei*, Boone, 1931). *Aquaculture*, **354**, 50–55.

Kanekiyo, K., Lee, J. B., Hayashi, K., Takenata, H., Hayakawa, Y., Endo, S., and Hayashi, T. (2005) Isolation of an antiviral polysaccharide, nosoflan, from a terrestrial Cyanobacterium, *Nostoc flagelliforme*. *Journal of Natural Products* **68**, 1037–1041.

Kang, K. H., Qian, Z. J., Ryu, B., Kim, D., and Kim, S. K. (2012) Protective effects of protein hydrolysate from marine microalgae Navicula incerta on ethanol-induced toxicity in HepG2/CYP2E1 cells. *Food Chemistry* **132(2)**, 677–685.

Kim, G. N., Shin, J. G., and Jang, H. D. (2009) Antioxidant and antidiabetic activity of Dangyuja (*Citrus grandis* Osbeck) extract treated with *Aspergillus saitoi*. *Food Chemistry* **117**, 35–41.

Li, H. B., Cheng, K. W., Wong, C. C., Fan, K. W., Chen, F., and Jiang, Y. (2007). Evaluation of antioxidant capacity and total phenolic content of different fractions of selected microalgae. *Food Chemistry* **102(3)**, 771–776.

Lin, J. Y. and Tang, C. Y. (2007) Determination of total phenolic and flavonoid contents in selected fruits and vegetables, as well as their stimulatory effects on mouse splenocyte proliferation. *Food Chemistry* **101(1)**, 140–147.

Macías-Sánchez, M., Mantell, C., Rodríguez, M., Martínez de la Ossa, E., Lubián, L., and Montero, O. (2007) Supercritical fluid extraction of carotenoids and chlorophyll a from *Synechococcus* sp. *The Journal of Supercritical Fluids* **39(3)**, 323–329.

Maeda, H., Hosokawa, M., Sashima, T., Funayama, K., and Miyashita, K. (2005) Fucoxanthin from edible seaweed, *Undaria pinnatifida*, shows antiobesity effect through UCP1 expression in white adipose tissues. *Biochemical and Biophysical Research Communications* **332(2)**, 392–397.

Mayfield, S. P., Manuell, A. L., Chen, S., Wu, J., Tran, M., Siefker, D., and Marin-Navarro, J. (2007) *Chlamydomonas reinhardtii* chloroplasts as protein factories. *Current Opinion in Biotechnology* **18(2)**, 126–133.

Melis, A., Seibert, M., and Happe, T. (2004) Genomics of green algal hydrogen research. *Photosynthesis Research* **82**, 277–288.

Melis, A., Zhang, L., Forestier, M., Ghirardi, M. L., and Seibert, M. (2000) Sustained photobiological hydrogen gas production upon reversible inactivation of oxygen evolution in the green alga *Chlamydomonas reinhardtii*. *Plant Physiology* **122**, 127–135.

Mendiola, J. A., Jaime, L., Santoyo, S., Reglero, G., Cifuentes, A., Ibañez, E., and Señoráns, F. J. (2007) Screening of functional compounds in supercritical fluid extracts from *Spirulina platensis*. *Food Chemistry* **102**, 1357–1367.

Miura, Y., Yagi, K., Shoga, M., and Miyamoto, K. (1982) Hydrogen production by a green alga, *Chlamydomonas reinhardtii*, in an alternating light/dark cycle. *Biotechnology and Bioengineering* **24**, 1555–1563.

Morimura, Y. and Tamiya, N. (1954) Preliminary experiments in the use of *Chlorella* as human food. *Food Technology* **8**, 179

Nakashima, Y., Ohsawa, I., Konishi, F., Hasegawa, T., Kumamoto, S., Suzuki, Y., and Ohta, S. (2009) Preventive effects of *Chlorella* on cognitive decline in age-dependent dementia model mice. *Neuroscience Letters* **464(3)**, 193–198.

Nose, T. (1972) Mineral requirements. *Suisan Zoshoku* **20**, 289–300.

Ozdemir, G., Ulku Karabay, N., Dalay, M. C., and Pazarbasi, B. (2004) Antibacterial activity of volatile component and various extracts of *Spirulina platensis*. *Phytotherapy Research* **18(9)**, 754–757.

Plaza, M., Herrero, M., Cifuentes, A., and Ibanez, E. (2009) Innovative natural functional ingredients from microalgae. *Journal of Agricultural and Food Chemistry* **57(16)**, 7159–7170.

Plaza, M., Santoyo, S., Jaime, L., Reina, G. G., Herrero, M., Senorans, F. J., and Ibáñez, E. (2010) Screening for bioactive compounds from algae. *Journal of Pharmaceutical and Biomedical Analysis* **51**, 450–455.

Ramírez-Fajardo, A., Esteban-Cerdan, L., Robles-Medina, A., Acién-Fernández, F. G., González-Moreno, P. A., and Molina-Grima, E. (2007) Lipid extraction from the microalga *Phaeodactylum tricornutum*. *European Journal of Lipid Science and Technology* **109**, 120–126.

Rasmussen, H. E., Blobaum, K. R., Park, Y. K., Ehlers, S. J., Lu, F., and Lee, J. Y. (2008) Lipid extract of Nostoc commune var. sphaeroides Kützing, a blue-green alga, inhibits the activation of sterol regulatory element binding proteins in HepG2 cells. *The Journal of Nutrition* **138(3)**, 476–481.

Ryu, B., Kang, K. H., Ngo, D. H., Qian, Z. J., and Kim, S. K. (2012) Statistical optimization of microalgae *Pavlova lutheri* cultivation conditions and its fermentation conditions by yeast, *Candida rugopelliculosa*. *Bioresource Technology* **107**, 307–313.

Sheih, I. C., Wu, T. K., and Fang, T. J. (2009) Antioxidant properties of a new antioxidative peptide from algae protein waste hydrolysate in different oxidation systems. *Bioresource Technology* **100**, 3419–3425.

Shim, J.-Y., Shin, H.-S., Han, J.-G., Park, H.-S., Lim, B.-L., Chung, K.-W., and Om, A.-S. (2008) Protective effects of *Chlorella vulgaris* on liver toxicity in cadmium-administered rats. *Journal of Medicinal Food* **11**, 479–485.

Simopoulos, A. P. (2002) The importance of the ratio of omega-6/omega-3 essential fatty acids. *Biomedicine & Pharmacotherapy* **56**, 365–379.

Specht, E., Miyake-Stoner, S., and Mayfield, S. (2010) Micro-algae come of age as a platform for recombinant protein production. *Biotechnology Letters* **32**, 1373–1383.

Spolaore, P., Joannis-Cassan, C., Duran, E., and Isambert, A. (2006) Commercial applications of microalgae. *Journal of Bioscience and Bioengineering* **101**, 87–96.

Stengel, D. B., S. Connan, and Popper, Z. A. (2011) Algal chemodiversity and bioactivity: Sources of natural variability and implications for commercial application. *Biotechnology Advances* **29**, 483–501.

Stolz, P. and Obermayer, B. (2005) Manufacturing microalgae for skin care. *Cosmetics and Toiletries* **120**, 99–106.

Tokuşoglu, Ö. and Üunal, M. K. (2003) Biomass nutrient profiles of three microalgae: *Spirulina platensis*, *Chlorella vulgaris*, and *Isochrisis galbana*. *Journal of Food Science* **68**, 1144–1148.

Tran, M., Henry, R. E., Siefker, D., Van, C., Newkirk, G., Kim, J., Bui, J., and Mayfield, S. P. (2013) Production of anti-cancer immunotoxins in algae: Ribosome inactivating proteins as fusion partners. *Biotechnology and Bioengineering* **110(11)**, 2826–2835.

Tsygankov, A., Kosourov, S., Seibert, M., and Ghirardi, M. L. (2002) Hydrogen photoproduction under continuous illumination by sulfur-deprived, synchronous *Chlamydomonas reinhardtii* cultures. *International Journal of Hydrogen Energy* **27**, 1239–1244.

Tumolo, T. and Lanfer-Marquez, U. M.(2012) Copper chlorophyllin: A food colorant with bioactive properties?. *Food Research International* **46**, 451–459.

Venugopal, V. (2009) *Marine Products for Healthcare: Functional and Bioactive Nutraceutical Compounds from the Ocean*. CRC Press, Boca Raton, FL.

Watanabe, F., Takenaka, S., Kittaka-Katsura, H., Ebara, S. and Miyamoto, E. (2002) Characterization and bioavailability of vitamin B12-compounds from edible algae. *Journal of Nutritional Science and Vitaminology* **48**, 325–331.

Yukino, T., Hayashi, M., Inoue, Y., Imamura, J., Nagano, N., and Murata, H. (2005) Preparation of docosahexaenoic acid fortified *Spirulina platensis* and its lipid and fatty acid compositions. *Nippon Suisan Gakkaishi* **71**, 74–79.

Zhang, L., Happe, T., and Melis, A. (2002) Biochemical and morphological characterization of sulfur-deprived and H_2-producing *Chlamydomonas reinhardtii* (green alga). *Planta* **214**, 552–561.

Index

D

E

G

H

P

Q

R

T

U

V

W

X

Z

Printed in the United States
by Baker & Taylor Publisher Services